THE ROUTLEDGE HANDBOOK ON BIOCHEMISTRY OF EXERCISE

From its early beginnings in the 1960s, the academic field of biochemistry of exercise has expanded beyond examining and describing metabolic responses to exercise and adaptations to training to include a wide understanding of molecular biology, cell signalling, interorgan communication, stem cell physiology, and a host of other cellular and biochemical mechanisms regulating acute responses and chronic adaptations related to exercise performance, human health/disease, nutrition, and cellular functioning.

The Routledge Handbook on Biochemistry of Exercise is the first book to pull together the full depth and breadth of this subject and to update a rapidly expanding field of study with current issues and controversies and a look forward to future research directions. Bringing together many experts and leading scientists, the book emphasizes the current understanding of the underlying metabolic, cellular, genetic, and cell signalling mechanisms associated with physical activity, exercise, training, and athletic performance as they relate to, interact with, and regulate cellular and muscular adaptations and consequent effects on human health/disease, nutrition and weight control, and human performance.

With more emphasis than ever on the need to be physically active and the role that being active plays in our overall health from a whole-body level down to the cell, this book makes an important contribution for scholars, medical practitioners, nutritionists, and coaches/trainers working in research and with a wide range of clients. This text is important reading for all students, scholars, and others with an interest in health, nutrition, and exercise/training in general.

Peter Tiidus is Dean of the Faculty of Applied Health Sciences and a Professor in Kinesiology at Brock University, St. Catharines, Ontario, Canada.

Rebecca E. K. MacPherson is an Assistant Professor in Health Sciences in the Faculty of Applied Health Sciences at Brock University, St. Catharines, Ontario, Canada.

Paul J. LeBlanc is a Professor in Health Sciences in the Faculty of Applied Health Sciences at Brock University, St. Catharines, Ontario, Canada.

Andrea R. Josse is an Assistant Professor in the School of Kinesiology and Health Science, Faculty of Health at York University, Toronto, Ontario, Canada.

THE ROUTLEDGE HANDBOOK ON BIOCHEMISTRY OF EXERCISE

Edited by
Peter M. Tiidus, Rebecca E. K. MacPherson,
Paul J. LeBlanc, and Andrea R. Josse

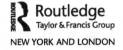

NEW YORK AND LONDON

First published 2021
by Routledge
52 Vanderbilt Avenue, New York, NY 10017

and by Routledge
2 Park Square, Milton Park, Abingdon, Oxon, OX14 4RN

Routledge is an imprint of the Taylor & Francis Group, an informa business

© 2021 Taylor & Francis

Library of Congress Cataloging-in-Publication Data
A catalogue record for this title has been requested

ISBN: 978-0-367-22383-0 (hbk)
ISBN: **978-0-367-64294-5 (pbk)**
ISBN: 978-1-003-12383-5 (ebk)

Typeset in Bembo
by KnowledgeWorks Global Ltd.

CONTENTS

List of Figures   *ix*

List of Tables   *xvi*

Contributors   *xviii*

SECTION I
Regulation of Metabolism and Responses to Acute Exercise   **1**

1   Whole-Body Regulation of Energy Expenditure, Exercise Fuel Selection, and Dietary Recommendations   3
Peter W.R. Lemon

2   Energy Provision, Fuel Use and Regulation of Skeletal Muscle Metabolism During the Exercise Intensity/Duration Continuum   15
Lawrence L. Spriet

3   Adipose Tissue (Adipokinome), Skeletal Muscle (Myokinome), and Liver (Hepatokinome) as Endocrine Regulators During Exercise   36
Logan K. Townsend, Greg L. McKie, Hesham Shamshoum, and David C. Wright

4   Regulation of Skeletal Muscle Reactive Oxygen Species During Exercise   51
Catherine A. Bellissimo and Christopher G.R. Perry

5   Biochemical Contributors to Exercise Fatigue   71
Arthur J. Cheng, Maja Schlittler, and Håkan Westerblad

6   Mechanotransduction Mechanisms of Hypertrophy and Performance with Resistance Exercise   85
Andrew C. Fry, Justin X. Nicoll, and Luke A. Olsen

7 Responses to Muscular Exercise, Heat Shock Proteins as Regulators
   of Inflammation, and Mitochondrial Quality Control   112
   Alex T. Von Schulze and Paige C. Geiger

8 Signalling Pathways in the Regulation of Cellular Responses to Exercise   124
   Anders Gudiksen, Stine Ringholm, and Henriette Pilegaard

SECTION II
Exercise Biochemistry, Chronic Training, and Athletic Performance   141

9 Exercise-Induced Mitochondrial Biogenesis: Molecular Regulation,
   Impact of Training, and Influence on Exercise Performance   143
   Hashim Islam, Jacob T. Bonafiglia, Cesare Granata, and Brendon J. Gurd

10 Resistance Exercise Training and the Regulation of Muscle Protein Synthesis   162
    Nathan Hodson, Daniel R. Moore, and Chris McGlory

11 Cellular Adaptations to High-Intensity and Sprint Interval Training   176
    Martin J. MacInnis and Lauren E. Skelly

12 Regulation of Muscle Satellite Cell Activation and Cycles Consequent
    to Various Forms of Training   193
    Sophie Joanisse and Gianni Parise

13 Biochemical and Metabolic Limitations to Athletic Performance   205
    Brendan M. Gabriel

14 Genetic Limitations to Athletic Performance   217
    Colin N. Moran and Guan Wang

15 The Role of Epigenetics in Skeletal Muscle Adaptations to Exercise
    and Exercise Training   232
    Sean L. McGee

16 Statistical Considerations and Biological Mechanisms Underlying Individual
    Differences in Adaptations to Exercise Training   242
    Jacob T. Bonafiglia, Hashim Islam, Nir Eynon, and Brendon J. Gurd

17 Effects of Hypoxia/Blood Flow Restriction on Cellular Adaptations
    to Training   260
    Scott J. Dankel and Jeremy P. Loenneke

SECTION III

Exercise Biochemistry/Nutrition Nexus in Physical Activity and Sport Performance   **275**

18 Exercise and Dietary Influences on the Regulation of Energy Balance
and Implications for Body Weight Control   277
Andrea M. Brennan and Robert Ross

19 Dietary Manipulation for Optimizing Endurance Training Adaptations
and Performance: Carbohydrate vs. Fat   292
Jamie Whitfield and Louise M. Burke

20 Dietary Influence on Muscle Protein Synthesis and Hypertrophy   304
James McKendry and Stuart M. Phillips

21 Micronutrients and Nutraceuticals: Effects on Exercise Performance   321
Stella L. Volpe and Quentin Nichols

22 Biochemistry of Buffering Capacity and Ingestion of Buffers in Exercise
and Athletic Performance   334
*Bryan Saunders, Guilherme G. Artioli, Eimear Dolan, Rebecca L. Jones, Joseph Matthews,
and Craig Sale*

23 Creatine Augmentation for Muscle and Bone Responses to Exercise   353
Philip D. Chilibeck

24 Biochemistry of Caffeine's Influence on Exercise Performance   363
Jane Shearer, Robyn F. Madden, and Jill A. Parnell

25 Nutrigenomics for Sport and Exercise Performance   375
Nanci S. Guest, Marc Sicova, and Ahmed El-Sohemy

SECTION IV

Exercise Biochemistry Relative to Health Through the Lifespan   **391**

26 Mitochondrial Dysfunction in Chronic Disease   393
Christopher Newell, Heather Leduc-Pessah, Aneal Khan, and Jane Shearer

27 Exercise Training, Mitochondrial Adaptations, and Aging   413
Nashwa Cheema, Matthew Triolo, and David A. Hood

28 Biochemistry of Exercise Effects in Type 2 Diabetes   433
Barry Braun, Karyn L. Hamilton, Dan S. Lark, and Alissa Newman

29 Biochemistry of Exercise Training and Mitigation of Cardiovascular Disease   455
    Barry A. Franklin and John C. Quindry

30 Biochemistry of Exercise Training and Type 1 Diabetes   479
    Sam N. Scott, Matt Cocks, Anton J. M. Wagenmakers, Sam O. Shepherd,
    and Michael C. Riddell

31 Biochemistry of Exercise Training: Mitigation of Cancers   499
    Brittany R. Counts, Jessica L. Halle, and James A. Carson

32 Biochemistry of Exercise Training: Effects on Bone   513
    Panagiota Klentrou and Rozalia Kouvelioti

33 Metabolic Effects of Exercise on Childhood Obesity   532
    Kristi B. Adamo, Taniya S. Nagpal, and Danilo F. DaSilva

Index   549

FIGURES

1.1	Fat oxidation estimates based on respiratory exchange ratio measures vs. exercise intensity in men and women (Ref. 1)	4
1.2a	Effect of exercise intensity on muscle glycogen use vs. time	8
1.2b	Effect of exercise intensity on muscle glycogen use vs. time	8
1.3a	Protein intake and $^{13}CO_2$ production from phenylalanine oxidation ($F^{13}CO_2$) in young male bodybuilders	11
1.3b	Protein intake and $^{13}CO_2$ production from phenylalanine oxidation ($F^{13}CO_2$) in young endurance-trained men	11
2.1	A schematic of the energy-producing pathways in skeletal muscle	16
2.2	Skeletal muscle lactate accumulation and phosphocreatine use during 10 min of exercise at 35%, 65%, and 90% and 30 s at ~250% VO_2 max (reproduced from 47, 65)	18
2.3	Skeletal muscle ATP content and free inorganic phosphate (Pi) accumulation during 10 min of exercise at 35%, 65%, and 90% and 30 s at ~250% VO_2 max (reproduced from 47, 65)	19
2.4	Skeletal muscle–free adenosine diphosphate (ADP) and adenosine monophosphate (AMP) accumulation during 10 min of exercise at 35%, 65%, and 90% and 30 s at ~250% VO_2 max (reproduced from 47, 65)	20
2.5	Contribution of phosphocreatine (PCr), anaerobic glycolysis, and oxidative phosphorylation to energy (ATP) provision during a 30 s all-out sprint at ~250% VO_2 max (reproduced from 65)	21
2.6	Pyruvate dehydrogenase (PDH) activation during 10 min of exercise at 35%, 65%, and 90% and 30 s at ~250% VO_2 max (reproduced from 47, 65)	21
2.7	Fuel use during exercise at 25%, 65%, and 85 VO_2 max (reproduced from 73)	22
2.8	Fuel use during exercise at 40%, 55%, and 75% W max (reproduced from 93)	23
2.9	Plasma free fatty acid (FFA) concentrations and whole-body carbohydrate and fat oxidation rates during 4 h of exercise at ~57% VO_2 max (reproduced from 99)	28
2.10	Fuel use during 4 h of exercise at ~57% VO_2 max (reproduced from 99)	28
2.11	Pyruvate dehydrogenase (PDHa) activation during 4 h of exercise at ~57% VO_2 max (reproduced from 99)	29
4.1	Major superoxide-producing sites and hydrogen peroxide (H_2O_2) generation in muscle during contraction	53
4.2	Glutathione and thioredoxin buffering systems and their response to exercise training	60

4.3 Examples of redox-sensitive proteins comprising the "redoxome"   •   61

5.1 Typical Ca^{2+}_i and force records obtained during fatigue induced by repeated tetanic stimulation in (A) a fatigue-resistant type 1 fibre from mouse soleus muscle and (B) a more easily fatigued type 2 fibre from mouse flexor digitorum brevis muscle   74

5.2 The rate of peripheral fatigue development critically depends on the extent of aerobic metabolism   75

5.3 Representative force and Ca^{2+}_i records of the 1st, 50th, and 100th fatiguing tetanic contractions (70 Hz, 350 ms duration given every 2 s) of individual flexor digitorum brevis type 2 fibres from a sedentary control mouse (A) and mouse with increased aerobic capacity after having access to a running wheel and running >10 km per 24 hours for 6 weeks (B). Figure adapted from (38)   76

5.4 Figure illustrating the various intracellular processes that are considered to have key roles in the development of skeletal muscle fatigue   76

6.1 Cellular mechanotransduction   93

6.2 Mechanotransduction following resistance exercise   95

7.1 Canonical HSP functions   113

7.2 Functions of HSPs post-exercise   116

7.3 HSF1–PGC1α–HSP70 and mitochondrial quality control   119

8.1 Initiation and response coupling in SkM with endurance exercise   119
The initiating stress induction (RED) leads to homeostatic perturbations in SkM, changes in Ca^{2+}, cellular energy status (AMP/ATP), and reactive oxygen species (ROS), as well as externally derived signals such as hormones and cytokines (ORANGE). Intracellular signalling events (YELLOW) transfer the signal inducing cellular responses including increased ATP production, substrate shift and gene regulation (GREEN) in order to re-establish cellular homeostasis.   125

8.2 Overview of intracellular signalling events in SkM induced by endurance exercise   126
Ca^{2+} activates conventional protein kinase C (cPKC) and binds to calmodulin (CaM) leading to activation of calcineurin (CaN) and calmodulin-dependent protein kinase (CaMK). Calcineurin dephosphorylates nuclear factor of activated T-cells (NFAT) and transcription factor EB (TFEB), which translocate to the nucleus, and CAMK phosphorylates myocyte enhancer factor 2 (MEF2) and cAMP response element binding protein (CREB). Ca^{2+} also activates pyruvate dehydrogenase (PDH). AMP-activated protein kinase (AMPK) is activated by elevated AMP/ATP resulting in phosphorylation and inactivation of AS160/TBC1D4 and acetyl–CoA carboxylase (ACC) inducing glucose transporter (GLUT) 4 translocation to the plasma membrane and fatty acid uptake into the mitochondria, respectively. Activation of p38, c-jun NH2-terminal kinase (JNK), and extracellular signal-regulated kinase (ERK)1/2 regulates transcription factors activator protein (AP)-1, activating transcription factor 2 (ATF2), MEF2, and CREB, inducing transcription of PGC-1α. Elevated levels of reactive oxygen species (ROS) result in translocation of nuclear factor erythroid-derived 2-like (Nrf)2 to the nucleus and enhanced transcription of antioxidant proteins. Adrenalin binds to the β2-adrenergic receptor at the plasma membrane, eliciting increases in cAMP, activation of protein kinase A (PKA) with concomitant regulation of phosphorylase kinase (PK), glycogen phosphorylase (GP), and glycogen synthase (GS), as well as PKA translocation to the nucleus to regulate gene expression. Binding of cytokines like IL-6 to the JAK/STAT receptor leads to activation of Janus kinase (JAK) and phosphorylation of signal transducer and phosphorylating activator of transcription (STAT)3, which translocates to the nucleus to induce transcription of target genes. Blue lines reflect interaction and/or post-translational modification, while green lines symbolize translocation.

9.1 Overview of the molecular events leading to mitochondrial biogenesis   145

10.1 Schematic overview of the molecular mechanisms governing skeletal muscle protein synthesis   166

10.2 A schematic depicting the mechanisms governing amino acid and resistance exercise–induced rates of muscle protein synthesis (MPS)   168

11.1 The annual number of publications related to interval training listed in PubMed between 1950 and 2019   177

11.2 A schematic outlining the key variables of an interval training session   178

11.3 A diagram outlining the cellular responses to exercise within a skeletal muscle cell that relate to mitochondrial biogenesis   180

12.1 A schematic representation of (A) the acute response of SCs to a bout of resistance exercise and (B) the impact of resistance exercise training on SC content   194

13.1 Post-exercise glycogen supercompensation as demonstrated in classic experiments by Bergström and Hultman (4, 5)   206

13.2 Illustration of elongated mitochondria with the ability to perform oxidative phosphorylation at the periphery of a myofiber and transfer proton gradient to areas with low O_2, hypothesized by Glancy et al. (17)   209

13.3 Illustration of intense exercise-induced build-up of ionic by-products, including Ca2+, H+, K+, Mg2+, and Pi (24), and reactive oxygen species (ROS) (46). Created with BioRender.   210

14.1 Images showing differences in physiology within one sport. Lionel Messi (1.7 m) and Cristiano Ronaldo (1.87 m), both renowned international footballers with markedly different statures   218

14.2 The importance of genetics in natural talent, genetics in trainability, and training. Athletes A and B have similar natural abilities (baseline genetics) and similar potential (trainability genetics), but athlete B trains harder, realizing more of their potential.   221

14.3 Graph showing the *ACTN3* R577X genotype frequencies in power athletes, endurance athletes, and controls   224

16.1 The molecular basis of skeletal muscle adaptation to exercise training   249

17.1 Adaptations resulting from acclimation to hypoxia independent of exercise   264

17.2 The impact of applying blood flow restriction on muscle mass   268

18.1 (A) Skeletal muscle, (B) adipose tissue, (C) central nervous system, and (D) gastrointestinal system. CCK, cholecystokinin; GLP-1, glucagon-like peptide-1; PYY, peptide YY; BDNF, brain-derived neurotrophic factor. Figure created with smart SERVIER MEDICAL ART https://smart.servier.com/).   285

19.1 Overview of skeletal muscle metabolic pathways. During exercise, skeletal muscle relies on both exogenous and endogenous sources of lipid (plasma FFA and IMTG, respectively) and carbohydrate (plasma glucose and glycogen, respectively) for energy production via mitochondrial oxidative phosphorylation. Both pathways rely on protein-mediated transport for exogenous substrate into the cytoplasm, utilizing glucose transporter 4 (GLUT4) as well as a family of fatty acid transporters (example used above, fatty acid translocase/CD36 (FAT/CD36)). Highlighted are key regulatory enzymes in the carbohydrate metabolic pathway resulting in ATP and reducing equivalent production/consumption including glycogen phosphorylase (PHOS), hexokinase (HK), phosphofructokinase (PFK), lactate dehydrogenase (LDH), and pyruvate dehydrogenase (PDH). Lipid metabolism is more heavily regulated by transport into the mitochondria. Free fatty acids (FFA) taken up from plasma or liberated from IMTG by adipose triglyceride lipase (ATGL) and hormone sensitive lipase (HSL), are converted to fatty Acyl-CoA by Acyl-CoA synthase (ACS), and subsequently moved across the mitochondrial membranes by the carnitine palmitoyltransferase complex, consisting of carnitine palmitoyltransferase (CPT-I), carnitine acylcarnitine transferase (CACT), and CPT-II. While each of these enzymes is subject to multiple levels of allosteric and covalent regulation, the inhibitory enzyme pyruvate dehydrogenase kinase (PDK) has been included as it is heavily upregulated in response to conditions of elevated intramuscular FFA such as a low-carbohydrate, high-fat diet, or training with reduced glycogen content. Additional sites of regulation modified by these nutritional interventions include beta(3)-hydroxyacyl-CoA dehydrogenase (β-HAD), a key enzyme in the β-oxidation pathway, as well as the fatty acid transporters FAT/CD36 and CPT-I. Figure created with https://biorender.com/ (licenced version).

19.2   Simplified schematic outlining the putative cell signalling cascades activated through exercise with low glycogen availability. Exercise will result in an increase in energy turnover, increasing the intracellular concentration of metabolites such as calcium (Ca^{2+}), AMP, and ADP, activating calcium/calmodulin-dependent protein kinase II (CaMKII) and the AMP protein kinase (AMPK). These kinases can then translocate to the nucleus in order to increase gene transcription. AMPK may also be bound to glycogen through a carbohydrate binding domain on its β-subunit. In conditions where intramuscular glycogen is decreased, AMPK is released, resulting in an increase in its activity, promoting phosphorylation of the downstream target PGC-1α as well as translocation to nucleus. PGC-1α can also translocate to the nucleus, where it autoregulates its own expression, and positively effects gene transcription through interactions with a variety of hormone receptors and transcription factors, including nuclear respiratory factors (NRF) 1 and 2. These two transcription factors promote the transcription of nuclear genes controlling the expression of cytochrome oxidase (COX) subunits. Additionally, NRF-1 also induces the expression of mitochondrial transcription factor A (Tfam), which is imported into the mitochondria in order to regulate the expression of mitochondrial (mt) DNA. AMPK can also increase the activity and alter the cellular localization of the tumor suppressor protein p53. Upon redistribution to the nucleus, both p53 and PGC-1α can coactivate Tfam to increase the expression of proteins that form subunits of the electron transport chain respiratory complexes. A decrease in glycogen content can induce cellular stress and increase the activity of p38 mitogen-activated protein kinase (p38 MAPK), promoting its translocation to the nucleus where it induces the expression of PGC-1α. Finally, exercise in a low glycogen state elevates circulating catecholamines increasing lipolysis and the breakdown of intramuscular triglycerides (IMTG). This increases the release of free fatty acids within muscle, activating the nuclear transcription factor peroxisome proliferator-activated receptor delta (PPARα), which controls the expression of key metabolic regulatory genes including fatty acid transporters (FAT/CD36 and CPT-I), and negative regulators of carbohydrate metabolism (PDK4). Figure created with https://biorender.com/ (licenced version).   297

20.1   Schematic representation of muscle protein synthesis and muscle protein breakdown throughout a typical daily protein feeding pattern [redrawn with permission from (84)].   306

20.2   A schematic overview of the cellular signalling pathways regulating skeletal muscle protein synthesis in response to AAs, growth factors, and muscular contraction from endurance and resistance exercise.   309

20.3   Schematic representation of a protein feeding pattern designed to maximize muscle protein synthesis and the muscle NBAL, subsequently facilitating skeletal muscle hypertrophy.   312

294

21.1   Vitamin D metabolism.   326
21.2   Whey protein and myofibrillar protein synthesis.   327
21.3   Nitric oxide production from foods.   329
22.1   Schematic representation of titration curves of pure water (A) and a buffered
        aqueous solution (B). In pure water, where there is no buffering system, the
        addition of small amounts of acid results in a large reduction in pH, whilst in a
        buffered system, there is a zone where the addition of large amounts of acid does
        not result in a reduced pH. The zone of effectiveness refers to the pH range around
        the pKa of that particular buffer, thereby varying according to the buffering agent.   337
22.2   Overview of beta-alanine supplementation to increase muscle buffering capacity
        during high-intensity exercise.   339
22.3   Overview of supplementation with extracellular buffers (sodium bicarbonate, sodium
        citrate, calcium lactate, and sodium lactate) to increase extracellular buffering
        capacity during high-intensity exercise.   342
23.1   Chemical structure of creatine.   354
23.2   The creatine shuttle system (adapted from 54).   354
23.3   Mechanisms by which creatine supplementation can lead to increased muscle mass.
        References are indicated in brackets to support different mechanisms.   357
23.4   Proposed mechanism by which creatine supplementation might activate osteoblasts
        to secrete osteoprotegerin (OPG). Osteoprotegerin acts as a decoy for receptor
        activator for the nuclear factor-kappaB ligand (RANKL), preventing its binding with
        RANK on osteoclast precursor cells. This prevents osteoclast differentiation and
        reduces bone resorption.   358
24.1   Metabolism of caffeine and its resulting metabolites. Chemical structures,
        metabolites, chemical name and approximate metabolite percentage are shown
        (53, 91). *Figures are taken from ChemSpider with permission (4).*   365
24.2   The impacts of caffeine are diverse and widespread throughout the body. Potential
        mechanisms by which caffeine exerts ergogenic benefit are listed. Adenosine receptor
        expression (ADORA2A) is widespread throughout the body as shown in this
        diagram from the *Human Protein Atlas (102).*   369
26.1   The mitochondria are a vastly complex organelle responsible for a host of functions
        regulating metabolic homeostasis   394
26.2   Mitochondrial dysfunction is implicated in a multitude of chronic diseases   402
27.1   Exercise-mediated mitochondrial biogenesis. Endurance exercise leads to the
        activation of intracellular signalling cascades that converge to induce biogenesis
        through the transcription and activation of PGC-1α. PGC-1α promotes the
        expression of NUGEMPs. Perturbations in cellular energy status, as measured by
        increased NAD:NADH and AMP:ATP, activate SIRT1 and AMPK, respectively.
        SIRT1 deacetylates, whereas AMPK phosphorylates PGC-1a, leading to its activation
        and nuclear localization. Second, oxygen consumption is enhanced in working
        muscle leading to elevations in absolute ROS production. ROS activate p38-MAPK,
        which phosphorylates and stabilizes PGC-1α. p38 also activates transcription factors
        such as USF1, ATF2, and MEF2, which drive the transcription of PGC-1α. Third,
        Ca^{2+} is released from the sarcoplasmic reticulum during contraction, which acts as
        a secondary messenger activating the phosphatase calcineurin and Ca-calmodulin
        kinase, ultimately activating transcription factors such as MEF2 and CREB that
        promote PGC-1α transcription. Proteins will be translated within the cytosol and
        imported into the mitochondria by the protein import machinery (PIM), where
        it will drive mtDNA expression or be incorporated into the organelle, ultimately
        leading to the expansion of the mitochondrial network within the muscle   416

27.2 Skeletal muscle deterioration with ageing. Muscle undergoes a vast number of changes as an individual becomes older. Muscle is composed of fascicles, which are bundles of muscle fibres. In older people, there are fewer fibres in a fibre bundle, and fibres have a smaller cross-sectional area in comparison to young fibres. Aged fibres are also prone to regions of atrophy that differ along fibre length, which is evident in a longitudinal view of the muscle. Muscle is also composed of connective tissue, fat, and other cell types. Satellite cells are the resident pool of muscle stem cells required for regeneration. There is an age-dependent decline in satellite cell number and function, which exacerbates muscle atrophy. Satellite cells are naturally in a quiescent state but when activated, they fuse with existing myofibres to repair damage. The nuclei of satellite cells become an extension of the multinucleated fibre. A decline in myonuclear number is seen with age, partly due to smaller satellite cell numbers and increasing cell death from stress signals within the fibre. The muscle fibre is composed of myofilaments and mitochondria. Mitochondria that lie underneath the sarcolemma are termed subsarcolemmal (SS), whereas the mitochondrial pool between myofilaments are intermyofibrillar mitochondria (IMF). In young fibres, IMF mitochondria are fused, whereas in aged fibres they are more fragmented. Aged mitochondria also exhibit a loss of internal structure of their cristae, increasing ROS levels, and damage to mtDNA and are more susceptible to apoptosis. The electron transport chain is less efficient in producing ATP. Regulation of mitochondrial biogenesis by the nucleus is also reduced, and with increasing mitophagy the consequence is that aged muscle has reduced mitochondrial content   421

28.1 Continuum of exercise adaptations in type 2 diabetes   434

29.1 Multiple mechanisms by which moderate-to-vigorous exercise training may reduce the risk for non-fatal and fatal cardiovascular events. BP, blood pressure; CACs, cultured/circulating angiogenic cells; EPC, endothelial progenitor cells; HR, heart rate; O_2, oxygen; ↑, increased; and ↓, decreased   456

29.2 Study design for ischemic pre-conditioning research   461

29.3 Study design for exercise pre-conditioning research   462

29.4 Conceptual overview of the dose-response association between exercise training volume and cardiovascular health outcomes in line with Panel A, the current dogma, and Panel B, and alternative hypothesis (reverse J-shaped or U-shaped curves)   468

29.5 Potential mechanisms and associated sequelae for atrial fibrillation induced by regular strenuous endurance exercise and competitive athletic events   468

30.1 Living with type 1 diabetes (T1D) is like walking a constant tightrope between hyperglycaemia and hypoglycaemia   481

30.2 Blood glucose trends caused by different types of exercise in individuals with type 1 diabetes (T1D)   482

30.3 (A) Glucoregulatory responses to moderate-intensity exercise (50–80% of $\dot{V}O_{2max}$) in a healthy individual without type 1 diabetes (T1D). (B) Glucoregulatory responses to high-intensity exercise (>80% of $\dot{V}O_{2max}$) in healthy individuals without diabetes.   483

30.4 (A) Glucoregulatory responses to moderate-intensity exercise (50–80% of $\dot{V}O_{2max}$) in individuals with T1D. (B) Glucoregulatory responses to high-intensity exercise in an individual with type 1 diabetes (T1D).   484

30.5 Summary of benefits of regular exercise in people with type 1 diabetes   486

31.1 Therapeutic efficacy of physical activity during anticancer treatment   504

31.2 Cancer and treatment's effect on skeletal muscle metabolic homeostasis   505

31.3   Mechanistic effect of cancer and anti-cancer treatment on mitochondrial
dysfunction and the control of proteostasis in muscle   508

33.1   Intergenerational cycle of obesity   534

33.2   Childhood obesity consequences   536

33.3   Main metabolic/physiological variables that improve after chronic exercise in
children and adolescents living with obesity   539

33.4   Potential mechanisms involved in the metabolic changes promoted by exercise in
childhood obesity   540

TABLES

1.1 Prevalence of obesity among Americans ages 20+ years (Ref. 20) 4

1.2 Typical carbohydrate stores in humans (Ref. 51) 5

2.1 Energy-producing pathways in skeletal muscle 16

6.1 Resistance exercise training–related variables important for mechanotransduction 88

12.1 Summary of studies examining the impact of resistance exercise training on the basal SC pool 196

12.2 Summary of studies examining the impact of aerobic exercise training on the basal SC pool 199

16.1 Genetic variants identified by Williams et al. (86) that are significantly associated with changes in VO_2 max following exercise training and have been replicated in different samples 248

18.1 Signals regulating energy intake. 280

21.1 Food sources of magnesium. 322

21.2 Food sources of iron. 323

21.3 Food sources of zinc. 324

21.4 Food sources of β-alanine. 330

22.1 Dissociation constant (Ka) and its negative log (pKa) of a few organic weak acids. 336

22.2 The pKa of ionizable groups of the amino acids. 338

24.1 Affinity of different adenosine receptors to caffeine in humans, adapted from (24). Affinity constant (K_D, μM) and primary tissues in which the receptor is found are listed. Caffeine expression (protein) levels were derived from the *Human Protein Atlas* (102). 370

25.1 Summary of genetic variants that modify the effect of dietary factors or biological molecules on performance-related outcomes. 384

26.1 Mitochondrial abnormalities associated with chronic diseases 403

28.1 Summary of published interactions between exercise and metformin treatment in people at risk for type 2 diabetes and in people with impaired glucose tolerance 442

29.1 The phenomenology of exercise pre-conditioning against ischemic insults in the heart. The key observations of exercise induced pre-conditioning include a biphasic time course for cardioprotection. Exercise pre-conditioning appears to be threshold-dependent, with various exercise modalities, intensities, and durations yielding equivalent levels of protection. Early findings suggest strength training protects

the heart in a similar fashion to aerobic exercise. Exercise pre-conditioning occurs
regardless of age or sex.   463

31.1   Role of physical activity during treatment and survival   506

32.1   Bone turnover markers: Characteristics, role, and function   518

32.2   Studies examining bone turnover markers and osteokine levels in response to exercise
training   523

33.1   Exercise prescription based on FITT principles to treat known adverse metabolic
effects of childhood obesity   543

CONTRIBUTORS

Kristi B. Adamo
School of Human Kinetics, University of Ottawa, Ottawa, Ontario, Canada

Guilherme G. Artioli
Applied Physiology and Nutrition Research Group, School of Physical Education and Sport; Rheumatology Division; Faculdade de Medicina FMUSP, University of São Paulo, São Paulo, Brazil

Catherine A. Bellissimo
School of Kinesiology and Health Science, York University, Toronto, Ontario, Canada

Jacob T. Bonafiglia
School of Kinesiology and Health Studies, Kingston, Ontario, Canada

Barry Braun
Department of Health and Exercise Science, Colorado State University, Fort Collins, CO, USA

Andrea M. Brennan
AdventHealth Research Institute, Translational Research Institute, Orlando, FL, USA

Louise M. Burke
Australian Institute of Sport, Bruce, ACT, Australia

James A. Carson
Division of Rehabilitation Sciences, University of Tennessee Health Science Center, Memphis, TN, USA

Nashwa Cheema
School of Kinesiology and Health Science, Muscle Health Research Centre, York University, Toronto, Ontario, Canada

Arthur J. Cheng
School of Kinesiology and Health Science, York University, Toronto, Ontario, Canada

Philip D. Chilibeck
College of Kinesiology, University of Saskatchewan, Saskatoon, Saskatchewan, Canada

Matt Cocks
Research Institute for Sport and Exercise Sciences, Liverpool John Moores University, Liverpool, UK

Brittany R. Counts
Division of Rehabilitation Sciences, University of Tennessee Health Science Center, Memphis TN, USA

Scott J. Dankel
Department of Health and Exercise Science, Exercise Physiology Laboratory, Rowan University, Glassboro, NJ, USA

Danilo F. DaSilva
School of Human Kinetics, University of Ottawa, Ottawa, Ontario, Canada

Eimear Dolan
Applied Physiology and Nutrition Research Group, School of Physical Education and Sport; Rheumatology Division; Faculdade de Medicina FMUSP, University of São Paulo, São Paulo, Brazil

Ahmed El-Sohemy
Department of Nutritional Sciences, Faculty of Medicine, University of Toronto, Toronto, Ontario, Canada

Nir Eynon
Institute for Health and Sport (iHeS), Victoria University, Melbourne, Victoria, Australia; Murdoch Children's Research Institute, Royal Children's Hospital, Melbourne, Victoria, Australia

Barry A. Franklin
William Beaumont Hospital, Royal Oak, MI & Oakland University William Beaumont School of Medicine, Rochester, MI, USA

Andrew Fry
Department of Health, Sport, and Exercise Sciences, School of Education, University of Kansas, Lawrence, KS, USA

Brendan M. Gabriel
Aberdeen Cardiovascular & Diabetes Centre, The Rowett Institute, University of Aberdeen, Aberdeen, UK; Metabolism, Obesity and Diabetes; Centre for Cardiovascular Science, University of Edinburgh, Edinburgh, UK; Integrative Physiology, Department of Physiology and Pharmacology, Karolinska Institutet, Stockholm, Sweden; Clinical Physiology, Department of Molecular Medicine and Surgery, Karolinska University Hospital, Stockholm, Sweden

Paige Geiger
University of Kansas Medical Center, Kansas City, KS, USA

Cesare Granata
Department of Diabetes, Central Clinical School, Faculty of Medicine, Nursing, and Health Sciences, Monash University, Melbourne, Victoria, Australia

Anders Gudiksen
Cell Biology and Physiology, University of Copenhagen, Copenhagen, Denmark

Nanci S. Guest
Department of Nutritional Sciences, Faculty of Medicine, University of Toronto, Toronto, Ontario, Canada

Brendon J. Gurd
School of Kinesiology and Health Studies, Kingston, Ontario, Canada

Jessica L. Halle
Division of Rehabilitation Sciences, University of Tennessee Health Science Center, Memphis, TN, USA

Karyn L. Hamilton
Department of Health and Exercise Science, Colorado State University, Fort Collins, CO, USA

Nathan Hodson
Faculty of Kinesiology and Physical Education, University of Toronto, Toronto, Ontario, Canada

David A. Hood
School of Kinesiology and Health Science, Muscle Health Research Centre, York University, Toronto, Ontario, Canada

Hashim Islam
School of Kinesiology and Health Studies, Kingston, Ontario, Canada

Sophie Joanisse
Department of Kinesiology, McMaster University, Hamilton, Ontario, Canada

Rebecca L. Jones
Institute for Sport and Physical Activity Research, School of Sport Science and Physical Activity, University of Bedfordshire, Bedford, UK

Aneal Khan
Department of Medical Genetics and Pediatrics, Alberta Children's Hospital Research Institute, Cumming School of Medicine, University of Calgary, Alberta, Canada

Panagiota Klentrou
Department of Kinesiology, Brock University, St. Catharines, Ontario, Canada

Rozalia Kouvelioti
Department of Kinesiology, Brock University, St. Catharines, Ontario, Canada

Dan S. Lark
Department of Health and Exercise Science, Colorado State University, Fort Collins, CO, USA

Heather Leduc-Pessah
Faculty of Medicine, Cumming School of Medicine, University of Calgary, Alberta, Canada

Peter W. Lemon
School of Kinesiology, Western University, London, Ontario, Canada

Jeremy P. Loenneke
Department of Health, Exercise Science, and Recreation Management, Kevser Ermin Applied Physiology Laboratory, University of Mississippi, University, MS, USA

Martin J. MacInnis
Faculty of Kinesiology, University of Calgary, Calgary, Alberta, Canada

Robyn F. Madden
Alberta Children's Hospital Research Institute, Cumming School of Medicine; Faculty of Kinesiology, University of Calgary, Calgary, Alberta, Canada

Joseph Matthews
Musculoskeletal Physiology Research Group, Sport, Health and Performance Enhancement (SHAPE) Research Centre, School of Science & Technology, Nottingham Trent University & Research Centre for Life and Sport Sciences (CLaSS), School of Health and Life Sciences, Department of Sport and Exercise, Birmingham City University, Birmingham, UK

Sean L. McGee
Metabolic Research Unit, School of Medicine, Deakin University, Waurn Ponds, Victoria, Australia

Chris McGlory
School of Kinesiology and Health Studies, Queens University, Kingston, Ontario, Canada

James McKendry
Exercise Metabolism Research Group, Department of Kinesiology, McMaster University, Hamilton, Ontario, Canada

Greg L. McKie
Human Health and Nutritional Sciences, College of Biological Science, University of Guelph, Guelph, Ontario, Canada

Daniel R. Moore
Faculty of Kinesiology and Physical Education, University of Toronto, Toronto, Ontario, Canada

Colin N Moran
Physiology, Exercise and Nutrition Research Group, Faculty of Health Sciences and Sport, University of Stirling, Scotland, UK

Taniya S. Nagpal
School of Human Kinetics, University of Ottawa, Ottawa, Ontario, Canada

Christopher Newell
Faculty of Medicine, Cumming School of Medicine, University of Calgary, Alberta, Canada

Alissa Newman
Department of Health and Exercise Science, Colorado State University, Fort Collins, CO, USA

Quentin Nichols
Department of Human Nutrition, Foods and Exercise, Virginia Tech, Blacksburg, Virginia, USA

Contributors

Justin X. Nicoll
Department of Kinesiology, California State University, Northridge, CA, USA

Luke A. Olsen
University of Kansas Medical Center, Kansas City, KS, USA

Gianni Parise
Department of Kinesiology, McMaster University, Hamilton, Ontario, Canada

Jill A. Parnell
Department of Health and Physical Education, Mount Royal University, Calgary, Alberta, Canada

Christopher Perry
School of Kinesiology and Health Science, York University, Toronto, Ontario, Canada

Stuart M. Phillips
Exercise Metabolism Research Group, Department of Kinesiology, McMaster University, Hamilton, Ontario, Canada

Henriette Pilegaard
Cell Biology and Physiology, University of Copenhagen, Copenhagen, Denmark

John C. Quindry
School of Integrative Physiology and Athletic Training, University of Montana, Missoula, MT, USA

Michael C. Riddell
School of Kinesiology and Health Sciences, York University, Toronto, Ontario, Canada

Stine Ringholm
Cell Biology and Physiology, University of Copenhagen, Copenhagen, Denmark

Robert Ross
School of Kinesiology and Health Studies, Queens University, Kingston, Ontario, Canada

Craig Sale
Musculoskeletal Physiology Research Group, Sport, Health and Performance Enhancement (SHAPE) Research Centre, School of Science & Technology, Nottingham Trent University, UK

Bryan Saunders
Applied Physiology and Nutrition Research Group, School of Physical Education and Sport; Rheumatology Division & Institute of Orthopaedics and Traumatology, Faculty of Medicine FMUSP, University of São Paulo, São Paulo, Brazil

Maja Schlittler
Department of Physiology & Pharmacology, Karolinska Institute, Stockholm, Sweden

Sam N. Scott
School of Kinesiology and Health Sciences, York University, Toronto Canada & Research Institute for Sport and Exercise Sciences, Liverpool John Moores University, Liverpool, UK

Hesham Shamshoum
Human Health and Nutritional Sciences, College of Biological Science, University of Guelph, Guelph, Ontario, Canada

Jane Shearer
Alberta Children's Hospital Research Institute, Cumming School of Medicine;
Faculty of Kinesiology, University of Calgary, Calgary, Alberta, Canada

Sam O. Shepherd
Research Institute for Sport and Exercise Sciences, Liverpool John Moores University, Liverpool, UK

Marc Sicova
Department of Nutritional Sciences, Faculty of Medicine, University of Toronto, Toronto, Ontario, Canada

Lauren E. Skelly
Faculty of Health, York University, Toronto, Ontario, Canada

Lawrence Spriet
Human Health and Nutritional Sciences, College of Biological Science, University of Guelph, Guelph, Ontario, Canada

Logan K. Townsend
Human Health and Nutritional Sciences, College of Biological Science, University of Guelph, Guelph, Ontario, Canada

Matthew Triolo
School of Kinesiology and Health Science, Muscle Health Research Centre, York University, Toronto Ontario, Canada

Alex T. Von Schulze
University of Kansas Medical Center, Kansas City, KS, USA

Stella L. Volpe
Department of Human Nutrition, Foods, and Exercise, Virginia Tech, Blacksburg, Virginia, USA

Anton J.M. Wagenmakers
Research Institute for Sport and Exercise Sciences, Liverpool John Moores University, Liverpool, UK

Guan Wang
Collaborating Centre of Sports Medicine, University of Brighton, Eastbourne, UK

Håkan Westerblad
Department of Physiology & Pharmacology, Karolinska Institute, Stockholm, Sweden

Jamie Whitfield
Mary MacKillop Institute for Health Research, Melbourne, VIC, Australia

David C. Wright
Human Health and Nutritional Sciences, College of Biological Science, University of Guelph, Guelph, Ontario, Canada

SECTION I

Regulation of Metabolism and Responses to Acute Exercise

Rebecca E.K. MacPherson

Exercise is a potent stimulus that results in a constellation of changes in signaling cascades and metabolism. These changes function to provide energy required for muscle contraction, as well as to stimulate adaptations to better respond to repeated exercise bouts. This section will provide a detailed understanding of the unique biochemical characteristics of an acute exercise stimulus.

The ability to exercise depends on the conversion of chemical energy to mechanical energy in skeletal muscle. The nature of the exercise challenge determines the acute metabolic and molecular responses, which ultimately lead to the long-term physiological adaptations of exercise training. With acute exercise, the contribution of metabolic pathways to energy provision is determined by the relative intensity and absolute power output of the exercise bout. The absolute power output determines the rate of adenosine triphosphate (ATP) demand and energy expenditure, whereas the relative exercise intensity influences the relative contributions of carbohydrate and lipid sources. Further, alterations in signaling cascades depend on the duration, intensity, and type of exercise (aerobic, anaerobic, resistance, etc.).

This chapter focuses on the underlying biochemical and regulatory mechanisms involved in the response to an acute bout of exercise. We begin with an understanding of whole-body regulation of energy expenditure and fuel selection, how energy utilization varies depending on exercise intensity and duration, and the role of endocrine regulators during exercise. This chapter further includes an examination of reactive oxygen species as signaling molecules during and following exercise, the biochemical contributors to exercise fatigue, mechanosensitive mechanisms and responses to resistance exercise, heat shock proteins, and multiple signaling pathways in the regulation of cellular responses to exercise.

1

WHOLE-BODY REGULATION OF ENERGY EXPENDITURE, EXERCISE FUEL SELECTION, AND DIETARY RECOMMENDATIONS

Peter W.R. Lemon

Introduction

Today's elite athletes train year-round and expend huge amounts of energy daily. Consequently, dietary recommendations must differ substantially compared to their sedentary counterparts, or both training adaptations and performance will be suboptimal (51). Of primary concern are energy and macronutrient (carbohydrate, fat, and protein) intake because when these needs are met, micronutrient (minerals and vitamins) requirements will also be covered.

To appreciate dietary recommendations fully, an understanding of energy metabolism during intense exercise is required.

Exercise Metabolism

It is well known that with maximal exercise in humans, the whole-body metabolic rate can increase from ~3–3.5 mL oxygen (O_2)•kilogram (kg) body mass (BM)$^{-1}$•minute (min)$^{-1}$ to perhaps 85 mL•kg^{-1}•min^{-1} (~20- to 25-fold), necessitating a huge increase in skeletal muscle substrate supply (3). This fuel consists of the macronutrients fat, protein, and carbohydrate (CHO); originates from one's diet; and is made available rapidly from existing body stores within skeletal muscle, liver, and adipose tissue.

Fat

Quantitatively, the largest supply of exercise substrate is fat [energy density = ~9 kcal•gram (g)$^{-1}$], located primarily in gender-specific adipose sites as triacylglycerol (31, 46) (i.e., abdominal area in men vs. hips and thighs in women). The magnitude of body fat stores can vary widely from perhaps single digits as a percentage of body mass (4%–9%) in young fit male athletes to values in excess of 50% in many otherwise healthy individuals (14, 18). Free fatty acids (FFAs) are mobilized and released from this triacylglycerol store into the bloodstream by the action of hormone-sensitive lipase when stress hormones are released with exercise. Once in the blood, the FFAs bind to the circulating protein albumin, as they are insoluble in blood, and are delivered to other body tissues via the vascular system. Much of these FFAs go to contracting skeletal muscle due to a rerouting (shunting) of blood flow, as well as a 3- to 5-fold increase in cardiac output (34). These circulating FFAs are rapidly taken up by contracting skeletal muscle [in proportion to their concentration (53, 62)] and oxidized. Fat contributes significantly to the substrate supply for most exercise bouts, except maximal exercise; its rate of use peaks at submaximal intensities (~45%–60% $\dot{V}O_2$max), and it appears to be absolutely greater for women at all exercise intensities (Figure 1.1).

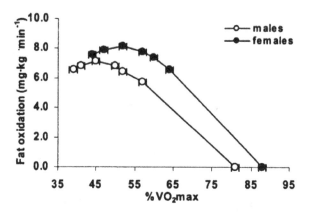

Figure 1.1 Fat oxidation estimates based on respiratory exchange ratio measures vs. exercise intensity in men and women (Ref. 1)

The adipose energy store totals at least 60,000 kilocalories (kcal) in a lean male individual, that is, 10% body fat for a 70-kg man would be ~63,000 kcal (0.1×70 kg $\times 9$ kcal•g^{-1}) to ~284,000 kcal for a 90-kg, 35% body fat female (0.35×90 kg $\times 9$ kcal•g^{-1}=283,500 kcal). To appreciate fully the vastness of this energy supply, even a 63,000-kcal energy store of fat could provide fuel for exercise to continue nonstop at a moderate pace (jogging pace of 2 litres (L) O_2•min^{-1}) for nearly 4.5 days (d) (63,000 kcal ÷ 10 kcal•min^{-1} ÷ 1,440 min•d^{-1} = 4.4 d), assuming 5 kcal energy•L O_2^{-1}! Obviously, storing energy as fat when the food supply is abundant is effective. However, without intermittent periods where food is scarce, this exceptional ability of humans to store dietary energy as fat, especially when combined with a sedentary lifestyle, has resulted in the unfortunate situation where perhaps ~50% of individuals in developed countries are overweight or obese [Table 1.1, (21)].

Typically, overweight is identified as having a body mass index (BMI) = 25–29.9 and obesity as ≥30, where BMI = body mass in kg ÷ height in m^2. Although quantification of body fat by dual energy absorptiometry or densitometry is more accurate in vivo, BMI is easily determined and is acceptable for most because overweight is highly correlated with obesity, except for elite athletes, who are often erroneously classified as obese with this method because of a preponderance of muscle and bone, not fat!

Fat can also be stored in skeletal muscle, and this supply provides additional exercise fuel, especially in exercise-trained individuals (65). However, the skeletal muscle fat energy store pales in comparison to that of adipose tissue, but is important nonetheless because it is readily available as a result of its location next to the contractile proteins. Further, these stores are increased with endurance exercise training and are not insignificant (~2,000–3,000 kcal).

Table 1.1 Prevalence of obesity among Americans ages 20+ years (Ref. 20)

	Age (y)			
	20+	20–39	40–59	60+
	Percent ± SEM			
Men	43.0 ± 2.7	40.3 ± 3.8	46.4 ± 3.2	42.2 ± 3.3
Women	41.9 ± 2.0	39.7 ± 2.7	43.3 ± 2.7	43.3 ± 3.0
Total	42.4 ± 1.8	40.0 ± 2.6	44.8 ± 1.9	42.8 ± 2.5

Source: National Health and Education Examination Survey, 2017–18

y = years, SEM = standard error of the mean

Protein

The next greatest energy store for humans is protein, perhaps 25,000–30,000 kcal in a 70-kg male. However, protein is a minimal contributor as a fuel for muscle contraction, typically because the vast majority of this protein energy is found in either structural (skeletal muscle) or functional (enzymes, hormones, etc.) protein. Protein is made up of amino acids (AAs), which can be oxidized (providing ~4 kcal•g^{-1}) for exercise fuel when other energy sources have become low, but this is a last resort, as it is like burning the walls of a house or the functional components of a furnace in order to keep the place warm. Experimental data indicate that AA oxidation contributes <5% of exercise energy in most exercise situations, increasing to perhaps a maximum of 10% with very prolonged exercise when CHO availability is reduced significantly (36, 37). Consequently, although substantial, protein energy typically does not contribute significantly to exercise fuel. However, meeting dietary protein requirements remains critical for athletes because AAs are needed to repair muscle contraction–induced structural damage, as well as to maximize the exercise training adaptative responses of both hormones and enzymes.

Carbohydrate

In terms of the magnitude of energy stored, the third exercise fuel source is CHO located in skeletal muscle and liver, as well as a small amount as glucose in extracellular fluid. In total, CHO energy (~4 kcal•g^{-1}) amounts to about 1,300–2,800 kcal for a 70-kg individual, depending on both prior exercise and dietary CHO [see Table 1.2 (52)]. Importantly, CHO is the major fuel for intense exercise and, in contrast to fat, its supply can run low or even be exhausted during a single exercise bout, assuming intense, continuous exercise of ~90–120 min duration, like with the 42.2-km marathon run or during repeated, brief, intense efforts over several hours, like those found in many sporting activities (i.e., soccer, football, hockey, tennis, etc.) (6, 20, 25).

Metabolic Pathways

Skeletal muscle uses glucose (glycolysis) from both skeletal muscle glycogen stores (glycogenolysis) and from blood glucose because muscle contraction has an insulin-like effect on muscle glucose uptake from the bloodstream (60). Initially, this circulating glucose is replaced via glucose provided by enhanced liver glycogenolysis. However, in due course, liver glycogen also becomes low or depleted, while muscle uptake continues at a very high rate, resulting in reduced blood glucose concentration with prolonged exercise (hypoglycemia). This needs to be avoided because it can cause disorientation due to a low glucose supply to the brain, as well as exercise fatigue.

Phosphagens: Finally, for intense, short exercise efforts of ~5 sec or less, skeletal muscle phosphagens [adenosine triphosphate (ATP; Reaction 1) and phosphocreatine (PCr; Reaction 2) stored within skeletal muscle contribute energy anaerobically (i.e., without O$_2$). These are especially important when the

Table 1.2 Typical carbohydrate stores in humans (Ref. 51)

Site	CHO (g)		
	Mixed Diet	*High CHO*	*Low CHO*
ECF	9–10	10–11	8–9
Liver	40–50	70–90	0–20
Skeletal Muscle	350	600	300

CHO = carbohydrate, g = grams, ECF = extracellular fluid

exercise intensity exceeds one's aerobic maximum, but these stores are small in magnitude, so a rapid reduction in maximal power output results after just a few seconds of intense effort (8) because the other metabolic pathways (glycolysis and oxidative phosphorylation) regenerate ATP at slower rates.

$$\text{ATP} \xrightarrow{\text{ATPase}} \text{ADP} + \text{Pi} + \text{energy} \qquad [\text{Reaction 1}]$$

$$\text{PCr} + \text{ADP} + \text{H}^+ \xrightarrow{\text{Creatine Kinase}} \text{ATP} + \text{Creatine} \qquad [\text{Reaction 2}]$$

The ATP reaction (Reaction 1) regenerates energy at the greatest rate (several times one's aerobic maximum), and the PCr reaction (Reaction 2) rapidly regenerates ATP. However, the total energy available is limited to a few seconds of maximal exercise due to the modest quantity of both ATP and PCr stored in skeletal muscle (15, 33). Thereafter, exercise can continue, but its intensity must decrease as the anaerobic regeneration of ATP via the breakdown of glucose (glycolysis; Reaction 3) ramps up (peaking by about 60–90 sec) but, as mentioned earlier, cannot match the maximal rate of energy availability from stored ATP breakdown.

$$\text{Glucose} + \text{NAD}^+ + \text{ADP} \rightarrow \text{Lactic Acid} + \text{NAD}^+ + \text{ATP} \qquad [\text{Reaction 3}]$$

Glycolysis: Anaerobic glycolysis occurs in the fluid portion of the muscle (sarcoplasm) and is the process where glucose (itself the end product of glycogenolysis) is converted into lactic acid, regenerating ATP and NAD^+ in the process (Reaction 3). The latter is necessary for glycolysis to continue, as it is needed in an earlier step in the process. Glycolysis regenerates ATP at the next fastest rate following that of the PCr reaction (Reaction 2) and therefore is utilized extensively as exercise intensity increases (becoming substantial at ~60%–70% $\dot{V}O_2$max and increasingly so as intensity exceeds one's aerobic maximum). The resulting increased CO_2 production from lactic acid buffering is thought to activate the respiratory centre in the brain, causing ventilation to increase out of proportion (hyperventilation) to the exercise workload (64), although there has been some debate about the mechanism responsible (49). After a modest delay, some lactic acid enters the bloodstream and is often used to assess the involvement of glycolysis to an exercise bout, as blood is easily collected. However, a blood concentration is only an estimate because some muscle lactic acid is oxidized by adjacent slow-twitch muscle fibres or perhaps even in the same muscle cell [lactate-malate-aspartate shuttle (30)] and therefore never gets into the blood. Further, circulating concentrations reflect the sum total of substance entry into and removal from the blood, so they are not always a good measure of production (i.e., a decrease in removal by the liver would increase blood lactic acid concentration independent of production in skeletal muscle).

Oxidative Phosphorylation: At rest or with exercise below the respiratory threshold (~60%–70% $\dot{V}O_2$max), aerobic glycolysis predominates. Here, pyruvic acid enters the mitochondria rather than being reduced to lactic acid and is converted into acetyl-CoA by the action of the pyruvate dehydrogenase complex, making the electron carrier nicotinamide adenine dinucleotide (NADH) available, as it is not needed to form lactic acid. The acetyl-CoA enters the citric acid cycle, where additional NADH and another electron carrier ($FADH_2$), CO_2, and a small amount of ATP (substrate phosphorylation) are formed. Ultimately, these carriers pass electrons along the electron transport chain (ETC), also located within the mitochondria, resulting in ATP synthesis, utilizing O_2, and forming H_2O as an end product. Since the 1960s this electron carrier oxidation coupling to ATP synthesis (chemiosmotic theory; 42) has been the prevailing explanation underlying how oxidative phosphorylation works, but data are accumulating that the torsional theory may more accurately explain the detail of this key step in oxidative metabolism (2, 45). Finally, aerobic metabolism predominates at rest and with low-to-moderate exercise intensities until the rate of pyruvic acid formation from accelerated glycolysis exceeds its maximal removal rate as acetyl-CoA into the citric acid cycle, at which point anaerobic glycolysis ramps up and muscle lactic acid production increases rapidly.

Glucose

Fatty Acids $+ ADP + NAD^+ + O_2 \rightarrow NAD^+ + CO_2 + H_2O + ATP$ [Reaction 4]

Amino Acids

Oxidative phosphorylation can utilize glucose, FFAs, or even AAs (but, as mentioned, AAs are only minor contributors to exercise energy). Aerobic metabolism is the most energy-efficient metabolic pathway, providing 36–39 ATP (about 18 times more ATP from a mol of glucose vs. anaerobic glycolysis) and much more from a mol of fatty acids, but more importantly, fat oxidation requires O_2 (Reaction 4). From a muscle performance standpoint, this O_2 requirement is critical because it means that the maximal aerobic ATP regeneration rate is determined by the ability to supply and utilize O_2 (i.e., one's $\dot{V}O_2$max). Therefore, possessing a high $\dot{V}O_2$max (at least 70–80 mL•kg^{-1}•min^{-1} for men and 60–70s for women) is one essential prerequisite for elite athletic efforts of ~2 min or longer. In addition, economy of the movement (i.e., $\dot{V}O_2$) required for a given exercise rate is critical (7). Moreover, although exercise training can improve both, genetics is a major determinant, so hard work, although necessary, is not sufficient for athletic success whenever the competition is elite. Finally, a common misconception exists that with intense exercise, these energy pathways are utilized independently and sequentially over time, that is, phosphagens first, then anaerobic glycolysis, and finally oxidative phosphorylation (the latter is delayed, as it takes a couple of min to ramp up the cardiovascular system to deliver the necessary O_2 to the exercising muscle). However, in reality, with intense exercise, all are activated instantaneously when the muscle ATP/ADP (adenosine diphosphate) ratio decreases, but in terms of percentage of energy supplied for the effort, each contributes disproportionally with time, that is, stored phosphagens predominate in the first few sec, anaerobic glycolysis ramps up (peaking at ~30–90 sec), and finally oxidative phosphorylation becomes the major contributor to ATP regeneration from ~2 min onwards (29). Obviously, the situation changes with submaximal exercise intensities. In other words, with moderate intensity exercise, the active skeletal muscle would not rely significantly on stored ATP breakdown or anaerobic glycolysis except briefly, very early in the exercise bout, because the energy requirement could be met by the aerobic capacity of the individual, that is, any stored phosphagen or anaerobic glycolysis involvement would occur only early on, before the cardiovascular system has time to adjust to the increased metabolic demand, and the magnitude of any anaerobic energy contribution would be small and increasingly so as exercise is prolonged. To illustrate, elite marathon runners (42.2 km) have very low circulating lactic acid concentrations (12, 26, 57).

Exercise Fuel Selection

Muscle fuel selection is determined by several factors (exercise intensity, exercise duration, exercise training adaptation, and prior diet). Basically, CHO becomes the predominate fuel with increasing exercise intensity because it is the only macronutrient that muscle can use anaerobically once the very limited stores of phosphagens have been utilized (Figure 1.1). Exercise duration is also a factor because of the limited store of CHO available. As a result, maximizing CHO stores (glycogen loading) prior to glycogen-depleting exercise is critical to performance outcome (9) because once these stores are exhausted, although exercise can continue using FFAs as fuel, it can only do so at a slower pace, which dramatically reduces the chances of success. This is due to the greater O_2 requirement for ATP regeneration from fat (i.e., at any given $\dot{V}O_2$, less ATP is regenerated from fat vs. CHO). Consequently, to perform intense exercise, O_2 utilization becomes the limiting factor to ATP production and not the fuel supply. Of course, this is unfortunate, as it means the vast energy supply in fat stores cannot be utilized fully when exercise becomes intense.

Carbohydrate Loading: Over the years, it has been determined that consuming ~6–10 g•kg^{-1}•d^{-1}, combined with a progressive reduction in exercise training load over several days with no training on the day before competition, increases CHO storage in both skeletal muscle and liver (to about 200%), resulting in enhanced performance in any exercise activity where glycogen stores are challenged (55). This enables one to exercise intensely longer, but it does not double exercise duration because skeletal muscle will use CHO preferentially when dietary CHO is high (1). Further, and more importantly, CHO loading can be accomplished in just 1 day (17) and even without any exercise depletion (10), so there is every reason to take advantage of this procedure whenever CHO depletion could limit performance. However, there is a caveat because this procedure also increases body mass by as much as a kg not only due to the increased onboard CHO but also due to the water stored along with it. Practically, this could affect performance adversely if utilized for activities where the additional CHO is not necessary (i.e., for activities where glycogen depletion is not limiting). This would include short-duration activities (<60 min), regardless of how intense they are. Importantly, this also means that a reduction in dietary CHO intake for a few days prior to shorter-duration events will enhance performance in many activities because less effort is needed when body mass is reduced. Of course, training bouts are often more intense than competitions, that is, 5- to 10-km runners train longer than it takes to race, so they can benefit from CHO loading in training and partial depletion for their races. Consequently, the goal should be to have sufficient CHO on board to maximize exercise intensity for the event duration but not any extra! As with any dietary manipulation, this requires trial and error experimentation, as considerable individual differences exist (Figure 1.2).

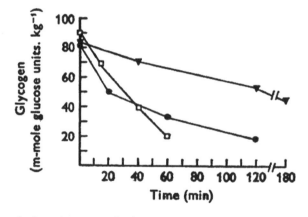

Figure 1.2a   Effect of exercise intensity on muscle glycogen use vs. time

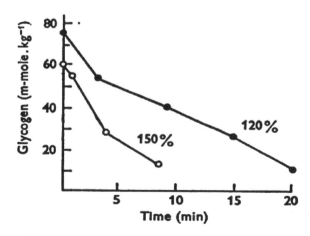

Figure 1.2b   Effect of exercise intensity on muscle glycogen use vs. time

Exercise training also affects fuel use largely because training-induced mitochondrial enzyme adaptations increase the contribution of fatty acid oxidation to any exercise bout (excluding maximal exercise), thereby reducing CHO use (glycogen-sparing effect of exercise training) (28, 44). This often enhances performance because it allows athletes to save their more limited CHO stores for a finishing kick, if needed.

Acute (pre-exercise) ingestion of macronutrient intake also influences the fuel mix used during exercise (47). For example, CHO ingestion and the resulting increase in blood glucose stimulate insulin release from the pancreas, which increases muscle glucose use and inhibits both fat mobilization and oxidation (13). Consequently, one must be careful when attempting to top up glycogen stores with pre-exercise CHO ingestion, as it could affect performance adversely by speeding up glycogen depletion or even causing a hypoglycemic response early in exercise long before glycogen is depleted. Practically, to avoid these concerns, some will need to have their last meal at least 1–4 h prior to the event, depending on individual differences in gut transit/absorption time.

Recently there has been considerable interest in whether a chronic high-fat (ketogenic; $\geq$70% fat) diet can enhance performance by increasing exercise fat use, but the exercise performance data are inconsistent except in very prolonged exercise (i.e., ultramarathons or ironman competitions where the exercise intensity is more modest) (22). Further, these diets are not very palatable, and adherence is often poor (54). However, decreases in body fat mass have been observed that could be advantageous indirectly for any events where body mass needs to be transported (i.e., running races). In particular, various attempts have been made to elevate circulating FFA via ingestion of a fatty pre-exercise meal or with a variety of nutritional supplements, and although several do so and can even reduce reliance on glycogen, exercise performance is seldom enhanced (23).

Dietary Recommendations vs Dietary Requirements

These terms are misunderstood routinely, and because this affects behavior, it is important to clarify each. Very simply, a requirement is the mean value determined in a representative experimental sample group. In contrast, a recommendation is this mean plus 2 standard deviations of the observed data. This means the recommendation contains a safety buffer to cover those in the population at large with greater-than-average requirements. Statistically, this buffer means ~98% of the population will be covered by the recommendation. Importantly, it also means that many will meet their requirement even if they consume less than the recommendation. Often an intake of ~67% of the recommendation is sufficient.

Dietary Recommendation for Athletes

The energy intake of athletes can exceed 50 kcal•kg^{-1}•d^{-1} and, even then, has been reported to be as much as 7%–19% below total daily expenditure in some individuals, depending on the training phase (event preparation vs. competition) (25). Undereating relative to the exercise training load is more prevalent in women (63) and often results in a decrease in metabolism in order to preserve body energy stores similar to how the body responds to starvation (56). This response prolongs life with starvation, but with intense exercise training leads to many adverse effects, including nutritional deficiencies, secondary amenorrhea, and diminished exercise performance (58). This phenomenon has become known as relative energy deficiency in sport (RED-S). Regular snacking will be needed for many athletes in order to attain an adequate daily energy intake, especially for women. Moreover, interindividual variability is substantial, suggesting that individuals should monitor body composition routinely and adjust food/snack/energy supplement intake to prevent energy imbalance.

Macronutrients: Often macronutrient intake is reported as a dietary percentage (i.e., % of energy intake), but this is problematic because, as indicated earlier, dietary intake varies considerably and is often insufficient to match expenditure. Therefore, while 50% dietary CHO would be sufficient for an athlete in training when energy intake is adequate, even 80% CHO would be inadequate when energy intake is low. Therefore, to be certain that a particular diet is sufficient, recommendations should always be expressed as g (for macronutrients) or kcal (for energy) per kg BM.

Carbohydrate: For optimal performance, daily CHO intake should be very high for many athletes (6–10 $g•kg^{-1}•d^{-1}$) because CHO is reduced significantly with most training sessions. Further, many will become satiated before this huge quantity of CHO has been consumed, often necessitating the use of liquid CHO supplementation and/or increased intake of sugar-sweetened snacks or beverages to prevent adverse effects on performance. Although such a practice is contraindicated for sedentary or less physically active individuals, because high sugar and/or energy intake is associated with a number of adverse health effects, including heart disease, diabetes, and obesity (43), the fate of these sugars is different for individuals who exercise and train regularly (i.e., exercise fuel), so this practice does not result in these concerns with athletes.

Protein: The protein needs of athletes have been debated for many years (35, 38), and some believe that regular exercise has little effect on protein requirements (27); however, most groups who work with athletes recognize that exercise training does in fact increase protein need (39, 51, 61). The underlying controversy is complex but centres on the fact that the traditional methodology used to access protein requirements (i.e., nitrogen balance) has several significant limitations (41). Moreover, it requires accurate quantification of nitrogen intake as well as excretion, which can be very difficult practically (36, 40). In contrast, athlete groups rely more on measures of performance, which are more definitive. Importantly, recent data using more precise measures [muscle protein synthesis (59) and the indicator AA technique (16, 48)] indicate clearly that protein needs are increased over their sedentary counterparts, that is, recent indicator AA technique data indicate that protein requirements are increased above current dietary recommendations by 100%–250% (4, 5, 32). The latter technique is minimally invasive, it is accepted as a valid measure of protein requirements (27), and it is more appropriate for athletes because it is performance related, that is, it assesses the protein intake necessary to maximize the adaptive responses to exercise training. Briefly, this technique is based on the partitioning of AA between protein synthesis and oxidation. Very simply, all AA are needed for protein synthesis, so when dietary protein is insufficient, fewer AA enter protein synthesis and, as a result, oxidation of all AA, including the indicator AA, will be significant. When dietary protein increases, oxidation of the indicator AA (like all AA) will decrease because more AA are involved in protein synthesis (i.e., incorporated into body protein). Once the dietary requirement is met, there is no further change in the oxidation of the indicator AA, and the resulting inflection, or "breakpoint," is thought to be the requirement (48). More study is needed with exercise-trained individuals, but recent indicator AA data over a range of protein intakes clearly are consistent with and even extend the earlier nitrogen balance data (39, 61) in support of increased protein recommendations (~2 $g•kg^{-1}•d^{-1}$) for anyone involved in regular exercise training (4, 5; Figure 1.3).

Practically, it is important to understand that despite these observations, protein deficiencies are not likely to be common among athletes. This is because the necessary quantities of protein can be obtained from one's diet without having to utilize supplemental protein, assuming the diet has sufficient energy and contains a wide variety of foods, that is, even a modest protein intake, say 15% of a 4,000-kcal energy intake would be 2.1 $g•kg^{-1}•d^{-1}$ (4,000 kcal × 0.15 ÷ 4 $kcal•g^{-1}$ ÷ 70 kg BM = 2.1 $g•kg^{-1}•d^{-1}$).

Fat: Dietary fat should be adequate to prevent a loss of BM (~1-2 $g•kg^{-1}•d^{-1}$) and could be very important for many athletes to ensure an adequate energy intake because of its energy density. Moreover, low-fat diets have been promoted since the 1960s because of the erroneous belief that fat intake promotes heart disease (50), and many still follow this advice. In contrast, high-fat (ketogenic) diets not only result in body fat and body mass losses, as mentioned, but they also promote a variety of beneficial health effects (11), especially when monounsaturated and polyunsaturated fats are consumed as opposed to saturated and trans fat. Therefore, there is no need for athletes to restrict overall fat intake.

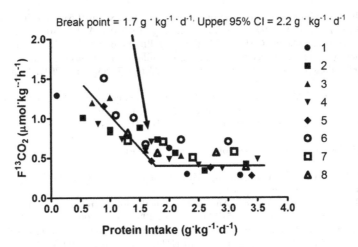

Figure 1.3a Protein intake and $^{13}CO_2$ production from phenylalanine oxidation ($F^{13}CO_2$) in young male bodybuilders

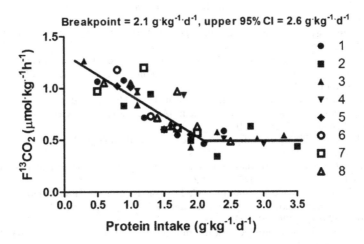

Figure 1.3b Protein intake and $^{13}CO_2$ production from phenylalanine oxidation ($F^{13}CO_2$) in young endurance-trained men

Summary

Elite athletes expend huge amounts of energy in training and often do not consume sufficient dietary energy and/or macronutrients to compensate. As a result, exercise performance is affected adversely. It is recommended that those who train regularly consume 6–10 g•kg^{-1}•d^{-1} of CHO, ~2 g•kg^{-1}•d^{-1} of protein, and 1–2 g•kg^{-1}•d^{-1} of fat. Moreover, energy intakes of 50 kcal•kg^{-1}•d^{-1} or greater are necessary to maintain energy balance. Substantial interindividual differences exist among athletes, so regular monitoring of body composition is recommended in order for individual adjustments to be made.

References

1. Achten J, Jeukendrup AE. Optimizing fat oxidation through exercise and diet. *Nutrition* 20: 716–727, 2004. https://doi.org/10.1016/j,nut2004.04.005
2. Agarwal B. Revisiting the 'chemiosmotic theory': Coupled transport of anion and proton for ATP synthesis. *Bioenergetics* 2:2 2013. https://doi.org/10.4172/2167-7662.1000e116

3. Ball D. Metabolic response and endocrine response to exercise: Sympathoadrenal integration with skeletal muscle. *J Endocrinol* 224: R79–R95, 2015. https://doi.org/10.1530/JOE-14-0408

4. Bandegan A, Courtney-Martin G, Rafii M, Pencharz PB, Lemon PWR. Indicator amino acid–derived estimate of dietary protein requirement for male bodybuilders on a nontraining day is several-fold greater than the current recommended dietary allowance. *J Nutr* 147: 850–857, 2017. https://doi.org/10.3945/jn.116.236331

5. Bandegan A, Courtney-Martin G, Rafii M, Pencharz PB, Lemon PWR. Indicator amino acid oxidation protein requirement estimate in endurance-trained men 24 h postexercise exceeds both the EAR and current athlete guidelines. *Am J Physiol (Enocrinol Metabol)* 316: E741–E748, 2019. https://doi.org/10.1152/ajpendo.00174.2018

6. Bangsbo J, Iaia FM, Krustrup P. Metabolic response and fatigue in soccer. *Int J Sports Physiol Perform* 2: 111–127, 2007. https://doi.org/10.1123/ijspp.2.2.111

7. Barnes KR, Kilding AE. Running economy: Measurement, norms, and determining factors. *Sports Med* 1: 8, 2015. https://doi.org/10.1186/s40798-015-0007-y

8. Bar-Or O. The Wingate anaerobic test: An update on methodology, reliability and validity. *Sports Medicine* 4: 381–394, 1987. https://doi.org/10.2165%2F00007256-198704060-00001

9. Bergström J, Hermansen L, Hultman E, Saltin B. Diet, muscle glycogen and physical performance. *Acta Physiol Scand* 71: 140–150, 1967. https://doi.org/10.1111/j.1748-1716.1967.tb03720.x

10. Bussau VA, Fairchild TJ, Rao A, Steele P, Fournier PA. Carbohydrate loading in human muscle: An improved 1 day protocol. *Eur J Appl Physiol* 87: 290–295, 2002. https://doi.org/10.1007/s00421-002-0621-5

11. Cavaleri F, Bashar E. Potential synergies of β-hydroxybutyrate and butyrate on the modulation of metabolism, inflammation, cognition, and general Health. *J Nutr Metab ecollection* 2018: 7195760, 2018. https://doi.org/10.1155/2018/7195760

12. Costill DL. Physiology of marathon running. *JAMA* 221: 1024–1029, 1972. https://doi.org/10.1001/jama.1972.03200220058013

13. Coyle EF, Jeukendrup AE, Wagenmakers A, Saris W. Fatty acid oxidation is directly regulated by carbohydrate metabolism during exercise. *Am J Physiol Endocrinol Metab* 273: E268–E275, 1997. https://doi.org/10.1152/ajpendo.1997.273.2.E268

14. Duda K, Majerczak J, Nieckarz Z, Heymsfield SB, Zoladz JA. Human body composition and muscle mass. In: *Muscle and Exercise Physiology*, edited by Zoladz JA. Amsterdam: Elsevier, 2019, p 3–26. https://doi.org/10.1016/B978-0-12-814593-7.00001-3

15. Ekblom B. The muscle biopsy technique. Historical and methodological considerations. *Scand J Med Sci Sports* 27: 458–461, 2017. https://doi.org/10.1111/sms.12808

16. Elango R, Ball RO, Pencharz PB. Indicator amino acid oxidation: Concept and application. *J Nutr* 138: 243–246, 2008. https://doi.org/10.1093/jn/138.2.243

17. Fairchild TJ, Fletcher S, Steele P, Goodman C, Dawson B, Fournier PA. Rapid carbohydrate loading after a short bout of near maximal-intensity exercise. *Med Sci Sports Exerc* 34: 980–986, 2002. https://doi.org/10.1097/00005768-200206000-00012

18. Fleck S. Body composition in elite American athletes. *Am J Sport Med* 11: 398–403, 1983. https://doi.org/10.1177/036354658301100604

19. Gollnick PD, Piehl K, Saltin B. Selective glycogen depletion pattern in human muscle fibres after exercise of varying intensity and at varying pedalling rates. *J Physiol* 241: 45–57, 1974. https://doi.org/10.1113/jphysiol.1974.sp010639

20. Green HJ, Daub BD, Painter DC, Thomson JA. Glycogen depletion patterns during ice hockey performance. *Med Sci Sports* 10: 289–293, 1978.

21. Hales CM, Carroll MD, Fryar CD, Ogden CL. Prevalence of obesity and severe obesity among adults: United States, 2017–2018. *NCHS Data Brief* No. 360, 2020. https://www.cdc.gov/nchs/products/databriefs/db360.htm

22. Harvey KL, Holcomb LE, Kolwicz SC Jr. Ketogenic diets and exercise performance. *Nutrients* 11: 2296, 2019. https://doi.org/10.3390/nu11102296

23. Hawley JA. Effect of increased fat availability on metabolism and exercise capacity. *Med Sci Sports Exerc* 2002; 34: 1485–1491, 2002. https://doi.org/10.1097/00005768-200209000-00014

24. Hearris MA, Hammond KM, Fell JM, Morton JP. Regulation of muscle glycogen metabolism during exercise: Implications for endurance performance and training adaptations. *Nutrients* 10: 298, 2018. https://doi.org/10.3390/nu10030298

25. Heydenreich J, Kayser B, Schutz Y, Melzer K. Total energy expenditure, energy intake, and body composition in endurance athletes across the training season: A systematic review. *Sports Med Open* 3: 8, 2017. https://doi.org/10.1186/s40798-017-0076-1

26. Hoff J, Støren Ø, Finstad A, Wang, E, Helgerud J. Increased blood lactate level deteriorates running economy in world class endurance athletes. *J Stren Cond Res* 30: 1373–1378, 2016. https://doi.org/10.1519/JSC.0000000000001349

27. Institute of Medicine. *Dietary Reference Intakes for Energy, Carbohydrate, Fiber, Fat, Fatty Acids, Cholesterol, Protein, and Amino Acids.* Washington, DC: National Academy Press, 2005. https://doi.org/10.17226/10490

28. James DE, Kraegen EW. The effect of exercise training on glycogen, glycogen synthase and phosphorylase in muscle and liver. *Eur J Appl Physiol Occup Physiol* 52: 276–281, 1984. https://doi.org/10.1007/bf01015209

29. Jeukendrup A, Gleeson M. *Sport Nutrition* (3rd Edition). Champaign, IL: Human Kinetics, 2019.

30. Kane DA. Lactate oxidation at the mitochondria: A lactate-malate-aspartate shuttle at work. *Front Neurosci* 8: 366, 2014. https://doi.org/10.3389/fnins.2014.00366

31. Karastergiou K, Smith SR, Greenberg AS, Fried SK. Sex differences in human adipose tissues – the biology of pear shape. *Biol Sex Differ* 3 :13, 2012. https://doi.org/10.1186/2042-6410-3-13

32. Kato H, Suzuki K, Bannai M, Moore DR. Protein requirements are elevated in endurance athletes after exercise as determined by the indicator amino acid oxidation method. *PLoS One* 11(6): e0157406, 2016. https://doi.org/10.1371/journal.pone.0157406

33. Kemp GJ, Meyerspeer M, Moser E. Absolute quantification of phosphorus metabolite concentrations in human muscle *in vivo* by ^{31}P MRS: A quantitative review. *NMR Biomed* 20: 555–565, 2007 .https://doi.org/10.1002/nbm.1192

34. Laughlin, MH. Cardiovascular response to exercise. *Adv Physiol Ed* 277: S245–S259, 1999. https://doi.org/10.1152/advances.1999.277.6.S244

35. Lemon PW. Protein and strength exercise: Historical perspectives. In: *Dietary Protein and Resistance Exercise*, edited by Lowery L &Antonio J. Boca Raton, FL :CRC Press: 2012, p 1–16.

36. Lemon PW. Protein and amino acids. In: *Sport and Exercise Nutrition*, edited by Lanham-New S, Stear SJ, Shirreffs SM &Collins AL. Oxford: Wiley-Blackwell, 2011, p 41–50.

37. Lemon PW, Mullin JP. Effect of initial muscle glycogen levels on protein catabolism during exercise. *J Appl Physiol* 48: 624–629, 1980. https://doi.org/10.1152/jappl.1980.48.4.624

38. Lemon PW, Nagle FJ. Effects of exercise on protein and amino acid metabolism. *Med Sci Sports Exerc* 13: 141–149, 1981.

39. Lemon PW, Tarnopolsky MA, MacDougall JD, Atkinson SA. Protein requirements and muscle mass/strength changes during intensive training in novice bodybuilders. *J Appl Physiol* 73: 767–775, 1992. https://doi.org/10.1152/jappl.1992.73.2.767

40. Lemon PW, Yarasheski KE. Feasibility of sweat collection by whole body washdown in moderate to high humidity environments. *Int J Sports Med* 6: 41–43, 1985. https://doi.org/10.1055/s-2008-1025811

41. Millward DJ. Methodological considerations. *Proc Nutr Soc* 60: 3–5, 2001. https://doi.org/10.1079/PNS200064

42. Mitchell P. Coupling of phosphorylation to electron and hydrogen transfer by a chemi-osmotic type of mechanism. *Nature* 191: 144–148, 1961. https://doi.org/10.1038/191144a0

43. Moore JB, Fielding BA. Sugar and metabolic health: Is there still a debate? *Curr Opin Clin Nutr Metab Care* 19: 303–309, 2016. https://doi.org/10.1097/MCO.0000000000000028

44. Nakatani A, Han D, Hansen PA, Nolte LA, Host HH, Hickner RC, Holloszy JO. Effect of endurance exercise training on muscle glycogen supercompensation in rats. *J. Appl. Physiol.* 82: 711–715, 1997. https://doi.org/10.1152/jappl.1997.82.2.711

45. Nath S, Siddhartha J. The detailed molecular mechanism of ATP synthesis in the F_0 portion of ATP synthase reveals a non-chemiosmotic mode of energy coupling. *Thermochim Acta* 394: 89–98, 2002. https://doi.org/10.1016/S0040-6031(02)00242-3

46. Nindl BC, Scoville CR, Sheehan KM, Leone CD, Mello RP. Gender differences in regional body composition and somatotrophic influences of IGF-I and leptin. *J Appl Physiol* 92: 1611–1618, 2002. https://doi.org/10.1152/japplphysiol.00892.2001

47. Ormsbee MJ, Bach CW, Baur DA. Pre-exercise nutrition: The role of macronutrients, modified starches and supplements on metabolism and endurance performance. *Nutrients* 6: 1782–1808, 2014. https://doi.org/10.3390/nu6051782

48. Pencharz PB, Ball RO. Different approaches to define individual amino acid requirements. *Annu Rev Nutr* 23: 101–16, 2003. https://doi.ord/10.1146/annurev.nutr.23.011702.073247

49. Péronnet F, Aguilaniu B. Lactic acid buffering, nonmetabolic CO_2 and exercise hyperventilation: A critical reappraisal. *Resp Physiol Neurobiol* 25: 4–18, 2006. https://doi.org/10.1016/j.resp.2005.04.005

50. Pett KD, Willett WC, Vartiainen E, Katz DL. The Seven Countries Study. *European Heart Journal* 38: 3119–3121, 2017. https://doi.org/10.1093/eurheartj/ehx603

51. Position of the Academy of Nutrition and Dietetics, Dietitians of Canada, and the American College of Sports Medicine: Nutrition and Athletic Performance. *J Acad Nutri Dietet* 116: 501–528, 2016. https://doi.org/10.1016/j.jand.2015.12.006

52. Saltin B, Gollnick PD. Fuel for muscular exercise: Role of carbohydrate. In: *Exercise, Nutrition and Exercise Metabolism*, edited by Horton ES & Terjung RL. New York, NY: MacMillian, 1988, p 45–71.

53. Schiffelers S, Saris W, van Baak, M. The effect of an increased free fatty acid concentration on thermogenesis and substrate oxidation in obese and lean men. *Int J Obes* 25: 33–38, 2001. https://doi.org/10.1038/sj.ijo.0801528

54. Schoeler NE, Cross, JH. Ketogenic dietary therapies in adults with epilepsy: A practical guide. *Pract Neurol* 16: 208–214, 2016. http://dx.doi.org/10.1136/practneurol-2015-001288

55. Sherman WM, Costill DL, Fink WJ, Miller JM. Effect of exercise-diet manipulation on muscle glycogen and its subsequent utilization during performance. *Int J Sports Med* 2: 114–118, 1981. https://doi.org/10.1055/s-2008-1034594

56. Shetty PS. Physiological mechanisms in the adaptive response of metabolic rates to energy restriction. *Nutr Res Rev* 3: 49–74, 1990. https://doi.org/10.1079/NRR19900006

57. Sjödin B, Jacobs I. Onset of blood lactate accumulation and marathon running performance. *Int J Sports Med* 2: 23–26, 1981. https://doi.org/10.1016/j.resp.2005.04.005

58. Statuta SM, Asi IM, Drezner JA. Relative energy deficiency in sport (RED-S). *Br J Sport Med* 51: 1570–1571, 2017. http://dx.doi.org/10.1136/bjsports-2017-097700

59. Stokes T, Hector AJ, Morton RW, McGlory C, Phillips SM. Recent perspectives regarding the role of dietary protein for the promotion of muscle hypertrophy with resistance exercise training. *Nutrients* 10: 180, 2018. https://doi.org/10.3390/nu10020180

60. Sylow L Kleinert M, Richter EA, Jensen TE. Exercise-stimulated glucose uptake - regulation and implications for glycaemic control .*Nat Rev Endocrinol* 13: 133–148, 2017. https://doi.org/10.1038/nrendo.2016.162

61. Tarnopolsky MA, MacDougall JD, Atkinson SA. Influence of protein intake and training status on nitrogen balance and lean body mass. *J Appl Physiol* 64: 187–193, 1988. https://doi.org/10.1152/jappl.1988.64.1.187

62. Turcotte LP, Richter EA, Kiens B. Increased plasma FFA uptake and oxidation during prolonged exercise in trained vs untrained humans. *Am J Physiol* 262: E791–E799, 1992. https://doi.org/10.1152/ajpendo.1992.262.6.E791

63. van Erp-Baart AMJ, Saris WHM, Binkhorst RA, Vos JA, Elvers JWH. Nationwide survey on nutritional habits in elite athletes part 1: Energy, carbohydrate, protein, and fat intake. *Int J Sports Med* 10: S3–S10, 1989. https://doi.org/10.1055/s-2007-1024947

64. Wasserman K. Dyspnea on exertion. Is it the heart or the lungs? *JAMA* 248: 2039–2043, 1982. https://doi.org/10.1001/jama.1982.03330160083033

65. Wolfe RR. Fat metabolism in exercise. In: *Skeletal Muscle Metabolism in Exercise and Diabetes. Advances in Experimental Medicine and Biology*, edited by Richter EA, Kiens B, Galbo H, Saltin B. Boston, MA: Springer, 1998, Vol 441, p 147–156. https://doi.org/10.1007/978-1-4899-1928-_14

2

ENERGY PROVISION, FUEL USE AND REGULATION OF SKELETAL MUSCLE METABOLISM DURING THE EXERCISE INTENSITY/DURATION CONTINUUM

Lawrence L. Spriet

Introduction

The provision of energy in the form of adenosine triphosphate (ATP) is essential for skeletal muscle contractions. The amount of ATP that is needed during exercise is determined primarily by the intensity and duration of the exercise. However, other factors can influence the need for energy, including the preceding diet, training status, age, sex, and environmental conditions. During exercise of any intensity, ATP is required for the processes involved in activating and contracting muscle. The enzymes involved in these processes include membrane excitability (Na^+-K^+ ATPase), sarcoplasmic reticulum calcium handling (Ca^{2+} ATPase), and myofilament cross-bridge cycling (myosin ATPase). An interesting characteristic of muscle cells is that the ATP store is small at ~25 mmol/kg dry muscle (dm) or ~5 mmol/kg wet muscle (wm), which means that contractions could not be sustained for very long without the generation of new ATP. For example, if exercising at a submaximal power output of ~200 W (~67% of maximal oxygen uptake [VO_2 max]), the rate of ATP utilization would be ~0.4 mmol ATP/kg wm/s and the muscle ATP store would last ~12–13 s! During an all-out 10 s sprint, where power output averages ~1,000 W (~333% of VO_2 max), the ATP utilization rate would be ~3.7 mmol ATP/kg wm/s and exercise would last <2 s if stored ATP was the only energy source. Remarkably, the skeletal muscle (ATP) is well defended and does not decrease during most exercise situations. This is explained by the existence of very well-developed metabolic pathways that can generate ATP at very high rates for short periods of time and lower rates for very long times.

The purpose of this chapter is to provide an overview of skeletal muscle energy utilization and metabolism during the exercise intensity/duration continuum. The metabolic responses to exercise and fuel use during exercise have been well studied and described since the early 20th century (6). Many previous review articles have been written on aspects of this topic, and the reader is encouraged to consult these resources for historical information and more detail than may be found here (21, 30, 31, 35, 39, 51, 71, 75, 76, 82, 83).

Overview of Metabolism and Fuel Use

To meet the ATP needs of exercise, skeletal muscle has an array of metabolic pathways that can synthesize ATP from adenosine diphosphate (ADP) and inorganic phosphate (Pi) at very high rates and for long periods of time (Figure 2.1). These ATP-producing pathways can be categorized as substrate-level

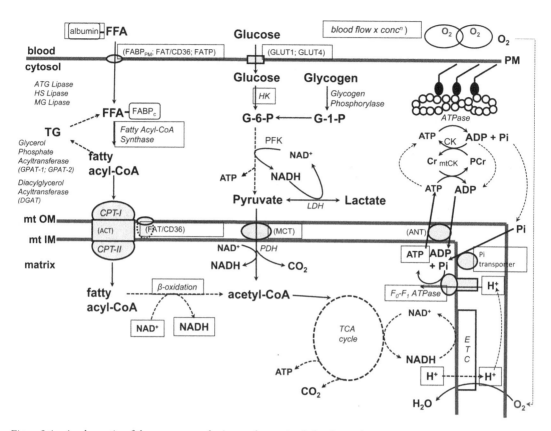

Figure 2.1   A schematic of the energy-producing pathways in skeletal muscle

phosphorylation (or "anaerobic") and oxidative phosphorylation (or "aerobic"). The so-called anaerobic energy pathways include the breakdown of phosphocreatine (PCr) to produce ATP and the generation of ATP in the glycolytic pathway, with muscle glycogen as the substrate and lactate as a by-product (Table 2.1). These pathways reside in the cytoplasm and have a much higher rate of ATP production but a smaller capacity for ATP production as compared to the aerobic pathways (77). The production of aerobic ATP in the mitochondria requires oxygen, ADP, and Pi and reducing equivalents (NADH, $FADH_2$) from the metabolism of primarily fat and carbohydrate (CHO). The produced ATP is then moved into the cytoplasm to the various sites of ATP utilization. Skeletal muscle is very dependent

Table 2.1 Energy-producing pathways in skeletal muscle

	ATP Utilization
	$ATP + H_2O \rightarrow ADP + Pi + energy$
	ATP Resynthesis
Substrate phosphorylation	$PCr + ADP + H^+ \rightarrow ATP + creatine$
	$2\,ADP \rightarrow ATP + AMP$
	$Glycogen + 3\,ADP \rightarrow 2\,lactate + 2H^+ + 3\,ATP$
Oxidative phosphorylation	$Glucose + 6O_2 + 36\text{–}38\,ADP \rightarrow 6CO_2 + 6H_2O + 36\text{–}8\,ATP$
	$Palmitate + 23O_2 + 136\text{–}8\,ADP \rightarrow 16CO_2 + 16H_2O + 136\text{–}8\,ATP$

ADP = adenosine diphosphate; ATP = adenosine triphosphate; AMP = adenosine monophosphate;
Pi = inorganic phosphate; PCr = phosphocreatine

on the respiratory and cardiovascular systems to deliver adequate oxygen for the maintenance of aerobic ATP provision, and the by-products of ATP breakdown in the cytoplasm (ADP, Pi) must also be transported back into the mitochondria. Most of the required reducing equivalents are produced directly in the mitochondria in the fat and CHO metabolic pathways and the tricarboxylic acid (TCA) cycle (Figure 2.1). A small amount of NADH produced in the glycolytic pathway can also be shuttled into the mitochondria. In terms of the fuel for oxidative metabolism, CHO oxidation can be activated quickly, has a higher power output, and is a more efficient fuel (kcal/L O_2 used) when compared to fat, but does have a lower capacity than fat oxidation. Given that CHO can also be used to provide anaerobic energy, it is clearly the dominant fuel for high-intensity exercise, whether it be in the aerobic or anaerobic (sprinting) domains.

High-Intensity, Short-Term Exercise

When very intense, sprint-like exercise lasting a few seconds begins, all the pathways associated with both anaerobic and aerobic ATP provision are activated, or "turned on." However, the rates of ATP provision from the anaerobic sources, PCr and anaerobic glycolysis, are much quicker than from aerobic pathways, as the latter needs time to fully activate. Direct measurements of muscle PCr and glycogen before, during, and after sprint exercise bouts (~250% VO_2 max) show significant decreases in these substrates and increases in lactate (26, 59, 60, 65) (Figure 2.2). The decreases in PCr and glycogen and increases in lactate are usually greater in type II compared with type I fibres (29). And as stated, the muscle (ATP) is reasonably well maintained, although it may decrease by ~20–40% during very intense exercise (Figure 2.3) (29, 65). PCr is a remarkable fuel source, as only one metabolic reaction is required to provide ATP (Table 2.1). The enzyme that catalyzes this reaction (creatine phosphokinase [CPK]) is in high abundance and only regulated by the concentration of its substrates and products—a so-called "near-equilibrium enzyme." So as soon as contractions begin and ATP is broken down and the ADP concentration increases, this reaction will move from left to right and ATP is regenerated in a few msec (Table 2.1).

At the same time, cellular Ca^{2+} (and to some extent epinephrine [EPI] from outside the cell) activates phosphorylase kinase to move glycogen phosphorylase from its less active "b" form to the more active "a" form in what is called covalent regulation. Increases in ADP and adenosine monophosphate (AMP) (Figure 2.4) also activate phosphorylase a directly (allosteric regulation) to degrade glycogen and combine with Pi to produce glucose 1-phosphate, glucose 6-phosphate (G-6-P), and fructose 6-phosphate (F-6-P) in the glycolytic pathway (19, 70). Phosphorylase is considered a "non-equilibrium enzyme," as it is controlled by external factors and not just substrates and products. This impressive combination of covalent and allosteric regulation explains how the flux through phosphorylase can increase from very low rates at rest to very high rates during intense exercise in only a few msec! The increases in allosteric regulators ADP, AMP, and Pi (which are by-products of ATP breakdown, Figure 2.4) and the accumulating substrate F-6-P activate the regulatory enzyme phosphofructokinase and flux through the reactions of the glycolytic pathway, which continues with a net production of 3 ATP and lactate formation.

Even though more reactions are involved in producing ATP in the glycolytic pathway compared to PCr, the production of ATP through anaerobic glycolysis is also activated over a msec time course. Lactate accumulation can be measured in the muscle after a 1 s contraction and the contribution of anaerobic energy from PCr and anaerobic glycolysis is essentially equivalent after 6–10 s of intense exercise (Figure 2.5) (26, 65, 84). When intense exercise is sustained and the demand for ATP is great, a small amount of energy can be produced in the near-equilibrium myokinase reaction, where 2 ADP generate ATP and AMP (Table 2.1).

The capacity of the PCr energy store is a function of its resting content (~75 mmol/kg dm) and can be mostly used up in 10–15 s of all-out exercise, whereas the anaerobic glycolytic capacity is about 3-fold higher (~225 mmol/kg dm) over exercise lasting 30–90 s and is limited not by glycogen substrate, but

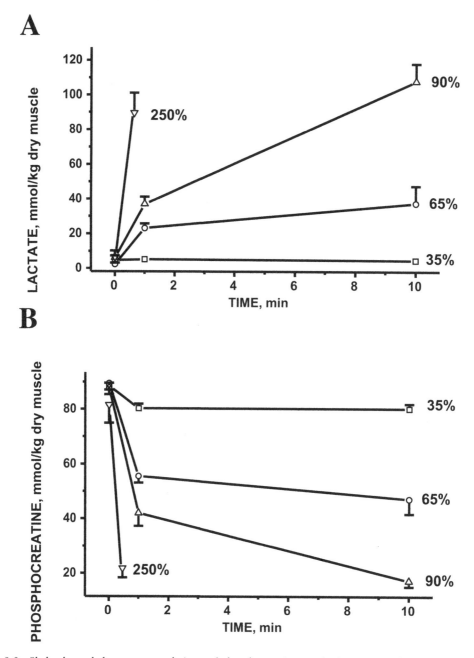

Figure 2.2 Skeletal muscle lactate accumulation and phosphocreatine use during 10 min of exercise at 35%, 65%, and 90% and 30 s at ~250% VO$_2$ max (reproduced from 47, 65)

the muscle's increasing acidity (7, 59, 60). The increases in ATP utilization, glycolysis, and strong ion fluxes during sprint exercise result in metabolic acidosis (52, 85). The decline in power output during single and repeated bouts of maximal exercise is associated with PCr depletion (17, 32, 85), accumulation of metabolic by-products (H$^+$, ADP, AMP, Pi) (17, 32), and hyperkalaemia (58) that decrease the excitation–contraction coupling processes within skeletal muscle (3). Much of this information was generated during all-out cycling sprints where the power output in the first 5–10 s was ~1,000 W

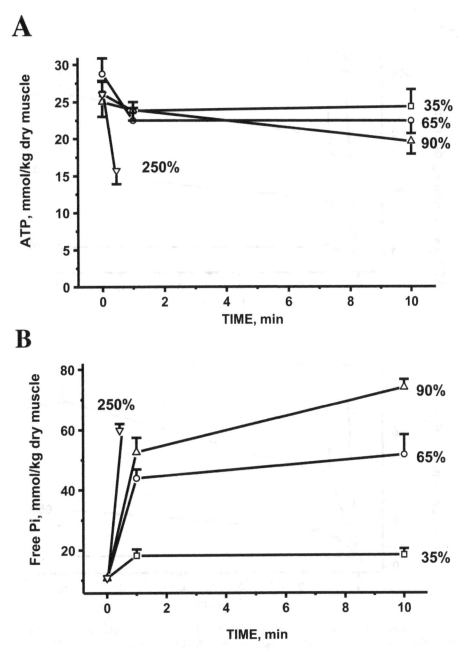

Figure 2.3 Skeletal muscle ATP content and free inorganic phosphate (Pi) accumulation during 10 min of exercise at 35%, 65%, and 90% and 30 s at ~250% VO$_2$ max (reproduced from 47, 65)

and despite maximal efforts, the power output decreased to ~400–500 W by 30 s. Sprinting efforts requiring lower-power outputs require lower rates of anaerobic energy production, and in fact most sprints in stop-and-go sports last only 2–5 s, although there will be many sprints in an entire training session or game (54).

It should also be pointed out that the production of aerobic ATP is turning on during very intense exercise and 70–100% of the VO$_2$ max can be reached in an all-out 30 s sprint (Figure 2.5) (52, 65).

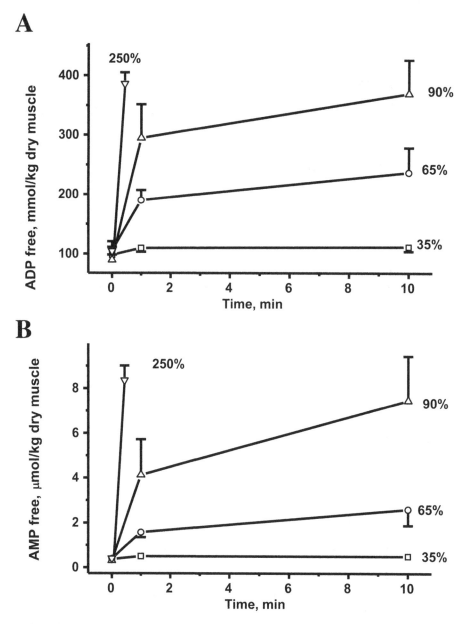

Figure 2.4 Skeletal muscle–free adenosine diphosphate (ADP) and adenosine monophosphate (AMP) accumulation during 10 min of exercise at 35%, 65%, and 90% and 30 s at ~250% VO_2 max (reproduced from 47, 65)

However, the time for aerobic ATP contribution is short, and while little is provided in the first 5–10 s, ~50% of the energy contribution in the last 5 s of the 30 s sprint is aerobic (65). If the exercise task lasts beyond about 1 min, oxidative phosphorylation becomes the major ATP-generating pathway (59). During the transition from rest to intense exercise, the substrate for the increasing aerobic ATP production is from muscle glycogen as a small amount of the produced pyruvate is transported into the mitochondria to produce acetyl-CoA and the reducing equivalent NADH in the pyruvate dehydrogenase (PDH) reaction (Figure 2.6). This enzyme is also under covalent control, existing in an inactive form at rest and moved to a fully active form by Ca^{2+} during exercise. The power of Ca^{2+}, with help from

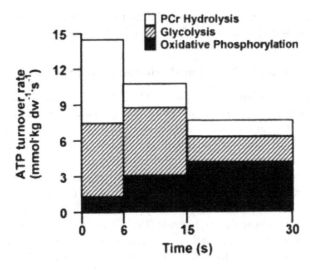

Figure 2.5 Contribution of phosphocreatine (PCr), anaerobic glycolysis, and oxidative phosphorylation to energy (ATP) provision during a 30 s all-out sprint at ~250% VO$_2$ max (reproduced from 65)

pyruvate, keeps the enzyme in the active form despite increases in acetyl-CoA that would normally inactivate the enzyme at rest (47).

Another important aspect of high-intensity, short-term energy production relates to the ability to rapidly resynthesize PCr when the exercise intensity falls to low levels or the athlete rests. This is common in stop-and-go sports where short sprints are interspersed with rest periods and where continued aerobic ATP production fuels the regeneration of PCr, such that the store can be completely recovered in 60–120 s (33, 48). This is extremely important for the ability to repeatedly sprint in stop-and-go or intermittent sports, as the recovery of the glycolytic system from prolonged sprinting (20–120 s) and the associated muscle acidity takes minutes, not seconds, and can limit performance (26, 65). The ability to buffer the produced acid is also paramount for success in one-off sprints and in stop-and-go sports, and buffering capacities are generally very high in these athletes due to a combination of genetic

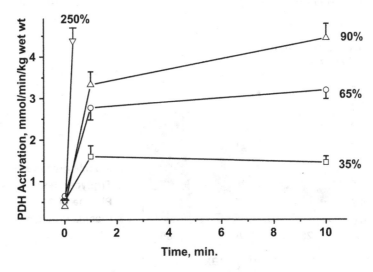

Figure 2.6 Pyruvate dehydrogenase (PDH) activation during 10 min of exercise at 35%, 65%, and 90% and 30 s at ~250% VO$_2$ max (reproduced from 47, 65)

endowment and adaptation to sprint training (10). In most stop-and-go sports, sprints are usually kept short such that increasing acidity is minimized and the PCr store is not completely exhausted (54).

Energy Provision During Aerobic Exercise

During exercise lasting several minutes through to ~2 h that is aerobic in nature (requiring less energy than at VO$_2$ max), the oxidative metabolism of CHO and fat provides almost all the ATP for contracting skeletal muscles. Other potential fuels like amino acids can contribute energy, but this contribution is usually very small in well-fed subjects. The initial transition from rest to exercise in the first 1–2 min and any transitions from one power output to a higher power output will still require some anaerobic energy while oxidative metabolism adjusts to the new higher power output. The amount of anaerobic energy required at the start of exercise increases as a function of the intensity of the exercise and is referred to as the oxygen deficit (46, 59, 60). The major substrates in the muscle for aerobic ATP production are glycogen and intramuscular triglyceride (IMTG) and from outside the cell (exogenous) are blood glucose (derived from liver glycogenolysis and gluconeogenesis and from the gut when CHO is ingested) and free fatty acids (FFAs) derived from adipose tissue triglyceride stores (Figure 2.1). The reliance on these substrates was accurately measured by two independent laboratories at varying exercise power outputs expressed as a percentage of VO$_2$ max or W max (Figures 2.7 and 2.8) (73, 93). These measurements were made on well-trained young male cyclists using indirect calorimetry, stable isotope techniques, and muscle biopsies. In the Romijn et al. (73) study, measurements were made in the final 30 min of 2-hour cycles at 25% and 65% VO$_2$ max and between 20 and 30 min at 85% VO$_2$ max. In the van Loon et al. (93) study, measurements were made during a 30-min cycle at each of the three workloads.

These data provide several important insights regarding fuel utilization with increasing exercise intensity. At rest and 25% VO$_2$ max, glucose and FFA can be transported into the cell at a rate that provides the required fuel, with FFA as the dominant fuel at 25% VO$_2$ max (low intensity). When the exercise intensity is increased to 40–55% W max and 65% VO$_2$ max (moderate intensities), the contribution from exogenous FFA is maintained, the exogenous glucose contribution increases, and significant amounts of muscle glycogen and IMTG are used to meet the increasing energy demand (73, 93). The contribution of fat reaches its max at these moderate power outputs, and the total contribution from fat and CHO is about 50/50 (Figures 2.7 and 2.8). When moving to 75% W max and 85% VO$_2$ max (high intensities), the contribution from FFA and IMTG decreases, reliance on blood-borne glucose increases,

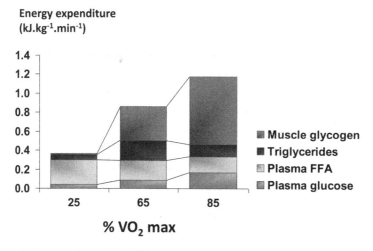

Figure 2.7   Fuel use during exercise at 25%, 65%, and 85 VO$_2$ max (reproduced from 73)

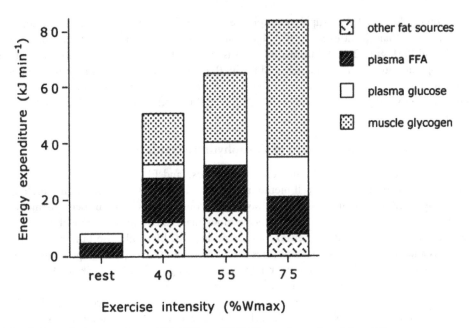

Figure 2.8 Fuel use during exercise at 40%, 55%, and 75% W max (reproduced from 93)

and use of muscle glycogen becomes the dominate provider of fuel. In both data sets, CHO provided ~75% of the fuel at these higher power outputs. To summarize, CHO oxidation, in particular from muscle glycogen, dominates at the higher exercise intensities, and fat oxidation is more important at lower intensities. Maximal rates of fat oxidation occur at moderate intensities (~60–65% VO_2 max) (1).

In a similar experiment with young well-trained women (74), the fuel use results at 25%, 65%, and 85% VO_2 max were essentially identical to those of the men (73). In less well-trained or untrained subjects, the reliance on CHO is higher at moderate and higher power outputs (20–22). In addition, less well-trained subjects cannot sustain exercise at power outputs of ~60% VO_2 max and above as long as trained subjects can, even though the absolute power outputs are much lower (47).

Regulation of Aerobic Energy Production

When examining the regulation of energy production during aerobic exercise, there is time to mobilize fat and CHO fuel not only from sources in the muscle but also from adipose tissue and the liver. To produce the required ATP, the respiratory or electron transport chain in the mitochondria needs the following substrates: reducing equivalents in the form of NADH and $FADH_2$, free ADP and Pi, and O_2. The respiratory and cardiovascular systems ensure the delivery of O_2 to the contracting muscles, and the by-products of ATP use in the cytoplasm (ADP, Pi) are transported back into the mitochondria for resynthesis. The processes that move ATP out of the mitochondria and ADP and Pi back into the mitochondria are being intensely studied and appear to be more heavily controlled than previously thought (62, 67). In the face of ample O_2, ADP, and Pi in the mitochondria, the increase in ADP with exercise is believed to activate the respiratory chain to produce ATP (37).

The TCA cycle in the mitochondria specializes in producing reducing equivalents and accepts acetyl-CoA from both CHO and fat (and to a minor extent other fuels) to achieve this. During aerobic exercise, increasing Ca^{2+} activates many regulatory sites of metabolism, starting with the isocitrate and alpha-ketoglutarate dehydrogenase enzymes in the TCA cycle (75). Substrate accumulation and local regulators fine-tune the flux through these dehydrogenases and a third enzyme, citrate synthase, to increase and control TCA cycle flux. Ca^{2+} also activates glycogen phosphorylase and PDH (Figure 2.6), but the glycolytic flux needed to supply enough acetyl-CoA from CHO and ultimately aerobic ATP production is lower than sprint exercise (47), due to smaller increases in the fine-tuners of metabolism, ADP, AMP, and Pi (Figure 2.3). Additional NADH is produced in the glycolytic pathway and shuttled from the cytoplasm into the mitochondria and in the PDH reaction, which is in the mitochondria. At the same time Ca^{2+} (and EPI) also activates the key enzymes regulating IMTG degradation, adipose triglyceride lipase (ATGL) and hormone sensitive lipase (HSL), and FFAs are provided in the cytoplasm (90, 100) (Figure 2.1).

Regulation of Carbohydrate Oxidation

Increased Ca^{2+} also contributes to the movement of glucose and FFAs into the muscle cell from the blood using transport proteins at the cell membranes and t-tubules (30, 31). Although muscle glycogen is quantitatively more important as a CHO fuel source for contracting skeletal muscle during moderate- and high-intensity aerobic exercise, blood glucose does make an important contribution to overall carbohydrate oxidation, especially when exercise is prolonged. Liver glucose output from both liver glycogenolysis and gluconeogenesis accompanies the increase in muscle glucose uptake such that blood (glucose) is generally maintained, unless exercise is very prolonged (2, 22, 95). Skeletal muscle glucose uptake occurs by facilitated diffusion with three sites of regulation: (1) glucose delivery, (2) sarcolemmal glucose transport mediated by a glucose transporter (GLUT4), and (3) glucose phosphorylation by hexokinase and subsequent metabolism (96). Although glucose transport is thought to be rate-limiting under resting conditions, the large increases in blood flow and glucose delivery and rapid GLUT4 translocation to surface membranes allow glucose transport to increase during exercise (45, 53, 104). While increasing Ca^{2+} is important for increasing glucose uptake during exercise (102), other factors may play a role in this process, including mechanical stress/force, metabolic perturbations (increased AMP, decreased PCr and glycogen), changes in the redox state associated with increased levels of reactive oxygen species (ROS), and increased nitric oxide (NO). For a detailed examination of these factors and the underlying signals and molecular control of glucose uptake, see Richter and Hargreaves (71) and Hargreaves and Spriet (31).

With increasing aerobic exercise intensities there is greater reliance on muscle glycogen for CHO fuel. As discussed in the previous section on high-intensity, short-term exercise, the flux through phosphorylase is activated by moving more of this enzyme to the active form (Ca^{2+} and, to some extent, EPI) and increasing its activity through direct allosteric regulation by ADP and AMP (47, 101). This assumes that ample glycogen and Pi are available as substrates. The enzyme PDH is also quickly activated (less than 1 min) by Ca^{2+} and increasing pyruvate levels, and the rates of CHO oxidation are increased with increasing exercise intensity in parallel with PDH activation (47) (Figure 2.6). However, the flux rates needed to provide the necessary pyruvate for transport into the mitochondria and CHO oxidation during aerobic exercise are much lower than during sprint exercise, where the emphasis is on producing ATP in the glycolytic pathway (47, 65). Despite the increased PDH activity, accelerated rates of glycolysis also result in production of some lactate that accumulates in muscle and blood (84). Although lactate is often simply considered a metabolic by-product, it is an important substrate for oxidative metabolism and gluconeogenesis, thereby providing a link between glycolytic and oxidative metabolism (14).

The regulation of skeletal muscle glycogenolysis is interesting in that it appears to serve two masters—the low-flux situation of aerobic exercise, where the majority of the produced pyruvate is moved into the mitochondria for further metabolism and aerobic energy production (~36–38 ATP/glucose moiety) and little needs to be converted to lactate and the high-flux situation associated with sprinting at power outputs above what the aerobic system can handle, where ATP is mainly produced in the glycolytic pathway and most of the produced pyruvate is converted to lactate to convert NADH to NAD to maintain the pathway flux at a high level (Figure 2.1). Since the ATP yield from each glucose moiety is only 3 ATP in this situation, the flux through the pathway must be very high to provide large amounts of ATP and do so rapidly.

Regulation of Fat Oxidation

On the fat side, we now understand that FFAs are moved across the muscle membrane and t-tubules via protein-mediated transport systems during exercise (11, 27, 40, 86). These transport proteins include the plasma membrane fatty acid–binding protein (FABPpm), fatty acid transport proteins (FATPs), and fatty acid translocase (FAT/CD36). And unique to fat metabolism, FFAs are bound to protein chaperones in order to be transported in the cytoplasm for storage as IMTG or delivery to the mitochondria (28). At the mitochondrial membranes, all the FFA transported into the cell and released from IMTG must be transported across the mitochondrial membranes with the help of the carnitine palmitoyl transferase I (CPT I) system and FATPs (mainly FAT/CD36) (9, 15, 80, 81). During exercise, FATPs are also moved to the muscle membrane (mainly FABPpm) and mitochondrial (mainly FAT/CD36) membranes to help bring fat into the cell, but this occurs over a slower time course (~15–30 min) than GLUT4 translocation (12, 13, 40). It is expected that Ca^{2+} and the factors related to the energy status of the cell (e.g., free ADP, AMP, Pi, and AMPK activation) are involved, as they play an important role in activating the transport and docking of GLUT4 into the muscle membrane. For more detail on the regulation of these processes see (25, 31, 49, 50).

The breakdown of IMTG in muscle can also provide FFA for oxidation during low- and moderate-intensity exercise, and skeletal muscle has a large amount of stored energy in lipid droplets, especially in physically trained individuals (55, 73, 88). The key enzymes involved in regulating lipolysis in skeletal muscle are ATGL, HSL, and monoglyceride lipase (MGL) that sequentially remove a fatty acid from the IMTG stored in lipid droplets (5, 97, 98). ATGL and HSL are highly regulated, while MGL is not (4, 97, 98). Other factors also play a role in IMTG breakdown, including lipid droplet size, droplet localization, and the fact that lipid droplets have a protein (perilipins) coating (55, 56).

The perilipin proteins appear to separate IMTG from ATGL and HSL, maintaining low rates of lipolysis at rest. During moderate-intensity exercise, Ca^{2+} and EPI-related events phosphorylate HSL (90, 100), and AMPK phosphorylation of perilipin is involved in recruiting both HSL and ATGL to the lipid droplet, collectively enhancing rates of IMTG hydrolysis (69). However, at higher power outputs, it appears that AMPK phosphorylates additional sites on HSL that inhibit the phosphorylation by EPI and Ca^{2+}, providing a potential mechanism for the lower rates of IMTG use reported at these higher intensities (100). Less is known about the role of ATGL, but exercise training increases ATGL content (4, 91), and lipolysis was maintained when HSL was pharmacologically inhibited or knocked out in rodent skeletal muscle (5). ATGL is activated by association with a protein called comparative gene identification-58 (CGI-58) and putatively inhibited by G(0)/G(1) switch gene-2 (G0S2) (57, 91, 92). Perilipins are a family of proteins involved in the storage and mobilization and use of fatty acids (FAs) in cells. PLIN1 has been implicated in regulating lipolysis in adipose tissue by interacting with the TG lipases. However, it has been reported that PLIN1 is not found in skeletal muscle, and it is not clear whether any of the PLINs found in skeletal muscle (PLIN 2, 3 and 5) are involved in regulating lipolysis in a manner similar to PLIN1 in adipose tissue (see 56 for review). Interestingly, all three PLINs interact with HSL and ATGL; PLIN 3 and 5 interact with CGI-58, and it has been suggested they act as locating and scaffolding proteins for ATGL until a lipolytic stimulus appears. In summary, while it is clear that IMTG lipolysis plays an important role in providing FA for oxidation during exercise (Figure 2.1), understanding the regulation that occurs at the level of the lipid droplet for FAs to be released and delivered to the surface of the mitochondria has not been clarified.

The transport of FAs into mitochondria is a key step in regulating the overall rate at which skeletal muscle can oxidize FAs (41, 43, 79, 81). At one time, the increases in mitochondrial FA transport and oxidation with exercise were solely attributed to the relationship between carnitine palmitoyl transferase I (CPTI) activity and malonyl-CoA (M-CoA) (61). M-CoA content was high and inhibitory in rodent skeletal muscle at rest and decreased with exercise to release CPTI inhibition and allow FFA transport. However, measurements of M-CoA in human skeletal muscle at rest and during exercise demonstrated that M-CoA content was unaffected by exercise at varying power outputs (35–100% VO_2 max) and rates of fat oxidation (64) or decreased only slightly during prolonged exercise (72). Work with human permeabilized skeletal muscle fibres also demonstrated that M-CoA inhibition of CPT1 was dependent on the palmitoyl-CoA content, suggesting that an increase in palmitoyl-CoA content at the onset of exercise could override any inhibitory effect of M-CoA and allow FA transport and oxidation to proceed (81). In keeping with the suggestion that the regulation of CPTI activity and FA transport across the mitochondrial membranes was more complex was the finding that FAT/CD36 also existed on skeletal muscle mitochondrial membranes (9, 15). It was also demonstrated that while FABPpm facilitated FA transport at the sarcolemma, it played no role at the mitochondria (42). FAT/CD36 appeared to regulate mitochondrial FA oxidation, as rates were lower in animals with no FAT/CD36 (41). In human skeletal muscle, moderate-intensity exercise acutely increased the mitochondrial membrane FAT/CD36 protein content and mitochondrial FA oxidation (40), FAT/CD36 co-immunoprecipitated with CPTI (78), and exercise training increased the FAT/CD36 content on the mitochondria membranes to a greater extent than the increase in mitochondrial volume (89). Smith et al. (79, 80) proposed that FAT/CD36 is located on the outer mitochondrial membrane upstream of the acyl-CoA synthase enzyme. This location, in some unexplained manner, appears to facilitate the delivery of long-chain fatty acids to this enzyme so they can proceed through the reaction and the CPT complex and into the mitochondria (80). Interestingly, there has been no evidence that Ca^{2+} plays a role in the direct regulation of fat transport at the level of the mitochondria, other than activating the movement of more FAT/CD36 to the location.

Once inside the mitochondria, fat enters the beta-oxidation pathway with the formation of acetyl-CoA and reducing equivalents (NADH, $FADH_2$), and the long-chain nature of FFA results in the production of large amounts of aerobic ATP (Table 2.1). Interestingly, there has been no concrete evidence that there is metabolic regulation in the beta-oxidation pathway—it simply responds to the provision of substrate (75). Given that the beta-oxidation pathway exists in the mitochondria, the mitochondrial volume of the muscle cell determines the overall capacity to oxidize fat during exercise (39, 66).

General Aspects of the Regulation of Aerobic Metabolism

The discussion on the regulation of fat and CHO fuel use supports the concept of "dual stage control" in skeletal muscle metabolism, with the first stage being the "gross control" by Ca^{2+} (and possibly EPI) activating key regulatory enzymes, followed by second stage, or "fine-tuning control," to adjust the production of ATP to the actual ATP demand. The by-products of ATP use, free ADP, AMP, and Pi (and many others at specific enzymes) are perfect to relay information about the severity of the ATP need (Figures 2.3 and 2.4). The gross control could be seen as an early warning or feed-forward control—as the Ca^{2+} that is released from the sarcoplasmic reticulum and binds to troponin to allow cross-bridge movement and contraction—and activates many key steps in the regulation of metabolic pathways that use CHO and fat to produce energy. Then the feedback regulators that accumulate as a function of ATP degradation fine-tune the rate of ATP production to meet the need (47).

It is important to remember that other fuels can also provide substrates for aerobic energy production in the cell during exercise, including amino acids, acetate, medium-chain triglycerides, and the ketones beta-hydroxybutyrate and acetoacetic acid. Consumption of low-CHO diets can also force contracting muscles to oxidize fat at high rates during exercise (15). While these fuels can be used to spare or substitute for the use of CHO in some moderate-intensity exercise situations, they cannot efficiently provide the rate of energy provision needed to fuel intense aerobic exercise. This is because the delivery of the fuel to the muscle is low, the metabolic machinery is not designed for rapid energy provision (transport proteins/enzyme contents controlling the use of these fuels are low), and/or the amount stored/available in the muscles is low. Nothing matches the rate of aerobic energy provision from CHO and, of course, these alternative fuels cannot be used to produce anaerobic energy (34)

The Relationship Between Fat and Carbohydrate Metabolism

At moderate exercise intensities of ~50–65% VO_2 max, both fat and CHO contribute substrate from stores inside and outside the muscle. However, during intense endurance events athletes are often competing at ~80–90% of their VO_2 max. In these situations, fuel use shifts to CHO and away from fat (Figures 2.7 and 2.8). From a performance point of view this fuel shift makes sense, as the energy yield from CHO oxidation production is about 7% more efficient than from fat. However, if the endurance event is too long, liver and skeletal muscle glycogen stores may exhaust, requiring the athlete to slow down. This is the reason why endurance athletes adapt to intense endurance training by increasing their resting or pre-exercise liver and glycogen stores (36) and also commonly ingest CHO during exercise to help the liver provide glucose to the contracting muscles and brain while maintaining the blood glucose concentration constant (18, 23, 87). Researchers have now identified several sites where fat metabolism is down-regulated at high aerobic exercise intensities, including decreased FFA release from adipose tissue, less transport to the muscles and therefore less FFA transport into cells, decreased activation of HSL and possibly ATGL and less IMTG breakdown, inhibition of CPT I activity due to small decreases in muscle pH, and decreased CPTI sensitivity to carnitine and possibly low levels of cytoplasmic carnitine reducing mitochondrial membrane transport (68, 83).

These discussions also emphasize the importance of CHO as a fuel for high-intensity exercise—whether in the high aerobic domain (~80–100% VO_2 max), during sprinting (typically referred to as a % above VO_2 max), or a combination of these in stop-and-go individual and team sports (34, 54, 63). In many team sports, a high aerobic ability is needed for the player to move about the field or playing surface at a fast pace, while sprints (and anaerobic ATP) are added as dictated by the game, on the back of the aerobic ATP contribution. This scenario is repeated many times during the game, and CHO provides most of the aerobic fuel and much of the anaerobic fuel. Not surprisingly, almost every regulatory aspect of CHO metabolism is designed for rapid provision of ATP. CHO is the only fuel that can be used for both aerobic and anaerobic ATP production, and both systems turn on very quickly during the transitions from rest to exercise and from one power output to a higher power output. CHO can also provide all the fuel when exercising at a power output that elicits ~100% VO_2 max and is a more efficient fuel than fat (as stated earlier). Fat-derived ATP production is designed to be a helper fuel during exercise and provides its maximum amount of fuel at power outputs of ~60–65% VO_2 max (1). In addition, the processes that provide FFA to the muscle are slower and the pathways that metabolize fat and provide ATP in the muscle are slower than CHO (82, 83). However, in events that require long periods of exercise at submaximal power outputs, fat can provide energy for long periods of time and has a much larger capacity than CHO. Fat also plays a role in recovery from exercise or rest periods between activity.

Prolonged Aerobic Exercise

Oxidation of muscle glycogen and FFA derived from IMTG is greatest during the early stages of exercise and declines as exercise duration is extended, coinciding with progressive increases in muscle glucose and FFA uptake and oxidation (2, 8, 73, 94, 99). Usually, the increases in glucose uptake are balanced by increases in liver glucose output from glycogenolysis and gluconeogenesis (2, 21, 22, 95). With prolonged exercise (4 h at 30% VO_2 max), liver glucose output may fall below muscle glucose uptake (2) resulting in hypoglycaemia that can be prevented by CHO ingestion (23). An increase in adipose tissue lipolysis supports the progressive increase in plasma FFA uptake and oxidation (44), but since lipolysis exceeds uptake and oxidation, there is a gradual increase in plasma FFA levels. Glycerol is released into the circulation from adipose tissue lipolysis and alanine is released from contracting muscle, and both can serve as liver gluconeogenic precursors during exercise (2).

Watt et al. (99) had well-trained cyclists ride for 4 h at ~57% VO_2 max and examined fuel use with indirect calorimetry and measurements of skeletal muscle IMTG and glycogen use from biopsy samples.

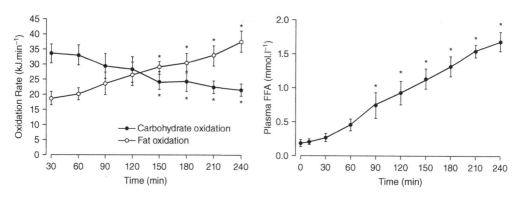

Figure 2.9 Plasma free fatty acid (FFA) concentrations and whole-body carbohydrate and fat oxidation rates during 4 h of exercise at ~57% VO$_2$ max (reproduced from 99)

CHO oxidation dominated fuel provision in the first 2 h, accounting for ~63% of the energy provision, with glycogen providing 45% and blood glucose 55% of the CHO oxidized (Figures 2.9 and 2.10). Fat accounted for 37% of the fuel, with plasma FFA oxidation accounting for 90% of the fat oxidized, and IMTG use only 10% in the first 2 hours. Plasma glucose provided slightly more of the blood-borne energy than plasma FFA in the initial 2 h of exercise. Fat oxidation increased over the 4 h and became the dominant fuel just past the 2-h mark as CHO oxidation steadily decreased over time (Figure 2.9). In hours 2–4, fat oxidation accounted for 58% of the fuel, with virtually all the substrate provided by plasma FFA. There was a steady increase in plasma FFA from ~0.2 mmol/L at rest to ~0.9 at 2 h and 1.66 + 0.32 mmol/L at 4 h (Figure 2.9). While CHO oxidation decreased in the final 2 h, it still supplied 42% of the energy, and most of the fuel (85%) was derived from plasma glucose uptake and little from

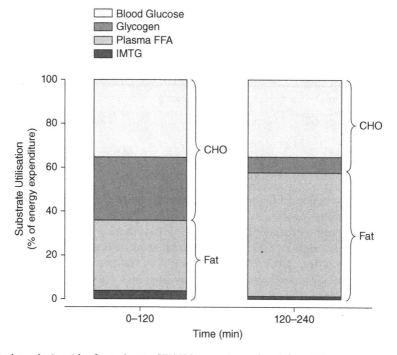

Figure 2.10   Fuel use during 4 h of exercise at ~57% VO$_2$ max (reproduced from 99)

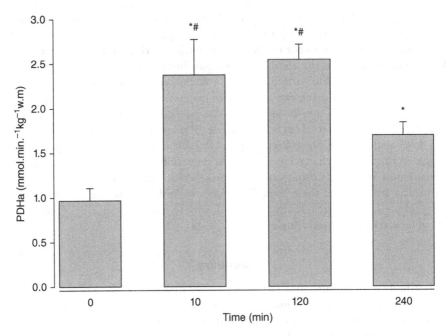

Figure 2.11   Pyruvate dehydrogenase (PDHa) activation during 4 h of exercise at ~57% VO$_2$ max (reproduced from 99)

muscle glycogen. Muscle PDH activity increased early in exercise and maintained at 120 min but markedly decreased at 240 min in line with the decreased CHO oxidation (Figure 2.11). Blood glucose was reasonably maintained as it decreased from 4.9 + 0.3 mmol/L at rest and 5.1 + 0.3 at 1 h to 4.0 mmol/L at 4 h. While blood lactate levels were very low throughout the entire cycle, plasma glycerol increased steadily from 119 + 18 umol/L at rest to 701 umol/L at 4 h, providing the liver with substrate for gluconeogenesis (99).

In the final 2 h of exercise at ~57% VO$_2$ max blood-borne fuel accounted for 92% of the oxidative energy, with FFA contributing 60% and blood glucose 40% (Figure 2.10). These data clearly demonstrate the shift away from intramuscular fuel use in the first half of prolonged exercise and the increase in reliance on blood-borne FFA and glucose in the latter half of the 4-h ride, with plasma FFA becoming the dominant fuel. Also impressive was the relative maintenance of blood glucose levels, as no exogenous CHO was consumed, suggesting that gluconeogenesis contributed to glucose production as the liver glycogen store approached depletion.

Future Directions

The understanding of exercise energy provision, regulation of metabolism, and the use of fat and CHO fuels during exercise has increased over the years based on studies employing various methods, including indirect calorimetry, metabolic tracer sampling, isolated skeletal muscle preparations, and analysis of whole-body and arteriovenous blood samples and tissue samples from contracting skeletal muscle. However, in virtually all areas of the regulation of fat and CHO metabolism, there is still much that is unknown. The introduction of molecular biology techniques provided a renaissance of experiments examining the time course of responses to acute and chronic exercise, but even these measures are limited by our ability to repeatedly sample muscle. We also continue to struggle with measures specific to the various compartments that exist in the cell, lack of knowledge about the physical structure and scaffolding that exists inside these compartments, and the communication that exists between proteins and metabolic pathways within compartments. An obvious example of these issues is studying the events that occur in the mitochondrion during exercise. One area that has not advanced as rapidly as needed is the ability to make non-invasive measures of the fuels, metabolites, proteins, etc., in the various compartment of the muscle cell that are important and involved in the regulation of metabolism during exercise. While magnetic resonance spectroscopy has been able to measure certain compounds non-invasively, we are generally not able to measure changes at the molecular and cellular level that occur with exercise. Researchers are investigating fuel use at the whole-body level with a more physiological approach, and others are examining the intricacies of cell signalling and molecular changes with a more reductionist approach to examine metabolism. There are many new approaches using genomics, proteomics, and metabolomics and system biology approaches to data analysis, and these should provide new insights into the molecular regulation of exercise metabolism. In conclusion, many avenues of work remain in every area of energy metabolism and the use of fat and CHO fuels during exercise.

Summary

The energy utilization of skeletal muscle at rest is very low. However, when exercise begins, the contracting muscles are called upon to provide energy at very high rates for short periods of time or at lower rates for longer time periods and everything in between. And to make things more complicated we store very little energy (ATP) in skeletal muscles at rest. To meet the energy needs of exercise, muscles have metabolic pathways that produce ATP that can be categorized as anaerobic (substrate phosphorylation, needing no oxygen) and aerobic (oxidative phosphorylation) systems. These pathways turn on together and work together from the onset of exercise and the transition from one power output to a higher one to precisely meet the demands of a given exercise situation. While the aerobic pathways are the default and dominate energy-producing pathways, they need some time to fully activate (s to min), and during this time the anaerobic systems rapidly (msec to s) provide the energy to cover what the aerobic system cannot provide. Anaerobic energy provision is most important in situations of high exercise intensity, where the requirement for energy far exceeds the ability of the aerobic systems to provide it. This is common in so-called stop-and-go sports where transitions from low to high energy needs and vice versa are numerous—and both aerobic and anaerobic energy provision are paramount for success.

Fat and CHO are the dominant fuels for exercise in well-fed individuals, and they are stored directly in skeletal muscle. CHO and fat are also delivered to skeletal muscles in the blood during exercise. CHO is a fuel for both aerobic and anaerobic energy production and is designed to be the dominant fuel during high-intensity exercise, whether in the high aerobic domain (~80–100% VO_2 max) or during sprinting (power outputs above 100% VO_2 max). PCr is also a large provider of anaerobic energy during intense exercise and recovers quickly during rest periods. Every aspect of CHO metabolism is designed for rapid provision of ATP, as the aerobic and anaerobic provision of CHO turns on very quickly during the transitions from rest to exercise and from one power output to a higher power output. CHO can also provide all the fuel when exercising at power outputs that elicit ~100% VO_2 max and is a more efficient fuel than fat (~7% more kcal/L O_2 consumed). Fat-derived ATP production is designed as a helper fuel during exercise and provides its maximum amount of energy at power outputs of ~60–65% VO_2 max. The processes that provide FFA to the muscle are slower, and the pathways that provide ATP are slower than CHO. However, in events that require long periods of exercise at submaximal power outputs, fat can provide energy for long periods of time and has a much larger capacity than CHO. Fat also plays a role in recovery from exercise or rest periods between activity. Together, aerobic energy production using fat and CHO as fuels and anaerobic energy provision from PCr and CHO use in the glycolytic pathway permits us to meet the energy needs of a wide variety of exercise demands.

References

1. Achten J, Jeukendrup AE. Maximal fat oxidation during exercise in trained men. *Int J Sports Med* 24: 603–608, 2003.
2. Ahlborg G, Felig P, Hagenfeldt L, Hendler R, Wahren J. Substrate turnover during prolonged exercise in man. *J Clin Invest* 53: 1080–1090, 1974.
3. Allen DG, Lamb GD, Westerbald H. Skeletal muscle fatigue: cellular mechanisms. *Physiol Rev* 88: 287–332, 2008.
4. Alsted TJ, Nybo L, Schweiger M, Fledelius C, Jacobsen P, Zimmermann R, Zechner R, Kiens B. Adipose triglyceride lipase in human skeletal muscle is upregulated by exercise training. *Am J Physiol* 296: E445–E453, 2009.
5. Alsted TJ, Ploug T, Prats C, Serup AK, Høeg L, Schjerling P, Holm C, et al. Contraction-induced lipolysis is not impaired by inhibition of hormone-sensitive lipase in skeletal muscle. *J Physiol* 591: 5141–5155, 2013.
6. Asmussen, E. Muscle metabolism during exercise in man. A historical survey. In: *Muscle Metabolism During Exercise*. New York: Plenum Press, pp. 1–11, 1971.
7. Bangsbo J, Gollnick PB, Graham TE, Juel C, Kiens B, Mizuno M, Saltin B. Anaerobic energy production and O_2 deficit - debt relationship during exhaustive exercise in humans. *J Physiol* 422: 539–559, 1990.
8. Bergström J. Hultman E. A study of the glycogen metabolism during exercise in man. *Scand J Clin Lab Invest* 19: 218–228, 1967.
9. Bezaire V, Bruce CR, Heigenhauser GJ, Tarendon NN, Glatz JFC, Luiken JJJF, Bonen A, Spriet LL. Identification of fatty acid translocase on human skeletal muscle mitochondrial membranes: essential role in fatty acid oxidation. *Am J Physiol* 290: E509–E515, 2006.
10. Bishop D, Edge J, Goodman C. Muscle buffer capacity and aerobic fitness are associated with repeated-sprint ability in women. *Eur J Appl Physiol* 92: 540–547, 2004.
11. Bonen A, Chabowski A, Luiken JJFP, Glatz JF. Is membrane transport of FFA mediated by lipid, protein, or both? Mechanisms and regulation of protein-mediated cellular fatty acid uptake: molecular, biochemical, and physiological evidence. *Physiologist* 22: 15–29, 2007.
12. Bonen, A, Luiken JJFP, Arumugam T, Glatz JF, Tandon NN. Acute regulation of fatty acid uptake involves the cellular redistribution of fatty acid translocase. *J Biol Chem* 275: 14501–14508, 2000.
13. Bradley NS, Snook LA, Jain SS, Heigenhauser, GJF, Bonen A, Spriet LL. Acute endurance exercise increases plasma membrane fatty acid transport proteins in rat and human skeletal muscle. *Am J Physiol* 302: E183–E189, 2012.
14. Brooks GA. Cell-cell and intracellular lactate shuttles. *J Physiol* 587: 5591–5600, 2009.
15. Burke LM, Ross ML, Garvican-Lewis LA, Welvaert M, Heikura IA, Forbes SG, Mirtschin JG, et al. Low carbohydrate, high fat diet impairs exercise economy and negates the performance benefit from intensified training in elite race walkers. *J Physiol* 595: 2785–2807, 2017.
16. Campbell SE, Tandon NN, Woldegiorgis G, Luiken JJFP, Glatz JFC, Bonen A. A novel function for fatty acid translocase (FAT)/CD36. *J Biol Chem* 279: 36235–36241, 2004.
17. Casey A, Constantin-Teodosiu D, Howell S, Hultman E, Greenhaff PL. Metabolic responses of type I and II muscle fibres during repeated bouts of maximal exercise in humans. *Am J Physiol* 271: E38–E43, 1996.
18. Cermak NM, van Loon LJ. The use of carbohydrates during exercise as an ergogenic aid. *Sports Med* 43: 1139–1155, 2013.
19. Chasiotis D, Sahlin K, Hultman E. Regulation of glycogenolysis in human muscle at rest and during exercise. *J Appl Physiol* 53: 788–715, 1982.
20. Coggan AR, Kohrt WM, Spina RJ, Bier DM, Holloszy JO. Endurance training decreases plasma glucose turnover and oxidation during moderate-intensity exercise in men. *J Appl Physiol* 68: 990–996, 1990.
21. Coggan AR, Raguso CA, Williams BD, Sidossis LS, Gastaldelli A. Glucose kinetics during high-intensity exercise in endurance-trained and untrained humans. *J Appl Physiol* 78: 1203–1207, 1995.
22. Coggan AR, Swanson SC, Mendenhall LA, Habash DL, Kien CL. Effect of endurance training on hepatic glycogenolysis and gluconeogenesis during prolonged exercise in men. *Am J Physiol* 268: E375–E383, 1995.
23. Coyle EF, Hagberg JM, Hurley BF, Martin WH, Ehsani AA, Holloszy JO. Carbohydrate feeding during prolonged strenuous exercise can delay fatigue. *J Appl Physiol* 55: 230–235, 1983.
24. Egan B, Zierath JR. Exercise metabolism and the molecular regulation of skeletal muscle adaptation. *Cell Metab* 17: 162–184, 2013.
25. Fentz J, Kjobsted R, Birk JB, Jeppesen J, Thorsen K, Schjerling P, Kiens B, Jessen N, Viollet B, Wojtaszewski, JF. AMPKα is critical for enhancing skeletal muscle fatty acid utilization during in vivo exercise in mice. *FASEB J* 29: 1725–1738, 2016.

26. Gaitanos GC, Williams C, Boobis LH, Brooks S. Human muscle metabolism during intermittent maximal exercise. *J Appl Physiol* 75: 712–719, 1993.

27. Glatz JF, Luiken JJ, Bonen A. Membrane fatty acid transporters as regulators of lipid metabolism: implications for metabolic disease. *Physiol Rev* 90: 367–417, 2010.

28. Glatz JF, Schapp FG, Binas B, Bonen A, van der Vusse GJ, Luiken JJ. Cytoplasmic fatty acid-binding protein facilitates fatty acid utilization by skeletal muscle. *Acta Physiol Scand* 178: 367–372, 2003.

29. Greenhaff PL, Nevill ME, Soderlund K, Bodin K, Boobis LH, Williams C, Hultman E. The metabolic responses of human type I and II muscle fibres during maximal treadmill sprinting. *J Physiol* 478: 149–155, 1994.

30. Hargreaves M. The metabolic systems: Carbohydrate metabolism. In: *Advanced Exercise Physiology*, 2nd Ed. Farrell PA, Joyner MJ, Caiozzo VJ (eds). Philadelphia: Lippincott, Williams and Wilkins, pp 408–422, 2012.

31. Hargreaves M, Spriet LL. Exercise metabolism: Fuels for the fire. In: *The Biology of Exercise*. Zierath JR, Joyner MJ and Hawley JA (eds). New York: Cold Spring Harbor Laboratory Press, Cold Spring Harbor, pp. 57–72, 2017.

32. Hargreaves M, McKenna MJ, Jenkins DG, Warmington SA, Li JL, Snow RJ, Febbraio MA. Muscle metabolites and performance during high intensity, intermittent exercise. *J Appl Physiol* 84: 1687–1691, 1998.

33. Harris RC, Edwards RH, Hultman E, Nordesjö LO, Nylind B, Sahlin K. The time course of phosphorylcreatine resynthesis during recovery of the quadriceps muscle in man. *Pflugers Arch* 367: 137–142, 1976.

34. Hawley JA. Leckey JJ. Carbohydrate dependence during prolonged, intense endurance exercise. *Sports Med.* 45: S5–S12, 2015.

35. Hawley JA, Hargreaves M, Joyner MJ, Zierath JR. Integrative biology of exercise. *Cell* 159: 738–749, 2014.

36. Hawley JA, Schabort EJ, Noakes TD, Dennis SC. Carbohydrate-loading and exercise performance: an update. *Sports Med* 24: 73–81, 1997.

37. Holloway GP. Nutrition and training influences on the regulation of mitochondrial adenosine diphosphate sensitivity and bioenergetics. *Sports Med.* 47(Suppl 1): 13–21, 2017.

38. Holloway GP, Spriet LL. Skeletal muscle metabolic adaptations to training. (Ch 5). In: *The IOC Textbook of Science in Sport* (1st Edition). Maughan RJ (ed). Oxford, UK: Wiley-Blackwell, pp. 70–83, 2009.

39. Holloway GP, Spriet LL. The metabolic systems: Interaction of lipid and carbohydrate metabolism. In: *Advanced Exercise Physiology*, 2nd Ed. Farrell PA, Joyner MJ, Caiozzo VJ (eds). Philadelphia: Lippincott, Williams and Wilkins, pp 408–422, 2012.

40. Holloway GP, Bezaire V, Heigenhauser GJF, Tarendon NN, Glatz JFC, Luiken JJFP, Bonen A, Spriet LL. Mitochondrial long chain fatty acid oxidation, fatty acid translocase/CD36 content and carnitine palmitoyltransferase I activity in human skeletal muscle during aerobic exercise. *J Physiol* 571: 201–210, 2006.

41. Holloway GP, Jain SS, Bezaire V, Han XX, Glatz JF, Luiken JJ, Harper ME, Bonen A. FAT/CD36 null mice reveal that mitochondrial FAT/CD36 is required to up-regulate mitochondrial fatty acid oxidation in contracting muscle. *Am J Physiol* 297: R960–R967, 2009.

42. Holloway GP, Lally J, Nickerson JG, Alkhateeb H, Snook LA, Heigenhauser GJF, Calles-Escandon J, et al. Fatty acid binding protein facilitates sarcolemmal fatty acid transport but not mitochondrial oxidation in rat and human skeletal muscle. *J Physiol* 582: 393–405, 2007.

43. Holloway GP, Luiken JJFP, Glatz JF, Spriet LL, Bonen A. Contribution of FAT/CD36 to the regulation of skeletal muscle fatty acid oxidation: an overview. *Acta Physiol* 194: 293–309, 2008.

44. Horowitz JF, Klein S. Lipid metabolism during endurance exercise. *Am J Clin Nutr* 72: S558–S563, 2000.

45. Howlett KF, Andrikopoulos S, Proietto J, Hargreaves M. Exercise-induced muscle glucose uptake in mice with graded, muscle-specific GLUT-4 deletion. *Physiol Reports* 1(3): e00065, 2013.

46. Howlett RA, Heigenhauser GJF, Spriet LL. Skeletal muscle metabolism during high-intensity sprint exercise is unaffected by dichloroacetate or acetate infusion. *J Appl Physiol* 87: 1747–1751, 1999.

47. Howlett RA, Parolin ML, Dyck DJ, Hultman E, Jones NL, Heigenhauser GJF, Spriet LL. Regulation of skeletal muscle glycogen phosphorylase and PDH at varying exercise power outputs. *Am J Physiol* 275: R418–R425, 1998.

48. Hultman E, Bergstrsm J, McLennan-Anderson N. Breakdown and resynthesis of phosphorylcreatine and adenosine triphosphate in connection with muscular work in man. *Scand J Clin Lab Invest* 19: 56–66, 1967.

49. Jain SS, Chabowski A, Snook LA, Schwenk RW, Glatz JFC, Luiken JJFP, Bonen A. Additive effects of insulin and muscle contraction on fatty acid transport and fatty acid transporters, FAT/CD36, FABPpm, FATP1, 4 and 6. *FEBS Lett* 583: 2294–2300, 2009.

50. Jain SS, Luiken JJ, Snook LA, Han XX, Holloway GP, Glatz JF, Bonen A. Fatty acid transport and transporters in muscle are critically regulated by Akt2. *FEBS Lett* 589: 2769–75, 2015.

51. Kiens B. Skeletal muscle lipid metabolism in exercise and insulin resistance. *Physiol Rev* 86: 205–243, 2006.

52. Kowalchuk JM, Heigenhauser GJ, Lindinger MI, Sutton JR, Jones NL. Factors influencing hydrogen ion concentration in muscle after intense exercise. *J Appl Physiol* 65: 2080–2089, 1988.

53. Kristiansen S, Hargreaves M, Richter EA. Progressive increase in glucose transport and GLUT4 in human sarcolemmal vesicles during moderate exercise. *Am J Physiol* 272: E385–E389, 1997.

54. Krustrup P, Mohr M, Steensberg A, Bencke J, Kjaer M, Bangsbo J. Muscle and blood metabolites during a soccer game: implications for sprint performance. *Med Sci Sports Exerc* 38: 1165–1174, 2006.

55. Loher H, Kreis R, Boesch C, Christ E. The flexibility of ectopic lipids. *Int J Mol Sci* 17: E1554, 2016.

56. MacPherson, RE, Peters SJ. Piecing together the puzzle of perilipin proteins and skeletal muscle lipolysis. *Appl Physiol Nutr Metab* 40: 641–651, 2015.

57. MacPherson, RE, Ramos SV, Vandenboom R, Roy BD, Peters SJ. Skeletal muscle PLIN proteins, ATGL and CGI-58, interactions at rest and following stimulated contraction. *Am J Physiol* 304: R644–R650, 2013.

58. Medbø JI, Sejersted OM. Plasma potassium changes with high intensity exercise. *J Physiol* 421: 105–122, 1990.

59. Medbø JI, Tabata I. Relative importance of aerobic and anaerobic energy release during short-lasting exhausting bicycle exercise. *J Appl Physiol* 67: 1881–1886, 1989.

60. Medbø JI, Tabata I. Anaerobic energy release in working muscle during 30 s to 3 min of exhausting bicycling. *J Appl Physiol* 75: 1654–1660, 1993.

61. McGarry JD, Brown NF. The mitochondrial carnitine palmitoyltransferase system. From concept to molecular analysis. *Eur J Biochem* 244: 1–14, 1997.

62. Miotto PM, Holloway GP. In the absence of phosphate shuttling, exercise reveals the in vivo importance of creatine-independent mitochondrial ADP transport. *Biochem J* 473: 2831–2843, 2016.

63. O'Brien MJ, Viguie CA, Mazzeo RS, Brooks GA. Carbohydrate dependence during marathon running. *Med Sci Sports Exerc* 25: 1009–1017, 1993.

64. Odland LM, Howlett RA, Heigenhauser GJF, Hultman E, Spriet LL. Skeletal muscle malonyl-CoA content at the onset of exercise at varying power outputs in humans. *Am J Physiol* 274: E1080–E1085, 1998.

65. Parolin ML, Chesley A, Matsos MP, Spriet LL, Jones NL, Heigenhauser GJF. Regulation of glycogen phosphorylase and PDH during maximal intermittent exercise. *Am J Physiol* 277: E890–E900, 1999.

66. Perry CGR, Heigenhauser GJF, Bonen A, Spriet LL. High-intensity aerobic interval training increases fat and carbohydrate metabolic capacities in human skeletal muscle. *Appl Physiol Nutr Metab* 33: 1112–1123, 2008.

67. Perry CGR, Kane DA, Herbst EA, Mukai K, Lark DS, Wright DC, Heigenhauser JGF, Neufer PD, Spriet LL, Holloway GP. Mitochondrial creatine kinase activity and phosphate shuttling are acutely regulated by exercise in human skeletal muscle. *J Physiol* 590: 5475–5486, 2012.

68. Petrick HL, Holloway GP. High intensity exercise inhibits carnitine palmitoyl transferase-1 sensitivity to L-carnitine. *Biochem J* 476: 547–558, 2019.

69. Prats C, Donsmark M, Qvortrup K, Londos C, Sztalryd C, Holm C, Galbo H, Ploug T. Decrease in intramuscular lipid droplets and translocation of HSL in response to muscle contraction and epinephrine. *Lipid Res* 47: 2392–2399, 2006.

70. Ren JM, Hultman E. Regulation of glycogenolysis in human skeletal muscle, *J Appl Physiol* 67: 2243–2248, 1989.

71. Richter EA, Hargreaves M. Exercise, GLUT4 and skeletal muscle glucose uptake. *Physiol Rev* 93: 993–1017, 2013.

72. Roepstorff C, Halberg N, Hillig T, Saha A, Ruderman NB, Wojtaszewski JF, Richter EA, Kiens B. Malonyl-CoA and carnitine in regulation of fat oxidation in human skeletal muscle during exercise. *Am J Physiol* 288: E133–E142, 2005.

73. Romijn JA, Coyle EF, Sidossis LS, Gastaldelli A, Horowitz JF, Endert E, Wolfe RR. Regulation of endogenous fat and carbohydrate metabolism in relation to exercise intensity and duration. *Am J Physiol* 265: E380–E391, 1993.

74. Romijn JA, Coyle EF, Sidossis LS, Rosenblatt J, Wolfe RR. Substrate metabolism during differentexercise intensities in endurance-trained women. *J Appl Physiol* 88: 1707–1714, 2000

75. Sahlin K. Control of lipid oxidation at the mitochondrial level. *Appl Physiol Nutr Metab* 34: 382–388, 2009.

76. Sahlin K. Muscle energetics during explosive activities and potential effects of nutrition and training. *Sports Med* 44(Suppl 2): S167–73, 2014.

77. Sahlin K, Tonkonogi M, Söderlund K. Energy supply and muscle fatigue in humans. *Acta Physiol Scand* 162: 261–266, 1998.

78. Schenk S, Horowitz JF. Coimmunoprecipitation of FAT/CD36 and CPT I in skeletal muscle increases proportionally with fat oxidation after endurance exercise training. *Am J Physiol* 291: E254–E260, 2006.

79. Smith BK, Bonen A, Holloway GP. A dual mechanism of action for skeletal muscle FAT/CD36 during exercise. *Exerc Sport Sci Rev* 40: 211–217, 2012.

80. Smith BK, Jain SS, Rimbaud S, Dam A, Quadrilatero J, Ventura-Clapier R, Bonen A, Holloway GP. FAT/CD36 is located on the outer mitochondrial membrane, upstream of long-chain acyl-CoA synthetase, and regulates palmitate oxidation. *Biochem J* 437: 125–34, 2011.

81. Smith BK, Perry CG, Koves TR, Wright DC, Smith JC, Neufer PD, Muoio DM, Holloway GP. Identification of a novel malonyl-CoA IC50 for CPT-1: implications for predicting in vivo fatty acid oxidation rates. *Biochem J* 448: 13–20, 2012.

82. Spriet LL. The metabolic systems: Lipid metabolism. In: *Advanced Exercise Physiology* (2nd Edition). Farrell PA, Joyner MJ, Caiozzo VJ, (eds). Philadelphia: Lippincott, Williams, Wilkins, pp. 392–407, 2012.

83. Spriet LL. New insights into the interaction of carbohydrate and fat metabolism during exercise. *Sports Med* 44: S87–S96, 2014.

84. Spriet LL, Howlett RA, Heigenhauser GJ. An enzymatic approach to lactate production in human skeletal muscle during exercise. *Med Sci Sports Exerc* 32: 756–763, 2000.

85. Spriet LL, Lindinger MI, McKelvie RS, Heigenhauser GJF, Jones NL. Muscle glycogenolysis and H^+ concentration during maximal intermittent cycling. *J Appl Physiol* 66: 8–13, 1989.

86. Stefanyk, LE, Bonen A, Dyck DJ. Insulin and contraction-induced movement of fatty acid transport proteins to skeletal muscle transverse tubules is distinctly different than to the sarcolemma. *Metabolism* 61: 1518–1522, 2012.

87. Stellingwerff T, Cox GR. Systematic review: carbohydrate supplementation on exercise performance or capacity of varying durations. *Appl Physiol Nutr Metab* 39: 998–1011, 2014.

88. Stellingwerff T, Boon H, Jonkers RA, Senden JM, Spriet LL, Koopman R, van Loon LJC. Significant intramyocellular lipid use during prolonged cycling in endurance-trained males as assessed by three different methodologies. *Am J Physiol* 292: E1715–E1723, 2007.

89. Talanian, JL, Holloway GP, Snook L, Heigenhauser GJF, Bonen A, Spriet LL. Exercise training increases sarcolemmal and mitochondrial fatty acid transport proteins in human skeletal muscle. *Am J Physiol* 299: E180–E188, 2010.

90. Talanian JL, Tunstall RJ, Watt MJ, Duong M, Perry CGR, Steinberg GR, Kemp B, Heigenhauser GJF, Spriet LL. Beta-adrenergic regulation of human skeletal muscle hormone sensitive lipase activity during exercise onset. *Am J Physiol* 291: R1094–R1099, 2006.

91. Turnbull PC, Longo AB, Ramos SV, Roy BD, Ward WE, Peters SJ. Increases in skeletal muscle ATGL and its inhibitor G0S2 following 8 weeks of endurance training in metabolically different rat skeletal muscles. *Am J Physiol* 310: R125–R133, 2016.

92. Turnbull PC, Ramos SV, MacPherson REK, Roy BD, Peters SJ. Characterization of lipolytic inhibitor G(0)/G(1) switch gene-2 protein (G0S2) expression in male Sprague Dawley rat skeletal muscle compared to relative content of adipose triglyceride lipase (ATGL) and comparative gene-idetification-58 (CGI-58). *PLoS One* 10: e120136, 2015.

93. Van Loon LJ, Greenhaff PL, Constantin-Teodosiu D, Saris WM, Wagenmakers AJ. The effects of increasing exercise intensity on muscle fuel utilisation in humans. *J Physiol* 536: 275–304, 2001.

94. Wahren J, Felig P, Ahlborg G, Jorfeldt L. Glucose metabolism during leg exercise in man. *J Clin Invest* 50: 15–25, 1971.

95. Wasserman DH. Four grams of glucose. *Am J Physiol* 296: E11–E21, 2009.

96. Wasserman DH, Kang L, Ayala JE, Fueger PT, Lee-Young RS. The physiological regulation of glucose flux into muscle *in vivo*. *J Exp Biol* 214: 254–262, 2011.

97. Watt MJ. Triglyceride lipases alter fuel metabolism and mitochondrial gene expression. *Appl Physiol Nutr Metab* 34: 340–347, 2009.

98. Watt M, Spriet, LL. Triacylglycerol lipases and metabolic control: implications for health and disease. *Am J Physiol* 299: E162–E168, 2010.

99. Watt MJ, Heigenhauser GJF, Dyck DJ, Spriet LL. Intramuscular triacylglycerol, glycogen and acetyl group metabolism during 4 h of moderate exercise in man. *J Physiol* 541: 969–978, 2002.

100. Watt MJ, Heigenhauser GJF, Spriet LL. Effects of dynamic exercise intensity on the activation of hormone-sensitive lipase in human skeletal muscle. *J Physiol* 547: 301–308, 2003.

101. Watt MJ, Howlett KF, Febbraio MA, Spriet LL, Hargreaves M. Adrenaline increases skeletal muscle glycogenolysis, PDH activation and carbohydrate oxidation during moderate exercise in humans. *J Physiol* 534: 269–278, 2001.

102. Wright DC, Hucker KA, Holloszy JO, Han DH. Ca^{2+} and AMPK both mediate stimulation of glucose transport by muscle contractions. *Diabetes* 53: 330–335, 2004.

103. Zimmermann R, Strauss JG, Haemmerle G, Schoiswohl G, Birner-Gruenberger R, Riederer M, Lass A, et al. Fat mobilization in adipose tissue is promoted by adipose triglyceride lipase. *Science* 306: 1383–1386, 2004.

104. Zinker BA, Lacy DB, Bracy DP, Wasserman DH. Role of glucose and insulin loads to exercising limb in increasing glucose uptake and metabolism. *J Appl Physiol* 74: 2915–2922, 1993.

3

ADIPOSE TISSUE (ADIPOKINOME), SKELETAL MUSCLE (MYOKINOME), AND LIVER (HEPATOKINOME) AS ENDOCRINE REGULATORS DURING EXERCISE

Logan K. Townsend, Greg L. McKie, Hesham Shamshoum, and David C. Wright

Introduction

Exercise has long been recognized to confer beneficial metabolic effects. These include increasing insulin-independent glucose transport into skeletal muscle, enhancing insulin sensitivity, and increasing the oxidative capacity of numerous tissues, including skeletal muscle, adipose, and liver. While the effects of exercise, at least in skeletal muscle, were largely believed to be driven by localized changes within the contracting skeletal muscle itself, such as spikes in intracellular calcium concentrations and fluctuations in high-energy phosphate (AMP, ADP, ATP, etc.) levels, there is a growing appreciation that systemic signalling factors released from muscle, adipose tissue, and liver play a role in mediating adaptations to exercise.

Myokines

Myokines are cytokines or peptides that are synthetized and released by muscle fibres and exert autocrine, paracrine, or endocrine effects in response to muscular contractions/exercise (106). The autocrine and paracrine effects of myokines are mostly involved in the regulation of muscle physiology, such as muscle growth and the regulation of carbohydrate and lipid metabolism. In contrast, the endocrine effects of myokines are thought to be important in mediating the systemic effects of exercise. To date it has been speculated that muscle communicates with distal tissues, including adipose tissue, liver, pancreas, bone, and the brain. In the following section, we will focus on some of the roles of myokines that have been discovered to date.

Interleukin-6

Interleukin-6 (IL-6) is a prototypical myokine that is secreted by contracting skeletal muscle during exercise. Contrary to its putative pro-inflammatory classification, IL-6 has been postulated to be involved in anti-inflammatory effects of exercise. In 1998, Ostrowski et al. first demonstrated that IL-6 messenger RNA (mRNA) in muscle and plasma levels of IL-6 are elevated during acute exercise (102). Previously it had been thought that the exercise-induced rise in IL-6 was a result of an immune response due to local damage in contracting muscles (96). However, it was demonstrated that IL-6 mRNA in monocytes did not increase as a result of bicycle exercise (133). In an attempt to determine which cells produce IL-6, Keller et al. (62) isolated nuclei from muscle biopsies obtained before, during, and after exercise. It was demonstrated that the transcription rate of IL-6 increases rapidly after exercise (62). During exercise, circulating IL-6 levels are elevated up to 100-fold, and this increase is associated with duration and intensity of exercise (33, 105). That is, the longer and the more intense the exercise, the greater the increase in IL-6.

Skeletal muscle cells produce IL-6 in response to numerous stimuli such as lipopolysaccharide (bacteria), reactive oxygen species, and inflammatory cytokines. On the other hand, exercise stimulates IL-6 release from skeletal muscle through a distinct pathway(s) that is not associated with increases in markers of inflammation (31, 61). The factors that lead to increases in IL-6 gene transcription, and ultimately release from muscle during contraction, are not fully understood but could be linked to the degree of metabolic stress that is induced during exercise. In this regard, reductions in muscle glycogen concentrations lead to a potentiated effect of exercise on the transcription (62) and release of IL-6 (125).

Work completed in both cultured muscle cells and in humans provides evidence that IL-6 can modulate skeletal muscle glucose metabolism. Exposure of muscle cells to IL-6 increases glucose uptake and the movement of glucose transporters to the plasma membrane (13). Likewise, infusing IL-6 into healthy subjects during a hyperinsulinemic-euglycaemic clamp increases whole-body insulin action (13). The effects of IL-6 on glucose metabolism in muscle are likely controlled, at least in part, by 5'AMP–activated protein kinase (AMPK) (13), an enzyme that is thought to regulate insulin-independent muscle glucose uptake.

Exercise-induced IL-6 is not limited to only regulating local muscle metabolism but has also been postulated to have an endocrine function. For example, prior studies suggest that IL-6 may affect liver glucose metabolism by inhibiting glycogen synthase (60) and increasing liver glucose production (132). Similarly, there is emerging evidence suggesting that IL-6 increases adipose tissue lipolysis. In cultured fat cells, IL-6 treatment causes small yet significant increases in lipolysis, whereas the infusion of IL-6 into human subjects increases circulating levels of fatty acids (126).

More recently, a randomized, double-blind, parallel group trial demonstrated that intact IL-6 signalling is required for the exercise-induced loss in visceral adipose tissue mass in obese men and women (135). Participants in this study either remained sedentary or performed a progressively more intense 45-min high-intensity interval training (HIIT) protocol (50–85% VO_2 max) on a cycle ergometer for 12 weeks. Additionally, participants either received tocilizumab, a humanized monoclonal IL-6 receptor antibody, or placebo infusions. Given the rigorous design of the trial, these authors were able to determine the effects of exercise on visceral adipose tissue independent of IL-6. Twelve weeks of training on its own induced a 142-g decrease (8% of pre-training) in visceral adipose tissue mass, but this effect was abolished in the group exercising and receiving tocilizumab, who actually increased visceral fat mass by 135 g (10% of pre-exercise values), effectively suggesting that IL-6 is required for the exercise-induced loss in visceral adipose tissue mass in obese men and women.

Interleukin-15

IL-15 is a four–α-helix cytokine that belongs to the IL-2 superfamily and is expressed in a wide range of tissues, including skeletal muscle. IL-15 is primarily known for its hypertrophic action in skeletal muscle. Previous studies demonstrated that circulating IL-15 levels are increased after an acute bout of resistance exercise in human subjects (8, 108, 116), an effect that is also present following aerobic exercise (16, 110). Using cultured muscle cells IL-15 has been shown to increase the content of proteins involved in the contractile apparatus (36, 114) and to stimulate muscle cell differentiation (112, 113). The ability of IL-15 to serve as a hypertrophic signal could be due to its effects on inhibiting the rate of proteolysis (12).

Irisin

Peroxisome proliferator–activated receptor-γ (PPARγ) coactivator-1α (PGC-1α) is a transcriptional co-activator and master regulator of mitochondrial biogenesis in skeletal muscle. PGC-1α is robustly induced with exercise and has been shown to increase the expression of fibronectin domain–containing protein 5 (FNDC5), the cleavage of which results in the production of a reputed myokine called irisin, which has been thought to drive exercise-mediated changes in adipose tissue metabolism such as "browning" (10). Browning is a process by which white adipocytes acquire features that are characteristic of brown adipocytes, such as the expression of uncoupling protein 1 (UCP1). Though not a universal finding, the browning of white adipose tissue has been thought to increase whole-body energy expenditure. While the discovery of irisin has received considerable attention, numerous studies examining irisin thereafter revealed inconsistent results, especially with respect to the circulating levels of irisin post-exercise (10, 28, 54, 57).

Myostatin

Myostatin is one of the only myokines that is reduced in response to exercise (84). Myostatin inhibits muscle cell proliferation and differentiation via an autocrine and paracrine mechanism. The genetic deletion of myostatin leads to muscle hypertrophy in mice and humans (74, 84, 115, 122). Myostatin inhibition positively regulates muscle growth, and myostatin expression is down-regulated after endurance and resistance exercise (1). Therefore, it has been proposed that myostatin inhibition could serve as a therapeutic agent for treatment of patients with muscular dystrophies (71). Myostatin has also been suggested to be a negative regulator of glucose and lipid metabolism (32, 39, 147). In high-fat diet-fed mice, it has been shown that inhibition of myostatin ameliorates obesity and the development of insulin resistance, and this associates with increases in the browning of white adipose tissue (145).

Adipokines

White adipose tissue (WAT) can no longer be viewed as an inert storage organ for excess triglycerides (TAGs), but rather a highly pliable endocrine organ capable of secreting various hormones known as adipokines (37). Adipokines exert pleiotropic effects on surrounding tissues to facilitate interorgan crosstalk and the regulation of various physiological processes (27, 37). The nature of their downstream effects ultimately dictates their function; however, adipokine secretion is dependent upon a number of factors, including nutrient availability and inflammation, both of which are either directly or indirectly manipulated by exercise (131). It is perhaps not surprising then that exercise induces the secretion of adipokines. True adipokines, such as leptin and adiponectin, are produced by pre-adipocytes and mature adipocytes (139, 146); however, other so-called adipokines are actually the product of resident immune cells within the stromal vascular fraction of adipose tissue. Nonetheless, this section will focus on adipose tissue–derived adipokines, with a specific focus on the ability of aerobic exercise to induce the secretion of the adipokines leptin, adiponectin, and TGFβ2. We will cover their discovery, cellular signalling, and metabolic actions in response to exercise.

Leptin

Humans have a remarkable capacity to regulate body weight despite marked fluctuations in energy intake over time. In the early 1950s it was hypothesized that there was a mechanism to explain how the body achieves this. Since adipose tissue maintains its mass over long periods, it was thought that there must be a homeostatic signal to decrease energy intake and increase energy expenditure in times of excessive energy storage (63). This mechanism is now commonly referred to as the lipostatic set-point theory, and the hypothesized regulatory signal is the adipose tissue–derived hormone leptin (from the Greek word *leptos* meaning thin).

Leptin was identified as the protein product of the *ob* gene in 1994 by Dr Friedman's laboratory (146). It is secreted predominantly from visceral WAT and subcutaneous WAT in rodents and humans, respectively (53). However, other adipose tissue depots, such as the epicardial (6),and mesenteric depots (38), along with the stromal vascular fraction of adipose tissue (22), all express leptin. Given that one of leptin's primary roles is as a lipostatic negative-feedback signal, leptin concentrations share a strong correlation with adipose tissue mass (11, 143), and thus weight loss results in a marked reduction in circulating leptin (80), whereas weight gain leads to increased circulating leptin and even leptin resistance in obesity (124). Leptin resistance in obesity is largely due to the fact that leptin acts centrally (i.e., on the brain) through a saturable transport mechanism at the blood–brain barrier (7). As body mass increases in obesity, so, too, does the secretion of leptin, yet the leptin transporters in the brain are already saturated; therefore, the body is less responsive to circulating leptin (i.e., leptin resistance).

Centrally, leptin is known to regulate glucose homeostasis (14), while in the periphery it acts on the liver to attenuate insulin signalling and down-regulate gluconeogenesis (18). In adipose tissue leptin suppresses lipogenesis (5), and in skeletal muscle leptin reduces lipogenesis (91) while also stimulating fatty acid oxidation (86).

Following an acute bout of moderate-intensity aerobic exercise, circulating concentrations of leptin do not appear to change (23, 24, 46, 70). However, there are reports that when plasma is sampled over a protracted period post-exercise, circulating leptin concentrations tend to decrease (30, 100), though sufficient evidence now demonstrates that this is likely due to diurnal variation (67) and not exercise per se. While acute exercise does not seem to appreciably alter circulating leptin levels, exercise training does (109). However, given the close relationship between leptin and energy balance, it is more than likely that reports of decreased leptin with aerobic training are not attributable to the direct effects of exercise per se, but rather secondary to the effects of exercise on causing weight loss.

Adiponectin

Adiponectin was originally identified as an adipose complement–related protein of 30 kDa (Acrp30) (121). Shortly thereafter a number of other laboratories made the same breakthrough but named the protein AdipoQ (51), apM1 (79), and GBP28 (93); to avoid confusion, the name adiponectin was agreed upon (3). Interestingly, adiponectin is the only adipokine whose plasma concentrations inversely correlate with body mass (83), yet plasma concentrations are unrelated to fitness level or sex (55, 81, 119). Adiponectin is secreted from adipocytes as a monomer but forms higher-order structures and circulates in human plasma as a high-molecular-weight (HMW) multimer or a low-molecular-weight (LMW) hexamer (103, 123). Though the HMW form is the better measure of insulin sensitivity, the globular head of the adiponectin C-terminal domain, which is produced via proteolytic cleavage, is much more biologically potent (35). Besides its autocrine functions in adipose tissue such as regulating macrophage polarization and up-regulating the anti-inflammatory cytokine IL-10 (69, 99), adiponectin exerts pleiotropic effects in the pancreas, on macrophages, in endothelial cells, and most notably in skeletal muscle and the liver. Administering exogenous adiponectin to healthy or obese diabetic mice results in decreased serum glucose concentrations (101) via a down-regulation of the key hepatic enzymes involved in gluconeogenesis (19). Adiponectin is also well known for its role in increasing skeletal muscle glucose uptake (140) and increasing skeletal muscle fatty acid oxidation (35).

The data regarding the effects of exercise on circulating adiponectin levels are inconsistent. Some reports studying human participants document increases in circulating concentrations of adiponectin post-exercise (65, 68, 77), while others fail to observe such effects (58, 94, 98). Similarly, in rodents, some studies have demonstrated increases in circulating adiponectin concentrations post-exercise

(72, 144), while others have not (9, 52, 72). While adiponectin has been shown to be required for the beneficial metabolic effects of insulin-sensitizing drugs such as thiazolidinediones (95), adiponectin does not appear necessary for the beneficial effects of exercise training. This has been demonstrated in studies showing that exercise-mediated improvements in glucose homeostasis are intact in adiponectin knockout mice (117, 118).

Transforming Growth Factor β2

Transforming growth factor β2 (TGFβ2) is a TGFβ receptor ligand and one of three mammalian TGFβ isoforms encoded by TGFβ genes (59). TGFβ2 is involved in a number of physiological functions, including the suppression of T-cell generation and proliferation, as well as the regulation of glucose and fatty acid metabolism (128, 137). TGFβ signal transduction relies primarily on SMAD proteins, ubiquitous intracellular transcription factors, to initiate the expression of target genes in the nucleus. Given that the TGFβ family of proteins plays an important role in cellular development, it is not surprising that impairments in the TGFβ signalling pathway are commonly associated with a number of diseased states (138).

While much is known about the cellular functions of TGFβ2 and its role in disease pathophysiology, there has been little work examining its effects on exercise metabolism. In one study examining the activation of extracellular matrix genes in skeletal muscle following endurance training, Timmons et al. (129) demonstrated that expression of TGFβ2 and the TGFβII receptor in skeletal muscle were markedly up-regulated in response to 6 weeks of supervised cycling at 75% of pre-training VO_2 max for 45 min/day 4 days/week. Interestingly, the up-regulation of TGFβ2 and the TGFβII receptor were only observed in the participants who had the greatest training-induced improvement in cardiorespiratory fitness, leading these authors to suggest that the skeletal muscle–derived increases in TGFβ2 mediated the improvements in cardiorespiratory fitness.

More recent work demonstrated that 11 days of voluntary wheel running in mice increased serum TGFβ2 concentrations and TGFβ2 gene expression in subcutaneous WAT (128). These authors further demonstrated that the exercise training increased adipose tissue–derived TGFβ2 through a muscle–adipose tissue crosstalk mechanism involving lactate and that 13 days of TGFβ2 treatment in vivo reversed the impairments in glucose tolerance brought about from high-fat diet feeding in mice. Interestingly, when these authors measured serum TGFβ2 from prior studies in humans, they found that several different exercise interventions did not increase serum TGFβ2 concentrations (90, 128, 141, 142). Clearly, more work is needed to definitively address the impact of exercise on circulating levels of TGFβ2 in humans.

Hepatokines

The liver plays a major role in regulating whole-body energy metabolism and contributes to both energy storage and utilization. Because of this, physiological challenges, like exercise, can profoundly affect liver metabolism (48). Similar to the bioactive signalling molecules secreted from skeletal muscle and adipose tissue, factors secreted primarily from the liver that enter circulation and affect distant tissues/organs have been termed "hepatokines." Identification of hepatokines is more recent than myokines and adipokines, and most research has focused on their role in metabolic diseases. For example, two hepatokines, fetuin-A (104) and selenoprotein P (87), are increased in obesity and contribute to the development of insulin resistance.

Recent work suggests that the liver may secrete up to 168 proteins that could potentially exert endocrine effects on distant tissues (85). Perhaps surprisingly, a single bout of non-exhaustive exercise causes more transcriptional alterations in the liver than skeletal muscle, at least in mice (47, 49); because the liver is essentially inaccessible in humans, much less is known about acute effects of exercise.

When focusing on the genes that encode proteins that may be secreted from the liver, 55 genes are up-regulated immediately post-exercise with 29 others being down-regulated (136). However, this form of analysis, namely transcriptomics, may underestimate the actual number of exercise-induced hepatokines because proteins can be secreted without any increase in transcript levels. This section will focus on only the hepatokines that have been consistently shown to be responsive to exercise and have established effects on distant tissues; it is likely that additional factors will emerge over time as this field progresses.

Fibroblast Growth Factor 21 (FGF21)

FGF21 is predominantly expressed in the liver, but is also present in white and brown adipose tissue, skeletal muscle, and the pancreas to lesser extents (97). Despite expression in other tissues, most, if not all, circulating FGF21 is from the liver (82), whereas FGF21 in other tissues most likely works in a paracrine/autocrine manner (26, 50). In both rodents and humans, circulating FGF21 is increased by acute exercise (41). In humans, moderate-to-intense aerobic exercise leads to transient increases in circulating FGF21 (41, 42, 120), and this has been shown to be derived from the liver and not contracting skeletal muscle (41). There has been little research on the effects of chronic aerobic exercise training on FGF21 or how FGF21 contributes to chronic training adaptations, and the results so far are conflicting; some studies show that chronic aerobic exercise training reduces circulating FGF21 in overweight and elderly people, whereas others show no effect or that daily physical activity is associated with increased circulating FGF21 (20).

Various mechanisms seem to regulate hepatic FGF21 expression and secretion. The predominant mechanism seems to be PPARγ, both in vivo and in vitro (4). Acute (4-hour) infusion of fatty acids, which are natural activators of PPARγ, in humans produce modest ~1.5-fold increases in circulating FGF21 (17). However, that fatty acids produce a modest (~1.5-fold) increase in circulating FGF21 compared to exercise (~3-fold) suggests that other mechanisms exist. These other factors could likely involve glucagon, which stimulates hepatic FGF21 secretion, and insulin, which inhibits it (41, 42). Infusing glucagon alone does not increase hepatic FGF21 secretion in humans, probably because glucagon increases blood glucose, which then drives an increase in insulin. But when glucagon and somatostatin (somatostatin prevents secretion of pancreatic hormones, including insulin and glucagon) were simultaneously infused, hepatic FGF21 secretion was similar to exercise (41). Preventing the exercise-associated increase in the glucagon-to-insulin ratio blunts the increase in FGF21 (42), but it does not completely block it, demonstrating that other factors still play a role. The lack of an increased glucagon-to-insulin ratio probably explains why resistance exercise has no effect on circulating FGF21 (89).

There is conflicting evidence on the contribution of FGF21 to the benefits of exercise. In one report, obese mice genetically bred to lack FGF21 experienced impaired exercise-induced adaptations, despite losing similar body weight and running the same amount (78). On the other hand, others have shown that the responses to chronic exercise training are intact in mice lacking FGF21 (34, 111). These differences could be explained by the use of obese (78) compared to lean animals (34, 111).

Follistatin (FST)

FST was discovered in ovarian follicular fluid and was primarily studied in relation to reproductive physiology (92). FST gets its name because it has the ability to suppress secretion of follicle-stimulating hormone. FST is expressed in various tissues, including the pituitary gland, ovary, testis, and skeletal muscle (2), but the liver has recently been identified as the main source of circulating FST (44).

Follistatin is a protein known to inhibit members of the TGFβ superfamily, including myostatin (2). By neutralizing circulating myostatin, FST can increase skeletal muscle mass (73, 74). Treating non-human primates with FST led to muscle hypertrophy (66). FST can also stimulate insulin and glucagon secretion from the pancreas (44).

In the initial hours after aerobic exercise, circulating FST is greatly increased in humans (40, 42, 120). Examination of various tissues in mice revealed that the liver exhibits a marked increase in FST mRNA expression immediately after an acute exercise bout (40). Similarly, it has been demonstrated that the exercise-induced increase in circulating FST concentrations is liver, not muscle, derived (44). Currently, the impact of exercise training on circulating FST levels has not been consistently demonstrated (29, 43, 136).

When looking for the exercise factor that regulates FST secretion, it appears that the glucagon-to-insulin ratio may play a prominent role, much like it does for FGF21. Mice that lack the glucagon receptor have greatly reduced exercise-induced hepatic FST expression immediately post-exercise, showing that glucagon can regulate FST expression with exercise (107). In humans there is a correlation between exercise-induced peak hepatic FST secretion and peak glucagon-to-insulin ratio (44). When glucagon is infused with somatostatin to resting humans, there is a large increase in hepatic FST secretion, showing that the glucagon-to-insulin ratio is an important regulator of hepatic FST secretion in humans (44). However, when the exercise-associated increase in the glucagon-to-insulin ratio was prevented, FST secretion was only blunted by ~50% (44), suggesting there are other important regulators.

Infusion of lipids into healthy males reduced circulating FST by ~50% (44), showing that fatty acids are not regulators of FST. Exercise increases circulating epinephrine, which acts on the liver via different receptors than glucagon but actually converge on the same intracellular pathways (134). Hepatic FST gene expression is increased in mice injected with epinephrine (107), but when epinephrine's activity was blocked (with propranolol) during exercise, there was no difference in hepatic FST expression (107), suggesting epinephrine may not contribute to exercise-induced FST.

FST works by inhibiting the TGFβ family, including myostatin. The TGFβ cascade phosphorylate the mothers against decapentaplegic homolog proteins (45). FST inhibits this activity. However, following exercise there is no evidence of altered SMAD phosphorylation in the liver of mice (107), whereas exercise-induced SMAD phosphorylation and gene expression occur in skeletal muscle of rats following running and in humans only after resistance exercise (75, 76). Together, it seems that exercise increases SMAD phosphorylation and thus TGF-β signalling in muscle, but not liver, suggesting an endocrine role of liver-derived FST.

Angiopoietin-Like Protein-4 (ANGPTL4)

In humans, ANGPTL4 is expressed in adipose tissue, intestine, skeletal muscle, and, by far most abundantly, in the liver (56). ANGPTL4 regulates plasma triglyceride levels by decreasing lipoprotein lipase (LPL) activity (25, 127). LPL is bound to the inside of capillaries and endothelial cells and hydrolyzes circulating triglycerides, thereby allowing the resulting free fatty acids to be taken up by underlying tissues.

Increased plasma ANGPTL4 in response to exercise was originally considered to be muscle derived, leading to the designation "myokine" (15). However, in humans performing one-legged exercise there is a robust increase in ANGPTL4 gene expression only in the resting leg, and this is hypothesized to inhibit fatty acid uptake by the resting leg, thereby allowing the exercising leg to take up greater fuel for exercise (15). During 2 hours of aerobic exercise there was a ~2-fold increase in circulating ANGPTL4 but at no point was there a difference in the arterial-venous difference across resting or exercising leg muscles, indicating that during exercise skeletal muscle does not secrete ANGPTL4 into circulation

(56). In these same subjects, there was a ~5-fold increase in the arterial-venous difference across the hepato-splanchnic bed demonstrating that the liver is the source of circulating ANGPTL4 during exercise (15, 56). Fat is an important fuel source during exercise, so it appears counterintuitive that ANGPTL4 should increase during exercise, ultimately blocking uptake of fatty acids into tissues. But it is possible that this serves as a way to regulate, or limit, fatty acid uptake, as excessive fatty acids can be harmful to skeletal muscle. This is similar to the explanation for why the rate of re-esterification in adipose tissue is also increased during exercise, since this also limits the release of fatty acids into circulation (130).

There has been little research into the chronic effects of exercise on ANGPTL4. But 2 weeks of alternating days of interval and endurance cycling did not alter circulating ANGPTL4 in young healthy males (15). Even following 12 weeks of three times a week exercise training there was no change in circulating ANGPTL4, again in healthy young males (15). There is only one report of increased circulating ANGPTL4 with training, and it came after 6 months of three times a week exercise in obese subjects (21). These results are surprising, since the training led to weight loss and obese people have increased circulating ANGPTL4.

Several regulatory mechanisms are suggested to increase the expression of ANGPTL4, including free fatty acids via PPAR activation (64) and glucagon via cyclic adenosine monophosphate/protein kinase A (cAMP/PKA) (56). The exercise-induced increase in plasma ANGPTL4 is at least partly due to the increase in circulating fatty acids, since exercise-induced ANGPTL4 is much greater in the fasted state, where circulating fatty acids are greater, than the fed state (64). Interestingly, insulin has an inhibitory effect on both ANGPTL4 gene transcription in rodent liver and plasma levels of ANGPTL4 in humans (88); this could be direct or secondary to insulin's ability to attenuate lipolysis (i.e., reduced circulating fatty acids). Pharmacologically inhibiting lipolysis also blocks increased circulating ANGPTL4 (64). As with the other hepatokines, the glucagon-to-insulin ratio seems to regulate exercise-induced hepatic ANGPTL4 secretion. When somatostatin was infused during exercise (inhibiting the increase in glucagon), there was a nearly complete inhibition of increased AGPTL4 (56), although this protocol also prevented the increase in circulating fatty acids during exercise, so it is not entirely clear what contribution the glucagon-to-insulin ratio made. However, when the glucagon-to-insulin ratio was increased in sedentary subjects by infusions of glucagon and somatostatin, there was a similar response in circulating ANGPTL4 to that of exercise, namely a ~33% increase ~3 hours into the infusion, about 1 hour after a spike in circulating fatty acid, then returning to baseline by ~6 hours (56), although again it is hard to tease out the effects of glucagon from the increase in fatty acids. Perhaps the best evidence that the glucagon-to-insulin ratio directly affects hepatic ANGPTL4 expression and secretion is from cell culture experiments where, independent of fatty acids, glucagon increases production of ANGPTL4 from hepatocytes (56).

Conclusion

In the end, exercise-induced myokines, adipokines, and hepatokines participate in crosstalk between different organs during exercise. In this chapter we discussed only cytokines with consistent exercise-inducible characteristics and is by no means a complete list of exercise-induced factors. At the same time, we described cytokines with clear biological roles (e.g., glucose and lipid uptake, adipose tissue browning), but it should be noted that these cytokines likely mediate only a small portion of the overall adaptation to exercise. Nevertheless, the field of tissue crosstalk is rapidly advancing, and additional exercise-induced factors are constantly being uncovered. Future work should examine the effects of different exercise interventions beyond aerobic exercise, including resistance training and the increasingly popular HIIT.

References

1. Allen DL, Hittel DS, McPherron AC. Expression and function of myostatin in obesity, diabetes, and exercise adaptation. *Med Sci Sports Exerc* 43: 1828–1835, 2011.
2. Amthor H, Nicholas G, McKinnell I, Kemp CF, Sharma M, Kambadur R, Patel K. Follistatin complexes Myostatin and antagonises Myostatin-mediated inhibition of myogenesis. *Dev Biol* 270: 19–30, 2004.
3. Arita Y, Kihara S, Ouchi N, Takahashi M, Maeda K, Miyagawa J, Hotta K, et al. Paradoxical decrease of an adipose-specific protein, adiponectin, in obesity. *Biochem Biophys Res Commun* 257: 79–83, 1999.
4. Badman MK, Pissios P, Kennedy AR, Koukos G, Flier JS, Maratos-Flier E. Hepatic fibroblast growth factor 21 is regulated by PPARalpha and is a key mediator of hepatic lipid metabolism in ketotic states. *Cell Metab* 5: 426–437, 2007.
5. Bai Y, Zhang S, Kim KS, Lee JK, Kim KH. Obese gene expression alters the ability of 30A5 preadipocytes to respond to lipogenic hormones. *J Biol Chem* 271: 13939–13942, 1996.
6. Baker AR, Silva NFD, Quinn DW, Harte AL, Pagano D, Bonser RS, Kumar S, McTernan PG. Human epicardial adipose tissue expresses a pathogenic profile of adipocytokines in patients with cardiovascular disease. *Cardiovasc Diabetol* 5(1): 2006.
7. Banks WA, Farrell CL. Impaired transport of leptin across the blood-brain barrier in obesity is acquired and reversible. *Am J Physiol Endocrinol Metab* 285: E10–E15, 2003.
8. Bazgir B, Salesi M, Koushki M, Amirghofran Z. Effects of eccentric and concentric emphasized resistance exercise on IL-15 serum levels and its relation to inflammatory markers in athletes and non-athletes. *Asian J Sports Med* 6: e27980, 2015.
9. Bhattacharya A, Rahman MM, Sun D, Lawrence R, Mejia W, McCarter R, O'Shea M, Fernandes G. The combination of dietary conjugated linoleic acid and treadmill exercise lowers gain in body fat mass and enhances lean body mass in high fat-fed male Balb/C mice. *J Nutr* 135: 1124–1130, 2005.
10. Boström P, Wu J, Jedrychowski MP, Korde A, Ye L, Lo JC, Rasbach KA, et al. A PGC1-α-dependent myokine that drives brown-fat-like development of white fat and thermogenesis. *Nature* 481: 463–468, 2012.
11. Bradley RL, Jeon JY, Liu F-F, Maratos-Flier E. Voluntary exercise improves insulin sensitivity and adipose tissue inflammation in diet-induced obese mice. *Am J Physiol Endocrinol Metab* 295: E586–E594, 2008.
12. Busquets S, Figueras MT, Meijsing S, Carbó N, Quinn LS, Almendro V, Argilés JM, López-Soriano FJ. Interleukin-15 decreases proteolysis in skeletal muscle: A direct effect. *Int J Mol Med* 16: 471–476, 2005.
13. Carey AL, Steinberg GR, Macaulay SL, Thomas WG, Holmes AG, Ramm G, Prelovsek O, et al. Interleukin-6 increases insulin-stimulated glucose disposal in humans and glucose uptake and fatty acid oxidation in vitro via AMP-activated protein kinase. *Diabetes* 55: 2688–2697, 2006.
14. Caron A, Lee S, Elmquist JK, Gautron L. Leptin and brain-adipose crosstalks. *Nat Rev Neurosci* 19: 153–165, 2018.
15. Catoire M, Alex S, Paraskevopulos N, Mattijssen F, Evers-van Gogh I, Schaart G, Jeppesen J, et al. Fatty acid-inducible ANGPTL4 governs lipid metabolic response to exercise. *Proc Natl Acad Sci USA* 111: E1043–E1052, 2014.
16. Christiansen T, Paulsen SK, Bruun JM, Pedersen SB, Richelsen B. Exercise training versus diet-induced weight-loss on metabolic risk factors and inflammatory markers in obese subjects: A 12-week randomized intervention study. *Am J Physiol Endocrinol Metab* 298: E824–E831, 2010.
17. Christodoulides C, Dyson P, Sprecher D, Tsintzas K, Karpe F. Circulating fibroblast growth factor 21 is induced by peroxisome proliferator-activated receptor agonists but not ketosis in man. *J Clin Endocrinol Metab* 94: 3594–3601, 2009.
18. Cohen B, Novick D, Rubinstein M. Modulation of insulin activities by leptin. *Science* 274: 1185–1188, 1996.
19. Combs TP, Berg AH, Obici S, Scherer PE, Rossetti L. Endogenous glucose production is inhibited by the adipose-derived protein Acrp30. *J Clin Invest* 108: 1875–1881, 2001.
20. Cuevas-Ramos D, Almeda-Valdes P, Gómez-Pérez FJ, Meza-Arana CE, Cruz-Bautista I, Arellano-Campos O, Navarrete-López M, Aguilar-Salinas CA. Daily physical activity, fasting glucose, uric acid, and body mass index are independent factors associated with serum fibroblast growth factor 21 levels. *Eur J Endocrinol* 163: 469–477, 2010.
21. Cullberg KB, Christiansen T, Paulsen SK, Bruun JM, Pedersen SB, Richelsen B. Effect of weight loss and exercise on angiogenic factors in the circulation and in adipose tissue in obese subjects. *Obesity (Silver Spring)* 21: 454–460, 2013.
22. Curat CA, Miranville A, Sengenès C, Diehl M, Tonus C, Busse R, Bouloumié A. From blood monocytes to adipose tissue-resident macrophages: Induction of diapedesis by human mature adipocytes. *Diabetes* 53: 1285–1292, 2004.

23. Desgorces FD, Chennaoui M, Gomez-Merino D, Drogou C, Bonneau D, Guezennec CY. Leptin, catecholamines and free fatty acids related to reduced recovery delays after training. *Eur J Appl Physiol* 93: 153–158, 2004.

24. Desgorces FD, Chennaoui M, Gomez-Merino D, Drogou C, Guezennec CY. Leptin response to acute prolonged exercise after training in rowers. *Eur J Appl Physiol* 91: 677–681, 2004.

25. Dijk W, Beigneux AP, Larsson M, Bensadoun A, Young SG, Kersten S. Angiopoietin-like 4 promotes intracellular degradation of lipoprotein lipase in adipocytes. *J Lipid Res* 57: 1670–1683, 2016.

26. Dutchak PA, Katafuchi T, Bookout AL, Choi JH, Yu RT, Mangelsdorf DJ, Kliewer SA. Fibroblast growth factor-21 regulates PPARγ activity and the antidiabetic actions of thiazolidinediones. *Cell* 148: 556–567, 2012.

27. Dyck DJ. Adipokines as regulators of muscle metabolism and insulin sensitivity. *Appl Physiol Nutr Metab* 34: 396–402, 2009.

28. Ellefsen S, Vikmoen O, Slettaløkken G, Whist JE, Nygaard H, Hollan I, Rauk I, et al. Irisin and FNDC5: effects of 12-week strength training, and relations to muscle phenotype and body mass composition in untrained women. *Eur J Appl Physiol* 114: 1875–1888, 2014.

29. Ennequin G, Sirvent P, Whitham M. Role of exercise-induced hepatokines in metabolic disorders. *Am J Physiol Endocrinol Metab* (April 9, 2019). doi: 10.1152/ajpendo.00433.2018.

30. Essig DA, Alderson NL, Ferguson MA, Bartoli WP, Durstine JL. Delayed effects of exercise on the plasma leptin concentration. *Metabolism* 49: 395–399, 2000.

31. Febbraio MA, Pedersen BK. Muscle-derived interleukin-6: Mechanisms for activation and possible biological roles. *FASEB J* 16: 1335–1347, 2002.

32. Feldman BJ, Streeper RS, Farese RV, Yamamoto KR. Myostatin modulates adipogenesis to generate adipocytes with favorable metabolic effects. *Proc Natl Acad Sci U S A* 103: 15675–15680, 2006.

33. Fischer CP. Interleukin-6 in acute exercise and training: What is the biological relevance? *Exerc Immunol Rev* 12: 6–33, 2006.

34. Fletcher JA, Linden MA, Sheldon RD, Meers GM, Morris EM, Butterfield A, Perfield JW, Thyfault JP, Rector RS. Fibroblast growth factor 21 and exercise-induced hepatic mitochondrial adaptations. *Am J Physiol Gastrointest Liver Physiol* 310: G832–G843, 2016.

35. Fruebis J, Tsao TS, Javorschi S, Ebbets-Reed D, Erickson MR, Yen FT, Bihain BE, Lodish HF. Proteolytic cleavage product of 30-kDa adipocyte complement-related protein increases fatty acid oxidation in muscle and causes weight loss in mice. *Proc Natl Acad Sci U S A* 98: 2005–2010, 2001.

36. Furmanczyk PS, Quinn LS. Interleukin-15 increases myosin accretion in human skeletal myogenic cultures. *Cell Biol Int* 27: 845–851, 2003.

37. Galic S, Oakhill JS, Steinberg GR. Adipose tissue as an endocrine organ. *Mol Cell Endocrinol* 316: 129–139, 2010.

38. Gálvez B, de Castro J, Herold D, Dubrovska G, Arribas S, González MC, Aranguez I, et al. Perivascular adipose tissue and mesenteric vascular function in spontaneously hypertensive rats. *Arterioscler Thromb Vasc Biol* 26: 1297–1302, 2006.

39. Guo T, Jou W, Chanturiya T, Portas J, Gavrilova O, McPherron AC. Myostatin inhibition in muscle, but not adipose tissue, decreases fat mass and improves insulin sensitivity. *PLOS ONE* 4: e4937, 2009.

40. Hansen J, Brandt C, Nielsen AR, Hojman P, Whitham M, Febbraio MA, Pedersen BK, Plomgaard P. Exercise induces a marked increase in plasma follistatin: Evidence that follistatin is a contraction-induced hepatokine. *Endocrinology* 152: 164–171, 2011.

41. Hansen JS, Clemmesen JO, Secher NH, Hoene M, Drescher A, Weigert C, Pedersen BK, Plomgaard P. Glucagon-to-insulin ratio is pivotal for splanchnic regulation of FGF-21 in humans. *Mol Metab* 4: 551–560, 2015.

42. Hansen JS, Pedersen BK, Xu G, Lehmann R, Weigert C, Plomgaard P. Exercise-induced secretion of FGF21 and follistatin are blocked by pancreatic clamp and impaired in type 2 diabetes. *J Clin Endocrinol Metab* (May 10, 2016). doi: 10.1210/jc.2016-1681.

43. Hansen JS, Plomgaard P. Circulating follistatin in relation to energy metabolism. *Mol Cell Endocrinol* 433: 87–93, 2016.

44. Hansen JS, Rutti S, Arous C, Clemmesen JO, Secher NH, Drescher A, Gonelle-Gispert C, et al. Circulating follistatin is liver-derived and regulated by the glucagon-to-insulin ratio. *J Clin Endocrinol Metab* 101: 550–560, 2016.

45. Hedger MP, Winnall WR, Phillips DJ, de Kretser DM. The regulation and functions of activin and follistatin in inflammation and immunity. *Vitam Horm* 85: 255–297, 2011.

46. Hickey MS, Considine RV, Israel RG, Mahar TL, McCammon MR, Tyndall GL, Houmard JA, Caro JF. Leptin is related to body fat content in male distance runners. *Am J Physiol* 271: E938–E940, 1996.

47. Hoene M, Franken H, Fritsche L, Lehmann R, Pohl AK, Häring HU, Zell A, Schleicher ED, Weigert C. Activation of the mitogen-activated protein kinase (MAPK) signalling pathway in the liver of mice is related to plasma glucose levels after acute exercise. *Diabetologia* 53: 1131–1141, 2010.

48. Hoene M, Lehmann R, Hennige AM, Pohl AK, Häring HU, Schleicher ED, Weigert C. Acute regulation of metabolic genes and insulin receptor substrates in the liver of mice by one single bout of treadmill exercise. *The Journal of Physiology* 587: 241–252, 2009.

49. Hoene M, Weigert C. The stress response of the liver to physical exercise. *Exerc Immunol Rev* 16: 163–183, 2010.

50. Hondares E, Iglesias R, Giralt A, Gonzalez FJ, Giralt M, Mampel T, Villarroya F. Thermogenic activation induces FGF21 expression and release in brown adipose tissue. *J Biol Chem* 286: 12983–12990, 2011.

51. Hu E, Liang P, Spiegelman BM. AdipoQ is a novel adipose-specific gene dysregulated in obesity. *J Biol Chem* 271: 10697–10703, 1996.

52. Huang H, Iida KT, Sone H, Ajisaka R. The regulation of adiponectin receptors expression by acute exercise in mice. *Exp Clin Endocrinol Diabetes* 115: 417–422, 2007.

53. Hube F, Lietz U, Igel M, Jensen PB, Tornqvist H, Joost HG, Hauner H. Difference in leptin mRNA levels between omental and subcutaneous abdominal adipose tissue from obese humans. *Horm Metab Res* 28: 690–693, 1996.

54. Huh JY, Panagiotou G, Mougios V, Brinkoetter M, Vamvini MT, Schneider BE, Mantzoros CS. FNDC5 and irisin in humans: I. Predictors of circulating concentrations in serum and plasma and II. mRNA expression and circulating concentrations in response to weight loss and exercise. *Metab Clin Exp* 61: 1725–1738, 2012.

55. Hulver MW, Zheng D, Tanner CJ, Houmard JA, Kraus WE, Slentz CA, Sinha MK, Pories WJ, MacDonald KG, Dohm GL. Adiponectin is not altered with exercise training despite enhanced insulin action. *Am J Physiol Endocrinol Metab* 283: E861–E865, 2002.

56. Ingerslev B, Hansen JS, Hoffmann C, Clemmesen JO, Secher NH, Scheler M, Hrabě de Angelis M, et al. Angiopoietin-like protein 4 is an exercise-induced hepatokine in humans, regulated by glucagon and cAMP. *Mol Metab* 6: 1286–1295, 2017.

57. Jedrychowski MP, Wrann CD, Paulo JA, Gerber KK, Szpyt J, Robinson MM, Nair KS, Gygi SP, Spiegelman BM. Detection and quantitation of circulating human irisin by tandem mass spectrometry. *Cell Metab* 22: 734–740, 2015.

58. Jürimäe J, Purge P, Jürimäe T. Effect of prolonged training period on plasma adiponectin in elite male rowers. *Horm Metab Res* 39: 519–523, 2007.

59. Kamato D, Burch ML, Piva TJ, Rezaei HB, Rostam MA, Xu S, Zheng W, Little PJ, Osman N. Transforming growth factor-β signalling: Role and consequences of Smad linker region phosphorylation. *Cell Signal* 25: 2017–2024, 2013.

60. Kanemaki T, Kitade H, Kaibori M, Sakitani K, Hiramatsu Y, Kamiyama Y, Ito S, Okumura T. Interleukin 1beta and interleukin 6, but not tumor necrosis factor alpha, inhibit insulin-stimulated glycogen synthesis in rat hepatocytes. *Hepatology* 27: 1296–1303, 1998.

61. Keller C, Hellsten Y, Steensberg A, Pedersen BK. Differential regulation of IL-6 and TNF-alpha via calcineurin in human skeletal muscle cells. *Cytokine* 36: 141–147, 2006.

62. Keller C, Steensberg A, Pilegaard H, Osada T, Saltin B, Pedersen BK, Neufer PD. Transcriptional activation of the IL-6 gene in human contracting skeletal muscle: Influence of muscle glycogen content. *FASEB J* 15: 2748–2750, 2001.

63. KENNEDY GC. The role of depot fat in the hypothalamic control of food intake in the rat. *Proc R Soc Lond, B, Biol Sci* 140: 578–596, 1953.

64. Kersten S, Lichtenstein L, Steenbergen E, Mudde K, Hendriks HFJ, Hesselink MK, Schrauwen P, Müller M. Caloric restriction and exercise increase plasma ANGPTL4 levels in humans via elevated free fatty acids. *Arterioscler Thromb Vasc Biol* 29: 969–974, 2009.

65. Kondo T, Kobayashi I, Murakami M. Effect of exercise on circulating adipokine levels in obese young women. *Endocr J* 53: 189–195, 2006.

66. Kota J, Handy CR, Haidet AM, Montgomery CL, Eagle A, Rodino-Klapac LR, Tucker D, et al. Follistatin gene delivery enhances muscle growth and strength in nonhuman primates. *Sci Transl Med* 1: 6ra15–6ra15, 2009.

67. Kraemer RR, Chu H, Castracane VD. Leptin and exercise. *Exp Biol Med (Maywood)* 227: 701–708, 2002.

68. Kriketos AD, Gan SK, Poynten AM, Furler SM, Chisholm DJ, Campbell LV. Exercise increases adiponectin levels and insulin sensitivity in humans. *Diabetes Care* 27: 629–630, 2004.

69. Kumada M, Kihara S, Ouchi N, Kobayashi H, Okamoto Y, Ohashi K, Maeda K, et al. Adiponectin specifically increased tissue inhibitor of metalloproteinase-1 through interleukin-10 expression in human macrophages. *Circulation* 109: 2046–2049, 2004.

70. Landt M, Lawson GM, Helgeson JM, Davila-Roman VG, Ladenson JH, Jaffe AS, Hickner RC. Prolonged exercise decreases serum leptin concentrations. *Metabolism* 46: 1109–1112, 1997.

71. Lebrasseur NK. Building muscle, browning fat and preventing obesity by inhibiting myostatin. *Diabetologia* 55: 13–17, 2012.

72. Lee S, Park Y, Dellsperger KC, Zhang C. Exercise training improves endothelial function via adiponectin-dependent and independent pathways in type 2 diabetic mice. *Am J Physiol Heart Circ Physiol* 301: H306–H314, 2011.

73. Lee S-J, Lee Y-S, Zimmers TA, Soleimani A, Matzuk MM, Tsuchida K, Cohn RD, Barton ER. Regulation of muscle mass by follistatin and activins. *Mol Endocrinol* 24: 1998–2008, 2010.

74. Lee SJ, McPherron AC. Regulation of myostatin activity and muscle growth. *Proc Natl Acad Sci USA* 98: 9306–9311, 2001.

75. Lessard SJ, MacDonald TL, Pathak P, Han MS, Coffey VG, EDGE J, Rivas DA, Hirshman MF, Davis RJ, Goodyear LJ. JNK regulates muscle remodeling via myostatin/SMAD inhibition. *Nature Communications* 9: 3030, 2018.

76. Lessard SJ, Rivas DA, Alves-Wagner AB, Hirshman MF, Gallagher IJ, Constantin-Teodosiu D, Atkins R, et al. Resistance to aerobic exercise training causes metabolic dysfunction and reveals novel exercise-regulated signaling networks. *Diabetes* 62: 2717–2727, 2013.

77. Lim S, Choi SH, Jeong I-K, Kim JH, Moon MK, Park KS, Lee HK, Kim Y-B, Jang HC. Insulin-sensitizing effects of exercise on adiponectin and retinol-binding protein-4 concentrations in young and middle-aged women. *J Clin Endocrinol Metab* 93: 2263–2268, 2008.

78. Loyd C, Magrisso IJ, Haas M, Balusu S, Krishna R, Itoh N, Sandoval DA, Perez-Tilve D, Obici S, Habegger KM. Fibroblast growth factor 21 is required for beneficial effects of exercise during chronic high-fat feeding. *J Appl Physiol* 121: 687–698, 2016.

79. Maeda K, Okubo K, Shimomura I, Funahashi T, Matsuzawa Y, Matsubara K. cDNA cloning and expression of a novel adipose specific collagen-like factor, apM1 (AdiPose Most abundant Gene transcript 1). *Biochem Biophys Res Commun* 221: 286–289, 1996.

80. Maffei M, Halaas J, Ravussin E, Pratley RE, Lee GH, Zhang Y, Fei H, Kim S, Lallone R, Ranganathan S. Leptin levels in human and rodent: Measurement of plasma leptin and ob RNA in obese and weight-reduced subjects. *Nat Med* 1: 1155–1161, 1995.

81. Marcell TJ, McAuley KA, Traustadóttir T, Reaven PD. Exercise training is not associated with improved levels of C-reactive protein or adiponectin. *Metabolism* 54: 533–541, 2005.

82. Markan KR, Naber MC, Ameka MK, Anderegg MD, Mangelsdorf DJ, Kliewer SA, Mohammadi M, Potthoff MJ. Circulating FGF21 is liver derived and enhances glucose uptake during refeeding and overfeeding. *Diabetes* 63: 4057–4063, 2014.

83. Mazaki-Tovi S, Kanety H, Sivan E. Adiponectin and human pregnancy. *Curr Diab Rep* 5: 278–281, 2005.

84. McPherron AC, Lawler AM, Lee SJ. Regulation of skeletal muscle mass in mice by a new TGF-beta super-family member. *Nature* 387: 83–90, 1997.

85. Meex RC, Hoy AJ, Morris A, Brown RD, Lo JCY, Burke M, Goode RJA, et al. Fetuin B is a secreted hepatocyte factor linking steatosis to impaired glucose metabolism. *Cell Metab* 22: 1078–1089, 2015.

86. Minokoshi Y, Kim Y-B, Peroni OD, Fryer LGD, Müller C, Carling D, Kahn BB. Leptin stimulates fatty-acid oxidation by activating AMP-activated protein kinase. *Nature* 415: 339–343, 2002.

87. Misu H, Takayama H, Saito Y, Mita Y, Kikuchi A, Ishii K-A, Chikamoto K, et al. Deficiency of the hepatokine selenoprotein P increases responsiveness to exercise in mice through upregulation of reactive oxygen species and AMP-activated protein kinase in muscle. *Nat Med* 23: 508–516, 2017.

88. Mizutani N, Ozaki N, Seino Y, Fukami A, Sakamoto E, Fukuyama T, Sugimura Y, Nagasaki H, Arima H, Oiso Y. Reduction of insulin signaling upregulates angiopoietin-like protein 4 through elevated free fatty acids in diabetic mice. *Exp Clin Endocrinol Diabetes* 120: 139–144, 2012.

89. Morville T, Sahl RE, Trammell SA, Svenningsen JS, Gillum MP, Helge JW, Clemmensen C. Divergent effects of resistance and endurance exercise on plasma bile acids, FGF19, and FGF21 in humans. *JCI Insight* 3: 990, 2018.

90. Motiani P, Virtanen KA, Motiani KK, Eskelinen JJ, Middelbeek RJ, Goodyear LJ, Savolainen AM, et al. Decreased insulin-stimulated brown adipose tissue glucose uptake after short-term exercise training in healthy middle-aged men. *Diabetes Obes Metab* 19: 1379–1388, 2017.

91. Muoio DM, Dohm GL, Fiedorek FT, Tapscott EB, Coleman RA, Dohn GL. Leptin directly alters lipid partitioning in skeletal muscle. *Diabetes* 46: 1360–1363, 1997.

92. Nakamura T, Takio K, Eto Y, Shibai H, Titani K, Sugino H. Activin-binding protein from rat ovary is follistatin. *Science* 247: 836–838, 1990.

93. Nakano Y, Tobe T, Choi-Miura NH, Mazda T, Tomita M. Isolation and characterization of GBP28, a novel gelatin-binding protein purified from human plasma. *J Biochem* 120: 803–812, 1996.

94. Nassis GP, Papantakou K, Skenderi K, Triandafillopoulou M, Kavouras SA, Yannakoulia M, Chrousos GP, Sidossis LS. Aerobic exercise training improves insulin sensitivity without changes in body weight, body fat, adiponectin, and inflammatory markers in overweight and obese girls. *Metabolism* 54: 1472–1479, 2005.

95. Nawrocki AR, Rajala MW, Tomas E, Pajvani UB, Saha AK, Trumbauer ME, Pang Z, et al. Mice lacking adiponectin show decreased hepatic insulin sensitivity and reduced responsiveness to peroxisome proliferator-activated receptor gamma agonists. *J Biol Chem* 281: 2654–2660, 2006.

96. Nieman DC, Nehlsen-Cannarella SL, Fagoaga OR, Henson DA, Utter A, Davis JM, Williams F, Butterworth DE. Influence of mode and carbohydrate on the cytokine response to heavy exertion. *Med Sci Sports Exerc* 30: 671–678, 1998.

97. Nishimura T, Nakatake Y, Konishi M, Itoh N. Identification of a novel FGF, FGF-21, preferentially expressed in the liver. *Biochim Biophys Acta* 1492: 203–206, 2000.

98. O'Leary VB, Jorett AE, Marchetti CM, Gonzalez F, Phillips SA, Ciaraldi TP, Kirwan JP. Enhanced adiponectin multimer ratio and skeletal muscle adiponectin receptor expression following exercise training and diet in older insulin-resistant adults. *Am J Physiol Endocrinol Metab* 293: E421–E427, 2007.

99. Ohashi K, Parker JL, Ouchi N, Higuchi A, Vita JA, Gokce N, Pedersen AA, et al. Adiponectin promotes macrophage polarization toward an anti-inflammatory phenotype. *J Biol Chem* 285: 6153–6160, 2010.

100. Olive JL, Miller GD. Differential effects of maximal- and moderate-intensity runs on plasma leptin in healthy trained subjects. *Nutrition* 17: 365–369, 2001.

101. Oshima K, Nampei A, Matsuda M, Iwaki M, Fukuhara A, Hashimoto J, Yoshikawa H, Shimomura I. Adiponectin increases bone mass by suppressing osteoclast and activating osteoblast. *Biochem Biophys Res Commun* 331: 520–526, 2005.

102. Ostrowski K, Rohde T, Zacho M, Asp S, Pedersen BK. Evidence that interleukin-6 is produced in human skeletal muscle during prolonged running. *The Journal of Physiology* 508: 949–953, 1998.

103. Pajvani UB, Hawkins M, Combs TP, Rajala MW, Doebber T, Berger JP, Wagner JA, et al. Complex distribution, not absolute amount of adiponectin, correlates with thiazolidinedione-mediated improvement in insulin sensitivity. *J Biol Chem* 279: 12152–12162, 2004.

104. Pal D, Dasgupta S, Kundu R, Maitra S, Das G, Mukhopadhyay S, Ray S, Majumdar SS, Bhattacharya S. Fetuin-A acts as an endogenous ligand of TLR4 to promote lipid-induced insulin resistance. *Nat Med* 18: 1279–1285, 2012.

105. Pedersen BK, Febbraio MA. Muscle as an endocrine organ: Focus on muscle-derived interleukin-6. *Physiol Rev* 88: 1379–1406, 2008.

106. Pedersen BK. Muscle as a secretory organ. *Compr Physiol* 3: 1337–1362, 2013.

107. Peppler WT, Castellani LN, Root-Mccaig J, Townsend LK, Sutton CD, Frendo-Cumbo S, Medak KD, MacPherson REK, Charron MJ, Wright DC. Regulation of hepatic follistatin expression at rest and during exercise in mice. *Med Sci Sports Exerc* 51(6): 1116–1125, 2019.

108. Pérez-López A, McKendry J, Martin-Rincon M, Morales-Alamo D, Pérez-Köhler B, Valadés D, Buján J, Calbet JAL, Breen L. Skeletal muscle IL-15/IL-15Rα and myofibrillar protein synthesis after resistance exercise. *Scand J Med Sci Sports* 28: 116–125, 2018.

109. Pérusse L, Collier G, Gagnon J, Leon AS, Rao DC, Skinner JS, Wilmore JH, Nadeau A, Zimmet PZ, Bouchard C. Acute and chronic effects of exercise on leptin levels in humans. *J Appl Physiol* 83: 5–10, 1997.

110. Pierce JR, Maples JM, Hickner RC. IL-15 concentrations in skeletal muscle and subcutaneous adipose tissue in lean and obese humans: local effects of IL-15 on adipose tissue lipolysis. *Am J Physiol Endocrinol Metab* 308: E1131–E1139, 2015.

111. Porter JW, Rowles JL, Fletcher JA, Zidon TM, Winn NC, McCabe LT, Park Y-M, et al. Anti-inflammatory effects of exercise training in adipose tissue do not require FGF21. *J Endocrinol* 235: 97–109, 2017.

112. Quinn LS, Anderson BG, Drivdahl RH, Alvarez B, Argilés JM. Overexpression of interleukin-15 induces skeletal muscle hypertrophy in vitro: Implications for treatment of muscle wasting disorders. *Exp Cell Res* 280: 55–63, 2002.

113. Quinn LS, Haugk KL, Damon SE. Interleukin-15 stimulates C2 skeletal myoblast differentiation. *Biochem Biophys Res Commun* 239: 6–10, 1997.

114. Quinn LS, Strait-Bodey L, Anderson BG, Argilés JM, Havel PJ. Interleukin-15 stimulates adiponectin secretion by 3T3-L1 adipocytes: Evidence for a skeletal muscle-to-fat signaling pathway. *Cell Biol Int* 29: 449–457, 2005.

115. Relizani K, Mouisel E, Giannesini B, Hourdé C, Patel K, Morales Gonzalez S, Jülich K, et al. Blockade of ActRIIB signaling triggers muscle fatigability and metabolic myopathy. *Mol Ther* 22: 1423–1433, 2014.

116. Riechman SE, Balasekaran G, Roth SM, Ferrell RE. Association of interleukin-15 protein and interleukin-15 receptor genetic variation with resistance exercise training responses. *J Appl Physiol* 97: 2214–2219, 2004.

117. Ritchie IRW, MacDonald TL, Wright DC, Dyck DJ. Adiponectin is sufficient, but not required, for exercise-induced increases in the expression of skeletal muscle mitochondrial enzymes. *J Physiol* 592: 2653–2665, 2014.

118. Ritchie IRW, Wright DC, Dyck DJ. Adiponectin is not required for exercise training-induced improvements in glucose and insulin tolerance in mice. *Physiol Rep* 2: e12146, 2014.

119. Ryan AS, Nicklas BJ, Berman DM, Elahi D. Adiponectin levels do not change with moderate dietary induced weight loss and exercise in obese postmenopausal women. *Int J Obes Relat Metab Disord* 27: 1066–1071, 2003.

120. Sargeant JA, Aithal GP, Takamura T, Misu H, Takayama H, Douglas JA, Turner MC, et al. The influence of adiposity and acute exercise on circulating hepatokines in normal-weight and overweight/obese men. *Appl Physiol Nutr Metab* 43: 482–490, 2018.

121. Scherer PE, Williams S, Fogliano M, Baldini G, Lodish HF. A novel serum protein similar to C1q, produced exclusively in adipocytes. *J Biol Chem* 270: 26746–26749, 1995.

122. Schuelke M, Wagner KR, Stolz LE, Hübner C, Riebel T, Kömen W, Braun T, Tobin JF, Lee S-J. Myostatin mutation associated with gross muscle hypertrophy in a child. *N Engl J Med* 350: 2682–2688, 2004.

123. Shapiro L, Scherer PE. The crystal structure of a complement-1q family protein suggests an evolutionary link to tumor necrosis factor. *Curr Biol* 8: 335–338, 1998.

124. Sledzinski T, Korczynska J, Hallmann A, Kaska L, Proczko-Markuszewska M, Stefaniak T, Sledzinski M, Swierczynski J. The increase of serum chemerin concentration is mainly associated with the increase of body mass index in obese, non-diabetic subjects. *J endocrinol Invest* 36: 428–434, 2013.

125. Steensberg A, Febbraio MA, Osada T, Schjerling P, van Hall G, Saltin B, Pedersen BK. Interleukin-6 production in contracting human skeletal muscle is influenced by pre-exercise muscle glycogen content. *J Physiol* 537: 633–639, 2001.

126. Stouthard JM, Romijn JA, Van der Poll T, Endert E, Klein S, Bakker PJ, Veenhof CH, Sauerwein HP. Endocrinologic and metabolic effects of interleukin-6 in humans. *Am J Physiol* 268: E813–E819, 1995.

127. Sukonina V, Lookene A, Olivecrona T, Olivecrona G. Angiopoietin-like protein 4 converts lipoprotein lipase to inactive monomers and modulates lipase activity in adipose tissue. *Proc Natl Acad Sci U S A* 103: 17450–17455, 2006.

128. Takahashi H, Alves CRR, Stanford KI, Middelbeek RJW, Pasquale Nigro, Ryan RE, Xue R, et al. TGF-β2 is an exercise-induced adipokine that regulates glucose and fatty acid metabolism. *Nat Metab* 1: 291–303, 2019.

129. Timmons JA, Jansson E, Fischer H, Gustafsson T, Greenhaff PL, Ridden J, Rachman J, Sundberg CJ. Modulation of extracellular matrix genes reflects the magnitude of physiological adaptation to aerobic exercise training in humans. *BMC Biol* 3: 19, 2005.

130. Townsend LK, Knuth CM, Wright DC. Cycling our way to fit fat. *Physiol Rep* 5: e13247, 2017.

131. Trayhurn P, Wood IS. Adipokines: Inflammation and the pleiotropic role of white adipose tissue. *Brit J Nutr* 92: 347–355, 2004.

132. Tsigos C, Papanicolaou DA, Kyrou I, Defensor R, Mitsiadis CS, Chrousos GP. Dose-dependent effects of recombinant human interleukin-6 on glucose regulation. *J Clin Endocrinol Metab* 82: 4167–4170, 1997.

133. Ullum H, Haahr PM, Diamant M, Palmø J, Halkjaer-Kristensen J, Pedersen BK. Bicycle exercise enhances plasma IL-6 but does not change IL-1 alpha, IL-1 beta, IL-6, or TNF-alpha pre-mRNA in BMNC. *J Appl Physiol* 77: 93–97, 1994.

134. Wasserman DH, Cherrington AD. Hepatic fuel metabolism during muscular work: Role and regulation. *Am J Physiol* 260: E811–E824, 1991.

135. Wedell-Neergaard A-S, Lang Lehrskov L, Christensen RH, Legaard GE, Dorph E, Larsen MK, Launbo N, et al. Exercise-induced changes in visceral adipose tissue mass are regulated by IL-6 signaling: A randomized controlled trial. *Cell Metab* 29: 844–855.e3, 2019.

136. Weigert C, Hoene M, Plomgaard P. Hepatokines-a novel group of exercise factors. *Pflugers Arch* 471: 383–396, 2019.

137. Weiss A, Attisano L. The TGFbeta superfamily signaling pathway. *Wiley Interdiscip Rev Dev Biol* 2: 47–63, 2013.

138. Yadav H, Quijano C, Kamaraju AK, Gavrilova O, Malek R, Chen W, Zerfas P, et al. Protection from obesity and diabetes by blockade of TGF-β/Smad3 signaling. *Cell Metab* 14: 67–79, 2011.

139. Yamauchi T, Kamon J, Ito Y, Tsuchida A, Yokomizo T, Kita S, Sugiyama T, et al. Cloning of adiponectin receptors that mediate antidiabetic metabolic effects. *Nature* 423: 762–769, 2003.

140. Yamauchi T, Kamon J, Minokoshi Y, Ito Y, Waki H, Uchida S, Yamashita S, et al. Adiponectin stimulates glucose utilization and fatty-acid oxidation by activating AMP-activated protein kinase. *Nat Med* 8: 1288–1295, 2002.

141. Yfanti C, Akerström T, Nielsen S, Nielsen AR, Mounier R, Mortensen OH, Lykkesfeldt J, Rose AJ, Fischer CP, Pedersen BK. Antioxidant supplementation does not alter endurance training adaptation. *Med Sci Sports Exerc* 42: 1388–1395, 2010.

142. Yfanti C, Nielsen AR, Akerström T, Nielsen S, Rose AJ, Richter EA, Lykkesfeldt J, Fischer CP, Pedersen BK. Effect of antioxidant supplementation on insulin sensitivity in response to endurance exercise training. *Am J Physiol Endocrinol Metab* 300: E761–E770, 2011.

143. Zachwieja JJ, Hendry SL, Smith SR, Harris RB. Voluntary wheel running decreases adipose tissue mass and expression of leptin mRNA in Osborne-Mendel rats. *Diabetes* 46: 1159–1166, 1997.

144. Zeng Q, Isobe K, Fu L, Ohkoshi N, Ohmori H, Takekoshi K, Kawakami Y. Effects of exercise on adiponectin and adiponectin receptor levels in rats. *Life Sci* 80: 454–459, 2007.

145. Zhang C, McFarlane C, Lokireddy S, Masuda S, Ge X, Gluckman PD, Sharma M, Kambadur R. Inhibition of myostatin protects against diet-induced obesity by enhancing fatty acid oxidation and promoting a brown adipose phenotype in mice. *Diabetologia* 55: 183–193, 2012.

146. Zhang Y, Proenca R, Maffei M, Barone M, Leopold L, Friedman JM. Positional cloning of the mouse obese gene and its human homologue. *Nature* 372: 425–432, 1994.

147. Zhao B, Wall RJ, Yang J. Transgenic expression of myostatin propeptide prevents diet-induced obesity and insulin resistance. *Biochem Biophys Res Commun* 337: 248–255, 2005.

4

REGULATION OF SKELETAL MUSCLE REACTIVE OXYGEN SPECIES DURING EXERCISE

Catherine A. Bellissimo and Christopher G.R. Perry

Introduction

Exercise poses an immediate challenge to multiple homeostatic functions within skeletal muscle. Left unchecked, the challenge posed by exercise would rapidly compromise vital processes such as energy balance, pH, temperature, ion homeostasis, and other functions and limit the ability to sustain contraction. Each of these critical variables are sensed by feedback loops that acutely correct the imbalance by altering the activity of rate-limiting proteins in a variety of cellular pathways. These disturbances also activate nuclear responses that mediate longer-term muscle adaptation to chronic exercise. The signals generated during exercise that trigger such feedback loops are typically an imbalance in the very factors that are essential to the cell (calcium, ADP/ATP, etc.) and are therefore "stress signals." In this light, the discoveries that reactive oxygen species (ROS) are generated during muscle (21, 67) led to a new direction of inquiry that has attempted to resolve whether ROS are damaging products of contraction, essential regulatory signals, or both.

The purpose of this chapter is to provide an overview of major advances that led to our current understanding of how exercise regulates ROS in skeletal muscle, as well as their potential role as regulatory signals. The chapter also provides a brief introduction to the paradigm of "redox signalling" in order to demonstrate the untapped potential for discovery of redox regulation of skeletal muscle function in response to exercise. Another key aspect of this chapter is to demonstrate how understanding differences in experimental techniques is essential for framing precise conclusions, avoiding generalization, and identifying remaining uncertainties. In so doing, common generalizations can be deconstructed to guide focused research directions aimed at completing our understanding of how ROS regulates muscle function in response to exercise.

While this chapter will focus primarily on known ROS responses to exercise in skeletal muscle, it should be noted that reactive nitrogen species (RNS) or reactive oxygen–nitrogen species (RONS), such as nitric oxide, are also increased during contraction (63). RNS/RONS are thought to be regulators of redox signalling through mechanisms such as S-nitrosylation of redox-sensitive proteins, as might also be the case for RONS like peroxynitrite (28). Other reviews address their role in skeletal muscle during exercise (17, 101). Likewise, there is a considerable literature on blood-based measures of ROS and oxidative stress, but these measures may reflect redox responses in other cell types related to inflammation that may be important for muscle adaptation. This topic is thoroughly addressed elsewhere (9).

ROS and Muscle Function During Exercise

Many excellent reviews have been written on the potential mechanisms of how ROS may regulate muscle function during exercise and as mediators of adaptation to training (16, 17, 66, 69, 81, 114, 117, 118). Briefly, the first discoveries that ROS affect muscle function focused on their relationship specifically to fatigue (5, 24, 75, 106, 122, 123, 135). ROS are also known to acutely regulate metabolism in certain conditions (2, 57) such that their role in regulating metabolism specifically during exercise is now being investigated. Another major area of research has focused on the role of ROS in triggering muscle adaptation to chronic exercise training, as discussed in this chapter. The precise signalling mechanisms by which ROS mediate these responses has not been investigated with direct assessments of regulatory proteins that become oxidized except in a few cases. For example, exercise and muscle contraction are known to regulate the ryanodine receptor through redox signalling, with profound effects on sarcoplasmic reticulum calcium release (17, 59, 81), while ROS can also alter proteins regulating myofibrillar calcium sensitivity (17, 81). This research highlights the power of using specialized techniques that determine whether specific proteins have been oxidized and serves as an example for unravelling additional ROS-signalling mechanisms for other cell functions (addressed in more detail later). To date, most ROS-signalling has been indirect by measuring the response of certain signalling pathways and gene expression that are known in general to be ROS sensitive, but exact protein oxidation networks in response to exercise remain a ripe area for future research.

A Primer on Redox Biology

ROS regulate a spectrum of cellular functions by directly modifying protein and membrane oxidation states through a concept referred to as "redox signalling." ROS serve as messengers that can facilitate ligand activation of receptors (e.g., hormones) to modulate downstream signalling cascades or serve as relay signals that communicate imbalances in a variety of cellular homeostatic systems (e.g., stress responses). Key to their roles as signals is the concept of compartmentation; ROS-generating systems are often spatially organized in micro-domains located precisely where they are needed (37, 70). Such organization serves to localize the concentration of ROS around redox-sensitive proteins. Redox buffering is central to this process whereby ROS can be scavenged to prevent excessive or unregulated protein and membrane oxidation, or used to facilitate intentional redox modifications of regulatory proteins (88, 103)—a framework that has been referred to as "redox circuits" (70). In this light, the process of "oxidative stress" has been proposed to focus on disruption of normal function of such redox circuits in a manner that causes detrimental effects to cell function (70, 71). This contemporary view extends the previous and common doctrine that oxidative stress occurs when ROS "exceeds" antioxidants by adding the critical focus of how ROS-mediated signalling pathways can lose their spatial and kinetic regulation that results in impaired cell functions. In so doing, this model guides specific lines of inquiry to understand how ROS can be either essential signals or toxic instruments to a cell by considering the enzymatic source of ROS, the location of ROS, the type of ROS, and the regulation of redox buffers and protein oxidation state (e.g., glutathione, GSH, and thioredoxin, which are Trx-based buffering nodes).

Of the various types of ROS, superoxide (O_2^-) is commonly produced from multiple sites, including nicotinamide adenine dinucleotide phosphate (NADPH) oxidases, xanthine oxidase, and mitochondria. Superoxide is also the source of hydrogen peroxide (H_2O_2), which is thought to be a major redox signal, given it is relatively stable and membrane permeable (71). As such, H_2O_2 derived from all sources, including mitochondria, has the potential to signal coordinated responses throughout the cell. Indeed, H_2O_2 is thought to be the major redox signal from the mitochondria that can diffuse rapidly across mitochondrial membranes and activate redox signalling throughout the cell (summarized in Figure 4.1) (70).

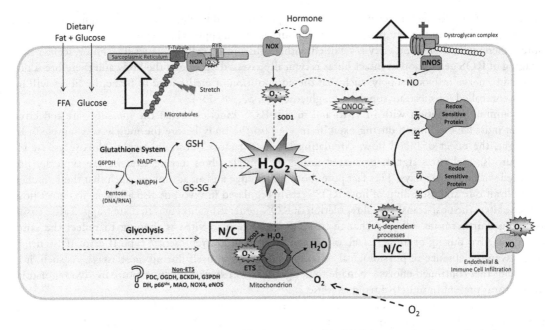

Figure 4.1 Major superoxide-producing sites and hydrogen peroxide (H_2O_2) generation in muscle during contraction

ROS production in skeletal muscle is highly regulated at specific sub-cellular locations, including the sarcolemma, cytoplasm, nucleus, and mitochondria (Figure 4.1). Most research on the regulation of ROS production in skeletal muscle has focused on NADPH oxidases (NOX) in multiple compartments and mitochondrial dehydrogenases, but some evidence supports extracellular xanthine oxidase (XO) as a source, as discussed later. Other sources remain largely unexplored during exercise, such as lipoxygenases and phospholipases (PLA), which are expressed in skeletal muscle (140, 160), although calcium-independent phospholipase A2 (iPLA2) did not alter superoxide production during isolated muscle contraction (130). As discussed in the next section, a variety of models have been used to answer these questions, such that a basic appreciation for the strengths and limitations of common experimental approaches is important for resolving discrepancies in the literature and reaching an informed conclusion on how and where exercise stimulates ROS production in muscle, as shown in Figure 4.1.

Regulation of ROS Generation in Skeletal Muscle During Exercise

Understanding Experimental Approaches: A Key Step in Framing Conclusions

Many technical challenges of measuring ROS production in skeletal muscle have been overcome in the past 30+ years, resulting in a variety of techniques that provide specific advantages and limitations (66). For example, many studies of skeletal muscle ROS during exercise used experimental assays that are performed in vitro on muscle specimens. In vitro approaches often use isolated subcellular components (e.g., isolated mitochondria or membrane fractions), permeabilized cells or tissues, or homogenate. The advantage of these experiments is that they permit the detection of kinetic rates of ROS production by allowing the controlled addition of substrates targeting specific enzymatic sources. By isolating such systems free from other physiological influences, they also create the limitation of eliminating potential regulatory factors that may be present in the blood (e.g., hormones, normal blends of glucose and fatty acid supply, etc.), the local environment (e.g., vascular-muscle crosstalk, inflammation, extracellular matrix components, etc.), or intracellular conditions such as physiological partial pressure of O_2, given most assays are performed under normobaric or hyperoxic conditions that are much higher than levels in vivo (specifically in the cytoplasm or mitochondria). In situ approaches typically assess intact muscle fibres whereby the fibre's integrity is retained without disrupting cellular structures. Fluorescent-based imaging of ROS generation in intact fibres is typically assessed outside of the body and therefore is not exposed to nerve or blood supply, such that the composition of media used to bathe the fibres will be highly controlled for substrate supply (e.g., glucose) (57, 58, 98, 130).

A common assumption with in vitro and in situ ROS kinetics is that the measures are reflective of what must have occurred during exercise in vivo (in the body before the muscle was sampled). In this light, the effect of blood flow, circulating humoral factors, substrate supply (glucose vs. fat vs. anapleurosis), and stress signals generated inside the muscle fibres during exercise are typically not captured with in vitro assays. This fact poses both a challenge and an advantage, such that their absence might limit our understanding of how ROS is truly regulated in vivo but also allow us to detect how exercise alters the post-translational regulation of ROS-generating enzymes that are trapped after tissue sampling. Furthermore, while a change in ROS generation in vitro is thought to reflect the same change in vivo during exercise, a lack of change in vitro might represent a type II error (false negative), given the absence of physiological systems or contraction itself during most assays. As such, it is important that continued efforts are made to design in vitro experiments to capture in vivo regulatory mechanisms present in muscle during exercise.

Another consideration relates to the type of fluorescent reporter used to detect ROS. Understanding the specificity of fluorescent reporter tools to target specific types of ROS and their sub-cellular locations is critical for guiding interpretations. The advantages and limitations of many probes are discussed elsewhere (15, 152), but a brief overview is provided here to help interpret key findings from the literature discussed in this chapter. For example, when using intact cells or fibres, certain fluorophores will accumulate in the cytoplasm to monitor superoxide production, as is the case with the common probe dihydroethidium (DHE) (25). This probe does not report the specific enzymatic source of superoxide. However, this can be inferred by monitoring decreases in its fluorescence when combined with specific inhibitors, as is often done to quantify NOX-derived superoxide. Mitochondrial-specific superoxide can be detected by a modified form of DHE known as "MitoSOX," which operates freely from the influence of cytoplasmic ROS when using intact cells or fibres. Alternatively, mitochondrial H_2O_2 emission can be detected with H_2O_2-specific fluorophores such as Amplex Ultrared in isolated mitochondria or permeabilized muscle fibres with the cytoplasm removed. This technique also targets mitochondria by adding mitochondrial-specific substrates (e.g., pyruvate for NADH, succinate for $FADH_2$) that avoids stimulation of non-mitochondrial sources (113). Another important limitation to these fluorescent probes is their specificity, as not all probes are specific to only a single type of ROS. For example, while DHE has very high specificity for superoxide, it also reacts somewhat with peroxynitrite ($ONOO^-$) or hydroxyl radicals (OH^-) (reviewed in [152]). Lastly, other tools include transgenic animal models where redox-sensitive proteins expressed in the compartment of interest alter their fluorescence based on the compartment's local redox state or specific types of ROS (18). A more detailed overview of methods used to detect ROS are also provided elsewhere (13, 25, 87, 126, 133, 139). The advantages and limitations of each approach should be kept in mind in the event that experimental observations might be explained by mechanisms other than the primary intention of the study, particularly in the case of fluorophores that react with multiple types of ROS (25, 152).

NADPH Oxidases vs. Mitochondria: What Is the Major Source During Exercise?

Historically, mitochondria were thought to be the major source of ROS during exercise in part because superoxide and downstream H_2O_2 emission are by-products of oxidative phosphorylation and because mitochondria are a major site of oxidant generation in cells in general. This idea followed the first report of free radical generation detected in muscle homogenate and intact muscle sampled immediately after exercise in rodents using electron paramagnetic resonance (21). As this technique detects a mixture of free radicals (e.g., superoxide, hydroxyl radicals and lipid radicals) located throughout the cell, this land-mark discovery inspired new directions of research that have examined the major types and sources of ROS formed during exercise.

The collective evidence since that discovery suggests that mitochondria are not the major source of ROS during exercise. This perspective is based on the following lines of evidence:

Mitochondrial ROS is lowered when oxidative phosphorylation increases: Fundamental principles of mito-chondrial bioenergetics predict that exercise should not increase mitochondrial ROS. Superoxide generation within the electron transport system (e.g., complex I and III) are governed by membrane potential (104) prior to its dismutation to H_2O_2. As reducing equivalents (NADH, $FADH_2$) supply electrons to the electron transport system, protons are pumped from the matrix to the inner mem-brane space. This process is interdependent, such that proton pumping cannot occur without electron flux to oxygen at complex IV, and electron flux cannot occur without proton pumping. Continual provision of reducing equivalents increases membrane potential across the inner membrane due to proton pumping, thereby creating a gradient that would theoretically slow further proton pumping, attenuate electron flux, and cause electron slip prematurely onto oxygen at complexes I and III (104). In the context of exercise, these principles predict that increases in free adenosine diphos-phate (ADP) and inorganic phosphate (Pi) from adenosine triphosphate (ATP) utilization during contraction will stimulate a re-entry of protons through ATP synthase to regenerate ATP, thereby lowering membrane potential, increasing electron flux, and lowering the rate of electron slip and superoxide generation. As such, the balance between the supply of electrons (NADH and $FADH_2$ from substrate catabolism) and "energy demand" (free ADP, Pi) determines superoxide generation and downstream H_2O_2 emission following its dismutation by superoxide dismutase. Indeed, ADP and Pi are routinely added to attenuate mitochondrial H_2O_2 emission during in vitro assays (44, 104), which models the increased energy demand of exercising muscle. Collectively, these principles and in vitro experimental evidence predict that the increased metabolic demand of contracting muscle will lower mitochondrial H_2O_2 emission. For visual demonstrations of the governance of ROS gen-eration by the electron transport system, the reader is referred to *Bioenergetics* by David Nicholls and *The Bioenergetics of Exercise* by P. Darrell Neufer (102, 104).

These principles focus on governance of superoxide production at the electron transport system by membrane potential (12, 44, 153). However, it is now known that other dehydrogenases such as the pyruvate dehydrogenase complex (31), certain enzymes in the tricarboxylic acid cycle (12, 44, 90), and branched-chain amino acid catabolic pathways (39, 120) are also sources of superoxide that dismutate to H_2O_2. Mitochondria also include NOX (NOX-4), several dehydrogenases, monoamine oxidases and other sources of superoxide that dismutate to H_2O_2 through superoxide dismutase (SOD), as well as endothelial nitric oxide synthase (eNOS) that generates nitric oxide (NO) (61, 77, 130). While these sources are expressed in muscle (Figure 4.1), the effect of exercise on these ROS-generating pathways remains to be fully characterized. Likewise, the effect of repetitious rest–exercise transitions, which may oscillate O_2 delivery and substrate supply, as occurs during interval-based exercise, has not been investigated nor has the relative effect of altering substrate availability during exercise, such as manipu-lating glucose to fat oxidation or transitions to fat oxidation during prolonged exercise. For example, a positive relationship was found between plasma free fatty acids and skeletal muscle mitochondrial H_2O_2 emission in humans after ultra-endurance exercise (129), suggesting that the increased H_2O_2 that occurs during fat oxidation might be an important factor in determining the mitochondrial ROS response to exercise (2, 129). Potential roles of hypoxia during exercise might also be considered in future research. For example, succinate accumulates in cardiac muscle following ischaemia, which increases electron provision ($FADH_2$) and superoxide generation in the electron transport system (ETS) (19), but whether this occurs in skeletal muscle during hypoxia remains to be determined. Most experimental approaches to date assess mitochondrial ROS generation in vitro (isolated mitochondria, permeabilized muscle fibres) or in situ (isolated intact muscle fibres) under conditions of normal oxygen levels (normobaric) or hyperoxia, such that the potential influences of hypoxia during the exercise bout before the sample was collected may no longer be captured by the assays. While future directions might consider new approaches that capture these and other potential stressors of exercise, the experimental evidence to date, as described next, does not support the idea that exercise increases mitochondrial ROS, which is in support of the principles described earlier.

Limited evidence of increased mitochondrial ROS during contraction: Some of the key studies that argued against mitochondria being a source of ROS used a redox sensitive mito-roGFP fluorescent protein to determine the effects of single-fibre contraction on mitochondrial redox potential (108). Changes in fluorescence of this protein reflect a change in either mitochondrial ROS generation or redox buffering activity. Following 15 minutes of contractions of mouse muscle fibres in situ, no changes in fluorescence were observed, suggesting contraction did not alter the fluorescence of this reporter protein (98). This same method was used following 20 minutes of moderate-intensity treadmill exercise, whereby no increase in mito-roGFP fluorescence was observed in mouse skeletal muscle (57). Similar conclusions were made by inhibiting superoxide-release channels on mitochondria while monitoring fluorescence of a superoxide-sensitive fluorophore loaded in the cytoplasm of mouse single muscle fibres (130). These inhibitors had no effect on cytoplasmic superoxide responses to contraction, indicating that mitochondrial superoxide release was not affected by contraction. However, mitochondrial superoxide can also be dismutated to membrane-permeable H_2O_2 that diffuses into the cytoplasm and is thought to do so at a very high rate independent of the exporting superoxide itself. As such, mitochondrial H_2O_2 emission is not monitored with this approach, although it is possible that a lack of change in superoxide export means it is also unlikely that there was an increase in superoxide sufficient to accelerate H_2O_2 emission. Overall, the results are consistent with the lack of change in mitochondrial redox potential (mito-roGFP fluorescence) after single-fibre contraction and suggests that mitochondrial ROS is not elevated after exercise.

In a similar light, emerging evidence suggests that mitochondrial ROS do not contribute to muscle adaptation to chronic exercise. The mitochondrial-targeted antioxidant MitoQ was ingested during 3 weeks of exercise training (3–5 days/week, 45 min stationary cycling at 50--65% VO_2 max) in young healthy adults (134). MitoQ did not alter the improvements of whole-body or leg VO_2 max after training, nor did it alter estimated mitochondrial oxidative capacity as measured indirectly with near-infrared spectroscopy in vivo. While skeletal muscle mitochondrial ROS was not measured directly, the results suggest that mitochondrial superoxide may not have been elevated during the exercise training sessions, given MitoQ prevents increases in mitochondrial superoxide, at least in diseases (36, 96, 127), and has high reactivity with superoxide relative to other free radicals (73, 93, 96). MitoQ specifically prevents superoxide from oxidizing mitochondrial membranes which could otherwise alter mitochondrial bioenergetics and indirectly change how mitochondria respond to exercise and contribute to stress signals mediating chronic adaptation. As such, these data suggest indirectly that chronic exercise training does not increase mitochondrial superoxide, or at least not to a sufficient level that might stimulate improvements in aerobic fitness.

Similar findings have been found in the heart after exercise training. Rodents that engaged in exercise training experienced less cardiac necrosis following experimental induction of myocardial infarction (14). This cardioprotective effect of exercise was not prevented by daily administration of the mitochondrial cardiolipin-targeted compound Bendavia, which prevents increases in mitochondrial ROS. This result suggests that cardiac mitochondrial ROS is not increased during exercise training, or at least that mitochondrial ROS does not mediate the cardioprotective effects of exercise. In contrast, NOX inhibition with apocynin or Vas2870, which inhibits multiple NOX isoforms (4), prevented the cardioprotective effect of exercise such that necrosis was similar to controls after a myocardial infarction. These results add to the lines of evidence outlined earlier that exercise may not increase mitochondrial ROS to a level sufficient to trigger adaptation, whereas NOX may be a more predominant source, as discussed later.

There is some evidence that mitochondrial H_2O_2 emission is elevated post-exercise when measured in isolated mitochondria or permeabilized muscle fibres (129, 145). Complex I–supported ROS (but not complex III) was increased after extreme ultra-endurance exercise in human muscle (129) that returned to normal 28 hours after exercise. In contrast, another study did not see an increase in H_2O_2 emission immediately after exercise of moderate-, high-, or sprint-intensity exercise but did report an increase 3 hours into recovery. A study using a mitochondrial-specific reporter dye in single fibres in mice found that exercise increased mitochondrial oxidative stress from 3 to 12 hours after exercise (80). It is challenging to reconcile these findings with the studies that showed no change in mitochondrial redox state (57, 98) or superoxide release (130) in single contracting fibres sampled immediately after exercise, as discussed earlier. One possibility is that these differences may be due to the timepoint of assessments, given two out of the three studies noted earlier observed an increase in mitochondrial ROS/oxidation state several hours after exercise. Indeed, repeated bouts of *in situ* contraction in single fibres also caused a slow and modest increase in mitochondrial superoxide in recovery (112).

It is also possible that the differences in observations are partially explained by the methodologies used in both cases. For example, targeting specific pathways to stimulate ROS production in vitro is typically performed with excess substrates that generate saturating concentrations of NADH and $FADH_2$, thereby maximizing electron flux into the electron transport system. These results demonstrate the *capacity* for ROS emission is altered by exercise, but the actual rates during contraction may be different under a blend of concentrations of various substrates that are far less than those used in experiments. As such, exercise may alter the *potential* to produce ROS in mitochondria, but this may not necessarily occur under all conditions during contraction. Nonetheless, these in vitro approaches offer the advantage of directly determining the capacity for ROS emission from specific pathways that is otherwise difficult to perform in intact tissue. Furthermore, using intact single fibres has the advantage of assessing mitochondrial redox markers during or immediately after in situ contraction. As described earlier, the evidence provided by this intact model suggests that mitochondrial ROS does not increase with contraction, regardless of its altered potential capacity.

NOX-derived superoxide is elevated following contraction and exercise: NOXs are highly abundant, exist in multiple isoforms, and are tightly coupled to specific cell functions regulated by redox signalling. For example, sarcolemmal-bound NOXs are thought to be activated by extracellular hormonal ligands (33, 40, 41, 89, 114, 121). NOX bound to the sarcoplasmic reticulum and t-tubules are also thought to contribute to exercise-induced ROS, given they are activated in response to muscle fibre stretch or contraction (74, 119). Intriguingly, microtubule-bound NOX are activated under mechanical stretch, suggesting that contraction may increase NOX activity through mechanotransduction (74, 119). NOX are also expressed in other cellular compartments, including mitochondria and nuclei (45, 47, 130, 136, 142), but their potential responses to exercise are unknown.

Multiple lines of evidence indicate that NOX are important sources of superoxide and potential regulators of cellular changes during exercise. In general, these studies monitored cellular or muscle function responses to NOX inhibition and serve as a foundation for future research to identify specific redox signalling targets, as discussed in later sections. For example, NOX inhibition with apocynin attenuated exercise activation of the stress signalling pathway and inflammatory responses to 60 min of swimming in rats (56). As discussed earlier, NOX inhibition prevented the cardioprotective benefits of exercise training, which indicates that myocardial NOX are activated by exercise (14). Likewise, deletion of NOX-4 (48) attenuated the activation of Nrf2—a transcription factor that activates genes encoding antioxidants that are normally triggered by exercise. In situ mouse skeletal muscle single-fibre contractions generated less cytoplasmic superoxide when NOX was inhibited with diphenyleneiodonium, which inhibits all NOX isoforms (98). However, later work found that this inhibitor also lowers force production during muscle contraction, which could limit the ability to test contraction-induced NOX activation at controlled force levels (130). Instead, other inhibitors, including apocynin, were later used successfully to prevent contraction-induced superoxide production without appreciable changes in force production compared to control (130). Collectively, these experiments with inhibitors of varying specificities indicate that contraction increases NOX-derived superoxide production. This is supported by a separate study that tracked the time course of cytosolic superoxide generation over 1 hour of repeated bouts of contraction in single fibres. In this study, cytosolic DHE fluorescence increased during contraction but returned to baseline in the periods of rest (112), which demonstrates the acute nature of cytosolic ROS responses that are most likely NOX dependent.

The development of a mouse model engineered to express a redox-sensitive green fluorescence protein linked to a subunit of NOX-2 made it possible to directly detect superoxide production from this source. As NOX-2 is expressed primarily on t-tubules near the sarcoplasmic reticulum junction (59, 119, 131), this model allows isolation of superoxide production from this specific sub-cellular location. Using this model, electrical stimulation of single muscle fibres showed increased fluorescence, which reflected greater activity of NOX-2. Using this same redox sensor, it was shown that treadmill exercise increases NOX-2 fluorescence in fibres sampled from mouse tibialis anterior (57). This same study demonstrated that exercise-induced muscle glucose uptake was impaired when NOX-2 was deleted from skeletal muscle, thereby showing one functional relevance of this source of ROS for muscle function during exercise. A similar study in NOX-2–deficient mice showed that muscle metabolic protein responses and maximal running capacity improvements were attenuated (58).

Collectively, the use of redox-sensitive chemical and protein fluorescent detectors have consistently demonstrated that muscle contraction or exercise stimulates ROS production from NOX. This work lays the foundation for examining their role in regulating specific muscle functions during exercise, the manner by which exercise activates NOX activity, and the mechanisms of how ROS signals through protein-based redox circuits to alter these functions. One intriguing possibility is that exercise may activate NOX-2 through mechanotransduction, given that mechanical stretch transduced through microtubules increases NOX-2 activity in the heart and is required for activating calcium release through ryanodine receptor activation (119) (Figure 4.1). The link between exercise, NOX-2, calcium-regulating proteins, and muscle function/adaptations remains to be investigated but may be one example by which ROS signalling mediates changes in various muscle functions in response to exercise.

Other Sources and Approaches of Targeting ROS in Muscle During Exercise

Xanthine oxidase (XO): XO is active in muscle endothelial cells and leucocytes (46, 54, 141). XO regulates catabolism of hypoxanthine to xanthine and xanthine to uric acid, with superoxide being produced in both cases. Hypoxanthine is a product of adenine nucleotide degradation, such that decreases in ATP during intense exercise have been linked to hypoxanthine release from muscle during and more so after intense exercise (52, 53, 55). This greater release suggests that exercise increases flux through XO, which might implicate this enzyme as a unique source of superoxide during exercise. However, there is limited direct evidence of XO-derived ROS in muscle to support this notion. One report suggested that inhibition of XO with allopurinol prevented plasma markers of muscle damage (creatine kinase, aspartate aminotransferase) in four Tour de France cyclists compared to five control cyclists (42). Given circulating creatine kinase (CK) is a marker of muscle damage, this finding suggests that muscle XO might contribute to exhaustive exercise-induced damage. This is supported by reductions in circulating CK in mice with allopurinol during exhaustive exercise along with faster restoration of glutathione (GSH) post-exercise, which indirectly suggests attenuated ROS production in muscle (26). However, no direct measures of muscle XO activity were reported.

In contrast, 60 minutes of high-intensity treadmill exercise (2 7m/min, 5% incline) in rodents did not increase maximal XO activity measured in vitro, nor did allopurinol affect this activity or prevent exercise-induced increases in oxidized glutathione (GS-SG)—a marker of ROS production (149). While this exercise intensity is considered to be high, ATP levels were not reported, and it is not clear if hypoxanthine or xanthine was released from muscle as an index of in vivo XO flux, although mixed venous xanthine did not increase. Nevertheless, certain signalling cascades that are known to be redox sensitive were inhibited by allopurinol, although muscle adaptation at the level of mitochondrial biogenesis was unaffected. This finding questions the importance of XO in mediating redox-dependent adaptations to exercise.

It is possible that XO has a more pronounced contribution to ROS production during contraction in aged muscle. Several days of in vivo plantar flexor contraction in rodents increased muscle XO activity and xanthine content in young and more so in aged gastrocnemius, all of which were prevented by allopurinol (128). Likewise, electron paramagnetic resonance was used to detect free radical production, which includes superoxide, albeit without delineating from other free radicals, and found a slight increase following repeated contractions in young muscle with a much larger increase in aged muscle. Allopurinol prevented these increases, which is perhaps the most direct evidence that contraction increases XO-derived superoxide in muscle, with even greater increases in aged muscle. Maximal force production was also increased by allopurinol but only in the aged muscle, as there was no effect in young muscle. Allopurinol also rescues muscle force production in mouse models of Duchenne muscular dystrophy (84), disuse atrophy (23), and possibly other myopathies (132), suggesting muscle dysfunctions are more prone to XO-derived superoxide similar to this study in aged muscle. It is also noteworthy that lifelong athletes have less circulating hypoxanthine and xanthine than untrained individuals (159), suggesting that regular exercise may actually attenuate XO activity, but extrapolating to an attenuation of XO-derived superoxide is speculative without direct measures. Overall, the evidence suggests that exercise may activate XO if sufficient muscle damage occurs or if muscle dysfunction is present, with little activity occurring at lighter intensities in healthy muscle.

In support of the possibility that XO is activated with damaging exercise protocols, an early pioneering study by Hellsten et al. (54) demonstrated increased XO in human skeletal muscle 1 to 4 days post-eccentric exercise. However, increases in XO content following exercise were restricted to endothelial cells and leucocytes in association with inflammation but not within the myofibres themselves. This is consistent with prior evidence that XO is present in rat myocardium but specifically in interstitial, capillary, and intriguingly, vascular smooth muscle cells (3), as well as pulmonary artery endothelial cells whereby neutrophils can activate XO (150). This evidence supports a role of XO-derived superoxide post-exercise and through an inflammatory link to muscle damage, at least in young healthy muscle, but the effect of aging or myopathies may alter this relationship. While it has been proposed that XO-derived superoxide may be damaging to skeletal muscle, given allopurinol prevents increases in circulating CK and other markers of muscle damage (147), it is well recognized that inflammation is critical for muscle repair in recovery (111). As such, it may be that XO-derived superoxide is an important signal in facilitating immune-mediated clearance of damaged muscle tissue and subsequent repair, consistent with emerging concerns that allopurinol may interfere with adaptations to exercise (132).

Vitamins and ROS: While other studies have used a variety of antioxidants to determine the effect of ROS on mediating muscle adaptation to exercise, these approaches generally did not consider specific targets of ROS per se. For example, vitamins E and C were shown to prevent training-induced increases in mitochondrial biogenesis in rat muscle (60), although this is not consistently reported (43). However, a study in humans demonstrated that both vitamins suppressed muscle adaptations to endurance training (125). With regard to strength training, a recent review noted that there is insufficient literature to make a firm conclusion (30), but most evidence to date suggests that vitamins do not impair adaptations (10, 11, 29, 110), although a detriment was found after strength training in the elderly (8).

Resolving the different findings in the literature might be possible if the mechanism of the vitamins' antioxidant activities is considered in future studies. For example, vitamin E lowers lipid peroxides and prevents oxidation of long-chain polyunsaturated fatty acids in membranes throughout the cell, thereby preserving membrane fluidity and structure (144). Based on this mechanism, vitamin E's potential effects on mediating adaptation to exercise might be linked directly or indirectly to lipid peroxide signalling or membrane instability, neither of which is fully understood with respect to mediating muscle adaptation to exercise. Vitamin C also protects against lipid peroxidation in concert with vitamin E and has some reactivity with other free radicals such as superoxide and peroxynitrite (79, 95, 105, 144). Vitamin C may also protect endothelial cells by preserving NO production in certain conditions (95). Whether these effects occur in healthy people supplemented with vitamins during exercise is unclear. Nevertheless, with such varied potential mechanisms of action (27, 95), it is difficult to interpret the literature regarding vitamin E and C's divergent effects on muscle adaptation to exercise with regard to the type and source of ROS being targeted during exercise. While most evidence indicates that vitamins do not enhance exercise training adaptations, their impact as experimental tools to understand how ROS mediate adaptation through redox signalling is somewhat limited until their mechanisms of action are considered in future investigations, which might differ in specific populations such as the elderly (8).

The Effects of Exercise on Redox Buffering

The regulation of the redox proteome is largely mediated by enzymatic systems centring around GSH and Trx (37, 38, 70, 88). Both redox buffers are present in multiple cellular compartments, including the cytoplasm, mitochondria, and nucleus. While each compartment expresses different isoforms of the major protein regulators, the general schematic for their regulation are shown in Figure 4.2, although additional regulatory components can be considered (22). Moreover, each system exists in sub-cellular compartments (e.g., cytoplasm, nucleus, mitochondria) through expression of different isoforms. Briefly, both GSH and Trx buffer H_2O_2 through GSH peroxidase and peroxiredoxins, respectively. As GSH and Trx become oxidized through this process (forming GS-SG or oxidized Trx), they themselves become "recycled" by reduction through GSH reductase (GR) and Trx reductase (TrxR), respectively. NADPH is the master reducing power of the cell through its role in providing the electrons necessary for these reductases to reduce GSH and Trx. Of interest, glucose is a major source of NADPH through the pentose phosphate pathway, although NADPH is also generated from isocitrate dehydrogenase in

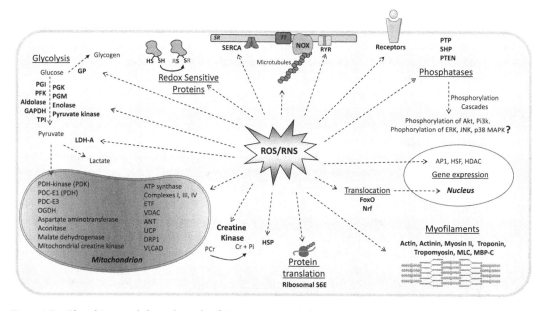

Figure 4.2   Glutathione and thioredoxin buffering systems and their response to exercise training

the tricarboxylic acid (TCA) cycle and other sources. Furthermore, the redox state of redox-sensitive proteins can be regulated by both systems through glutaredoxins (Grx) coupled to GSH or directly by Trx themselves, as appears to be the case with certain transcription factors and apoptosis-regulating proteins (62, 72, 85). Trx can also "recycle" the redox state of peroxiredoxins (Prx), which directly scavenge H_2O_2. Trx itself can be inhibited by Trx interacting protein (TXNIP) (88). As reviewed by Lu and Holmgren, crosstalk between the GSH and Trx systems also occurs, whereby Trx can reduce oxidized GSH, and GSH with Grx can reduce oxidized Trx, as well as other examples (88). The list of potential redox-sensitive proteins subject to regulation by these redox couples is growing but remains largely unexplored in the context of muscle responses to exercise (see Figure 4.3 for potential research directions, as discussed later).

Some studies have examined the effects of exercise on the expression or activity of certain components in the GSH and Trx redox buffering systems. First, it should be noted that blood-based measures of antioxidant responses to exercise may not reflect the same pathways in muscle but may be involved in inflammatory responses, given the role of ROS in regulating immune cell function. In addition, it should be considered that redox regulators such as Trx can be released as chemotactic signals to recruit immune responses (7). Still, more evidence is required to link such blood-based responses to muscle adaptation to exercise.

With respect to muscle-specific responses in redox buffering systems, it is generally regarded that exercise increases antioxidant buffering capacity, including GSH content and glutathione peroxidase (GPx) activities, through redox stress signals, as reviewed in detail elsewhere (115–117). However, total GSH does not always change after training despite changes in glutathione reductase (GR) activity or content, as discussed later (32, 34). This might suggest that assessments of GSH content and GSH/GS-SG ratios measured post-exercise may not reflect their altered regulation during exercise, which is

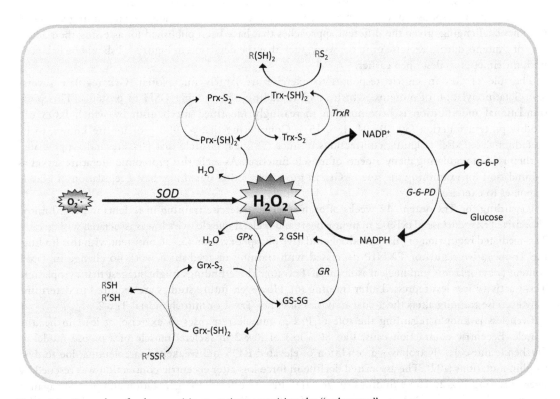

Figure 4.3 Examples of redox-sensitive proteins comprising the "redoxome"

expected to be improved following training. For now, monitoring GSH/GS-SG responses in real time during exercise in vivo are not possible with current techniques.

More recent studies have demonstrated alterations in additional components of these redox buffering systems, as shown in Figure 4.2. For example, an intriguing study demonstrated that acute exercise (assessed immediately after 10 days of training) increases GR activity in mouse heart, which is mediated by NOX-dependent ROS activation (34), thereby demonstrating a redox-signalling mechanism by which exercise activates the glutathione couple (GSH and GS-SG). This activation was associated with decreased ratios of GSH/GS-SG consistent with ROS production by NOX during exercise. Collectively, these observations support the notion of a feedback loop between NOX-derived ROS activating GR to counteract the decline in GSH/GS-SG during exercise, which is an important example of a potential role of ROS signalling in regulating a critical cell parameter—in this case, glutathione homeostasis. Contrary to acute exercise resulting in increased GR activity, another study showed that GR activity decreases in rat heart but not skeletal muscle 15 hours after the last session of 12 weeks of high-intensity exercise training (32). The reason for decreased GR activity after this longer-term training protocol is not clear but might suggest that trained muscle generates less ROS (less activation of GR) during exercise, or at least in recovery from exercise when it was measured, or other redox buffers become more active in trained muscle, as is the case with greater activity of the thioredoxin system, as noted later (32). Future studies could compare how exercise training alters the degree of NOX-derived ROS production in comparison to the activity of the GSH redox buffer (and indeed Trx, as discussed later) to understand how the system interacts in specific sub-cellular compartments to regulate redox homeostasis during exercise, and of course link such ROS-buffering cycles to redox-sensitive proteins that regulate specific cell functions. Based on the available literature, one possible model could be that ROS generated during acute exercise activates GR, presumably to maintain GSH/GS-SG, whereas chronic training may have more dynamic effects on the regulation of GSH-mediated redox buffering by increasing GSH and GPx activities, as noted earlier, or sharing the load with a more enhanced Trx system (115). Lastly, summarizing the responses of each redox buffer component to exercise (long-term training vs. acute) becomes challenging, given the different approaches that have been published for assessing their activities or contents during exercise or in recovery, such that the depiction in Figure 4.2 should be balanced with the timepoints described earlier.

The role of Grx in muscle responses to exercise are largely unexplored. Grx regulate reversible glutathionylation of proteins, which involves adding or removing GSH to proteins. This post-translational modification is becoming an increasingly identified mechanism by which ROS can modify protein function (50, 91, 94, 156, 157). Considering that >2,000 proteins are known to be glutathionylated after fatiguing contractions in mice (78), it is possible that Grx are underappreciated in their role in regulating many aspects of muscle function. As such, this proteomic literature serves as a foundation for examining the role of Grx in mediating redox signalling–based regulation of muscle responses to exercise.

Regarding the Trx system, 12 weeks of high-intensity exercise training in rodents increased mitochondrial Trx reductase (TrxR)-2 in mouse heart and skeletal muscle, which was associated with greater Trx-mediated regulation of mitochondrial oxidative phosphorylation (32). Consistent with this finding, the Tr- negative regulator TXNIP decreased with training in aged mice, with no change in Trx-1 content (a cytoplasmic and nuclear isoform of Trx) (6). These findings might suggest that cytoplasmic Trx-1 activity was less repressed after training (6). However, future studies are required to determine how exercise training alters the actual activities of either Trx-1 or mitochondrial Trx-2.

Even less is known regarding the role of Prx in muscle responses to exercise, at least in healthy muscle. Eccentric contraction caused an 80% loss of Prx-2 in skeletal muscle of a mouse model of Duchenne muscular dystrophy—a condition of elevated ROS and weakened sarcolemma due to dystrophin mutations (107). The associated decline in force loss after eccentric contraction was rescued by overexpressing Prx-2. These findings suggest that Prx-2 buffers ROS generation and protects against muscle weakness, at least in this disease model. The loss of Prx-2 during eccentric contraction is similar to the loss seen in contracting C2C12 myotubes (92) and may be related to dimerization of this protein following reaction with H_2O_2 (148). Given Prx can activate inflammation by binding to toll-like receptors (TLRs) on immune cells (124), these observations of peroxiredoxin release from damaged muscle raises the intriguing possibility that ROS generated during contraction can signal inflammation-mediated muscle repair by oxidizing peroxiredoxins that are then exported to the extracellular compartment, as suggested previously (148). This proposal represents a potentially fruitful area for future research to understand the role of Prx in muscle responses to exercise, as well as in the context of how Trx regulate their redox state (Figure 4.2).

Lastly, integrating glucose flux to NADPH generation (Figure 4.2) linked to reductase activities for both GSH and Trx redox couples remains a virtually untapped area of research. Such directions would likely give new perspectives on how glucose metabolism is linked to the maintenance of redox conditions across the redoxome and membranes during exercise, and may give new insight into how altered metabolism contributes to fatigue, recovery, or regeneration after damaging exercise. In general, measures of the pentose phosphate pathway in muscle focus on intermediate metabolite concentrations as an index of activity of this pathway, but concentrations do not always reflect flux. As such, flux assessments with radioactive tracers would likely be required, as has been performed cell culture, or in isolated mouse livers (100), but it appears that no such attempt has been performed in muscle specimens.

The Future: Mapping Precise Redox Signalling Networks That Regulate Acute and Chronic Responses to Exercise in Muscle

As noted at the beginning of the chapter, ROS and RNS/RONS are likely primary regulators of multiple cell functions within skeletal muscle in response to exercise (17, 66, 68, 81, 114, 118). Many proteins have been identified as redox-sensitive (1, 13, 20, 33, 35, 49, 51, 68, 76, 82, 83, 86, 97, 99, 109, 137, 138, 146, 151, 155, 158) across categories that include metabolism, gene expression, ion homeostasis, stress signalling, receptor-linked signalling, cytoskeletal, and protein translation (Figure 4.3). However, the vast majority of these proteins have not been investigated for their potential roles in redox signalling during exercise. Rather, indirect indices of ROS signalling have generally been measured, such as phosphorylation of "ROS-sensitive" signalling cascades, such that future investigations can now map such networks. Likewise, a common approach has been to study the effects of antioxidants on signalling, metabolic, and transcriptional responses to exercise. In many cases, the antioxidants alter muscle responses to exercise, but the precise protein-oxidation signalling mechanisms are typically not identified. With the advancement of numerous redox proteomics techniques in recent years (35, 64, 65, 137, 143, 154), there are many examples of redox-sensitive proteins, listed in Figure 4.3, that might serve as regulators of muscle function through redox signalling. To date, there is an incomplete foundation of knowledge on how ROS alters the activity of these proteins. In other words, the growing identification of redox-sensitive proteins alone does not prove that they are regulated by ROS/RNS. Once this basic knowledge is available, the field of exercise physiology could map such redox-dependent pathways by comparing their redox states with redox proteomics to their activities. Such combined approaches would unravel the role of the "redoxome" to understanding how muscle function is truly regulated by ROS and RNS during and after exercise.

Perspectives and Concluding Remarks

Since it was first identified that exercise increases skeletal muscle free radicals (21), major challenges emerged in the ability to identify the precise source and type of ROS. It now appears that NOX are activated by exercise, with XO activated in recovery from high-intensity exercise. Their precise roles in regulating muscle responses to exercise so far include calcium regulation by SERCA and RYR (74, 119), with other functions, such as glucose uptake (57) and associations with muscle recovery (54), being identified but not yet mapped through redox signalling. Mitochondrial ROS is not activated during single-fibre contraction, but the response during exercise or recovery in vivo under conditions of altered oxygen and substrate availability could be further investigated.

The role of ROS in mediating adaptation to chronic exercise has also received much attention. ROS-sensitive pathways were shown to be activated in response to exercise to mediate chronic adaptations, including mitochondrial biogenesis and increased antioxidant production. However, little is known regarding the precise oxidative modifications that occur on proposed transcriptional regulators or upstream redox-signalling cascades. With the array of redox proteomic detection methods available, it is possible to expand the field by exploring how GSH- and Trx-based systems regulate redox state on specific proteins that control gene expression during adaptation to exercise training. Similarly, the precise mechanisms by which ROS/RNS regulate proteins controlling metabolic and other homeostatic mechanisms during acute exercise could also be explored, as has been done with SERCA and RYR, mentioned earlier. The role of membrane oxidation in signalling stress responses during exercise also remains virtually unexplored with direct measures of redox signalling.

Applying concepts of redox biology to understanding muscle responses to exercise will likely require careful consideration of location, type, and timing of ROS generation within muscle during and following contraction. From a translational perspective, current guidelines of taking or avoiding "antioxidants" could be refined in the future by considering the specific mechanism of action of various supplements. As noted earlier, viewing ROS as signals within a grander redox-regulatory network (Figures 4.1–4.3) provides an exciting framework for new lines of inquiry that could greatly improve our understanding of how redox switches regulate muscle function and adaptation in response to acute and chronic exercise.

References

1. Ahn SG, Thiele DJ. Redox regulation of mammalian heat shock factor 1 is essential for Hsp gene activation and protection from stress. *Genes Dev* 17: 516–528, 2003.
2. Anderson EJ, Lustig ME, Boyle KE, Woodlief TL, Kane DA, Lin CT, et al. Mitochondrial H2O2 emission and cellular redox state link excess fat intake to insulin resistance in both rodents and humans. *J Clin Invest* 119: 573–581, 2009.
3. Ashraf M, Samra ZQ. Subcellular distribution of xanthine oxidase during cardiac ischemia and reperfusion: an immunocytochemical study. *J Submicrosc Cytol Pathol* 25: 193–201, 1993.
4. Augsburger F, Filippova A, Rasti D, Seredenina T, Lam M, Maghzal G, et al. Pharmacological characterization of the seven human NOX isoforms and their inhibitors. *Redox Biol* 26: 101272, 2019.
5. Barclay JK, Hansel M. Free radicals may contribute to oxidative skeletal muscle fatigue. *Can J Physiol Pharmacol* 69: 279–284, 1991.
6. Belaya I, Suwa M, Chen T, Giniatullin R, Kanninen KM, Atalay M, Kumagai S. Long-term exercise protects against cellular stresses in aged mice. *Oxid Med Cell Longev* 2018: 2894247, 2018.
7. Bertini R, Howard OM, Dong HF, Oppenheim JJ, Bizzarri C, Sergi R, et al. Thioredoxin, a redox enzyme released in infection and inflammation, is a unique chemoattractant for neutrophils, monocytes, and T cells. *J Exp Med* 189: 1783–1789, 1999.
8. Bjornsen T, Salvesen S, Berntsen S, Hetlelid KJ, Stea TH, Lohne-Seiler H, et al. Vitamin C and E supplementation blunts increases in total lean body mass in elderly men after strength training. *Scand J Med Sci Sports* 26: 755–763, 2016.
9. Bloomer RJ, Cole B, Fisher-Wellman KH. Racial differences in postprandial oxidative stress with and without acute exercise. *Int J Sport Nutr Exerc Metab* 19: 457–472, 2009.
10. Bobeuf F, Labonte M, Dionne IJ, Khalil A. Combined effect of antioxidant supplementation and resistance training on oxidative stress markers, muscle and body composition in an elderly population. *J Nutr Health Aging* 15: 883–889, 2011.
11. Bobeuf F, Labonte M, Khalil A, Dionne IJ. Effects of resistance training combined with antioxidant supplementation on fat-free mass and insulin sensitivity in healthy elderly subjects. *Diabetes Res Clin Pract* 87: e1–3, 2010.
12. Brand MD. The sites and topology of mitochondrial superoxide production. *Exp Gerontol* 45: 466–472, 2010.

13. Brewer TF, Garcia FJ, Onak CS, Carroll KS, Chang CJ. Chemical approaches to discovery and study of sources and targets of hydrogen peroxide redox signaling through NADPH oxidase proteins. *Annu Rev Biochem* 84: 765–790, 2015.
14. Brown DA, Hale SL, Baines CP, del Rio CL, Hamlin RL, Yueyama Y, et al. Reduction of early reperfusion injury with the mitochondria-targeting peptide bendavia. *J Cardiovasc Pharmacol Ther* 19: 121–132, 2014.
15. Chen J, Mathews CE. Use of chemical probes to detect mitochondrial ROS by flow cytometry and spectrofluorometry. *Methods Enzymol* 542: 223–241, 2014.
16. Cheng AJ, Jude B, Lanner JT. Intramuscular mechanisms of overtraining. *Redox Biol* 101480, 2020.
17. Cheng AJ, Yamada T, Rassier DE, Andersson DC, Westerblad H, Lanner JT. Reactive oxygen/nitrogen species and contractile function in skeletal muscle during fatigue and recovery. *J Physiol* 594: 5149–5160, 2016.
18. Chiu WK, Towheed A, Palladino MJ. Genetically encoded redox sensors. *Methods Enzymol* 542: 263–287, 2014.
19. Chouchani ET, Pell VR, Gaude E, Aksentijevic D, Sundier SY, Robb EL, et al. Ischaemic accumulation of succinate controls reperfusion injury through mitochondrial ROS. *Nature* 515: 431–435, 2014.
20. Dansen TB, Smits LM, van Triest MH, de Keizer PL, van Leenen D, Koerkamp MG, et al. Redox-sensitive cysteines bridge p300/CBP-mediated acetylation and FoxO4 activity. *Nat Chem Biol* 5: 664–672, 2009.
21. Davies KJ, Quintanilha AT, Brooks GA, Packer L. Free radicals and tissue damage produced by exercise. *Biochem Biophys Res Commun* 107: 1198–1205, 1982.
22. DeBalsi KL, Wong KE, Koves TR, Slentz DH, Seiler SE, Wittmann AH, et al. Targeted metabolomics connects thioredoxin-interacting protein (TXNIP) to mitochondrial fuel selection and regulation of specific oxidoreductase enzymes in skeletal muscle. *J Biol Chem* 289: 8106–8120, 2014.
23. Derbre F, Ferrando B, Gomez-Cabrera MC, Sanchis-Gomar F, Martinez-Bello VE, Olaso-Gonzalez G, et al. Inhibition of xanthine oxidase by allopurinol prevents skeletal muscle atrophy: role of p38 MAPKinase and E3 ubiquitin ligases. *PLOS ONE* 7: e46668, 2012.
24. Diaz PT, Brownstein E, Clanton TL. Effects of N-acetylcysteine on in vitro diaphragm function are temperature dependent. *J Appl Physiol (1985)* 77: 2434–2439, 1994.
25. Dikalov SI, Harrison DG. Methods for detection of mitochondrial and cellular reactive oxygen species. *Antioxid Redox Signal* 20: 372–382, 2014.
26. Duarte JA, Appell HJ, Carvalho F, Bastos ML, Soares JM. Endothelium-derived oxidative stress may contribute to exercise-induced muscle damage. *Int J Sports Med* 14: 440–443, 1993.
27. Duarte TL, Lunec J. Review: When is an antioxidant not an antioxidant? A review of novel actions and reactions of vitamin C. *Free Radic Res* 39: 671–686, 2005.
28. Dutka TL, Mollica JP, Lamb GD. Differential effects of peroxynitrite on contractile protein properties in fast- and slow-twitch skeletal muscle fibers of rat. *J Appl Physiol (1985)* 110: 705–716, 2011.
29. Dutra MT, Alex S, Mota MR, Sales NB, Brown LE, Bottaro M. Effect of strength training combined with antioxidant supplementation on muscular performance. *Appl Physiol Nutr Metab* 43: 775–781, 2018.
30. Dutra MT, Martins WR, Ribeiro ALA, Bottaro M. The effects of strength training combined with vitamin C and E supplementation on skeletal muscle mass and strength: A systematic review and meta-analysis. *J Sports Med (Hindawi Publ Corp)* 2020: 3505209, 2020.
31. Fisher-Wellman KH, Lin CT, Ryan TE, Reese LR, Gilliam LA, Cathey BL, et al. Pyruvate dehydrogenase complex and nicotinamide nucleotide transhydrogenase constitute an energy-consuming redox circuit. *Biochem J* 467: 271–280, 2015.
32. Fisher-Wellman KH, Mattox TA, Thayne K, Katunga LA, La Favor JD, Neufer PD, et al. Novel role for thioredoxin reductase-2 in mitochondrial redox adaptations to obesogenic diet and exercise in heart and skeletal muscle. *J Physiol* 591: 3471–3486, 2013.
33. Fisher-Wellman KH, Neufer PD. Linking mitochondrial bioenergetics to insulin resistance via redox biology. *Trends Endocrinol Metab* 23: 142–153, 2012.
34. Frasier CR, Moukdar F, Patel HD, Sloan RC, Stewart LM, Alleman RJ, et al. Redox-dependent increases in glutathione reductase and exercise preconditioning: role of NADPH oxidase and mitochondria. *Cardiovasc Res* 98: 47–55, 2013.
35. Fu C, Hu J, Liu T, Ago T, Sadoshima J, Li H. Quantitative analysis of redox-sensitive proteome with DIGE and ICAT. *J Proteome Res* 7: 3789–3802, 2008.
36. Gioscia-Ryan RA, LaRocca TJ, Sindler AL, Zigler MC, Murphy MP, Seals DR. Mitochondria-targeted antioxidant (MitoQ) ameliorates age-related arterial endothelial dysfunction in mice. *J Physiol* 592: 2549–2561, 2014.
37. Go YM, Jones DP. The redox proteome. *J Biol Chem* 288: 26512–26520, 2013.
38. Go YM, Roede JR, Walker DI, Duong DM, Seyfried NT, Orr M, et al. Selective targeting of the cysteine proteome by thioredoxin and glutathione redox systems. *Mol Cell Proteomics* 12: 3285–3296, 2013.

39. Goldberg EJ, Buddo KA, McLaughlin KL, Fernandez RF, Pereyra AS, Psaltis CE, et al. Tissue-specific characterization of mitochondrial branched-chain keto acid oxidation using a multiplexed assay platform. *Biochem J* 476: 1521–1537, 2019.

40. Goldstein BJ, Mahadev K, Wu X. Redox paradox: insulin action is facilitated by insulin-stimulated reactive oxygen species with multiple potential signaling targets. *Diabetes* 54: 311–321, 2005.

41. Goldstein BJ, Mahadev K, Wu X, Zhu L, Motoshima H. Role of insulin-induced reactive oxygen species in the insulin signaling pathway. *Antioxid Redox Signal* 7: 1021–1031, 2005.

42. Gomez-Cabrera MC, Pallardo FV, Sastre J, Vina J, Garcia-del-Moral L. Allopurinol and markers of muscle damage among participants in the Tour de France. *JAMA* 289: 2503–2504, 2003.

43. Gomez-Cabrera MC, Salvador-Pascual A, Cabo H, Ferrando B, Vina J. Redox modulation of mitochondriogenesis in exercise. Does antioxidant supplementation blunt the benefits of exercise training? *Free Radic Biol Med* 86: 37–46, 2015.

44. Goncalves RL, Quinlan CL, Perevoshchikova IV, Hey-Mogensen M, Brand MD. Sites of superoxide and hydrogen peroxide production by muscle mitochondria assessed ex vivo under conditions mimicking rest and exercise. *J Biol Chem* 290: 209–227, 2015.

45. Gordillo G, Fang H, Park H, Roy S. Nox-4-dependent nuclear H2O2 drives DNA oxidation resulting in 8-OHdG as urinary biomarker and hemangioendothelioma formation. *Antioxid Redox Signal* 12: 933–943, 2010.

46. Grum CM, Gross TJ, Mody CH, Sitrin RG. Expression of xanthine oxidase activity by murine leukocytes. *J Lab Clin Med* 116: 211–218, 1990.

47. Hahn NE, Meischl C, Wijnker PJ, Musters RJ, Fornerod M, Janssen HW, et al. NOX2, p22phox and p47phox are targeted to the nuclear pore complex in ischemic cardiomyocytes colocalizing with local reactive oxygen species. *Cell Physiol Biochem* 27: 471–478, 2011.

48. Hancock M, Hafstad AD, Nabeebaccus AA, Catibog N, Logan A, Smyrnias I, et al. Myocardial NADPH oxidase-4 regulates the physiological response to acute exercise. *Elife* 7: 2018.

49. Handy DE, Loscalzo J. Redox regulation of mitochondrial function. *Antioxid Redox Signal* 16: 1323–1367, 2012.

50. Hanschmann EM, Godoy JR, Berndt C, Hudemann C, Lillig CH. Thioredoxins, glutaredoxins, and peroxiredoxins—molecular mechanisms and health significance: from cofactors to antioxidants to redox signaling. *Antioxid Redox Signal* 19: 1539–1605, 2013.

51. Hansen JM, Watson WH, Jones DP. Compartmentation of Nrf-2 redox control: regulation of cytoplasmic activation by glutathione and DNA binding by thioredoxin-1. *Toxicol Sci* 82: 308–317, 2004.

52. Hellsten-Westing Y, Kaijser L, Ekblom B, Sjodin B. Exchange of purines in human liver and skeletal muscle with short-term exhaustive exercise. *Am J Physiol* 266: R81–86, 1994.

53. Hellsten Y, Ahlborg G, Jensen-Urstad M, Sjodin B. Indication of in vivo xanthine oxidase activity in human skeletal muscle during exercise. *Acta Physiol Scand* 134: 159–160, 1988.

54. Hellsten Y, Frandsen U, Orthenblad N, Sjodin B, Richter EA. Xanthine oxidase in human skeletal muscle following eccentric exercise: a role in inflammation. *J Physiol* 498 (Pt 1): 239–248, 1997.

55. Hellsten Y, Richter EA, Kiens B, Bangsbo J. AMP deamination and purine exchange in human skeletal muscle during and after intense exercise. *J Physiol* 520 Pt 3: 909–920, 1999.

56. Henriquez-Olguin C, Diaz-Vegas A, Utreras-Mendoza Y, Campos C, Arias-Calderon M, Llanos P, et al. NOX2 inhibition impairs early muscle gene expression induced by a single exercise bout. *Front Physiol* 7: 282, 2016.

57. Henriquez-Olguin C, Knudsen JR, Raun SH, Li Z, Dalbram E, Treebak JT, et al. Cytosolic ROS production by NADPH oxidase 2 regulates muscle glucose uptake during exercise. *Nat Commun* 10: 4623, 2019.

58. Henriquez-Olguin C, Renani LB, Arab-Ceschia L, Raun SH, Bhatia A, Li Z, et al. Adaptations to high-intensity interval training in skeletal muscle require NADPH oxidase 2. *Redox Biol* 24: 101188, 2019.

59. Hidalgo C, Sanchez G, Barrientos G, Aracena-Parks P. A transverse tubule NADPH oxidase activity stimulates calcium release from isolated triads via ryanodine receptor type 1 S -glutathionylation. *J Biol Chem* 281: 26473–26482, 2006.

60. Higashida K, Kim SH, Higuchi M, Holloszy JO, Han DH. Normal adaptations to exercise despite protection against oxidative stress. *Am J Physiol Endocrinol Metab* 301: E779–784, 2011.

61. Himms-Hagen J, Irwin C. Monamine oxidase in outer membrane of skeletal muscle mitochondria. *Biochim Biophys Acta* 437: 498–504, 1976.

62. Hirota K, Matsui M, Iwata S, Nishiyama A, Mori K, Yodoi J. AP-1 transcriptional activity is regulated by a direct association between thioredoxin and Ref-1. *Proc Natl Acad Sci U S A* 94: 3633–3638, 1997.

63. Hirschfield W, Moody MR, O'Brien WE, Gregg AR, Bryan RM, Jr., Reid MB. Nitric oxide release and contractile properties of skeletal muscles from mice deficient in type III NOS. *Am J Physiol Regul Integr Comp Physiol* 278: R95–R100, 2000.

64. Hurd TR, James AM, Lilley KS, Murphy MP. Chapter 19 Measuring redox changes to mitochondrial protein thiols with redox difference gel electrophoresis (redox-DIGE). *Methods Enzymol* 456: 343–361, 2009.

65. Hurd TR, Prime TA, Harbour ME, Lilley KS, Murphy MP. Detection of reactive oxygen species-sensitive thiol proteins by redox difference gel electrophoresis: implications for mitochondrial redox signaling. *J Biol Chem* 282: 22040–22051, 2007.

66. Jackson MJ. Recent advances and long-standing problems in detecting oxidative damage and reactive oxygen species in skeletal muscle. *J Physiol* 594: 5185–5193, 2016.

67. Jackson MJ, Edwards RH, Symons MC. Electron spin resonance studies of intact mammalian skeletal muscle. *Biochim Biophys Acta* 847: 185–190, 1985.

68. Jackson MJ, McArdle A. Role of reactive oxygen species in age-related neuromuscular deficits. *J Physiol* 594: 1979–1988, 2016.

69. Ji LL. Redox signaling in skeletal muscle: role of aging and exercise. *Adv Physiol Educ* 39: 352–359, 2015.

70. Jones DP. Radical-free biology of oxidative stress. *Am J Physiol Cell Physiol* 295: C849–868, 2008.

71. Jones DP. Redefining oxidative stress. *Antioxid Redox Signal* 8: 1865–1879, 2006.

72. Kelleher ZT, Sha Y, Foster MW, Foster WM, Forrester MT, Marshall HE. Thioredoxin-mediated denitrosylation regulates cytokine-induced nuclear factor kappaB (NF-kappaB) activation. *J Biol Chem* 289: 3066–3072, 2014.

73. Kelso GF, Porteous CM, Coulter CV, Hughes G, Porteous WK, Ledgerwood EC, et al. Selective targeting of a redox-active ubiquinone to mitochondria within cells: antioxidant and antiapoptotic properties. *J Biol Chem* 276: 4588–4596, 2001.

74. Khairallah RJ, Shi G, Sbrana F, Prosser BL, Borroto C, Mazaitis MJ, et al. Microtubules underlie dysfunction in duchenne muscular dystrophy. *Sci Signal* 5: ra56, 2012.

75. Khawli FA, Reid MB. N-acetylcysteine depresses contractile function and inhibits fatigue of diaphragm in vitro. *J Appl Physiol (1985)* 77: 317–324, 1994.

76. Kim JH, Choi TG, Park S, Yun HR, Nguyen NNY, Jo YH, et al. Mitochondrial ROS-derived PTEN oxidation activates PI3K pathway for mTOR-induced myogenic autophagy. *Cell Death Differ* 25: 1921–1937, 2018.

77. Kobzik L, Stringer B, Balligand JL, Reid MB, Stamler JS. Endothelial type nitric oxide synthase in skeletal muscle fibers: mitochondrial relationships. *Biochem Biophys Res Commun* 211: 375–381, 1995.

78. Kramer PA, Duan J, Gaffrey MJ, Shukla AK, Wang L, Bammler TK, et al. Fatiguing contractions increase protein S-glutathionylation occupancy in mouse skeletal muscle. *Redox Biol* 17: 367–376, 2018.

79. Kuzkaya N, Weissmann N, Harrison DG, Dikalov S. Interactions of peroxynitrite, tetrahydrobiopterin, ascorbic acid, and thiols: implications for uncoupling endothelial nitric-oxide synthase. *J Biol Chem* 278: 22546–22554, 2003.

80. Laker RC, Drake JC, Wilson RJ, Lira VA, Lewellen BM, Ryall KA, et al. Ampk phosphorylation of Ulk1 is required for targeting of mitochondria to lysosomes in exercise-induced mitophagy. *Nat Commun* 8: 548, 2017.

81. Lamb GD, Westerblad H. Acute effects of reactive oxygen and nitrogen species on the contractile function of skeletal muscle. *J Physiol* 589: 2119–2127, 2011.

82. Leichert LI, Gehrke F, Gudiseva HV, Blackwell T, Ilbert M, Walker AK, et al. Quantifying changes in the thiol redox proteome upon oxidative stress in vivo. *Proc Natl Acad Sci U S A* 105: 8197–8202, 2008.

83. Leonard SE, Reddie KG, Carroll KS. Mining the thiol proteome for sulfenic acid modifications reveals new targets for oxidation in cells. *ACS Chem Biol* 4: 783–799, 2009.

84. Lindsay A, McCourt PM, Karachunski P, Lowe DA, Ervasti JM. Xanthine oxidase is hyper-active in Duchenne muscular dystrophy. *Free Radic Biol Med* 129: 364–371, 2018.

85. Liu H, Nishitoh H, Ichijo H, Kyriakis JM. Activation of apoptosis signal-regulating kinase 1 (ASK1) by tumor necrosis factor receptor-associated factor 2 requires prior dissociation of the ASK1 inhibitor thioredoxin. *Mol Cell Biol* 20: 2198–2208, 2000.

86. Liu P, Zhang H, Yu B, Xiong L, Xia Y. Proteomic identification of early salicylate- and flg22-responsive redox-sensitive proteins in Arabidopsis. *Sci Rep* 5: 8625, 2015.

87. Logan A, Cocheme HM, Li Pun PB, Apostolova N, Smith RA, Larsen L, et al. Using exomarkers to assess mitochondrial reactive species in vivo. *Biochim Biophys Acta* 1840: 923–930, 2014.

88. Lu J, Holmgren A. The thioredoxin antioxidant system. *Free Radic Biol Med* 66: 75–87, 2014.

89. Mahadev K, Wu X, Zilbering A, Zhu L, Lawrence JT, Goldstein BJ. Hydrogen peroxide generated during cellular insulin stimulation is integral to activation of the distal insulin signaling cascade in 3T3-L1 adipocytes. *J Biol Chem* 276: 48662–48669, 2001.

90. Mailloux RJ, McBride SL, Harper ME. Unearthing the secrets of mitochondrial ROS and glutathione in bioenergetics. *Trends Biochem Sci* 38: 592–602, 2013.

91. Mailloux RJ, Xuan JY, McBride S, Maharsy W, Thorn S, Holterman CE, et al. Glutaredoxin-2 is required to control oxidative phosphorylation in cardiac muscle by mediating deglutathionylation reactions. *J Biol Chem* 289: 14812–14828, 2014.

92. Manabe Y, Takagi M, Nakamura-Yamada M, Goto-Inoue N, Taoka M, Isobe T, et al. Redox proteins are constitutively secreted by skeletal muscle. *J Physiol Sci* 64: 401–409, 2014.

93. Maroz A, Anderson RF, Smith RA, Murphy MP. Reactivity of ubiquinone and ubiquinol with superoxide and the hydroperoxyl radical: implications for in vivo antioxidant activity. *Free Radic Biol Med* 46: 105–109, 2009.

94. Mashamaite LN, Rohwer JM, Pillay CS. The glutaredoxin mono- and di-thiol mechanisms for deglutathionylation are functionally equivalent: implications for redox systems biology. *Biosci Rep* 35: 2015.

95. May JM. How does ascorbic acid prevent endothelial dysfunction? *Free Radic Biol Med* 28: 1421–1429, 2000.

96. McManus MJ, Murphy MP, Franklin JL. Mitochondria-derived reactive oxygen species mediate caspase-dependent and -independent neuronal deaths. *Mol Cell Neurosci* 63: 13–23, 2014.

97. Meng TC, Fukada T, Tonks NK. Reversible oxidation and inactivation of protein tyrosine phosphatases in vivo. *Mol Cell* 9: 387–399, 2002.

98. Michaelson LP, Shi G, Ward CW, Rodney GG. Mitochondrial redox potential during contraction in single intact muscle fibers. *Muscle Nerve* 42: 522–529, 2010.

99. Moen RJ, Cornea S, Oseid DE, Binder BP, Klein JC, Thomas DD. Redox-sensitive residue in the actin-binding interface of myosin. *Biochem Biophys Res Commun* 453: 345–349, 2014.

100. Moreno KX, Harrison CE, Merritt ME, Kovacs Z, Malloy CR, Sherry AD. Hyperpolarized delta-[1-(13) C] gluconolactone as a probe of the pentose phosphate pathway. *NMR Biomed* 30: 2017.

101. Nemes R, Koltai E, Taylor AW, Suzuki K, Gyori F, Radak Z. Reactive oxygen and nitrogen species regulate key metabolic, anabolic, and catabolic pathways in skeletal muscle. *Antioxidants (Basel)* 7: 2018.

102. Neufer PD. The bioenergetics of exercise. *Cold Spring Harb Perspect Med* 8: 2018.

103. Ng CF, Schafer FQ, Buettner GR, Rodgers VG. The rate of cellular hydrogen peroxide removal shows dependency on GSH: mathematical insight into in vivo H2O2 and GPx concentrations. *Free Radic Res* 41: 1201–1211, 2007.

104. Nicholls DG, Ferguson SJ. *Bioenergetics (4th Edition)*. Waltham, MA: Academic Press, 2013, p. 434.

105. Niki E. Action of ascorbic acid as a scavenger of active and stable oxygen radicals. *Am J Clin Nutr* 54: 1119S–1124S, 1991.

106. Novelli GP, Bracciotti G, Falsini S. Spin-trappers and vitamin E prolong endurance to muscle fatigue in mice. *Free Radic Biol Med* 8: 9–13, 1990.

107. Olthoff JT, Lindsay A, Abo-Zahrah R, Baltgalvis KA, Patrinostro X, Belanto JJ, et al. Loss of peroxiredoxin-2 exacerbates eccentric contraction-induced force loss in dystrophin-deficient muscle. *Nat Commun* 9: 5104, 2018.

108. Pal R, Basu Thakur P, Li S, Minard C, Rodney GG. Real-time imaging of NADPH oxidase activity in living cells using a novel fluorescent protein reporter. *PLOS ONE* 8: e63989, 2013.

109. Paulsen CE, Carroll KS. Orchestrating redox signaling networks through regulatory cysteine switches. *ACS Chem Biol* 5: 47–62, 2010.

110. Paulsen G, Hamarsland H, Cumming KT, Johansen RE, Hulmi JJ, Borsheim E, et al. Vitamin C and E supplementation alters protein signalling after a strength training session, but not muscle growth during 10 weeks of training. *J Physiol* 592: 5391–5408, 2014.

111. Peake JM, Neubauer O, Della Gatta PA, Nosaka K. Muscle damage and inflammation during recovery from exercise. *J Appl Physiol (1985)* 122: 559–570, 2017.

112. Pearson T, Kabayo T, Ng R, Chamberlain J, McArdle A, Jackson MJ. Skeletal muscle contractions induce acute changes in cytosolic superoxide, but slower responses in mitochondrial superoxide and cellular hydrogen peroxide. *PLoS One* 9: e96378, 2014.

113. Perry CG, Kane DA, Lanza IR, Neufer PD. Methods for assessing mitochondrial function in diabetes. *Diabetes* 62: 1041–1053, 2013.

114. Powers SK, Ji LL, Kavazis AN, Jackson MJ. Reactive oxygen species: impact on skeletal muscle. *Compr Physiol* 1: 941–969, 2011.

115. Powers SK, Ji LL, Leeuwenburgh C. Exercise training-induced alterations in skeletal muscle antioxidant capacity: a brief review. *Med Sci Sports Exerc* 31: 987–997, 1999.

116. Powers SK, Lennon SL. Analysis of cellular responses to free radicals: focus on exercise and skeletal muscle. *Proc Nutr Soc* 58: 1025–1033, 1999.

117. Powers SK, Radak Z, Ji LL. Exercise-induced oxidative stress: past, present and future. *J Physiol* 594: 5081–5092, 2016.

118. Powers SK, Talbert EE, Adhihetty PJ. Reactive oxygen and nitrogen species as intracellular signals in skeletal muscle. *J Physiol* 589: 2129–2138, 2011.

119. Prosser BL, Ward CW, Lederer WJ. X-ROS signaling: rapid mechano-chemo transduction in heart. *Science* 333: 1440–1445, 2011.

120. Quinlan CL, Goncalves RL, Hey-Mogensen M, Yadava N, Bunik VI, Brand MD. The 2-oxoacid dehydrogenase complexes in mitochondria can produce superoxide/hydrogen peroxide at much higher rates than complex I. *J Biol Chem* 289: 8312–8325, 2014.

121. Rahman MM, El Jamali A, Halade GV, Ouhtit A, Abou-Saleh H, Pintus G. Nox2 activity is required in obesity-mediated alteration of bone remodeling. *Oxid Med Cell Longev* 2018: 6054361, 2018.

122. Reid MB, Haack KE, Franchek KM, Valberg PA, Kobzik L, West MS. Reactive oxygen in skeletal muscle. I. Intracellular oxidant kinetics and fatigue in vitro. *J Appl Physiol (1985)* 73: 1797–1804, 1992.

123. Reid MB, Stokic DS, Koch SM, Khawli FA, Leis AA. N-acetylcysteine inhibits muscle fatigue in humans. *J Clin Invest* 94: 2468–2474, 1994.

124. Riddell JR, Wang XY, Minderman H, Gollnick SO. Peroxiredoxin 1 stimulates secretion of proinflammatory cytokines by binding to TLR4. *J Immunol* 184: 1022–1030, 2010.

125. Ristow M, Zarse K, Oberbach A, Kloting N, Birringer M, Kiehntopf M, et al. Antioxidants prevent health-promoting effects of physical exercise in humans. *Proc Natl Acad Sci U S A* 106: 8665–8670, 2009.

126. Roma LP, Deponte M, Riemer J, Morgan B. Mechanisms and applications of redox-sensitive green fluorescent protein-based hydrogen peroxide probes. *Antioxid Redox Signal* 29: 552–568, 2018.

127. Rossman MJ, Santos-Parker JR, Steward CAC, Bispham NZ, Cuevas LM, Rosenberg HL, et al. Chronic supplementation with a mitochondrial antioxidant (MitoQ) improves vascular function in healthy older adults. *Hypertension* 71: 1056–1063, 2018.

128. Ryan MJ, Jackson JR, Hao Y, Leonard SS, Alway SE. Inhibition of xanthine oxidase reduces oxidative stress and improves skeletal muscle function in response to electrically stimulated isometric contractions in aged mice. *Free Radic Biol Med* 51: 38–52, 2011.

129. Sahlin K, Shabalina IG, Mattsson CM, Bakkman L, Fernstrom M, Rozhdestvenskaya Z, et al. Ultraendurance exercise increases the production of reactive oxygen species in isolated mitochondria from human skeletal muscle. *J Appl Physiol (1985)* 108: 780–787, 2010.

130. Sakellariou GK, Vasilaki A, Palomero J, Kayani A, Zibrik L, McArdle A, Jackson MJ. Studies of mitochondrial and nonmitochondrial sources implicate nicotinamide adenine dinucleotide phosphate oxidase(s) in the increased skeletal muscle superoxide generation that occurs during contractile activity. *Antioxid Redox Signal* 18: 603–621, 2013.

131. Sanchez G, Escobar M, Pedrozo Z, Macho P, Domenech R, Hartel S, Hidalgo C, Donoso P. Exercise and tachycardia increase NADPH oxidase and ryanodine receptor-2 activity: possible role in cardioprotection. *Cardiovasc Res* 77: 380–386, 2008.

132. Sanchis-Gomar F, Pareja-Galeano H, Perez-Quilis C, Santos-Lozano A, Fiuza-Luces C, Garatachea N, et al. Effects of allopurinol on exercise-induced muscle damage: new therapeutic approaches? *Cell Stress Chaperones* 20: 3–13, 2015.

133. Schwarzlander M, Dick TP, Meyer AJ, and Morgan B. Dissecting redox biology using fluorescent protein sensors. *Antioxid Redox Signal* 24: 680–712, 2016.

134. Shill DD, Southern WM, Willingham TB, Lansford KA, McCully KK, Jenkins NT. Mitochondria-specific antioxidant supplementation does not influence endurance exercise training-induced adaptations in circulating angiogenic cells, skeletal muscle oxidative capacity or maximal oxygen uptake. *J Physiol* 594: 7005–7014, 2016.

135. Shindoh C, DiMarco A, Thomas A, Manubay P, Supinski G. Effect of N-acetylcysteine on diaphragm fatigue. *J Appl Physiol (1985)* 68: 2107–2113, 1990.

136. Sipkens JA, Krijnen PA, Hahn NE, Wassink M, Meischl C, Smith DE, et al. Homocysteine-induced cardiomyocyte apoptosis and plasma membrane flip-flop are independent of S-adenosylhomocysteine: a crucial role for nuclear p47(phox). *Mol Cell Biochem* 358: 229–239, 2011.

137. Smith NT, Soriano-Arroquia A, Goljanek-Whysall K, Jackson MJ, McDonagh B. Redox responses are preserved across muscle fibres with differential susceptibility to aging. *J Proteomics* 177: 112–123, 2018.

138. Son Y, Kim S, Chung HT, Pae HO. Reactive oxygen species in the activation of MAP kinases. *Methods Enzymol* 528: 27–48, 2013.

139. Staudacher V, Trujillo M, Diederichs T, Dick TP, Radi R, Morgan B, et al. Redox-sensitive GFP fusions for monitoring the catalytic mechanism and inactivation of peroxiredoxins in living cells. *Redox Biol* 14: 549–556, 2018.

140. Steinbacher P, Eckl P. Impact of oxidative stress on exercising skeletal muscle. *Biomolecules* 5: 356–377, 2015.

141. Suzuki M, Grisham MB, Granger DN. Leukocyte-endothelial cell adhesive interactions: role of xanthine oxidase-derived oxidants. *J Leukoc Biol* 50: 488–494, 1991.

142. Ter Horst EN, Hahn NE, Geerts D, Musters RJP, Paulus WJ, van Rossum AC, et al. p47phox-Dependent Reactive Oxygen Species Stimulate Nuclear Translocation of the FoxO1 Transcription Factor During Metabolic Inhibition in Cardiomyoblasts. *Cell Biochem Biophys* 76: 401–410, 2018.

143. Thamsen M, Jakob U. The redoxome: Proteomic analysis of cellular redox networks. *Curr Opin Chem Biol* 15: 113–119, 2011.
144. Traber MG, Atkinson J. Vitamin E, antioxidant and nothing more. *Free Radic Biol Med* 43: 4–15, 2007.
145. Trewin AJ, Parker L, Shaw CS, Hiam DS, Garnham A, Levinger I, et al. Acute HIIE elicits similar changes in human skeletal muscle mitochondrial H2O2 release, respiration, and cell signaling as endurance exercise even with less work. *Am J Physiol Regul Integr Comp Physiol* 315: R1003–R1016, 2018.
146. Verschoor ML, Wilson LA, Singh G. Mechanisms associated with mitochondrial-generated reactive oxygen species in cancer. *Can J Physiol Pharmacol* 88: 204–219, 2010.
147. Vina J, Gimeno A, Sastre J, Desco C, Asensi M, Pallardo FV, et al. Mechanism of free radical production in exhaustive exercise in humans and rats; role of xanthine oxidase and protection by allopurinol. *IUBMB Life* 49: 539–544, 2000.
148. Wadley AJ, Aldred S, Coles SJ. An unexplored role for Peroxiredoxin in exercise-induced redox signalling? *Redox Biol* 8: 51–58, 2016.
149. Wadley GD, Nicolas MA, Hiam DS, McConell GK. Xanthine oxidase inhibition attenuates skeletal muscle signaling following acute exercise but does not impair mitochondrial adaptations to endurance training. *Am J Physiol Endocrinol Metab* 304: E853–862, 2013.
150. Ward PA. Mechanisms of endothelial cell killing by H2O2 or products of activated neutrophils. *Am J Med* 91: 89S–94S, 1991.
151. Weibrecht I, Bohmer SA, Dagnell M, Kappert K, Ostman A, Bohmer FD. Oxidation sensitivity of the catalytic cysteine of the protein-tyrosine phosphatases SHP-1 and SHP-2. *Free Radic Biol Med* 43: 100–110, 2007.
152. Wojtala A, Bonora M, Malinska D, Pinton P, Duszynski J, Wieckowski MR. Methods to monitor ROS production by fluorescence microscopy and fluorometry. *Methods Enzymol* 542: 243–262, 2014.
153. Wong HS, Dighe PA, Mezera V, Monternier PA, Brand MD. Production of superoxide and hydrogen peroxide from specific mitochondrial sites under different bioenergetic conditions. *J Biol Chem* 292: 16804–16809, 2017.
154. Xiao H, Jedrychowski MP, Schweppe DK, Huttlin EL, Yu Q, Heppner DE, et al. A quantitative tissue-specific landscape of protein redox regulation during aging. *Cell* 2020.
155. Yan LJ, Sumien N, Thangthaeng N, Forster MJ. Reversible inactivation of dihydrolipoamide dehydrogenase by mitochondrial hydrogen peroxide. *Free Radic Res* 47: 123–133, 2013.
156. Young A, Gardiner D, Kuksal N, Gill R, O'Brien M, Mailloux RJ. Deletion of the glutaredoxin-2 gene protects mice from diet-induced weight gain, which correlates with increased mitochondrial respiration and proton leaks in skeletal muscle. *Antioxid Redox Signal* 31: 1272–1288, 2019.
157. Young A, Gill R, Mailloux RJ. Protein S-glutathionylation: The linchpin for the transmission of regulatory information on redox buffering capacity in mitochondria. *Chem Biol Interact* 299: 151–162, 2019.
158. Zhang J, Jin B, Li L, Block ER, Patel JM. Nitric oxide-induced persistent inhibition and nitrosylation of active site cysteine residues of mitochondrial cytochrome-c oxidase in lung endothelial cells. *Am J Physiol Cell Physiol* 288: C840–849, 2005.
159. Zielinski J, Slominska EM, Krol-Zielinska M, Krasinski Z, Kusy K. Purine metabolism in sprint- vs endurance-trained athletes aged 2090 years. *Sci Rep* 9: 12075, 2019.
160. Zuo L, Christofi FL, Wright VP, Bao S, Clanton TL. Lipoxygenase-dependent superoxide release in skeletal muscle. *J Appl Physiol (1985)* 97: 661–668, 2004.

5

BIOCHEMICAL CONTRIBUTORS TO EXERCISE FATIGUE

Arthur J. Cheng, Maja Schlittler, and Håkan Westerblad

Introduction

Most everyday activities such as walking and running involve brief, repeated activation of muscles. During locomotion, the rate at which energy in the form of adenosine triphosphate (ATP) is delivered to energy-consuming ion pumps and molecular motors, i.e., the myosin cross-bridges, increases dramatically in skeletal muscle. In fact, the rate of ATP turnover can increase more than 100-fold when a muscle goes from the resting to the fully activated contracting state, and this can occur within a few milliseconds and without any major change in the cellular ATP concentration (74). However, this effective metabolic system comes with a price: Highly energy-demanding physical exercise requires a rate of ATP delivery that exceeds the capacity of aerobic energy metabolism of the muscle fibres, and the additional anaerobic metabolism results in end products that make contractions weaker and slower; that is, *peripheral fatigue* develops. In addition, the performance during physical exercise can be limited by impaired neuronal activation of muscles, and this is referred to as *central fatigue* (31).

In this chapter we will describe the unique metabolic and contractile properties of different muscle fibre types and how these allow for muscles to cope with the energy demands of diverse exercise tasks. We will also describe the contribution of the various metabolic systems that allow for maintained energy turnover during strenuous exercise. Thereafter, we will discuss the key cellular mechanisms of skeletal muscle fatigue and recovery and how fatigue actually plays an important role in preventing critical energy depletion in skeletal muscle during intense exercise. Finally, we will describe how endurance training can trigger adaptations resulting in improved fatigue resistance.

Muscle Fibre Types

Skeletal muscles must be able to perform a large variety of activities, ranging from prolonged upright standing to instantaneous ballistic movements when, for instance, throwing a ball. In order to perform such divergent activities, muscles are composed of specialized muscle fibre types that differ in metabolic properties, contractile speed, intracellular Ca^{2+} handling, and fatigue resistance (8, 80). Muscle fibre types in mammalian skeletal muscle are typically classified based on their myosin heavy-chain (MyHC) isoforms: type 1, 2A, 2X, and 2B (76). Note that the MyHC 2B protein is not detectable in human muscle, although the corresponding *MYH4* gene is present in the genome, and human fibres typed as 2B based on ATPase staining are in fact MyHC 2X fibres (79). In addition, some fibres express more than one MyHC isoform, suggesting that a spectrum of fibre types can co-exist (76).

The rate of cross-bridge cycling, and hence the speed of contraction, is determined by the MyHC isoform and in human muscle type 1 is the slowest, type 2A intermediate, and type 2X the fastest; type 2B, which is not expressed in human muscle, is faster than type 2X. The expression pattern of numerous other protein isoforms also differs between muscle fibres. For some protein isoforms there is a pattern of gene co-expression where, for instance, the slow MyHC type 1 is co-expressed with "slow" isoforms of other proteins. However, this is not always the case, and gene expression of different protein isoforms is controlled by multiple interacting mechanisms (80).

The fibre type classification based on MyHC isoforms is relevant from an energy metabolic perspective because the speed of cross-bridge cycling is directly related to the speed of ATP consumption. In addition, there are other important differences between fibre types related to energy metabolism. The density of the other major ATP-consuming protein in skeletal muscles, the sarcoplasmic reticulum (SR) Ca^{2+} pumps, is much higher in fast than in slow fibres, and these pumps exist in two isoforms: SERCA1, mainly expressed in fast type 2 fibres, and SERCA2, mainly expressed in slow type 1 fibres (8, 65). Moreover, type 2 fibres generally have a lower oxidative capacity than type 1 fibres.

In summary, skeletal muscle fibres show substantial differences in their contractile and metabolic properties, which serve the purpose of allowing a range of activities from explosive ballistic movements to energy-preserving endurance activities.

Energy Metabolism

The massive increase in energy consumption during contractions is the ultimate mechanism underlying acute muscle fatigue. The major energy-consuming entities within skeletal muscle are the molecular motors, the cross-bridges, and the SR Ca^{2+} pumps (37), which are essential for muscle relaxation. The extent of energy utilized by the cross-bridges vs. the SR Ca^{2+} pumps depends on the type of exercise performed (e.g., sustained vs. intermittent contractions, maximal vs. submaximal), and their relative importance for the total energy consumption is currently debated (6, 83, 94).

ATP is the immediate energy source for muscle contraction. The ATP stored within muscle fibres is very limited and can be depleted within 2 s during a maximal contraction. (74). Thus, other metabolic pathways are required to rapidly replenish ATP to meet the energy demands of exercise. Critical to supplying the necessary ATP are the anaerobic and aerobic metabolic pathways, with anaerobic metabolism dominating during high-intensity exercise, whereas aerobic metabolism is the predominate source during prolonged endurance exercise (74).

Anaerobic Metabolism

The dominating anaerobic pathways to replenish ATP are the degradation of phosphocreatine (PCr) and the breakdown of muscle glycogen to lactate and hydrogen ions. A minor additional source of ATP comes from adenylate kinase that converts adenosine diphosphate (ADP) to ATP and adenosine monophosphate (AMP) (2 ADP $\leftrightarrow$ ATP + AMP), and the AMP produced in this reaction will be deaminated to inosine monophosphate (IMP) + NH_4^+.

Creatine kinase (CK) catalyzes the near-equilibrium reaction: PCr + ADP $\leftrightarrow$ Cr + ATP. This reaction is driven to the right during periods of high ATP consumption, with the net effects being a reduction in PCr and increases in the concentrations of creatine (Cr) and inorganic phosphate ions (Pi), whereas ATP remains almost constant (PCr + ADP $\rightarrow$ Cr + ATP $\rightarrow$ Cr + ADP + Pi + energy). Conversely, during the recovery after periods of high ATP consumption, energy provided mainly by aerobic metabolism (see later) refills the PCr store (energy + P_i + ADP + Cr $\rightarrow$ ATP + Cr $\rightarrow$ ADP + PCr). When PCr reaches low levels, ATP starts to fall and ADP and AMP show transient increases, which are reflected in a gradual accumulation of IMP (96). Studies on whole muscles or muscle homogenates suggest that intracellular ATP does not decrease below ~60% of the resting value during intense exercise, whereas studies on individual muscle fibres suggest that markedly larger changes can occur. For instance, in type 2X fibres

ATP was reduced to ~20% of the resting value and IMP increased from undetectable levels to ~5 mM after maximal cycling exercise (42).

Glycogen breakdown is controlled by glycogen phosphorylase, which is regulated by covalent phosphorylation, allosteric regulation, and substrate availability (44). Phosphorylase exists in two forms: a phosphorylated form (referred to as phosphorylase a) that is considered to be constitutively active and a non-phosphorylated form (referred to as phosphorylase b) that is fully dependent on AMP for activation and is considered to be essentially inactive in resting muscle (13). Phosphorylation (activation) and dephosphorylation (inactivation) of phosphorylase are catalyzed by specific kinases and phosphatases, respectively (39). Glycogen synthesis is catalyzed by glycogen synthase, and the activity of this enzyme is controlled by phosphorylation in a complex manner (72).

The end point of anaerobic glycogen breakdown is lactate ions and H^+. The rate of anaerobic glycogen breakdown depends on O_2 availability and mitochondrial capacity relative to the energy demand, which means that lactate accumulation occurs mainly during intensive exercise when the rate of ATP consumption is high. The H^+ generated in parallel with the lactate ions causes acidosis, and during intense exercise, intracellular pH in muscle cells can fall from ~7.0 to ~6.5 (27). A major disadvantage with rapid lactate formation is that this yields much less ATP per glucosyl unit as compared to aerobic glycogen breakdown (theoretically 3 vs. 38 ATP/glucosyl unit), and it is well documented that depletion of intramuscular glycogen stores can limit muscle performance during prolonged exercise (2, 7, 98).

Aerobic Metabolism

Oxidative metabolism of carbohydrates and lipids is the dominating ATP-producing system during prolonged exercise (81). The dominating carbohydrate substrate during short-term exercise is muscle glycogen, and the contribution of extracellular glucose increases with exercise duration (43).

The control of glucose uptake in muscle fibres during exercise occurs mainly via an insulin-independent pathway (36). Numerous recent studies have implicated the activation of AMP-dependent protein kinase (AMPK) as a key process in the activation of contraction-mediated glucose uptake in muscle (33). An increase in AMP is believed to play a major role in the activation of AMPK during exercise, but the increase in AMP is generally small and transient (96), and additional mechanisms are probably involved (33). For instance, the production of reactive oxygen–nitrogen species (RONS) increases during exercise (70), and RONS has been shown to play an important role in contraction-mediated glucose uptake, although it remains uncertain whether this occurs via signalling that is AMPK dependent or independent (35, 75).

The major lipid source fuelling aerobic energy metabolism is free fatty acids derived from triglyceride stored in muscle or adipose tissue. The relative contribution of carbohydrate vs. lipid metabolism depends on, for instance, the exercise intensity and the training status. It is worth noting that the relative contribution of fatty acids to aerobic ATP production is largest at low-intensity exercise and at exercise intensities above ~ 60% of the maximal oxygen uptake, fatty acid oxidation actually decreases (73, 74).

Amino acids derived from muscle protein degradation constitute an additional substrate for aerobic metabolism, but their contribution to the overall energy metabolism is small during prolonged exercise: ~5% with carbohydrates available and ~10% in the almost complete absence of carbohydrates (49).

Fatigue

Acute peripheral fatigue with weaker and slower contractions develops when the rate of ATP consumption required to sustain the energy demands of exercise exceeds the ability of the muscle to produce ATP via aerobic metabolism. Thus, acute fatigue is closely related to the link between the energy consumed during contractions and the aerobic capacity of the contracting muscle fibre:

A. Type 1 fibres have slow MyHC, relatively few SR Ca^{2+} pumps, and a high aerobic capacity and are therefore fatigue resistant (Figure 5.1A).

B. Type 2 fibres have faster MyHC, more SR Ca^{2+} pumps, and a lower aerobic capacity; hence, they fatigue more rapidly than type 1 fibres (Figure 5.1B).

Experiments performed on isolated type 1 fibres from mouse soleus muscles demonstrate the importance of aerobic metabolism for fatigue development (Figure 5.2). Under normal conditions, force is well maintained during repeated tetanic stimulation, whereas force falls at about the same rate as in type 2 fibres when mitochondrial respiration is inhibited with cyanide (95). It is worth noting that due to limited O_2 diffusion, deeper parts of isolated whole muscles will become hypoxic during contractile activities (5), and hence the rate of fatigue development in isolated whole soleus muscles is similar to

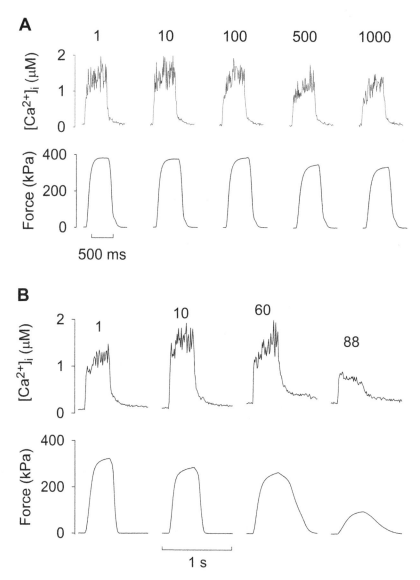

Figure 5.1 Typical Ca^{2+}_i and force records obtained during fatigue induced by repeated tetanic stimulation in (A) a fatigue-resistant type 1 fibre from mouse soleus muscle and (B) a more easily fatigued type 2 fibre from mouse flexor digitorum brevis muscle

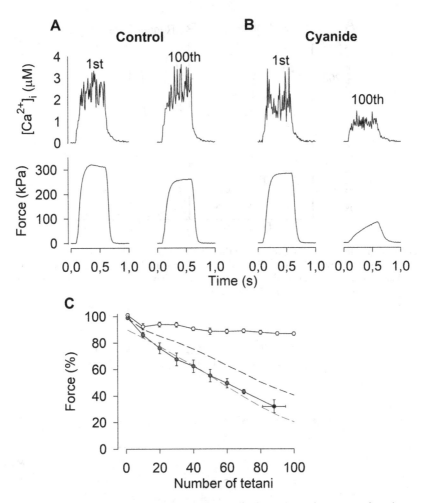

Figure 5.2 The rate of peripheral fatigue development critically depends on the extent of aerobic metabolism

that of cyanide-exposed single soleus fibres (Figure 5.2C). Conversely, endurance training results in an increased aerobic capacity, and fast-twitch type 2 fibres of endurance-trained mice are more fatigue resistant than fibres of sedentary mice (Figure 5.3).

Muscle contraction is linked by a series of events, and fatigue can potentially be attributed to failure at any of the cellular sites involved in the activation and contraction of the muscle fibres (Figure 5.4). The activation of skeletal muscle contraction starts at the central nervous system, thereby activating α-motor neurons, and action potentials propagate along the axons of these neurons out to the muscle fibres. The smallest functional unit of the central motor system, the motor unit, consists of one α-motor neuron and the muscle fibres it activates. The number of muscle fibres in a motor unit varies from muscle to muscle. For instance, in the hand an α-motor neuron generally activates fewer than 100 muscle fibres, whereas for the lower leg a single motor unit may contain up to 1,000 muscle fibres (12). Generally, the larger the number of muscle fibres in a motor unit, the less precise the associated movements.

Central Fatigue

The activation of motor units by the central nervous system and its role in the regulation of skeletal muscle force generation is highly complex, which makes it difficult to identify mechanisms within the

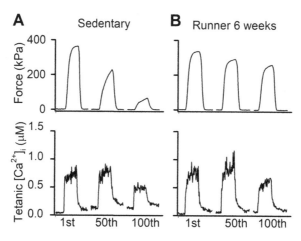

Figure 5.3 Representative force and Ca^{2+}_i records of the 1st, 50th, and 100th fatiguing tetanic contractions (70 Hz, 350 ms duration given every 2 s) of individual flexor digitorum brevis type 2 fibres from a sedentary control mouse (A) and mouse with increased aerobic capacity after having access to a running wheel and running >10 km per 24 hours for 6 weeks (B). Figure adapted from (38)

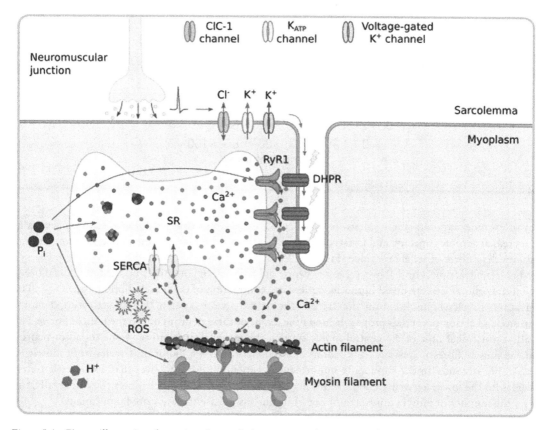

Figure 5.4 Figure illustrating the various intracellular processes that are considered to have key roles in the development of skeletal muscle fatigue

central nervous system that contribute to fatigue during various types of exercise (31). Nevertheless, recent evidence has linked central fatigue mechanisms to intramuscular metabolic changes, implicating that metabolic disturbances within fatiguing muscles provide afferent feedback to the central nervous system, which results in down-regulated voluntary drive that may prevent critical intramuscular energy depletion (3, 78).

Peripheral Fatigue

Within skeletal muscle, activation of the muscle fibres starts at the neuromuscular junction, where an action potential arriving at the presynaptic terminal of an α-motor neuron causes acetylcholine release, which binds to receptors on the motor end plate of the sarcolemma. This initiates an action potential that propagates along the sarcolemma and down into the transverse tubular (t-tubular) system, where it activates the t-tubular voltage-sensing protein, the dihydropyridine receptor (DHPR). DHPR then activates the SR Ca^{2+} release channel, the ryanodine receptor type 1 (RyR1), which releases Ca^{2+} into the cytosol, thereby increasing the cytosolic free Ca^{2+} (Ca^{2+}_i). Ca^{2+} then binds to troponin C causing tropomyosin to unwind, which opens the binding sites on actin for myosin heads to attach, resulting in ATP-dependent cross-bridge cycling and muscle contraction. Increased pumping of Ca^{2+} back into the SR by the ATP-consuming SERCA is commenced as soon as Ca^{2+}_i is raised, and relaxation occurs when SR Ca^{2+} release stops and Ca^{2+}_i declines towards the resting value. All of these steps can be adversely affected by metabolic changes, thereby causing peripheral fatigue. Nevertheless, some steps are more susceptible than others, and these will now be discussed (Figure 5.4).

Impaired Action Potential Propagation

Repeated depolarization of the sarcolemma causes an increase in extracellular K^+ (K^+_o) that is regarded as a potential cause of fatigue. During exercise of increasing intensity in humans, an elevation in blood plasma K^+_o of up to 8 mM has been observed, and local concentrations surrounding muscle fibres may even reach 15 mM (59). When resting muscle fibres are exposed to such elevations of K^+_o, the resulting depolarization will inactivate the voltage-gated Na^+ channels whereby action potential generation and propagation, especially into the t-tubular system, will be impaired, resulting in decreased SR Ca^{2+} release and reduced force production (58). Lactate and H^+ are also produced during intense exercise requiring anaerobic metabolism, that is, under the same exercise conditions that cause increased K^+_o. Intriguingly, the ensuing intracellular acidosis decreases the sarcolemmal chloride ion conductance, which facilitates action potential propagation into the t-tubular system, and SR Ca^{2+} release is better maintained (63, 64). Thus, an intracellular acidification due to increased anaerobic metabolism may actually counteract, or even prevent, a fatigue-induced decline in force due to impaired action potential propagation.

Decreased SR Ca^{2+} Release via RyR1

Intrinsic processes exist to prevent critical energy depletion within skeletal muscle, which would result in formation of rigor cross-bridges and inability to pump Ca^{2+} into the SR. Decreased SR Ca^{2+} release is an effective way to reduce the cellular energy consumption, because inhibiting SR Ca^{2+} release reduces the number of ATP-consuming cycling cross-bridges and lessens the demand to actively pump Ca^{2+} back into the SR. There are several mechanisms by which SR Ca^{2+} release can be reduced via inhibition of RyR1.

RyR1 opening is facilitated by ATP, and its breakdown products, ADP and AMP, act as weak competitive agonists. In cells, ATP generally exists as MgATP, which means that a decrease in cytosolic ATP is accompanied by an increase in the free cytosolic Mg^{2+} (Mg^{2+}_i), and Mg^{2+} inhibits RyR1 opening (25, 46, 47, 53). Large changes in ATP and Mg^{2+}_i are required to induce a substantial inhibition of voltage-activated RyR1 Ca^{2+} release (25); hence, this mechanism would only affect SR Ca^{2+} release during very intense physical activities.

Early studies on isolated RyR1 incorporated in artificial planar lipid bilayers showed a marked inhibition of the RyR1 open probability when pH was lowered to values observed in fatigued muscle fibres (50). However, subsequent studies have shown that normal action potential–induced SR Ca^{2+} release is little, if at all, affected by lowering pH to values observed in acute fatigue (10, 46, 89). In fact, a recent study showed increased tetanic Ca^{2+}_i in acidified human intercostal muscle fibres (61).

Skinned fibre experiments have shown that increased Pi can inhibit depolarization-induced SR Ca^{2+} release by acting on the RyR1 (23, 82). This fits with the finding that inhibition of CK, and hence no major increase in Pi during fatiguing contractions, reduces the rate of fatigue-induced decrease in tetanic Ca^{2+}_i in mouse skeletal muscle (19).

Reduced SR Ca^{2+} Available for Release

Some of the Pi produced during fatiguing contractions may enter the Ca^{2+}-rich SR, where the Ca^{2+}–Pi solubility product might be exceeded, resulting in Ca^{2+}–Pi precipitation and a decreased amount of Ca^{2+} available for release (30) (Figure 5.4). Although direct experimental evidence of this proposed SR Ca^{2+}–Pi precipitation is missing, indirect evidence exists both from experiments on skinned fibres with intact SR exposed to high Pi (23, 24, 30) and intact fibres injected with Pi (88). Moreover, the Ca^{2+}_i increase with high doses of caffeine or 4-chloro-m-cresol (compounds that directly stimulate Ca^{2+} release via RyR1) was reduced in fatigued muscle fibres, indicating decreased Ca^{2+} available for rapid release (40, 87) and the SR free Ca^{2+}, as assessed with low-affinity Ca^{2+} indicators, showed a decline during fatiguing stimulation in both isolated toad muscle fibres and mouse muscle studied in situ (1, 41).

Glycogen Depletion

Exercise capacity is severely compromised when muscle glycogen stores become depleted (98). Within muscle fibres, glycogen is preferentially located in three distinct sub-cellular compartments: subsarcolemmal, intermyofibrillar (i.e., between myofibrils and close to the mitochondria and SR), and intramyofibrillar (i.e., within the contracting myofibrils) (51, 57, 98). Studies using electron microscopy show a preferential depletion of intramyofibrillar glycogen in fatigued muscle fibres from rodents (55, 57) and humans (52, 56, 97). A correlation between reduced SR Ca^{2+} release and depletion in intramyofibrillar, and to some extent intermyofibrillar, glycogen has been observed in fatigued mouse muscle fibres (55), but the exact underlying mechanism(s) remains to be established.

Impaired Myofibrillar Function

During fatiguing isometric contractions, impairments in myofibrillar function are manifested as decreased ability of the actomyosin cross-bridges to generate force and reduced myofibrillar Ca^{2+} sensitivity (2, 20, 87). These two impairments occur early during fatiguing stimulation and decrease force by ~20% at saturating Ca^{2+}_i. The decreased myofibrillar Ca^{2+} sensitivity has a much larger force-depressing effect when Ca^{2+}_i starts to decline in later stages of fatigue, hence entering the steep part of the force–Ca^{2+}_i relationship (2, 20).

Anaerobic metabolism results in accumulation of lactate ions and H^+, mainly due to glycogen breakdown, and of creatine ions and Pi, due to PCr breakdown. Lactate and creatine ions have no major impact on force production (54, 68), whereas increased cytoplasmic concentrations of both H^+ and Pi can inhibit myofibrillar contractile function. Traditionally, the acidosis accompanying "lactic acid" accumulation was considered the major cause of acute fatigue, but this viewpoint is challenged by many studies where acidosis has been shown to be of limited importance (10, 22, 61, 62, 93). Instead increased

Pi is proposed to be the dominant cause of the impaired myofibrillar force production during acute fatigue (1, 17, 90). However, this topic remains controversial, with a major unresolved issue being whether or not the force-reducing effects of elevated Pi in fatigue are amplified by the concomitant acidosis (28, 86).

In addition to reducing force-generating capacity, fatigue-induced impairments in myofibrillar contractile function include a reduced rate of cross-bridge cycling resulting in slowed relaxation and decreased muscle-shortening velocity (2). Both these impairments can have large impact on exercise performance. A slowed relaxation can, for instance, be caused by intracellular acidosis (61), and it may hinder physical exercises involving alternating movements, which includes most types of locomotor activities, since active movements in a joint can be counteracted by continued contractile activity in muscles acting in the opposite direction. A reduced shortening velocity can, for instance, be due to a transiently increased cytoplasmic ADP during contraction of fatigued muscle fibres (91). Acidosis has been shown to decrease the shortening velocity in skinned muscle preparations (21), but it remains controversial whether or not intracellular acidosis is an important mechanism in intact mammalian muscle fibres contracting at physiological temperatures (90). A reduced shortening velocity will, together with a decreased force production, impede the power output (i.e., velocity × force) of the muscle, which will decrease the speed of locomotor activities. It is worth noting that the maximum power produced by muscles occurs at a velocity of ~30% of the maximum shortening velocity. This means that fatigue-induced changes in the curvature of the force–velocity relationship will affect the decline of maximum power output in fatigued muscle; both increased and decreased curvatures have been observed in fatigued muscle, which exaggerate and counteract the decline in maximum power, respectively (45).

Recovery

The decline in contractile force during fatiguing exercise is reversible, although it may take several hours to days for complete recovery. Recovery of contractile force in fatigued muscle can be tested with electrical stimulation in vivo and in vitro. Such tests have revealed that during recovery, the reduction in contractile force is typically more pronounced at low (10–20 Hz) than at high (>70 Hz) stimulation frequencies. This phenomenon was first described in human adductor pollicis muscles (26) and has since been observed in numerous in vivo and in vitro studies (2, 67). It was originally named "low frequency fatigue," but this term has become imprecise because it has been used for many different conditions. Thus, most prefer using the term "prolonged low frequency force depression" (PLFFD). In general, PLFFD can be explained by long-lasting decreases in SR Ca^{2+} release and/or myofibrillar Ca^{2+} sensitivity (2, 67).

Restitution of muscular glycogen stores is essential for recovery after prolonged exercise, and PLFFD is not reversed in the absence of glucose (15). Along the same line, increasing the temperature accelerates glycogen re-synthesis as well as recovery of tetanic Ca^{2+}_i and force in fatigued muscle (15).

The production of RONS in skeletal muscle increases during physical exercise (70). Acutely fatigued type 2 muscle fibres display a marked PLFFD that is mainly caused by decreased SR Ca^{2+} release (11, 14, 84, 85, 92). Intriguingly, the cause of PLFFD changed towards reduced myofibrillar Ca^{2+} sensitivity in genetically modified muscle fibres overexpressing the mitochondrial matrix redox enzyme superoxide dismutase 2 (11) and in muscle fibres exposed to pharmacological antioxidants (14, 84). Thus, these results imply that antioxidants do not prevent PLFFD, but they change the underlying mechanism from impaired SR Ca^{2+} release to reduced myofibrillar Ca^{2+} sensitivity.

Adaptations

Skeletal muscle is a multifaceted tissue which adapts to a wide range of external stimuli (29). Physical exercise induces muscular adaptations that improve contractile performance, whereas physical inactivity causes muscle weakness and reduced contractility. A frequently discussed issue related to muscular adaptation is whether or not physical exercise causes a change in MyHC fibre type, which would be accompanied by altered metabolic and contractile properties as well as fatigue resistance. MyHC switches are commonplace during development and in regenerating muscle cells (77). In order to undergo fibre type changes, adult muscle requires severe stimuli, such as changes in thyroid hormone status or paralysis due to spinal cord injury (66, 77). Training intervention studies, on the other hand, show little to no exercise-induced changes in MyHC fibre type composition, especially between type 1 and type 2 fibres (34). Instead, exercise stimulates several other muscular adaptations that improve contractility and/or reduce fatigability. Resistance training induces muscle fibre hypertrophy, resulting in a larger cross-sectional area and hence higher contractile force due to an increased number of parallel myofibrils (60).

Endurance training mainly causes beneficial adaptations in muscle energy metabolism, including (1) mitochondrial biogenesis and increased oxidative capacity; (2) facilitated fatty acid metabolism, hence preserving glycogen stores during prolonged exercise; (3) enhanced glucose uptake and insulin sensitivity, thereby counteracting deleterious changes associated with the metabolic syndrome and type 2 diabetes; and (4) angiogenesis resulting in improved oxygen delivery to muscle fibres (4, 29). These muscular adaptations can be triggered by hypoxia, increased Ca^{2+}_i at rest, increased reactive oxygen species (ROS) production, and/or changes in the concentration of high energy phosphates (e.g., AMP and ATP) in the muscle fibres (4, 29, 38, 69). Recent studies indicate a central role of RONS signalling in endurance training adaptations, since antioxidant supplementation was found to hamper the beneficial effects of endurance training (32, 69, 71, 75).

A key player in endurance exercise adaptations is the peroxisome proliferator–activated receptor gamma coactivator 1α (PGC-1α), which detects changes in the previously mentioned signalling pathways and interacts with transcription factors to induce protein changes (4, 16). In addition, there is PGC-1α-independent signalling because endurance training–induced changes are also observed in muscles of PGC-1α deficient mice (48).

Conclusions

Acute fatigue develops when energy demand by exercising muscle exceeds aerobic metabolism capacity. Human skeletal muscle contains three MyHC-classified fibre types: type 1, type 2A, and type 2X. These fibre types show substantial differences in their contractile and metabolic properties, which serve the purpose of allowing a range of activities from explosive ballistic movements to energy-preserving endurance activities. Within skeletal muscle, various steps in the activation and contraction processes can fail during induction of fatigue, with decreased SR Ca^{2+} release playing a dominant role in preventing critical ATP depletion within the muscle fibres. Finally, RONS play an important role in the development of PLFFD after fatiguing exercise, as well as in triggering endurance training adaptations in skeletal muscle. By and large, the accumulated experimental evidence forces us to conclude that most aspects of energy metabolism, fatigue development, and muscle adaptations involve multiple and overlapping pathways, which highlights that these processes are too intricate and important to depend on one single molecule or mechanism.

References

1. Allen DG, Clugston E, Petersen Y, Röder IV, Chapman B, Rudolf R. Interactions between intracellular calcium and phosphate in intact mouse muscle during fatigue. *J Apl Physiol* 111: 358–366, 2011.
2. Allen DG, Lamb GD, Westerblad H. Skeletal muscle fatigue: cellular mechanisms. *Physiol Rev* 88: 287–332, 2008.
3. Amann M, Proctor LT, Sebranek JJ, Pegelow DF, Dempsey JA. Opioid-mediated muscle afferents inhibit central motor drive and limit peripheral muscle fatigue development in humans. *J Physiol* 587: 271–283, 2009.

4. Arany Z. PGC-1 coactivators and skeletal muscle adaptations in health and disease. *Curr Opin Genet Dev* 18: 426–434, 2008.
5. Barclay CJ. Modelling diffusive O_2 supply of isolated preparations of mammalian skeletal and cardiac muscle. *J Muscle Res Cell Motil* 26: 225–235, 2005.
6. Barclay CJ, Woledge RC, Curtin NA. Energy turnover for Ca^{2+} cycling in skeletal muscle. *J Muscle Res Cell Motil* 28: 259–274, 2007.
7. Bergström J, Hermansen L, Hultman E, Saltin B. Diet, muscle glycogen and physical performance. *Acta Physiol Scand* 71: 140–150, 1967.
8. Bottinelli R, Reggiani C. Human skeletal muscle fibres: molecular and functional diversity. *Prog Biophys Mol Biol* 73: 195–262, 2000.
9. Bruton J, Tavi P, Aydin J, Westerblad H, and Lännergren J. Mitochondrial and myoplasmic $[Ca^{2+}]$ in single fibres from mouse limb muscles during repeated tetanic contractions. *J Physiol* 551: 179–190, 2003.
10. Bruton JD, Lännergren J, Westerblad H. Effects of CO_2-induced acidification on the fatigue resistance of single mouse muscle fibers at 28°C. *J Appl Physiol* 85: 478–483, 1998.
11. Bruton JD, Place N, Yamada T, Silva JP, Andrade FH, Dahlstedt AJ, et al. Reactive oxygen species and fatigue-induced prolonged low-frequency force depression in skeletal muscle fibres of rats, mice and SOD2 overexpressing mice. *J Physiol* 586: 175–184, 2008.
12. Buchthal F, Schmalbruch H. Motor unit of mammalian muscle. *Physiol Rev* 60: 90–142, 1980.
13. Chasiotis D. The regulation of glycogen phosphorylase and glycogen breakdown in human skeletal muscle. *Acta PhysiolScandSuppl* 518: 1–68, 1983.
14. Cheng AJ, Bruton JD, Lanner JT, Westerblad H. Antioxidant treatments do not improve force recovery after fatiguing stimulation of mouse skeletal muscle fibres. *J Physiol* 593: 457–472, 2015.
15. Cheng AJ, Willis SJ, Zinner C, Chaillou T, Ivarsson N, Ørtenblad N, et al. Post-exercise recovery of contractile function and endurance in humans and mice is accelerated by heating and slowed by cooling skeletal muscle. *J Physiol* 595: 7413–7426, 2017.
16. Correia JC, Ferreira DM, Ruas JL. Intercellular: local and systemic actions of skeletal muscle PGC-1s. *Trends Endocrinol Metab* 26: 305–314, 2015.
17. Dahlstedt A, Katz A, Westerblad H. Role of myoplasmic phosphate in contractile function of skeletal muscle: studies on creatine kinase-deficient mice. *J Physiol* 533: 379–388, 2001.
18. Dahlstedt AJ, Katz A, Wieringa B, Westerblad H. Is creatine kinase responsible for fatigue? Studies of skeletal muscle deficient of creatine kinase. *FASEB J* 14: 982–990, 2000.
19. Dahlstedt AJ, Westerblad H. Inhibition of creatine kinase reduces the rate of fatigue-induced decrease in tetanic $[Ca^{2+}]_i$ in mouse skeletal muscle. *J Physiol* 533: 639–649, 2001.
20. Debold EP. Decreased myofilament calcium sensitivity plays a significant role in muscle fatigue. *Exerc Sport Sci Rev* 44: 144–149, 2016.
21. Debold EP, Fitts RH, Sundberg CW, Nosek TM. Muscle fatigue from the perspective of a single crossbridge. *Med Sci Sports Exerc* 48: 2270–2280, 2016.
22. Degroot M, Massie BM, Boska M, Gober J, Miller RG, Weiner MW. Dissociation of $[H^+]$ from fatigue in human muscle detected by high time resolution ^{31}P-NMR. *Muscle Nerve* 16: 91–98, 1993.
23. Duke AM, Steele DS. Mechanisms of reduced SR Ca^{2+} release induced by inorganic phosphate in rat skeletal muscle fibers. *Am J Physiol Cell Physiol* 281: C418–C429, 2001.
24. Dutka TL, Cole L, Lamb GD. Calcium-phosphate precipitation in the sarcoplasmic reticulum reduces action potential-mediated Ca^{2+} release in mammalian skeletal muscle. *Am J Physiol Cell Physiol* 289: C1502–C1512, 2005.
25. Dutka TL, Lamb GD. Effect of low cytoplasmic [ATP] on excitation-contraction coupling in fast-twitch muscle fibres of the rat. *J Physiol* 560: 451–468, 2004.
26. Edwards RH, Hill DK, Jones DA, Merton PA. Fatigue of long duration in human skeletal muscle after exercise. *J Physiol* 272: 769–778, 1977.
27. Fitts RH. Cellular mechanisms of muscle fatigue. *Physiol Rev* 74: 49–94, 1994.
28. Fitts RH. The role of acidosis in fatigue: pro perspective. *Med Sci Sports Exerc* 48: 2335–2338, 2016.
29. Flück M. Functional, structural and molecular plasticity of mammalian skeletal muscle in response to exercise stimuli. *J Exp Biol* 209: 2239–2248, 2006.
30. Fryer MW, Owen VJ, Lamb GD, Stephenson DG. Effects of creatine phosphate and P_i on Ca^{2+} movements and tension development in rat skinned skeletal muscle fibres. *J Physiol* 482: 123–140, 1995.
31. Gandevia SC. Spinal and supraspinal factors in human muscle fatigue. *Physiol Rev* 81: 1725–1789, 2001.
32. Gomez-Cabrera MC, Domenech E, Romagnoli M, Arduini A, Borras C, Pallardo FV, et al. Oral administration of vitamin C decreases muscle mitochondrial biogenesis and hampers training-induced adaptations in endurance performance. *Am J Clin Nutr* 87: 142–149, 2008.

33. Hardie DG, Sakamoto K. AMPK: a key sensor of fuel and energy status in skeletal muscle. *Physiology (Bethesda)* 21: 48–60, 2006.

34. Harridge SD. Plasticity of human skeletal muscle: gene expression to *in vivo* function. *Exp Physiol* 92: 783–797, 2007.

35. Henriquez-Olguin C, Knudsen JR, Raun SH, Li Z, Dalbram E, Treebak JT, et al. Cytosolic ROS production by NADPH oxidase 2 regulates muscle glucose uptake during exercise. *Nat Commun* 10: 4623, 2019.

36. Holloszy JO. A forty-year memoir of research on the regulation of glucose transport into muscle. *Am J Physiol Endocrinol Metab* 284: E453–E467, 2003.

37. Homsher E. Muscle enthalpy production and its relationship to actomyosin ATPase. *Annu Rev Physiol* 49: 673–690, 1987.

38. Ivarsson N, Mattsson CM, Cheng AJ, Bruton JD, Ekblom B, Lanner JT, et al. SR Ca^{2+} leak in skeletal muscle fibers acts as an intracellular signal to increase fatigue resistance. *J Gen Physiol* 151: 567–577, 2019.

39. Johnson LN. The regulation of protein phosphorylation. *Biochem Soc Trans* 37: 627–641, 2009.

40. Kabbara AA, Allen DG. The role of calcium stores in fatigue of isolated single muscle fibres from the cane toad. *J Physiol* 519: 169–176, 1999.

41. Kabbara AA, Allen DG. The use of fluo-5N to measure sarcoplasmic reticulum calcium in single muscle fibres of the cane toad. *J Physiol* 534: 87–97, 2001.

42. Karatzaferi C, de Haan A, Ferguson RA, van Mechelen W, Sargeant AJ. Phosphocreatine and ATP content in human single muscle fibres before and after maximum dynamic exercise. *Pflügers Arch* 442: 467–474, 2001.

43. Katz A, Sahlin K, Broberg S. Regulation of glucose utilization in human skeletal muscle during moderate dynamic exercise. *Am J Physiol* 260: E411–E415, 1991.

44. Katz A, Westerblad H. Regulation of glycogen breakdown and its consequences for skeletal muscle function after training. *Mamm Genome* 25: 464–472, 2014.

45. Kristensen AM, Nielsen OB, Pedersen TH, Overgaard K. Fatiguing stimulation increases curvature of the force-velocity relationship in isolated fast-twitch and slow-twitch rat muscles. *J Exp Biol* 222: In press, 2019.

46. Lamb GD, Stephenson DG. Effects of intracellular pH and $[Mg^{2+}]$ on excitation-contraction coupling in skeletal muscle fibres of the rat. *J Physiol* 478: 331–339, 1994.

47. Laver DR, Lenz GKE, Lamb GD. Regulation of the calcium release channel from rabbit skeletal muscle by the nucleotides ATP, AMP, IMP and adenosine. *J Physiol* 537: 763–778, 2001.

48. Leick L, Wojtaszewski JF, Johansen ST, Kiilerich K, Comes G, Hellsten Y, et al. PGC-1alpha is not mandatory for exercise- and training-induced adaptive gene responses in mouse skeletal muscle. *Am J Physiol Endocrinol Metab* 294: E463–E474, 2008.

49. Lemon PW, Mullin JP. Effect of initial muscle glycogen levels on protein catabolism during exercise. *J Appl Physiol* 48: 624–629, 1980.

50. Ma J, Fill M, Knudson CM, Campbell KP, Coronado R. Ryanodine receptor of skeletal muscle is a gap junction-type channel. *Science* 242: 99–102, 1988.

51. Marchand I, Chorneyko K, Tarnopolsky M, Hamilton S, Shearer J, Potvin J, et al. Quantification of subcellular glycogen in resting human muscle: granule size, number, and location. *J Appl Physiol* 93: 1598–1607, 2002.

52. Marchand I, Tarnopolsky M, Adamo KB, Bourgeois JM, Chorneyko K, Graham TE. Quantitative assessment of human muscle glycogen granules size and number in subcellular locations during recovery from prolonged exercise. *J Physiol* 580: 617–628, 2007.

53. Meissner G, Darling E, Eveleth J. Kinetics of rapid Ca^{2+} release by sarcoplasmic reticulum. Effects of Ca^{2+}, Mg^{2+}, and adenine nucleotides. *Biochemistry (Mosc)* 25: 236–244, 1986.

54. Murphy RM, Stephenson DG, Lamb GD. Effect of creatine on contractile force and sensitivity in mechanically skinned single fibers from rat skeletal muscle. *Am J Physiol Cell Physiol* 287: C1589–C1595, 2004.

55. Nielsen J, Cheng AJ, Ørtenblad N, Westerblad H. Subcellular distribution of glycogen and decreased tetanic Ca^{2+} in fatigued single intact mouse muscle fibres. *J Physiol* 592: 2003–2012, 2014.

56. Nielsen J, Holmberg HC, Schrøder HD, Saltin B, Ørtenblad N. Human skeletal muscle glycogen utilization in exhaustive exercise: role of subcellular localization and fibre type. *J Physiol* 589: 2871–2885, 2011.

57. Nielsen J, Schrøder HD, Rix CG, Ørtenblad N. Distinct effects of subcellular glycogen localization on tetanic relaxation time and endurance in mechanically skinned rat skeletal muscle fibres. *J Physiol* 587: 3679–3690, 2009.

58. Nielsen OB, de Paoli F, Overgaard K. Protective effects of lactic acid on force production in rat skeletal muscle. *J Physiol* 536: 161–166, 2001.

59. Nielsen OB, de Paoli FV. Regulation of Na^+-K^+ homeostasis and excitability in contracting muscles: implications for fatigue. *Appl Physiol Nutr Metab* 32: 974–984, 2007.

60. Norrbrand L, Fluckey JD, Pozzo M, Tesch PA. Resistance training using eccentric overload induces early adaptations in skeletal muscle size. *Eur J Appl Physiol* 102: 271–281, 2008.

61. Olsson K, Cheng AJ, Al-Ameri M, Wyckelsma VL, Rullman E, Westerblad H, et al. Impaired sarcoplasmic reticulum Ca^{2+} release is the major cause of fatigue-induced force loss in intact single fibres from human skeletal muscle. *J Physiol* Accepted: 2020.

62. Pate E, Bhimani M, Franks-Skiba K, Cooke R. Reduced effect of pH on skinned rabbit psoas muscle mechanics at high temperatures: implications for fatigue. *J Physiol* 486: 689–694, 1995.

63. Pedersen TH, de Paoli F, Nielsen OB. Increased excitability of acidified skeletal muscle: role of chloride conductance. *J Gen Physiol* 125: 237–246, 2005.

64. Pedersen TH, Nielsen OB, Lamb GD, Stephenson DG. Intracellular acidosis enhances the excitability of working muscle. *Science* 305: 1144–1147, 2004.

65. Periasamy M, Kalyanasundaram A. SERCA pump isoforms: their role in calcium transport and disease. *Muscle Nerve* 35: 430–442, 2007.

66. Pette D, Staron RS. Myosin isoforms, muscle fiber types, and transitions. *Microsc Res Tech* 50: 500–509, 2000.

67. Place N, Yamada T, Bruton JD, Westerblad H. Muscle fatigue: from observations in humans to underlying mechanisms studied in intact single muscle fibres. *Eur J Appl Physiol* 110: 1–15, 2010.

68. Posterino GS, Dutka TL, Lamb GD. L. (+)-lactate does not affect twitch and tetanic responses in mechanically skinned mammalian muscle fibres. *Pflügers Arch* 442: 197–203, 2001.

69. Powers SK, Duarte J, Kavazis AN, Talbert EE. Reactive oxygen species are signalling molecules for skeletal muscle adaptation. *Exp Physiol* 95: 1–9, 2010.

70. Powers SK, Jackson MJ. Exercise-induced oxidative stress: cellular mechanisms and impact on muscle force production. *Physiol Rev* 88: 1243–1276, 2008.

71. Ristow M, Zarse K, Oberbach A, Klöting N, Birringer M, Kiehntopf M, et al. Antioxidants prevent health-promoting effects of physical exercise in humans. *Proc Natl Acad Sci U S A* 106: 8665–8670, 2009.

72. Roach PJ. Glycogen and its metabolism. *Curr Mol Med* 2: 101–120, 2002.

73. Sahlin K. Metabolic changes limiting muscle performance. *Int Series Sport Sci* 16: 323–343, 1986.

74. Sahlin K, Tonkonogi M, Söderlund K. Energy supply and muscle fatigue in humans. *Acta Physiol Scand* 162: 261–266, 1998.

75. Sandström ME, Zhang SJ, Bruton J, Silva JP, Reid MB, Westerblad H, et al. Role of reactive oxygen species in contraction-mediated glucose transport in mouse skeletal muscle. *J Physiol* 575: 251–262, 2006.

76. Schiaffino S, Reggiani C. Fiber types in mammalian skeletal muscles. *Physiol Rev* 91: 1447–1531, 2011.

77. Schiaffino S, Sandri M, Murgia M. Activity-dependent signaling pathways controlling muscle diversity and plasticity. *Physiology (Bethesda)* 22: 269–278, 2007.

78. Sidhu SK, Weavil JC, Mangum TS, Jessop JE, Richardson RS, Morgan DE, et al. Group III/IV locomotor muscle afferents alter motor cortical and corticospinal excitability and promote central fatigue during cycling exercise. *Clin Neurophysiol* 128: 44–55, 2017.

79. Smerdu V, Karsch-Mizrachi I, Campione M, Leinwand L, Schiaffino S. Type IIx myosin heavy chain transcripts are expressed in type IIb fibers of human skeletal muscle. *Am J Physiol* 267: C1723–C1728, 1994.

80. Spangenburg EE, Booth FW. Molecular regulation of individual skeletal muscle fibre types. *Acta Physiol Scand* 178: 413–424, 2003.

81. Spriet LL, Watt MJ. Regulatory mechanisms in the interaction between carbohydrate and lipid oxidation during exercise. *Acta Physiol Scand* 178: 443–452, 2003.

82. Steele DS, Duke AM. Metabolic factors contributing to altered Ca^{2+} regulation in skeletal muscle fatigue. *Acta Physiol Scand* 179: 39–48, 2003.

83. Szentesi P, Zaremba R, van Mechelen W, Stienen GJ. ATP utilization for calcium uptake and force production in different types of human skeletal muscle fibres. *J Physiol* 531: 393–403, 2001.

84. Watanabe D, Aibara C, Wada M. Treatment with EUK-134 improves sarcoplasmic reticulum Ca^{2+} release but not myofibrillar Ca^{2+} sensitivity after fatiguing contraction of rat fast-twitch muscle. *Am J Physiol Regul Integr Comp Physiol* 316: R543–R551, 2019.

85. Watanabe D, Kanzaki K, Kuratani M, Matsunaga S, Yanaka N, Wada M. Contribution of impaired myofibril and ryanodine receptor function to prolonged low-frequency force depression after in situ stimulation in rat skeletal muscle. *J Muscle Res Cell Motil* 36: 275–286, 2015.

86. Westerblad H. Acidosis is not a significant cause of skeletal muscle fatigue. *Med Sci Sports Exerc* 48: 2339–2342, 2016.

87. Westerblad H, Allen DG. Changes of myoplasmic calcium concentration during fatigue in single mouse muscle fibers. *J Gen Physiol* 98: 615–635, 1991.

88. Westerblad H, Allen DG. The effects of intracellular injections of phosphate on intracellular calcium and force in single fibres of mouse skeletal muscle. *Pflügers Arch* 431: 964–970, 1996.

89. Westerblad H, Allen DG. The influence of intracellular pH on contraction, relaxation and $[Ca^{2+}]_i$ in intact single fibres from mouse muscle. *J Physiol* 466: 611–628, 1993.

90. Westerblad H, Allen DG, Lännergren J. Muscle fatigue: lactic acid or inorganic phosphate the major cause? *News Physiol Sci* 17: 17–21, 2002.

91. Westerblad H, Dahlstedt AJ, Lännergren J. Mechanisms underlying reduced maximum shortening velocity during fatigue of intact, single fibres of mouse muscle. *J Physiol* 510: 269–277, 1998.

92. Westerblad H, Duty S, Allen DG. Intracellular calcium concentration during low-frequency fatigue in isolated single fibers of mouse skeletal muscle. *J Appl Physiol* 75: 382–388, 1993.

93. Wiseman RW, Kushmerick MJ. Creatine kinase equilibration follows solution thermodynamics in skeletal muscle. 31P NMR studies using creatine analogs. *J Biol Chem* 270: 12428–12438, 1995.

94. Zhang SJ, Andersson DC, Sandström ME, Westerblad H, Katz A. Cross-bridges account for only 20% of total ATP consumption during submaximal isometric contraction in mouse fast-twitch skeletal muscle. *Am J Physiol Cell Physiol* 291: C147–C154, 2006.

95. Zhang SJ, Bruton JD, Katz A, Westerblad H. Limited oxygen diffusion accelerates fatigue development in mouse skeletal muscle. *J Physiol* 572: 551–559, 2006.

96. Zhang SJ, Sandström ME, Aydin J, Westerblad H, Wieringa B, Katz A. Activation of glucose transport and AMP-activated protein kinase during muscle contraction in adenylate kinase-1 knockout mice. *Acta Physiol (Oxf)* 192: 413–420, 2008.

97. Ørtenblad N, Nielsen J, Saltin B, Holmberg HC. Role of glycogen availability in sarcoplasmic reticulum Ca2+ kinetics in human skeletal muscle. *J Physiol* 589: 711–725, 2011.

98. Ørtenblad N, Westerblad H, Nielsen J. Muscle glycogen stores and fatigue. *J Physiol* 591: 4405–4413, 2013.

6

MECHANOTRANSDUCTION MECHANISMS OF HYPERTROPHY AND PERFORMANCE WITH RESISTANCE EXERCISE

Andrew C. Fry, Justin X. Nicoll, and Luke A. Olsen

Introduction

When the world-renowned Italian scientist Luigi Galvani discovered that an electrical spark could cause a frog muscle to contract, the flood gates opened on the world of skeletal muscle physiology (51). While at first glance it may seem that Galvani's famous experiment from the late 1700s has only led to slow progress over the last quarter-millennium, one must realize what the prevailing theories had previously been concerning how muscle works. Over the centuries, scientists had struggled with numerous ideas as to how skeletal muscle could function as efficiently as it does within the human body. By the time of Galvani's experiment, the dominant thought was that nervous aethers would fill the muscles, thus causing contraction and relaxation (113). What exactly these aethers were was unknown, but clearly the nerves were contributing to a muscle action. As with many ground-breaking discoveries, Galvani's findings led to much progress in many related scientific disciplines. For example, Alessandro Volta took some of Galvani's concepts and eventually developed the electric battery. Also, as you might imagine, Galvani's work inspired impassioned debate among members of the scientific community, as many found his novel theory of muscle activation unbelievable. Nonetheless, we can clearly see in retrospect that much has evolved in our understanding of skeletal muscle physiology, and much remains to be discovered.

This chapter will take a close look at the rapidly emerging field of mechanotransduction in skeletal muscle. The term "transduction" refers to the conversion of a message or energy from one form to another. Since the function of skeletal muscle is specifically to contract and develop force, how does the muscle cell convert these mechanical forces to an intracellular signal? And how might these signals influence the muscle phenotype, size, and performance? In this chapter, we will specifically examine the muscle forces that are developed during resistance exercise. As you will soon read, we will first present an overview of what is currently known about mechanotransduction in skeletal muscle. This is followed by a brief presentation of what resistance exercise is in its many forms, followed by a description of what current research tells us about how resistance exercise uses mechanotransduction in the adaptation process. Finally, we will attempt to integrate the mechanotransduction system with other well-studied physiological systems that help regulate the activity of skeletal muscle. It is imperative that we not examine mechanotransduction in isolation, especially since the successful performance of skeletal muscle is so dependent on numerous physiological systems working in highly organized synchrony with each other.

Andrew C. Fry, Justin X. Nicoll, and Luke A. Olsen

Overview of Mechanotransduction

Life on earth has evolved in the presence of a constant gravitational force, 9.8 m/s^2 to be exact. Like all evolutionary selective pressures, this specific stimulus necessitated both unicellular and multicellular organisms to sense and respond to its physical environment in a concerted, functional manner. Throughout time, the human body has done just that; it has developed structures such as the otoliths in hair cells to sense gravity and maintain equilibrium; it has equipped cells with a structural framework to sense and transmit changes in cellular tension such as the cytoskeleton; and it has developed small contractile units, such as the sarcomere, as a means to overcome gravitational force and allow locomotion through muscle contraction (127). Thus, the evolution of mechanosensation and transduction is at the foundation of cellular communication. While the significance of cellular mechanotransduction is readily agreed, the mechanisms through which the cell, and more specifically the muscle cell, can respond to an external stimulus is still under intense investigation. Mechanotransduction, defined as the ability of a cell to sense and respond to a mechanical stimulus (78), can be separated into two non-exclusive pathways; specifically, biochemical and biophysical mechanotransduction.

Biophysical mechanotransduction can be viewed as the cell's ability to sense a mechanical stimulus and propagate that stimulus throughout the interior of the cell through its structural network, most notably the cytoskeleton (86). The cytoskeleton can be thought of as the cell's scaffolding system, which provides physical support, maintains cellular integrity, and allows for physical continuity with the cell's exterior. The cytoskeleton is a dynamic structure composed of microtubules, actin filaments, and intermediate filaments, all of which change their orientation and content dependent upon internal and external cues (26). Along with enhanced structural integrity, the cytoskeleton permits a mode of rapid force propagation along its framework, allowing force transmission from one part of the cell to opposing ends within a matter of milliseconds, all in lieu of biochemical signalling. First, however, the cell must sense this mechanical perturbation. This is made possible by transmembrane proteins housed at the cellular plasma membrane, such as the integrin.

The family of integrin proteins, 24 in all, are heterodimeric consisting of 18 α and 8 β subunits (13). As transmembrane proteins, the integrin physically connects the extracellular matrix to the intracellular space. Within the cell, the integrin indirectly connects to the actin cytoskeleton through scaffolding proteins positioned at the integrin's cytoplasmic tail such as talin, kindlin, and paxillin. Thus, through its transmembrane nature, the integrin allows communication in a bidirectional manner—both in an inside-out and outside-in fashion (96). Interestingly, research has shed light upon the extended physical continuity from the cytoskeleton into the nucleus, made possible by the linker of the nucleoskeleton and cytoskeleton (LINC) complex (109). This continuous physical link from the extracellular space, through the integrin to the cytoskeleton, and into the nucleus via the LINC complex, directly influences gene expression in a matter of seconds upon mechanical activity, such as muscle tension produced with exercise.

While the role of biophysical mechanotransduction has proven integral to cellular signalling, technical analysis has just recently become available to test this phenomenon in vivo. Thus, its exact mode of dynamics following muscle activity has yet to be delineated. An area with greater research is the field of biochemical mechanotransduction which, compared to biophysical mechanotransduction, is the conversion of a mechanical stimulus into an intracellular biochemical response. Like their ability to transmit force, integrins work in a similar biochemical signalling fashion. Upon elevated mechanical tension and subsequent integrin activation, a number of signalling proteins translocate to the integrin's cytoplasmic tail and form focal adhesion complexes. These focal adhesions can comprise hundreds of proteins, both structural and signalling alike, with many influencing intracellular metabolism, primarily through regulating protein synthesis via mechanistic target of rapamycin complex 1 (mTORC1), coined the master regulator of protein synthesis (101). However, others have shown that mechanically sensitive proteins can work in an mTORC1-independent fashion, lending biochemical mechanotransduction as an incredibly intricate, yet diverse, means of cellular signalling.

These forms of mechanotransduction, whether biophysical or biochemical, do not work in isolation from one another. Rather, they are highly integrated, resulting in a functional response. Of specific interest in this chapter is the role that resistance exercise has upon these two forms of mechanotransduction, ultimately influencing cellular metabolism.

What is Resistance Exercise?

Any time a physiological system's responses to a stimulus are studied, it is imperative to understand and describe the properties of the stimulus. This holds true for heavy resistance exercise. It is not unusual that responses to resistance exercise sessions or chronic training programs are simply all grouped together, with little to no appreciation for the unique characteristics of the original stimuli. Since mechanotransduction is the process of converting mechanical stimuli into cellular and molecular responses, this is particularly critical for our discussion of the mechanotransduction system of skeletal muscle.

Performance Variables

To correctly study the cellular responses to mechanical forces, we must first know the exact kinetics and kinematics of the training programme. Although these properties are not always readily apparent or easy to discern, the following are a few of the performance factors to account for:

- Force (including torque)
- Power
- Velocity
- Rate of force development
- Explosive strength deficit (aka, dynamic strength deficit, dynamic strength index; compares task-specific strength with maximal strength)
- Reactive strength index (measure of ability to transition from eccentric to concentric muscle actions rapidly; requires high eccentric strength)

Acute and Chronic Training Variables

The actual resistance exercise training stimulus, both for a single session and for long-term or chronic training, are many and varied. Table 6.1 lists some of the factors to consider, and which in many cases, appear to be critical for the resulting physiological responses. While most practitioners (i.e., coaches, trainers, therapists) have a practical appreciation of these options, it is vital that the scientists studying mechanotransduction appreciate the idiosyncrasies of the various resistance exercise protocols as well. However, the multiple types of resistance exercises possible are too many and varied to describe in detail in this chapter, so the reader is referred to several excellent sources for detailed study (10, 46, 62, 143, 162, 186). Table 6.1 lists several factors believed to be particularly important, which must be considered or accounted for when studying the role of mechanotransduction during resistance exercise.

Table 6.1 Resistance exercise training–related variables important for mechanotransduction

Variables	Considerations
Performance measures	Force (including torque), power, velocity, rate of force development, explosive strength deficit, reactive strength index
Choice of exercise	
Muscle involvement	1° movers, 2° movers, antagonists
Modality	Free weights, machines, isokinetic, other devices, body weight
Velocity of movement	Normal, fast, slow, stretch-shortening cycle
Muscle actions	Concentric, eccentric, isometric, isokinetic, isoinertial, impact
Order of exercise	Can influence fatigue and neural activation patterns
Volume of exercise	Total repetitions, volume-load (reps × weight), work (J)
Intensity of exercise (load)	Absolute load (kg or lb), relative (% RM)
Interset rest interval	Long (>2 or 3 min), typical (approx. 1 min), short (<30 sec), no rest
Chronic training variables	Frequency, duration, periodized and type of periodization, auto-regulation
Purpose of the training	Hypertrophy, strength, power, speed, rehabilitation/therapy, general fitness, peak performance
Other factors	Animal or human subjects, subject training status (prior history), age, sex, activities outside the study, diet and nutrition, metabolic demands and fatigue, endocrine responses and adaptations, diurnal factors, presence of PEDs, correct exercise techniques

Adaptations to Resistance Exercise

Hypertrophy

Chronic resistance exercise increases muscular hypertrophy, strength, contraction velocity, and structural architecture (47). These phenotypic adaptations improve sport and occupational performances, as well as quality of living and successful aging. While a plethora of research supports the use of resistance exercise to improve muscular adaptations for sport and quality of daily living, the molecular underpinnings of these adaptations remain less clear. The foremost studied of these pathways is the protein kinase B (Akt)/mechanistic target of rapamycin (mTOR) cascade (155). Relevant data from the last two decades have established this pathway as a central regulator of nutrient sensitivity, protein synthesis, and mechanotransduction (70). Another family of signalling proteins called the mitogen-activated protein kinase (MAPK) pathway converge on Akt/mTOR and regulate many of its downstream substrates (45, 100, 111, 118, 148, 175, 181). However, investigations in humans and intact skeletal muscle require further elucidation, since the crosstalk between these two pathways has not been clearly defined. Recent evidence indicates differential MAPK/mTOR signalling depends on the resistance exercise load, volume (i.e., number of contractions), and rest intervals (17, 56, 114, 169). Further, their responses also depend on the training status of the individual (i.e., untrained vs. highly trained) (30, 59). The differential activation of these pathways may be related to the altered differential rates of protein synthesis, recovery, and translational capacity reported between resistance training–naïve and resistance training–accustomed individuals (167, 179).

Early studies have primarily utilized insulin-like growth factor-1 (IGF-1) administration to investigate the role MAPK and mTOR signalling may contribute to adaptation (61). In particular, the responses of MAPK suggest they might be involved in mechanotransduction and contraction-mediated muscle hypertrophy (21, 112, 183). Of these, extracellular signal–regulated kinase (ERK) has been the most investigated MAPK in relation to muscle hypertrophy. While the primary regulator of protein synthesis appears to be mTOR downstream substrates, including p70S6K and S6 protein, the ERK pathway can phosphorylate the aforementioned proteins during signal transduction (188). Although there have been correlations between p70S6K phosphorylation and muscle hypertrophy (169), there have been no direct correlations between the ERK pathway and muscle growth in humans. Instead, it appears that contraction-induced activation of ERK may "prime" the translational machinery for translation initiation and elongation (181). It should also be noted that hypertrophy of muscle fibres may not always be synonymous with proportional increases in sarcomere components (i.e., actin and myosin), since high-volume resistance training in trained men reportedly resulted in fibre hypertrophy but dilution of contractile components (change in fibre size was not proportional to a change in myofibrillar proteins) (68). Hypertrophy of the sarcoplasm (but not contractile components) was previously reported in a cross-sectional study of contractile properties of untrained subjects, bodybuilders, and power athletes (115). Furthermore, the degree of fibre hypertrophy to a resistance training programme may be partially determined by the nature of the resistance training programme (50), and possibly the predominant fibre type and the size of those fibres prior to training (69). Further work is needed to examine the concepts of compartmentalized hypertrophy (i.e., sarcoplasmic vs. myofibrillar).

Fibre Composition

Specificity of resistance training elicits specific adaptations in skeletal muscle (136). Myosin heavy chain (MHC) isoform expression changes following chronic resistance training (50). Normally there is an isoform shift from MHC IIx to MHC IIa following chronic training (3, 158). Cell culture models indicate MAPK may mediate MHC isoform expression (116, 117). Immobilization or decreased contractile activity increases MHC IIx expression. High-velocity resistance exercise with increasing amounts of fatigue decreases MHC IIx expression (136). However, decreased MHC IIx expression also increases in response to muscle hypertrophy due to the increased total training volume performed (136).

Murgia et al. (125) showed that low-frequency electrical stimulation increases ERK activity and in conjunction with a constitutively active Ras (upstream of ERK) promotes a slow fibre program. Given that ERK activity is sensitive to the amount and pattern of imposed demands on muscle, these authors suggested ERK might serve as an "activity sensor" that regulates transcriptional events that coordinate slow phenotype adaptations. Conversely, Shi et al. (149) reported greater ERK expression in fast muscle fibres, and more importantly, the presence of ERK signalling actually promoted the fast phenotype (153). Additionally, fibre-specific hypertrophy in response to ERK signalling is influenced by β-agonist activity (152). Thus, the role of ERK in muscle phenotype expression is not clear. It is likely that coordination with other signalling mechanisms and factors contributes to these responses.

Myonuclei

Chronic resistance training increases the hypertrophy of muscle fibres (50). Muscle fibre hypertrophy stimulates the accretion of new myonuclei into the fibre (139). The addition of myonuclei originates from resident stem cells called satellite cells. Satellite cells respond to muscle disruption or damage, and their expansion serves to assist in fibre repair from injury and support hypertrophy as newly incorporated myonuclei following chronic resistance training (35). The threshold of hypertrophy required for the incorporation of a new myonuclei into the fibre is unclear, since myonuclear accretion has been reported in hypertrophy ranges of 10–22% increase in size from pre-training (31). Thus, the myonuclear domain appears to be more flexible than originally hypothesized (123). Furthermore, the accretion of myonuclei, hypertrophy, and the activation of satellite cells are genetically determined, since there is evidence of high versus low responders of muscle hypertrophy that is partly mediated by satellite cell content and expansion (139). Individuals who displayed the greatest hypertrophy to a resistance training programme also had the greatest number of satellite cells prior to training and were able to recruit more satellite cells during the training period. Furthermore, most, but not all, evidence suggests that myonuclei gained during growth are not lost after a period of detraining and atrophy (151). The ability for newly gained myonuclei to persist after a period of atrophy or deconditioning may contribute to faster hypertrophic responses observed upon retraining.

Ribosome Biogenesis

Besides the mechanism of increasing ribosome assembly and translation initiation, the activation of early immediate genes from MAPK further regulates increases in ribosomal biogenesis (14, 161). Thus, the short-term activation post exercise to increase indices and assembly of ribosomal proteins for protein synthesis also activates translational capacity. This increase in ribosome biogenesis from mechanical overload appears to be partially mTOR independent (60, 175) and suggestive of ERK/ MAPK involvement. Importantly, the MAPK pathway appears necessary for the maintenance of muscle mass via ERK and c-Jun N-terminal kinases (JNK) by sensitizing and integrating contraction and IGF-1 mediated stimuli into muscle hypertrophy (61, 111, 154). Although it is clear now that increased ribosome biogenesis from chronic resistance exercise supports enhanced translational capacity (14, 45), in vitro data suggest ribosome biogenesis alone is not the sole determinant of IGF-1-mediation of muscle hypertrophy (33). Finally, like satellite cell responses to resistance training, the expansion of ribosome biogenesis following chronic resistance exercise appears to be genetically determined, since recent data suggest older individuals who experience the greatest hypertrophy to a resistance training programme have faster ribosome biogenesis responses early in the training programme (159).

Mechanotransduction Responses to Resistance Exercise

What hopefully is now readily apparent is the complex nature of resistance exercise. More specifically, the harmonious nature through which the body responds to exercise and the many variables that must be taken into consideration. We will now specifically highlight resistance exercise-driven mechanotransduction within the muscle fibre (Figure 6.1). At any point in time, humans must overcome an overload stimulus. Even gravity (9.8 m/s^2), as discussed earlier, provides a stimulus influencing mechanical tension within individual muscle fibres. A readily apparent example of this are the postural muscles of the spine (paraspinal) and lower limbs (soleus), which are chronically active to support the body in an upright position when walking, sitting, and, in some cases, while lying down. Thus, even in what would be considered a relaxed state, mechanical tension and, hence, mechanotransduction within our muscle fibres, is taking place. However, resistance exercise presents a unique mechanical stimulus, capable of creating an ever-increasing load one must overcome and, subsequently, increasing the degree to which mechanotransduction plays a role.

Resistance exercise is well-known to increase muscle size, force production, and improve tissue integrity. Research spanning decades has actively pursued the underlying mechanisms regulating such adaptations. The majority have focused on dynamic intracellular biochemical signalling cascades, many of which arise from endocrine and paracrine factors such as insulin and testosterone, as previously mentioned. However, work has shed light on the largely permissive nature of these signalling factors upon exercise and muscle growth (177). Indeed, the degree of mechanical tension generated within a given muscle fibre has gained in popularity concerning its role as the primary regulator of muscle growth following resistance exercise.

Biochemical Mechanotransduction

Mechanical tension resulting from resistance exercise and subsequent muscle fibre anabolism takes place through two primary mechanisms influencing protein synthesis: an mTORC1-dependent pathway and an mTORC1-independent pathway. Following elevated mechanical tension and subsequent recruitment of the transmembrane $\alpha 7\beta 1$ integrin, both mTORC1-dependent and -independent signalling ensue (13). mTORC1-dependent signalling following resistance exercise works in part through the focal adhesion kinase (FAK) protein (88). With mechanical tension, FAK translocates to the cytoplasmic tail of the beta-1 integrin subunit. While the integrin lacks catalytic activity, the increased mechanical tension leads to FAK autophosphorylation at residue Thr397. Phosphorylated FAK can then translocate to the lysosome and indirectly activate mTORC1 via phosphorylating and subsequently inhibiting the protein tuberous sclerosis complex 2 (TSC2). TSC2 is a well-documented antagonist of mTORC1 through maintaining the protein ras homologue enriched in brain (Rheb) in a GDP-bound state, unable to activate mTORC1 (94). In a GTP-bound state, mTORC1 and Rheb interact, positively regulating mTORC1 signalling, much of which takes place upon the previously mentioned lysosome. Thus, with heightened mechanical tension and integrin-induced FAK phosphorylation and subsequent translocation, TSC2 can become inhibited leading to Rheb transitioning from a GDP- to GTP-bound state, ultimately activating mTORC1. However, recent findings question this proposed role of integrin-induced FAK autophosphorylation and mTORC1 activation, thus requiring further investigation. Interestingly, novel mechanically sensitive phosphorylation sites upon TSC2 have been revealed following eccentric muscle contractions, all of which were necessary for mTORC1 signalling and protein synthesis (82). The enzymes responsible for this phosphorylation of TSC2 have yet to be identified. Nonetheless, it is clear that maximal mechanical tension activates mTORC1 through the phosphorylation and inhibition of TSC2 and subsequent mTORC1-induced increase in protein synthesis.

Mechanotransduction not only influences lysosome-mediated protein signalling, such as the TSC2–Rheb–mTORC1 complex, but also regulates the spatial characteristics of the lysosome. Maximal muscle contraction stimulates lysosomal translocation to the muscle membrane through an unestablished mechanism (72). It is likely, however, that this positioning is partially driven via microtubule dynamics following resistance exercise–induced mechanical stimulation. This lysosomal movement allows lysosome-bound proteins, namely mTORC1, Rheb, and other mTORC1-regulating proteins, to reside in close proximity to the influx of amino acids and growth-related hormones: a demonstration of mechanotransduction and endocrine/paracrine and nutrient integration.

The recruitment of mTORC1 to the lysosome may influence its activity through other mechanisms than those mentioned previously; specifically, through the lipid second messenger phosphatidic acid (PA). PA can directly activate mTORC1 through binding to its FKBP12-binding domain (184). Interestingly, phosphatidic acid increases following exercise and accumulates through the mechanosensitive properties of its upstream enzyme diacylglycerol kinase zeta (DGKζ) and phospholipase D (PLD). Indeed, the inhibition of these two enzymes attenuated mechanically driven muscle growth, while the overexpression of either PLD or DGKζ resulted in muscle hypertrophy. Moreover, PA localizes around the lysosome rendering it in close proximity to mTORC1. Outside of its ability to interact with mTORC1, PA also mediates the activity of the energy-sensing HIPPO pathway via indirect activation of yes-associated protein (YAP) through inhibition of its downstream inhibitor, long-acting thyroid stimulator (LATS) (65). Following this physical activity–induced decrease in YAP inhibition, YAP can then translocate to the nucleus, directly regulating the expression of hypertrophic genes.

While mTORC1 is coined the master regulator of protein synthesis and is required for muscle growth following resistance exercise, other means of fine-tuning the highly dynamic and diverse protein synthesis machinery in an mTORC1-independent manner is becoming increasingly appreciated. One such mechanism is the biophysical mechanotransducing properties of the cytoskeleton. The cytoskeleton is an incredibly dynamic system altering structural orientation dependent upon both internal (sarcomeric force generation) and external (extracellular matrix force propagation) mechanical stimuli. Early work from the Ingber Lab at Harvard University demonstrated cytoskeletal reorientation following physical stimulation of the integrin (109). It was also revealed that messenger ribonucleic acid (mRNA), ribosomal RNA (rRNA), and proteins are immobilized upon the cytoskeleton and focal adhesion complex, ultimately becoming activated following integrin-mediated mechanical stimulation (26).

Post-translation modifications appear to similarly be regulated by cytoskeletal tension, such as phosphorylation of Src proteins (a cytoplasmic protein–tyrosine kinase) within milliseconds of integrin-driven cytoskeletal tension and force propagation (126). Heightened cytoskeletal tension also influences the mechanotransducer YAP in a similar fashion as that mentioned with PA. Upon increased cytoskeletal tension, YAP dephosphorylates and subsequently translocates to the nucleus increasing transcription of a subset of anabolic genes (64).

Not only does the plasma membrane house transmembrane proteins, such as the integrins, to physically connect the intracellular space with the extracellular matrix (ECM), the nucleus and its double membrane are also composed of transmembrane protein complexes, termed LINC. These allow for the direct physical continuity between the cytoskeleton and the deoxyribonucleic acid (DNA) (49). Thus, taking a distant view of the muscle cell, a continuous physical link can be observed from the ECM through the integrin to the cytoskeleton, and then from the cytoskeleton to the DNA via the nuclear membrane LINC complex. With this in mind, resistance exercise is likely to influence transcription dramatically through force propagation sensed through the structural framework of the muscle fibre. This biophysical communication system was elegantly demonstrated by pulling on the integrin and observing nuclear chromatin remodelling (163). Indeed, upon integrin stimulation, chromatin stretching was observed with rapid transcription ensuing. Thus, the ability of a cell to sense a mechanical perturbation at its membrane and propagate this signal to the nucleus in a tension-dependent manner is crucial. The cytoskeleton plays an integral role in nuclear mechanotransduction, as the ablation of the most abundant skeletal muscle cytoskeletal filament desmin leads to a reduced nuclear flattening upon muscle fibre stretching (135). This area of biophysical mechanotransduction appears paramount, as resistance exercise increases both integrin and cytoskeletal protein content, ultimately influencing cellular tension–based signalling and biophysical nuclear signalling.

Sarcomeric Mechanotransduction

The sarcomere, while readily apparent as a force generator, can equally be viewed as a mechanosensor and ultimate signaller influencing gene expression and protein synthesis in response to resistance exercise. The sarcomere physically connects both the nuclear and cellular membrane via the cytoskeletal protein desmin (4), rendering each cross-bridge cycle generated from a given sarcomere to be sensed throughout the nucleus, sarcoplasm, and ECM via desmin–transmembrane protein complexes and hence, sarcomeric-induced biophysical mechanotransduction. On the other hand, sarcomeric-driven biochemical mechanotransduction is proposed to largely work through proteins immobilized upon the z-disc (147). For example, during a cross-bridge cycle, a myriad of proteins become active and translocate away from the sarcomeric z-disc to both the cellular membrane and the nucleus so as to induce a signalling cascade and/or provide structural support. Of the proteins translocating to the nucleus, the protein Trip22 was found to co-localize with Mef2c, and this protein complex provided a link from the DNA to the nuclear pore complex (NPC) (34). The NPC is the site of mRNA export. Thus, providing close proximity of a given DNA sequence to the NPC renders improved nuclear cytoplasmic shuttling and subsequent mRNA translation. Moreover, this specific means of DNA tethering to the NPC, as revealed by D'Angelo (34), is required for muscle growth. This ability of the nucleus to sense sarcomeric mechanical stimuli and convert them into genomic reorganization so as to positively regulate a subset of muscle development genes gives direct insight into the highly integrated cellular mechanotransducing system (27).

Skeletal Muscle Force Transmission

The ability of a single muscle fibre to produce force is largely dependent upon many of the structural proteins previously discussed. As mentioned earlier, the force-generating unit of the skeletal muscle is the sarcomere. The sarcomere can transmit force in two directions, laterally (perpendicular to the

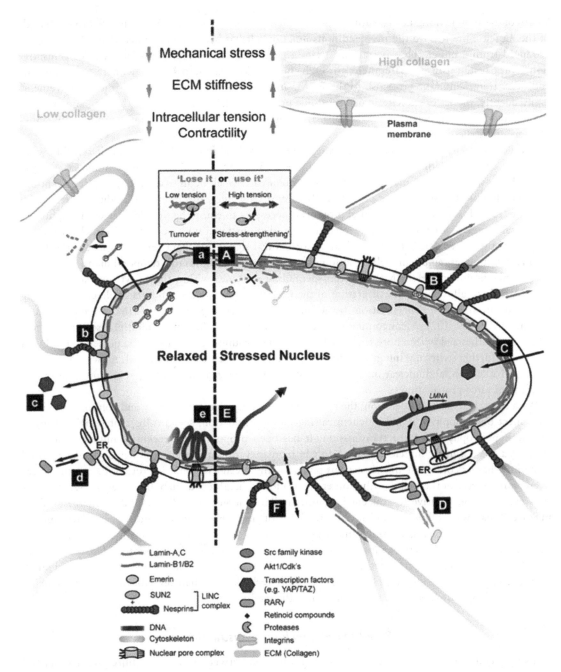

Figure 6.1 Cellular mechanotransduction

Schematic representation of continuity between thee extracellular matrix, cytoskeleton, and nuclear matrix. Emphasis is placed on nuclear mechanotransduction in both a "stressed" and "relaxed" state and how this may influence internuclear signaling dynamics. From Cho S, Irianto J, Discher DE. Mechanosensing by the nucleus: From pathways to scaling relationships. J Cell Biol 216(2):305–315, 2017

length of the muscle fibre, i.e., toward the plasma membrane) and longitudinally (parallel to the length of the muscle fibre toward the myotendinous junction). It has been demonstrated that ~80% of force produced from a muscle fibre is transmitted in a lateral direction (142). This lateral force transmission is propagated from the sarcomere, through the cytoskeleton, across the costamere (i.e., integrins and other transmembrane proteins), to the ECM, and ultimately to the tendon to initiate movement. Consequently, modes of exercise which reinforce proteins within these lateral pathways, namely those most active during eccentric muscle actions, are proposed to improve muscle force production, transmission, and structural integrity.

Eccentric exercise produces a rapid decrease in the cytoskeletal protein desmin immediately following resistance exercise, with a subsequent 3-fold increase 5–7 days later (5). Woolstenhulme et al. (182) similarly showed a gradual increase in desmin content each week of an 8-week training intervention. The muscle fibre transmembrane protein $\alpha 7\beta 1$ integrin also increases following traditional resistance exercise (13). This increase in structural proteins is necessary to equip the muscle fibre with heightened structural integrity for further force propagation, as demonstrated with conditional knockout models revealing augmented force transmission and biochemical signalling characteristics. Indeed, the ECM similarly undergoes rapid remodelling following a mechanical stimulus in a temporal manner. Initially, matrix metalloproteinases (MMPs), protein-degrading enzymes within the ECM, increase in abundance largely to allow necessary migration of the fibroblast, satellite cell, and macrophages. Following this acute rise in MMP concentration, tissue inhibitors of metalloproteinases (TIMPs) are elevated to inhibit MMPs (89, 107). A concomitant increase in ECM proteins, such as multiple isoforms of collagen, are synthesized within both the muscle fibre and surrounding cells and are exported to the ECM to provide further structural integrity. This enhanced protein content of the ECM, muscle fibre membrane, cytoskeleton, and nuclear membrane allow for an improved means of rapid communication via biophysical force propagation.

With this taken into consideration, the mode of exercise concerning intensity and volume will markedly affect both biophysical and biochemical mechanotransduction, specifically, that which relates to muscle hypertrophy and force transmission. It has been proposed that eccentric muscle actions, as compared to concentric muscle actions, result in increased transmembrane and cytoskeletal structural proteins, whereas concentric muscle actions preferentially recruit sarcomeric proteins due to the active overcoming forces of the muscle. Eliasson et al. (42) found heightened anabolic signalling with eccentric muscle actions relative to concentric. Similarly, Hornberger et al. (75) found an increase of the mTORC1 pathway following multiaxial stretching of myotubes, which simulates eccentric muscle action relative to uniaxial stretching simulating concentric. There are many likely mechanisms driving this differential response between mode of muscle action, such as muscle disruption or damage, levels of circulating inflammatory cytokines, canonical intracellular anabolic signalling, and the proposed direct force transmission to the nucleus. However, one often overlooked mechanism is the mechanotransducing properties of the muscle-specific stem cell termed the satellite cell.

Satellite Cell Mechanotransduction

In its quiescent state, the satellite cell remains positioned between the muscle fibre sarcolemma and basal lamina. Upon stimulation, the satellite cell initially proliferates, with a subset of these cells differentiating into a phenotype similar to a myoblast, ultimately fusing with the muscle fibre (124). The satellite cell, similar to the muscle fibre, is composed of integrins spanning its membrane, and these, too, are highly sensitive to mechanical perturbation leading to cytoskeletal rearrangement and an altered tension state (55). Interestingly, the cytoskeletal-sensitive protein YAP regulates satellite cell fate primarily through influencing satellite cell proliferation, enhancing muscle fibre regeneration (83). As previously mentioned, YAP is highly responsive to change in cytoskeletal tension such that an increase in tension leads to YAP translocation to the nucleus and a subsequent increase in muscle growth–related genes. Similarly, the dystrophin–glycoprotein complex which, similar to the integrin protein spans the cell membrane and provides structural integrity, is required for satellite cell activation (24). Thus, mechanical tension plays an integral role in muscle tissue regeneration and growth via the satellite cell, and these biophysical mechanotransducing properties of the satellite cell may be one mechanism through which satellite cells are preferentially recruited following eccentric exercise.

Role of Resistance Exercise Intensity on Mechanotransduction

Exercise intensity, here defined as the percentage of a person's one-repetition maximum (1RM), directly influences the response and ultimate adaptation of skeletal muscle (Figure 6.2). Indeed, mechanotransducing pathways are thought to be minimally active following low-intensity resistance exercise (less than 50% of the 1RM), whereas high-intensity exercise (greater than 75% of the 1RM) is required for mechanotransduction. In support of this, the beta-1 integrin subunit was shown to be phosphorylated exclusively following maximal resistance exercise, whereas integrin phosphorylation remained unaffected following low-intensity exercise (66). Similarly, the steroidogenic acute regulatory protein (STAR) pathway, a key regulator of cytoskeletal turnover, also increased to a greater degree following acute resistance exercise relative to endurance exercise (93). However, while this was observed in trained subjects, untrained subjects showed no difference in STAR dynamics whether performing endurance or resistance exercise, thus demonstrating one's training status, whether novice or advanced, as a likely contributor. Moreover, a small heat shock protein integral to cytoskeletal integrity, αB-crystallin (CRYAB), was phosphorylated in an intensity-specific manner (81). Specifically, while endurance exercise increased CRYAB to a similar degree as high-intensity exercise, specifically in slow-twitch muscle fibres, CRYAB phosphorylation within fast-twitch fibres was found to be greater following high-intensity exercise. With this in mind, low-intensity exercise carried out to

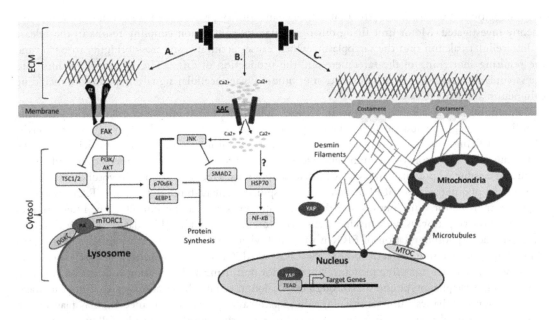

Figure 6.2   Mechanotransduction following resistance exercise

Schematic representation of resistance exercise-mediated mechanotransduction. A: Demonstration of biochemical mechanotransduction via integrin activation and subsequent FAK-mTORC1 signaling. B: Calcium stretch-activated channels regulating MAPK and heat shock proteins. C: Biophysical mechanotransduction via force propagation through transmembrane complexes (costameres) along microtubules and intermediate filaments, to surrounding organelles such as the mitochondria and nucleus

failure has recently shown to recruit both slow- and fast-twitch muscle fibres (121), leading to speculation as to whether maximal loads are required for heightened muscle fibre mechanotransduction. It may be that the degree to which exercise intensity influences mechanotransduction drastically differs between biophysical and biochemical mechanotransduction, with the latter being more responsive to a range of exercise intensity, whereas biophysical mechanotransduction requires a heightened stimulus for activation.

Thus, the role of resistance exercise–initiated mechanotransduction upon cellular anabolism and muscle hypertrophy cannot be understated. While most research has focused on biochemical signalling driven by various hormones, the muscle fibre is equipped with an intrinsic capacity to respond and transduce mechanical perturbation. Future work is required to extrapolate the effect of different modes of exercise, namely intensity, volume, and muscle action, and the likely ability of the muscle fibre to uniquely sense these diverse stimuli. Similarly, the mechanotransducing characteristics of the muscle fibre progenitors, termed satellite cells, is likely crucial for their responsiveness

Mechanotransduction Integration with Other Physiological Systems

It may be easy for the reader to conclude that mechanotransduction is the major contributor to skeletal muscle hypertrophy and adaptation. However, it is important to note that, as with many physiological systems, there is much integration and synergy among the numerous mechanisms of biological adaptation. Indeed, it would be naïve to think that mechanotransduction functions in isolation in the intact human body. The following are several potential areas for such synergy.

Neural

The integration of the nervous system on the mechanosensory properties of skeletal muscle is less frequently investigated. Motor unit firing during excitation–contraction coupling results in the release of intracellular calcium into the sarcoplasm, which causes actin–myosin cross-bridging to occur and the resulting shortening of the sarcomere and the production of force. The release of calcium into the sarcoplasm increases the phosphorylation of numerous intracellular signalling pathways, including calmodulin and MAPK cascades.

Calmodulin acts as a calcium sensor in muscle cells. Both calmodulin and calcineurin signalling coordinate to regulate muscle fibre phenotype, fibre size, apoptosis, and inflammatory responses. Motor unit firing patterns coordinate the duration and magnitude of the release of calcium into the cell. Thus, the activation of calcium-sensitive signalling proteins, and their interaction with other mechanotransducive proteins, influences muscle adaptations. Depolarization of myotube membranes increase the phosphorylation of ERK and cAMP-response element-binding protein (CREB) that subsequently increase the transcription of early immediate genes c-fos and c-jun (20). The integration of calcium-sensitive pathways with mechanosensitive proteins is exemplified by data reporting the static stretch-induced phosphorylation of ERK is inhibited when p38 and calcineurin signalling is blocked (144). This evidence suggests activation of the ERK/MAPK pathway is regulated in part via calcium homeostasis and other signalling proteins. Thus, motor unit firing and excitation contraction coupling modulates muscle phenotype and size through both calcium and mechanosensitive signalling pathways. It should be noted that calcium-sensitive signalling pathways (specifically calcineurin) may play a more prominent role in fibre type switching as opposed to regulating fibre hypertrophy following mechanical overload, as the genetic loss of calcineurin prevents slow to fast fibre transitions following mechanical overload but does not attenuate increases in fibre size (137). Contrary to genetic deletion of calcineurin, inhibition of calcineurin via administration of cyclosporin A (a calcineurin inhibitor) in response to functional overload of rat plantaris blunted the shift of fast to slow MHC isoforms and partially attenuated increases in fibre size (133).

Denervation attenuates the activity of ERK in both fast and slow muscles (54). Furthermore, denervation studies suggest that the interruption of neuron innervation with muscle fibres regulates protein synthesis and degradation pathways in the basal state (54). Denervation also decreases myostatin expression and increases basal mTOR signalling in mouse muscle despite decreasing markers of ribosome biogenesis (106). Thus, it appears that nervous system integration in skeletal muscle not only helps regulate fibre type transitions and size, it also controls, at least in part, basal translational capacity in the absence of mechanical load.

Immune and Inflammatory Responses

Immune cell response and acute elevations of inflammatory proteins contribute to regulation of skeletal muscle adaptations to exercise. Cytokines secreted from skeletal muscle during muscular contractions are called myokines (160). Although numerous myokines have been described in the literature, interleukin (IL)-6, IL-8, IL-10, and IL-15 and tumour necrosis factor-α (TNF-α) are most frequently investigated. Some cytokines such as IL-6 are released from muscle independent of the degree of muscle disruption or damage (23), and the IL-6 response to resistance exercise remains preserved following chronic training (172). Others, such as IL-15, appear to play an important role in anabolism after resistance exercise (138, 146). Indeed, recent data indicate the post-exercise response of IL-15 signalling was associated with post-exercise myofibrillar protein synthesis rates, and IL-15 receptor protein content was significantly related to leg press maximal strength (138).

Following muscle contraction, it is generally well regarded that inflammation plays a contributory role in muscle adaptations. However, the degree of inflammation during the recovery period and its subsequent role in regulating muscular adaptations appear to be population specific. In young healthy individuals, the consumption of high-dose anti-inflammatory medication impairs adaptations in muscular hypertrophy (99). On the contrary, in older individuals who are reported to express low-grade systemic inflammation, the consumption of non-steroidal anti-inflammatory drugs (NSAIDs) and cyclooxygenase 2 (COX-2) inhibitors appears to enhance muscular training adaptations (171). In younger individuals, the consumption of ibuprofen before and after a single bout of resistance exercise impaired the post-exercise increase in the phosphorylation of the ERK pathway (110), suggesting ibuprofen consumption may blunt some anabolic pathways. The inflammatory response also appears to be important for the activation and recruitment of satellite cells, since consumption of anti-inflammatory medication interferes with the myogenic process during recovery from bouts of exercise (103). The activation of satellite cells during regeneration involves the recruitment of monocytes and macrophages to satellite cells that support chemotaxis and regulate fibre hypertrophy (25).

Muscle Disruption and Damage

Clearly, muscle disruption and remodelling are critical to adaptation. Extreme disruption actually damages the muscle, in some cases to the point of dysfunction or even cell death. It is postulated by some that muscle damage is necessary for optimal muscle adaptation in response to resistance exercise. However, we suggest that cellular damage is not necessary for optimal muscle adaptations, but that carefully titrated cellular disruption and subsequent remodelling can be important contributors.

Muscular damage or disruption in response to mechanical overload is influenced by a multitude of factors, including structural deformation of actin–myosin filaments, disruption of z-bands and sarcomere alignment, elevated reactive oxygen species (ROS), and activation of calcium-dependent injury pathways (36, 128, 149, 164, 165). Muscle-damaging exercise causes the release of inflammatory cytokines such as TNF-α from muscle tissue (98). TNF-α is involved in the recovery of injured muscle and may regulate genes associated with regeneration, including gene expression of MyoD (174). It appears eccentric muscle actions induce greater indices of muscle damage than concentric muscle actions, and the damage observed during early and late recovery is mechanical and chemical in origin, respectively (128). Although both concentric and eccentric muscle actions are capable of inducing muscle hypertrophy, it appears eccentric actions induce greater anabolic signalling (47) and markers of satellite cell activation (77). In vitro stretching of muscle fibres also activates myogenic stem cells via a hepatocyte growth factor mechanism (168). Furthermore, although both types of muscle actions increase hypertrophy, concentric actions primarily increase anatomical cross-sectional area (ACSA) in the middle but not distal portion of muscle. Conversely, eccentric actions increase hypertrophy at middle and distal portions of trained muscle (47). Molecular data also indicate there is region-specific regulation of phosphorylated FAK in response to eccentric-only training. The increase in phosphorylated FAK occurred in the distal portion of muscle where only distal growth was seen in the eccentric-only condition (48).

The repeated-bout effect attenuates muscle damage following repeated exposure to exercise training. Thus, indices of muscle damage are attenuated following chronic training. Indeed, resistance-trained subjects exhibited fewer markers of muscle damage and a more rapid return of performance than untrained individuals (9). The mechanotransducer α7β1-integrin increases following exercise and protects muscle fibres from injury (12). The consequence of increased integrin expression is attenuated phosphorylation of MAPKs ERK, JNK, and p38. Indeed, heavy eccentric exercise activates the JNK pathway and is related to muscle damage after resistance exercise (11, 165). However, repeated bouts of resistance exercise attenuate the JNK phosphorylation response post-exercise (165). Recently, JNK has been implicated as the "molecular switch" that regulates fibre size following resistance and endurance exercise training. Acute activation of JNK is required for muscle growth, whereas inhibition of this response blunts hypertrophic responses (97). The contraction-induced increase in JNK is still preserved in trained individuals (59), and repeated bouts of resistance exercise attenuate inflammatory responses and increase (or specify) anabolic signalling (84). In fact, rodent models support the notion that muscle previously exposed to injurious exercise actually enhances muscle protein synthesis and anabolic signalling of the mTOR pathway (84, 165). It could be that muscle damage is inhibitory to muscle adaptation during cases of excessive exercise. Insufficient rest between exercise bouts impairs adaptation in damaged muscle during recovery, possibly through exacerbated inflammatory or degradative signalling pathways (2, 28, 129, 131, 166)

Endocrine

Hormones interact with their respective receptors at the cell membrane or intracellularly. Collectively, testosterone and cortisol are thought to primarily regulate muscle adaptations through their cellular receptors, the androgen and glucocorticoid receptors, respectively. However, a growing body of literature suggests these hormones and their receptors interact with and signal through mechanotransductive proteins of the Akt/mTOR and MAPK pathways. While very little data have specifically investigated how these hormones contribute to mechanosignalling, the following section will elaborate on how these endocrine factors and their receptors may modulate hypertrophic adaptations through signal transduction proteins.

The physiological role exercise-induced elevations in testosterone contribute to muscle hypertrophy has been contested (67, 120). The magnitude of hormonal responses is certainly not the sole determinant of hypertrophic adaptations (120); however, the presence of any testosterone response to acute or chronic training is related to muscular adaptations (108). Indeed, significant correlations have been reported between basal (158) and acute (120) testosterone and cortisol responses to resistance exercise and changes in muscle fibre cross-sectional areas.

Suppression of endogenous testosterone attenuates, but does not completely abolish, the hypertrophic response to resistance training. This indicates mechanotransduction plays a role in muscle growth in the absence of circulating testosterone (92). Thus, it seems the presence of testosterone is permissive, but not required, for muscle hypertrophic adaptations. It may be that circulating testosterone regulates muscle growth in the late stages of recovery from resistance exercise, since overnight muscle protein synthesis is correlated with the nocturnal plasma concentration of total testosterone (8). However, acute exercise-induced hypertrophic responses are more clearly regulated by intramuscular signalling proteins. Decreased p70S6K phosphorylation following resistance exercise, despite an increase in anabolic hormones, was observed in a group of untrained men. The authors hypothesized that the decreased p70S6K response was due to elevated cortisol in the high hormone condition (155). Interestingly, in that same cohort but a different analysis, Spiering et al. (156) reported that the resistance exercise–induced increase of testosterone in the high hormone condition potentiated and sustained androgen receptor content, whereas the low hormone condition saw a decrease in androgen receptor content. Taken together, it might be speculated that in conditions where metabolic stress and cortisol are high, testosterone may potentiate androgen receptor signalling to compensate for decreased Akt/p70S6K activity. Conversely, in conditions where metabolic stress is low but intensity (%1RM) is high, signalling may be maintained through mechanosensitive events (56), as high-load, low-volume, long-rest resistance exercise does not usually produce increases in testosterone or cortisol (155, 156). In trained men, different resistance exercise protocols activate different pathways that regulate translation initiation (104). Thus, it is possible that androgen and glucocorticoid receptors integrate hormonal and contractile stimuli synergistically to regulate skeletal muscle adaptations. Recent reports show that the androgen receptor can be phosphorylated at serine210/213 in response to exercise (187). Phosphorylation at this site is related to cell growth and is regulated by MAPK signalling (85). There have been no studies to specifically investigate if phosphorylation at this site from exercise is mediated by MAPK, and it remains speculative that there may be integration of these systems, given that activation of this site can occur in the absence of androgens (187). To date, only Nicoll et al. (131) have investigated androgen receptor phosphorylation in response to exercise. Their results reported specific sites on the androgen receptor are phosphorylated in response to resistance exercise (ser213, ser515), and the phosphorylation of these sites occurred in tandem with MAPK phosphorylation. However, those authors did not perform co-immunoprecipition studies to determine if exercise-induced MAPK phosphorylation was the specific kinase phosphorylating the androgen receptors at those sites. It has also been suggested that androgen receptor content and phosphorylation depend in part on the training status of the individual. Finally, in myotubes testosterone has been shown to regulate hypertrophy and calcium handling through Akt, mTOR, ERK, and the androgen receptor, effects which involve fast non-genomic and slower genomic effects (6, 43, 178).

The glucocorticoid receptor is less investigated in relation to resistance exercise adaptation; however, like the androgen receptor, the glucocorticoid receptor is regulated by ligands and intracellular signalling proteins like MAPK. The phosphorylation of glucocorticoid receptors at ser226 has been shown to influence its nuclear/cytoplasmic shuttling (79). Furthermore, MAPK/JNK specifically regulates phosphorylation at this serine. Increasing the activity and expression of JNK increases phosphorylation of glucocorticoid receptors on ser226. The increase in phosphorylation on ser226 decreases glucocorticoid receptor transcriptional activity via regulating nuclear export (79). Muscular contraction activates JNK early during an exercise session (52) and in a load-dependent manner (56). Currently, it is speculative if the contraction-induced phosphorylation of JNK influences shuttling or transcriptional activity of the glucocorticoid receptors in response to resistance exercise.

Metabolism and Energy

Substrate utilization during high-intensity muscle contraction produces metabolites that create an acidic cellular environment. An increase in intramuscular H^+ concentration is considered a contributing factor of fatigue during exercise (15). The role that acidosis and metabolic stress contribute to adaptations following chronic resistance training remains less clear. The limited data investigating the role of metabolic stress and muscular adaptations after resistance exercise suggest metabolic stress may blunt the early translation initiation steps of protein synthesis (29). In murine and human models, prolonged states of an acidic muscular environment decrease basal muscle protein synthesis (22, 87), although one report of oral ingestion of a lactate- and caffeine-containing compound induced post-exercise satellite cell activity and enhanced anabolic signalling (134). However, resistance exercise responses are conflicting, since a high-volume, short-rest interval resistance exercise protocol increased ERK and p70S6K phosphorylation more than a high-load, long-rest interval protocol in untrained men (76). Further complicating this topic is that short interset rest intervals blunt anabolic signalling and muscle protein synthesis during the early, but not late, recovery period (114). Training studies on the role of short versus long rest intervals during resistance exercise (and therefore indicative of metabolic stress) remain inconclusive, with some studies reporting an advantage to long rest intervals (150), while others report no difference in hypertrophy between short and long rest periods (39).

The specificity of the resistance training protocol implemented dictates the anabolic signalling response during recovery (76). High-resistance exercise volume (1, 76, 90, 169) and short interset rest intervals (90, 114) increase lactate concentrations during and after resistance exercise more than low-volume and long-rest interval protocols. Metabolic stress and an elevated lactate concentration after resistance exercise are correlated to the activation of ERK during late recovery (140). Furthermore, the increase in ERK post exercise was independent of load or time under tension, indicating that at least in their study design, metabolic stress was sufficient to increase ERK phosphorylation after resistance exercise (140). To our knowledge, there have been no human studies specifically reporting positive correlations between the activation of ERK signalling and muscle protein synthesis. However, recently in vitro studies indicate lactate and succinate are able to induce hypertrophy of myotubes via activation of the ERK pathway (132, 185). It may be that metabolic perturbation impairs translation initiation and elongation signals early in recovery, yet the system is "primed" to sustain protein synthesis at later time points. A growing body of literature points to the involvement of the ERK pathway in regulating protein synthesis during the late recovery period (18, 175). p38 phosphorylation is sensitive to the force–time integral during high-frequency electrical stimulation muscle contraction, and this response is coordinated with mTOR and independent of metabolic stress (141). Interestingly when C2C12 muscle cells are exposed to high concentrations of lactate (20 mM), there is a blunting of p38 phosphorylation and late myogenic differentiation genes (180). In vivo, a high-intensity resistance training protocol with elevated lactate concentration suppressed post-exercise p38 phosphorylation, indicating that this protein is indeed influenced by metabolic stress in response to resistance exercise in humans (180).

Depletion of energetic substrates increases the phosphorylation of AMPK (57). Early data with in vitro and in vivo murine models indicated increased AMPK activity as a regulatory protein that reduces mTOR signalling and muscle protein synthesis. Elevated AMPK levels have been shown to increase FAK phosphorylation, ultimately affecting cell metabolism (95). While data do suggest overactivation of AMPK signalling impairs proteins regulating translation initiation and elongation (170), research in humans indicates the activation of this protein may not blunt the hypertrophic responses to chronic resistance training (102). Collectively, data suggest metabolic stress may attenuate anabolic phosphorylation events in the early recovery period, but eventual training adaptations in muscle hypertrophy may not be impaired.

Nutrition and Dietary Supplementation

Mechanosensitive proteins respond to contractile stress and integrate with other signalling nutrient-sensitive proteins. The availability of nutrients and/or supplementation with dietary ergogenic aids has received considerable attention. The ingestion of protein after a resistance exercise bout prolongs anabolic signalling and the muscle protein synthetic response after exercise. The availability of nutrients after resistance exercise influences mTOR localization with the lysosome and may serve as a focal point for integrating and coordinating mechanical stress, feeding, and anabolic signalling with the translational machinery (71). While feeding alone can stimulate anabolic signalling (58), protein phosphorylation and muscle protein synthesis are amplified when resistance exercise is performed prior to feeding (119). Furthermore, the sensitivity of amino acid uptake into muscle persists for at least 24 hours after resistance exercise (19), highlighting the role mechanical loading has on muscle-adaptive responses. The consumption of amino acids after resistance exercise suggests whey protein may accelerate satellite cell proliferation following muscle-damaging exercise (44).

Creatine is another popular dietary ergogenic aid that is used to improve muscle strength and hypertrophy responses to resistance exercise. Acute supplementations with creatine for 5 days does not improve the anabolic signalling responses to resistance exercise, but did increase gene expression of glucose-transporter 4 (GLUT-4) and MHC-I mRNA (37). In vitro work has shown that creatine enhances MHC-II expression and differentiation in myotubes, an effect that may be mediated by Akt and p38 (38). Since in vitro work suggested creatine may be efficacious in enhancing differentiation, further work sought to investigate the effect of creatine on regeneration of muscle after injury and reported that creatine had no influence on regeneration in muscle injury in rats (32). A limitation of this study was that injury was induced by notexin injection, and muscle damage was not due to contraction-mediated stress.

Training Status

Cumulatively, exercise-induced responses in the trained state appear different relative to the untrained state (167, 179). Further, muscle metabolism at rest in the trained state also indicates enhanced resting rates of muscle protein synthesis and reduced protein breakdown (74, 145). Chronic resistance exercise increases in ribosome biogenesis (45). At the same time, satellite cells proliferate and are incorporated into the muscle fibres as new myonuclei following chronic resistance exercise (7, 139). Long-term (many years) resistance training decreases total protein content of anabolic signalling proteins ERK and eEF2 (53, 105). The down-regulation of these anabolic proteins may serve as a negative-feedback loop to regulate the pronounced hypertrophy observed following many years of chronic resistance training. Similarly, the acute exercise response to chronic resistance training indicates there is a much more specific and potent anabolic signalling response in trained muscle compared to untrained muscle (105). Furthermore, unlike untrained muscle that may have a "generalized" signalling response to a novel acute resistance exercise protocol (30), highly trained muscle appears to use different signalling cascades to regulate translation initiation and elongation (104). Lysenko et al. (104) reported that in highly resistance-trained men a high-volume, moderate-load resistance exercise protocol specifically activated the p70s6K signalling axis, while a high-load, low-volume protocol specifically activated the ERK signalling pathway. More importantly, the peak activation and total duration of these signalling pathways differed, suggesting that as one accumulates more training experience, specificity of the resistance exercise protocol may require greater attention to see continued adaptations via activation of specific anabolic pathways. This concept is also evident in reference to testosterone responses and interactions with the AR after acute resistance exercise. In untrained men, the acute elevation of testosterone may be important for stabilization or potentiation of the AR (156), while in trained men the AR can increase activity and DNA binding without an exercise-induced increase in testosterone concentrations (157). Unfortunately, the importance of the specifics of the resistance training programme is not always fully appreciated (16).

For muscle hypertrophy, numerous intracellular adaptations may sustain enhanced hypertrophy. Further, changes in satellite cell activation, ribosome biogenesis, and translational efficiency may occur independently of each other at different time courses as one goes from untrained to trained. Increased phosphorylation and a generalized protein synthetic response may occur early in resistance training history followed by increases in ribosome biogenesis to sustain enhanced translational capacity. Finally, satellite cell expansion and incorporation into the myofibre may ultimately sustain muscle hypertrophy and enhance the regeneration properties following in the trained state.

Sex

The role that sex contributes to mechanotransduction and anabolism following resistance exercise has not been well investigated. Although males possess larger circulating concentrations of androgens compared to females, the acute resistance exercise MPS response indicates similar rates of protein synthesis between the sexes. At rest, basal states of MPS between the sexes appear to be similar (41, 176). Although males typically express greater muscle mass compared to females, their relative increase in response to resistance training is similar (63, 158). Although West et al. (176) reported greater Akt and mTOR phosphorylation in males during the early recovery period after resistance exercise, females had higher p70S6K phosphorylation during the late recovery period (28 hours post exercise) following feeding. The early recovery phosphorylation responses reported by West et al. (176) conflict with those of Dreyer and colleagues (41), who found no differences in signalling proteins in the mTOR pathway following resistance exercise. Thus, there appears there may be a difference between the acute phosphorylation responses and MPS responses between sexes. Possible differences in the myostatin genotype for men and women may also contribute to sex differences in the hypertrophic response to resistance exercise (80). Recently Nicoll and colleagues (130) reported a greater ratio of phosphorylation at ser81 and ser515 on the androgen receptor in females compared to males, but when accounting for differences in total receptor content at this site (males > females), the phosphorylation was similar between sexes. It has also been reported that post-resistance exercise total content of androgen and glucocorticoid receptors differ between men and women (173). Considering the information mentioned in the previous sections, it is likely that metabolic, hormonal, and mechanosensing mechanisms fine-tune the muscle-adaptive responses for each sex.

Type of Resistance Exercise Stimulus

The design of the acute resistance exercise bout can influence the activation of mechanotransduction pathways. High-intensity overload has been shown to enhance neuromuscular junction morphology in rats (40). Of particular importance is the fact the total duration and peak activation of protein phosphorylation depend on the resistance exercise protocol implemented (56). In general, low- to moderate-load voluminous exercise, low-repetition and high-load, and high-power development regimens have all been shown to induce phosphorylation of MAPK and mTOR signalling pathways, albeit to varying degrees of activation (17, 52, 73, 91). While hypertrophic and strength-focused protocols have primarily been utilized when investigating mechanotransduction responses, to our knowledge only two investigations have studied the molecular responses to high-power ballistic exercises (52, 91). The relative change in the phosphorylation of MAPK is of a much smaller magnitude than what is commonly reported in high-volume or high-load protocols, and this may be due to the absence of metabolic stress or use of longer rest periods to avoid muscular fatigue while maintaining high movement velocities. Considering that high-velocity movements or high-power development is an essential component of athletic success in various sports, understanding the molecular responses to high-power protocols deserves further investigation.

Summary

By this point, it should be readily apparent that the process of mechanotransduction in skeletal muscle is complex and multifaceted. The overview of the various mechanotransducing pathways presented in this chapter makes it abundantly clear that the muscle cell is a robust and adaptable system, ready to respond to many stimuli and conditions. It must also be noted here that this is a still emerging field where we have likely only scratched the surface. To complicate matters, the stimuli discussed in the previous pages are also very complex. It is easy to think that all resistance exercise is the same, yet we have briefly described how variable just a single training session can be. On top of that is the fact that the long-term training programme can also be quite diverse. Even if one is following a well-planned periodized resistance exercise training programme, the prolonged stimulus can vary considerably, thus complicating study of the mechanotransduction process. Besides the acute and chronic resistance exercise training variables, one must be reminded of the actual stimulus presented in the muscle cell. Obviously, the mechanical properties created in the muscle cell include the developed forces, but these forces can come in many forms. Whether it is the magnitude, the duration, or the rates of force development, these forces appear to be critical. It is also important to distinguish the differences between muscle disruption and remodelling that occur from a well-designed training programme from actual muscle damage and injury. Non-contractile forces may be present as well, such as when cell volume is affected. Finally, it is imperative to remember that mechanotransduction mechanisms do not function in isolation. It is only through a careful understanding of the fantastic synergy with other physiological processes that the muscle cell can fully take advantage of all its adaptive capabilities. Too often it is easy to oversimplify complex physiological adaptations, thus missing the amazing coordination between the many aspects of biological adjustments. Perhaps the muscle cell is like a large orchestra playing a beautiful symphony. Individually, the various instrument sections make disjointed, nonsensical musical sounds, but when the entire orchestra works together, a beautiful masterpiece results. As stated as long ago as 1911 by the renowned Scottish American naturalist, John Muir, "When we try to pick out anything by itself, we find it hitched to everything else in the universe" (122). Likewise, the mechanotransduction mechanisms of the muscle cell must work in harmony with the rest of the cell to optimize muscle adaptation.

References

1. Ahtianen JP, Walker S, Silvennoinen M, Kyröläinen H, Nindl BC, Häkkinen K, Nyman K, Selänne H, Hulmi, JJ. Exercise type and volume alter signaling pathways regulating skeletal muscle glucose uptake and protein synthesis. *Eur J Appl Physiol* 115: 835–845, 2015.
2. Alves Souza RW, Aguiar AF, Vechetti-Júnior IJ, Piedade WP, Rocha Campos GE, Dal-Pai-Silva M. Resistance training with excessive training load and insufficient recovery alters skeletal muscle mass-related protein expression. *J Strength Condit Res* 28: 2338–2345, 2014.
3. Andersen JL, Gruschy-Knudsen T. Rapid switch-off of the human myosin heavy chain IIX gene after heavy load muscle contractions is sustained for at least four days. *Scand J Med Sci Sports* 28: 371–380, 2018.
4. Bamman MM, Roberts BM, Adams GR. Molecular regulation of exercise-induced muscle fiber hypertrophy. *Cold Spring Harb Perspect Med* 8: a029751, 2018.
5. Barash IA, Peters D, Friden J, Lutz GJ, Lieber RL. Desmin cytoskeletal, modifications after a bout of eccentric exercise in the rat. *Am J Physiol: Reg, Integr Comp Physiol* 283: 958–963, 2002.
6. Basualto-Alarco NC, Jorquera G, Altamirano F, Jaimovich E, Estrada M. Testosterone signals through mTOR and androgen receptor to induce muscle hypertrophy. *Med Sci Sports Exerc* 45: 1712–1720, 2013.
7. Bellamy LM, Joanisse S, Grubb A, Mitchell CJ, McKay BR, Phillips SM, Baker S, Parise G. The acute satellite cell response and skeletal muscle hypertrophy following resistance training. *PLOS ONE* 9: e109739, 2014.
8. Betts JA, Beelen M, Stokes KA, Saris WHM, van Loon LJC. Endocrine responses during overnight recovery from exercise: impact of nutrition and relationships with muscle protein synthesis. *Int J Sport Nutri Exerc Metabol* 21: 398–409, 2011.
9. Bloomer RJ, Fry AC, Schilling BK, Chiu LZF, Hori N, Weiss LW. Astaxanthin supplementation does not attenuate markers of muscle injury following eccentric exercise. *Int J Sports Nutri Exerc Metabol* 15: 401–412, 2005.
10. Bompa T, Haff GG. *Periodization: Theory and Methodology of Training* (5th Edition). Champaign, IL: Human Kinetics, 2009.
11. Boppart MD, Aronson D, Gibson L, Roubenoff R, Abad LW, Bean J, Goodyear LJ, Fielding RA. Eccentric exercise markedly increases c-Jun NH$_2$-terminal kinase activity in human skeletal muscle. *J Appl Physiol* 87: 1668–1673, 1999.
12. Boppart MD, Durkin DJ, Kaufman SJ. Alpha7beta1-integrin regulates mechanotransduction and prevents skeletal muscle injury. *Am J Physiol: Cell Physiol* 290: C1660–C1665, 2006.
13. Boppart MD, Mahmassani ZS. Integrin signaling: linking mechanical stimulation to skeletal muscle hypertrophy. *Am J Physiol: Cell Physiol* 317: C629–C641, 2019.

14. Brook MS, Wilkinson DJ, Mitchell WK, Lund JN, Phillips BE, Szewczyk NJ, Greenhaff PL, Smith K, Atherton PJ. Synchronous deficits in cumulative muscle protein synthesis and ribosomal biogenesis underline age-related anabolic resistance to exercise in humans. *J Physiol* 594: 7399–7417, 2016.

15. Broxterman RM, Layec G, Hureau TJ, Amann M, Richardson RS. Skeletal muscle bioenergetics during all-out exercise: mechanistic insight into the oxygen uptake slow component and neuromuscular fatigue. *J Appl Physiol* 122: 1208–1217, 2017.

16. Buckner SL, Jessee MB, Mouser JG, Dankel SJ, Mattocks KT, Bell ZW, Abe T, Loenneke JP. The basics of training for muscle size and strength. *Med Sci Sports Exerc* 52: 645–653, 2019.

17. Burd NA, Holwerda AM, Selby KC, West DW, Staples AW, Cain NE, Cashaback JG, Potvin JR, Backer SK, Phillips SM. Resistance exercise volume affects myofibrillar protein synthesis and anabolic signaling molecule phosphorylation in young men. *J Physiol* 588: 3119–3130, 2010.

18. Burd NA, Andrews RJ, West DW, Little JP, Cochran AJ, Hector AJ, Cashaback JG, et al. Muscle time under tension during resistance exercise stimulates differential muscle protein sub-fractional synthetic responses in men. *J Physiol* 590: 351–362, 2012.

19. Burd NA, West DW, Moore DR, Atherton PJ, Staples AW, Prior T, Tang JE, Ressie MJ, Baker SK, Phillips SM. Enhanced amino acid sensitivity of myofibrillar protein synthesis persists for up to 24 h after resistance exercise in young men. *J Nutri* 141: 568–573, 2011.

20. Carrasco MA, Riveros N, Rios J, Müller M, Torres F, Pineda J, Lantadilla S, Jaimovich E. Depolarization-induced slow calcium transients activate early genes in skeletal muscle cells. *Am J Physiol: Cell Physiol* 284: C1438–C1447, 2003.

21. Carlson CJ, Fan Z, Gordon SE, Booth FW. Time course of the MAPK and PI3 kinase response within 24h of skeletal muscle overload. *J Appl Physiol* 91: 2079–2087, 2001.

22. Caso G, Garlick BA, Casella GA, Sasvary D, Garlick PJ. Acute metabolic acidosis inhibits muscle protein synthesis in rats. *Am J Physiol: Endocrinol Metabol* 287: E90–E96, 2004.

23. Chan MHS, Carey AL, Watt MJ, Febbraio MA. Cytokine gene expression in human skeletal muscle during concentric contraction: evidence that IL-8, like IL-6, is influenced by glycogen availability. *Am J Physiol: Reg Integr Comp Physiol* 287: 322–327, 2004.

24. Chang NC, Sincennes MC, Chevalier FP, Brun CE, Lacaria M, Segalés J, Muñoz-Cánoves P, Ming H, Rudnicki MA. The dystrophin glycoprotein complex regulates the epigenetic activation of muscle stem cell commitment. *Cell Stem Cell*, 22(5), 755–768, 2018.

25. Chazaud B, Sonnet C, Lafuste P, Bassez G, Rimaniol AC, Poron F, Authier FJ, Dreyfus PA, Gheradri RK. Satellite cells attract monocytes and use macrophages as a support to escape apoptosis and enhance muscle growth. *J Cell Biol* 163: 1133–43, 2003.

26. Chicurel ME, Singer RH, Meyer CJ, Ingber DE. Integrin binding and mechanical tension induce movement of mRNA and ribosomes to focal adhesions. *Nature* 392: 730–733, 1998.

27. Cho S, Irianto J, Discher DE. Mechanosensing by the nucleus: From pathways to scaling relationships. *J Cell Biol* 216: 305–315, 2017.

28. Coffey VG, Reeder DW, Lancaster GI, Yeo WK, Febbraio MA, Yaspelkis III BB, Hawley JA. Effect of high-frequency resistance exercise on adaptive responsive in skeletal muscle. *Med Sci Sports Exerc* 39: 2135–2144, 2007.

29. Coffey VG, Jemiolo B, Edge J, Garnham AP, Trappe SW, Hawley JA. Effect of consecutive repeated sprint and resistance exercise bouts on acute adaptive responses in human skeletal muscle. *Am J Physiol: Reg Integr Comp Physiol* 297: R1441–51, 2009.

30. Coffey VG, Zhong Z, Shield A, Canny BJ, Chibalin AV, Zierath JR, Hawley JA. Early signaling responses to divergent exercise stimuli in skeletal muscle from well-trained humans. *FASEB J* 20: 190–2, 2006.

31. Conceição MS, Vechin FC, Lixandrão M, Damas F, Libardi CA, Tricoli V, Roschel H, Camera D, Urgrinowitsch C. Muscle fiber hypertrophy and myonuclei addition: A systematic review and meta-analysis. *Med Sci Sports Exerc* 50: 1385–1393, 2018.

32. Crassous B, Richard-Bulteau H, Deldicque L, Serrurier B, Pasdeloup M, Francaux M, Bigard X, Koulmann N. Lack of effects of creatine on the regeneration of soleus muscle after injury in rats. *Med Sci Sports Exerc* 41: 1761–9, 2009.

33. Crossland H, Timmons JA, Atherton PJ. A dynamic ribosomal biogenesis response is not required for IGF-1 mediated hypertrophy of human primary myotubes. *FASEB J* 31: 5196–5207, 2017.

34. D'Angelo MA. Nuclear pore complexes as hubs for gene regulation. *Nucleus* 9: 142–148, 2018.

35. Damas F, Libardi CA, Ugrinowitsch C, Vechin FC, Lixandrão ME, Snijders T, Nederveen JP, et al. Early- and later-phases satellite cell responses and myonuclear content with resistance training in young men. *PLOS ONE* 13: e0191039, 2018.

36. Damas F, Phillips SM, Libardi CA, Vechin FC, Lixandrão ME, Janning PR, Costa LA, et al. Resistance training-induced changes in integrated myofibrillar protein synthesis are related to hypertrophy only after attenuation of muscle damage. *J Physiol* 594: 5209–22, 2016.

37. Deldicque L, Atherton P, Patel R, Theisen D, Nielens H, Rennie MJ, Francaux M. Effects of resistance exercise with and without creatine supplementation on gene expression and cell signaling in human skeletal muscle. *J Appl Physiol* 104: 371–8, 2008.

38. Deldicque L, Theisen D, Betrand L, Hespel P, Hue L, Francaux M. Creatine enhances differentiation of mygenic C2C12 cells by activating both p38 and Akt/PKB pathways. *Am J Physiol: Cell Physiol* 293: C1263–71, 2007.

39. de Souza Jr TP, Fleck SJ, Simão R, Dubas JP, Pereira B, de Brito Pacheco EM, da Silva AC, de Oliveira PR. Comparison between constant and decreasing rest intervals: influence on maximal strength and hypertrophy. *J Strength Condit Res* 24: 1843–1850, 2010.

40. Deschenes MR, Maresh CM, Crivello JF, Armstrong LE, Kraemer WJ, Covault J. The effects of exercise training of different intensities on neuromuscular junction morphology. *J Neurocytol* 22: 603–15, 1993.

41. Dreyer, HC, Fujita S, Glynn EL, Drummond MJ, Volpi E, Rasmussen BB. Resistance exercise increase leg muscle protein synthesis and mTOR signaling independent of sex. *Acta Physiol (Oxf)* 199: 71–81, 2010.

42. Eliasson J, Elfegoun T, Nilsson J, Köhnke R, Ekblom B, Blomstrand E. Maximal lengthening contractions increase p70 S6 kinase phosphorylation in human skeletal muscle in the absence of nutritional supply. *Am J Physiol: Endocrinol Metabol* 291: E1197–E1205, 2006.

43. Estrada M, Espinosa A, Müller M, Jaimovich E. Testosterone stimulates intracellular calcium release and mitogen-activated protein kinases via a G protein-coupled receptor in skeletal muscle cells. *Endocrinol* 144: 3586–97, 2003.

44. Farup J, Rahbek SK, Knudsen IS, de Paoli F, Mackey AL, Vissing K. Whey protein supplementation accelerates satellite cell proliferation during recovery from eccentric exercise. *Amino Acids* 46: 2503–16, 2014.

45. Figueiredo VC, Caldow MK, Massie V, Markworth JF, Cameron-Smith D, Blazevich AJ. Ribosome biogenesis adaptation in resistance training-induced human skeletal muscle hypertrophy. *Am J Physiol: Endocrinol Metabol* 309: E72–83, 2015.

46. Fleck SJ, Kraemer WJ. *Designing Resistance Training Programs* (4th Edition). Champaign, IL: Human Kinetics, 2014.

47. Franchi MV, Atherton PJ, Reeves ND, Flück M, Williams J, Mitchell WK, Selby A, Beltran Valls RM, Narici MV. Architectural, functional and molecular responses to concentric and eccentric loading in human skeletal muscle. *Acta Physiol (Oxf)* 210: 642–654, 2014.

48. Franchi MV, Ruoss S, Valdiviseo P, Mitchell KW, Smith K, Atherton PJ, Narici MV, Flück M. Regional regulation of focal adhesion kinase after concentric and eccentric loading is related to remodeling of human skeletal muscle. *Acta Physiol (Oxf)* 223: e13056, 2018.

49. Fruleux A, Hawkins RJ. Physical role for the nucleus in cell migration. *J Physics: Cond Matter* 28: 363002, 2016.

50. Fry AC. The role of resistance exercise intensity on muscle fibre adaptations. *Sports Med* 34: 663–79, 2004.

51. Fry AC, Newton RU. A brief history of strength training and basic principles and concepts. In: *Strength Training for Sport*, edited by Kraemer WJ, Häkkinen K. London, UK: Blackwell Scientific, 2002, p. 1–19.

52. Galpin AJ, Fry AC, Chiu LZF, Thomason DB, Schilling BK. High-power resistance exercise induces MAPK phosphorylation in weightlifting trained men. *Appl Physiol Nutri Metabol* 37: 80–7, 2012.

53. Galpin AJ, Fry AC, Nicoll JX, Moore CA, Schilling BK, Thomason DB. Resting extracellular signal-regulated protein kinase 1/2 expression following a continuum of chronic resistance exercise training paradigms. *Res Sports Med* 24: 298–303, 2016.

54. Gao H, Li Y. Distinct signal transductions in fast- and slow- twitch muscles upon denervation. *Physiol Reports* 6: e13606, 2018.

55. Gattazzo F, Urciuolo A, Bonaldo P. Extracellular matrix: a. dynamic microenvironment for stem cell niche. *Biochim Biophys Acta* 1840: 2506–2519, 2014.

56. Gehlert S, Suhr F, Gutsche K, Willkomm L, Kern J, Jacko D, Knicker A, Schiffer T, Wackerhage H, Bloch W. High force development augments skeletal muscle signaling in resistance exercise modes equalized for time under tension. *Pflüg Archiv* 467: 1343–56, 2015.

57. Gibala MJ, McGee SL, Garnham AP, Howlett KF, Snow RJ, Hargreaves M. Brief intense interval exercise activates AMPK and p38 MAPK signaling and increases the expression of PGC-1alpha in human skeletal muscle. *J Appl Physiol* 106: 929–34, 2009.

58. Glover EI, Oates BR, Tang JE, Moore DR, Tarnopolsky MA, Phillips SM. Resistance exercise decreases eIF2Bepsilon phosphorylation and potentiates the feeding-induced stimulation of p70S6K1 and rpS6 in young men. *Am J Physiol: Reg Integr Comp Physiol* 295: R604–10, 2008.

59. Gonzalez AM, Hoffman JR, Townsend JR, Jajtner AR, Boone CH, Beyer KS, Baker KM, et al. Intramuscular MAPK signaling following high volume and high intensity resistance exercise protocols in trained men. *Eur J Appl Physiol* 116: 1663–70, 2016.

60. Goodman CA, Frey JW, Mabrey DM, Jacobs BL, Lincoln HC, You JS, Hornberger TA. The role of skeletal muscle mTOR in the regulation of mechanical load-induced growth. *J Physiol* 589: 5485–501, 2011.

61. Haddad F, Adams GR. Inhibition of MAPK/ERK kinase prevents IGF-1-induced hypertrophy in rat muscles. *J Physiol* 96: 203–210, 2004.

62. Haff GG, Triplett NT. *Essentials of Strength Training and Conditioning* (4th Edition). Champaign, IL: Human Kinetics, 2016.

63. Hagan FT, Sale DG, MacDougall JD, Garner SH. Response to resistance training in young women and men. *Int J Sports Med* 16: 314–21, 1995.

64. Halder G, Dupont S, Piccolo S. Transduction of mechanical and cytoskeletal cues by YAP and TAZ. *Nature Rev: Mol Cell Biol* 13: 591–600, 2012.

65. Han H, Qi R, Zhou JJ, Ta AP, Yang B, Nakaoka HJ, Seo G, Guan KL, Luo R, Wang W. Regulation of the HIPPO pathway by phosphatidic acid-mediated lipid-protein interaction. *Mol Cell* 72: 328–340, 2018.

66. Hansson B, Olsen LA, Nicoll JX, von Walden F, Melin M, Stromberg A, Rullman E, et al. Skeletal muscle signaling responses to resistance exercise of the elbow extensors are not compromised by a preceding bout of aerobic exercise. *Am J Physiol: Reg Integr Comp Physiol* 317: R83–R92, 2019.

67. Hansen S, Kvorning T, Kjaer M, Sjøgaard G. The effect of short-term strength training on human skeletal muscle: the importance of physiologically elevated hormone levels. *Scand J Med Sci Sports* 11: 347–54, 2001.

68. Haun CT, Vann CG, Osburn SC, Mumford PW, Roberson PA, Romero MA, Fox CD, et al. (2019a). Muscle fiber hypertrophy in response to 6 weeks of high-volume resistance training in trained young men is largely attributed to sarcoplasmic hypertrophy. *PLOS ONE* 14: e0215267, 2019.

69. Haun CT, Vann CG, Mobley CB, Osburn SC, Mumford PW, Roberson PA, Romero MA, et al. Pre-training skeletal muscle fiber size and predominant fiber type best predict hypertrophic responses to 6 weeks of resistance training in previously trained young men. *Front Physiol* 10: 297, 2019.

70. Hawley JA, Hargreaves M, Joyner MJ, Zierath JR. Integrative biology of exercise. *Cell* 159: 738–749, 2014.

71. Hodson N, McGlory C, Oikawa SY, Jeromson S, Song Z, Rüegg MA, Hamilton DL, Phillips SM, Philp A. Differential localization and anabolic responsiveness of mTOR complexes in human skeletal muscle in response to feeding and exercise. *Am J Physiol: Cell Physiol* 313: C604–C611, 2017.

72. Hodson N, Andrew P. The importance of mTOR trafficking for human skeletal muscle translational control. *Exerc Sport Sci Rev* 47: 46–53, 2019.

73. Holm L, van Hall G, Rose AJ, Miller BF, Doessing S, Richter EA. Contraction intensity and feeding affect collagen and myofibrillar protein synthesis rates differently in human skeletal muscle. *Am J Physiol: Endocrinol Metabol* 298: E257–E269, 2010.

74. Holwerda AM, Paulessen KJM, Overkamp M, Smeets JSJ, Gijsen AP, Goessens JPB, Verdijk LB, van Loon LJC. Daily resistance-typr exercise stimulates muscle protein synthesis in vivo in young men. *J Appl Physiol* 124: 66–75, 2018.

75. Hornberger TA, Armstrong DD, Koh TJ, Burkholder TJ, Esser KA. Intracellular signaling specificity in response to uniaxial vs. multiaxial stretch: implications for mechanotransduction. *Am J Physiol: Cell Physiol* 288: C185–C194, 2005.

76. Hulmi JJ, Walker S, Ahtiainen JP, Nymen K, Kraemer WJ, Häkkinen K. Molecular signaling in muscle is affected by the specificity of resistance exercise protocol. *Scand J Med Sci Sports* 22: 240–248, 2012.

77. Imaoka Y, Kawai M, Mori F, Miyata H. Effect of eccentric contraction on satellite cell activation in human vastus lateralis muscle. *J Physiol Sci* 65: 461–469, 2015.

78. Ingber DE. Cellular mechanotransduction: putting all the pieces together again. *FASEB J* 20: 811–827, 2006.

79. Itoh M, Adachi M, Yasui H, Takekawa M, Tanaka H, Imai K. Nuclear export of glucocorticoid receptor is enhanced by c-Jun N-terminal kinase-mediated phosphorylation. *Mol Endocrinol* 16: 2382–2392, 2002.

80. Ivey FM, Roth SM, Ferrell RE, Tracy BL, Lemmer JT, Hurlbut DE, Martel GF, et al. Effects of age, gender, and myostatin genotype on the hypertrophic response to heavy resistance strength training. *J Gerontol: Series A Biol Sci Med Sci* 55: M641–M648, 2000.

81. Jacko D, Bersiner K, Hebchen J, de Marees M, Bloch W, Gehlert S. Phosphorylation of αB-crystallin and its cytoskeleton association differs in skeletal myofiber types depending on resistance exercise intensity and volume. *J Appl Physiol* 123: 1607–1618, 2019.

82. Jacobs BL, You J-S, Frey JW, Goodman CA, Gundermann DM, Hornberger TA. Eccentric contractions increase the phosphorylation of tuberous sclerosis complex-2 (TSC2) and alter the targeting of TSC2 and the mechanistic target of rapamycin to the lysosome. *J Physiol* 591: 4611–4620, 2013.

83. Judson RN, Tremblay AM, Knopp P, White RB, Urcia R, De Bari C, Zammit PS, Camargo FD, Wackerhage H. The hippo pathway member Yap plays a key role in influencing fate decisions in muscle satellite cells. *J Cell Sci* 125: 6009–6019, 2012.

84. Karagounis LG, Yaspelkis BB, Reeder DW, Lancaster GI, Hawley JA, Coffey VG. Contraction-induced changes in TNFalpha and Akt-mediated signaling are associated with increased myofibrillar protein in rat skeletal muscle. *Eur J Appl Physiol* 109: 839–848, 2010.

85. Kim HJ, Lee WJ. Ligand-independent activation of the androgen receptor by insulin-like growth factor-1 and the role of the MAPK pathway in skeletal muscle cells. *Mol Cells* 28: 589–593, 2009.

86. Kirby TJ. Mechanosensitive pathways controlling translation regulatory processes in skeletal muscle and implications for adaptation. *J Appl Physiol* 127: 608–618, 2019.

87. Kleger GR, Turgay M, Imoberdorf R, McNurlan MA, Garlick PJ, Ballmer PE. Acute metabolic acidosis decreases muscle protein synthesis but not albumin synthesis in humans. *Am J Kidney Dis* 38: 1199–1207, 2001.

88. Klossner S, Durieux AC, Freyssenet D, Flueck M. Mechano-transduction to muscle protein synthesis is modulated by FAK. *Eur J Appl Physiol* 106: 389–398, 2009.

89. Koskinen SO, Ahtikoski AM, Komulainen J, Hesselink MK, Drost MR, Takala TE. Short-term effects of forced eccentric contractions on collagen synthesis and degradation in rat skeletal muscle. *Pflüg Arch* 444: 59–72, 2002.

90. Kraemer WJ, Marchitelli L, Gordon SE, Harman E, Dziados JE, Mello R, Frykman P, McCurry D, Fleck SJ. Hormonal and growth factor responses to heavy resistance exercise protocols. *J Appl Physiol* 69: 1442–1450, 1990.

91. Kudrna RA, Fry AC, Nicoll JX, Gallagher PM, Prewitt MR. Effect of three different maximal concentric velocity squat protocols on MAPK phosphorylation and endocrine responses. *J Strength Condit Res* 33: 1692–1702, 2019.

92. Kvorning T, Andersen M, Brixen K, Madsen K. Suppression of endogenous testosterone production attenuates the response to strength training: a randomized, placebo-controlled, and blinded intervention study. *Am J Physiol: Endocrinol Metabol* 291: 1325–32, 2006.

93. Lamon S, Wallace MA, Russell AP. The STARS signaling pathway: A key regulator of skeletal muscle function. *Pflüg Archiv* 466: 1659–1671, 2014.

94. Laplante M, Sabatini DM. mTOR signaling at a glance. *J Cell Sci* 122: 3589–3594, 2009.

95. Lassiter DG, Nylén C, Sjögren RJO, Chibalin AV, Wallberg-Henriksson H, Näslund E, Krook A, Zierath JR. FAK tyrosine phosphorylation is regulated by AMPK and controls metabolism in human skeletal muscle. *Diabetologia* 61: 424–432, 2018.

96. Legate KR, Wickstrom SA, Fassler R. Genetic and cell biological analysis of integrin outside-in signaling. *Genes Develop* 23: 397–418, 2009.

97. Lessard SJ, MacDonald TL, Pathak P, Han MS, Coffey VG, Edge J, Rivas DA, Hirshman MF, Davis RJ, Goodyear LJ. JNK regulates muscle remodeling via myostatin/SMAD inhibition. *Nature Comm* 9: 3030, 2018.

98. Liao P, Zhou J, Ji LL, Zhang Y. Eccentric contraction induces inflammatory responses in rat skeletal muscle: role of tumor necrosis factor-alpha. *Am J Physiol: Reg Integr Comp Physiol* 298: R599–R607, 2010.

99. Lilja M, Mandić M, Apró W, Melin M, Olsson K, Rosenborg S, Gustafsson T, Lundberg TR. High doses of anti-inflammatory drugs compromise muscle strength and hypertrophic adaptations to resistance training in young adults. *Acta Physiol (Oxf)* 222: e12948, 2018.

100. Liu Y, Vertommen D, Rider MH, Lai YC. Mammalian target of rapamycin-independent S6K1 and 4E-BP1 phosphorylation during contraction in rat skeletal muscle. *Cell Signal* 25: 1877–1886, 2013.

101. Lueders TN, Zou K, Huntsman HD, Meador B, Mahmassani Z, Abel M, Valero MC, Huey KA, Boppart MD. The alpha7beta1-integrin accelerates fiber hypertrophy and myogenesis following a single bout of eccentric exercise. *Am J Physiol: Cell Physiol* 301: C938–C946, 2011.

102. Lundberg TR, Fernandez-Gonzalo R, Tesch PA. Exercise-induced AMPK activation does not interfere with muscle hypertrophy in response to resistance training in men. *J Appl Physiol* 116: 611–620, 2014.

103. Lundberg TR, Howatson G. Analgesic and anti-inflammatory drugs in sports: Implications for exercise performance and training adaptations. *Scand J Med Sci Sports* 28: 2252–2262, 2018.

104. Lysenko EA, Popov DV, Vepkhvadze TF, Sharova AP, Vinogradova OL. Signaling responses to high and moderate load strength exercise in trained muscle. *Physiol Reports* 7: e14100, 2019.

105. Lysenko EA, Popov DV, Vepkhvadze TF, Sharova AP, Vinogradova OL. Moderate-Intensity Strength Exercise to Exhaustion Results in More Pronounced Signaling Changes in Skeletal Muscles of Strength-Trained Compared With Untrained Individuals. *J Strength Condit Res* 34: 1103–1112, 2020.

106. Machida M, Takeda K, Yokono H, Ikemune S, Taniguchi Y, Kiyosawa H, Takemasa T. Reduction of ribosome biogenesis with activation of the mTOR pathway in denervated atrophic muscle. *J Cell Physiol* 227: 1569–76, 2012.

107. Mackey AL, Donnelly AE, Turpeenniemi-Hujanen T, Roper HP. Skeletal muscle collagen content in humans after high-force eccentric contractions. *J Appl Physiol* 97: 197–203, 2004.

108. Mangine GT, Hoffman JR, Gonzalez AM, Townsend JR, Wells AJ, Jajtner AR, Beyer KS, et al. Exercise-induced hormone elevations are related to muscle growth. *J Strength Condit Res* 31: 45–53, 2017.

109. Maniotis AJ, Chen CS, Ingber DE. Demonstration of mechanical connections between integrins, cytoskeletal filaments, and nucleoplasm that stabilize nuclear structure. *Proc Natl Acad Sci* 94: 849–854, 1997.

110. Markworth JF, Vella LD, Figueiredo VC, Cameron-Smith D. Ibuprofen treatment blunts early translational signaling responses in human skeletal muscle following resistance exercise. *J Appl Physiol* 117: 20–28 2014.

111. Martin TD, Dennis MD, Gordon BS, Kimball SR, Jefferson LS. mTORC1 and JNK coordinate phosphorylation of the p70S6K1 autoinhibitory domain in skeletal muscle following functional overloading. *Am J Physiol: Endocrinol Metabol* 306: E1397–E1405, 2014.

112. Martineau LC, Gardiner PF. Insight into skeletal muscle mechanotransduction: MAPK activation is quantitatively related to tension. *J Appl Physiol* 91: 693–702, 2011.

113. Martyn J. Chapter I – Zoology and the anatomy of animals. In: *The Philosophical Transactions Abridged. Part III Anatomical and Medical Papers*. London, UK: The Royal Society, p. 799–926, 1756.

114. McKendry J, Pérez-López A, McLeod M, Luo D, Dent JR, Smeuninx B, Yu J, Taylor AE, Philp A, Breen L. Short inter-set rest blunts resistance exercise-induced increases in myofibrillar protein synthesis and intracellular signaling in young males. *Exp Physiol* 101: 866–82, 2016.

115. Meijer JP, Jaspers RT, Rittweger J, Seynnes OR, Kamandulis S, Brazaitis M, Skurvydas A, et al. Single muscle fibre contractile properties differ between body-builders, power athletes and control subjects. *Exp Physiol* 100: 1331–41, 2015.

116. Meissner JD, Chang KC, Kubis HP, Nebreda AR, Gros G, Scheibe RJ. The p38alpha/beta mitogen-activated protein kinases mediate recruitment of CREB-binding protein to preserve fast myosin heavy chain IId/x gene activity in myotubes. *J Biol Chem* 282: 7265–75, 2007.

117. Meissner JD, Freund R, Krone D, Umeda PK, Chang KC, Gros G, Scheibe RJ. Extracellular signal-regulated kinase ½ – mediated phosphorylation of p300 enhances myosin heavy chain I/beta gene expression via acetylation of nuclear factor of activated T cells c1. *Nucl Acids Res* 39: 5907–5925, 2011.

118. Miyazaki M, McCarthy JJ, Fedele MJ, Esser KA. Early activation of mTORC1 signaling in response to mechanical overload is independent of phosphoinositide 3-kinase/Akt signaling. *J Physiol* 589: 1831–1846, 2011.

119. Moore DR, Atherton PJ, Rennie MJ, Tarnopolsky MA, Phillips SM. Resistance exercise enhances mTOR and MAPK signaling in human muscle over that seen at rest after bolus protein ingestion. *Acta Physiol (Oxf)* 201: 365–372, 2011.

120. Morton RW, Oikawa SY, Wavell CG, Mazara N, McGlory C, Quadrilatero J, Baechler BL, Baker SK, Phillips SM. Neither load nor systemic hormones determine resistance training-mediated hypertrophy or strength gains in resistance-trained young men. *J Appl Physiol* 121: 129–138, 2016.

121. Morton RW, Sonne MW, Farias Zuniga A, Mohammad IYZ, Jones A, McGlory C, Keir PJ, Potvin JR, Phillips SM. Muscle fibre activation is unaffected by load and repetition duration when resistance exercise is performed to task failure. *J Physiol* 597: 4601–4613, 2019.

122. Muir J. *My First Summer in the Sierra*. Boston, MA: Houghton Mifflin, 1911, p. 110.

123. Murach KA, Englund DA, Dupont-Versteegden EE, McCarthy JJ, Peterson CA. Myonuclear domain flexibility challenges rigid assumptions on satellite cell contribution to skeletal muscle fiber hypertrophy. *Front Physiol* 9: 635, 2018.

124. Murach KA, Fry CS, Kirby TJ, Jackson JR, Lee JD, White SH, Dupont-Versteegden EE, McCarthy JJ, Peterson CA. Starring or supporting role? Satellite cells and skeletal muscle fiber size regulation. *Physiol* 33: 26–38, 2018.

125. Murgia M, Serrano AL, Calabria E, Pallafacchina G, Lomo T, Schiaffino S. Ras is involved in nerve-activity-dependent regulation of muscle genes. *Nature Cell Biol* 2: 142–147, 2000.

126. Na S, Collin O, Chowdhury F, Tay B, Ouyang M, Wang Y, Wang N. Rapid signal transduction in living cells is a unique feature of mechanotransduction. *Proc Natl Acad Sci* 105: 6626–6631, 2008.

127. Najrana T, Sanchez-Esteban J. Mechanotransduction as an adaptation to gravity. *Front Pediatrics* 4: 140, 2016.

128. Newham DJ, McPhail G, Mills KR, Edwards RH. Ultrastructural changes after concentric and eccentric contractions of human muscle. *J Neurosci* 61: 109–122, 1983.

129. Nicoll JX, Fry AC, Galpin AJ, Sterczala AJ, Thomason DB, Moore CA, Weiss LW, Chiu LZF. Changes in resting mitogen-activated protein kinases following resistance exercise overreaching and overtraining. *Eur J Appl Physiol* 116: 2401–2413, 2016

130. Nicoll JX, Fry AC, Mosier EM. Sex-based differences in resting MAPK, androgen, and glucocorticoid receptor phosphorylation in human skeletal muscle. *Steroids* 141: 23–29, 2019a.

131. Nicoll JX, Fry AC, Mosier EM, Olsen LA, Sontag SA. MAPK, androgen, and glucocorticoid receptor phosphorylation following high-frequency resistance exercise non-functional overreaching. *Eur J Appl Physiol* 119: 2237–2253, 2019b.

132. Ohno Y, Oyama A, Kaneko H, Egawa T, Yokoyama S, Sugiura T, Ohira Y, Yoshioka T, Goto K. Lactate increases myotube diameter via activation of MEK/ERK pathway in C2C12 cells. *Acta Physiol (Oxf)* 223: e13042, 2018.

133. Oishi Y, Ogata T, Ohira Y, Taniguchi K, Roy RR. Calcineurin and heat shock protein 72 in functionally overloaded rat plantaris muscle. *Biochem Biophysl Res Comm* 330: 706–713, 2005.

134. Oishi Y, Tsukamoto H, Yokokawa T, Hirotsu K, Shimazu M, Uchida K, Tomi H, Higashida K, Iwanaka N, Hashimoto T. Mixed lactate and caffeine compound increases satellite cell activity and anabolic signals for muscle hypertrophy. *J Appl Physiol* 118: 742–749, 2015.

135. Palmisano MG, Bremner SN, Hornberger TA, Meyer GA, Domenighetti AA, Shah SB, Kiss B, Kellermayer M, Ryan AF, Lieber RL. Skeletal muscle intermediate filaments form a stress-transmitting and stress-signaling network. *J Cell Sci* 128: 219–24, 2015.

136. Pareja-Blanco F, Rodriguez-Rosell D, Sánchez-Medina L, Sanchis-Moysi J, Dorado C, Mora-Custodio R, Yáñez-Garcia JM, et al. Effects of velocity loss during resistance training on athletic performance, strength gains and muscle adaptations. *Scand J Med Sci Sports* 27: 724–735, 2017.

137. Parsons SA, Millay DP, Wilkins BJ, Bueno OF, Tsika GL, Neilson JR, Liberatore CM, et al. Genetic loss of calcineurin blocks mechanical overload-induced skeletal muscle fiber type switching but not hypertrophy. *J Biol Chem* 279: 26192–26200, 2004.

138. Pérez-López A, McKendry J, Martin-Rincon M, Morales-Alamo D, Pérez-Köhler B, Valadés D, Buján J, Calbet JAL, Breen L. Skeletal muscle IL-15/IL-15Ra and myofibrillar protein synthesis after resistance exercise. *Scand J Med Sci Sports* 28: 116–125, 2018.

139. Petrella JK, Kim JS, Mayhew DL, Cross JM, Bamman MM. Potent myofiber hypertrophy during resistance training in humans is associated with satellite cell-mediated myonuclear addition: a cluster analysis. *J Appl Physiol* 104: 1736–1742, 2008.

140. Popov DV, Lysenko EA, Bachinin AV, Miller TF, Kurochkina NS, Kravchenko IV, Furalyov VA, Vinogradova OL. Influence of resistance exercise intensity and metabolic stress on anabolic signaling and expression of myogenic genes in skeletal muscle. *Muscle Nerve* 51: 434–442, 2015.

141. Rahnert JA, Burkholder TJ. High-frequency electrical stimulation reveals a p38-mTOR signaling module correlated with force-time integral. *J Exp Biol* 216: 2619–2631, 2013.

142. Ramaswamy KS, Palmer ML, van der Meulen JH, Renoux A, Kostrominova TY, Michele DE, Faulkner JA. Lateral transmission of force is impaired in skeletal muscles of dystrophic mice and very old rats. *J Physiol* 589: 1195–1208, 2011.

143. Ratamess N. *ACSM's Foundations of Strength Training and Conditioning*. Philadelphia, PA: Lippincott Williams & Wilkins, 2012.

144. Rauch C, Loughna PT. Strech-induced activation of ERK in myocytes is p38 and calcineurin-dependent. *Cell Biochem Funct* 26: 866–869, 2008.

145. Reidy PT, Porack MS, Markofski MM, Dickinson JM, Fry CS, Deer RR, Volpi E, Rasmussen BB. Post-absorptive muscle protein turnover affects resistance training hypertrophy. *Eur J Appl Physiol* 117: 853–866, 2017.

146. Riechman SE, Balasekaran G, Roth SM, Ferrell RE. Association of interleukin-15 protein and inter-leukin-15 receptor genetic variation with resistance exercise training responses. *J Appl Physiol* 97: 2214–2219, 2004.

147. Rindom E, Vissing K. Mechanosensitive molecular networks involved in transducing resistance exercise-signals into muscle protein accretion. *Front Physiol* 7: 547, 2016.

148. Roux PP, Shahbazian D, Vu H, Holz MK, Cohen MS, Taunton J, Soenberg N, Blenis J. RAS/ERK signaling promotes site-specific ribosomal protein S6 phosphorylation via RSK and stimulates cap-dependent translation. *J Biol Chem* 282: 14056–14064, 2007.

149. Schoenfeld BJ. Does exercise-induced muscle damage play a role in skeletal muscle hypertrophy? *J Strength Condit Res* 26: 1441–1453, 2012.

150. Schoenfeld BJ, Pope ZK, Benik FM, Hester GM, Sellers J, Nooner JL, Schnaiter JA, et al. Longer interset rest periods enhance muscle strength and hypertrophy in resistance-trained men. *J Strength Condit Res* 30: 1805–1812, 2016.

151. Schwartz LM. Skeletal muscles do not undergo apoptosis during either atrophy or programmed cell death-revisiting the myonuclear domain hypothesis. *Front Physiol* 9: 1887, 2019.

152. Shi H, Zeng C, Ricome A, Hannon K, Grant A, Gerrard DE. Extracellular signal-regulated kinase pathway is differentially involved in beta agonist-induced hypertrophy in slow and fast muscles. *Am J Physiol* 292: C1681–C1689, 2007.

153. Shi H, Scheffler JM, Pleitner JM, Zeng C, Park S, Hannon KM, Grant AL, Gerrard DE. Modulation of skel-etal muscle fiber type by mitogen-activated protein kinase signaling. *FASEB J* 8: 2990–3000, 2008.

154. Shi H, Scheffler JM, Zeng C, Pleitner JM, Hannon KM, Grant AL, Gerrard DE. Mitogen-activated protein kinase signaling is necessary for maintenance of skeletal muscle mass. *Am J Physiol: Cell Physiol* 296: C1040–C1048, 2009.

155. Spiering BA, Kraemer WJ, Anderson JM, Armstrong LE, Nindl BC, Volek JS, Judelson DAet al. Effects of elevated circulating hormones on resistance exercise-induced Akt signaling. *Med Sci Sports Exerc* 40: 1039–1048, 2008.

156. Spiering BA, Kraemer WJ, Vingren JL, Ratamess NA, Anderson JM, Armstrong LE, Nindl BC, Volek JS, Häkkinen K, Maresh CM. Elevated endogenous testosterone concentrations potentiate muscle androgen receptor responses to resistance exercise. *J Steroid Biochem Mol Biol* 114: 195–199, 2009.

157. Spillane M, Schwarz N, Willoughby DS. Upper-body resistance exercise vastus lateralis androgen receptor-DNA binding and canonical Wnt/B-catenin signaling compared to lower-body resistance exercise in resistance-trained men without an increase in serum testosterone. *Steroids* 98: 63–71, 2015.

158. Staron RS, Karapondo DL, Kraemer WJ, Fry AC, Gordon SE, Falkel JE, Hagerman FC, Hikida RS. Skeletal muscle adaptations during early phase of heavy-resistance training in men and women. *J Appl Physiol* 76: 1247–1255, 1994.

159. Stec MJ, Kelly NA, Many GM, Windham ST, Tuggle SC, Bamman MM. Ribosome biogenesis may augment resistance training-induced myofiber hypertrophy and is required for myotube growth in vitro. *Am J Physiol: Endocrinol Metabol* 310: E652–E661, 2016.

160. Steensberg A, Keller C, Starkie RL, Osada T, Febbraio MA, Pedersen BK. IL-6 and TNF-alpha expression in, and release from, contracting human skeletal muscle. *Am J Physiol: Endocrinol Metabol* 283: E1272–E1278, 2002.

161. Stefanovsky VY, Pelletier G, Hannan R, Gagnon-Kugler T, Rothblum LI, Moss T. An immediate response of ribosomal transcription to growth factor stimulation in mammals is mediated by ERK phosphorylation of UBF. *Mol Cell* 8: 1063–1073, 2001.

162. Stone MH, Stone M, Sands WA. *Principles and Practice of Resistance Training*. Champaign, IL: Human Kinetics, 2007.

163. Tajik A, Zhang Y, Wei F, Sun J, Jia Q, Zhou W, Wang N. Transcription upregulation via force-induced direct stretching of chromatin. *Nat Mater* 15: 1287–1296, 2016.

164. Takagi R, Ogasawara R, Takegaki J, Tamura Y, Tsutaki A, Nakazato K, Ishii N. Past injurious exercise attenuates activation of primary calcium-dependent injury pathways in skeletal muscle during subsequent exercise. *Physiol Reports* 6: e13660, 2018.

165. Takagi R, Ogasawara R, Takegaki J, Tsutaki A, Nakazato K, Ishii N. Influence of past injurious exercise on fiber-type specific acute anabolic response to resistance exercise in skeletal muscle. *J Appl Physiol* 124: 16–22, 2018.

166. Takegaki J, Ogaswara R, Tamura Y, Takagi R, Arihara Y, Tsutaki A, Nakazato K, Ishii N. Repeated bouts of resistance exercise with short recovery periods activates mTOR signaling, not protein synthesis in mouse skeletal muscle. *Physiol Reports* 5: e13515, 2017.

167. Tang JE, Perco JG, Moore DR, Wilkinson SB, Phillips SM. Resistance training alters the response of fed state mixed muscle protein synthesis in young men. *Am J Physiol: Reg Integr Comp Physiol* 294: R172–R178, 2008.

168. Tatsumi R. Mechano-biology of skeletal muscle hypertrophy and regeneration: possible mechanism of stretch-induced activation of resident myogenic stem cells. *Anim Sci J* 81: 11–20, 2010.

169. Terzis G, Spengos K, Mascher H, Georgiadis G, Manta P, Bloomstrand E. The degree of p70S6k and S6 phosphorylation in human skeletal muscle in response to resistance exercise depends on the training volume. *Eur J Appl Physiol* 110: 835–843, 2010.

170. Thomson DM, Fick CA, Gordon SE. AMPK activation attenuates S6K1, 4E-BP1, and eEF2 signaling responses to high-frequency electrically stimulated skeletal muscle contractions. *J Appl Physiol* 104: 625–632, 2008.

171. Trappe TA, Carroll CC, Dickinson JM, LeMoine JK, Haus JM, Sullivan BE, Lee JD, Jemiolo B, Weinheimer EM, Hollon CJ. Influence of acetaminophen and ibuprofen on skeletal muscle adaptations to resistance exercise in older adults. *Am J Physiol: Reg Integr Comp Physiol* 300: R655–R662, 2011.

172. Trenerry MK, Della Gatta PA, Larsen AE, Garnham AP, Cameron-Smith D. Impact of resistance exercise training on interleukin-6 and JAK/STAT in young men. *Muscle Nerve* 43: 385–392, 2011.

173. Vingren JL, Kraemer WJ, Hatfield DL, Volek JS, Ratamess NA, Anderson JM, Häkkinen K, et al. Effect of resistance exercise on muscle steroid receptor protein content in strength-trained men and women. *Steroids* 74: 1033–1039, 2009.

174. Warren GL, Hulderman T, Jensen N, McKinstry M, Mishra M, Luster MI, Simeonova PP. Physiological role of tumor necrosis factor alpha in traumatic muscle injury. *FASEB J* 16: 1630–1632, 2002.

175. West DW, Baehr LM, Marcotte GR, Chason CM, Tolento L, Gomes AV, Bodine SC, Baar K. Acute resistance exercise activates rapamycin-sensitive and -insensitive mechanisms that control translational activity and capacity in skeletal muscle. *J Physiol* 594: 453–468, 2016.

176. West DW, Burd NA, Churchward-Venne TA, Camera DM, Mitchell CJ, Baker SK, Hawley JA, Coffey VG, Phillips SM. Sex-based comparisons of myofibrillar protein synthesis after resistance exercise in the fed state. *J Appl Physiol* 112: 1805–1813, 2012.

177. West DW, Burd NA, Staples AW, Phillips SM. Human exercise-mediated skeletal muscle hypertrophy is an intrinsic process. *Int J Biochem Cell Biol* 42: 1371–1375, 2010.

178. White JP, Gao S, Puppa MJ, Sato S, Welle SL, Carson JA. Testosterone regulation of Akt/mTORC1/Foxo signaling in skeletal muscle. *Mol Cell Endocrinol* 365: 174–186, 2013.

179. Wilkinson SB, Phillips SM, Atherton PJ, Patel R, Yarasheski KE, Tarnopolsky MA, Rennie MJ. Differential effects of resistance and endurance exercise in the fed state on signaling molecule phosphorylation and protein synthesis in human muscle. *J Physiol* 586: 3701–3717, 2008.

180. Willkomm L, Gehlert S, Jacko D, Schiffer T, Bloch W. p38MAPK activation and H3K4 trimethylation is decreased by lactate in vitro and high intensity resistance training in human skeletal muscle. *PLOS ONE* 12: e0176609, 2017.

181. Williamson DL, Kubica N, Kimball SR, Jefferson LS. Exercise-induced alterations in extracellular signal-related kinase ½ and mammalian target of rapamycin (mTOR) signaling to regulatory mechanisms of mRNA translation in mouse muscle. *J Physiol* 573: 497–510, 2006.

182. Woolstenhulme MT, Conlee RK, Drummond MJ, Stites AW, Parcell AC. Temporal response of desmin and dystrophin proteins to progressive resistance exercise in human skeletal muscle. *J Appl Physiol* 100: 1876–1882, 2006.

183. Wretman,C, Lionikas A, Widegren U, Lännergren J, Westerblad H, Henriksson J. Effects of concentric and eccentric contractions on phosphorylation of MAPKerk1/2 and MAPKp38 in isolated rate skeletal muscle. *J Physiol* 535: 155–164, 2001.

184. You J-S, Lincoln HC, Kim CR, Frey JW, Goodman CA, Zhong XP, Hornberger TA. The role of diacylglycerol kinase ζ and phosphatidic acid in the mechanical activation of mammalian target of rapamycin (mTOR) signaling and skeletal muscle hypertrophy. *J Biol Chem* 289: 1551–1563, 2014.

185. Yuan Y, Xu Y, Xu J, Liang B, Cai X, Zhu C, Wang L, et al. Succinate promotes skeletal muscle protein synthesis via Erk1/2 signaling pathway. *Mol Med Reports* 16: 7361–7366, 2017.

186. Zatsiorsky, V, Kraemer WJ, Fry AC. *Science and Practice of Strength Training* (3rd Edition). Champaign, IL: Human Kinetics, 2021.

187. Zeng F, Zhao H, Liao J. Androgen interacts with exercise through the mTOR pathway to induce skeletal muscle hypertrophy. *Biol Sport* 34: 313–321, 2017.

188. Zhang Z, Liu R, Townsend PA, Proud CG. p90RSKs mediate activation of ribosomal RNA synthesis by hypertrophic agonist phenylephrine in adult cardiomyocytes. *J Mol Cell Cardiol* 59: 139–147, 2013.

7

RESPONSES TO MUSCULAR EXERCISE, HEAT SHOCK PROTEINS AS REGULATORS OF INFLAMMATION, AND MITOCHONDRIAL QUALITY CONTROL

Alex T. Von Schulze and Paige C. Geiger

Background

While we often think of muscular exercise as beneficial to health, it remains important to remember that acute exercise bouts are an intense bioenergetic stress at the molecular level. For instance, aerobic exercise is known to increase cellular oxidative stress (71), cause alterations in mitochondrial respiratory capacity (35), and induce the unfolded protein response (95). Despite these acute stressors, it is well-established that exercise is a net-positive in terms of overall cellular health. One may ask how these acute stressors lead to a positive net effect over time. The answer may lie within a highly conserved set of proteins named heat shock proteins (HSPs), which are induced by exercise and oxidative stress (46, 51).

Molecular Chaperones: Heat Shock Proteins

Like many great discoveries in science, HSPs were first discovered by accident. Ferruccio Ritossa, the investigator credited in part with the discovery of HSPs, recounts from the 1960s when a member of his lab increased the temperature on an incubator housing *Drosophila* and he noticed a distinct "puffing pattern" on their chromosomes (75). This chromosomal puffing pattern was later determined to be messenger ribonucleic acid (mRNA) transcription sites for a distinct set of stress chaperones, aptly named HSPs, acting to protect the cell from apoptosis (90). From their discovery in the 1960s to now, HSPs have become commonplace when studying diseases that cause metabolic and/or proteotoxic stress in cells. The reason for this is that HSPs can act as molecular chaperones, ultimately reducing inflammation, apoptotic signalling, and proteotoxic stress.

Broadly defined, molecular chaperones are a key set of proteins that help "guide" various proteins within the cell to remain functional and/or get targeted for degradation under stressful conditions. In this way, molecular chaperones such as HSPs allow cells to survive under stress. HSPs specifically facilitate the folding of new proteins, the refolding of damaged proteins, the targeting on non-functional proteins/organelles for degradation, intracellular signalling, and the import/export of proteins into/out of the mitochondria (Figure 7.1) (15, 24, 29, 92). Importantly, different HSPs (characterized by their molecular weight in kilodaltons) have varying functions. For the purposes

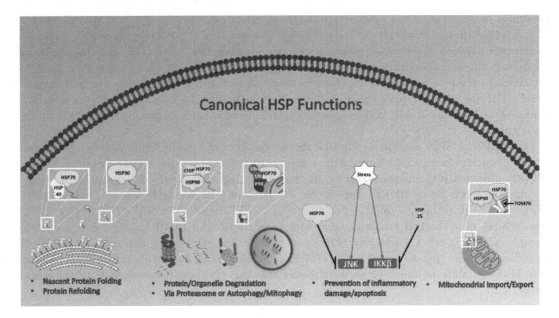

Figure 7.1   Canonical HSP functions

of this chapter, we will focus on four well-characterized HSP families: HSP70, HSP40, HSP90, and HSP25.

Initiation

As mentioned previously, HSP induction occurs as a cellular stress response to stimuli such as exercise or oxidative stress. This induction is first initiated by the primary transcription factor for HSPs, heat shock factor 1 (HSF1), which trimerizes and undergoes nuclear translocation under stress (53, 78). In combination with the transcriptional co-activator peroxisome proliferator-activated receptor gamma coactivator 1-alpha (PGC1α), HSF1 binds to its canonical DNA docking sites known as heat shock elements (HSEs), which act as promoter regions for HSP-related genes (78, 97). Upon the HSF1–PGC1α complex binding, HSF1 is phosphorylated and transcription is initiated (78). As with many other proteins, HSF1's activity is dependent on HSP content. Specifically, once enough HSPs (specifically HSP70) are translated, they in turn bind to HSF1, removing it from its DNA docking site and returning it to its monomeric form in the cytoplasm (78). PGC1α can also counter-regulate HSF1 through transcriptional repression (60). In this way, the stress response is a tightly regulated process coupled to cellular HSP and PGC1α content. Moreover, this increase in intracellular HSP content is critical for cell survival and proteostasis under stress.

Cell Survival and Intracellular Signalling

Cellular stress in the form of oxidative injury, structural damage, or bioenergetic disruption can lead to the activation of cell death, or apoptotic, signalling pathways. Fortunately, under normal physiologic circumstances, cells have the ability to override that signalling via the activation of cell survival and anti-inflammatory signalling pathways. Not surprisingly, molecular chaperones such as HSPs are critical mediators of this cell survival process.

Under stress conditions, an adaptive mechanism of the cell is to suppress protein synthesis, cell cycle progression, and cell differentiation and to instigate inflammatory signalling. The canonical mediators of this "hard-stop" pathway are the mitogen-activated protein kinases (MAPKs) such as C-jun-NH2-terminal kinase (JNK) and p38 (91). More specifically, the activation of JNK causes the nuclear translocation of the transcription factor c-Jun via phosphorylation (37). Upon nuclear translocation, c-Jun increases transcriptional activity of pro-apoptotic and oncogenic genes (6, 7, 81, 100). However, in the presence of HSP70, this pro-apoptotic and oncogenic stimulus can be repressed. HSP70 directly inhibits c-Jun's upstream kinase JNK by preventing its activation by its respective kinase SEK1 (67). In this way, HSP70 re-routes signalling away from apoptotic pathways to cell survival pathways.

Like HSP70, HSP25 is known to inhibit the activation of the pro-inflammatory transcriptional complex, nuclear factor kappa-light-chain-enhancer of activated B cells (NF-κB). HSP25-induced NF-κB inhibition is thought to occur by preventing the degradation NF-κB's upstream inhibitory regulator, the IκB kinase (IKK) complex (25, 45). It is believed that HSP25 blocks the phosphorylation of IKKβ, whose phosphorylation is critical for the degradation of the IKK complex (68). This inhibition of the IκB kinase complex formation (IKKα and IKKβ) causes a decrease in the phosphorylation of NF-κB inhibitor, IκB, which ultimately suppresses the activation of the NF-κB signalling pathway (45). As with HSP70, HSP25 can shift the cell away from inflammatory signalling. However, shifts in signalling are not the only ways that HSPs can prevent cell death and restore homeostasis.

Protein Folding and Degradation

HSPs are critical in cell proteostasis through their ability to fold nascent proteins and refold damaged proteins. Importantly, HSP70, HSP40, and HSP90 are all critical in ensuring proteostasis by facilitating proper folding of newly translated proteins exiting ribosomes at the endoplasmic reticulum (ER) (24, 29, 92). Ribosome-associated co-chaperones (MPP1 and HSPA14) transfer nascent proteins to non-ribosomal HSP70 chaperone complexes (HSP70 and HSP40), which facilitate the native folding of proteins requiring a high degree of complex co-translational folding (some subsets may be transferred to HSP90 for further processing via Hsp70-Hsp90 Organizing Protein (HOP)) (88, 92). In addition to the folding of nascent proteins, these HSPs are involved in the refolding of damaged or unfolded proteins. After recognition, recruitment, and transfer of unfolded proteins via co-chaperone HSP40, protein-bound HSP70 undergoes adenosine triphosphate (ATP) cycling via nucleotide exchange factors to cause conformational changes in HSP70—ultimately enabling native folding based on amino acid characteristics (i.e., polarity) (29). If proteins are unable to refold via HSP70, they can be passed along to chaperonins (i.e., HSP60 and HSP10) and/or HSP90 for extended processing. If it is not possible for the protein to fold into its native form via its interactions with these chaperones, it is likely to be tagged for degradation via the ubiquitin–proteasome system (UPS).

HSPs have the additional ability to tag and initiate the degradation of damaged proteins via the UPS. The UPS tags damaged or aggregated proteins with ubiquitin to target them for degradation via the proteasome (22). HSP70 and HSP90 are linked to the UPS via the co-chaperone carboxyl terminus of Hsc70 interacting protein (CHIP) and ubiquitin conjugating enzyme E2 N (UBE2N) (20, 98). CHIP, an E3 ubiquitin ligase, contains N-terminal binding domains for both HSP70 and HSP90. Upon HSP70 or HSP90 binding with the damaged target protein, the protein-bound HSP complexes are recruited to CHIP (12). This CHIP:HSP:Protein complex then interacts with the UBEN2, allowing for the transfer and ligation of ubiquitin onto target proteins (98). Once the substrate protein is tagged with ubiquitin, the nucleotide exchange factor, Bcl-2-associated athanogene 1 (BAG1), binds to the CHIP:HSP:Protein-ub complex allowing for proteasomal recruitment and eventual substrate release (54). In this way, HSP40, HSP70, and HSP90 work with CHIP synergistically to degrade proteins that are beyond repair.

Mitochondrial Import

In addition to their roles in signalling and protein folding/degradation, HSPs facilitate the translocation of precursor proteins into the mitochondria. HSP70 and HSP90 translocate precursor proteins with mitochondrial localization sequences to the outer mitochondrial membrane, transferring them to the translocase receptor TOM70 for mitochondrial import (13, 99). Upon import through the TOM and TIM complexes on the outer and inner mitochondrial membrane, respectively, intramitochondrial HSP70 folds the protein into its native functional form (13). As most mitochondrial proteins are encoded by nuclear deoxyribonucleic acid (DNA) and made in the ER, cytoplasmic transport and mitochondrial import of mitochondrial target proteins are critical for overall mitochondrial health and function. In this way, HSPs are indirectly or directly involved in energy homeostasis.

HSPs and Chronic Disease

Considering all the critical functions that HSPs play in cell homeostasis and survival, it is not surprising that overall HSP function is associated with human health and disease. For instance, HSP function is tightly coupled to insulin resistance and type 2 diabetes (25). Specifically, HSP expression declines with type 2 diabetes in humans, and rodents have increased susceptibility to insulin resistance when the gene for HSP70 is knocked out (11, 15). Conversely, HSP induction via transgenic overexpression, pharmacologic intervention, or heat protects against diet-induced obesity and insulin resistance in rodent studies (11, 27, 76). It is hypothesized that this association is due in part to the anti-inflammatory/anti-apoptotic signalling roles of HSPs during disease-induced stress (25). For instance, type 2 diabetes and insulin resistance increase oxidative stress, instigating c-Jun and NF-κB activation—ultimately increasing inflammation and inhibiting a critical component of the insulin signalling pathway: insulin receptor substrate-1 (IRS-1) (30, 42). As noted earlier, HSP70 and HSP25 are shown to reduce c-Jun and NF-κB activity, respectively (25), thus relieving repression on the insulin signalling cascade to allow for proper substrate utilization. Of note, this protective effect of HSPs extends to diseases far beyond type 2 diabetes such as cardiovascular disease, Alzheimer disease, Parkinson disease, autoimmune diseases, and cancer (10, 63, 70, 74, 94). Thus, HSPs are proving to provide therapeutic potential in nearly all diseases with an inflammatory, proteostatic, and/or metabolic component, making them an increasingly interesting area of research.

HSPs and Exercise

As mentioned previously, exercise is an acute bioenergetic and metabolic stress; thus, it is not surprising that stress proteins such as HSPs up-regulate after exercise. It is well known that the HSP70 and HSP20 families increase transcription and content after bouts of physical exercise (18, 43, 47, 84, 85). Importantly, HSP70 is responsive to both high-intensity endurance (59) and resistance training (62), whereas HSP20 is more responsive to resistance training (eccentric) (23). This response is critical for exercise adaptation and recovery (32, 40).

Interestingly, the primary stressor responsible for HSP synthesis post-exercise is not known. It is known that common effects of exercise such as increased temperature, ischemia, acidosis, intracellular calcium, and oxidation can all independently induce HSPs in a variety of tissues/models (8, 33, 51, 56, 89). In addition, it is known that ATP and glycogen depletion (which are primary outcomes during exercise) instigate HSP synthesis (17, 19). Put simply, the milieu of stressors associated with exercise likely all contribute to HSP induction and, importantly, the degree to which these stressors are at play appear to act as a rheostat for HSP expression. A summary of the role of HSP induction post-exercise can be found in Figure 7.2.

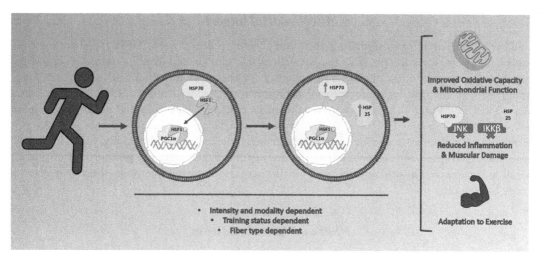

Figure 7.2 Functions of HSPs post–exercise

Intensity Is the Primary Driver of the HSP Response to Exercise

As with most adaptations to exercise, the HSP response to an exercise bout is dependent on duration and intensity (32). However, it appears that intensity is a greater factor driving HSP induction than duration per se. For instance, when exercise protocols have equal volumes and differing intensities, varying levels of HSP70 expression are attributed to the degree of intensity at which the exercise is performed (49). This positive correlation between exercise intensity (both aerobic and strength training) and HSP70 induction has been noted in numerous studies (18, 49, 50, 72). Interestingly, the addition of heat to exercise bouts leads to a potentiated increase in HSP70 expression compared to either stressor alone (80). Therefore, exercise intensity appears to be a more potent regulator of HSP70 expression than overall volume. Put another way, the more stress that is incurred on the system, the greater the stress response. In this light, it would be correct to assume that the HSP response is also dependent on training status (i.e., trained versus sedentary).

The HSP Response is Dependent on Training Status

It is well established that a repeated bout of identical or similar training loads results in muscular adaptations that reduce symptoms associated with muscle damage compared to the original bout (57). This process of adaptation is referred to as the repeated bout effect (64) and can last anywhere from 4 weeks (83) to 6 months after just one bout of damaging exercise (66). Therefore, it would seem appropriate that the stress response to similar exercise bouts would diminish over time. Indeed, a compensatory adaptation to chronic exercise training is a constitutive up-regulation of basal HSP expression and only a modest induction of HSPs post-exercise, as opposed to acute training in untrained subjects (26, 83, 85). Conversely, detraining reduces basal HSPs to levels similar to pre-training (26). In summary, exposure to high-intensity exercise can provide a positive physiologic adaptation in terms of basal HSP content level and reduced muscular damage.

HSPs Involvement in Muscular Remodelling

Intensive exercise, specifically eccentric contractions, are extremely destructive to the structural components of muscle cells and fibres, often causing apoptotic signalling (2, 3, 93). Interestingly, increases in HSP70 expression only increase with exercise that contains lengthening contractions, and there is a positive correlation between force-generating capacity and increased HSP70 expression (36, 69). Thus, it appears that structural damage and pro-apoptotic signalling are the primary inducers of HSP expression, not just muscular work alone. Indeed, sarcoplasmic destruction increases pro-apoptotic cleaved caspase-3 activity, which is mediated in part by JNK signalling (9, 93). Recalling that HSP70 is a potent inhibitor of JNK (67), it is plausible that the primary instigator of exercise-induced HSP content is pro-apoptotic signalling.

Like the repeated bout effect, overexpression or induction of HSP70 prior to exercise can mitigate the degree of damage induced in skeletal muscle (61, 65, 87). Therefore, it appears that having chaperones around prior to exercise can mitigate the amount of damage to muscle cells and/or aid in the regeneration process. Indeed, many have suggested that HSPs are required for muscle regeneration post-injury (39, 79, 87). This regeneration is thought to occur through HSP70-modulated satellite cell proliferation and protein synthesis (39). These data suggest that HSPs are a critical component to exercise adaptation. However, the HSP response and subsequent adaptation appear to be fibre type–dependent.

HSP Expression is Fibre Type Specific

Numerous studies show a direct association between HSP content and skeletal muscle fibre type (34, 44, 52). For instance, at rest HSPs (HSP72 and HSP25) are constitutively expressed in the predominantly type I fibre soleus, but not in the type IIA-B fibre white gastrocnemius and extensor digitorum longus (EDL) (44, 52). Similarly, during exercise HSP expression increases in the soleus but gradually declines in the EDL (34). However, within the hours following exercise, there is a greater HSP response in the EDL compared to the soleus (34). This potentiated response in type II fibre muscles could be due to their inherently low basal HSP content, rendering the tissue less equipped for any stress imposed. In this way, HSP expression and response to exercise correlate to the proportion of type I fibre and oxidative capacity of the muscle involved (52).

HSPs and Oxidative Capacity

Oxidative capacity is directly linked to muscle fibre type and therefore linked to basal HSP content and the HSP response (5). Moreover, fibre type/oxidative capacity are linked to mitochondrial content and function capacity in skeletal muscle (5). Thus, it would be safe to hypothesize that HSP content is associated with muscle oxidative capacity and mitochondrial function. Indeed, transgenic overexpression of HSP72 in skeletal muscle also increases mitochondrial enzyme activity, mitochondrial content, and endurance running capacity (5, 8), whereas mitochondrial function is compromised in the absence of HSP72 (1, 15). Additionally, it has been shown that intrinsic aerobic capacity is inherently coupled to muscle HSP content and the HSP response in rodents selectively bred for running capacity (76). However, the direct role of HSP content in muscle oxidative capacity and mitochondrial functions remains unknown.

HSPs and Mitochondrial Quality Control

Mitochondrial quality control ([MitoQC], defined as adequate or enhanced mitochondrial oxidative capacity) is critical in bioenergetic homeostasis both at rest and during exercise. MitoQC is often characterized by two coordinated steps: (1) the degradation of damaged mitochondria (mitophagy) and (2) the synthesis of new healthy mitochondria (mitochondrial biogenesis) (41, 82). Importantly, mitophagy alleviates oxidative stress by reducing the accumulation of damaged reactive oxygen species (ROS)–producing mitochondria (14). ROS is also simultaneously reduced via improved mitochondrial coupling efficiency in newly synthesized "healthy" mitochondria (21). As mentioned previously, exercise induces mitochondrial ROS production (71); thus, exercise likely triggers MitoQC.

Indeed, endurance exercise is shown to increase mitochondrial enzyme activity and content, as well as mitophagy, in humans (4, 35).

HSPs and Mitophagy

As we know that exercise induces HSP expression and that HSPs are involved in mitochondrial function, it is tempting to speculate that HSPs are directly involved in exercise-induced mitophagy. Indeed, HSP72 is thought to be a critical binding partner for the mitochondrial recruitment and action of the mitophagy-associated E3 ubiquitin ligase, parkin (15). Briefly, parkin regulates mitophagy through ubiquitination of outer mitochondrial membrane proteins, which are subsequently targeted for autophagosome recruitment (38). In this way, HSP72 may be directly involved in skeletal muscle mitophagy. Indeed, muscle cells lacking HSP72 demonstrate a reduced ability to degrade mitochondria through mitophagy (15). Additionally, these mice exhibit enlarged dysmorphic mitochondria with reduced muscle respiratory capacity and increased lipid accumulation (15). Importantly, mitochondrial dysfunction associated with the lack of HSP72 extends beyond skeletal muscle and occurs in the liver (1). Thus, it is possible that the activation of HSP72 may improve mitochondrial quality by enhancing the degradation of dysfunctional mitochondria via mitophagy. However, as mitophagy is only one component of MitoQC, the role of HSP72 in the coordination between mitophagy and mitochondrial biogenesis remains ill-defined.

HSF1, PGC1α, and HSPs in Coordinating MitoQC

An additional regulator governing both mitochondrial biogenesis and mitophagy is the HSP transcription factor, HSF1 (31, 55, 73, 77, 101). Specifically, the consensus sequence for the HSF1–DNA binding element (heat shock response element) is overrepresented in the promoters of both PGC1α and HSPs (16, 55). Importantly, PGC1α is the primary transcriptional co-activator responsible for mitochondrial biogenesis (96). Previous reports do suggest that this interaction elevates mitochondrial content in a variety of tissues (i.e. adipose, muscle, and liver tissue) (31, 55, 101). Additional data suggest that HSF1 activation elevates adipocyte oxygen consumption (via increased mitochondrial content and PGC1α-dependent transactivation of uncoupling protein 1 [UCP1]) and increases the expression of metabolic genes encoding for sirtuin 1 (SIRT1), carnitine palmitoyltransferase 1a (CPT1a), medium-chain acyl-CoA dehydrogenase (MCAD), and superoxide dismutase 2 (SOD2) (55, 86, 101).

As exercise induces HSF1, PGC1α, and HSPs, this transcriptional axis may coordinate the yin and yang between mitophagy and mitochondrial biogenesis (28, 48, 58). As mentioned previously, HSP70 and PGC1α can counter-regulate HSF1—ultimately reducing its activity when homeostasis is regained (60, 78). Therefore, a possible pathway could exist in which HSF1 becomes active, translocates to the nucleus, binds to PGC1α, and activates HSP expression—triggering mitophagy and other proteostatic functions. Later in this process, HSF1 could increase PGC1α content to up-regulate mitochondrial biogenesis. Finally, the excess of both HSPs and PGC1α would turn off HSF1. In this way, the HSF1–PGC1α–HSP72 transcriptional access could coordinate MitoQC following exercise (Figure 7.3).

Conclusion

While exercise is a net-positive event for metabolic and cardiovascular health, we must remember that it is also a very intense bioenergetic stress. In order to gain the net-positive effect of exercise for our health, our cells must adapt to this stress over time. HSPs are key in this adaptive process. As mentioned earlier, HSPs are critical for the folding of new proteins, the refolding and/or degradation of damaged proteins/organelles, prevention of oxidative damage and inflammatory signalling, and the import/

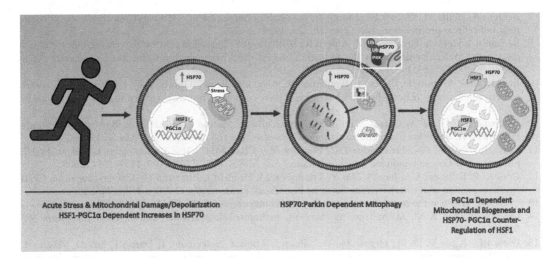

Figure 7.3   HSF1–PGC1α–HSP70 and mitochondrial quality control

export of proteins into and out of the mitochondria—all functions necessary to maintain homeostasis and recover during and after exercise (24, 29, 92). In addition, HSPs are critical for mitochondrial and systemic metabolic health both in exercise and during disease states (15, 25). Thus, HSPs are not only critical for the adaptation for exercise but are also a key component of any disease with a metabolic or inflammatory component.

Despite our immense knowledge regarding the functions of HSPs, much more research is needed to determine how HSPs coordinate with other proteins to facilitate their various functions. For instance, we know that HSF1, PGC1α, and HSPs are all involved in MitoQC and metabolic homeostasis (31, 55, 73, 77, 101). However, the direct coordination between these proteins remains ill-defined. As exercise instigates this HSF1–PGC1α–HSP transcriptional axis and is a primary treatment modality for metabolic disease, it is critical that this pathway becomes well understood. Developments in this area could lead to novel therapeutics aimed at tackling diseases with metabolic or inflammatory components. While there is still much work to be done, HSPs offer a unique target for exercise and metabolic researchers to consider when designing and completing their studies—they may offer key insights into metabolic health and disease.

References

1. Archer AE, Rogers RS, Von Schulze AT, Wheatley JL, Morris EM, McCoin CS, Thyfault JP, Geiger PC. Heat shock protein 72 regulates hepatic lipid accumulation. *Am J Physiol Regul Integr Comp Physiol* 315: R696–R707, 2018.

2. Armstrong R, Ogilvie R, Schwane J. Eccentric exercise-induced injury to rat skeletal muscle. *J Appl Physiol* 54: 80–93, 1983.

3. Armstrong R, Warren G, Warren J. Mechanisms of exercise-induced muscle fibre injury. *Sports Med* 12: 184–207, 1991.

4. Balan E, Schwalm C, Naslain D, Nielens H, Francaux M, Deldicque L. Regular endurance exercise promotes fission, mitophagy, and oxidative phosphorylation in human skeletal muscle independently of age. *Front Physiol* 10: 1088, 2019.

5. Baldwin K, Klinkerfuss G, Terjung R, Mole P, Holloszy J. Respiratory capacity of white, red, and intermediate muscle: adaptive response to exercise. *Am J Physiol Cell Physiol Legacy Content* 222: 373–378, 1972.

6. Bang O-S, Ha B-G, Park EK, Kang S-S. Activation of Akt is induced by heat shock and involved in suppression of heat-shock-induced apoptosis of NIH3T3 cells. *Biochem Biophys Res Commun* 278: 306–311, 2000.

7. Behrens A, Sibilia M, Wagner EF. Amino-terminal phosphorylation of c-Jun regulates stress-induced apoptosis and cellular proliferation. *Nat Genet* 21: 326, 1999.

8. Benjamin I, Horie S, Greenberg M, Alpern R, Williams RS. Induction of stress proteins in cultured myogenic cells. Molecular signals for the activation of heat shock transcription factor during ischemia. *J Clin Investig* 89: 1685–1689, 1992.

9. Boppart MD, Aronson D, Gibson L, Roubenoff R, Abad LW, Bean J, Goodyear LJ, Fielding RA. Eccentric exercise markedly increases c-Jun NH2-terminal kinase activity in human skeletal muscle. *J Appl Physiol* 87: 1668–1673, 1999.

10. Campanella C, Pace A, Caruso Bavisotto C, Marzullo P, Marino Gammazza A, Buscemi S, Palumbo Piccionello A. Heat shock proteins in alzheimer's disease: role and targeting. *Int J Mol Sci* 19: 2603, 2018.

11. Chung J, Nguyen AK, Henstridge DC, Holmes AG, Chan MH, Mesa JL, Lancaster GI, et al. HSP72 protects against obesity-induced insulin resistance. *Proc Natl Acad Sci U S A* 105: 1739–1744, 2008.

12. Connell P, Ballinger CA, Jiang J, Wu Y, Thompson LJ, Hohfeld J, Patterson C. The co-chaperone CHIP regulates protein triage decisions mediated by heat-shock proteins. *Nat Cell Biol* 3: 93–96, 2001.

13. Craig EA. Hsp70 at the membrane: driving protein translocation. *BMC Biol* 16: 11–11, 2018.

14. Ding W-X, Yin X-M. Mitophagy: mechanisms, pathophysiological roles, and analysis. *Biol Chem* 393: 547–564, 2012.

15. Drew BG, Ribas V, Le JA, Henstridge DC, Phun J, Zhou Z, Soleymani T, Daraei P, Sitz D, Vergnes L. HSP72 is a mitochondrial stress sensor critical for Parkin action, oxidative metabolism, and insulin sensitivity in skeletal muscle. *Diabetes* 63: 1488–1505, 2014.

16. Eastmond DL, Nelson HCM. Genome-wide analysis reveals new roles for the activation domains of the saccharomyces cerevisiae heat shock transcription factor (Hsf1) during the transient heat shock response. *J Biol Chem* 281: 32909–32921, 2006.

17. Ecochard L, Roussel D, Sempore B, Favier R. Stimulation of HSP72 expression following ATP depletion and short-term exercise training in fast-twitch muscle. *Acta Physiologica Scandinavica* 180: 71–78, 2004.

18. Febbraio M, Koukoulas I. HSP72 gene expression progressively increases in human skeletal muscle during prolonged, exhaustive exercise. *J Appl Physiol* 89: 1055–1060, 2000.

19. Febbraio MA, Steensberg A, Walsh R, Koukoulas I, Hall Gv, Saltin B, Pedersen BK. Reduced glycogen availability is associated with an elevation in HSP72 in contracting human skeletal muscle. *J physiol* 538: 911–917, 2002.

20. Fernández-Fernández MR, Gragera M, Ochoa-Ibarrola L, Quintana-Gallardo L, Valpuesta JM. Hsp70 – a master regulator in protein degradation. *FEBS Letters* 591: 2648–2660, 2017.

21. Finck BN, Kelly DP. PGC-1 coactivators: inducible regulators of energy metabolism in health and disease. *J Clin Invest* 116: 615–622, 2006.

22. Finley D. Recognition and processing of ubiquitin-protein conjugates by the proteasome. *Annu Rev Biochem* 78: 477–513, 2009.

23. Folkesson M, Mackey AL, Holm L, Kjaer M, Paulsen G, Raastad T, Henriksson J, Kadi F. Immunohistochemical changes in the expression of HSP27 in exercised human vastus lateralis muscle. *Acta Physiologica* 194: 215–222, 2008.

24. Frydman J. Folding of newly translated proteins in vivo: the role of molecular chaperones. *Ann Rev Biochem* 70: 603–647, 2001.

25. Geiger PC, Gupte AA. Heat shock proteins are important mediators of skeletal muscle insulin sensitivity. *Exerc Sport Sci Rev* 39: 34–42, 2011.

26. Gjøvaag TF, Dahl HA. Effect of training and detraining on the expression of heat shock proteins in m. triceps brachii of untrained males and females. *European J Appl Physiol* 98: 310–322, 2006.

27. Gupte AA, Bomhoff GL, Swerdlow RH, Geiger PC. Heat treatment improves glucose tolerance and prevents skeletal muscle insulin resistance in rats fed a high-fat diet. *Diabetes* 58: 567–578, 2009.

28. Handschin C, Spiegelman BM. Peroxisome proliferator-activated receptor gamma coactivator 1 coactivators, energy homeostasis, and metabolism. *Endocr Rev* 27: 728–735, 2006.

29. Hartl FU, Bracher A, Hayer-Hartl M. Molecular chaperones in protein folding and proteostasis. *Nature* 475: 324–332, 2011.

30. Hemi R, Paz K, Wertheim N, Karasik A, Zick Y, Kanety H. Transactivation of ErbB2 and ErbB3 by tumor necrosis factor-alpha and anisomycin leads to impaired insulin signaling through serine/threonine phosphorylation of IRS proteins. *J Biol Chem* 277: 8961–8969, 2002.

31. Henstridge DC, Bruce CR, Drew BG, Tory K, Kolonics A, Estevez E, Chung J, et al. Activating HSP72 in rodent skeletal muscle increases mitochondrial number and oxidative capacity and decreases insulin resistance. *Diabetes* 63: 1881–1894, 2014.

32. Henstridge DC, Febbraio MA, Hargreaves M. Heat shock proteins and exercise adaptations. Our knowledge thus far and the road still ahead. *J Appl Physiol* 120: 683–691, 2015.

33. Hernández-Santana A, Pérez-López V, Zubeldia JM, Jiménez-del-Rio M. A Rhodiola rosea root extract protects skeletal muscle cells against chemically induced oxidative stress by modulating heat shock protein 70 (HSP70) expression. *Phytother Res* 28: 623–628, 2014.

34. Hernando R, Manso R. Muscle fibre stress in response to exercise: synthesis, accumulation and isoform transitions of 70-kDa heat-shock proteins. *Eur J Biochem* 243: 460–467, 1997.

35. Holloszy JO. Biochemical adaptations in muscle. Effects of exercise on mitochondrial oxygen uptake and respiratory enzyme activity in skeletal muscle. *J Biol Chem* 242: 2278–2282, 1967.

36. Holwerda AM, Locke M. Hsp25 and Hsp72 content in rat skeletal muscle following controlled shortening and lengthening contractions. *Appl Physiol Nutr Metab* 39: 1380–1387, 2014.

37. Ip YT, Davis RJ. Signal transduction by the c-Jun N-terminal kinase (JNK)—from inflammation to development. *Curr Opin Cell Biol* 10: 205–219, 1998.

38. Jin SM, Youle RJ. PINK1- and Parkin-mediated mitophagy at a glance. *J Cell Sci* 125: 795–799, 2012.

39. Kojima A, Goto K, Morioka S, Naito T, Akema T, Fujiya H, Sugiura T, Ohira Y, Beppu M, Aoki H. Heat stress facilitates the regeneration of injured skeletal muscle in rats. *J Orthop Sci* 12: 74, 2007.

40. Kruger K, Reichel T, Zeilinger C. Role of heat shock proteins 70/90 in exercise physiology and exercise immunology and their diagnostic potential in sports. *J Appl Physiol (1985)* 126: 916–927, 2019.

41. Kubli DA, Gustafsson ÅB. Mitochondria and mitophagy: the yin and yang of cell death control. *Circ res* 111: 1208–1221, 2012.

42. Kyriakis JM, Avruch J. Sounding the alarm: protein kinase cascades activated by stress and inflammation. *J Biol Chem* 271: 24313–24316, 1996.

43. Lappalainen Z, Lappalainen J, Oksala N, Laaksonen D, Khanna S, Sen C, Atalay M. Exercise training and experimental diabetes modulate heat shock protein response in brain. *Scand J Med Sci Sports* 20: 83–89, 2010.

44. Larkins NT, Murphy RM, Lamb GD. Absolute amounts and diffusibility of HSP72, HSP25, and αB-crystallin in fast-and slow-twitch skeletal muscle fibers of rat. *Am. J. Physiol., Cell Physiol* 302: C228–C239, 2011.

45. Lee FS, Peters RT, Dang LC, Maniatis T. MEKK1 activates both IκB kinase α and IκB kinase β. *Proc Natl Acad Sci U S A* 95: 9319–9324, 1998.

46. Lee YJ, Corry PM. Metabolic oxidative stress-induced HSP70 gene expression is mediated through SAPK pathway. role of Bcl-2 and c-Jun NH2-terminal kinase. *J Biol Chem* 273: 29857–29863, 1998.

47. Lewis EJ, Ramsook AH, Locke M, Amara CE. Mild eccentric exercise increases Hsp72 content in skeletal muscles from adult and late middle-aged rats. *Cell Stress Chaperones* 18: 667–673, 2013.

48. Lira VA, Benton CR, Yan Z, Bonen A. PGC-1alpha regulation by exercise training and its influences on muscle function and insulin sensitivity. *Am. J. Physiol. Endocrinol. Metab* 299: E145–E161, 2010.

49. Liu Y, Lormes W, Baur C, Opitz-Gress A, Altenburg D, Lehmann M, Steinacker JM. Human skeletal muscle HSP70 response to physical training depends on exercise intensity. *Int J Sports Med* 21: 351–355, 2000.

50. Liu Y, Lormes W, Wang L, Reissnecker S, Steinacker JM. Different skeletal muscle HSP70 responses to high-intensity strength training and low-intensity endurance training. *European J Appl Physiol* 91: 330–335, 2004.

51. Locke M, Noble EG. Stress proteins: the exercise response. *Can J Appl Physiol* 20: 155–167, 1995.

52. Locke M, Noble EG, Atkinson BG. Inducible isoform of HSP70 is constitutively expressed in a muscle fiber type specific pattern. *Am. J. Physiol., Cell Physiol* 261: C774–C779, 1991.

53. Locke M, Noble EG, Tanguay RM, Feild MR, Ianuzzo SE, Ianuzzo CD. Activation of heat-shock transcription factor in rat heart after heat shock and exercise. *Am J Physiol* 268: C1387–1394, 1995.

54. Luders J, Demand J, Hohfeld J. The ubiquitin-related BAG-1 provides a link between the molecular chaperones Hsc70/Hsp70 and the proteasome. *J Biol Chem* 275: 4613–4617, 2000.

55. Ma X, Xu L, Alberobello AT, Gavrilova O, Bagattin A, Skarulis M, Liu J, Finkel T, Mueller E. Celastrol protects against obesity and metabolic dysfunction through activation of a HSF1-PGC1alpha transcriptional axis. *Cell Metab* 22: 695–708, 2015.

56. Marber MS, Latchman DS, Walker JM, Yellon DM. Cardiac stress protein elevation 24 hours after brief ischemia or heat stress is associated with resistance to myocardial infarction. *Circulation* 88: 1264–1272, 1993.

57. McHugh MP. Recent advances in the understanding of the repeated bout effect: the protective effect against muscle damage from a single bout of eccentric exercise. *Scand J Med Sci Sports* 13: 88–97, 2003.

58. Melling CW, Thorp DB, Milne KJ, Krause MP, Noble EG. Exercise-mediated regulation of Hsp70 expression following aerobic exercise training. *Am J Physiol Heart Circ Physiol* 293: H3692–3698, 2007.

59. Milne KJ, Noble EG. Exercise-induced elevation of HSP70 is intensity dependent. *J Appl Physiol* 93: 561–568, 2002.

60. Minsky N, Roeder RG. Direct link between metabolic regulation and the heat-shock response through the transcriptional regulator PGC-1α. *Proc Natl Acad Sci U S A* 112: E5669–E5678, 2015.

61. Miyabara EH, Martin JL, Griffin TM, Moriscot AS, Mestril R. Overexpression of inducible 70-kDa heat shock protein in mouse attenuates skeletal muscle damage induced by cryolesioning. *Am. J. Physiol., Cell Physiol* 290: C1128–C1138, 2006.

62. Murlasits Z, Cutlip RG, Geronilla KB, Rao KMK, Wonderlin WF, Alway SE. Resistance training increases heat shock protein levels in skeletal muscle of young and old rats. *Exp Gerontol* 41: 398–406, 2006.

63. Murphy ME. The HSP70 family and cancer. *Carcinogenesis* 34: 1181–1188, 2013.

64. Nosaka K, Clarkson PM. Muscle damage following repeated bouts of high force eccentric exercise. *Med Sci Sports Exerc* 27: 1263–1269, 1995.

65. Nosaka K, Muthalib M, Lavender A, Laursen PB. Attenuation of muscle damage by preconditioning with muscle hyperthermia 1-day prior to eccentric exercise. *European J Appl Physiol* 99: 183–192, 2007.

66. Nosaka K, Sakamoto K, Newton M, Sacco P. How long does the protective effect on eccentric exercise-induced muscle damage last? *Med Sci Sports Exerc* 33: 1490–1495, 2001.

67. Park H-S, Lee J-S, Huh S-H, Seo J-S, Choi E-J. Hsp72 functions as a natural inhibitory protein of c-Jun N-terminal kinase. *EMBO J* 20: 446–456, 2001.

68. Park K-J, Gaynor RB, Kwak YT. Heat shock protein 27 association with the IκB kinase complex regulates tumor necrosis factor α-induced NF-κB activation. *J Biol Chem* 278: 35272–35278, 2003.

69. Paulsen G, Vissing K, Kalhovde JM, Ugelstad I, Bayer ML, Kadi F, Schjerling P, Hallén J, Raastad T. Maximal eccentric exercise induces a rapid accumulation of small heat shock proteins on myofibrils and a delayed HSP70 response in humans. *Am J Physiol Regul Integr Comp Physiol* 293: R844–R853, 2007.

70. Pockley AG. Heat shock proteins, inflammation, and cardiovascular disease. *Circulation* 105: 1012–1017, 2002.

71. Powers SK, Nelson WB, Hudson MB. Exercise-induced oxidative stress in humans: cause and consequences. *Free Radic Biol Med* 51: 942–950, 2011.

72. Puntschart A, Vogt M, Widmer H, Hoppeler H, Billeter R. Hsp70 expression in human skeletal muscle after exercise. *Acta Physiologica Scandinavica* 157: 411–417, 1996.

73. Qiao A, Jin X, Pang J, Moskophidis D, Mivechi NF. The transcriptional regulator of the chaperone response HSF1 controls hepatic bioenergetics and protein homeostasis. *J Cell Biol* 216: 723–741, 2017.

74. Raska M, Weigl E. Heat shock proteins in autoimmune diseases. *Biomed Pap Med Fac Univ Palacky Olomouc Czech Repub* 49: 243–249, 2005.

75. Ritossa F. Discovery of the heat shock response. *Cell Stress Chaperones* 1: 97–98, 1996.

76. Rogers RS, Morris EM, Wheatley JL, Archer AE, McCoin CS, White KS, Wilson DR, et al. Deficiency in the heat stress response could underlie susceptibility to metabolic disease. *Diabetes* 65: 3341–3351, 2016.

77. Sammut IA, Jayakumar J, Latif N, Rothery S, Severs NJ, Smolenski RT, Bates TE, Yacoub MH. Heat stress contributes to the enhancement of cardiac mitochondrial complex activity. *Am J Patholy* 158: 1821–1831, 2001.

78. Sarge KD, Murphy SP, Morimoto RI. Activation of heat shock gene transcription by heat shock factor 1 involves oligomerization, acquisition of DNA-binding activity, and nuclear localization and can occur in the absence of stress. *Mol Cell Biol* 13: 1392–1407, 1993.

79. Senf SM, Howard TM, Ahn B, Ferreira LF, Judge AR. Loss of the inducible Hsp70 delays the inflammatory response to skeletal muscle injury and severely impairs muscle regeneration. *PLOS ONE* 8: e62687, 2013.

80. Skidmore R, Gutierrez JA, Guerriero Jr V, Kregel K. HSP70 induction during exercise and heat stress in rats: role of internal temperature. *Am J Physiol Regul Integr Comp Physiol* 268: R92–R97, 1995.

81. Smeal T, Binetruy B, Mercola DA, Birrer M, Karin M. Oncogenic and transcriptional cooperation with Ha-Ras requires phosphorylation of c-Jun on serines 63 and 73. *Nature* 354: 494, 1991.

82. Tatsuta T, Langer T. Quality control of mitochondria: protection against neurodegeneration and ageing. *Embo j* 27: 306–314, 2008.

83. Thompson H, Clarkson P, Scordilis S. The repeated bout effect and heat shock proteins: intramuscular HSP27 and HSP70 expression following two bouts of eccentric exercise in humans. *Acta Physiol Scand* 174: 47–56, 2002.

84. Thompson H, Maynard E, Morales E, Scordilis S. Exercise-induced HSP27, HSP70 and MAPK responses in human skeletal muscle. *Acta Physiol Scand* 178: 61–72, 2003.

85. Thompson H, Scordilis S, Clarkson P, Lohrer W. A single bout of eccentric exercise increases HSP27 and HSC/HSP70 in human skeletal muscle. *Acta Physiol Scand* 171: 187–193, 2001.

86. Tiraby C, Tavernier G, Lefort C, Larrouy D, Bouillaud F, Ricquier D, Langin D. Acquirement of brown fat cell features by human white adipocytes. *J Biol Chem* 278: 33370–33376, 2003.

87. Touchberry CD, Gupte AA, Bomhoff GL, Graham ZA, Geiger PC, Gallagher PM. Acute heat stress prior to downhill running may enhance skeletal muscle remodeling. *Cell Stress Chaperones* 17: 693–705, 2012.

88. Wandinger SK, Richter K, Buchner J. The Hsp90 chaperone machinery. *J Biol Chem* 283: 18473–18477, 2008.

89. Weitzel G, Pilatus U, Rensing L. Similar dose response of heat shock protein synthesis and intracellular pH change in yeast. *Exp Cell Res* 159: 252–256, 1985.

90. Welch WJ. How cells respond to stress. *Sci Am* 268: 56–64, 1993.

91. Widegren U, Ryder JW, Zierath JR. Mitogen-activated protein kinase signal transduction in skeletal muscle: effects of exercise and muscle contraction. *Acta Physiol Scand* 172: 227–238, 2001.

92. Willmund F, del Alamo M, Pechmann S, Chen T, Albanèse V, Dammer Eric B, Peng J, Frydman J. The Cotranslational function of ribosome-associated Hsp70 in eukaryotic protein homeostasis. *Cell* 152: 196–209, 2013.

93. Willoughby DS, Rosene J, Myers J. HSP-72 and ubiquitin expression and caspase-3 activity after a single bout of eccentric exercise. *J Exerc Physiol Online* 6: 96–104, 2003.

94. Witt SN. Hsp70 molecular chaperones and Parkinson's disease. *Biopolymers* 93: 218–228, 2010.

95. Wu J, Ruas JL, Estall JL, Rasbach KA, Choi JH, Ye L, Bostrom P, et al. The unfolded protein response mediates adaptation to exercise in skeletal muscle through a PGC-1alpha/ATF6alpha complex. *Cell Metab* 13: 160–169, 2011.

96. Wu Z, Puigserver P, Andersson U, Zhang C, Adelmant G, Mootha V, Troy A, Cinti S, Lowell B, Scarpulla RC, Spiegelman BM. Mechanisms controlling mitochondrial biogenesis and respiration through the thermogenic coactivator PGC-1. *Cell* 98: 115–124, 1999.

97. Xu L, Ma X, Bagattin A, Mueller E. The transcriptional coactivator PGC1α protects against hyperthermic stress via cooperation with the heat shock factor HSF1. *Cell Death Dis* 7: e2102–e2102, 2016.

98. Ye Y, Rape M. Building ubiquitin chains: E2 enzymes at work. *Nat Rev Mol Cell Biol* 10: 755–764, 2009.

99. Young JC, Hoogenraad NJ, Hartl FU. Molecular chaperones Hsp90 and Hsp70 deliver preproteins to the mitochondrial import receptor Tom70. *Cell* 112: 41–50, 2003.

100. Zanke BW, Boudreau K, Rubie E, Winnett E, Tibbles LA, Zon L, Kyriakis J, Liu F-F, Woodgett JR. The stress-activated protein kinase pathway mediates cell death following injury induced by cis-platinum, UV irradiation or heat. *Curr Biol* 6: 606–613, 1996.

101. Zhang Y, Geng C, Liu X, Li M, Gao M, Liu X, Fang F, Chang Y. Celastrol ameliorates liver metabolic damage caused by a high-fat diet through Sirt1. *Mol Metab* 6: 138–147, 2017.

8

SIGNALLING PATHWAYS IN THE REGULATION OF CELLULAR RESPONSES TO EXERCISE

Anders Gudiksen, Stine Ringholm, and Henriette Pilegaard

Introduction

Skeletal muscle (SkM) is characterized by the ability to promptly increase adenosine triphosphate (ATP) production to cover the large energy demand for muscle contractions. Moreover, SkM is exceptionally metabolically flexible, as shown by the capability to rapidly switch between carbohydrate and lipid utilization in accordance with changes in substrate availability and energy demand during metabolic challenges (46). Such adjustments in ATP production and substrate utilization during prolonged exercise involve the acute regulation of multiple metabolic enzymes and localization of membrane transporters in SkM.

SkM is also defined by an extraordinary plasticity enabling SkM tissue to adapt structurally and functionally to changes in the degree and pattern of muscle activity. Thus, endurance exercise training (repeated sessions of exercise) is known to enhance the capacity and efficiency of SkM oxidative metabolism. These cellular adaptations in SkM are thought at least in part to stem from cumulative effects of repeated bouts of exercise (96). This emphasizes that a crucial cellular response behind metabolic adaptations to endurance exercise training is the exercise-induced regulation of gene transcription.

The initiating event leading to SkM adaptations, alterations in energy production, and substrate utilization is disturbed homeostasis, and the purpose of the induced cellular response is to re-establish cellular homeostasis. The perturbation in homeostasis is reflected by intracellular changes in Ca^{2+}, cellular energy status (AMP/ATP), and reactive oxygen species (ROS), as well as externally derived signals such as hormones and cytokines, each of which elicits intracellular signalling. Moreover, each intracellular signalling pathway may mediate both exercise-induced gene regulation and exercise-induced metabolic regulation (Figure 8.1).

This chapter will focus on intracellular signalling pathways in SkM induced by a single bout of endurance exercise. Following are detailed separate presentations of the main exercise-regulated intracellular signalling pathways in SkM, with descriptions of the cellular responses of the pathway and presentation of research findings on exercise-induced regulation of key factors in the specific signalling pathway. It should be noted that this chapter is not an exhaustive account on research findings within the topic, but a selection applicable to the confines of this chapter.

Ca^{2+} Signalling

Muscle contractions are associated with oscillating changes in the cellular distribution of Ca^{2+} that play an essential role in regulating actin–myosin cross-bridge cycling. However, Ca^{2+} is also a key intracellular second messenger regulating both metabolic processes and gene transcription. Ca^{2+} binds to and

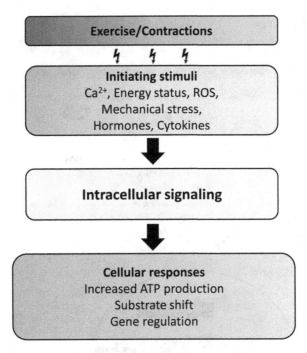

Figure 8.1 Initiation and response coupling in SkM with endurance exercise

The initiating stress induction (RED) leads to homeostatic perturbations in SkM, changes in Ca²⁺, cellular energy status (AMP/ATP), and reactive oxygen species (ROS), as well as externally derived signals such as hormones and cytokines (ORANGE). Intracellular signalling events (YELLOW) transfer the signal inducing cellular responses including increased ATP production, substrate shift and gene regulation (GREEN) in order to re-establish cellular homeostasis.

activates Ca^{2+}-sensitive enzymes, including protein kinase C (PKC) and calmodulin (CaM), resulting in several signalling branches (Figure 8.2).

PKC exists as several isoforms, where the conventional (c) isoforms constitute a PKC subfamily, which is responsive to Ca^{2+} and diacylglycerol (DAC). This includes PKCα, which is the dominant isoform in mouse SkM (60). Electrically induced muscle contractions in rats in vivo resulted in translocation and a marked increase in maximal PKC activity (representing all PKC isoforms) in a membrane fraction of the samples (101). This was confirmed using a similar experimental setup showing a time-dependent translocation of PKC activity. Moreover, this regulation of PKC was associated with an increase in DAC concentration, which occurred earlier than the PKC activity translocation (18), suggesting that DAG and Ca^{2+} together may regulate PKC translocation. Studies using pharmacological inhibitors have indicated that cPKC contributes to regulating contraction-induced glucose uptake in SkM (19, 56, 60), but the use of PKCα knockout (KO) mice revealed that cPKCα is not required for contraction-stimulated glucose uptake in mouse SkM (60).

Ca^{2+}-bound CaM activates the phosphatase calcineurin, which has been shown to dephosphorylate nuclear factor of activated T-cells (NFAT), leading to translocation of NFAT to the nucleus (73, 99). Several gene promoters have the NFAT binding site in their regulatory region, and NFAT may be involved in the transcription of cytokines, as well as lysosomal and autophagic gene transcription through transcription factor EB (TFEB) (77). In addition, both contractile activity in myotubes and exercise to exhaustion in mice have indicated that calcineurin dephosphorylates TFEB Ser211 and Ser142, enabling TFEB to translocate to the nucleus (27, 75, 77). This suggests that calcineurin–TFEB interactions are important in metabolic gene transcription in response to exercise (Figure 8.2).

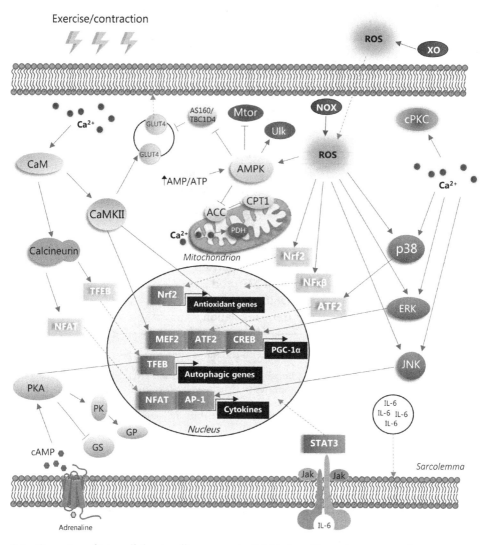

Figure 8.2 Overview of intracellular signalling events in SkM induced by endurance exercise

Ca^{2+} activates conventional protein kinase C (cPKC) and binds to calmodulin (CaM) leading to activation of calcineurin (CaN) and calmodulin-dependent protein kinase (CaMK). Calcineurin dephosphorylates nuclear factor of activated T-cells (NFAT) and transcription factor EB (TFEB), which translocate to the nucleus, and CAMK phosphorylates myocyte enhancer factor 2 (MEF2) and cAMP response element binding protein (CREB). Ca^{2+} also activates pyruvate dehydrogenase (PDH). AMP-activated protein kinase (AMPK) is activated by elevated AMP/ATP resulting in phosphorylation and inactivation of AS160/TBC1D4 and acetyl-CoA carboxylase (ACC) inducing glucose transporter (GLUT) 4 translocation to the plasma membrane and fatty acid uptake into the mitochondria, respectively. Activation of p38, c-jun NH2-terminal kinase (JNK), and extracellular signal-regulated kinase (ERK)1/2 regulates transcription factors activator protein (AP)-1, activating transcription factor 2 (ATF2), MEF2, and CREB, inducing transcription of PGC-1α. Elevated levels of reactive oxygen species (ROS) result in translocation of nuclear factor erythroid-derived 2-like (Nrf)2 to the nucleus and enhanced transcription of antioxidant proteins. Adrenalin binds to the β2-adrenergic receptor at the plasma membrane, eliciting increases in cAMP, activation of protein kinase A (PKA) with concomitant regulation of phosphorylase kinase (PK), glycogen phosphorylase (GP), and glycogen synthase (GS), as well as PKA translocation to the nucleus to regulate gene expression. Binding of cytokines like IL-6 to the JAK/STAT receptor leads to activation of Janus kinase (JAK) and phosphorylation of signal transducer and phosphorylating activator of transcription (STAT)3, which translocates to the nucleus to induce transcription of target genes. Blue lines reflect interaction and/or post-translational modification, while green lines symbolize translocation.

Activated CaM also leads to phosphorylation and activation of the calmodulin-dependent protein kinase (CaMK) of which CaMKII is the main isoform in human SkM (102). CaMKII consists of a number of intricately interacting subunits that can autophosphorylate each other, exhibiting a deciphering property that translates the given Ca^{2+} signal into subtle phases of graded kinase activity depending on the amplitude and frequency of the exercise-driven Ca^{2+} bursts (17, 24). CaMKII phosphorylates transcription factors such as cAMP response element-binding protein (CREB) and myocyte enhancer factor 2 (MEF2), as well as type II histone deacetylases (HDACs) turning on transcription of genes involved in glucose metabolism and mitochondrial biogenesis. CAMK has also been shown to regulate glucose transport (128, 134) as well as fatty acid uptake and oxidation (1, 98) in contracting mouse and rat SkM (Figure 8.2).

CaMKII phosphorylation has been shown to be elevated in human SkM during prolonged exercise, with a marked peak already after 1 minute of exercise (102), and the exercise-induced CAMKII phosphorylation in human SkM has been reported to be intensity dependent (26). The finding that transgenic mice expressing a constitutively active form of CAMKIV in SkM had elevated messenger RNA (mRNA) levels of the transcriptional coactivator PGC-1α mRNA (135) suggested that Ca^{2+} regulates PGC-1α transcription in response to acute exercise. In accordance, the PGC-1α mRNA increased in primary rat SkM cells when the cytosolic Ca^{2+} concentration was raised by incubation in the Ca^{2+} ionophore, ionomycin, or ryanodine receptor agonis, caffeine (70). These responses were prevented by treatment with the calcineurin inhibitor cyclosporine A and reduced by the CAMK inhibitor KN-62 (70). In accordance, prior treatment with cyclosporine A or KN-62 also prevented a contraction-induced increase in PGC-1α mRNA in rat EDL muscle ex vivo (70). Similarly, 5 days of incubation of L6 myotubes in ionomycin or caffeine increased cytochrome oxidase I (COXI), cytochrome c, and citrate synthase protein content and incubation in the ryanodine receptor inhibitor, dantrolene, or the Ca^{2+} chelator EGTA (90) or the CAMK inhibitor KN93 (89) prevented these effects. This indicates that both calcineurin and CAMK are involved in gene regulation. However, an increased cytochrome c mRNA content in myotubes incubated in the Ca^{2+} ionophore A23187 was prevented by simultaneous incubation in the PKC inhibitor staurosporine, but not the CAMK inhibitor KN-62. Moreover, incubation with a mitogen-activated protein kinase (MAPK) inhibitor prevented the Ca^{2+}-induced increase in cytochrome c transcriptional activity, and extracellular signal-regulated kinase (ERK)1/2 phosphorylation showed an early increase (32). This suggests that a Ca^{2+} PKA ERK-dependent pathway is involved in regulation of gene expression of mitochondrial proteins, but it should be noted that not all PKC isoforms are activated by Ca^{2+}, as mentioned earlier. Together these studies indicate that Ca^{2+} plays an important role in transcriptional regulation of PGC-1α and oxidative proteins in SkM through ERK1/2, calcineurin and CAMK-mediated regulation. Because PGC-1α has been shown to regulate the transcription of a broad range of mitochondrial proteins and mitochondrial volume in mouse SkM (44, 72), Ca^{2+} signalling is thought to be central in exercise training–induced mitochondrial biogenesis in SkM through effects on PGC-1α transcription. Ca^{2+} has also been suggested to regulate the transcription of the myokine interleukin (IL)-6 in SkM, which is supported by an observed increase in IL-6 mRNA in myotubes incubated in the Ca^{2+} ionophore calcimycin A23187 (124) (Figure 8.2).

Acute exercise has been shown to increase mitochondrial Ca^{2+} concentrations in human (74) and mouse SkM (8), supporting the theory that Ca^{2+} also regulates metabolic enzymes within the mitochondria. In accordance, Ca^{2+} has been shown to activate the pyruvate dehydrogenase (PDH) phosphatase 1 (PDP1), which dephosphorylates and activates PDH in the mitochondria (55). The observation that the activity of PDH in the active form (PDHa) increased in human SkM within 6 seconds of maximal isokinetic cycling exercise (93) demonstrates an exceptionally fast regulation likely executed by Ca^{2+}-mediated regulation of PDP1. Because the PDH complex catalyzes the irreversible conversion of pyruvate to acetyl-CoA in the mitochondria, this suggests that Ca^{2+} signalling plays a key role in rapidly increasing carbohydrate oxidation in skeletal muscle at the onset of exercise (Figure 8.2).

AMPK Signalling

Conserving cellular ATP levels during muscle contractions is vital to maintain cell function. Adenosine monophosphate (AMP)-activated protein kinase (AMPK) is highly responsive to metabolic perturbations and is acutely activated to re-establish cellular energy homeostasis through phosphorylation of key metabolic enzymes. AMPK activation turns on catalytic ATP-generating processes while inhibiting anabolic processes such as lipid and protein synthesis. The highly conserved AMPK is a heterotrimeric kinase consisting of a catalytic α as well as a regulatory β and γ subunit, all of which are found in multiple isoform complexes (45, 111). AMP-binding sites and a glycogen-binding domain are contained within the β subunit, which presumably acts to inhibit the activity of the kinase when glycogen stores are abundant (97). AMPK is allosterically inhibited by creatine phosphate and activated several-fold by an increase in cytosolic AMP/ATP ratio (11, 31). Binding of AMP to AMPK allows exposure of the threonine residue on the α subunit, which is phosphorylated by the upstream AMPK kinases constitutively active tumour suppressor liver kinase B1 (LKB1)(133) and CAMK kinase β (48, 132) (Figure 8.2).

Numerous studies have shown that a single bout of exercise increases AMPK activity in human, rat, and mouse SkM (15, 34, 131) and that AMPK^{Thr172} phosphorylation reflects AMPK activity (47, 103). Exercise-induced AMPK phosphorylation in human SkM has been shown to be both intensity and duration dependent (100, 131) but generally only observable at exercise intensities from 60% VO$_2$ max and upwards (16, 113, 131).

AMPK appears to be directly linked to the signalling cascade initiating mitochondrial biogenesis. Thus AMPK has been proposed to activate PGC-1α, both through direct phosphorylation, as shown in vitro (59), and possibly indirectly through AMPK-mediated activation of SIRT1, which has been suggested to deacetylate PGC-1α (9). Furthermore, AICAR-induced PGC-1α mRNA induction was absent in AMPKα2 KO mice, and although the exercise-induced PGC-1α mRNA response was similar in AMPKα2 KO and WT mice, PGC-1α transcription was markedly lower in AMPKα2 KO mice than WT mice at rest and after exercise (63). Together this provides evidence for AMPK-mediated regulation of both PGC-1α transcription and activity in SkM during exercise.

AMPK has been demonstrated to regulate contraction-induced glucose uptake in mouse SkM using AICAR as well as in mice lacking AMPK (94, 130). Moreover, AS160/TBC1D4 has been identified as central in contraction-induced glucose uptake in SkM. The observations that AICAR-induced AS160/TBC1D4 phosphorylation was markedly reduced in AMPKα2 KO mice, AMPKα2 kinase-dead, and γ3 AMPK KO mice and that contraction-induced AS160/TBC1D4 phosphorylation was lower in AMPKα2 KO and AMPK α2 kinase-dead mice than in control mice (117) clearly demonstrated that TBC1D4 is a target for AMPK during exercise. Later studies identified serine 711 as a novel phosphorylation site on TBC1D4 and showed that contractions and AICAR increased phosphorylation of TBC1D4Ser711 in SkM of control mice but not AMPKα2 kinase-dead mice (118). In accordance, AS160 phosphorylation measured by the PAS antibody increased in human SkM at 60 min and 90 min of moderate-intensity exercise, but not in response to exercise at higher intensity and of shorter duration (116). However, TBC1D4Ser711 phosphorylation, measured by phospho-specific antibodies, increased in human SkM immediately after 20 min of high-intensity exercise (118). This supports the theory that AMPK stimulates recruitment of the GLUT4 transporters to the plasma membrane during exercise by phosphorylating AS160/TBC1D4, allowing for the marked increase in insulin-independent glucose uptake in SkM (Figure 8.2).

AMPK has also been implicated in enhancing fat oxidation in SkM during exercise (115). Moreover, by use of giant vesicles the fatty acid transporter FAT/CD36 was shown to translocate to the plasma membrane during muscle contractions enhancing the capacity of fatty acid uptake (6). The observation that the AICAR-stimulated increase in palmitate uptake and palmitate oxidation by perfused hind limb muscles was reduced by 50% in FAT/CD36 KO mice suggests that AMPK regulates contraction-induced translocation of CD36 to the plasma membrane (6). In addition, AMPK has been reported to phosphorylate and inactivate acetyl-CoA carboxylase 2 (ACC2) (127). Upon inactivation,

ACC2 ceases to convert acetyl-CoA to malonyl-CoA, which inhibits the mitochondrial carnitine-palmitoyltransferase 1 (CPT1) that in turn controls the transport of fatty acids into mitochondria. In accordance, endurance exercise has been shown to increase SkM ACC2 phosphorylation in mice (Ser212) and humans (Ser221) (35, 78). This induction occurs typically in parallel with an increased AMPK phosphorylation, supporting the theory that AMPK regulates ACC during exercise, although dissociations between exercise-induced regulation of AMPK and ACC phosphorylation have been demonstrated in human SkM during prolonged exercise (129). The findings that an exercise-induced ACC phosphorylation observed in SkM of WT mice was absent in AMPKα2 KO mice (62) further underlines the impact of AMPK on fatty acid uptake into the mitochondria during muscle contractions (Figure 8.2).

SkM PDHa activity has been shown to increase during exercise and decrease towards resting levels during prolonged exercise (83). The observation that PDHa activity was higher and PDH phosphorylation lower in AMPKα2 KO mice than WT mice after 1 hour of treadmill running (69) may suggest that AMPK also contributes to limiting carbohydrate oxidation during prolonged exercise through effects on PDH phosphorylation status. However, this could not be confirmed by the use of AICAR in vitro (69), and further studies are warranted to clarify this potential relationship (Figure 8.2).

MAPK Signalling

Mechanical stress and Ca^{2+} also turn on the MAPK signalling cascade in SkM. Exercise was first shown to increase phosphorylation and/or activity of the three distinct kinases of the MAPK family p38, c-jun NH2-terminal kinase (JNK), and ERK1/2 in rat SkM (39), but shortly after also in human SkM (4, 125). Exercise-induced ERK phosphorylation in human muscle has been shown to be intensity dependent (4, 126), although the regulation of ERK phosphorylation and activation by contraction still remain unclear. ERK is responsible for activating a number of transcription factors, amongst others CREB (Figure 8.2). It has been reported that exercise modality (continuous low intensity, sprints, or high intensity bouts) did not influence the exercise-induced increase in p38 MAPK phosphorylation in human SkM (92). On the other hand, with matched total work performed, p38 phosphorylation was higher in SkM when 40 min moderate-intensity exercise was followed by 20 min of 30-sec sprints than when performing continuous moderate-intensity cycling with or without sprints distributed over the exercise period (7). This may indicate that exercise-induced p38 regulation is influenced by the exercise intensity. Moreover, training status has been shown to modify the exercise-mediated regulation of the MAPK (21) (Figure 8.2).

p38 has been shown to directly phosphorylate three different serine residues on PGC-1α, increasing PGC-1α activity in vitro (2), as well as to phosphorylate activating transcription factor 2 (ATF2) and MEF2, thus also promoting PGC-1α transcription (2, 76). ATF2 is a member of the CREB/ATF family of transcription factors that binds to the PGC-1α promoter and induces its transcription (Figure 8.2). Prolonged exercise (marathon running) has been shown to increase p38 and ERK1/2 phosphorylation together with enhancing DNA binding of MEF2 in human SkM (137). Moreover, it has been demonstrated that binding of ATF2 and MEF2 to PGC-1α increases 3 hours into recovery from an exercise bout (107), which may lead to transcription of genes encoding oxidative proteins (22, 105). In addition, MEF2 associated with HDAC5 decreased (indicating a nuclear export of HDAC5 and increased transcription) and MEF2 associated with PGC-1α increased in human SkM in response to 1 hour of moderate-intensity exercise (76) (Figure 8.2). Taken together, this establishes a firm connection between exercise-induced p38 regulation and regulation of mitochondrial biogenesis (Figure 8.2).

JNK has been implicated in the regulation of the myokine IL-6. Electrical stimulation of C2C12 myotubes increased JNK phosphorylation, the reporter activity of transcription factor activator protein (AP)-1, and IL-6 mRNA (124). In addition, inhibition of JNK by use of BMS-345541 prevented the contraction-induced increase in IL-6 mRNA in the myotubes and IL-6 protein in the cell culture medium, and an exercise-induced increase in IL-6 mRNA in mouse SkM was absent in JNK KO mice (124). Together this provides evidence for a JNK-mediated regulation of IL-6 transcription in SkM with potential concomitant IL-6 release and IL-6 mediated organ crosstalk (Figure 8.2).

ROS Signalling

Reactive oxygen species (ROS) are produced at multiple sites in SkM, including the electron transport system, the NADPH oxidase (NOX), and the xanthine oxidase (XO) (38, 58). Transient increases in low to moderate concentrations of ROS (including superoxide, H_2O_2 and OH-) are thought to elicit beneficial cellular responses in SkM, while high and/or constantly elevated ROS levels will damage cellular components.

Muscle contractions have been reported to increase ROS production in SkM, as first reported by Davies et al. (23). This increase has later been shown unlikely to derive from the mitochondrial complexes (38), but rather from the NADPH oxidase (58) and xanthine oxidase (37, 51). Redox-sensitive signalling pathways use ROS to transfer signals to intracellular locations with an effect on gene transcription and modification of enzyme activities. Superoxide has a short half-life and is rapidly converted to H_2O_2, which with a longer half-life and the ability to cross membranes, can act as a second messenger in ROS signalling over longer distances reacting with various targets in the cell (28).

ERK, JNK, and p38, as well as nuclear factor kappa-light-chain-enhancer of activated B cells (NFkB), are in particular thought to be important in mediating ROS signalling in SkM. Treatment with the XO inhibitor allopurinol prevented an exercise-induced increase in p38 and ERK1 phosphorylation in rat SkM (36, 122), as well as NFκB nuclear localization (36, 64). Moreover, an exercise-induced increase in JNK phosphorylation in human SkM was blunted by N-acetylcysteine (NAC) treatment, while the increase in p38 phosphorylation was unaffected by NAC and NFκB phosphorylation was unchanged by exercise (95). Treatment with the NOX2 inhibitor apocynin for 3 days reduced exercise-induced phosphorylation and hence activation of p38, ERK1/2, and NFkB, as well as the increase in superoxide dismutase (SOD), glutathione peroxidase (Gpx), and citrate synthase mRNA in mouse SkM (52). Together this provides evidence that p38, ERK, JNK, and NFKB mediate exercise-induced ROS signalling towards gene regulation of oxidative and antioxidant proteins in SkM (Figure 8.2).

Most antioxidant enzymes have antioxidant response elements (ARE) in the promoter for interaction with redox-sensitive transcription factors (3). The transcription factor nuclear factor erythroid-derived 2-like 2 (NFE2L2 or Nrf2) has been reported to be regulated by ROS and to induce the transcription of antioxidant enzymes. Thus, Nrf2 is kept in the cytosol bound to Kelch-like ECH associated protein (Keap)1, but increases in ROS lead to dissociation of Keap1 and Nrf2 with concomitant translocation of Nrf2 to the nucleus (67). A single 6-hour exercise bout has been shown to increase Nrf2 localization in the nucleus as well as Nrf2 binding to ARE with an associated increase in the mRNA content of SOD1 and 2 ,as well as catalase in mouse SkM (71). Moreover, Nrf2 was required for exercise-induced mRNA responses of antioxidant proteins in mouse SkM (79). Together these findings support that Nrf2 mediates transcriptional regulation of antioxidant enzymes in SkM in response to exercise-induced ROS signalling (Figure 8.2).

Several studies provide evidence that ROS production contributes to exercise training–induced mitochondrial biogenesis in SkM. Of notice these effects are initiated during each single exercise bout through exercise-induced ROS signalling targeting redox-sensitive transcription factors. Incubation of C2C12 cells in H_2O_2 increased the PGC-1α mRNA content, while treatment with the antioxidant NAC prevented this (57). Moreover, electrical stimulation of primary rat SkM cells increased PGC-1α mRNA, which was prevented by incubation with a mixture of antioxidants (108). On the other hand, pharmacological inhibition of NOS using L-NAME in rats as well as NOS deletion in mice did not prevent an exercise-induced PGC-1α mRNA increase in SkM (120, 121). Moreover, while one study did not observe effects of allopurinol-induced XO inhibition on the exercise-induced PGC-1α mRNA response in rat SkM (122), another study demonstrated reduced PGC-1α mRNA response after exercise when rats were treated with allopurinol (64). These differences may be due to a more marked reduction in protein oxidation by allopurinol in the latter study. Similarly, 4 weeks of vitamin C and E supplementation (82) or NAC infusion (95) did not prevent an exercise-induced increase the PGC-1α mRNA content in human SkM. On the other hand, a reported tendency to increase GSSG in response to exercise was not affected by the vitamin C and E supplementation (82), suggesting that exercise-induced ROS signalling may not have been blunted sufficiently by the treatment to observe effects on the PGC-1α response. Taken together, these findings suggest that ROS signalling may contribute to exercise-induced transcriptional regulation of PGC-1α in SkM, but further studies are needed to clarify potential differences between ROS sources and use of different antioxidants in human experiments.

Studies in C2C12 myotubes have shown that H_2O_2 incubation increased IL-6 mRNA together with increased NFκB signalling and binding of the NFκB p65 subunit to the IL-6 promoter (124). In accordance, treating mice with the NOX inhibitor apocynin prevented the exercise-induced increase in SkM IL-6 mRNA and reduced the plasma IL-6 level after exercise relative to control mice (52). However, supplementation with vitamin C and E for 4 weeks (136) or NAC infusion prior to and during exercise did not affect the exercise-induced IL-6 mRNA in human SkM. Together this indicates that ROS signalling may target SkM IL-6 transcription, but whether such a mechanism takes place in humans is unclear.

The observation that NAC reduced contraction-induced glucose uptake in isolated mouse EDL muscle (104) suggests that ROS are involved in regulating SkM glucose uptake during exercise. Similarly, using antioxidants, including NAC, indicated that stretch-induced glucose uptake in isolated mouse EDL muscle is mediated by ROS (13). On the other hand, NAC infusion in humans did not affect exercise-induced glucose uptake during prolonged moderate-intensity cycling (80). However, it has been suggested that the lack of effect was related to the intensity of the exercise and the dose of NAC being low relative to animal studies (65). Together this may suggest that ROS contribute to the contraction-induced increase in SkM glucose uptake, but additional clarifications are warranted.

ROS signalling may be affected by ROS-induced ROS release, where mitochondrial-derived ROS affects NADPH oxidase or NADPH oxidase-derived ROS influences ROS production by the mitochondria (30). ROS signalling also interacts with the other well-characterized signalling pathways. Hence, ROS have been shown to alter Ca^{2+} release from the sarcoplasmic reticulum as well as the Ca^{2+} ATPase and hence Ca^{2+} reuptake in the sarcoplasmic reticulum (29, 106), suggesting a link between ROS and Ca^{2+} signalling. Furthermore, allopurinol treatment has been shown to prevent an exercise-induced increase in CREB phosphorylation (64) indicating an overlap between β-adrenergic signalling and ROS signalling. In addition, incubation in NAC reduced the contraction-induced increase in AMPK activity and phosphorylation together with preventing an increase in GSSG and GSSG/TGSH in isolated mouse SkM (104) providing evidence for an association between ROS and AMPK signalling. This is supported by observations in HEK cells and using recombinant AMPK that oxidation of AMPKα at cysteine residues 130 and 174 interfered with AMPK phosphorylation, while S-glutathionylation of Cys299 abd304 in AMPKα1/2 subunits increased the AMPK activity (138). Together these findings emphasize the complexity of exercise-induced ROS intracellular signalling.

β-Adrenergic Signalling

Exercise is known to increase circulating adrenaline/epinephrine concentrations with concomitant effects in numerous tissues, including SkM. Thus, previous studies using adrenaline infusion and/or adrenalectomized human subjects have shown that adrenaline contributes to regulating the activity of SkM glycogen phosphorylase (14, 68), glycogen synthase (14), and hormone-sensitive lipase (68, 123) in humans. In addition, the use of β-adrenergic agonists and antagonists has indicated that adrenaline regulates PGC-1α gene expression (81).

Adrenalin signalling is initiated when adrenaline binds to the G-coupled β2-adrenergic receptor in SkM leading to increased activity of adenylate cyclase with generation of cyclic AMP (cAMP). This is followed by activation of protein kinase A (PKA) through cAMP-induced dissociation of the catalytic and regulatory PKA subunits. The activated catalytic PKA phosphorylates glycogen phosphorylase kinase, which by phosphorylation converts glycogen phosphorylase from the inactive to the active form. Moreover, PKA has been reported to inactivate glycogen synthase by direct phosphorylation of site 2, 1a and 1b (87). In addition, PKA translocates to the nucleus with concomitant phosphorylation of target proteins, including CREB. Phosphorylated and activated CREB binds to the cAMP response element in the promoter region of target genes, which has been suggested to include PGC-1α, resulting in enhanced transcriptional activity (Figure 8.2).

Adrenaline infusion has been shown to increase the cAMP concentration by 2- to 3-fold in human SkM within 5 min of infusion (14). Moreover, a single adrenaline injection in rats enhanced p38, ERK, CREB, and PKA substrate, but not AMPK, with phosphorylation in triceps muscle demonstrating induction of a broad adrenergic signalling cascade (33). Moreover, inhalation of the β2 agonist formoterol increased PKA substrate phosphorylation in human muscle (54), indicating β2-adrenergic-induced PKA signalling in human SkM. In accordance, increased phosphorylation of PKA substrates was demonstrated in response to a single bout of high-intensity cycling to exhaustion using global analysis of protein phosphorylation on human SkM biopsies (53). Furthermore, as presented earlier for p38 and ERK, previous studies have shown that acute exercise increases CREB phosphorylation in human SkM in the recovery period after both low- and high-intensity exercise, while a decline has been reported immediately after exercise (7, 26, 114). However, an enhanced plasma adrenaline level immediately after exercise was not consistently associated with higher CREB phosphorylation in human SkM after exercise (7). Similarly, the exercise-induced PGC-1α mRNA response in SkM was not affected when CREB phosphorylation was elevated by fasting (114). Together this provides evidence for β-adrenergic signalling towards metabolic regulation in SkM during exercise, while the impact of β-adrenergic signalling in exercise-induced regulation of PGC-1α transcription in human SkM remains to be clarified.

Cytokine Signalling

Cytokines are produced in multiple tissues and exert autocrine, paracrine, and endocrine effects on various organs. Cytokines released from SkM, termed myokines, generate a diverse response that has an impact on metabolic regulation both during and following a single exercise bout. IL-6 is the most well-known and studied exercise-induced myokine. IL-6 has been shown to increase in the circulation during endurance exercise in both humans and rodents (25, 86, 91) and has been reported to regulate both glucose and fat metabolism (10, 50, 119).

IL-6 signals through the IL-6 receptor system composed of the ligand-binding IL-6 receptor α (IL-6Rα) and a homodimer of the signal transducing β-subunit, gp130, also functioning as a scaffold (84). Upon activation of the receptor, IL-6 signals through the Janus kinase 2 (JAK2) that autophosphorylates, activating a cytoplasmic domain on gp130 allowing recruitment of signal transducer and phosphorylating activator of transcription 3 (STAT3). In turn, STAT3 dimerizes and relocates to the nucleus inducing transcription of target genes (40). This includes suppressor of cytokine signalling 3 (SOCS3), which as a negative feedback control results in inhibition of the JAK/STAT pathway (61, 85, 110) quenching the IL-6 signalling pathway (Figure 8.2).

Human cell culture studies have demonstrated elevated STAT3 phosphorylation in response to physiological concentrations of IL-6 (61), and a single IL-6 injection in mice increased STAT3 phosphorylation in SkM (5). In accordance, an exercise-induced increase in STAT3 phosphorylation has been shown in human SkM of untrained subjects during incremental endurance exercise, where plasma IL-6 increased (41). A single injection of IL-6 in rats has been reported to increase AMPK phosphorylation proposedly through the cAMP pathway (66). This has been confirmed in mice during fasting, but not fed, conditions (5), and other studies in humans and in mouse KO models have also contested an IL-6–mediated regulation of AMPK (42, 49, 88). Additional studies are needed to clarify the relationship between IL-6 and AMPK. In addition, muscle-specific IL-6 KO mice have been shown to have higher respiratory exchange ratio during exercise and in accordance higher PDHa activity in SkM at rest and during exercise than control mice (42). This suggests that IL-6 enhances SkM fat utilization by inhibiting PDH. However, the molecular mechanism behind this regulation remains to be determined.

Future Perspectives

ROS Signalling and Exercise-Induced Autophagy

Autophagy serves to remove dysfunctional proteins and cellular components, and a single exercise bout has been suggested to increase autophagy in SkM. For example, microtubule-associated protein 1A/1B-light chain 3 (LC3)II protein content was increased in mouse SkM in recovery from a single treadmill exercise bout, suggesting an increased number of autophagosomes and hence autophagy. Moreover, this was associated with reduced protein carbonylation in SkM (44) potentially indicating that enhanced autophagy had removed oxidized proteins. AMPK has been demonstrated to play a role in regulation of autophagy (43), but it has also been suggested that ROS signalling induces autophagy. Although inhibition of mitochondrial ROS production has been shown to prevent a contraction-induced increase in mRNA of key autophagy genes (109), the link between ROS signalling and induction of autophagy remains to be resolved.

ROS-Mediated Post-Translational Modifications During Exercise

Exercise has been shown to increase global glutathionylation and carbonylation in rat SkM (36), supporting the finding that a single exercise bout elicits oxidation of proteins. In accordance, the effects of ROS signalling on gene transcription have been suggested to be executed through post-translational modifications and localization of transcription factors such as NFkB and Nrf2 (3, 36, 37, 109, 122). Calcineurin has been shown to be susceptible to oxidation, which disrupts enzyme activation, indicating that also phosphatases in SkM are redox sensitive (12). In addition, endogenously produced ROS has been reported to target numerous redox active cysteine residues in proteins via S-glutathionylation (protein-SSG), disulfide bond formation (S-S), and S-nitrosation (protein-SNO) post-translational modifications indicating ROS-dependent regulation of enzyme activity (20). Together this provides evidence that ROS signalling involves multiple post-translational modifications of proteins. However, the potential ROS-mediated regulation of redox-sensitive cysteine residues in selected proteins in response to exercise would be very interesting to pursue in future studies.

Exercise-Induced PKA Regulation

Numerous studies have reported adrenaline-mediated effects on metabolic enzymes, and some have demonstrated exercise-induced regulation of CREB phosphorylation in SkM (7, 26, 114), indicating β-adrenergic signalling in SkM in response to acute exercise. Although this is in general interpreted as PKA-mediated effects, only a few studies have provided measures of PKA substrate phosphorylation. Direct measures of exercise-regulated PKA activity or translocation of PKA in SkM would also be relevant for the understanding of β-adrenergic signalling in SkM and cAMP signalling in general.

Regulation of Myokine Release During Exercise

IL-6 has been shown to be released from human SkM during prolonged exercise (91, 112). In line with this, numerous studies have shown that exercise increases the mRNA content of IL-6 in SkM, which may be translated to IL-6 protein and released from the muscle cell. Ca^{2+} has been suggested to contribute to the exercise-induced IL-6 gene expression in SkM (124), but further details in this regulation could be examined. Moreover, additional stimuli are required for inducing the translocation of IL-6–containing vesicles to the plasma membrane, but the knowledge on the intracellular signalling pathway leading to vesicle translocation and IL-6 release from muscle cells during exercise is scarce. Resolving this mechanism would be an interesting task to pursue in the future.

References

1. Abbott MJ, Edelman AM, Turcotte LP. CaMKK is an upstream signal of AMP-activated protein kinase in regulation of substrate metabolism in contracting skeletal muscle. *Am J Physiol Regul Integr Comp Physiol* 297: R1724–R1732, 2009.
2. Akimoto T, Pohnert SC, Li P, Zhang M, Gumbs C, Rosenberg PB, et al. Exercise stimulates Pgc-1alpha transcription in skeletal muscle through activation of the p38 MAPK pathway. *J Biol Chem* 280: 19587–19593, 2005.
3. Allen RG, Tresini M. Oxidative stress and gene regulation. *Free Radic Biol Med* 28: 463–499, 2000.
4. Aronson D, Violan MA, Dufresne SD, Zangen D, Fielding RA, Goodyear LJ. Exercise stimulates the mitogen-activated protein kinase pathway in human skeletal muscle. *J Clin Invest* 99: 1251–1257, 1997.
5. Bienso RS, Knudsen JG, Brandt N, Pedersen PA, Pilegaard H. Effects of IL-6 on pyruvate dehydrogenase regulation in mouse skeletal muscle. *Pflugers Arch* 466: 1647–1657, 2014.
6. Bonen A, Han XX, Habets DD, Febbraio M, Glatz JF, Luiken JJ. A null mutation in skeletal muscle FAT/CD36 reveals its essential role in insulin- and AICAR-stimulated fatty acid metabolism. *Am J Physiol Endocrinol Metab* 292: E1740–E1749, 2007.
7. Brandt N, Gunnarsson TP, Hostrup M, Tybirk J, Nybo L, Pilegaard H et al. Impact of adrenaline and metabolic stress on exercise-induced intracellular signaling and PGC-1alpha mRNA response in human skeletal muscle. *Physiol Rep* 4: 2016.
8. Bruton J, Tavi P, Aydin J, Westerblad H, Lannergren J. Mitochondrial and myoplasmic [Ca2+] in single fibres from mouse limb muscles during repeated tetanic contractions. *J Physiol* 551: 179–190, 2003.
9. Canto C, Jiang LQ, Deshmukh AS, Mataki C, Coste A, Lagouge M, et al. Interdependence of AMPK and SIRT1 for metabolic adaptation to fasting and exercise in skeletal muscle. *Cell Metab* 11: 213–219, 2010.
10. Carey AL, Steinberg GR, Macaulay SL, Thomas WG, Holmes AG, Ramm G, et al. Interleukin-6 increases insulin-stimulated glucose disposal in humans and glucose uptake and fatty acid oxidation in vitro via AMP-activated protein kinase. *Diabetes* 55: 2688–2697, 2006.
11. Carling D, Clarke PR, Zammit VA, Hardie DG. Purification and characterization of the AMP-activated protein kinase. Copurification of acetyl-CoA carboxylase kinase and 3-hydroxy-3-methylglutaryl-CoA reductase kinase activities. *Eur J Biochem* 186: 129–136, 1989.
12. Carruthers NJ, Stemmer PM. Methionine oxidation in the calmodulin-binding domain of calcineurin disrupts calmodulin binding and calcineurin activation. *Biochemistry* 47: 3085–3095, 2008.
13. Chambers MA, Moylan JS, Smith JD, Goodyear LJ, Reid MB. Stretch-stimulated glucose uptake in skeletal muscle is mediated by reactive oxygen species and p38 MAP-kinase. *J Physiol* 587: 3363–3373, 2009.
14. Chasiotis D, Sahlin K, Hultman E. Regulation of glycogenolysis in human muscle in response to epinephrine infusion. *J Appl Physiol Respir Environ Exerc Physiol* 54: 45–50, 1983.
15. Chen ZP, McConell GK, Michell BJ, Snow RJ, Canny BJ, Kemp BE. AMPK signaling in contracting human skeletal muscle: acetyl-CoA carboxylase and NO synthase phosphorylation. *Am J Physiol Endocrinol Metab* 279: E1202–E1206, 2000.
16. Chen ZP, Stephens TJ, Murthy S, Canny BJ, Hargreaves M, Witters LA, et al. Effect of exercise intensity on skeletal muscle AMPK signaling in humans. *Diabetes* 52: 2205–2212, 2003.
17. Chin ER. Intracellular Ca2+ signaling in skeletal muscle: decoding a complex message. *Exerc Sport Sci Rev* 38: 76–85, 2010.
18. Cleland PJ, Appleby GJ, Rattigan S, Clark MG. Exercise-induced translocation of protein kinase C and production of diacylglycerol and phosphatidic acid in rat skeletal muscle in vivo. Relationship to changes in glucose transport. *J Biol Chem* 264: 17704–17711, 1989.

19. Cleland PJ, Rattigan S, Clark MG. Glucose-induced loss of exercise-mediated 3-0-methyl glucose uptake by isolated rat soleus and epitrochlearis muscles. *Horm Metab Res* 22: 121–122, 1990.

20. Cobley JN, McHardy H, Morton JP, Nikolaidis MG, Close GL. Influence of vitamin C and vitamin E on redox signaling: implications for exercise adaptations. *Free Radic Biol Med* 84: 65–76, 2015.

21. Coffey VG, Zhong Z, Shield A, Canny BJ, Chibalin AV, Zierath JR, et al. Early signaling responses to divergent exercise stimuli in skeletal muscle from well-trained humans. *FASEB J* 20: 190–192, 2006.

22. Czubryt MP, McAnally J, Fishman GI, Olson EN. Regulation of peroxisome proliferator-activated receptor gamma coactivator 1 alpha (PGC-1 alpha) and mitochondrial function by MEF2 and HDAC5. *Proc Natl Acad Sci U S A* 100: 1711–1716, 2003.

23. Davies KJ, Quintanilha AT, Brooks GA, Packer L. Free radicals and tissue damage produced by exercise. *Biochem Biophys Res Commun* 107: 1198–1205, 1982.

24. Dolmetsch RE, Lewis RS, Goodnow CC, Healy JI. Differential activation of transcription factors induced by Ca2+ response amplitude and duration. *Nature* 386: 855–858, 1997.

25. Drenth JP, Van Uum SH, Van DM, Pesman GJ, Van dV, Van der Meer JW. Endurance run increases circulating IL-6 and IL-1ra but downregulates ex vivo TNF-alpha and IL-1 beta production. *J Appl Physiol (1985)* 79: 1497–1503, 1995.

26. Egan B, Carson BP, Garcia-Roves PM, Chibalin AV, Sarsfield FM, Barron N, et al. Exercise intensity-dependent regulation of peroxisome proliferator-activated receptor coactivator-1 mRNA abundance is associated with differential activation of upstream signalling kinases in human skeletal muscle. *J Physiol* 588: 1779–1790, 2010.

27. Erlich AT, Brownlee DM, Beyfuss K, Hood DA. Exercise induces TFEB expression and activity in skeletal muscle in a PGC-1alpha-dependent manner. *Am J Physiol Cell Physiol* 314: C62–C72, 2018.

28. Espinosa A, Henriquez-Olguin C, Jaimovich E. Reactive oxygen species and calcium signals in skeletal muscle: a crosstalk involved in both normal signaling and disease. *Cell Calcium* 60: 172–179, 2016.

29. Favero TG, Zable AC, Abramson JJ. Hydrogen peroxide stimulates the Ca2+ release channel from skeletal muscle sarcoplasmic reticulum. *J Biol Chem* 270: 25557–25563, 1995.

30. Ferreira LF, Laitano O. Regulation of NADPH oxidases in skeletal muscle. *Free Radic Biol Med* 98: 18–28, 2016.

31. Ferrer A, Caelles C, Massot N, Hegardt FG. Activation of rat liver cytosolic 3-hydroxy-3-methylglutaryl coenzyme a reductase kinase by adenosine 5'-monophosphate. *Biochem Biophys Res Commun* 132: 497–504, 1985.

32. Freyssenet D, Di CM, Hood DA. Calcium-dependent regulation of cytochrome c gene expression in skeletal muscle cells. Identification of a protein kinase c-dependent pathway. *J Biol Chem* 274: 9305–9311, 1999.

33. Frier BC, Wan Z, Williams DB, Stefanson AL, Wright DC. Epinephrine and AICAR-induced PGC-1alpha mRNA expression is intact in skeletal muscle from rats fed a high-fat diet. *Am J Physiol Cell Physiol* 302: C1772–C1779, 2012.

34. Fujii N, Hayashi T, Hirshman MF, Smith JT, Habinowski SA, Kaijser L, et al. Exercise induces isoform-specific increase in 5'AMP-activated protein kinase activity in human skeletal muscle. *Biochem Biophys Res Commun* 273: 1150–1155, 2000.

35. Fullerton MD, Galic S, Marcinko K, Sikkema S, Pulinilkunnil T, Chen ZP, et al. Single phosphorylation sites in Acc1 and Acc2 regulate lipid homeostasis and the insulin-sensitizing effects of metformin. *Nat Med* 19: 1649–1654, 2013.

36. Gomez-Cabrera MC, Borras C, Pallardo FV, Sastre J, Ji LL, Vina J. Decreasing xanthine oxidase-mediated oxidative stress prevents useful cellular adaptations to exercise in rats. *J Physiol* 567: 113–120, 2005.

37. Gomez-Cabrera MC, Close GL, Kayani A, McArdle A, Vina J, Jackson MJ. Effect of xanthine oxidase-generated extracellular superoxide on skeletal muscle force generation. *Am J Physiol Regul Integr Comp Physiol* 298: R2–R8, 2010.

38. Goncalves RL, Quinlan CL, Perevoshchikova IV, Hey-Mogensen M, Brand MD. Sites of superoxide and hydrogen peroxide production by muscle mitochondria assessed ex vivo under conditions mimicking rest and exercise. *J Biol Chem* 290: 209–227, 2015.

39. Goodyear LJ, Chang PY, Sherwood DJ, Dufresne SD, and Moller DE. Effects of exercise and insulin on mitogen-activated protein kinase signaling pathways in rat skeletal muscle. *Am J Physiol* 271: E403–E408, 1996.

40. Guadagnin E, Mazala D, Chen YW. STAT3 in Skeletal muscle function and disorders. *Int J Mol Sci* 19: 2018.

41. Gudiksen A, Bertholdt L, Stankiewicz T, Tybirk J, Plomgaard P, Bangsbo J, et al. Effects of training status on PDH regulation in human skeletal muscle during exercise. *Pflugers Arch* 469: 1615–1630, 2017.

42. Gudiksen A, Schwartz CL, Bertholdt L, Joensen E, Knudsen JG, Pilegaard H. Lack of skeletal muscle IL-6 affects pyruvate dehydrogenase activity at rest and during prolonged exercise. *PLoS One* 11: e0156460, 2016.

43. Halling JF, Pilegaard H. Autophagy-dependent beneficial effects of exercise. *Cold Spring Harb Perspect Med* 7: 2017.

44. Halling JF, Ringholm S, Olesen J, Prats C, Pilegaard H. Exercise training protects against aging-induced mitochondrial fragmentation in mouse skeletal muscle in a PGC-1alpha dependent manner. *Exp Gerontol* 96: 1–6, 2017.

45. Hardie DG, Carling D, Carlson M. The AMP-activated/SNF1 protein kinase subfamily: metabolic sensors of the eukaryotic cell? *Annu Rev Biochem* 67: 821–855, 1998.

46. Hawley JA. Adaptations of skeletal muscle to prolonged, intense endurance training. *Clin Exp Pharmacol Physiol* 29: 218–222, 2002.

47. Hawley SA, Davison M, Woods A, Davies SP, Beri RK, Carling D, et al. Characterization of the AMP-activated protein kinase kinase from rat liver and identification of threonine 172 as the major site at which it phosphorylates AMP-activated protein kinase. *J Biol Chem* 271: 27879–27887, 1996.

48. Hawley SA, Pan DA, Mustard KJ, Ross L, Bain J, Edelman AM, et al. Calmodulin-dependent protein kinase kinase-beta is an alternative upstream kinase for AMP-activated protein kinase. *Cell Metab* 2: 9–19, 2005.

49. Helge JW, Klein DK, Andersen TM, van HG, Calbet J, Boushel R, et al. Interleukin-6 release is higher across arm than leg muscles during whole-body exercise. *Exp Physiol* 96: 590–598, 2011.

50. Helge JW, Stallknecht B, Pedersen BK, Galbo H, Kiens B, Richter EA. The effect of graded exercise on IL-6 release and glucose uptake in human skeletal muscle. *J Physiol* 546: 299–305, 2003.

51. Hellsten Y, Ahlborg G, Jensen-Urstad M, Sjodin B. Indication of in vivo xanthine oxidase activity in human skeletal muscle during exercise. *Acta Physiol Scand* 134: 159–160, 1988.

52. Henriquez-Olguin C, Diaz-Vegas A, Utreras-Mendoza Y, Campos C, Arias-Calderon M, Llanos P, et al. NOX2 inhibition impairs early muscle gene expression induced by a single exercise bout. *Front Physiol* 7: 282, 2016.

53. Hoffman NJ, Parker BL, Chaudhuri R, Fisher-Wellman KH, Kleinert M, Humphrey SJ, et al. Global phosphoproteomic analysis of human skeletal muscle reveals a network of exercise-regulated kinases and AMPK substrates. *Cell Metab* 22: 922–935, 2015.

54. Hostrup M, Narkowicz CK, Habib S, Nichols DS, Jacobson GA. Beta2 -adrenergic ligand racemic formoterol exhibits enantioselective disposition in blood and skeletal muscle of humans, and elicits myocellular PKA signaling at therapeutic inhaled doses. *Drug Test Anal* 11: 1048–1056, 2019.

55. Huang B, Gudi R, Wu P, Harris RA, Hamilton J, Popov KM. Isoenzymes of pyruvate dehydrogenase phosphatase. DNA-derived amino acid sequences, expression, and regulation. *J Biol Chem* 273: 17680–17688, 1998.

56. Ihlemann J, Galbo H, Ploug T. Calphostin C is an inhibitor of contraction, but not insulin-stimulated glucose transport, in skeletal muscle. *Acta Physiol Scand* 167: 69–75, 1999.

57. Irrcher I, Ljubicic V, Hood DA. Interactions between ROS and AMP kinase activity in the regulation of PGC-1alpha transcription in skeletal muscle cells. *Am J Physiol Cell Physiol* 296: C116–C123, 2009.

58. Jackson MJ, Vasilaki A, McArdle A. Cellular mechanisms underlying oxidative stress in human exercise. *Free Radic Biol Med* 98: 13–17, 2016.

59. Jager S, Handschin C, St-Pierre J, Spiegelman BM. AMP-activated protein kinase (AMPK) action in skeletal muscle via direct phosphorylation of PGC-1alpha. *Proc Natl Acad Sci U S A* 104: 12017–12022, 2007.

60. Jensen TE, Maarbjerg SJ, Rose AJ, Leitges M, Richter EA. Knockout of the predominant conventional PKC isoform, PKCalpha, in mouse skeletal muscle does not affect contraction-stimulated glucose uptake. *Am J Physiol Endocrinol Metab* 297: E340–E348, 2009.

61. Jiang LQ, Duque-Guimaraes DE, Machado UF, Zierath JR, Krook A. Altered response of skeletal muscle to IL-6 in type 2 diabetic patients. *Diabetes* 62: 355–361, 2013.

62. Jorgensen SB, Viollet B, Andreelli F, Frosig C, Birk JB, Schjerling P, et al. Knockout of the alpha2 but not alpha1 5'-AMP-activated protein kinase isoform abolishes 5-aminoimidazole-4-carboxamide-1-beta-4-ribofuranosidebut not contraction-induced glucose uptake in skeletal muscle. *J Biol Chem* 279: 1070–1079, 2004.

63. Jorgensen SB, Wojtaszewski JF, Viollet B, Andreelli F, Birk JB, Hellsten Y, et al. Effects of alpha-AMPK knockout on exercise-induced gene activation in mouse skeletal muscle. *FASEB J* 19: 1146–1148, 2005.

64. Kang C, O'Moore KM, Dickman JR, Ji LL. Exercise activation of muscle peroxisome proliferator-activated receptor-gamma coactivator-1alpha signaling is redox sensitive. *Free Radic Biol Med* 47: 1394–1400, 2009.

65. Katz A. Role of reactive oxygen species in regulation of glucose transport in skeletal muscle during exercise. *J Physiol* 594: 2787–2794, 2016.

66. Kelly M, Gauthier MS, Saha AK, Ruderman NB. Activation of AMP-activated protein kinase by interleukin-6 in rat skeletal muscle: association with changes in cAMP, energy state, and endogenous fuel mobilization. *Diabetes* 58: 1953–1960, 2009.

67. Keum YS, Choi BY. Molecular and chemical regulation of the Keap1-Nrf2 signaling pathway. *Molecules* 19: 10074–10089, 2014.
68. Kjaer M, Howlett K, Langfort J, Zimmerman-Belsing T, Lorentsen J, Bulow J, et al. Adrenaline and glycogenolysis in skeletal muscle during exercise: a study in adrenalectomised humans. *J Physiol* 528 Pt 2: 371–378, 2000.
69. Klein DK, Pilegaard H, Treebak JT, Jensen TE, Viollet B, Schjerling P, et al. Lack of AMPKalpha2 enhances pyruvate dehydrogenase activity during exercise. *Am J Physiol Endocrinol Metab* 293: E1242–E1249, 2007.
70. Kusuhara K, Madsen K, Jensen L, Hellsten Y, Pilegaard H. Calcium signalling in the regulation of PGC-1alpha, PDK4 and HKII mRNA expression. *Biol Chem* 388: 481–488, 2007.
71. Li T, He S, Liu S, Kong Z, Wang J, Zhang Y. Effects of different exercise durations on Keap1-Nrf2-ARE pathway activation in mouse skeletal muscle. *Free Radic Res* 49: 1269–1274, 2015.
72. Lin J, Wu H, Tarr PT, Zhang CY, Wu Z, Boss O, et al. Transcriptional co-activator PGC-1 alpha drives the formation of slow-twitch muscle fibres. *Nature* 418: 797–801, 2002.
73. Loh C, Shaw KT, Carew J, Viola JP, Luo C, Perrino BA, et al. Calcineurin binds the transcription factor NFAT1 and reversibly regulates its activity. *J Biol Chem* 271: 10884–10891, 1996.
74. Madsen K, Ertbjerg P, Djurhuus MS, Pedersen PK. Calcium content and respiratory control index of skeletal muscle mitochondria during exercise and recovery. *Am J Physiol* 271: E1044–E1050, 1996.
75. Mansueto G, Armani A, Viscomi C, D'Orsi L, De CR, Polishchuk EV, et al. Transcription factor EB controls metabolic flexibility during exercise. *Cell Metab* 25: 182–196, 2017.
76. McGee SL, Hargreaves M. Exercise and myocyte enhancer factor 2 regulation in human skeletal muscle. *Diabetes* 53: 1208–1214, 2004.
77. Medina DL, Di PS, Peluso I, Armani A, De SD, Venditti R, et al. Lysosomal calcium signalling regulates autophagy through calcineurin and TFEB. *Nat Cell Biol* 17: 288–299, 2015.
78. Merrill GF, Kurth EJ, Hardie DG, Winder WW. AICA riboside increases AMP-activated protein kinase, fatty acid oxidation, and glucose uptake in rat muscle. *Am J Physiol* 273: E1107–E1112, 1997.
79. Merry TL Ristow M. Nuclear factor erythroid-derived 2-like 2 (NFE2L2, Nrf2) mediates exercise-induced mitochondrial biogenesis and the anti-oxidant response in mice. *J Physiol* 594: 5195–5207, 2016.
80. Merry TL, Wadley GD, Stathis CG, Garnham AP, Rattigan S, Hargreaves M, et al. N-Acetylcysteine infusion does not affect glucose disposal during prolonged moderate-intensity exercise in humans. *J Physiol* 588: 1623–1634, 2010.
81. Miura S, Kawanaka K, Kai Y, Tamura M, Goto M, Shiuchi T, et al. An increase in murine skeletal muscle peroxisome proliferator-activated receptor-gamma coactivator-1alpha (PGC-1alpha) mRNA in response to exercise is mediated by beta-adrenergic receptor activation. *Endocrinology* 148: 3441–3448, 2007.
82. Morrison D, Hughes J, Della Gatta PA, Mason S, Lamon S, Russell AP, et al. Vitamin C and E supplementation prevents some of the cellular adaptations to endurance-training in humans. *Free Radic Biol Med* 89: 852–862, 2015.
83. Mourtzakis M, Saltin B, Graham T, Pilegaard H. Carbohydrate metabolism during prolonged exercise and recovery: interactions between pyruvate dehydrogenase, fatty acids, and amino acids. *J Appl Physiol (1985)* 100: 1822–1830, 2006.
84. Murakami M, Hibi M, Nakagawa N, Nakagawa T, Yasukawa K, Yamanishi K, et al. IL-6-induced homodimerization of gp130 and associated activation of a tyrosine kinase. *Science* 260: 1808–1810, 1993.
85. Naka T, Narazaki M, Hirata M, Matsumoto T, Minamoto S, Aono A, et al. Structure and function of a new STAT-induced STAT inhibitor. *Nature* 387: 924–929, 1997.
86. Nielsen HB, Secher NH, Christensen NJ, Pedersen BK. Lymphocytes and NK cell activity during repeated bouts of maximal exercise. *Am J Physiol* 271: R222–R227, 1996.
87. Nielsen JN Wojtaszewski JF. Regulation of glycogen synthase activity and phosphorylation by exercise. *Proc Nutr Soc* 63: 233–237, 2004.
88. O'Neill HM, Palanivel R, Wright DC, MacDonald T, Lally JS, Schertzer JD, et al. IL-6 is not essential for exercise-induced increases in glucose uptake. *J Appl Physiol (1985)* 114: 1151–1157, 2013.
89. Ojuka EO, Jones TE, Han DH, Chen M, Holloszy JO. Raising Ca2+ in L6 myotubes mimics effects of exercise on mitochondrial biogenesis in muscle. *FASEB J* 17: 675–681, 2003.
90. Ojuka EO, Jones TE, Han DH, Chen M, Wamhoff BR, Sturek M, et al. Intermittent increases in cytosolic Ca2+ stimulate mitochondrial biogenesis in muscle cells. *Am J Physiol Endocrinol Metab* 283: E1040–E1045, 2002.
91. Ostrowski K, Rohde T, Zacho M, Asp S, Pedersen BK. Evidence that interleukin-6 is produced in human skeletal muscle during prolonged running. *J Physiol* 508 (Pt 3): 949–953, 1998.
92. Parker L, Trewin A, Levinger I, Shaw CS, Stepto NK. The effect of exercise-intensity on skeletal muscle stress kinase and insulin protein signaling. *PLoS One* 12: e0171613, 2017.

93. Parolin ML, Chesley A, Matsos MP, Spriet LL, Jones NL, Heigenhauser GJ. Regulation of skeletal muscle glycogen phosphorylase and PDH during maximal intermittent exercise. *Am J Physiol* 277: E890–E900, 1999.

94. Pehmoller C, Treebak JT, Birk JB, Chen S, Mackintosh C, Hardie DG, et al. Genetic disruption of AMPK signaling abolishes both contraction- and insulin-stimulated TBC1D1 phosphorylation and 14-3-3 binding in mouse skeletal muscle. *Am J Physiol Endocrinol Metab* 297: E665–E675, 2009.

95. Petersen AC, McKenna MJ, Medved I, Murphy KT, Brown MJ, Della GP, et al. Infusion with the antioxidant N-acetylcysteine attenuates early adaptive responses to exercise in human skeletal muscle. *Acta Physiol (Oxf)* 204: 382–392, 2012.

96. Pilegaard H, Ordway GA, Saltin B, Neufer PD. Transcriptional regulation of gene expression in human skeletal muscle during recovery from exercise. *Am J Physiol Endocrinol Metab* 279: E806–E814, 2000.

97. Polekhina G, Gupta A, Michell BJ, van DB, Murthy S, Feil SC, et al. AMPK beta subunit targets metabolic stress sensing to glycogen. *Curr Biol* 13: 867–871, 2003.

98. Raney MA, Turcotte LP. Evidence for the involvement of CaMKII and AMPK in Ca2+-dependent signaling pathways regulating FA uptake and oxidation in contracting rodent muscle. *J Appl Physiol (1985)* 104: 1366–1373, 2008.

99. Rao A, Luo C, Hogan PG. Transcription factors of the NFAT family: regulation and function. *Annu Rev Immunol* 15: 707–747, 1997.

100. Rasmussen BB, Winder WW. Effect of exercise intensity on skeletal muscle malonyl-CoA and acetyl-CoA carboxylase. *J Appl Physiol (1985)* 83: 1104–1109, 1997.

101. Richter EA, Cleland PJ, Rattigan S, Clark MG. Contraction-associated translocation of protein kinase C in rat skeletal muscle. *FEBS Lett* 217: 232–236, 1987.

102. Rose AJ, Kiens B, Richter EA. Ca2+-calmodulin-dependent protein kinase expression and signalling in skeletal muscle during exercise. *J Physiol* 574: 889–903, 2006.

103. Sakamoto K, Goransson O, Hardie DG, Alessi DR. Activity of LKB1 and AMPK-related kinases in skeletal muscle: effects of contraction, phenformin, and AICAR. *Am J Physiol Endocrinol Metab* 287: E310–E317, 2004.

104. Sandstrom ME, Zhang SJ, Bruton J, Silva JP, Reid MB, Westerblad H, et al. Role of reactive oxygen species in contraction-mediated glucose transport in mouse skeletal muscle. *J Physiol* 575: 251–262, 2006.

105. Scarpulla RC. Transcriptional paradigms in mammalian mitochondrial biogenesis and function. *Physiol Rev* 88: 611–638, 2008.

106. Scherer NM, Deamer DW. Oxidative stress impairs the function of sarcoplasmic reticulum by oxidation of sulfhydryl groups in the Ca2+-ATPase. *Arch Biochem Biophys* 246: 589–601, 1986.

107. Shute RJ, Heesch MW, Zak RB, Kreiling JL, Slivka DR. Effects of exercise in a cold environment on transcriptional control of PGC-1alpha. *Am J Physiol Regul Integr Comp Physiol* 314: R850–R857, 2018.

108. Silveira LR, Pilegaard H, Kusuhara K, Curi R, Hellsten Y. The contraction induced increase in gene expression of peroxisome proliferator-activated receptor (PPAR)-gamma coactivator 1alpha (PGC-1alpha), mitochondrial uncoupling protein 3 (UCP3) and hexokinase II (HKII) in primary rat skeletal muscle cells is dependent on reactive oxygen species. *Biochim Biophys Acta* 1763: 969–976, 2006.

109. Smuder AJ, Sollanek KJ, Nelson WB, Min K, Talbert EE, Kavazis AN, et al. Crosstalk between autophagy and oxidative stress regulates proteolysis in the diaphragm during mechanical ventilation. *Free Radic Biol Med* 115: 179–190, 2018.

110. Spangenburg EE, Brown DA, Johnson MS, Moore RL. Exercise increases SOCS-3 expression in rat skeletal muscle: potential relationship to IL-6 expression. *J Physiol* 572: 839–848, 2006.

111. Stapleton D, Mitchelhill KI, Gao G, Widmer J, Michell BJ, Teh T, et al. Mammalian AMP-activated protein kinase subfamily. *J Biol Chem* 271: 611–614, 1996.

112. Steensberg A, van HG, Osada T, Sacchetti M, Saltin B, Klarlund PB. Production of interleukin-6 in contracting human skeletal muscles can account for the exercise-induced increase in plasma interleukin-6. *J Physiol* 529 Pt 1: 237–242, 2000.

113. Stephens TJ, Chen ZP, Canny BJ, Michell BJ, Kemp BE, McConell GK. Progressive increase in human skeletal muscle AMPKalpha2 activity and ACC phosphorylation during exercise. *Am J Physiol Endocrinol Metab* 282: E688–E694, 2002.

114. Stocks B, Dent JR, Ogden HB, Zemp M, Philp A. Postexercise skeletal muscle signaling responses to moderate- to high-intensity steady-state exercise in the fed or fasted state. *Am J Physiol Endocrinol Metab* 316: E230–E238, 2019.

115. Thomson DM, Winder WW. AMP-activated protein kinase control of fat metabolism in skeletal muscle. *Acta Physiol (Oxf)* 196: 147–154, 2009.

116. Treebak JT, Birk JB, Rose AJ, Kiens B, Richter EA, Wojtaszewski JF. AS160 phosphorylation is associated with activation of alpha2beta2gamma1- but not alpha2beta2gamma3-AMPK trimeric complex in skeletal muscle during exercise in humans. *Am J Physiol Endocrinol Metab* 292: E715–E722, 2007.

117. Treebak JT, Glund S, Deshmukh A, Klein DK, Long YC, Jensen TE, et al. AMPK-mediated AS160 phosphorylation in skeletal muscle is dependent on AMPK catalytic and regulatory subunits. *Diabetes* 55: 2051–2058, 2006.

118. Treebak JT, Taylor EB, Witczak CA, An D, Toyoda T, Koh HJ, et al. Identification of a novel phosphorylation site on TBC1D4 regulated by AMP-activated protein kinase in skeletal muscle. *Am J Physiol Cell Physiol* 298: C377–C385, 2010.

119. van HG, Steensberg A, Sacchetti M, Fischer C, Keller C, Schjerling P, et al. Interleukin-6 stimulates lipolysis and fat oxidation in humans. *J Clin Endocrinol Metab* 88: 3005–3010, 2003.

120. Wadley GD, Choate J, McConell GK. NOS isoform-specific regulation of basal but not exercise-induced mitochondrial biogenesis in mouse skeletal muscle. *J Physiol* 585: 253–262, 2007.

121. Wadley GD, McConell GK. Effect of nitric oxide synthase inhibition on mitochondrial biogenesis in rat skeletal muscle. *J Appl Physiol (1985)* 102: 314–320, 2007.

122. Wadley GD, Nicolas MA, Hiam DS, McConell GK. Xanthine oxidase inhibition attenuates skeletal muscle signaling following acute exercise but does not impair mitochondrial adaptations to endurance training. *Am J Physiol Endocrinol Metab* 304: E853–E862, 2013.

123. Watt MJ, Stellingwerff T, Heigenhauser GJ, Spriet LL. Effects of plasma adrenaline on hormone-sensitive lipase at rest and during moderate exercise in human skeletal muscle. *J Physiol* 550: 325–332, 2003.

124. Whitham M, Chan MH, Pal M, Matthews VB, Prelovsek O, Lunke S, et al. Contraction-induced interleukin-6 gene transcription in skeletal muscle is regulated by c-Jun terminal kinase/activator protein-1. *J Biol Chem* 287: 10771–10779, 2012.

125. Widegren U, Jiang XJ, Krook A, Chibalin AV, Bjornholm M, Tally M, et al. Divergent effects of exercise on metabolic and mitogenic signaling pathways in human skeletal muscle. *FASEB J* 12: 1379–1389, 1998.

126. Widegren U, Wretman C, Lionikas A, Hedin G, Henriksson J. Influence of exercise intensity on ERK/MAP kinase signalling in human skeletal muscle. *Pflugers Arch* 441: 317–322, 2000.

127. Winder WW, Wilson HA, Hardie DG, Rasmussen BB, Hutber CA, Call GB, et al. Phosphorylation of rat muscle acetyl-CoA carboxylase by AMP-activated protein kinase and protein kinase A. *J Appl Physiol (1985)* 82: 219–225, 1997.

128. Witczak CA, Jessen N, Warro DM, Toyoda T, Fujii N, Anderson ME, et al. CaMKII regulates contraction- but not insulin-induced glucose uptake in mouse skeletal muscle. *Am J Physiol Endocrinol Metab* 298: E1150–E1160, 2010.

129. Wojtaszewski JF, Mourtzakis M, Hillig T, Saltin B, Pilegaard H. Dissociation of AMPK activity and ACCbeta phosphorylation in human muscle during prolonged exercise. *Biochem Biophys Res Commun* 298: 309–316, 2002.

130. Wojtaszewski JF, Nielsen JN, Jorgensen SB, Frosig C, Birk JB, Richter EA. Transgenic models—a scientific tool to understand exercise-induced metabolism: the regulatory role of AMPK (5'-AMP-activated protein kinase) in glucose transport and glycogen synthase activity in skeletal muscle. *Biochem Soc Trans* 31: 1290–1294, 2003.

131. Wojtaszewski JF, Nielsen P, Hansen BF, Richter EA, Kiens B. Isoform-specific and exercise intensity-dependent activation of 5'-AMP-activated protein kinase in human skeletal muscle. *J Physiol* 528 Pt 1: 221–226, 2000.

132. Woods A, Dickerson K, Heath R, Hong SP, Momcilovic M, Johnstone SR, et al. Ca2+/calmodulin-dependent protein kinase kinase-beta acts upstream of AMP-activated protein kinase in mammalian cells. *Cell Metab* 2: 21–33, 2005.

133. Woods A, Johnstone SR, Dickerson K, Leiper FC, Fryer LG, Neumann D, et al. LKB1 is the upstream kinase in the AMP-activated protein kinase cascade. *Curr Biol* 13: 2004–2008, 2003.

134. Wright DC, Fick CA, Olesen JB, Lim K, Barnes BR, Craig BW. A role for calcium/calmodulin kinase in insulin stimulated glucose transport. *Life Sci* 74: 815–825, 2004.

135. Wu H, Kanatous SB, Thurmond FA, Gallardo T, Isotani E, Bassel-Duby R, et al. Regulation of mitochondrial biogenesis in skeletal muscle by CaMK. *Science* 296: 349–352, 2002.

136. Yfanti C, Fischer CP, Nielsen S, Akerstrom T, Nielsen AR, Veskoukis AS, et al. Role of vitamin C and E supplementation on IL-6 in response to training. *J Appl Physiol (1985)* 112: 990–1000, 2012.

137. Yu M, Blomstrand E, Chibalin AV, Krook A, Zierath JR. Marathon running increases ERK1/2 and p38 MAP kinase signalling to downstream targets in human skeletal muscle. *J Physiol* 536: 273–282, 2001.

138. Zmijewski JW, Banerjee S, Bae H, Friggeri A, Lazarowski ER, Abraham E. Exposure to hydrogen peroxide induces oxidation and activation of AMP-activated protein kinase. *J Biol Chem* 285: 33154–33164, 2010.

SECTION II

Exercise Biochemistry, Chronic Training, and Athletic Performance

Paul J. LeBlanc

No matter the motivation, be it to win a medal at the Olympic Games or successfully complete a locally organized triathlon, exercise training is a necessity. With each exercise training session, various systems are stressed by disrupting homeostasis in an attempt to prepare the body for future challenges. Duration, modality, and intensity are all important variables that must be considered when formulating exercise training programmes.

Despite exercise training classically being associated with athletics and performance, chronic exercise training is an important contributor to overall health and health maintenance. In fact, in 2007, the American College of Sports Medicine and the American Medical Association co-launched Exercise is Medicine. Since that time, this initiative has extended globally, reaching over 40 countries, promoting the vast benefits of exercise training and physical activity.

Be it endurance or resistance exercise training, the following chapters examine the underlying biochemical and regulatory mechanisms associated with chronic exercise adaptations, specifically in skeletal muscle, and propose areas for future research. These include increased mitochondrial content to support elevated energy demand during exercise, the role of protein metabolic homeostasis and satellite cells in resistance exercise–mediated hypertrophy, alternative training approaches (e.g., various forms of interval training, systemic hypoxia, and blood flow restriction) compared to traditional programmes, and various factors that may be implicated in limits to these adaptive responses (e.g., biochemical, metabolic, genetic, and epigenetic), with a chapter focused on "responders" and "low-responders."

Regardless if the goal is to attain peak athletic performance, maintain health, or complement strategies to treat/prevent disease, this section will help the reader understand and appreciate the biochemical basis, and limits, of chronic exercise training adaptations.

9

EXERCISE-INDUCED MITOCHONDRIAL BIOGENESIS: MOLECULAR REGULATION, IMPACT OF TRAINING, AND INFLUENCE ON EXERCISE PERFORMANCE

Hashim Islam, Jacob T. Bonafiglia, Cesare Granata,
and Brendon J. Gurd

Introduction

Mitochondrial Structure and Function __Within__ Skeletal Muscle

Mitochondria are double membrane–bound organelles composed of inner and outer membranes, an intermembrane space, and the mitochondrial matrix (54). Embedded in the inner and outer membranes is the protein import machinery that regulates the entry of nuclear-encoded and cytosolic protein into the organelle, while the inner membrane also houses the electron transport chain (ETC) enzymes required for cellular respiration (105). The mitochondrial matrix contains enzymes of the tricarboxylic acid (TCA) cycle and fatty acid oxidation, as well as the mitochondrial DNA (mtDNA). Skeletal muscle mitochondria exist as a reticular network that can be divided into two morphologically and biochemically distinct (yet interconnected) subpopulations (14). Specifically, the subsarcolemmal (SS) mitochondria (~20% of total mitochondrial content) provide energy for active transport and transcriptional processes, whereas the intermyofibrillar (IMF) mitochondria (~80%) sustain the energetic demands of the contractile machinery (54, 105). The total content of mitochondria typically falls within 3–10% depending on muscle group and training status, with type I fibres possessing the largest fraction of mitochondria (54). In addition to their established role in the provision of cellular adenosine triphosphate (ATP), the mitochondria are integral for cell survival and programmed cell death, heme and nucleotide biosynthesis, ion homeostasis, and signal transduction (105). Due to the broad spectra of functions in which mitochondria are involved, their dysfunction has been linked with a series of diseases, although not necessarily specific to skeletal muscle, and they are therefore considered pivotal players in health and disease (83).

The Mitochondrial Genome

Although the majority of the >1500 mitochondrial proteins (113) are nuclear-encoded, mtDNA encodes 13 essential subunits of the respiratory chain, 22 transfer RNAs, and 2 ribosomal RNAs that constitute the mitochondrial translational machinery (9). Consequently, mitochondrial proliferation necessitates the cooperation between the nuclear and mitochondrial genomes (51). The core human mitochondrial transcriptional machinery comprises the mitochondrial RNA polymerase (POLRMT) and the mitochondrial transcription factors A (TFAM), B1 (TFB1M), and B2 (TFB2M) (all nuclear-encoded) that collectively initiate transcription from the heavy- and light-strand promoters located within the regulatory D-loop region of mtDNA (9). mtDNA-encoded genes are transcribed as a single polycistronic transcript from each of the two promoters; however, the steady-state levels of the mitochondrial mRNAs can vary substantially due to differences in the post-transcriptional processes that control mRNA maturation and stability (81). Although the content of mtDNA associates closely with tissue oxidative capacity (26), mtDNA copy number itself is considered a poor biomarker of mitochondrial content in human skeletal muscle (69). However, mtDNA copy number is increased in trained relative to untrained skeletal muscle (99), suggesting some level of regulation at the pre-transcriptional level. For an in-depth review on the regulation of mitochondrial transcription and translation, the reader is referred to an excellent review (9).

Key Terminology

Skeletal muscle mitochondria are highly malleable in their ability to adapt to a plethora of environmental stimuli (49, 51). Depending on the type of stimulus, these adaptations may involve alterations in mitochondrial morphology, protein content, enzymatic activities, or respiratory function. As such, before discussing the molecular mechanisms that underpin mitochondrial adaptations to exercise training, it is important to understand key terms that are used to describe the adaptive remodelling of skeletal muscle mitochondria.

Mitochondrial Biogenesis

Since the first in vivo observation of a training-induced increase in mitochondrial protein content in rat skeletal muscle by John Holloszy (48), a significant body of research has been devoted to understanding the adaptive phenomenon now known as *mitochondrial biogenesis* (87). Despite its prevalent use in exercise physiology literature for several decades (26, 51), the term does not appear to have a widely accepted or standardized definition. Experts in the field have recently proposed to define mitochondrial biogenesis as "the making of new components of the mitochondrial reticulum" (38, 105), which seems appropriate because the expansion of the mitochondrial reticulum does not appear to be a consequence of de novo organelle synthesis, but instead the incorporation of newly formed protein (both nuclear- and mitochondrial-encoded) into existing mitochondrial sub-fractions (51, 105). Given the complex and multistep nature of mitochondrial biogenesis (discussed later), a variety of different approaches have been used to characterize this adaptive response, including changes in gene expression, protein synthetic rates, steady-state protein content, enzymatic activities, mtDNA copy number, and histological methods (e.g., electron or fluorescent microscopy). While each measure provides important information regarding various steps of mitochondrial remodelling, it is generally well accepted that a combination of the aforementioned indices is best suited to comprehensively assess mitochondrial biogenesis (79).

Mitochondrial Respiratory Function

Adaptive remodelling of skeletal muscle mitochondrial also involves qualitative changes in organelle function (e.g., enhanced bioenergetics) that may dissociate from changes in mitochondrial content (37). As such, coupling the assessment of mitochondrial biogenesis with indices of mitochondrial respiratory function can provide a more holistic view of mitochondrial remodelling versus either component alone. Presently, the measurement of oxygen consumption in permeabilized skeletal muscle fibres is considered the gold-standard index of mitochondrial respiratory function (37), though other indices (e.g., reactive oxygen species [ROS] emission) have also been employed (52). A more detailed discussion on the measurement of skeletal muscle mitochondrial function can be found in previous reviews (38, 52).

Molecular Regulation of Exercise-Induced Mitochondrial Biogenesis

Current Dogma: Signalling → mRNA → Protein

Changes in skeletal muscle phenotype arise from the disruption of myocellular homeostasis by various molecules generated during contractile activity. These include changes in intramuscular metabolites/ions, redox status, and mechanical disturbances that serve as primary messengers for the activation of intracellular signal transduction pathways (24). The convergence of these signalling pathways on downstream transcription factors and co-activators alters the activity and subcellular localization of these transcriptional regulators, thereby facilitating DNA binding and the initiation of gene transcription (24). Contraction-induced changes in gene transcription manifest as transient "bursts" of mRNA expression that occur following each single exercise bout and precede changes in protein content and enzyme activity that occur following successive exercise bouts (89). Replication of this temporal/correlational relationship between exercise-induced changes in mRNA expression and training-induced changes in skeletal muscle function (8, 23) has led to the widespread notion that exercise-induced remodelling is initiated at the transcriptional level (24). Thus, despite the absence of direct evidence linking exercise-induced changes in mRNA expression to training-induced adaptive outcomes (37), exercise studies frequently use transcriptional responses to a single session of exercise as primary outcome measures when evaluating the adaptive potential or effectiveness of an exercise training stimulus.

Although the early manifestation of mitochondrial biogenesis may be most apparent by the robust changes in mRNA expression observed in the post-exercise period (i.e., 0–48 h) (38), regulatory steps distal to gene transcription (e.g., mRNA stabilization, translation and post-translational processing, protein import) are also important determinants of training-induced changes in steady-state protein content and cellular function (51). Nevertheless, since the available evidence largely consists of signalling and transcriptional events that contribute to mitochondrial biogenesis, these events will be the focus of subsequent sections. An overview of underexplored regulatory events distal to gene transcription is also discussed to hopefully simulate future work in this area. A summary of the molecular pathways discussed in this section are depicted in Figure 9.1.

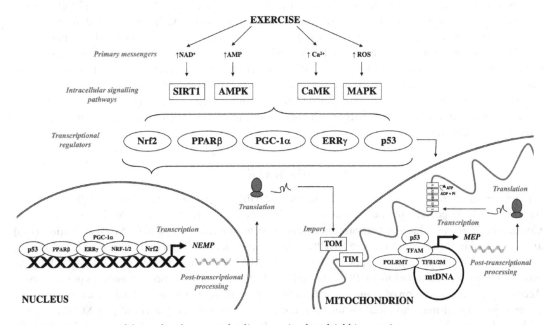

Figure 9.1   Overview of the molecular events leading to mitochondrial biogenesis

Intracellular Signalling Pathways Involved in Mitochondrial Biogenesis

Only a brief overview of key signalling events involved in the transcriptional activation of mitochondrial biogenesis is presented in this chapter. For a comprehensive discussion on this topic, the reader is referred to an excellent review (24).

AMPK

The cellular energy sensor AMP-activated protein kinase (AMPK) has an established role in the molecular regulation of mitochondrial biogenesis (reviewed in 100). During exercise, contraction-induced changes in myocellular phosphorylation potential (i.e., [AMP]/[ATP]) facilitate the binding of AMP to the g subunit of AMPK (36). The subsequent increase in AMPK phosphorylation (Thr172) leads to the activation and/or altered subcellular localization of its downstream targets that include regulatory proteins involved in transcriptional control of mitochondrial biogenesis, including peroxisome proliferator-activated receptor gamma co-activator 1-alpha (PGC-1a; discussed later), which is regarded as the "master regulator of mitochondrial biogenesis" (5, 65, 114). Accordingly, chronic pharmacological activation of AMPK leads to a robust increase in mitochondrial protein content and enzyme activity in rodent skeletal muscle (5, 122). Although these findings highlight the importance of AMPK for promoting mitochondrial biogenesis, AMPK does not seem to be required for the exercise-induced up-regulation of key regulatory proteins involved in mitochondrial biogenesis (66). These observations underscore the ability of contractile activity to activate additional signalling pathways leading to mitochondrial biogenesis.

Calcium Signalling

The link between intracellular calcium levels and mitochondrial biogenesis has been demonstrated in early muscle cell experiments where induced elevations in cytosolic calcium (e.g., ionophore treatment) increased mitochondrial biogenic gene expression, mitochondrial protein content, and enzymatic activities (28, 84). Moreover, genetic ablation of the calcium-sequestering protein parvalbumin is associated with a robust increase in mitochondrial content in murine skeletal muscle, further highlighting the importance of calcium for promoting mitochondrial biogenesis (13). Calcium-induced alterations in mitochondrial phenotype are partly mediated by the calcium/calmodulin serine/threonine kinase (CaMK) (125) and protein kinase C (28). Both CaMK and the related calcium/calmodulin-dependent serine/threonine phosphatase, calcineurin (111), interact with downstream transcription factors and co-activators involved in mitochondrial biogenesis (46, 125). Similar to AMPK, calcium signalling does not seem to be required for the exercise-induced increase in mitochondrial biogenesis (29), highlighting the overlapping and multifaceted nature of contraction-induced signalling cascades in mitochondrial remodelling following exercise.

p38 MAPK

Of the various mitogen-activated protein kinase (MAPK) family members, p38 MAPK appears to be particularly important in the regulation of mitochondrial biogenesis in skeletal muscle (1, 123). Contractile activity–induced elevations in cellular ROS production (127) and CaMKII activation (123) are implicated in the activation of p38 MAPK, which subsequently phosphorylates transcription factors controlling PGC-1a gene transcription (1, 123). p38 MAPK can also induce mitochondrial biogenesis via direct phosphorylation of PGC-1a and the induction of downstream gene expression (97). Accordingly, overexpression of a constitutively active p38 activator in rodent skeletal muscle is associated with an increase in mitochondrial protein content (1) and the gamma isoform of p38 MAPK appears to be indispensable for exercise-induced mitochondrial biogenesis in murine skeletal muscle (95).

Altogether, hese observations underscore the importance of p38 MAPK as an additional signalling pathway leading to mitochondrial biogenesis.

SIRT1/GCN5

The deacetylase enzyme sirtuin 1 (SIRT1) links changes in cellular redox potential ([NAD$^+$]/[NADH]) to alterations in skeletal muscle phenotype (42, 92). Fasting- and exercise-induced increases in cellular NAD$^+$ levels enhance SIRT1-mediated deacetylation of lysine residues on downstream transcriptional regulators involved in the control of oxidative metabolism (42, 92). For instance, SIRT1 deacetylates PGC-1a in rodent skeletal muscle and is required for the induction of mitochondrial gene transcription in muscle cells (30). Paradoxically, while SIRT1 is essential for basal mitochondrial content and respiratory function (77), SIRT1 overexpression reduces mitochondrial protein content and enzyme activities in rodent skeletal muscle (44). Although it has been proposed that SIRT1 activity (rather than protein content) is a more important determinant of exercise-induced mitochondrial biogenesis (45), this notion has also been refuted by observations of preserved mitochondrial biogenesis in exercised murine skeletal muscle lacking SIRT1 (91).

In experiments involving muscle-specific SIRT1 knockout mice, exercise-induced PGC-1a deacetylation coincides with a reduction in nuclear protein content of the acetyltransferase GCN5 (general control of amino acid synthesis 5) and reduced GCN5-PGC-1a interaction (91). Because GCN5 acetylation of PGC-1a opposes SIRT1 action by inhibiting PGC-1a's transcriptional activity (30), it has been suggested that changes in GCN5 acetyltransferase activity may be more important for mitochondrial biogenesis than SIRT1-mediated deacetylation of PGC-1a (91). However, recent work involving muscle-specific GCN5 knockout mice has demonstrated the preservation of both basal mitochondrial protein content and exercise-induced mitochondrial biogenesis in skeletal muscle (20). Collectively, these findings highlight the complexity surrounding SIRT1 and GCN5's involvement in mitochondrial biogenesis and discrepancies between in vitro and in vivo experiments (43).

Endogenous Gases (NO, CO)

Endogenous gas production has also been implicated in the regulation of mitochondrial biogenesis (96). For example, production of the vasodilator nitric oxide (NO) by NO synthases (NOS) leads to the transcriptional activation of mitochondrial biogenesis in vitro (82), while NOS inhibition in rat skeletal muscle reduces basal mitochondrial protein content and enzyme activity (120). Although the precise mechanisms of NO-induced mitochondrial remodelling have not been fully elucidated, experiments in adipocytes and myocytes suggest that AMPK or PGC-1a may be involved (71, 82).

Production of carbon monoxide (CO) by heme oxygenases (HO) can also promote mitochondrial biogenesis via stimulation of ROS production (93). In murine cardiomyocytes, CO production promotes the nuclear translocation of nuclear factor erythroid 2-related factor 2 (Nrf2) (93), where Nrf2 binds to the promotor of nuclear respiratory factor 1 (NRF-1; discussed later) leading to the transcriptional activation of mitochondrial biogenesis via TFAM (93). These observations are corroborated by human studies where CO breathing for 5 days increased mitochondrial content, mitochondrial protein content, and oxidative enzyme activities via induction of the HO-1/CO pathway (101). Altogether, these findings implicate endogenous gas production as an additional upstream signal leading to the transcriptional activation of mitochondrial biogenesis.

Transcription Factors and Co-Activators Involved in Mitochondrial Biogenesis

The next step in the induction of mitochondrial biogenesis is the convergence of the upstream signalling pathways (as previously discussed) on key transcriptional regulators. Importantly, as the cooperation between the nuclear and mitochondrial genomes is a prerequisite for the synthesis of functional mitochondria (51), these regulators must be collectively capable of upregulating nuclear- and mitochondrial-encoded gene expression in a coordinated fashion. It is important to note that the list of proteins covered here is not exhaustive, and many other regulatory proteins are undoubtedly involved, some of which likely remain to be discovered. We also refer the reader to several in-depth reviews covering established transcriptional regulators involved in the control of mitochondrial biogenesis (52, 110).

TFAM

TFAM is regarded as the most important regulator of mtDNA transcription and replication in humans (52). Increases in TFAM gene transcription, mRNA stability, and mitochondrial localization occur in parallel with augmentation of mtDNA copy number and cytochrome c oxidase (COX) transcripts during muscle cell differentiation (15), a process associated with a marked increase in mitochondrial biogenesis. Importantly, several signalling protein and transcriptional regulators that are activated in skeletal muscle by exercise have been identified as important upstream regulators of TFAM activity or TFAM gene and protein expression in vitro and in vivo (15, 85, 108, 119, 126). Accordingly, electrical stimulation of rat skeletal muscle augments mitochondrial gene expression and enzyme activity subsequent to an increase in TFAM import and mtDNA binding in IMF mitochondria (34). Similarly, skeletal muscle TFAM mRNA and protein expression are enhanced in response to exercise in both rodents (85, 108) and humans (4, 89, 94). Given that alternations in TFAM protein content/localization parallel changes in mitochondrial gene expression and oxidative capacity under various physiological conditions (e.g., denervation, differentiation, contractile activity) (51), higher cellular levels of TFAM may be an important adaptation that contributes to exercise-induced mitochondrial remodelling in skeletal muscle.

NRF-1/2

Binding sites for NRF-1/2 can be found on nuclear genes encoding essential components of all five respiratory complexes, mitochondrial import protein, and mitochondrial translation and assembly factors (110). Importantly, NRF-1/2 activates the promoters of TFAM (119, 126), TFB1M, and TFB2M (32) (essential components of the mitochondrial transcriptional machinery), thereby allowing for the coordination of nuclear- and mitochondrial-encoded gene transcription. In rodent skeletal muscle, a single session of exercise enhances NRF-1/2 DNA binding on the promoters of their respective target genes (2, 124) prior to an increase in mitochondrial protein content (2). Moreover, serine phosphorylation of NRF-1 enhances its DNA binding and transactivation of its target genes (110). This may explain why chronic AMPK activation increases NRF-1 binding activity and mitochondrial protein content in rat skeletal muscle (5). Alternatively, several other stress-responsive transcriptional regulators are capable of coactivating NRF-1's transcriptional function (126) and enhancing NRF-1 gene or protein expression (67, 93), thereby supporting the exercise-induced increases in NRF-1 activity/expression observed in rodent muscle (2, 124). Contrarily, the majority of studies show no change in NRF-1/2 mRNA and protein expression in exercised human skeletal muscle (38). In this regard, it is possible that the coactivation of existing NRF-1/2 protein by transcriptional co-regulators is sufficient to drive the induction of mitochondrial biogenic gene expression.

PGC-1a

Frequently designated as the "master regulator" of mitochondrial biogenesis, the transcriptional coactivator PGC-1a integrates environmental signals to coordinately up-regulate nuclear- and mitochondrial-encoded gene transcription via co-activation of multiple transcription factors (e.g., NRF-1/2, PPARs, ERRs) (98, 110, 126). Accordingly, numerous loss- and gain-of-function experiments have demonstrated the importance of PGC-1a for basal mitochondrial content/respiratory function and oxidative remodelling in skeletal muscle (52, 110). Of note, PGC-1a autoregulates its own expression via co-activation of the myocyte enhancer factor 2 (MEF2) on the PGC-1a promoter, providing a mechanism by which sufficient levels of PGC-1a are maintained in tissues of high metabolic demand or in response to exercise-mediated stress (46).

A particularly important attribute of PGC-1a is its responsiveness to multiple upstream pathways that are activated by contractile activity. For instance, AMPK, CaMK, p38 MAPK, SIRT1, and NO/CO have all been implicated in the transcriptional activation of PGC-1a gene expression or post-translational control of PGC-1a protein activity (52). It is therefore unsurprising that contractile activity robustly increases PGC-1a gene and protein expression in both rodent (2) and human (61, 94) skeletal muscle. Moreover, the exercise-dependent accumulation of PGC-1a in nuclear (108, 124) and mito-chondrial (114) fractions occurs in concert with the up-regulation of nuclear- and mitochondrial-encoded gene expression in rodents (108, 124). Although exercise also increases nuclear PGC-1a protein in human skeletal muscle (41), there is conflicting evidence for the accumulation of PGC-1a protein in the mitochondria of exercised human skeletal muscle. Specifically, one study reported an increase in PGC-1a protein in SS mitochondria (114), whereas another study reported no change in mitochon-drial PGC-1a protein content (116) in response to a single exercise session. Of note, the dispensability of PGC-1a for training-induced mitochondrial remodelling in rodent skeletal muscle (104) highlights the notion that PGC-1a is one of many regulatory proteins involved in the control of exercise-induced mitochondrial biogenesis.

p53

Early experiments demonstrated that the loss of the tumour suppressor protein p53 reduces mitochon-drial respiration and COX activity in murine liver and human cancer cells (76). Confirmation of these findings in vivo came from a series of experiments using whole-body p53 knockout mice, where p53 ablation was associated with reductions in basal mitochondrial content or respiratory function (85), as well as compromised structural integrity of the organelle in skeletal muscle (106). Consistent with the presence of putative p53 binding sites on the PGC-1a promoter (58) and the regulation of TFAM promoter by p53 (85), p53 knockout animals exhibit reductions in basal PGC-1a protein content (106) as well as NRF-1 and TFAM mRNA expression (107). In contrast to these compelling findings from whole-body knockout models, subsequent studies involving muscle-specific p53 deletion in mice have provided evidence both for (6) and against (115) an essential role for p53 in the maintenance of basal mitochondrial content and respiratory function.

Similar to PGC-1a, p53 can be activated by numerous upstream kinases/deacetylases that are respon-sive to exercise (52). Accordingly, treadmill running enhances p53's interaction with TFAM in the mitochondria and promotes a concerted increase in nuclear- and mitochondrial-encoded gene expres-sion in murine skeletal muscle (108). Moreover, genetic ablation of p53 attenuates (AMPK, CaMKII) or abolishes (p38 MAPK) kinase activation, prevents the nuclear accumulation of PGC-1a, and diminishes the increase in mitochondrial biogenic gene expression in exercised rodent muscle (107). The exercise-induced activation of p53 is also apparent in human studies where increased p53 phosphorylation and downstream mRNA expression are observed in response to a single session of exercise (3). However, in contrast to rodents, a single bout of exercise increases nuclear (41, 116) but not mitochondrial (116) p53 protein content in human skeletal muscle. Nevertheless, the observation that p53 protein content increases in parallel with training-induced improvements in mitochondrial content (40) and respira-tory function (39) supports a potential role for p53 in training-induced mitochondrial remodelling in human skeletal muscle. Like PGC-1a, p53 does not appear to be required for training-induced increases in mitochondrial content and respiratory function in murine skeletal muscle (6, 106).

Emerging Regulatory Proteins

A recurring theme in the preceding sections is the notion that while each of the aforementioned proteins play an important role in the control of exercise-induced mitochondrial biogenesis, genetic ablation of a single protein rarely results in absolute abolishment of the mitochondrial adaptive response to exercise. This is perhaps unsurprising given the complex and overlapping nature of the molecular circuits that underpin mitochondrial biogenesis, the inherent redundancies in adaptive pathways that defend metabolic homeostasis, and the multitude of pathways that are activated with contractile activity (52). Accordingly, additional regulatory proteins involved in the control of mitochondrial biogenesis continue to emerge (62).

The redox-sensitive transcription factor Nrf2 (not to be confused with the nuclear respiratory factors 1 and 2 [NRF-1/2]) has recently been implicated as an important regulator of mitochondrial biogenesis in a number of in vitro and transgenic rodent studies. The transcriptional control of mitochondrial biogenesis by Nrf2 is based largely on its ability to regulate the promoter of NRF-1 (93) in murine cardiomyocytes. Moreover, Nrf2 is activated in response to a single exercise bout in rodent skeletal muscle (17, 78), presumably due to the ability of several stress-induced signalling pathways to activate Nrf2 (62). In addition, Nrf2 appears to be required for the maintenance of basal mitochondrial respiratory function (17), and its deletion at the whole-body level blunts (17) or abolishes (78) training-induced increases in mitochondrial protein content in rodent skeletal muscle. The role of Nrf2 for exercised-induced mitochondrial remodelling in human skeletal muscle was recently examined in a study reporting a strong positive correlation between training-induced changes in Nrf2 and NRF-1 protein content (59). In this study, individuals who experienced large increases in mitochondrial content (assessed using citrate synthase [CS] maximal activity) also exhibited large increases in Nrf2 protein (59), thereby supporting the potential involvement of Nrf2 in exercise-induced mitochondrial biogenesis in humans.

Although the peroxisome proliferator-activated receptor (PPAR) family of nuclear hormone receptors have established roles in the control of oxidative gene expression and lipid metabolism, PPARβ has emerged as being particularly important in the context of skeletal muscle mitochondrial biogenesis (62). Muscle-specific overexpression of PPARβ in mice boosts markers of mitochondrial content, whereas its knockdown/deletion reduces several transcriptional regulators of mitochondrial biogenesis and subunits of the ETC at the mRNA and protein level (62). The control of mitochondrial content by PPARβ appears to be mediated by stabilization of existing PGC-1a protein (67), as well as the transcriptional control of PGC-1a (112) and NRF-1 (67) gene expression. Importantly, PPARβ expression increases at the mRNA or protein level in exercised rodent and human skeletal muscle (89), and its partial knockdown diminishes training-induced increases in mitochondrial protein in murine skeletal muscle (67). Altogether, these findings underscore the importance of PPARβ in the maintenance of mitochondrial content and its ability to promote oxidative remodelling in skeletal muscle via multiple pathways.

Similar to PPARβ, the oestrogen-related receptor (ERR) family of nuclear receptors are known regulators of oxidative metabolism, and their transcriptional activity is dependent on their interactions with various co-regulators (e.g., PGC-1a) (62). However, transgenic rodent studies suggest that oxidative remodelling of skeletal muscle by the gamma-isoform of this family (ERRg) may also occur independently from PGC-1a (25). Overexpression of ERRg in murine skeletal muscle increases mitochondrial content, oxidative enzyme activities, and exercise capacity (62). Most compellingly, ERRg overexpression in murine skeletal muscle devoid of both PGC-1 isoforms (PGC-1a/β) significantly improves defects in mitochondrial content and respiratory function associated with the loss of PGC-1a/β both basally and in response to exercise training (25). These findings implicate ERRg as an additional player in the transcriptional control of mitochondrial biogenesis beyond its established role as a downstream binding partner of PGC-1a.

Underexplored Regulatory Events Beyond Transcription

Thus far, the regulation of mitochondrial biogenesis has been described predominantly in the context of signalling and transcriptional events that contribute to improvements in mitochondrial content and respiratory function. This is because the field of exercise physiology as a whole has focused largely on signalling/transcriptional responses following a single exercise session, and these responses are often used to make inferences about more distal events in the adaptive process and the effectiveness of an exercise stimulus. Due to this emphasis on early molecular events, information regarding regulatory steps downstream of signalling/transcription that are also critical determinants of steady-state protein content (and thus tissue functionality) is comparatively lacking, particularly in studies involving exercised human skeletal muscle. Notably, transcript levels are only partially predictive of cellular protein abundance across a variety of organisms (19), highlighting an important role for regulatory events downstream of transcription.

In the context of mitochondrial biogenesis, important regulatory steps downstream of signalling and gene transcription include post-transcriptional processing of newly transcribed mRNAs, translation of mitochondrial protein from existing or newly formed mRNAs, post-translation processing and trafficking of newly synthesized protein to the mitochondria, translocation of protein across the outer and inner mitochondrial membranes, and redistribution of these proteins to their final destinations within the mitochondria (26, 51). In an effort to promote future investigation of these processes in the context of exercise-induced mitochondrial remodelling, some of these regulatory events are now discussed using data from in vitro and animal studies.

Post-Transcriptional Control of mRNA Stability

The stability of newly transcribed mRNAs is dependent on their interaction with various RNA-binding proteins that either destabilize or stabilize the transcript via binding to specific structural elements of the mRNA (e.g., poly-[A] tail, 3' untranslated region) (51). Although changes in gene expression are frequently attributed to enhanced mRNA synthesis (i.e., transcription), early experiments revealed an important role for mRNA stability in the initial adaptive response to contractile activity (27). For instance, increases in cytochrome c mRNA expression in electrically stimulated rat skeletal muscle are primarily attributed to the increase in mRNA stability (2–4 days) that precedes the increase in cytochrome c transcription observed after 5 days of stimulation (27). Additionally, the mRNA decay rates of key mitochondrial biogenic regulators (e.g., PGC-1a, TFAM) appear to be accelerated in contracted rat skeletal muscle; this response has been hypothesized to contribute to enhanced turnover of regulatory protein to facilitate a rapid adaptive response to environmental stress (68). Together, these observations highlight the importance of mRNA stability as an important and modifiable regulatory step in the regulation of mitochondrial phenotype, warranting future research in this area (particularly in humans).

Translational Control of Mitochondrial Protein Synthesis

The translation of mature mRNA into precursor protein provides an additional regulatory step that can contribute to steady-state protein content and therefore altered cellular function (26, 51). Two intriguing observations from early rodent studies that point to the importance of translational control in the regulation of exercise-induced mitochondrial remodelling are (1) an increase in cytochrome c protein content that exceeded the increase in its mRNA expression (27) and (2) an increase in COX activity that exceeded corresponding mRNA levels of its nuclear- and mitochondrial-encoded subunits (53). These observations are consistent with the "translation on demand" hypothesis, where induced translation of pre-existing transcripts increases cellular protein levels, thereby circumventing the time delay between gene transcription and increased functional protein levels (72). Indeed, such a mechanism would ensure rapid adaptive changes to cellular protein composition in response to stress and is congruent with the increased cytochrome c synthesis despite unchanged cytochrome c mRNA content (10) reported in electrically stimulated muscle early in the adaptation period.

With regard to exercised human skeletal muscle, studies have reported enhanced rates of mitochondrial protein synthesis following a single session of exercise (121) and a training intervention (102) and that the acute synthetic response appears to depend on both exercise intensity (21) and sex (109). However, there is presently no information regarding the impact of exercise on mitochondrial fraction-specific synthetic rates in human skeletal muscle. Moreover, it would be intriguing to examine the importance of mitochondrial protein synthesis and degradation during mitochondrial remodelling over the course of a training intervention. Addressing these questions by replicating some of the aforementioned experimental approaches used in rodents should shed further light on the regulation of mitochondrial biogenesis with training.

Protein Trafficking and Import

The final steps leading to mitochondrial biogenesis involve the targeting of cytosolic precursor protein to the mitochondria and their subsequent import and redistribution to their final destination within the organelle (51, 52). Given the nuclear origin of the vast majority of mitochondrial proteins, these terminal steps are particularly important for ensuring that earlier adaptive events (e.g., signalling, gene transcription, protein synthesis) are successfully converted into alterations in mitochondrial phenotype. In this regard, cytosolic chaperones unfold and direct precursor protein to specific compartments within the organelle based on the presence of a cleavable target sequence (51, 52). The transport of mitochondrial-destined protein is accomplished by translocase complexes of the outer and (for matrix-destined protein) inner membranes (TOM and TIM, respectively) (51, 52). Upon its arrival to the appropriate mitochondrial sub-compartment (e.g., matrix), the target sequence is removed from the precursor protein, which is subsequently refolded and directed to its final destination by mitochondrial chaperones, leading to the expansion of the mitochondrial reticulum (51, 52).

Several lines of evidence support the notion that mitochondrial import is an important regulatory step in the determination of mitochondrial phenotype and is modifiable with exercise (51, 52). For instance, electrical stimulation of rat muscle increases mtDNA promoter binding, mitochondrial transcript levels, and COX activity subsequent to an increase in TFAM import into IMF mitochondria (35). Similar to distinct respiratory and protein synthetic rates (14, 16), SS and IMF mitochondria also differ in their ability to take up cytosolic protein, with greater rates of protein import observed in IMF fractions (118). However, protein import into both fractions can be augmented in response to contractile activity (117), and the adaptability of various components of the import system has been demonstrated in exercised or electrically stimulated rodent skeletal muscle (51, 52). Together, the aforementioned evidence clearly implicates protein import as a key step in the adaptive process leading to mitochondrial biogenesis. Unfortunately, there has been little to no investigation into the adaptability of the mitochondrial import system components to exercise in humans, providing an important area of future research.

Mitochondrial Adaptations to Training and Their Influence on Exercise Performance

Up until this point, we have discussed the mechanisms by which a single session of exercise activates the molecular events that contribute to the enhancement of skeletal muscle mitochondrial content and respiratory function. What remains unclear is the extent to which each molecular event (e.g., signalling, gene transcription, protein synthesis) contributes to phenotypic changes in mitochondrial content and respiratory function. In this regard, there is no available evidence supporting a direct relationship between exercise-induced changes in signalling/gene expression and training-induced mitochondrial adaptations (37). An obvious explanation for this is the complex and intricate nature of mitochondrial biogenesis, which makes it difficult to ascribe complex phenotypic changes to a single regulatory step in the adaptive process. Another reason is the confounding influence of random variability on observed molecular responses to a single exercise session, making it difficult to discern true responses to exercise from technical artifacts or biological variation (60). Lastly and perhaps most importantly, studies that have comprehensively examined the time course of changes in multiple regulatory events (particularly those occurring after gene transcription) over the course of a training period (similar to 89) are presently limited.

Although the importance of each regulatory step in the adaptive process remains to be established, the ability of repeated bouts of exercise to promote mitochondrial remodelling over an extended training period is well established in both animal and human skeletal muscle (50, 54). Furthermore, the magnitude and type of adaptation that occurs are influenced by the nature of the exercise stimulus (e.g., exercise intensity, duration, frequency). As such, this section will provide an overview of the literature examining training-induced changes in mitochondrial content and respiratory function in skeletal muscle—see (37) for a recent in-depth review of the literature. The physiological consequences of training-induced changes in mitochondrial phenotype for exercise performance are also discussed.

Training-Induced Changes in Mitochondrial Content

Early clues into the oxidative remodelling of skeletal muscle came from observations in land animals and birds that sustained long periods of activity. The muscles of these active animals exhibited enhanced levels of mitochondria and oxidative enzyme activities as compared to more sedentary species, pointing towards an effect of physical activity (86). This hypothesis was tested in the pioneering work of John Holloszy, who subjected young rats to a 12-week training period (5 days of intense treadmill running/week) to examine the impact of exercise on biochemical adaptations in skeletal muscle (48). A 2-fold increase in the ability to oxidize pyruvate was observed in the hindlimb muscles from these rats, concomitant with a doubling of respiratory chain enzyme activities and a robust increase in exercise performance (48). The high degree of respiratory control and tight coupling of oxidative phosphorylation observed in skeletal muscle indicated that the improvement in endurance performance was attributable to a proportional enhancement of ATP synthesis via oxidative phosphorylation. Importantly, cytochrome c concentration in skeletal muscle was increased by 2-fold and the total protein content of the mitochondrial fraction by 60%, indicating that the oxidative remodelling of muscle was due to a training-induced increase in mitochondrial biogenesis.

These initial observations by Holloszy paved the way for subsequent work in the 1960s and 1970s demonstrating the ability of endurance exercise training to promote mitochondrial biogenesis in both human and rodent skeletal muscle (reviewed in 50 and 54). These findings were later corroborated by human studies employing exercise training interventions (33) and cross-sectional analyses of trained and untrained individuals (56). In these human studies, an increase in mitochondrial content (up to ~40%) and oxidative enzyme activities (up to ~150%) was consistently observed in trained muscle. Notably, the proliferation of skeletal muscle mitochondria in response to training appeared to be more pronounced in the SS compared with IMF fractions (56). However, the greater absolute amount of IMF mitochondria in skeletal muscle makes this sub-fraction the major contributor to the overall increase in mitochondrial content with training. Moreover, while an increase in mitochondrial content was observed across all fibre types, it occurred to a slightly greater extent in fast oxidative glycolytic type IIA fibres (12). Since these early studies, an expansive body of literature has been devoted towards characterizing and understanding the proliferation of skeletal muscle mitochondria, making it one of the most well-studied adaptations to exercise training (51, 87).

Training-Induced Changes in Mitochondrial Respiratory Function

Although the majority of studies examining training-induced mitochondrial remodelling have focused on quantitative aspects (probably because these are relatively easier to characterize than qualitative changes to mitochondria), experiments in isolated mitochondria and permeabilized muscle fibres have demonstrated that mitochondrial respiratory function is also enhanced with exercise training (37). This is evident from cross-sectional analyses where close associations are observed between training status (i.e., fitness levels) and mitochondrial respiratory capacity (e.g., maximal rate of oxygen consumption and/or ATP production) of skeletal muscle (64, 128), and studies where an increase in mitochondrial respiratory function is observed following a period of structured exercise training (37) . The training-induced improvement in respiratory function appears to be due to both an enhanced ability of the mitochondria to oxidize fatty acids and via increases in complex I- and complex I+II-linked respiration (37). While it is generally believed that the enhancement of mitochondrial respiratory function in trained skeletal muscle is attributable to a greater mitochondrial content (since both have often been reported to increase simultaneously; 37), a dissociation between the two variables has also been reported (39, 40) suggesting that an exercise stimulus capable of robustly enhancing mitochondrial content may not be best suited for improving mitochondrial respiratory function or vice versa (discussed in more detail in the next section). Perhaps more importantly, the dissociation between mitochondrial content and respiratory function underscores the importance of assessing both quantitative and qualitative aspects of mitochondrial adaptations to achieve a more comprehensive understanding of how mitochondria adapt to repeated bouts of exercise (37, 79).

Optimal Exercise Prescription for Improving Mitochondrial Content and Respiratory Function

As mentioned, certain exercise-related variables may be more important for optimizing quantitative improvements to the mitochondria, whereas others may be better suited for enhancing mitochondrial respiratory function. In this regard, recent debate has focused on the role of exercise intensity and volume in training-induced mitochondrial remodelling (7, 74). Although limited in number, studies utilizing gold-standard morphometric indices of mitochondrial content (i.e., transmission electron microscopy) appear to support an important role for exercise training volume for maximizing increases in skeletal muscle mitochondrial content (37). This notion is further supported by pooled analyses of 56 studies (albeit of varying characteristics) showing a moderate-to-strong relationship ($r = 0.59\text{-}0.71$) between training volume and training-induced changes in CS maximal activity (a validated biomarker of mitochondrial content) (37, 69). On the other hand, studies involving high-intensity and sprint interval training (HIIT and SIT, respectively) protocols appear to also suggest an important role for exercise intensity (73). These studies reported that HIIT seems to be superior to traditional moderate-intensity continuous training (MICT) when training volume is matched (75) and that SIT results in similar improvements to MICT despite a significantly lower training volume (one-fifth of that in MICT) (31). An important caveat to this debate is that despite the availability of between-study comparisons of exercise intensity and volume (37), no single study has directly compared the impact of manipulating *both* exercise intensity and volume on mitochondrial content when equating the total amount of work performed. Thus, while a definitive answer to the exercise intensity versus volume debate remains to be established, there is support for a beneficial role of both exercise intensity and volume for increasing mitochondrial content following training (see 7 and 74 for a recent discussion on this topic).

In contrast to the uncertainty surrounding the superiority of exercise intensity or volume for augmenting mitochondrial content, improvements in mitochondrial respiratory function appear to be more responsive to higher exercise intensities (37). For instance, a study involving SIT, HIIT, and MICT reported improvements in mitochondrial respiratory function (independent of mitochondrial content) following SIT only (despite a ~3-fold greater exercise volume in the HIIT and SIT groups) (39). This observation is supported by work-matched comparisons of different exercise intensity protocols demonstrating a greater improvement of mitochondrial respiratory function following HIIT compared to MICT (18, 75). Moreover, improvements in mitochondrial respiratory function can be observed after only six sessions of HIIT in 2 weeks (63) and are sometimes absent even with much larger (~22 sessions in 6 weeks) MICT interventions (80). Although a greater increase in mitochondrial respiratory function following significantly higher- versus lower-volume training of similar relative exercise intensities has been reported, this effect appeared to be primarily attributable to an increase in mitochondrial content as opposed to improved respiratory function per se (40). Altogether, it appears that exercise intensity is an important contributor to training-induced improvements in mitochondrial respiratory function and that these improvements can occur independent of alterations in mitochondrial content.

Impact of Training-Induced Mitochondrial Remodelling on Exercise Performance

Despite strong correlations between indices of mitochondrial content/respiratory function and whole-body aerobic capacity (e.g., VO_2 max) (55, 56, 64), it is generally well accepted that maximal exercise performance is limited by central (i.e., cardiovascular and haematological) factors controlling oxygen delivery as opposed to peripheral factors that determine oxygen extraction/utilization (50). In this regard, mitochondrial respiratory capacity is in excess of the ability of the circulatory system to deliver oxygen to working muscle (11). This observation corroborates early studies demonstrating greater training-induced increases in mitochondrial content and enzyme activities (55), as well as a faster post-training decline of skeletal muscle oxidative enzyme activities in relation to VO_2 max (47). While maximal human exercise performance may not be dependent on skeletal muscle respiratory capacity, the metabolic changes associated with enhanced mitochondrial content and respiratory function are still critical determinants of endurance performance at submaximal workloads. These metabolic changes include an improved sensitivity of respiratory control, preservation of muscle glycogen, and increased reliance on fat utilization (50). Collectively, these changes delay the accumulation of local factors (e.g., H^+, ADP, Pi) contributing to the development of fatigue and allow for higher intensities of submaximal exercise to be sustained for longer periods.

Increased Sensitivity of Respiratory Control

The breakdown of ATP during exercise increases intramuscular [ADP] and [Pi], stimulating the creatine kinase reaction towards the formation of ATP and creatine (Cr). As the phosphocreatine (PCr) system becomes progressively depleted, the ensuing accumulation of cellular [ADP] serves as a primary signal for the activation of oxidative phosphorylation within the mitochondria (22). With a higher mitochondrial content, a given exercise workload (i.e., ATP demand) will require a lower rate of oxidative phosphorylation per mitochondrion such that a smaller increase in [ADP] is required to elicit the same level of oxygen consumption (50). This phenomenon has been described as an increased sensitivity of respiratory control and is apparent by an attenuated increase in free [ADP] in trained muscle with a high mitochondrial content when exercising at the same absolute workload (22, 70).

Reduced Glycogen Depletion

Because the formation of ADP, Pi, and adenosine monophosphate (AMP) (via adenylate kinase) also results in the allosteric activation of key enzymes of the glycogenolytic (phosphorylase) and glycolytic (phosphofructokinase) pathways, an increased sensitivity of respiratory control will also decrease flux through these metabolic pathways (50). Consequently, the breakdown of carbohydrate to pyruvate and its subsequent conversion to lactate (via lactate dehydrogenase) is also attenuated in trained muscle (70, 90). The reduction in carbohydrate utilization in trained muscle is further aided by inhibition at the level of pyruvate dehydrogenase (PDH), presumably due to the alleviation of pyruvate- and ADP-induced inhibition of pyruvate dehydrogenase kinase (PDK), a negative regulator of PDH activity (70).

Increased Fat Utilization

The preservation of skeletal muscle glycogen is paralleled by a ~2-fold increase in the rate of intramuscular triglyceride breakdown, such that fat utilization contributes to more than half of the total caloric expenditure during submaximal exercise in the trained state (57). This shift in substrate utilization favouring fat oxidation is presumably aided by the training-induced increase in enzymes involved in lipid transport and beta oxidation (88). Importantly, as carbohydrates are the predominant fuel source at higher (>65% VO_2 max) exercise intensities (103), the conservation of skeletal muscle glycogen via enhanced fat oxidation is an important contributor to the ability to sustain higher workloads (particularly later in the exercise bout) in the trained state.

Summary and Future Directions

Mitochondrial biogenesis involves the integrated induction of nuclear- and mitochondrial-encoded gene transcription and the subsequent synthesis, import, and assembly of newly formed protein into the mitochondria, culminating in the expansion of the mitochondrial reticulum. Research to date has identified a number of signalling proteins and transcriptional regulators involved in the regulation of mitochondrial biogenesis, many of which are activated in response to exercise. Although a significant amount of research has been devoted towards the examination of signalling and transcriptional events involved in exercise-induced mitochondrial biogenesis, relatively little research has focused on regulatory events beyond transcription, particularly in human studies. Therefore, the importance of each of these regulatory events in chronic adaptive responses remains presently unclear. In this regard, future studies examining multiple events in the adaptive process over the course of a training period would be beneficial. Relatedly, as our understanding of key molecular regulators involved in mitochondrial biogenesis advances and novel candidates continue to emerge, examination of multiple regulatory proteins (as opposed to single "nodal" regulators) using emerging "-omics" platforms should provide a greater understanding of the redundancies and crosstalk between pathways leading to mitochondrial biogenesis. Finally, as the optimal exercise prescription for maximizing training-induced increases in mitochondrial content remains to be established, comparison of multiple exercise variables (e.g., intensity, volume) within a single study is warranted. Importantly, quantitative assessments of mitochondrial remodelling should be coupled with qualitative markers of mitochondrial respiratory function to provide a more comprehensive understanding of the phenotypic changes that occur with training.

References

1. Akimoto T, Pohnert SC, Li P, Zhang M, Gumbs C, Rosenberg PB, et al. Exercise stimulates Pgc-1alpha transcription in skeletal muscle through activation of the p38 MAPK pathway. *J Biol Chem* 280: 19587–19593, 2005.
2. Baar K, Wende AR, Jones TE, Marison M, Nolte LA, Chen M, et al. Adaptations of skeletal muscle to exercise: rapid increase in the transcriptional coactivator PGC-1. *FASEB J* 16: 1879–1886, 2002.
3. Bartlett JD, Hwa Joo C, Jeong T-S, Louhelainen J, Cochran AJ, Gibala MJ, et al. Matched work high-intensity interval and continuous running induce similar increases in PGC-1α mRNA, AMPK, p38, and p53 phosphorylation in human skeletal muscle. *J Appl Physiol* 112: 1135–1143, 2012.
4. Bengtsson J, Gustafsson T, Widegren U, Jansson E, Sundberg C. Mitochondrial transcription factor A and respiratory complex IV increase in response to exercise training in humans. *Pflüg Arch* 443: 61–66, 2001.

5. Bergeron R, Ren JM, Cadman KS, Moore IK, Perret P, Pypaert M, et al. Chronic activation of AMP kinase results in NRF-1 activation and mitochondrial biogenesis. *Am J Physiol* 281: E1340–E1346, 2001.

6. Beyfuss K, Erlich AT, Triolo M, Hood DA. The role of p53 in determining mitochondrial adaptations to endurance training in skeletal muscle. *Sci Rep* 8: 14710, 2018.

7. Bishop DJ, Botella J, Granata C. CrossTalk opposing view: exercise training volume is more important than training intensity to promote increases in mitochondrial content. *J Physiol* 597: 4115–4118, 2019.

8. Bonafiglia JT, Edgett BA, Baechler BL, Nelms MW, Simpson CA, Quadrilatero J, et al. Acute upregulation of *PGC-1α* mRNA correlates with training-induced increases in SDH activity in human skeletal muscle. *Appl Physiol Nutr Metab* 42: 656–666, 2017.

9. Bonawitz ND, Clayton DA, Shadel GS. Initiation and beyond: multiple functions of the human mitochondrial transcription machinery. *Mol Cell* 24: 813–825, 2006.

10. Booth FW. Cytochrome c protein synthesis rate in rat skeletal muscle. *J Appl Physiol* 71: 1225–1230, 1991.

11. Boushel R, Gnaiger E, Calbet JAL, Gonzalez-Alonso J, Wright-Paradis C, Sondergaard H, et al. Muscle mitochondrial capacity exceeds maximal oxygen delivery in humans. *Mitochondrion* 11: 303–307, 2011.

12. Bylund AC, Bjurö T, Cederblad G, Holm J, Lundholm K, Sjöstroöm M, et al. Physical training in man. Skeletal muscle metabolism in relation to muscle morphology and running ability. *Eur J Appl Physiol* 36: 151–169, 1977.

13. Chen G, Carroll S, Racay P, Dick J, Pette D, Traub I, et al. Deficiency in parvalbumin increases fatigue resistance in fast-twitch muscle and upregulates mitochondria. *Am J Physiol* 281: C114–C122, 2001.

14. Cogswell AM, Stevens RJ, Hood DA. Properties of skeletal muscle mitochondria isolated from subsarcolemmal and intermyofibrillar regions. *Am J Physiol* 264: C383–C389, 1993.

15. Collu-Marchese M, Shuen M, Pauly M, Saleem A, Hood D. The regulation of mitochondrial transcription factor A (Tfam) expression during skeletal muscle cell differentiation. *Biosci Rep* 35: e00221.

16. Connor MK, Bezborodova O, Escobar CP, Hood DA. Effect of contractile activity on protein turnover in skeletal muscle mitochondrial subfractions. *J Appl Physiol* 88: 1601–1606, 2000.

17. Crilly MJ, Tryon LD, Erlich AT, Hood DA. The role of Nrf2 in skeletal muscle contractile and mitochondrial function. *J Appl Physiol* 121: 730–740, 2016.

18. Daussin FN, Zoll J, Dufour SP, Ponsot E, Lonsdorfer-Wolf E, Doutreleau S, et al. Effect of interval versus continuous training on cardiorespiratory and mitochondrial functions: relationship to aerobic performance improvements in sedentary subjects. *Am J Physiol* 295: R264–R272, 2008.

19. de Sousa Abreu R, Penalva LO, Marcotte EM, Vogel C. Global signatures of protein and mRNA expression levels. *Mol Biosyst* 5: 1512–1526, 2009.

20. Dent JR, Martins VF, Svensson K, LaBarge SA, Schlenk NC, Esparza MC, et al. Muscle-specific knockout of general control of amino acid synthesis 5 (GCN5) does not enhance basal or endurance exercise-induced mitochondrial adaptation. *Mol Metab* 6: 1574–1584, 2017.

21. Di Donato DM, West DWD, Churchward-Venne TA, Breen L, Baker SK, Phillips SM. Influence of aerobic exercise intensity on myofibrillar and mitochondrial protein synthesis in young men during early and late postexercise recovery. *Am J Physiol* 306: E1025–E1032, 2014.

22. Dudley GA, Tullson PC, Terjung RL. Influence of mitochondrial content on the sensitivity of respiratory control. *J Biol Chem* 262: 9109–9114, 1987.

23. Egan B, O'Connor PL, Zierath JR, O'Gorman DJ. Time course analysis reveals gene-specific transcript and protein kinetics of adaptation to short-term aerobic exercise training in human skeletal muscle. *PLoS ONE* 8: e74098, 2013.

24. Egan B, Zierath JR. Exercise metabolism and the molecular regulation of skeletal muscle adaptation. *Cell Metab* 17: 162–184, 2013.

25. Fan W, He N, Lin CS, Wei Z, Hah N, Waizenegger W, et al. ERRγ promotes angiogenesis, mitochondrial biogenesis, and oxidative remodeling in PGC1α/β-deficient muscle. *Cell Rep* 22: 2521–2529, 2018.

26. Freyssenet D, Berthon P, Denis C. Mitochondrial biogenesis in skeletal muscle in response to endurance exercises. *Arch Physiol Biochem* 104: 129–141, 1996.

27. Freyssenet D, Connor MK, Takahashi M, Hood DA. Cytochrome c transcriptional activation and mRNA stability during contractile activity in skeletal muscle. *Am J Physiol* 277: E26–E32, 1999.

28. Freyssenet D, Di Carlo M, Hood DA. Calcium-dependent regulation of cytochrome c gene expression in skeletal muscle cells. Identification of a protein kinase c-dependent pathway. *J Biol Chem* 274: 9305–9311, 1999.

29. Garcia-Roves PM, Huss J, Holloszy JO. Role of calcineurin in exercise-induced mitochondrial biogenesis. *Am J Physiol* 290: E1172–E1179, 2006.

30. Gerhart-Hines Z, Rodgers JT, Bare O, Lerin C, Kim S-H, Mostoslavsky R, et al. Metabolic control of muscle mitochondrial function and fatty acid oxidation through SIRT1/PGC-1alpha. *EMBO J* 26: 1913–1923, 2007.

31. Gillen JB, Martin BJ, MacInnis MJ, Skelly LE, Tarnopolsky MA, Gibala MJ. Twelve weeks of sprint interval training improves indices of cardiometabolic health similar to traditional endurance training despite a five-fold lower exercise volume and time commitment. *PLOS ONE* 11: e0154075, 2016.

32. Gleyzer N, Vercauteren K, Scarpulla RC. Control of mitochondrial transcription specificity factors (TFB1M and TFB2M) by nuclear respiratory factors (NRF-1 and NRF-2) and PGC-1 family coactivators. *Mol Cell Biol* 25: 1354–1366, 2005.

33. Gollnick PD, Armstrong RB, Saltin B, Saubert CW, Sembrowich WL, Shepherd RE. Effect of training on enzyme activity and fiber composition of human skeletal muscle. *J Appl Physiol* 34: 107–111, 1973.

34. Gordon JW, Rungi AA, Inagaki H, Hood DA. Effects of contractile activity on mitochondrial transcription factor A expression in skeletal muscle. *J Appl Physiol* 90: 389–396, 2001.

35. Gordon JW, Rungi AA, Inagaki H, Hood DA. Selected contribution: effects of contractile activity on mitochondrial transcription factor a expression in skeletal muscle. *J Appl Physiol* 90: 389–396, 2001.

36. Gowans GJ, Hawley SA, Ross FA, Hardie DG. AMP is a true physiological regulator of AMP-activated protein kinase by both allosteric activation and enhancing net phosphorylation. *Cell Metab* 18: 556–566, 2013.

37. Granata C, Jamnick NA, Bishop DJ. Training-induced changes in mitochondrial content and respiratory function in human skeletal muscle. *Sports Med* 48: 1809–1828, 2018.

38. Granata C, Jamnick NA, Bishop DJ. Principles of exercise prescription, and how they influence exercise-induced changes of transcription factors and other regulators of mitochondrial biogenesis. *Sports Med* 48: 1541–1559, 2018.

39. Granata C, Oliveira RSF, Little JP, Renner K, Bishop DJ. Training intensity modulates changes in PGC-1α and p53 protein content and mitochondrial respiration, but not markers of mitochondrial content in human skeletal muscle. *FASEB J* 30: 959–970, 2016.

40. Granata C, Oliveira RSF, Little JP, Renner K, Bishop DJ. Mitochondrial adaptations to high-volume exercise training are rapidly reversed after a reduction in training volume in human skeletal muscle. *FASEB J* 30: 3413–3423, 2016.

41. Granata C, Oliveira RSF, Little JP, Renner K, Bishop DJ. Sprint-interval but not continuous exercise increases PGC-1α protein content and p53 phosphorylation in nuclear fractions of human skeletal muscle. *Sci Rep* 7: 44227, 2017.

42. Gurd BJ. Deacetylation of PGC-1α by SIRT1: importance for skeletal muscle function and exercise-induced mitochondrial biogenesis. *Appl Physiol Nutr Metab* 36: 589–597, 2011.

43. Gurd BJ, Little JP, Perry CGR. Does SIRT1 determine exercise-induced skeletal muscle mitochondrial biogenesis: differences between in vitro and in vivo experiments?. *J Appl Physiol* 112: 926–928, 2012.

44. Gurd BJ, Yoshida Y, Lally J, Holloway GP, Bonen A. The deacetylase enzyme SIRT1 is not associated with oxidative capacity in rat heart and skeletal muscle and its overexpression reduces mitochondrial biogenesis. *J Physiol* 587: 1817–1828, 2009.

45. Gurd BJ, Yoshida Y, McFarlan JT, Holloway GP, Moyes CD, Heigenhauser GJF, et al. Nuclear SIRT1 activity, but not protein content, regulates mitochondrial biogenesis in rat and human skeletal muscle. *Am J Physiol* 301: R67–R75, 2011.

46. Handschin C, Rhee J, Lin J, Tarr PT, Spiegelman BM. An autoregulatory loop controls peroxisome proliferator-activated receptor coactivator 1 expression in muscle. *Proc Natl Acad Sci USA* 100: 7111–7116, 2003.

47. Henriksson J, Reitman JS. Time course of changes in human skeletal muscle succinate dehydrogenase and cytochrome oxidase activities and maximal oxygen uptake with physical activity and inactivity. *Acta Physiol Scand* 99: 91–97, 1977.

48. Holloszy JO. Biochemical adaptations in muscle. Effects of exercise on mitochondrial oxygen uptake and respiratory enzyme activity in skeletal muscle. *J Biol Chem* 242: 2278–2282, 1967.

49. Holloszy JO. Regulation by exercise of skeletal muscle content of mitochondria and GLUT4. *J Physiol Pharmacol* 59 Suppl 7: 5–18, 2008.

50. Holloszy JO, Coyle EF. Adaptations of skeletal muscle to endurance exercise and their metabolic consequences. *J Appl Physiol* 56: 831–838, 1984.

51. Hood DA. Invited Review: contractile activity-induced mitochondrial biogenesis in skeletal muscle. *J Appl Physiol* 90: 1137–1157, 2001.

52. Hood DA, Tryon LD, Carter HN, Kim Y, Chen CCW. Unravelling the mechanisms regulating muscle mitochondrial biogenesis. *Biochem J* 473: 2295–2314, 2016.

53. Hood DA, Zak R, Pette D. Chronic stimulation of rat skeletal muscle induces coordinate increases in mitochondrial and nuclear mRNAs of cytochrome-c-oxidase subunits. *Eur J Biochem* 179: 275–280, 1989.

54. Hoppeler H. Exercise-induced ultrastructural changes in skeletal muscle. *Int J Sports Med* 7: 187–204, 1986.

55. Hoppeler H, Howald H, Conley K, Lindstedt SL, Claassen H, Vock P, et al. Endurance training in humans: aerobic capacity and structure of skeletal muscle. *J Appl Physiol* 59: 320–327, 1985.

56. Hoppeler H, Lüthi P, Claassen H, Weibel ER, Howald H. The ultrastructure of the normal human skeletal muscle. A morphometric analysis on untrained men, women and well-trained orienteers. *Pflugers Arch* 344: 217–232, 1973.

57. Hurley BF, Nemeth PM, Martin WH, Hagberg JM, Dalsky GP, Holloszy JO. Muscle triglyceride utilization during exercise: effect of training. *J Appl Physiol* 60: 562–567, 1986.

58. Irrcher I, Ljubicic V, Kirwan AF, Hood DA. AMP-activated protein kinase-regulated activation of the PGC-1α promoter in skeletal muscle cells. *PLoS ONE* 3: e3614, 2008.

59. Islam H, Bonafiglia JT, Turnbull PC, Simpson CA, Perry CGR, Gurd BJ. The impact of acute and chronic exercise on Nrf2 expression in relation to markers of mitochondrial biogenesis in human skeletal muscle. *Eur J Appl Physiol* 120: 149–160, 2020.

60. Islam H, Edgett BA, Bonafiglia JT, Shulman T, Ma A, Quadrilatero J, et al. Repeatability of exercise-induced changes in mRNA expression and technical considerations for qPCR analysis in human skeletal muscle. *Exp Physiol* 104: 407–420, 2019.

61. Islam H, Edgett BA, Gurd BJ. Coordination of mitochondrial biogenesis by PGC-1α in human skeletal muscle: a re-evaluation. *Metabolism* 79: 42–51, 2018.

62. Islam H, Hood DA, Gurd BJ. Looking beyond PGC-1α: emerging regulators of exercise-induced skeletal muscle mitochondrial biogenesis and their activation by dietary compounds. *Appl Physiol Nutr Metab* 45: 11–23, 2020.

63. Jacobs RA, Flück D, Bonne TC, Bürgi S, Christensen PM, Toigo M, et al. Improvements in exercise performance with high-intensity interval training coincide with an increase in skeletal muscle mitochondrial content and function. *J Appl Physiol* 115: 785–793, 2013.

64. Jacobs RA, Lundby C. Mitochondria express enhanced quality as well as quantity in association with aerobic fitness across recreationally active individuals up to elite athletes. *J Appl Physiol* 114: 344–350, 2013.

65. Jäger S, Handschin C, St-Pierre J, Spiegelman BM. AMP-activated protein kinase (AMPK) action in skeletal muscle via direct phosphorylation of PGC-1alpha. *Proc Natl Acad Sci USA* 104: 12017–12022, 2007.

66. Jørgensen SB, Wojtaszewski JFP, Viollet B, Andreelli F, Birk JB, Hellsten Y, et al. Effects of alpha-AMPK knockout on exercise-induced gene activation in mouse skeletal muscle. *FASEB J* 19: 1146–1148, 2005.

67. Koh J-H, Hancock CR, Terada S, Higashida K, Holloszy JO, Han D-H. PPARβ is essential for maintaining normal levels of PGC-1α and mitochondria and for the increase in muscle mitochondria induced by exercise. *Cell Metab* 25: 1176–1185, 2017.

68. Lai RYJ, Ljubicic V, D'souza D, Hood DA. Effect of chronic contractile activity on mRNA stability in skeletal muscle. *Am J Physiol* 299: C155–C163, 2010.

69. Larsen S, Nielsen J, Hansen CN, Nielsen LB, Wibrand F, Stride N, et al. Biomarkers of mitochondrial content in skeletal muscle of healthy young human subjects. *J Physiol* 590: 3349–3360, 2012.

70. LeBlanc PJ, Howarth KR, Gibala MJ, Heigenhauser GJF. Effects of 7 wk of endurance training on human skeletal muscle metabolism during submaximal exercise. *J Appl Physiol* 97: 2148–2153, 2004.

71. Lira VA, Brown DL, Lira AK, Kavazis AN, Soltow QA, Zeanah EH, et al. Nitric oxide and AMPK cooperatively regulate PGC-1α in skeletal muscle cells: NO/AMPK-dependent regulation of PGC-1α. *J Physiol* 588: 3551–3566, 2010.

72. Liu Y, Beyer A, Aebersold R. On the dependency of cellular protein levels on mRNA abundance. *Cell* 165: 535–550, 2016.

73. MacInnis MJ, Gibala MJ. Physiological adaptations to interval training and the role of exercise intensity. *J Physiol* 595: 2915–2930, 2017.

74. MacInnis MJ, Skelly LE, Gibala MJ. CrossTalk proposal: exercise training intensity is more important than volume to promote increases in human skeletal muscle mitochondrial content. *J Physiol* 597: 4111–4113, 2019.

75. MacInnis MJ, Zacharewicz E, Martin BJ, Haikalis ME, Skelly LE, Tarnopolsky MA, et al. Superior mitochondrial adaptations in human skeletal muscle after interval compared to continuous single-leg cycling matched for total work: aerobic exercise intensity mediates skeletal muscle adaptations. *J Physiol* 595: 2955–2968, 2017.

76. Matoba S, Kang J-G, Patino WD, Wragg A, Boehm M, Gavrilova O, et al. p53 regulates mitochondrial respiration. *Science* 312: 1650–1653, 2006.

77. Menzies KJ, Singh K, Saleem A, Hood DA. Sirtuin 1-mediated effects of exercise and resveratrol on mitochondrial biogenesis. *J Biol Chem* 288: 6968–6979, 2013.

78. Merry TL, Ristow M. Nuclear factor erythroid-derived 2-like 2 (NFE2L2, Nrf2) mediates exercise-induced mitochondrial biogenesis and the anti-oxidant response in mice: NFE2L2 and mitochondrial biogenesis. *J Physiol* 594: 5195–5207, 2016.

79. Miller BF, Hamilton KL. A perspective on the determination of mitochondrial biogenesis. *Am J Physiol* 302: E496–E499, 2012.

80. Montero D, Cathomen A, Jacobs RA, Flück D, de Leur J, Keiser S, et al. Haematological rather than skeletal muscle adaptations contribute to the increase in peak oxygen uptake induced by moderate endurance training: central and peripheral adaptations to training affecting V̇O2 peak. *J Physiol* 593: 4677–4688, 2015.

81. Nagao A, Hino-Shigi N, Suzuki T. Measuring mRNA decay in human mitochondria. *Methods Enzymol* 447: 489–499, 2008.

82. Nisoli E, Clementi E, Paolucci C, Cozzi V, Tonello C, Sciorati C, et al. Mitochondrial biogenesis in mammals: the role of endogenous nitric oxide. *Science* 299: 896–899, 2003.

83. Nunnari J, Suomalainen A. Mitochondria: in sickness and in health. *Cell* 148: 1145–1159, 2012.

84. Ojuka EO, Jones TE, Han D-H, Chen M, Holloszy JO. Raising Ca2+ in L6 myotubes mimics effects of exercise on mitochondrial biogenesis in muscle. *FASEB J* 17: 675–681, 2003.

85. Park J-Y, Wang PY, Matsumoto T, Sung HJ, Ma W, Choi JW, et al. p53 improves aerobic exercise capacity and augments skeletal muscle mitochondrial DNA content. *Circ Res* 105: 705–712, 2009.

86. Paul MH, Sperling E. Cyclophorase system. XXIII. Correlation of cyclophorase activity and mitochondrial density in striated muscle. *Proc Soc Exp Biol Med* 79: 352–354, 1952.

87. Perry CGR, Hawley JA. Molecular basis of exercise-induced skeletal muscle mitochondrial biogenesis: historical advances, current knowledge, and future challenges. *Cold Spring Harb Perspect Med* 8: a029686, 2018.

88. Perry CGR, Heigenhauser GJF, Bonen A, Spriet LL. High-intensity aerobic interval training increases fat and carbohydrate metabolic capacities in human skeletal muscle. *Appl Physiol Nutr Metab* 33: 1112–1123, 2008.

89. Perry CGR, Lally J, Holloway GP, Heigenhauser GJF, Bonen A, Spriet LL. Repeated transient mRNA bursts precede increases in transcriptional and mitochondrial proteins during training in human skeletal muscle: molecular responses during mitochondrial biogenesis. *J Physiol* 588: 4795–4810, 2010.

90. Phillips SM, Green HJ, Tarnopolsky MA, Heigenhauser GJ, Grant SM. Progressive effect of endurance training on metabolic adaptations in working skeletal muscle. *Am J Physiol* 270: E265–272, 1996.

91. Philp A, Chen A, Lan D, Meyer GA, Murphy AN, Knapp AE, et al. Sirtuin 1 (SIRT1) deacetylase activity is not required for mitochondrial biogenesis or peroxisome proliferator-activated receptor-gamma coactivator-1alpha (PGC-1alpha) deacetylation following endurance exercise. *J Biol Chem* 286: 30561–30570, 2011.

92. Philp A, Schenk S. Unraveling the complexities of SIRT1-mediated mitochondrial regulation in skeletal muscle. *Exerc Sport Sci Rev* 41: 174–181, 2013.

93. Piantadosi CA, Carraway MS, Babiker A, Suliman HB. Heme oxygenase-1 regulates cardiac mitochondrial biogenesis via Nrf2-mediated transcriptional control of nuclear respiratory factor-1. *Circ Res* 103: 1232–1240, 2008.

94. Pilegaard H, Saltin B, Neufer PD. Exercise induces transient transcriptional activation of the PGC-1alpha gene in human skeletal muscle. *J Physiol* 546: 851–858, 2003.

95. Pogozelski AR, Geng T, Li P, Yin X, Lira VA, Zhang M, et al. p38gamma mitogen-activated protein kinase is a key regulator in skeletal muscle metabolic adaptation in mice. *PloS One* 4: e7934, 2009.

96. Powers SK, Talbert EE, Adhihetty PJ. Reactive oxygen and nitrogen species as intracellular signals in skeletal muscle. *J Physiol* 589: 2129–2138, 2011.

97. Puigserver P, Rhee J, Lin J, Wu Z, Yoon JC, Zhang CY, et al. Cytokine stimulation of energy expenditure through p38 MAP kinase activation of PPARgamma coactivator-1. *Mol Cell* 8: 971–982, 2001.

98. Puigserver P, Wu Z, Park CW, Graves R, Wright M, Spiegelman BM. A cold-inducible coactivator of nuclear receptors linked to adaptive thermogenesis. *Cell* 92: 829–839, 1998.

99. Puntschart A, Claassen H, Jostarndt K, Hoppeler H, Billeter R. mRNAs of enzymes involved in energy metabolism and mtDNA are increased in endurance-trained athletes. *Am J Physiol* 269: C619–C625, 1995.

100. Reznick RM, Shulman GI. The role of AMP-activated protein kinase in mitochondrial biogenesis: AMPK in mitochondrial biogenesis. *J Physiol* 574: 33–39, 2006.

101. Rhodes MA, Carraway MS, Piantadosi CA, Reynolds CM, Cherry AD, Wester TE, et al. Carbon monoxide, skeletal muscle oxidative stress, and mitochondrial biogenesis in humans. *Am J Physiol* 297: H392–H399, 2009.

102. Robinson MM, Dasari S, Konopka AR, Johnson ML, Manjunatha S, Esponda RR, et al. Enhanced protein translation underlies improved metabolic and physical adaptations to different exercise training modes in young and old humans. *Cell Metab* 25: 581–592, 2017.

103. Romijn JA, Coyle EF, Sidossis LS, Gastaldelli A, Horowitz JF, Endert E, et al. Regulation of endogenous fat and carbohydrate metabolism in relation to exercise intensity and duration. *Am J Physiol* 265: E380–391, 1993.

104. Rowe GC, El-Khoury R, Patten IS, Rustin P, Arany Z. PGC-1α is dispensable for exercise-induced mitochondrial biogenesis in skeletal muscle. *PLoS ONE* 7: e41817, 2012.

105. Ryan MT, Hoogenraad NJ. Mitochondrial-nuclear communications. *Annu Rev Biochem* 76: 701–722, 2007.

106. Saleem A, Adhihetty PJ, Hood DA. Role of p53 in mitochondrial biogenesis and apoptosis in skeletal muscle. *Physiol Genomics* 37: 58–66, 2009.

107. Saleem A, Carter HN, Hood DA. p53 is necessary for the adaptive changes in cellular milieu subsequent to an acute bout of endurance exercise. *Am J Physiol* 306: C241–C249, 2014.

108. Saleem A, Hood DA. Acute exercise induces tumour suppressor protein p53 translocation to the mitochondria and promotes a p53-Tfam-mitochondrial DNA complex in skeletal muscle: Exercise and mitochondrial p53. *J Physiol* 591: 3625–3636, 2013.

109. Scalzo RL, Peltonen GL, Binns SE, Shankaran M, Giordano GR, Hartley DA, et al. Greater muscle protein synthesis and mitochondrial biogenesis in males compared with females during sprint interval training. *FASEB J* 28: 2705–2714, 2014.

110. Scarpulla RC. Transcriptional paradigms in mammalian mitochondrial biogenesis and function. *Physiol Rev* 88: 611–638, 2008.

111. Schaeffer PJ, Wende AR, Magee CJ, Neilson JR, Leone TC, Chen F, et al. Calcineurin and calcium/calmodulin-dependent protein kinase activate distinct metabolic gene regulatory programs in cardiac muscle. *J Biol Chem* 279: 39593–39603, 2004.

112. Schuler M, Ali F, Chambon C, Duteil D, Bornert J-M, Tardivel A, et al. PGC1α expression is controlled in skeletal muscles by PPARβ, whose ablation results in fiber-type switching, obesity, and type 2 diabetes. *Cell Metab* 4: 407–414, 2006.

113. Smith AC, Robinson AJ. MitoMiner v3.1, an update on the mitochondrial proteomics database. *Nucleic Acids Res* 44: D1258–D1261, 2016.

114. Smith BK, Mukai K, Lally JS, Maher AC, Gurd BJ, Heigenhauser GJF, et al. AMP-activated protein kinase is required for exercise-induced peroxisome proliferator-activated receptor γ co-activator 1α translocation to subsarcolemmal mitochondria in skeletal muscle: Translocation of PGC-1α to mitochondria. *J Physiol* 591: 1551–1561, 2013.

115. Stocks B, Dent JR, Joanisse S, McCurdy CE, Philp A. Skeletal muscle fibre-specific knockout of p53 does not reduce mitochondrial content or enzyme activity. *Front Physiol* 8: 941, 2017.

116. Tachtsis B, Smiles WJ, Lane SC, Hawley JA, Camera DM. Acute endurance exercise induces nuclear p53 abundance in human skeletal muscle. *Front Physiol* 7: 144, 2016.

117. Takahashi M, Chesley A, Freyssenet D, Hood DA. Contractile activity-induced adaptations in the mitochondrial protein import system. *Am J Physiol* 274: C1380–1387, 1998.

118. Takahashi M, Hood DA. Protein import into subsarcolemmal and intermyofibrillar skeletal muscle mitochondria. Differential import regulation in distinct subcellular regions. *J Biol Chem* 271: 27285–27291, 1996.

119. Virbasius JV, Scarpulla RC. Activation of the human mitochondrial transcription factor A gene by nuclear respiratory factors: a potential regulatory link between nuclear and mitochondrial gene expression in organelle biogenesis. *Proc Natl Acad Sci USA* 91: 1309–1313, 1994.

120. Wadley GD, Choate J, McConell GK. NOS isoform-specific regulation of basal but not exercise-induced mitochondrial biogenesis in mouse skeletal muscle: Regulation of mitochondrial biogenesis by NOS. *J Physiol* 585: 253–262, 2007.

121. Wilkinson SB, Phillips SM, Atherton PJ, Patel R, Yarasheski KE, Tarnopolsky MA, et al. Differential effects of resistance and endurance exercise in the fed state on signalling molecule phosphorylation and protein synthesis in human muscle. *J Physiol* 586: 3701–3717, 2008.

122. Winder WW, Holmes BF, Rubink DS, Jensen EB, Chen M, Holloszy JO. Activation of AMP-activated protein kinase increases mitochondrial enzymes in skeletal muscle. *J Appl Physiol* 88: 2219–2226, 2000.

123. Wright DC, Geiger PC, Han D-H, Jones TE, Holloszy JO. Calcium induces increases in peroxisome proliferator-activated receptor gamma coactivator-1alpha and mitochondrial biogenesis by a pathway leading to p38 mitogen-activated protein kinase activation. *J Biol Chem* 282: 18793–18799, 2007.

124. Wright DC, Han D-H, Garcia-Roves PM, Geiger PC, Jones TE, Holloszy JO. Exercise-induced mitochondrial biogenesis begins before the increase in muscle PGC-1alpha expression. *J Biol Chem* 282: 194–199, 2007.

125. Wu H, Kanatous SB, Thurmond FA, Gallardo T, Isotani E, Bassel-Duby R, et al. Regulation of mitochondrial biogenesis in skeletal muscle by CaMK. *Science* 296: 349–352, 2002.

126. Wu Z, Puigserver P, Andersson U, Zhang C, Adelmant G, Mootha V, et al. Mechanisms controlling mitochondrial biogenesis and respiration through the thermogenic coactivator PGC-1. *Cell* 98: 115–124, 1999.

127. Zhang Y, Uguccioni G, Ljubicic V, Irrcher I, Iqbal S, Singh K, et al. Multiple signaling pathways regulate contractile activity-mediated PGC-1α gene expression and activity in skeletal muscle cells. *Physiol Rep* 2, 2014.

128. Zoll J, Sanchez H, N'Guessan B, Ribera F, Lampert E, Bigard X, et al. Physical activity changes the regulation of mitochondrial respiration in human skeletal muscle. *J Physiol* 543: 191–200, 2002.

10

RESISTANCE EXERCISE TRAINING AND THE REGULATION OF MUSCLE PROTEIN SYNTHESIS

Nathan Hodson, Daniel R. Moore, and Chris McGlory

Introduction

Skeletal muscle is a highly plastic tissue demonstrating immense capacity to increase and decrease in mass and size in response to a variety of environmental stimuli (114). Skeletal muscle mass and quality are influenced by its rate of "turnover" governed by the intricate balance of two concurrent physiological processes: the breakdown of old/damaged proteins (muscle protein breakdown [MPB]) and the re-synthesis of new functional proteins (muscle protein synthesis [MPS]) (13). In times when MPS exceeds MPB, such as following a protein-rich meal, net protein balance (NPB) is positive and muscle proteins are accrued. Conversely, when MPB exceeds MPS, such as in the absence of dietary amino acids (AA) (i.e., postabsorptive state), NPB will be negative with a resultant loss of muscle proteins. In situations of stable lean body mass, these periods of muscle protein accretion and loss are equal across a 24-hour period and therefore skeletal muscle mass remains constant (9). However, maintaining a high rate of "turnover" even in the absence of changes in total skeletal muscle mass is important to ensure optimal skeletal muscle function. Notwithstanding the technical challenges of measuring MPB, in healthy humans, MPS is generally the more physiologically responsive variable (73) and has a greater impact on skeletal muscle mass regulation than MPB, resulting in the majority of research focusing on how diet and exercise regulate this arm of the NPB equation. The aim of this chapter is to discuss and critically evaluate current knowledge regarding how resistance exercise regulates rates of MPS and skeletal muscle mass, as well as the underpinning cellular and molecular mechanisms.

Modifiable Resistance Training Factors and Their Effects on MPS

Resistance exercise is a potent stimulator of MPS which in turn imparts a robust anabolic influence towards skeletal muscle. Indeed, in young healthy men a single bout of resistance exercise will result in increased rates of MPS that remain elevated even at 48 hours post-exercise, whilst rates of MPB are returned to baseline at 48 hours (74). The consumption of protein/AAs also results in increased rates of MPS, but this increase in response to protein feeding is far more transient than those observed following exercise as it returns to baseline ~3 hours following intake (64). However, the ingestion of dietary protein (or the essential AAs) is vital to maximize the exercise-induced stimulation of MPS during recovery, with ~0.3 g/kg representing a saturating single acute dose of intact high-quality protein (60). Over time, the repeated stimulation of MPS by resistance exercise with concomitant protein ingestion (up to ~1.6 g/kg/d) ultimately translates to training-induced increases in muscle and fat-free mass (66). Whilst these acute studies (60, 62, 74) have provided important information for the field, it is important to acknowledge that the acute (i.e., <6 hour) rise in rates of MPS following resistance exercise and feeding do not necessarily quantitatively predict the gains in skeletal muscle mass seen with chronic (weeks to months) resistance exercise training (57). The reason underlying this phenomenon is multifaceted and can be related to the training status of participants, extraneous environmental influences experienced in a free-living setting, and the relative contribution of MPS to remodelling vs. growth, which is particularly apparent during the early phase of training (21). Nevertheless, what these studies do provide is a qualitative readout as to the potential effectiveness, or "proof of principle" of a given intervention to promote muscle anabolism. They also enable key mechanistic insight regarding the cellular and molecular factors that regulate translational control and rates of MPS.

Resistance Exercise Load

Classically, it has been proposed that in order to induce skeletal muscle hypertrophy, the repetition load lifted during each set of resistance exercise should be ~70–80% of maximal strength (one repetition maximum [1RM]) for ~8–12 repetitions (122). As changes in rates of myofibrillar (contractile fraction of skeletal muscle) protein synthesis (MyoPS) following exercise training are thought to underpin the hypertrophic response, it would be logical to assume that these loads would also elicit the greatest effect on MyoPS. This thesis was ostensibly supported by Kumar et al. (49), who demonstrated using work-matched exercise conditions (15–75% 1RM) that a plateau MyoPS response over 4 hours of post-exercise recovery occurred at 60% 1RM in both young and older males, which agrees with the recommendations of the American College of Sports Medicine (122). However, it is now known that similar post-exercise rates of MPS can be achieved with both high and low repetition loads, provided exercise is completed to volitional failure. For instance, Burd et al. (14) demonstrated that lifting either 30% 1RM or 90% 1RM to volitional failure elicited similar elevations in mixed MPS and MyoPS in early (4 hours) and later (24 hours) windows of post-exercise recovery. Importantly, these acute MPS data qualitatively predicted chronic adaptations, as a follow-up study demonstrated that 10 weeks of resistance exercise training with low loads (~30% 1RM) to volitional failure elicited similar hypertrophic gains (58) as heavier loads (~80% 1RM). Therefore, resistance exercise load only seems to determine acute MPS responses and the subsequent hypertrophic response if resistance exercise is not completed to volitional failure. The primary mechanism underlying this effect is that performing resistance exercise to volitional failure will induce the recruitment of fast-twitch type II fibres and subsequent stimulation of translational processes irrespective of load lifted (68). This is analogous to the observation that light load blood-flow restricted exercise, which enhances muscle fibre recruitment secondary to an accelerated local metabolic fatigue, elicits a robust post-exercise stimulation of mixed MPS (30) and muscle hypertrophy (103).

Resistance Exercise Volume

Another factor that affects the MyoPS response to resistance exercise is the volume of mechanical work completed. Resistance exercise volume is typically more difficult to isolate from other variables, as it may be influenced by both repetitions per set and/or sets per exercise (14). To investigate the impact of exercise volume, Burd et al. (12) utilized a unique within-participant study design whereby one leg completed one set of resistance exercise whilst the contralateral leg completed three sets of resistance exercise at 70% 1RM to volitional fatigue in order to induce a ~2.3-fold difference in total exercise volume. While both resistance exercise regimens enhanced MyoPS in the fed state (i.e., 25 g of protein) over 5 hours post-exercise, three sets elicited a ~30% greater stimulation of MyoPS that persisted for up to 24 hours (12). Although not directly assessing the effect of resistance exercise volume, several other studies that report differences in volume between groups (albeit also with other exercise variables being altered) have nonetheless shown elevated MyoPS responses in the cohorts who completed greater work volume (14, 54). These acute studies complement the findings of others who have identified a dose-response relationship between exercise volume and gains in skeletal muscle mass (94), but not strength (93), during a period of resistance exercise training that appears to plateau at ~10 weekly sets per muscle group. There is evidence that more experienced resistance exercisers demonstrate reduced relative gains in skeletal muscle size with exercise training, suggesting that there are diminishing returns and even a plateau in muscle hypertrophy with higher volumes of training (71).

Contraction Mode

Skeletal muscle can generate greater force (and thus mechanical strain) during lengthening contractions as compared to shortening contractions. As muscle strain and/or "damage" (e.g., sarcomere "popping") have been suggested as important stimuli for muscle remodelling and growth, it has been postulated that the type of muscle contraction may influence MPS and the hypertrophic response to resistance exercise training (82). Phillips et al. (74) first demonstrated that there was no difference in the stimulation of mixed MPS up to 48 hours after submaximal, work-matched shortening and lengthening contractions. Furthermore, other studies have corroborated this finding with similar elevations in MyoPS (18, 28) with either contraction modality. However, because lengthening contractions can generate greater force than shortening contractions, matching total repetitions at submaximal loads would result in less muscle fibre recruitment for lengthening contractions, whereas matching total effort (e.g., maximal contractions) and repetitions would result in greater total work. When both exercise intensity and total work are equivalent, maximal lengthening contractions may induce a more rapid rise (i.e., over 4.5 hours) in MyoPS than shortening contractions (63). Although these acute MyoPS differences did not translate into statistically greater increases in muscle hypertrophy over 8 weeks in lengthening compared to shortening contractions, there was a moderate effect in favour of the former (65). This qualitative difference would generally align with meta-analytical data that suggest lengthening contractions may have a small benefit to enhancing resistance exercise–induced gains in skeletal muscle mass (95). However, this small effect did not reach statistical significance, highlighting both shortening and lengthening contractions can stimulate MyoPS and enhance muscle hypertrophy with resistance exercise training (95).

Sex Differences in MPS and Hypertrophic Responses to Resistance Exercise

Across all age ranges, men generally present with larger muscle mass and strength in an absolute sense compared to women (51). However, the force produced relative to muscle cross-sectional area (55) and the relative hypertrophic response to resistance exercise training (17, 117) are similar between young men and women. Although older women exhibit higher basal rates of MPS and a reduced MPS response to feeding (99), sexual dimorphism in MPS in younger individuals has not been observed (112). Given that men possess greater circulating concentrations of testosterone compared to women, the fact that younger women exhibit a similar hypertrophic response to resistance exercise training compared to younger men is perplexing. Importantly, in contrast to the provision of exogenous supraphysiological doses, it is known that in adult humans, exercise-induced changes in the concentration of so-called anabolic hormones (i.e., testosterone, growth hormone, insulin-like growth factor-1) play little to no role in mediating either the acute MyoPS response to a single bout of resistance exercise (112) or skeletal muscle hypertrophy following exercise training (67). Moreover, in women it has been shown that there is no effect of menstrual phase on rates of MyoPS after single-leg resistance exercise (56). Taken together, these studies (56, 112) suggest that there is little, if any, sex-specific differences in anabolic response of skeletal muscle to resistance exercise training in young adults.

Heterogeneity of Response to Resistance Exercise: Responders vs. Non-Responders

The increase in skeletal muscle mass with resistance exercise training is typically presented as an average response, which belies the substantial heterogeneity of responses that is characteristic of nonhomogeneous populations. For example, Hubal et al. (45) studied the effects of 12 weeks of progressive resistance training of the biceps brachii in a large cohort of individuals ($n = 585$) and reported that changes in muscle strength ranged from 0% to 250% and changes in muscle volume, measured via magnetic resonance imaging, varied from −2% to +59%. This typical training variation is also evidenced in acute studies. For example, Mitchell et al. (57) observed that MyoPS responses to a single bout of resistance exercise in 23 healthy untrained men at the same relative intensity varied between 0.02%/hour and 0.11%/hour at 1–3 hours post-exercise and 0.01%/hour and 0.10%/hour at 3–6 hours post-exercise. This high level of interindividual variability to a single bout of exercise suggests other factors may be implicated in the stimulation of MyoPS. These data therefore imply that a "one size fits all" approach to resistance exercise, both acutely and chronically, may not maximize skeletal muscle adaptations on an individual basis, although recent evidence suggests systematically manipulating resistance exercise variables on an individual basis also leads to high variation in hypertrophic responses (20). Interestingly, it seems that acute (≤5 hours) MyoPS responses to a single bout of resistance exercise do not correlate with gains in muscle mass as a result of prolonged resistance training (57). This suggests that not only is there large interindividual variations in responses to acute resistance exercise but within-subject adaptations are also highly variable. The exact mechanisms underlying the heterogeneity in the response of skeletal muscle to resistance exercise remain largely unknown, with genetic and environmental factors believed to confer significant influence. However, what is known is that key molecular factors within skeletal muscle are activated following resistance exercise and protein feeding, which initiate translational control and an increase in rates of MPS.

Mechanistic Regulation of MPS

The coordination of MPS involves the translation of a strand of messenger ribonucleic acid (mRNA) into a fully functioning protein by ribosomes within a muscle cell (41). This process begins in the nucleus, where a strand of mRNA corresponding to the gene to be expressed is produced from deoxyribonucleic acid (DNA) by RNA polymerases. This strand is then exported from the nucleus into the cytosol where various translation initiation factors bind and recruit ribosomal subunits (32). Once the full ribosome has been assembled around a strand of mRNA, the process of translation begins, whereby transfer RNA (tRNA) structures, bound to an AA, are recruited to the ribosome. Here, a peptide bond is formed between the carboxyl group of one AA and the amino group of the next (6, 41). This process is continued as the ribosome moves along the length of the mRNA strand until it reaches a stop codon (29). At this point, the newly formed peptide chain is released from the ribosome and undergoes various folding steps until it reaches its final, functional form (24). A schematic depicting the basic molecular mechanisms governing MPS can be seen in Figure 10.1.

mTORC1-Dependent Mechanisms

Originally, at the molecular level, MPS was believed to be entirely governed by the activity of one kinase complex, the mechanistic target of rapamycin complex 1 (mTORC1). This belief was founded upon pioneering research utilizing the mTORC1 inhibitor rapamycin, which blocked muscle contraction- and pharmacological-induced hypertrophy in rodents (8). This seminal work subsequently also has support in humans, whereby rapamycin ablated increases in MPS following resistance exercise or essential AA ingestion (23, 26). The main component of mTORC1 is the evolutionarily conserved serine/threonine kinase mTOR, which catalyzes the phosphorylation of mTORC1's downstream targets. In addition to mTOR, mTORC1 is composed of several regulatory proteins: regulatory-associated protein

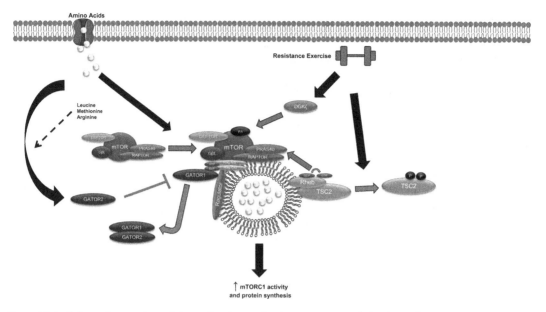

Figure 10.1 Schematic overview of the molecular mechanisms governing skeletal muscle protein synthesis

of mTOR (RAPTOR), proline-rich AKT substrate of 40kDa (PRAS40), DEP domain–containing mTOR-interacting protein (DEPTOR), and mammalian lethal with SEC13 protein 8/G protein beta subunit-like (mLST8/GβL), each of which is essential for the proper functionality of the kinase complex (35, 48, 88, 121). This kinase complex becomes activated when associated with the lysosome (46, 86), an organelle both rich in AAs and a direct activator of mTORC1, Rheb, and phosphatidic acid (PA) (47, 118). Interestingly, both AA ingestion and resistance exercise seem to activate mTORC1 by differential mechanisms, thereby explaining the potential synergy of these two anabolic stimuli on mTORC1 activity and subsequent MPS (7, 43). Following AA ingestion (or increased AA availability), mTORC1 is believed to be recruited to the lysosomal membrane through an interaction between Rag proteins and the mTORC1 subunit RAPTOR (87). This then places mTORC1 in close proximity to both AAs and Rheb/PA. Further research has also suggested that several individual AAs, namely leucine, arginine, and methionine, further mediate this process through the release of the inhibition of GATOR2, allowing this protein complex to inhibit GATOR1 and activate Rag proteins to recruit mTORC1 (15, 34, 115). Conversely, resistance exercise (or mechanical strain) seems to mediate mTORC1 activation through its direct activators Rheb and PA. In the basal state, Rheb is bound to tuberous sclerosis complex 2 (TSC2), which maintains Rheb in its inactive GDP-bound state (52). In response to contraction, TSC2 becomes phosphorylated and disassociates from Rheb, allowing Rheb to become active (GTP-bound) (47). In this state, Rheb can bind directly to the catalytic domain of mTORC1 and elevate its kinase capabilities (52). The production of PA is also elevated in response to contraction, as mechanical stimuli have been observed to elevate the activity of diacylglycerol kinase ζ, an enzyme which produces PA from the phosphorylation of diacylglycerol (119). This elevation in the content of PA seems to occur close to the lysosome, thereby placing PA in close proximity to bind to the FRB domain of mTOR and further enhance its kinase activity (119). Recent research has also proposed a new mechanism of mTORC1 activation in human skeletal muscle. Here, anabolic stimuli (resistance exercise and/or AA feeding) elicits the translocation of mTORC1-lysosomal complexes toward the cell periphery where they are closer to blood vessels, AA transporters, translation initiation factors, and a second pool of Rheb (42–44, 101). This research niche, however, is still in its infancy, and further research is therefore required to fully elucidate the true role of this novel mechanism.

The most well-characterized substrate of mTORC1 implicated in translational regulation is ribosomal protein S6 kinase 1 (S6K1) (3). Upon activation mTORC1 will phosphorylate S6K1 at threonine residue 389, resulting in an elevation of S6K1 kinase activity (39). This enhanced kinase activity of S6K1 then allows S6K1 to phosphorylate its own downstream targets, most of which are implicated in the regulation of MPS. The first target of S6K1 is ribosomal protein subunit 6 (rpS6), which is phosphorylated at either Ser235/236 or Ser240/244 by S6K1 (39, 85). This phosphorylation event was initially believed to regulate the translation of 5'TOP mRNA strands, as the two processes were closely correlated (105); however, this is now under some debate (97, 104). S6K1 is also able to phosphorylate eukaryotic initiation factor 4B (eIF4B), a component of the translation pre-initiation complex (39, 79). The role of this post-translational modification is more widely accepted, allowing eIF4B to associate with the other components of the pre-initiation complex and activate the helicase activity of eIF4A (32). At this point the translation of mRNA strands that have a secondary/helix–like structure will be elevated (32). Another downstream target of S6K1 is eukaryotic elongation factor 2 (eEF2) kinase (eEF2K), which unlike the other targets of S6K1, is inhibited following phosphorylation (11, 80, 81). This inhibition then causes a reduction in the phosphorylation of eEF2K's downstream target, eEF2, which in turn elevates translation elongation (i.e., the rate at which the ribosome travels along an mRNA strand (80, 81).

A second direct target of mTORC1 is eukaryotic translation initiation factor 4E-binding protein 1 (4EBP1), which is inhibited by mTORC1-dependent phosphorylation (31). Upon inhibition, 4EBP1 is removed from its association with eukaryotic initiation factor 4E (eIF4E), a further translation initiation factor that binds to the 5' cap of mRNA strands to recruit the pre-initiation complex to this area to begin translation (39, 40). The removal of 4EBP1 from eIF4E reveals the binding site for the pre-initiation complex and thereby elevates the rate at which translation of a particular mRNA strand can begin (40). mTORC1 is also able to phosphorylate the component of the translation pre-initiation complex, which associates with eIF4E, eukaryotic initiation factor 4G (eIF4G) (78). This initiation factor is phosphorylated at three different residues by mTORC1, and these post-translational modifications are suggested to induce conformational changes in this protein, which allow for more efficient assembly of the pre-initiation complex (78, 100). A final target of mTORC1 is protein phosphatase 2A (PP2A) whose predominant action is to remove phosphate groups from proteins (2). mTORC1-dependent phosphorylation of this phosphatase reduces its activity, resulting in a reduction in the rate that phosphate molecules are removed from other downstream targets of mTORC1 (72, 116). Therefore, through this mechanism mTORC1 is also able to indirectly affect protein translation by reducing the inhibition of the process by PP2A (72). Thus, overall, mTORC1-dependent mechanisms can control several aspects of MPS, including translation initiation and elongation. A schematic depicting the mechanisms governing AA and resistance exercise–induced rates of MPS can be seen in Figure 10.2.

mTORC1-Independent Mechanisms

Although initially it was believed that MPS could be entirely regulated through an mTORC1-dependent mechanism, recent research predominantly in rodent skeletal muscle has suggested MPS can still be elevated in response to anabolic stimuli in the presence of mTORC1 inhibitors (70, 111). Therefore, it has now been postulated that several mTORC1-independent mechanisms may be implicated in the regulation of protein synthesis, the majority of which appear to be coordinated through the mitogen-activated protein kinase/extracellular signal–regulated kinases 1/2 (MAPK/ERK1/2) pathway (22). In contrast to mTORC1-dependent mechanisms, which are sensitive to both mechanical and nutrient stimuli (59, 61, 109), this pathway seems to be predominantly mechanically regulated in human skeletal muscle (61). This intricate signalling pathway is initiated at the cell membrane via the binding of a ligand to its receptor or via the activation of focal adhesion kinase or integrins by mechanical stimuli (89, 91). Following this, several phosphorylation events occur, leading to the activation of ERK1/2 (50, 83, 96), a kinase which has several substrates implicated in the control of protein synthesis.

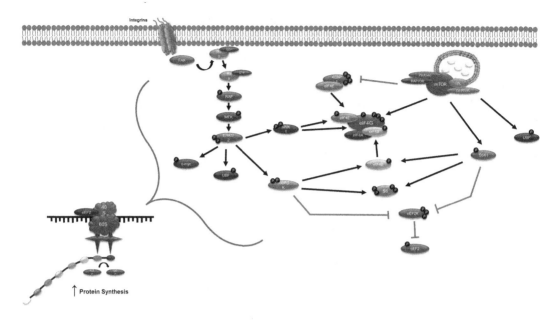

Figure 10.2 A schematic depicting the mechanisms governing amino acid and resistance exercise–induced rates of muscle protein synthesis (MPS)

This first of these substrates is p90 ribosomal protein S6 kinase (p90RSK), which shares a similar set of substrates to that of S6K1. Upon activation by ERK1/2, p90RSK will phosphorylate these downstream substrates (i.e., rpS6, eIF4B and eEF2K), eliciting elevations in the rates of translation initiation and elongation (19). Interestingly, however, the use of the mTORC1 inhibitor rapamycin, in vitro or in rodent skeletal muscle, completely ablates phosphorylation of these substrates (76, 84, 111, 120), suggesting that mTORC1-dependent mechanisms are the predominant regulators of these post-translational modifications. Findings in human skeletal muscle are more equivocal, with rapamycin administration seemingly having less of an effect on the phosphorylation of these substrates following resistance exercise (26). As such, more research is likely needed to understand the true effects of p90RSK activity on MPS in human skeletal muscle.

A second substrate of ERK1/2 is MAP kinase-interacting kinase 1 (MNK1), which is also phosphorylated and activated by p38MAPK (110). Once activated, this kinase will bind to and phosphorylate eIF4G (77, 98), a component of the translation pre-initiation complex. This phosphorylation event serves to stabilize the association between MNK1 and eIF4G (25, 107), allowing MNK1 to phosphorylate a second component of the pre-initiation complex eIF4E at serine residue 209 (77). Phosphorylation at this site is associated with elevated protein synthesis; however, its precise role in the process has yet to be determined (39). Interestingly, this mechanism of mTORC1-independent stimulation of MPS may actually rely on mTORC1 activation. When mTORC1 activity is low, eIF4E is bound to 4EBP1, which prevents its interaction with eIF4G and the pre-initiation complex. Therefore, it is possible that mTORC1 activity must be high to remove 4EBP1 from eIF4E in order for MNK1 to exhibit its full effects on eIF4E (31).

Ribosomal Biogenesis

Broadly speaking, the processes underlying an increase in rates of MPS at the molecular level can be separated into two processes: that of *translational efficiency* and *translational capacity*. Translational efficiency refers to the amount of protein yield per unit of mRNA/ribosome, whereas translational capacity typically means the amount of translational machinery (i.e., mRNA/ribosome abundance) available to build more muscle protein (27). In the previous section we primarily focused on how resistance exercise and AA feeding affect signalling events that regulate translational efficiency. However, there is recent evidence that translational capacity also may play a crucial role in resistance exercise–induced hypertrophy (27, 36).

Ribosomes are organelles which act to produce peptide chains corresponding to an mRNA strand, and therefore an increase in their content or capacity would elevate the rates at which new muscle proteins could be produced. The two predominant ways this may occur are through (1) an increase in the number of ribosomes bound to a single mRNA strand, that is, upon full activation the distance between ribosomes on an mRNA strand can shorten from ~90 to ~30 nucleotides (106) and (2) an elevated total content of ribosomes, both of which increase the protein yield per strand of mRNA. Mechanistically, ribosomal biogenesis is regulated by a series of transcription factors which act to elevate the rates at which ribosomal RNA (rRNA) and mRNA corresponding to ribosomal proteins are transcribed (106). One such transcription factor is c-myc which regulates both rRNA and ribosomal protein mRNA expression (33, 92). Overexpression of this transcription factor elevates rRNA levels and ribosomal protein content (92), whereas its inhibition elicits reductions in such parameters (33). Research regarding the upstream regulation of this transcription factor is slightly contentious, with data suggesting both mTORC1-dependent (53) and -independent (5) post-translational modifications. Nevertheless, this mechanism is implicated in the regulation of ribosomal biogenesis and is reported to be sensitive to contraction, albeit in rodent skeletal muscle (111).

A second transcription factor which is implicated in the control of ribosomal biogenesis is upstream binding factor (UBF) (37), which works alongside RNA polymerase transcription factor I (SL1) to regulate the synthesis of new rRNA (4). The depletion of this transcription factor causes silencing of several ribosomal-associated genes (90); however, this did not affect overall rRNA synthesis rates. Conversely, overexpression of UBF elevates rates of rDNA transcription, suggesting an important role for this transcription factor in ribosomal adaptations (38). At the post-translation level UBF activity can be regulated by several phosphorylation events. Phosphorylation at serine residue 388 is reported to be needed for UBF to interact with RNA polymerases and increases transcription of rDNA (108), and a similar observation has been made regarding phosphorylation at Ser484 (108). Interestingly, mTORC1 activity seemingly can regulate rDNA transcription rates through UBF phosphorylation; however, this post-translational modification occurs between AAs 675 and 765 on the UBF peptide chain (37). In rodent muscle, one phosphorylation site (Ser637) on UBF is rapamycin-sensitive following muscle contractions (111), and as this AA residue is located close to the region which affects UBF activity in an mTORC1-dependent manner, this may provide a mechanism whereby mTORC1 regulates ribosomal biogenesis. Moreover, in the same study, UBF[Ser388] phosphorylation was rapamycin-insensitive, suggesting both mTORC1-dependent and -independent mechanisms can regulate this transcription factor, and thereby rDNA transcription (111).

To date, the majority of research focused on elucidating the molecular mechanisms governing resistance exercise and feeding-induced changes in MPS and hypertrophy have centred on factors that affect translational efficiency. However, there is now a growing body of research showing that translational capacity (i.e., ribosomal biogenesis) may also play a fundamental role in mediating the hypertrophic response to resistance exercise training [reviewed by (27)]. Indeed, initial reports from rodents demonstrated robust increases in various readouts of ribosomal biogenesis concomitant with marked skeletal muscle hypertrophy following synergist ablation (1, 27, 69). Recent data in humans have also shown that increases in markers of ribosomal biogenesis are highly correlated with resistance exercise training–induced muscle hypertrophy in both younger (36) and older (102) adults. It is important to acknowledge that in many instances changes in static readouts of ribosomal biogenesis (e.g., total RNA, immunoblotting of ribosomal proteins) are used as a surrogate of ribosomal biogenesis as opposed to a direct measurement of ribosomal biogenesis per se. However, application of novel tracer approaches using deuterated water to directly quantify RNA turnover (10) in combination with assessment of changes in ribosomal protein contents, as described in this chapter, will no doubt significantly enhance existing knowledge in this field.

Summary

In summary, resistance exercise represents a robust non-pharmacological means to enhance rates of MyoPS/MPS and skeletal muscle hypertrophy. Whilst the minutiae of resistance exercise prescription, such as the manipulation of repetition load and contraction mode, have received significant experimental attention, for the general population performing sufficient resistance exercise volume is often the primary barrier to maximizing gains in skeletal muscle mass with resistance exercise training (16, 75). However, it is known that there is large heterogeneity in the response of skeletal muscle size to resistance exercise training between individuals, even with high-volume resistance exercise training. In this regard, future work that aims to reveal the underlying mechanisms responsible for this "responder/non-responder" phenomenon would provide important information for the field. Although it is important to note that when examining a range of outcomes (i.e., changes in lean body mass, strength, and size), it is known that individuals will exhibit a positive adaptive response to resistance exercise training in at least one of these variables (16). Thus, from a public health standpoint, engagement in resistance exercise should be encouraged with the confidence that at the very least one aspect of musculoskeletal health will be improved (75). Additionally, recent evidence in rodents has challenged the long-established thesis that resistance exercise–induced gains in skeletal muscle mass are mTORC1-dependent. Future work using novel technologies such as phosphoproteomics and transcriptomics in humans will no doubt help elucidate novel molecular signals that regulate contraction-mediated up-regulation of translational control and rates of MPS (in all fractions of skeletal muscle) (113). Such information would not only assist with the design of post-exercise nutritional interventions aimed at maximizing muscle mass but also the development of targeted pharmacological interventions to combat musculoskeletal disease.

References

1. Adams GR, Haddad F, Baldwin KM. Time course of changes in markers of myogenesis in overloaded rat skeletal muscles. *J Appl Physiol* 87: 1705–1712, 1999.
2. Andjelkovic N, Zolnierowicz S, Van Hoof C, Goris J, Hemmings BA. The catalytic subunit of protein phosphatase 2A associates with the translation termination factor eRF1. *EMBO J* 15: 7156–7167, 1996.
3. Baar K, Esser K. Phosphorylation of p70(S6k) correlates with increased skeletal muscle mass following resistance exercise. *Am J Physiol* 276: C120–C127, 1999.
4. Bell SP, Learned RM, Jantzen HM, Tjian R. Functional cooperativity between transcription factors UBF1 and SL1 mediates human ribosomal RNA synthesis. *Science* 241: 1192–1197, 1988.
5. Benassi B, Fanciulli M, Fiorentino F, Porrello A, Chiorino G, Loda M, et al. c-Myc phosphorylation is required for cellular response to oxidative stress. *Mol Cell* 21: 509–519, 2006.
6. Berg J, Tymoczko J, Stryer L. *Biochemistry* (5th Edition). New York: W H Freeman.
7. Biolo G, Tipton KD, Klein S, Wolfe RR. An abundant supply of amino acids enhances the metabolic effect of exercise on muscle protein. *Am J Physiol* 273: E122–E129, 1997.
8. Bodine SC, Stitt TN, Gonzalez M, Kline WO, Stover GL, Bauerlein R, et al. Akt/mTOR pathway is a crucial regulator of skeletal muscle hypertrophy and can prevent muscle atrophy in vivo. *Nat Cell Biol* 3: 1014–1019, 2001.
9. Breen L, Phillips SM. Interactions between exercise and nutrition to prevent muscle waste during ageing. *Br J Clin Pharmacol* 75: 708–715, 2013.
10. Brook MS, Wilkinson DJ, Mitchell WK, Lund JL, Phillips BE, Szewczyk NJ, et al. A novel D2O tracer method to quantify RNA turnover as a biomarker of de novo ribosomal biogenesis, in vitro, in animal models, and in human skeletal muscle. *Am J Physiol* 313: E681–E689, 2017.
11. Browne GJ, Proud CG. A novel mTOR-regulated phosphorylation site in elongation factor 2 kinase modulates the activity of the kinase and its binding to calmodulin. *Mol Cell Biol* 24: 2986–2997, 2004.

12. Burd NA, Holwerda AM, Selby KC, West DWD, Staples AW, Cain NE, et al. Resistance exercise volume affects myofibrillar protein synthesis and anabolic signalling molecule phosphorylation in young men. *J Physiol* 588: 3119–3130, 2010.

13. Burd NA, Tang JE, Moore DR, Phillips SM. Exercise training and protein metabolism: influences of contraction, protein intake, and sex-based differences. *J Appl Physiol* 106: 1692–1701, 2009.

14. Burd NA, West DW, Staples AW, Atherton PJ, Baker JM, Moore DR, et al. Low-load high volume resistance exercise stimulates muscle protein synthesis more than high-load low volume resistance exercise in young men. *PLOS ONE* 5: e12033, 2010.

15. Chantranupong L, Scaria SM, Saxton RA, Gygi MP, Shen K, Wyant GA, et al. The CASTOR proteins are arginine sensors for the mTORC1 pathway. *Cell* 165: 153–164, 2016.

16. Churchward-Venne TA, Tieland M, Verdijk LB, Leenders M, Dirks ML, de Groot LCPGM, et al. There are no nonresponders to resistance-type exercise training in older men and women. *J Am Med Dir Assoc* 16: 400–411, 2015.

17. Cureton KJ, Collins MA, Hill DW, McElhannon FMJ. Muscle hypertrophy in men and women. *Med Sci Sports Exerc* 20: 338–344, 1988.

18. Cuthbertson DJ, Babraj J, Smith K, Wilkes E, Fedele MJ, Esser K, et al. Anabolic signaling and protein synthesis in human skeletal muscle after dynamic shortening or lengthening exercise. *Am J Physiol* 290: E731–E738, 2006.

19. Dalby KN, Morrice N, Caudwell FB, Avruch J, Cohen P. Identification of regulatory phosphorylation sites in mitogen-activated protein kinase (MAPK)-activated protein kinase-1a/p90rsk that are inducible by MAPK. *J Biol Chem* 273: 1496–1505, 1998.

20. Damas F, Angleri V, Phillips SM, Witard OC, Ugrinowitsch C, Santanielo N, et al. Myofibrillar protein synthesis and muscle hypertrophy individualized responses to systematically changing resistance training variables in trained young men. *J Appl Physiol* 127: 806–815, 2019.

21. Damas F, Phillips SM, Libardi CA, Vechin FC, Lixandrao ME, Jannig PR, et al. Resistance training-induced changes in integrated myofibrillar protein synthesis are related to hypertrophy only after attenuation of muscle damage. *J Physiol* 594: 5209–5222, 2016.

22. De Luca A, Maiello MR, D'Alessio A, Pergameno M, Normanno N. The RAS/RAF/MEK/ERK and the PI3K/AKT signalling pathways: role in cancer pathogenesis and implications for therapeutic approaches. *Expert Opin Ther Targets* 16 Suppl 2: S17–27, 2012.

23. Dickinson JM, Fry CS, Drummond MJ, Gundermann DM, Walker DK, Glynn EL, et al. Mammalian target of rapamycin complex 1 activation is required for the stimulation of human skeletal muscle protein synthesis by essential amino acids. *J Nutr* 141: 856–862, 2011.

24. Dill KA, Ozkan SB, Shell MS, Weikl TR. The protein folding problem. *Annu Rev Biophys* 37: 289–316, 2008.

25. Dobrikov M, Dobrikova E, Shveygert M, Gromeier M. Phosphorylation of eukaryotic translation initiation factor 4G1 (eIF4G1) by protein kinase C{alpha} regulates eIF4G1 binding to Mnk1. *Mol Cell Biol* 31: 2947–2959, 2011.

26. Drummond MJ, Fry CS, Glynn EL, Dreyer HC, Dhanani S, Timmerman KL, et al. Rapamycin administration in humans blocks the contraction-induced increase in skeletal muscle protein synthesis. *J Physiol* 587: 1535–1546, 2009.

27. Figueiredo VC. Revisiting the roles of protein synthesis during skeletal muscle hypertrophy induced by exercise. *Am J Physiol* 317: R709–R718, 2019.

28. Franchi MV, Wilkinson DJ, Quinlan JI, Mitchell WK, Lund JN, Williams JP, et al. Early structural remodeling and deuterium oxide-derived protein metabolic responses to eccentric and concentric loading in human skeletal muscle. *Physiol Rep* 3, 2015.

29. Frolova LY, Merkulova TI, Kisselev LL. Translation termination in eukaryotes: polypeptide release factor eRF1 is composed of functionally and structurally distinct domains. *RNA* 6: 381–390, 2000.

30. Fry CS, Glynn EL, Drummond MJ, Timmerman KL, Fujita S, Abe T, et al. Blood flow restriction exercise stimulates mTORC1 signaling and muscle protein synthesis in older men. *J Appl Physiol* 108: 1199–1209, 2010.

31. Gingras AC, Gygi SP, Raught B, Polakiewicz RD, Abraham RT, Hoekstra MF, et al. Regulation of 4E-BP1 phosphorylation: a novel two-step mechanism. *Genes Dev* 13: 1422–1437, 1999.

32. Gingras AC, Raught B, Sonenberg N. eIF4 initiation factors: effectors of mRNA recruitment to ribosomes and regulators of translation. *Annu Rev Biochem* 68: 913–963, 1999.

33. Grandori C, Gomez-Roman N, Felton-Edkins ZA, Ngouenet C, Galloway DA, Eisenman RN, et al. c-Myc binds to human ribosomal DNA and stimulates transcription of rRNA genes by RNA polymerase I. *Nat Cell Biol* 7: 311–318, 2005.

34. Gu X, Orozco JM, Saxton RA, Condon KJ, Liu GY, Krawczyk PA, et al. SAMTOR is an S-adenosylmethionine sensor for the mTORC1 pathway. *Science* 358: 813–818, 2017.

35. Guertin DA, Stevens DM, Thoreen CC, Burds AA, Kalaany NY, Moffat J, et al. Ablation in mice of the mTORC components raptor, rictor, or mLST8 reveals that mTORC2 is required for signaling to Akt-FOXO and PKCalpha, but not S6K1. *Dev Cell* 11: 859–871, 2006.

36. Hammarström D, Øfsteng S, Koll L, Hanestadhaugen M, Hollan I, Apro W, et al. Benefits of higher resistance-training volume are related to ribosome biogenesis. *J Physiol* 598: 543–565, 2019.

37. Hannan KM, Brandenburger Y, Jenkins A, Sharkey K, Cavanaugh A, Rothblum L, et al. mTOR-dependent regulation of ribosomal gene transcription requires S6K1 and is mediated by phosphorylation of the carboxy-terminal activation domain of the nucleolar transcription factor UBF. *Mol Cell Biol* 23: 8862–8877, 2003.

38. Hannan RD, Stefanovsky V, Taylor L, Moss T, Rothblum LI. Overexpression of the transcription factor UBF1 is sufficient to increase ribosomal DNA transcription in neonatal cardiomyocytes: implications for cardiac hypertrophy. *Proc Natl Acad Sci U S A* 93: 8750–8755, 1996.

39. Hay N, Sonenberg N. Upstream and downstream of mTOR. *Genes Dev* 18: 1926–1945, 2004.

40. Heesom KJ, Denton RM. Dissociation of the eukaryotic initiation factor-4E/4E-BP1 complex involves phosphorylation of 4E-BP1 by an mTOR-associated kinase. *FEBS Lett* 457: 489–493, 1999.

41. Hershey JWB, Sonenberg N, Mathews MB. Principles of translational control. *Cold Spring Harb Perspect Biol* 11: a032607, 2019.

42. Hodson N, Brown T, Joanisse S, Aguirre N, West DWD, Moore DR, et al. Characterisation of L-type amino acid transporter 1 (LAT1) expression in human skeletal muscle by immunofluorescent microscopy. *Nutrients* 10, 2017.

43. Hodson N, McGlory C, Oikawa SY, Jeromson S, Song Z, Ruegg MA, et al. Differential localization and anabolic responsiveness of mTOR complexes in human skeletal muscle in response to feeding and exercise. *Am J Physiol* 313: C604–C611, 2017.

44. Hodson N, Philp A. The importance of mTOR trafficking for human skeletal muscle translational control. *Exerc Sport Sci Rev* 47: 46–53, 2019.

45. Hubal MJ, Gordish-Dressman H, Thompson PD, Price TB, Hoffman EP, Angelopoulos TJ, et al. Variability in muscle size and strength gain after unilateral resistance training. *Med Sci Sports Exerc* 37: 964–972, 2005.

46. Jacobs BL, Goodman CA, Hornberger TA. The mechanical activation of mTOR signaling: an emerging role for late endosome/lysosomal targeting. *J Muscle Res Cell Motil* 35: 11–21, 2014.

47. Jacobs BL, You JS, Frey JW, Goodman CA, Gundermann DM, Hornberger TA. Eccentric contractions increase the phosphorylation of tuberous sclerosis complex-2 (TSC2) and alter the targeting of TSC2 and the mechanistic target of rapamycin to the lysosome. *J Physiol* 591: 4611–4620, 2013.

48. Kim DH, Sarbassov DD, Ali SM, King JE, Latek RR, Erdjument-Bromage H, et al. mTOR interacts with raptor to form a nutrient-sensitive complex that signals to the cell growth machinery. *Cell* 110: 163–175, 2002.

49. Kumar V, Selby A, Rankin D, Patel R, Atherton P, Hildebrandt W, et al. Age-related differences in the dose-response relationship of muscle protein synthesis to resistance exercise in young and old men. *J Physiol* 587: 211–217, 2009.

50. Lavoie H, Therrien M. Regulation of RAF protein kinases in ERK signalling. *Nat Rev Mol Cell Biol* 16: 281–298, 2015.

51. Lee SJ, Janssen I, Heymsfield SB, Ross R. Relation between whole-body and regional measures of human skeletal muscle. *Am J Clin Nutr* 80: 1215–1221, 2004.

52. Long X, Lin Y, Ortiz-Vega S, Yonezawa K, Avruch J. Rheb binds and regulates the mTOR kinase. *Curr Biol* 15: 702–713, 2005.

53. Lynch M, Fitzgerald C, Johnston KA, Wang S, Schmidt EV. Activated eIF4E-binding protein slows G1 pro-gression and blocks transformation by c-myc without inhibiting cell growth. *J Biol Chem* 279: 3327–3339, 2004.

54. McKendry J, Perez-Lopez A, McLeod M, Luo D, Dent JR, Smeuninx B, et al. Short inter-set rest blunts resistance exercise-induced increases in myofibrillar protein synthesis and intracellular signalling in young males. *Exp Physiol* 101: 866–882, 2016.

55. Miller AE, MacDougall JD, Tarnopolsky MA, Sale DG. Gender differences in strength and muscle fiber characteristics. *Eur J Appl Physiol Occup Physiol* 66: 254–262, 1993.

56. Miller BF, Hansen M, Olesen JL, Flyvbjerg A, Schwarz P, Babraj JA, et al. No effect of menstrual cycle on myofibrillar and connective tissue protein synthesis in contracting skeletal muscle. *Am J Physiol* 290: E163–E168, 2006.

57. Mitchell CJ, Churchward-Venne TA, Parise G, Bellamy L, Baker SK, Smith K, et al. Acute post-exercise myofibrillar protein synthesis is not correlated with resistance training-induced muscle hypertrophy in young men. *PLoS One* 9: e89431, 2014.

58. Mitchell CJ, Churchward-Venne TA, West DWD, Burd NA, Breen L, Baker SK, et al. Resistance exercise load does not determine training-mediated hypertrophic gains in young men. *J Appl Physiol* 113: 71–77, 2012.

59. Moberg M, Apro W, Ekblom B, van Hall G, Holmberg HC, Blomstrand E. Activation of mTORC1 by leucine is potentiated by branched-chain amino acids and even more so by essential amino acids following resistance exercise. *Am J Physiol* 310: C874–84, 2016.

60. Moore DR. Maximizing post-exercise anabolism: the case for relative protein intakes. *Front Nutr* 6: 147, 2019.

61. Moore DR, Atherton PJ, Rennie MJ, Tarnopolsky MA, Phillips SM. Resistance exercise enhances mTOR and MAPK signalling in human muscle over that seen at rest after bolus protein ingestion. *Acta Physiol (Oxf)* 201: 365–372, 2011.

62. Moore DR, Churchward-Venne TA, Witard O, Breen L, Burd NA, Tipton KD, et al. Protein ingestion to stimulate myofibrillar protein synthesis requires greater relative intakes in healthy older versus younger men. *J Gerontol A Biol Sci Med Sci* 70: 57–62, 2015.

63. Moore DR, Phillips SM, Babraj JA, Smith K, Rennie MJ. Myofibrillar and collagen protein synthesis in human skeletal muscle in young men after maximal shortening and lengthening contractions. *Am J Physiol* 288: E1153–9, 2005.

64. Moore DR, Tang JE, Burd NA, Rerecich T, Tarnopolsky MA, Phillips SM. Differential stimulation of myofibrillar and sarcoplasmic protein synthesis with protein ingestion at rest and after resistance exercise. *J Physiol* 587: 897–904, 2009.

65. Moore DR, Young M, Phillips SM. Similar increases in muscle size and strength in young men after training with maximal shortening or lengthening contractions when matched for total work. *Eur J Appl Physiol* 112: 1587–1592, 2012.

66. Morton RW, Murphy KT, McKellar SR, Schoenfeld BJ, Henselmans M, Helms E, et al. A systematic review, meta-analysis and meta-regression of the effect of protein supplementation on resistance training-induced gains in muscle mass and strength in healthy adults. *Br J Sports Med* 52: 376–384, 2018.

67. Morton RW, Oikawa SY, Wavell CG, Mazara N, McGlory C, Quadrilatero J, et al. Neither load nor systemic hormones determine resistance training-mediated hypertrophy or strength gains in resistance-trained young men. *J Appl Physiol* 121: 129–138, 2016.

68. Morton RW, Sonne MW, Farias Zuniga A, Mohammad IYZ, Jones A, McGlory C, et al. Muscle fibre activation is unaffected by load and repetition duration when resistance exercise is performed to task failure. *J Physiol* 597: 4601–4613, 2019.

69. Nakada S, Ogasawara R, Kawada S, Maekawa T, Ishii N. Correlation between ribosome biogenesis and the magnitude of hypertrophy in overloaded skeletal muscle. *PLOS ONE* 11: e0147284, 2016.

70. Ogasawara R, Suginohara T. Rapamycin-insensitive mechanistic target of rapamycin regulates basal and resistance exercise-induced muscle protein synthesis. *FASEB J* [Epub ahead of print], 2018

71. Peterson MD, Rhea MR, Alvar BA. Applications of the dose-response for muscular strength development: a review of meta-analytic efficacy and reliability for designing training prescription. *J Strength Cond Res* 19: 950–958, 2005.

72. Peterson RT, Desai BN, Hardwick JS, Schreiber SL. Protein phosphatase 2A interacts with the 70-kDa S6 kinase and is activated by inhibition of FKBP12-rapamycinassociated protein. *Proc Natl Acad Sci U S A* 96: 4438–4442, 1999.

73. Phillips SM, McGlory C. CrossTalk proposal: the dominant mechanism causing disuse muscle atrophy is decreased protein synthesis. *J Physiol* 592: 5341–5343, 2014.

74. Phillips SM, Tipton KD, Aarsland A, Wolf SE, Wolfe RR. Mixed muscle protein synthesis and breakdown after resistance exercise in humans. *Am J Physiol* 273: E99–107, 1997.

75. Phillips SM, Winett RA. Uncomplicated resistance training and health-related outcomes: evidence for a public health mandate. *Curr Sports Med Rep* 9: 208–213, 2010.

76. Philp A, Schenk S, Perez-Schindler J, Hamilton DL, Breen L, Laverone E, et al. Rapamycin does not prevent increases in myofibrillar or mitochondrial protein synthesis following endurance exercise. *J Physiol* 593: 4275–4284, 2015.

77. Pyronnet S, Imataka H, Gingras AC, Fukunaga R, Hunter T, Sonenberg N. Human eukaryotic translation initiation factor 4G (eIF4G) recruits mnk1 to phosphorylate eIF4E. *EMBO J* 18: 270–279, 1999.

78. Raught B, Gingras AC, Gygi SP, Imataka H, Morino S, Gradi A, et al. Serum-stimulated, rapamycin-sensitive phosphorylation sites in the eukaryotic translation initiation factor 4GI. *EMBO J* 19: 434–444, 2000.

79. Raught B, Peiretti F, Gingras AC, Livingstone M, Shahbazian D, Mayeur GL, et al. Phosphorylation of eucaryotic translation initiation factor 4B Ser422 is modulated by S6 kinases. *EMBO J* 23: 1761–1769, 2004.

80. Redpath NT, Foulstone EJ, Proud CG. Regulation of translation elongation factor-2 by insulin via a rapamycin-sensitive signalling pathway. *EMBO J* 15: 2291–2297, 1996.
81. Redpath NT, Price NT, Severinov KV, Proud CG. Regulation of elongation factor-2 by multisite phosphorylation. *Eur J Biochem* 213: 689–699, 1993.
82. Roig M, O'Brien K, Kirk G, Murray R, McKinnon P, Shadgan B, et al. The effects of eccentric versus concentric resistance training on muscle strength and mass in healthy adults: a systematic review with meta-analysis. *Br J Sports Med* 43: 556–568, 2009.
83. Roskoski RJ. MEK1/2 dual-specificity protein kinases: structure and regulation. *Biochem Biophys Res Commun* 417: 5–10, 2012.
84. Ruvinsky I, Meyuhas O. Ribosomal protein S6 phosphorylation: from protein synthesis to cell size. *Trends Biochem Sci* 31: 342–348, 2006.
85. Ruvinsky I, Sharon N, Lerer T, Cohen H, Stolovich-Rain M, Nir T, et al. Ribosomal protein S6 phosphorylation is a determinant of cell size and glucose homeostasis. *Genes Dev* 19: 2199–2211, 2005.
86. Sancak Y, Bar-Peled L, Zoncu R, Markhard AL, Nada S, Sabatini DM. Ragulator-Rag complex targets mTORC1 to the lysosomal surface and is necessary for its activation by amino acids. *Cell* 141: 290–303, 2010.
87. Sancak Y, Peterson TR, Shaul YD, Lindquist RA, Thoreen CC, Bar-Peled L, et al. The rag GTPases bind raptor and mediate amino acid signaling to mTORC1. *Science* 320: 1496–1501, 2008.
88. Sancak Y, Thoreen CC, Peterson TR, Lindquist RA, Kang SA, Spooner E, et al. PRAS40 is an insulin-regulated inhibitor of the mTORC1 protein kinase. *Mol Cell* 25: 903–915, 2007.
89. Sanders MA, Basson MD. Collagen IV-dependent ERK activation in human Caco-2 intestinal epithelial cells requires focal adhesion kinase. *J Biol Chem* 275: 38040–38047, 2000.
90. Sanij E, Poortinga G, Sharkey K, Hung S, Holloway TP, Quin J, et al. UBF levels determine the number of active ribosomal RNA genes in mammals. *J Cell Biol* 183: 1259–1274, 2008.
91. Schlaepfer DD, Hunter T. Focal adhesion kinase overexpression enhances ras-dependent integrin signaling to ERK2/mitogen-activated protein kinase through interactions with and activation of c-Src. *J Biol Chem* 272: 13189–13195, 1997.
92. Schlosser I, Holzel M, Murnseer M, Burtscher H, Weidle UH, Eick D. A role for c-Myc in the regulation of ribosomal RNA processing. *Nucleic Acids Res* 31: 6148–6156, 2003.
93. Schoenfeld BJ, Contreras B, Krieger J, Grgic J, Delcastillo K, Belliard R, et al. Resistance training volume enhances muscle hypertrophy but not strength in trained men. *Med Sci Sports Exerc* 51: 94–103, 2019.
94. Schoenfeld BJ, Ogborn D, Krieger JW. Dose-response relationship between weekly resistance training volume and increases in muscle mass: a systematic review and meta-analysis. *J Sports Sci* 35: 1073–1082, 2017.
95. Schoenfeld BJ, Ogborn DI, Vigotsky AD, Franchi MV, Krieger JW. Hypertrophic effects of concentric vs. eccentric muscle actions: a systematic review and meta-analysis. *J Strength Cond Res* 31: 2599–2608, 2017.
96. Sears R, Nuckolls F, Haura E, Taya Y, Tamai K, Nevins JR. Multiple Ras-dependent phosphorylation pathways regulate Myc protein stability. *Genes Dev* 14: 2501–2514, 2000.
97. Shima H, Pende M, Chen Y, Fumagalli S, Thomas G, Kozma SC. Disruption of the p70(s6k)/p85(s6k) gene reveals a small mouse phenotype and a new functional S6 kinase. *EMBO J* 17: 6649–6659, 1998.
98. Shveygert M, Kaiser C, Bradrick SS, Gromeier M. Regulation of eukaryotic initiation factor 4E (eIF4E) phosphorylation by mitogen-activated protein kinase occurs through modulation of Mnk1-eIF4G interaction. *Mol Cell Biol* 30: 5160–5167, 2010.
99. Smith GI, Reeds DN, Hall AM, Chambers KT, Finck BN, Mittendorfer B. Sexually dimorphic effect of aging on skeletal muscle protein synthesis. *Biol Sex Differ* 3: 11, 2012.
100. Sonenberg N, Hinnebusch AG. Regulation of translation initiation in eukaryotes: mechanisms and biological targets. *Cell* 136: 731–745, 2009.
101. Song Z, Moore DR, Hodson N, Ward C, Dent JR, O'Leary MF, et al. Resistance exercise initiates mechanistic target of rapamycin (mTOR) translocation and protein complex co-localisation in human skeletal muscle. *Sci Rep* 7: 5028, 2017.
102. Stec MJ, Kelly NA, Many GM, Windham ST, Tuggle SC, Bamman MM. Ribosome biogenesis may augment resistance training-induced myofiber hypertrophy and is required for myotube growth in vitro. *Am J Physiol* 310: E652–E661, 2016.
103. Takarada Y, Takazawa H, Sato Y, Takebayashi S, Tanaka Y, Ishii N. Effects of resistance exercise combined with moderate vascular occlusion on muscular function in humans. *J Appl Physiol* 88: 2097–2106, 2000.
104. Tang H, Hornstein E, Stolovich M, Levy G, Livingstone M, Templeton D, et al. Amino acid–induced translation of TOP mRNAs is fully dependent on phosphatidylinositol 3-kinase-mediated signaling, is partially inhibited by rapamycin, and is independent of S6K1 and rpS6 phosphorylation. *Mol Cell Biol* 21: 8671–8683, 2001.

105. Thomas G. An encore for ribosome biogenesis in the control of cell proliferation. *Nat Cell Biol* 2: E71–2, 2000.
106. Thomson E, Ferreira-Cerca S, Hurt E. Eukaryotic ribosome biogenesis at a glance. *J Cell Sci* 126: 4815–4821, 2013.
107. Ueda T, Watanabe-Fukunaga R, Fukuyama H, Nagata S, Fukunaga R. Mnk2 and Mnk1 are essential for constitutive and inducible phosphorylation of eukaryotic initiation factor 4E but not for cell growth or development. *Mol Cell Biol* 24: 6539–6549, 2004.
108. Voit R, Grummt I. Phosphorylation of UBF at serine 388 is required for interaction with RNA polymerase I and activation of rDNA transcription. *Proc Natl Acad Sci U S A* 98: 13631–13636, 2001.
109. Walker DK, Dickinson JM, Timmerman KL, Drummond MJ, Reidy PT, Fry CS, et al. Exercise, amino acids, and aging in the control of human muscle protein synthesis. *Med Sci Sport Exerc* 43: 2249–2258, 2011.
110. Waskiewicz AJ, Flynn A, Proud CG, Cooper JA. Mitogen-activated protein kinases activate the serine/threonine kinases Mnk1 and Mnk2. *EMBO J* 16: 1909–1920, 1997.
111. West DW, Baehr LM, Marcotte GR, Chason CM, Tolento L, Gomes AV, et al. Acute resistance exercise activates rapamycin-sensitive and -insensitive mechanisms that control translational activity and capacity in skeletal muscle. *J Physiol* 594: 453–468, 2016.
112. West DWD, Burd NA, Churchward-Venne TA, Camera DM, Mitchell CJ, Baker SK, et al. Sex-based comparisons of myofibrillar protein synthesis after resistance exercise in the fed state. *J Appl Physiol* 112: 1805–1813, 2012.
113. Wilson GM, Blanco R, Coon JJ, Hornberger TA. Identifying novel signaling pathways: an exercise scientists guide to phosphoproteomics. *Exerc Sport Sci Rev* 46: 76–85, 2018.
114. Wolfe RR. Skeletal muscle protein metabolism and resistance exercise. *J Nutr* 136: 525s–528s, 2006.
115. Wolfson RL, Chantranupong L, Saxton RA, Shen K, Scaria SM, Cantor JR, et al. Sestrin2 is a leucine sensor for the mTORC1 pathway. *Science* 351: 43–48, 2016.
116. Wong PM, Feng Y, Wang J, Shi R, Jiang X. Regulation of autophagy by coordinated action of mTORC1 and protein phosphatase 2A. *Nat Commun* 6: 8048, 2015.
117. Yasuda N, Glover EI, Phillips SM, Isfort RJ, Tarnopolsky MA. Sex-based differences in skeletal muscle function and morphology with short-term limb immobilization. *J Appl Physiol* 99: 1085–1092, 2005.
118. Yoon MS, Du G, Backer JM, Frohman MA, Chen J. Class III PI-3-kinase activates phospholipase D in an amino acid-sensing mTORC1 pathway. *J Cell Biol* 195: 435–447, 2011.
119. You JS, Lincoln HC, Kim CR, Frey JW, Goodman CA, Zhong XP, et al. The role of diacylglycerol kinase zeta and phosphatidic acid in the mechanical activation of mammalian target of rapamycin (mTOR) signaling and skeletal muscle hypertrophy. *J Biol Chem* 289: 1551–1563, 2014.
120. You JS, McNally RM, Jacobs BL, Privett RE, Gundermann DM, Lin KH, et al. The role of raptor in the mechanical load-induced regulation of mTOR signaling, protein synthesis, and skeletal muscle hypertrophy. *FASEB J* 33: 4021–4034, 2019.
121. Zhang HR, Chen JM, Zeng ZY, Que WZ. Knockdown of DEPTOR inhibits cell proliferation and increases chemosensitivity to melphalan in human multiple myeloma RPMI-8226 cells via inhibiting PI3K/AKT activity. *J Int Med Res* 41: 584–595, 2013.
122. American College of Sports Medicine position stand. Progression models in resistance training for healthy adults. *Med Sci Sports Exerc* 41: 687–708, 2009.

11

CELLULAR ADAPTATIONS TO HIGH-INTENSITY AND SPRINT INTERVAL TRAINING

Martin J. MacInnis and Lauren E. Skelly

Introduction

Whether it is children running on a playground, hockey players taking shifts on the ice, or older adults alternating between periods of brisk and slow walking, intermittent exercise is ubiquitous. The rationale for intermittent exercise is obvious to most observers: It is difficult to maintain high-intensity exercise for a prolonged period of time, but one's capacity to exercise recovers at lower exercise intensities or with rest. What the casual observer might not realize is the potency of intermittent exercise for improving skeletal muscle fitness and whole-body exercise capacity. This chapter focuses on the acute responses and chronic adaptations that occur within (and around) skeletal muscle cells in response to interval exercise and training, respectively. Overall, the goals of this chapter are to (1) provide a brief overview of interval exercise definitions, nomenclature, and prescription; (2) summarize and discuss the available literature related to some of the key skeletal muscle cellular adaptations that occur in response to interval training; and (3) highlight future topics for research in interval training.

Interval Training Definitions, Nomenclature, and Prescription

Whereas intermittent exercise could be defined as any type of exercise that involves alternating between different exercise intensities, we define "interval training" as *structured* exercise that alternates between two or more exercise intensities. While the requirement for structure does not necessarily increase the efficacy of intermittent exercise (3, 62), the vast majority of skeletal muscle studies involving intermittent exercise employed structured exercise. Secondly, although it is often implicit, terms like "interval training" and "intermittent exercise" do not exclusively refer to exercise performed at high intensities. To clarify, the present chapter focuses on interval exercise involving bouts of high-intensity exercise, as we suggest that the exercise intensity is the attribute most directly responsible for the beneficial effects of interval training on skeletal muscle (70, 71). With that point in mind, it should be emphasized that intermittent exercise is not radically different from continuous exercise with respect to its acute and chronic effects on skeletal muscle: Adaptations to both forms of exercise training are similar in nature. In contrast, the time course and magnitude of the changes, as well as the molecular pathways involved in orchestrating these changes, may differ between interval and continuous exercise (70, 71). Finally, interval training could theoretically involve many different exercise modalities, including resistance training (46) and body-weight training (74); however, this chapter focuses on "aerobic" interval training, with a particular emphasis on studies involving cycling, as this is the predominant exercise mode in the literature.

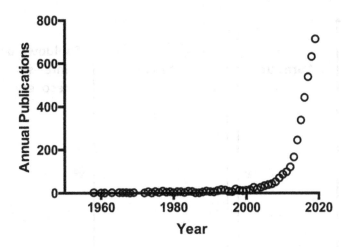

Figure 11.1 The annual number of publications related to interval training listed in PubMed between 1950 and 2019

With its use as a training strategy documented in the early 1900s (7) and its emergence as a research topic in the mid-1900s (1, 17), interval exercise is not new; however, the number of published studies investigating interval exercise has increased rapidly over the past two decades (Figure 11.1), and high-intensity interval training (HIIT) was ranked among the top five fitness trends by the American College of Sports Medicine from 2014 to 2020 (102). Although it is difficult to pinpoint the watershed moment for interval training research, this form of training clearly gained momentum in the 1990s and early 2000s. This was due, in part, to influential studies that reported short intense bouts of exercise elicited adaptations that were typically associated with classic (i.e., prolonged and continuous) endurance training (69, 100), studies demonstrating the benefits of HIIT in patient populations (103, 111), and studies demonstrating that low volumes of interval training could be as effective as much larger volumes of endurance exercise, particularly with respect to mitochondrial content, cardiorespiratory fitness, and performance (13, 34).

The definition of interval training appears simple, but a number of factors need to be considered when designing an interval training session (Figure 11.2). In addition to the exercise mode, the primary factors to consider are the intensity and duration of the work bouts and recovery periods and the number of repetitions that will be performed. Secondary factors to consider include the number of sets that are performed, and if multiple sets are performed, the between-set recovery duration and intensity. Finally, tertiary factors to consider include factors such as the environment (e.g., temperature and altitude) and the individual's current status (e.g., nutrition and fatigue). Collectively, these factors determine the nature of the training stress, which likely influences the acute and chronic physiological and metabolic responses/adaptations incurred (10, 48, 70).

Given that there is an infinite variety of interval training protocols, researchers have attempted to group similar protocols together. In the research context, interval training is often divided into HIIT, sprint interval training (SIT), and repeated sprint training (RST) (70). Note that there is no universal classification scheme for interval training: HIIT has also been referred to as aerobic interval training (AIT; 112); SIT is sometimes referred to as speed endurance training (33), reduced exertion high-intensity interval training (REHIT; 76), or simply not differentiated from HIIT or RST.

Interval training formats are generally differentiated by the intensity and duration of the work bouts. Weston et al. (108) defined HIIT as interval exercise eliciting ≥80% of maximal heart rate (HR$_{max}$) and SIT as interval exercise that is performed in an "all-out" manner. In contrast, Buchheit and Laursen (10)

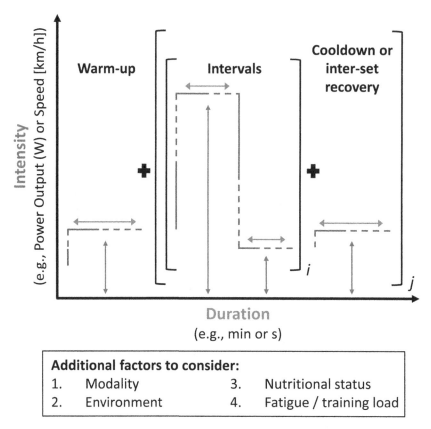

Figure 11.2 A schematic outlining the key variables of an interval training session

suggested that HIIT should be performed above the critical intensity of exercise (i.e., maximal lactate steady state [MLSS], critical power [CP], or critical speed) implying that work bouts must be performed in the severe intensity domain (84). Furthermore, these authors also suggested that, at least for running, SIT should be performed at 85–100% of maximum sprint speed (or above 160% of the minimal speed required to elicit maximal oxygen uptake, $\dot{V}O_2$max), which largely agrees with the general recommendation that the effort should simply be "all-out." Typically, work bouts for HIIT range from 1 to 5 min (68, 73), whereas work bouts for SIT are 20–30s (14, 36). For HIIT and SIT, a single set of 4–10 repetitions is common, and recovery periods for HIIT and SIT are generally, but not always, ~1–3 min and ~2–4.5 min, respectively (14, 36, 68, 73). In contrast, RST typically involves repeated efforts lasting <10 s interspersed with recovery periods generally <60s (39). While Buchheit and Laursen (10) suggested that the intensity of RST should be between the intensity of HIIT and SIT, other studies report that RST is performed "all-out" (32). Often, RST involves a similar or greater number of repetitions than HIIT and SIT and consists of multiple sets (32).

Interval training is often compared to exercise performed at a constant and lower intensity. Classically, this style of training has simply been termed aerobic or endurance training; however, given that interval training induces adaptations typically associated with endurance (13, 34, 69) and that interval training relies heavily on oxidative phosphorylation to resynthesize adenosine triphosphate (ATP) (80), this style of training has more recently been termed moderate-intensity continuous training (MICT; 109). Based on the available and proposed definitions of HIIT, MICT should be performed below the critical intensity of exercise (84); however, note that the intensity of MICT may fall in either the moderate or heavy domains. Other terms for MICT include sub-lactate threshold continuous training (42), lactate threshold training (49), and long slow distance training (49), among others. For many investigations, researchers match the total amount of work performed in continuous and interval exercise to remove the influence of this variable; however, studies comparing SIT and MICT generally do not match for total volume (70).

In addition to the different names and classification schemes, different approaches are used to prescribe high-intensity exercise. For example, exercise may be prescribed according to HR_{max} or heart rate reserve, ratings of perceived exertion, peak power output, $\dot{V}O_2$ reserve, $\dot{V}O_2max$, MLSS, CP, or critical speed. The marked variability in the design and prescription of exercise complicates interpretations of research studies.

Cellular Adaptations to Interval Training

The dramatically increased metabolic rates of contracting skeletal muscles challenge local and whole-body homeostasis. With repeated exercise training bouts, skeletal muscle cellular adaptations limit disruptions in local homeostasis, which has a cascading effect on the "service" organs (47). That is, with regular exercise training, skeletal muscle adaptations can attenuate whole-body disruptions in response to exercise, reducing the perceived exertion and increasing the sustainability of a given workload. Thus, the mechanisms through which exercise elicits skeletal muscle adaptations and the manner in which these mechanisms respond to different exercise training protocols are of significant importance to understanding exercise physiology and exercise performance. The focus of this section will be on the effects of acute and chronic high-intensity interval exercise—in comparison to continuous exercise, where possible—on cellular, biochemical, and metabolic responses and adaptations in skeletal muscle. In this context, this section discusses indices of mitochondrial biogenesis and mitochondrial content; fuel transport, storage, and use; and capillarization. Of these variables, there is considerably more data related to mitochondria, so this topic will be presented in more detail than other topics. Comparisons of interval and continuous exercise are supplemented with studies of relatively high- and low-intensity continuous exercise where appropriate.

Mitochondria: An Overview

The capacity of skeletal muscle to oxidize fuels to meet the demands of exercise depends in part on the density of skeletal muscle mitochondria (54). Exercise training can markedly increase the abundance of mitochondria in skeletal muscle (24, 53, 78), which can be measured through electron microscopy, respiration, enzyme activity, and protein content, among other methods (64). Expansion of the mitochondrial reticulum through de novo protein synthesis—termed mitochondria biogenesis (Figure 11.3)—is stimulated by exercise through a series of molecular events (29, 56, 70). Individual bouts of exercise create metabolic signals, such as increased [Ca^{2+}] and greater ratios of [ADP]:[ATP] and [AMP]:[ATP], which activate signalling cascades that increase the expression of relevant genes from the nuclear and mitochondrial genomes (27, 29, 82). Subsequently, the rate of mitochondrial protein synthesis is increased (26), elevating the abundance of mitochondrial proteins and (eventually, with regular training) the density of skeletal muscle mitochondria (76). The metabolic consequences of increased mitochondrial density include a greater capacity to aerobically resynthesize ATP (i.e., greater oxidative phosphorylation and lower lactate accumulation), increased fat oxidation and decreased carbohydrate oxidation at a given submaximal intensity of exercise, and the capacity to sustain greater exercise intensities (24, 55). Overall, increased mitochondrial density is associated with improved exercise performance. For a more in-depth review of the molecular mechanisms related to mitochondrial biogenesis, see elsewhere (29, 56).

Mitochondrial biogenesis in response to interval training

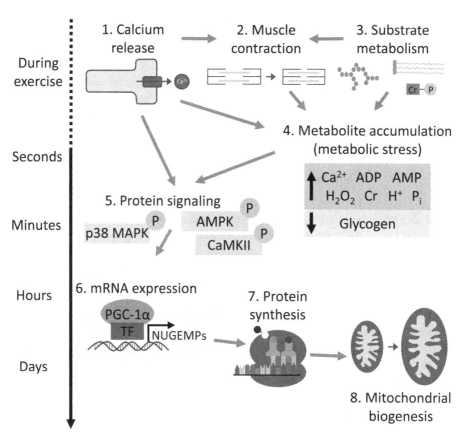

Figure 11.3 A diagram outlining the cellular responses to exercise within a skeletal muscle cell that relate to mitochondrial biogenesis

Mitochondria: Intensity Influences Acute Metabolic Responses to Exercise

ATP demand is positively related to exercise intensity and can increase as much as 100-fold relative to rest when maximal exercise is performed (91). Various metabolic processes regulate substrate metabolism such that ATP synthesis closely matches ATP hydrolysis. In studies that have compared equal durations of exercise performed at different intensities, muscle biopsy samples revealed that greater exercise intensities elicit markedly higher metabolic stress, due to a greater reliance on substrate-level phosphorylation and anaerobic metabolism as the concentration of skeletal muscle metabolites, such as H^+, ADP, AMP, P_i, creatine, and lactate, increase with exercise intensity (57, 89, 90). Although it could be argued that the greater concentration of metabolites in these studies is a result of a greater amount of work being performed—not the rate of work, per se—these variables seem to reach a steady state, at least at lower intensities (57). Thus, exercise intensity appears to be the key factor dictating the skeletal muscle metabolic response to exercise. For example, even short bursts of "all-out" exercise involving low amounts of total work cause large disruptions to metabolic homeostasis (80).

When comparisons have been made between interval and continuous exercise, they mostly agree with studies that have compared low and high intensities of exercise. For example, Fiorenza et al. (33)

recently demonstrated that SIT (6 × 20s sprints) and RST (5 × 18s) protocols decreased muscle [ATP], [PCr], and pH and increased muscle [lactate] to a greater extent than an MICT protocol involving eight times more work. Note that the SIT protocol elicited a greater increase in muscle [lactate] and a greater decrease in muscle pH compared to RST, despite the two protocols involving sprints and being work-matched, demonstrating that not all interval training protocols are identical and that exercise intensity is not the only relevant factor influencing metabolic stress. This point is supported by a recent ^{31}P magnetic resonance spectroscopy study in which exercise was performed at the same intensity and work:recovery ratio; however, decreases in [PCr] and pH were more pronounced for longer duration intervals (25). Thus, although the metabolic disturbance is dependent on intensity, bout duration influences the disturbance. Finally, in another work-matched comparison, Kristensen et al. (61) demonstrated that interval exercise (6 × [1.5 min at 100% $\dot{V}O_2$peak + 2.5 min at 40% $\dot{V}O_2$peak]) increased muscle [lactate] and [creatine] to a greater extent than continuous exercise (30 min at ~70% $\dot{V}O_2$peak).

The profound effect of high-intensity exercise on skeletal muscle metabolites is apparent in studies that have collected muscle biopsies before, during, and after one or more short (30s) maximal sprints (15, 80). For example, Cheetham et al. (15) demonstrated that a single maximal 30-s sprint performed on a nonmotorized treadmill reduced muscle [glycogen], [PCr], and [ATP] by 25%, 64%, and 37%, respectively, and increased muscle [pyruvate] and [lactate] 19 and 29 times, respectively. Despite the heavy reliance on anaerobic processes for a single bout of maximal exercise, the contributions of glycogenolysis, lactate production, and PCr breakdown to the overall synthesis of ATP decreased within and across a set of maximal sprints, whereas the relative contribution of oxidative phosphorylation increased (80).

Overall, it is clear that exercise intensity is a major determinant of the acute metabolic response to exercise. Whether work is matched or not, high-intensity interval exercise generally elicits greater metabolic stress than lower-intensity continuous exercise.

Mitochondria: Acute Molecular Responses to Exercise

Changes in the concentrations of muscle metabolites, indicative of contractile activity and metabolic demand, activate and regulate molecular pathways involved in mitochondrial biogenesis (29, 70). Thus, molecular pathways are also sensitive to exercise intensity (27).

As previously reviewed (29), numerous signalling proteins and genes are involved in mitochondrial biogenesis that are activated by exercise. In the present section, we will focus on the following proteins: AMP-activated protein kinase (AMPK), p38 mitogen activated protein kinase (p38-MAPK), and Ca^{2+}/calmodulin-dependent protein kinase II (CaMKII) (Figure 11.3). These signalling proteins are typically studied because they respond to exercise and modulate the expression and/or activity of the peroxisome proliferator-activated receptor gamma coactivator 1α (PGC-1α), a protein that coordinates the expression of mitochondrial genes from the nuclear and mitochondrial genome (29, 56). Phosphorylation of acetyl-CoA carboxylase (ACC), a downstream target of AMPK, is often used as a surrogate of AMPK activity (110).

AMPK (or ACC), p38-MAPK, and CaMKII are generally, but not always, phosphorylated to a greater extent with higher intensities of constant-load exercise (16, 27, 88, 112). While some of these studies did not match for total volume of exercise performed at each intensity (i.e., each intensity was performed for equal durations), Egan et al. (27) demonstrated that AMPK, ACC, and CaMKII were phosphorylated to a greater extent by high- compared to low-intensity continuous exercise when work was matched. Yet in contrast, comparisons of work-matched interval and continuous exercise protocols generally demonstrate similar protein signalling responses across different exercise intensities. For example, Bartlett et al. (5), Kristensen et al. (61), Parker et al. (79), and Trewin et al. (105) reported mostly similar protein signalling responses for HIIT and MICT protocols, matched for total work. Low-volume SIT activates these same protein signalling responses in skeletal muscle (33, 35, 75). However, in contrast to work-matched studies of HIIT and MICT, similar (5, 79, 95, 105) or even greater (33, 43) responses in protein signalling have been observed for SIT compared to MICT, despite large differences in the total volume of work.

Subsequent to the activation of signalling proteins and the nuclear translocation of relevant proteins, exercise increases the transcription of many genes involved in mitochondrial biogenesis (29). Egan et al. (27) demonstrated that when work is matched, continuous high-intensity exercise elicited larger increases in the expression of *PGC-1α* mRNA, which the authors attributed to greater activation of activating transcription factor-2 and class IIa histone deacetylases, as well as reduced methylation in the promoter regions of *PGC-1α* and related genes (4). In a review, Granata et al. (41) reported a moderate-strength, positive association between exercise intensity and *PGC-1α* mRNA expression over a large number of studies, which supports interval training eliciting greater increases in the expression of this gene than lower intensities of continuous exercise; however, as with signalling protein activation, *PGC-1α* expression is often similar across HIIT and MICT protocols when work is matched (5, 105, 106). Interestingly, *PGC-1α* gene expression has also been reported to be comparable for low-volume SIT in comparison to higher volumes of MICT and/or HIIT (18, 33, 43, 85, 105).

The synthetic rate of new mitochondrial proteins can also be measured as an acute marker of mitochondrial biogenesis (76). Di Donato et al. (26) demonstrated that a higher-intensity stimulus resulted in a greater mitochondrial fractional synthetic rate (FSR) 24–28 hours post-exercise than a lower-intensity stimulus matched for total work. From the same laboratory, Bell et al. (6) reported that HIIT increased sarcoplasmic FSR, a probable surrogate of mitochondrial protein synthesis (109), 1 day after exercise in older adults, whereas MICT did not. Both studies suggest that greater rates of mitochondrial biogenesis occur in response to higher compared to lower intensities of exercise, even when work is not matched (6). However, insufficient data are available to make strong conclusions on the effect of interval training, as compared to continuous training, on rates of mitochondrial protein synthesis in humans.

Overall, the acute outcomes discussed in this section are upstream of the phenotype of interest: mitochondrial content (Figure 11.3). Studies comparing changes in mitochondrial content provide the most direct evidence for understanding the efficacy of interval training for increasing this cellular attribute.

Mitochondria: Interval Training–Induced Changes in Content

Interval training is a potent exercise stimulus that elicits rapid improvements in mitochondrial content (70). For example, the maximal activity of citrate synthase (CS) is reported to increase following a single session of SIT (67) or three sessions of HIIT (82), which is similar to results for MICT (28). Training-induced increases in the maximal activity and protein content of mitochondrial enzymes have also been found following as few as 2 weeks of HIIT (73, 101) or SIT (12, 14, 34, 59, 63, 68). In work-matched comparisons over 2–8 weeks, HIIT has shown to increase the maximal activity of succinate dehydrogenase (SDH) or CS to a similar (2, 51) or greater (73) extent as MICT. Superior improvements in mitochondrial respiration within permeabilized fibres have also been shown following lower-volume (42) or work-matched (23, 73) interval training compared to MICT. Note that mitochondrial respiration is correlated to mitochondrial volume, density, and other measures of mitochondrial content (64). However, it is at times considered as a measure of mitochondrial function, not content. Numerous studies also reported similar increases in mitochondrial content following low-volume SIT and high-volume MICT using a variety of methods, including mitochondrial volume (96), maximal activities of CS (2, 13, 36) and SDH (95), and cytochrome *c* oxidase (COX) maximal activity or content (34, 96, 97). Furthermore, a recent study reported that 8 weeks of MICT increased CS and COX subunit IV (COXIV) protein content only if 30-s sprints were performed every 10 min during the 60-min training sessions (45). This result occurred despite the two protocols being work-matched and eliciting similar acute increases in *PGC-1α* expression. Overall, low-volume SIT is as effective as MICT, whereas HIIT seems to be equally as, or more effective than, MICT for increasing mitochondrial content. However, there are still relatively few studies comparing changes in mitochondrial content between HIIT and MICT, and most interventions are relatively short in duration.

Increases in the content of mitochondrial dynamic proteins, which have critical roles in remodelling and maintaining a healthy mitochondrial reticulum in skeletal muscle (56), have also been reported following interval training. Specifically, increases in the content of the mitochondrial fusion proteins mitofusin 1 (MFN1) and 2 (MFN2) and the fission proteins dynamin-related protein 1 and fission protein-1 are sometimes found following short-term SIT and HIIT (42, 66, 73, 82, 113). Moreover, two studies have shown similar increases in the protein content of MFN2 following interval training and MICT (42, 73).

Substrate Transport, Oxidation, and Storage

Interval training can also affect key proteins involved in substrate metabolism. Several investigations have measured interval training–induced increases in glucose transporter 4 (GLUT4) protein content and/or activity (11, 38, 68, 81), with similar increases following low-volume SIT and MICT (9, 36). In addition, the activity and protein content of glycolytic enzymes, including phosphofructokinase, hexokinase, and lactate dehydrogenase, are increased following interval training (44, 58, 65, 69, 87, 99), and short-term HIIT has demonstrated increases in the protein content of glycogen synthase (99). With respect to fat metabolism, 2 weeks of HIIT increased the protein content of fatty acid–binding protein (FABPpm) but not fatty acid translocase (FAT/CD36) (101), whereas 6 weeks of HIIT demonstrated increases in FABPpm and FAT/CD36 (81, 99). In contrast, there was no effect of 6 weeks of low-volume SIT on either FABPpm or FATCD/36 protein content (11). Interval training also increased the content of proteins involved in lipid droplet metabolism, as evidenced by similar increases in the expression of perilipin 2 and 5 following 4–6 weeks of low-volume SIT and MICT (96, 97). Lastly, both HIIT (37, 81, 101) and low-volume SIT (38, 86) increased the maximal activity of 3-β-hydroxyacyl CoA dehydrogenase, the rate-limiting enzyme in β-oxidation.

Higher resting skeletal muscle glycogen is reported following short-term HIIT (81, 99) and SIT (14, 68, 87, 95), with similar increases in type I–specific glycogen content found following 6 weeks of SIT and MICT (95). There were also similar increases in intramuscular triglyceride content following the same duration of SIT and MICT (95, 97). In addition to adaptations within resting skeletal muscle, there is evidence that low-volume SIT and MICT reduced glycogen use (13) and enhanced intramuscular triglyceride breakdown (97) during submaximal exercise to a similar extent.

Overall, there are relatively few studies comparing changes in the content of proteins involved in substrate transport, oxidation (aside from the mitochondrial proteins discussed earlier), and storage among different training protocols. However, the limited studies available suggest interval and continuous training protocols elicit similar adaptations.

Skeletal Muscle Capillarization

Capillaries are the site of gas, nutrient, and by-product exchange between muscles and blood. Growth of the capillary network within skeletal muscle (i.e., increased capillarization) provides a greater surface area for exchange and reduces the oxygen diffusion distance. The primary stimuli to increase capillary density in humans, which occurs in response to aerobic training over a period of weeks to months, are mechanical (i.e., shear stress and passive muscle stretch) and metabolic (i.e., muscle contractions). As described by Hellsten and Nyberg (50), capillary growth is regulated by transient changes in the concentration of pro-angiogenic (e.g., vascular endothelial growth factor [VEGF], angiopoietin-2) and anti-angiogenic (e.g., endostatin) compounds elicited by exercise.

The influence of exercise intensity and interval exercise on skeletal muscle capillarization has not been researched extensively. One study has reported that 8 weeks of MICT increased capillary density nearly twice as much as HIIT (matched for total work), although the arteriovenous oxygen difference increased similarly across these two protocols, suggesting that the HIIT condition was not disadvantaged despite the lower capillary density (23). When low-volume SIT has been compared to MICT, similar increases in capillary density were observed in several studies (19, 20, 95). Yet in another comparison, 4 weeks of SIT did not increase capillary density, whereas 4 weeks of MICT significantly increased capillary density (52). From the same data set, the authors reported that a single bout of SIT, compared to MICT, induced greater increases in *VEGF* mRNA but lower concentrations of interstitial VEGF protein. Furthermore, the application of interstitial fluid collected during MICT to human umbilical vein endothelial cells increased the proliferation of these cells more than interstitial fluid collected during SIT (52). Although Gliemann (40) suggested that these data provide evidence for a "Janus-faced coin," with short bouts of high-intensity favouring cardiac remodelling and mitochondrial biogenesis and prolonged, moderate-intensity exercise favouring capillarization, it should be noted that the MICT programme preceded the SIT programme for all participants. Considering this limitation, along with data from other studies comparing SIT and MICT (19, 20, 95), the reduced impact of SIT on capillary density from the study by Hoier et al. (52) could be interpreted as attenuated capillary growth with continued training (50) rather than evidence that SIT is less effective than MICT. Additional evidence from Jensen et al. (60) suggests that performing single-leg knee extensor exercise at 90% or 150% of $\dot{V}O_2$max increases capillarization similarly. In comparison, low-intensity exercise (45% $\dot{V}O_2$max) did not induce capillarization in another study (93). Aside from SIT data from Hoier (52), all other protocols discussed earlier, representing a range of intensities—and both interval and continuous training— were effective in increasing capillary density. Given the importance of capillary density for exercise performance (22) and maximal oxygen uptake (50) and the limited number of protocols that have been compared, more research is needed to determine whether interval training and/or exercise intensity mediates the extent to which exercise training augments capillarization.

Limitations to Studies of Cellular Adaptation

While exercise intensity clearly influences acute metabolic stress, signalling protein activation and gene expression are similar for interval and continuous exercise, despite differences in intensity. There is evidence that exercise intensity is the most important variable to consider for increasing mitochondrial content (71), with others arguing against this perspective (8). Increases in the abundance of proteins related to substrate transport, storage, and oxidation, as well as skeletal muscle capillarization, are generally similar across interval and continuous protocols, although there are limited studies to consider. That many variables respond similarly to MICT, HIIT, and SIT could indicate different forms of metabolic stress lead to similar skeletal muscle adaptations. To better resolve differences between interval and continuous training, we suggest that (1) more studies comparing cellular adaptations between interval and continuous training are needed, (2) more attention needs to be paid to extraneous factors that could influence cellular adaptations, (3) the relationship between acute signals and cellular adaptations may be more complex than currently recognized (77), and (4) technical errors in measurement hinder comparisons of cellular adaptations across protocols, particularly for between-participant designs. Studies employing larger sample sizes may also help resolve the influence of interval training, relative to MICT, on cellular adaptations to exercise.

Future Questions

While the amount of research related to interval training continues to grow rapidly (Figure 11.1), there are still many unanswered questions. We suggest several topics for future research.

The Influence of Continuity on Mitochondrial Adaptations to Interval Exercise

One could hypothesize that the intermittent nature of interval exercise, not the higher exercise intensity, is responsible for the augmented molecular responses to acute sessions of interval training. Combes et al. (21) tested this hypothesis by comparing 30 min of continuous exercise to exercise at the same intensity that was separated into 30 × 1-min intervals. These authors reported greater phosphorylation of AMPK, p38 MAPK, and CaMKII in response to the intermittent exercise. However, whether these results were related to the intermittent nature of the exercise per se—as opposed to the intermittent and potentially large effort needed to restart the flywheel at the beginning of each interval or the extended total duration of the exercise session —was not addressed. Regardless, it is unknown whether breaking MICT into intervals would influence changes in mitochondrial content, and future studies should examine the potential for "moderate-intensity interval training" to improve mitochondrial content relative to MICT.

Rather than directly augmenting mitochondrial adaptations to exercise, the intermittent nature of interval training may be important because it permits higher intensities of exercise to be performed relative to continuous training. Cochran et al. (18) compared the acute signalling response elicited by a typical SIT session to a work-matched continuous effort lasting ~4 min (i.e., half the average intensity but twice the duration of four repeated Wingate tests). In that study, the two protocols elicited similar phosphorylation of p38 MAPK and ACC and similar increases in *PGC-1α* gene expression. However, whereas the SIT protocol used in that experiment typically increases CS activity (13, 14), Cochran et al. (18) reported no change in CS activity in response to the brief, high-intensity continuous protocol when it was performed three times per week for 6 weeks. A recent study from MacInnis et al. (72) confirmed that six sessions of a typical HIIT protocol increased CS activity, but that six sessions involving a single 5-min bout of continuous high-intensity exercise did not (72). Collectively, this pair of studies suggests that when the total amount of work performed is low, dividing the exercise into intervals to permit greater intensities (as with SIT) seems necessary for increasing mitochondrial content. However, given the acute data from Combes et al. (21), additional research is warranted to clarify the relative importance of the intermittent nature of interval training.

Sex-Based Differences

A few studies have found sex-specific cellular responses to interval training. A SIT protocol involving 3 × 30-sec sprints interspersed with 20 min of recovery decreased glycogen content and increased blood lactate, plasma catecholamines, and ATP breakdown products (e.g., inosine) to a greater extent in males compared to females (30). However, the authors also found no sex-specific changes in [ATP], [ADP], [IMP], or [PCr] during each 30-sec sprint but did report a faster recovery of [ATP] during recovery periods in females vs. males (30). In contrast, other studies have found no sex-based differences in glycogen content, the response of signalling proteins, or the mRNA expression of *PGC-1α* following interval training (98, 104).

Some chronic responses to short-term interval training are reported to be greater in males relative to females. Specifically, males have demonstrated greater improvements in the protein content of GLUT4 and the maximal activity of β-HAD (38) and elevated rates of muscle protein synthesis and mitochondrial biogenesis (92) over short-term SIT compared to females. Despite the observed higher rates of mitochondrial biogenesis in males (92), SIT increased markers of mitochondrial content to a similar extent in men and women (38, 92). Another investigation found interval training–induced increases in type II fibre cross-sectional area and muscle glycogen in females but not males (31). Discrepancies regarding whether sex-based differences exist in cellular responses to interval training may be related to differences in the initial fitness level of the groups of males and females studied. Studies investigating potential sex-specific cellular adaptations to interval training while controlling for potential confounding factors, including baseline cardiorespiratory fitness and menstrual cycle phase timing, in larger cohorts of males and females are warranted.

Fibre Type–Specific Adaptations

One hypothesis for how interval training elicits comparable adaptations to MICT is by greater recruitment and remodelling of type II fibres as a result of the inherent higher exercise intensity. In support of this hypothesis, glycogen depletion and the phosphorylation of AMPK and ACC were greater in type IIa compared to type I fibres following a single session of HIIT (61, 104), whereas work-matched MICT did not induce a differential response across fibre types (61). In contrast to these divergent initial fibre type–specific responses, work-matched SIT and MICT elicited comparable increases in the mRNA expression of *PGC-1α* in type I and II fibres (107). Acute fibre type–specific comparisons of low-volume SIT vs. MICT are limited. One study showed similar fibre type–specific glycogen depletion and no changes in the phosphorylation of AMPK in either fibre type following low-volume SIT and MICT (95).

A few studies have compared fibre type–specific adaptations across different protocols. Work-matched HIIT and MICT did not change type I or IIa COXIV protein content over 2 weeks (73); however, longer, low-volume SIT and MICT comparisons demonstrated similar increases in COX or SDH activity within both fibre types (95–97). Scribbans et al. (95) found that 6 weeks of low-volume SIT increased α-glycerophosphate dehydrogenase, a marker of glycolytic potential, to a similar extent in type I fibres and a greater extent in type IIa fibres compared to MICT. There is also some evidence of divergent fibre type–specific responses when SIT is added to a MICT protocol. For example, an 8-week period of combined SIT and MICT increased the protein content of CS in type II, but not type I, fibres, whereas the MICT protocol did not elicit changes in either fibre type (45).

Overall, there is limited and conflicting evidence for whether interval training elicits superior responses in type II fibres compared to MICT. Additional investigations that examine responses in type IIx fibres and compare fibre type–specific adaptations between MICT and low-volume SIT or work-matched HIIT over longer periods of training may provide greater insight into this area of research.

Novel Mechanisms Involved in Mitochondrial Biogenesis

While the earlier sections described the general process through which the stress of exercise is transduced into signals to promote mitochondrial biogenesis (Figure 11.3), other processes have been proposed. Firstly, Place et al. (83) demonstrated that a single session of SIT caused fragmentation of the ryanodine receptor 1 protein (RYR1) 24 hours post-exercise. The authors suggested that this fragmentation leads to elevated Ca^{2+} leak from the sarcoplasmic reticulum, signalling the activation of mitochondrial biogenesis. Additional experiments demonstrated that this response was reactive oxygen species (ROS)–dependent and that well-trained humans did not demonstrate RYR1 fragmentation following a bout of SIT, potentially due to a greater abundance of endogenous antioxidant proteins (83). This result was further supported by Schlittler et al. (94), who reported decreased fragmentation following 3 weeks of SIT. Another potential ROS-dependent mechanism for exercise training–induced mitochondrial biogenesis was described by Larsen et al. (63). The authors' findings suggested that ROS-induced inactivation of aconitase contributed to SIT-induced increases in mitochondrial content. Although these mechanisms are intriguing, as they potentially explain the potency of SIT for increasing the oxidative capacity of skeletal muscle, future studies should investigate whether these mechanisms are specific to SIT or have a more general role in regulating mitochondrial adaptations to exercise: Do HIIT and MICT increase mitochondrial content through these mechanisms?

Conclusion

Interval training is a popular and effective method to increase exercise performance in humans, and many varieties of interval training have been examined. Overall, responses to HIIT and SIT are highly similar to traditional endurance training (i.e., MICT). In skeletal muscle, higher exercise intensities induce greater acute metabolic stress, which translates into greater activation of the mitochondrial biogenesis pathway. HIIT and SIT induce similar or greater protein signalling and gene expression responses compared to MICT, leading to similar or greater increases in skeletal muscle mitochondrial content. The abundance of proteins related to the transport, storage, and oxidation of substrates and skeletal muscle capillarization increase similarly across protocols. Improving our basic understanding of the mechanisms regulating cellular responses to exercise may expose the mechanisms through which interval training improves skeletal muscle fitness; however, increasing sample sizes and reducing technical and confounding errors will also help advance this field. In an effort to better understand the efficacy of interval training relative to MICT, we suggest that future research consider the impact of other training variables and molecular mechanisms, as well as the extent to which adaptations to interval training are sex- and fibre type–dependent.

References

1. Astrand I, Astrand PO, Christensen EH, Hedman R. Intermittent muscular work. *Acta Physiol Scand* 48: 448–453, 1960.
2. Baekkerud FH, Solberg F, Leinan IM, Wisloff U, Karlsen T, Rognmo O. Comparison of three popular exercise modalities on VO2max in overweight and obese. *Med Sci Sport Exerc* 48: 491–498, 2016.
3. Bangsbo J, Nielsen JJ, Mohr M, Randers MB, Krustrup BR, Brito J, et al. Performance enhancements and muscular adaptations of a 16-week recreational football intervention for untrained women. *Scand J Med Sci Sport* 20 Suppl 1: 24–30, 2010.
4. Barres R, Yan J, Egan B, Treebak JT, Rasmussen M, Fritz T, et al. Acute exercise remodels promoter methylation in human skeletal muscle. *Cell Metab* 15: 405–411, 2012.
5. Bartlett JD, Hwa Joo C, Jeong TS, Louhelainen J, Cochran AJ, Gibala MJ, et al. Matched work high-intensity interval and continuous running induce similar increases in PGC-1α mRNA, AMPK, p38, and p53 phosphorylation in human skeletal muscle. *J Appl Physiol* 112: 1135–1143, 2012.
6. Bell KE, Séguin C, Parise G, Baker SK, Phillips SM. Day-to-day changes in muscle protein synthesis in recovery from resistance, aerobic, and high- intensity interval exercise in older men. *J Gerontol A Biol Sci Med Sci* 70: 1024–1029, 2015.
7. Billat LV. Interval training for performance: a scientific and empirical practice. Special recommendations for middle- and long-distance running. Part I: aerobic interval training. *Sport Med* 31: 13–31, 2001.
8. Bishop DJ, Botella J, Granata C. CrossTalk opposing view: exercise training volume is more important than training intensity to promote increases in mitochondrial content. *J Physiol* 597: 4115–4118, 2019.
9. Bradley H, Shaw CS, Worthington PL, Shepherd SO, Cocks M, Wagenmakers AJM. Quantitative immunofluorescence microscopy of subcellular GLUT4 distribution in human skeletal muscle: effects of endurance and sprint interval training. *Physiol Rep* 2: e12085, 2014.
10. Buchheit M, Laursen PB. High-intensity interval training, solutions to the programming puzzle: part I: cardiopulmonary emphasis. *Sport Med* 43: 313–338, 2013.
11. Burgomaster KA, Cermak NM, Phillips SM, Benton CR, Bonen A, Gibala MJ. Divergent response of metabolite transport proteins in human skeletal muscle after sprint interval training and detraining. *Am J Physiol* 292: R1970–R1976, 2007.
12. Burgomaster KA, Heigenhauser GJ, Gibala MJ. Effect of short-term sprint interval training on human skeletal muscle carbohydrate metabolism during exercise and time-trial performance. *J Appl Physiol* 100: 2041–2047, 2006.
13. Burgomaster KA, Howarth KR, Phillips SM, Rakobowchuk M, Macdonald MJ, McGee SL, et al. Similar metabolic adaptations during exercise after low volume sprint interval and traditional endurance training in humans. *J Physiol* 586: 151–160, 2008.
14. Burgomaster KA, Hughes SC, Heigenhauser GJ, Bradwell SN, Gibala MJ. Six sessions of sprint interval training increases muscle oxidative potential and cycle endurance capacity in humans. *J Appl Physiol* 98: 1985–1990, 2005.
15. Cheetham ME, Boobis LH, Brooks S, Williams C. Human muscle metabolism during sprint running. *J Appl Physiol* 61: 54–60, 1986.
16. Chen Z, Stephens TJ, Murthy S, Canny BJ, Hargreaves M, Witters LA, et al. Effect of exercise intensity on skeletal muscle AMPK signaling in humans. *Diabetes* 52: 2205–2212, 2003.

17. Christensen EH, Hedman R, Saltin B. Intermittent and continuous running. (a further contribution to the physiology of intermittent work.). *Acta Physiol Scand* 50: 269–286, 1960.

18. Cochran AJ, Percival ME, Tricarico S, Little JP, Cermak N, Gillen JB, et al. Intermittent and continuous high-intensity exercise training induce similar acute but different chronic muscle adaptations. *Exp Physiol* 99: 782–791, 2014.

19. Cocks M, Shaw CS, Shepherd SO, Fisher JP, Ranasinghe A, Barker TA, et al. Sprint interval and moderate-intensity continuous training have equal benefits on aerobic capacity, insulin sensitivity, muscle capillarisation and endothelial eNOS/NAD(P)Hoxidase protein ratio in obese men. *J Physiol* 594: 2307–21, 2016.

20. Cocks M, Shaw CS, Shepherd SO, Fisher JP, Ranasinghe AM, Barker TA, et al. Sprint interval and endurance training are equally effective in increasing muscle microvascular density and eNOS content in sedentary males. *J Physiol* 591: 641–656, 2013.

21. Combes A, Dekerle J, Webborn N, Watt P, Bougault V, Daussin FN. Exercise-induced metabolic fluctuations influence AMPK, p38-MAPK and CaMKII phosphorylation in human skeletal muscle. *Physiol Rep* 3: e12462, 2015.

22. Coyle EF, Feltner ME, Kautz SA, Hamilton MT, Montain SJ, Baylor AM, et al. Physiological and biomechanical factors associated with elite endurance cycling performance. *Med Sci Sport Exerc* 23: 93–107, 1991.

23. Daussin FN, Zoll J, Dufour SP, Ponsot E, Lonsdorfer-Wolf E, Doutreleau S, et al. Effect of interval versus continuous training on cardiorespiratory and mitochondrial functions: relationship to aerobic performance improvements in sedentary subjects. *Am J Physiol* 295: R264–R272, 2008.

24. Davies KJA, Packer L, Brooks GA. Biochemical adaptation of mitochondria, muscle, and whole-animal respiration to endurance training. *Arch Biochem Biophys* 209: 539–554, 1981.

25. Davies MJ, Benson AP, Cannon DT, Marwood S, Kemp GJ, Rossiter HB, et al. Dissociating external power from intramuscular exercise intensity during intermittent bilateral knee-extension in humans. *J Physiol* 595: 6673–6686, 2017.

26. Di Donato DM, West DW, Churchward-Venne TA, Breen L, Baker SK, Phillips SM. Influence of aerobic exercise intensity on myofibrillar and mitochondrial protein synthesis in young men during early and late postexercise recovery. *Am J Physiol* 306: E1025–E1032, 2014.

27. Egan B, Carson BP, Garcia-Roves PM, Chibalin AV, Sarsfield FM, Barron N, et al. Exercise intensity-dependent regulation of peroxisome proliferator-activated receptor coactivator-1 mRNA abundance is associated with differential activation of upstream signalling kinases in human skeletal muscle. *J Physiol* 588: 1779–1790, 2010.

28. Egan B, O'Connor PL, Zierath JR, O'Gorman DJ. Time course analysis reveals gene-specific transcript and protein kinetics of adaptation to short-term aerobic exercise training in human skeletal muscle. *PLoS One* 8: e74098, 2013.

29. Egan B, Zierath JR. Exercise metabolism and the molecular regulation of skeletal muscle adaptation. *Cell Metab* 17: 162–184, 2013.

30. Esbjörnsson-Liljedahl M, Bodin K, Jansson E. Smaller muscle ATP reduction in women than in men by repeated bouts of sprint exercise. *J Appl Physiol* 93: 1075–1083, 2002.

31. Esbjörnsson Liljedahl M, Holm I, Sylven C, Jansson E. Different responses of skeletal muscle following sprint training in men and women. *Eur J Appl Physiol Occup Physiol* 74: 375–383, 1996.

32. Faiss R, Léger B, Vesin JM, Fournier PE, Eggel Y, Dériaz O, et al. Significant molecular and systemic adaptations after repeated sprint training in hypoxia. *PLOS ONE* 8: e56522, 2013.

33. Fiorenza M, Gunnarsson TP, Hostrup M, Iaia FM, Schena F, Pilegaard H, et al. Metabolic stress-dependent regulation of the mitochondrial biogenic molecular response to high-intensity exercise in human skeletal muscle. *J Physiol* 596: 2823–2840, 2018.

34. Gibala MJ, Little JP, van Essen M, Wilkin GP, Burgomaster KA, Safdar A, et al. Short-term sprint interval versus traditional endurance training: similar initial adaptations in human skeletal muscle and exercise performance. *J Physiol* 575: 901–911, 2006.

35. Gibala MJ, McGee SL, Garnham AP, Howlett KF, Snow RJ, Hargreaves M. Brief intense interval exercise activates AMPK and p38 MAPK signaling and increases the expression of PGC-1α in human skeletal muscle. *J Appl Physiol* 106: 929–934, 2009.

36. Gillen JB, Martin BJ, MacInnis MJ, Skelly LE, Tarnopolsky MA, Gibala MJ. Twelve weeks of sprint interval training improves indices of cardiometabolic health similar to traditional endurance training despite a five-fold lower exercise volume and time commitment. *PLOS ONE* 11: e0154075, 2016.

37. Gillen JB, Percival ME, Ludzki A, Tarnopolsky MA, Gibala MJ. Interval training in the fed or fasted state improves body composition and muscle oxidative capacity in overweight women. *Obesity* 21: 2249–2255, 2013.

38. Gillen JB, Percival ME, Skelly LE, Martin BJ, Tan RB, Tarnopolsky MA, et al. Three minutes of all-out intermittent exercise per week increases skeletal muscle oxidative capacity and improves cardiometabolic health. *PLoS One* 9: e111489, 2014.

39. Girard O, Mendez-Villanueva A, Bishop D. Repeated-sprint ability – Part I. *Sport Med* 41: 673–694, 2011.

40. Gliemann L. Training for skeletal muscle capillarization: a Janus-faced role of exercise intensity? *Eur J Appl Physiol* 116: 1443–1444, 2016.

41. Granata C, Jamnick NA, Bishop DJ. Principles of exercise prescription, and how they influence exercise-induced changes of transcription factors and other regulators of mitochondrial biogenesis. *Sport Med* 48: 1541–1559, 2018.

42. Granata C, Oliveira RS, Little JP, Renner K, Bishop DJ. Training intensity modulates changes in PGC-1α and p53 protein content and mitochondrial respiration, but not markers of mitochondrial content in human skeletal muscle. *FASEB J* 30: 959–970, 2016.

43. Granata C, Oliveira RSF, Little JP, Renner K, Bishop DJ. Sprint-interval but not continuous exercise increases PGC-1α protein content and p53 phosphorylation in nuclear fractions of human skeletal muscle. *Sci Rep* 7: 44227, 2017.

44. Green HJ, Burnett M, Carter S, Jacobs I, Ranney D, Smith I, et al. Role of exercise duration on metabolic adaptations in working muscle to short-term moderate-to-heavy aerobic-based cycle training. *Eur J Appl Physiol* 113: 1965–1978, 2013.

45. Gunnarsson TP, Brandt N, Fiorenza M, Hostrup M, Pilegaard H, Bangsbo J. Inclusion of sprints in moderate intensity continuous training leads to muscle oxidative adaptations in trained individuals. *Physiol Rep* 7: e13976, 2019.

46. Harber MP, Fry AC, Rubin MR, Smith JC, Weiss LW. Skeletal muscle and hormonal adaptations to circuit weight training in untrained men. *Scand J Med Sci Sport* 14: 176–185, 2004.

47. Hawley JA, Hargreaves M, Joyner MJ, Zierath JR. Integrative biology of exercise. *Cell* 159: 738–749, 2014.

48. Hawley JA, Lundby C, Cotter JD, Burke LM. Maximizing cellular adaptation to endurance exercise in skeletal muscle. *Cell Metab* 27: 962–976, 2018.

49. Helgerud J, Hoydal K, Wang E, Karlsen T, Berg P, Bjerkaas M, et al. Aerobic high-intensity intervals improve VO2max more than moderate training. *Med Sci Sport Exerc* 39: 665–671, 2007.

50. Hellsten Y, Nyberg M. Cardiovascular adaptations to exercise training. *Compr Physiol* 6: 1–32, 2016.

51. Henriksson J, Reitman JS. Quantitative measures of enzyme activities in type I and type II muscle fibres of man after training. *Acta Physiol Scand* 97: 392–397, 1976.

52. Hoier B, Passos M, Bangsbo J, Hellsten Y. Intense intermittent exercise provides weak stimulus for vascular endothelial growth factor secretion and capillary growth in skeletal muscle. *Exp Physiol* 98: 585–597, 2013.

53. Holloszy JO. Biochemical adaptations in muscle. Effects of exercise on mitochondrial oxygen uptake and respiratory enzyme activity in skeletal muscle. *J Biol Chem* 242: 2278–2282, 1967.

54. Holloszy JO. Adaptation of skeletal muscle to endurance exercise. *Med Sci Sport* 7: 155–164, 1975.

55. Holloszy JO, Coyle EF. Adaptations of skeletal-muscle to endurance exercise and their metabolic consequences. *J Appl Physiol* 56: 831–838, 1984.

56. Hood DA, Memme JM, Oliveira AN, Triolo M. Maintenance of skeletal muscle mitochondria in health, exercise, and aging. *Annu Rev Physiol* 81: 19–41, 2019.

57. Howlett RA, Parolin ML, Dyck DJ, Hultman E, Jones NL, Heigenhauser GJF, et al. Regulation of skeletal muscle glycogen phosphorylase and PDH at varying exercise power outputs. *Am J Physiol* 275: R418–R425, 1998.

58. Jacobs I, Esbjornsson M, Sylven C, Ingemar H, Jansson E. Sprint training effects on muscle myoglobin, enzymes, fiber types, and blood lactate. *Med Sci Sport Exerc* 19: 368–374, 1987.

59. Jacobs RA, Fluck D, Bonne TC, Burgi S, Christensen PM, Toigo M, et al. Improvements in exercise performance with high-intensity interval training coincide with an increase in skeletal muscle mitochondrial content and function. *J Appl Physiol* 115: 785–793, 2013.

60. Jensen L, Bangsbo J, Hellsten Y. Effect of high intensity training on capillarization and presence of angiogenic factors in human skeletal muscle. *J Physiol* 557: 571–582, 2004.

61. Kristensen DE, Albers PH, Prats C, Baba O, Birk JB, Wojtaszewski JFP. Human muscle fibre type-specific regulation of AMPK and downstream targets by exercise. *J Physiol* 593: 2053–2069, 2015.

62. Krustrup P, Christensen JF, Randers MB, Pedersen H, Sundstrup E, Jakobsen MD, et al. Muscle adaptations and performance enhancements of soccer training for untrained men. *Eur J Appl Physiol* 108: 1247–1258, 2010.

63. Larsen FJ, Schiffer TA, Ortenblad N, Zinner C, Morales-Alamo D, Willis SJ, et al. High-intensity sprint training inhibits mitochondrial respiration through aconitase inactivation. *FASEB J* 30: 417–427, 2016.

64. Larsen S, Nielsen J, Hansen CN, Nielsen LB, Wibrand F, Stride N, et al. Biomarkers of mitochondrial content in skeletal muscle of healthy young human subjects. *J Physiol* 590: 3349–3360, 2012.

65. Linossier MT, Dormois D, Perier C, Frey J, Geyssant A, Denis C. Enzyme adaptations of human skeletal muscle during bicycle short-sprint training and detraining. *Acta Physiol Scand* 161: 439–445, 1997.

66. Little JP, Gillen JB, Percival ME, Safdar A, Tarnopolsky MA, Punthakee Z, et al. Low-volume high-intensity interval training reduces hyperglycemia and increases muscle mitochondrial capacity in patients with type 2 diabetes. *J Appl Physiol* 111: 1554–1560, 2011.

67. Little JP, Safdar A, Bishop D, Tarnopolsky MA, Gibala MJ. An acute bout of high-intensity interval training increases the nuclear abundance of PGC-1α and activates mitochondrial biogenesis in human skeletal muscle. *Am J Physiol* 300: R1303–R1310, 2011.

68. Little JP, Safdar A, Wilkin GP, Tarnopolsky MA, Gibala MJ. A practical model of low-volume high-intensity interval training induces mitochondrial biogenesis in human skeletal muscle: potential mechanisms. *J Physiol* 588: 1011–1022, 2010.

69. Macdougall JD, Hicks AL, Macdonald JR, Mckelvie RS, Green HJ, Smith KM. Muscle performance and enzymatic adaptations to sprint interval training. *J Appl Physiol* 84: 2138–2142, 1998.

70. MacInnis MJ, Gibala MJ. Physiological adaptations to interval training and the role of exercise intensity. *J Physiol* 595: 2915–2930, 2017.

71. MacInnis MJ, Skelly LE, Gibala MJ. CrossTalk proposal: exercise training intensity is more important than volume to promote increases in human skeletal muscle mitochondrial content. *J Physiol* 597: 4111–4113, 2019.

72. MacInnis MJ, Skelly LE, Godkin FE, Martin BJ, Tripp TR, Tarnopolsky MA, et al. The effect of short-term, high-intensity exercise training on human skeletal muscle citrate synthase maximal activity: single versus multiple bouts per session. *Appl Physiol Nutr Metab* 1394: 1391–1394, 2019.

73. MacInnis MJ, Zacharewicz E, Martin BJ, Haikalis ME, Skelly LE, Tarnopolsky MA, et al. Superior mitochondrial adaptations in human skeletal muscle after interval compared to continuous single-leg cycling matched for total work. *J Physiol* 595: 2955–2968, 2017.

74. McRae G, Payne A, Zelt JG, Scribbans TD, Jung ME, Little JP, et al. Extremely low volume, whole-body aerobic-resistance training improves aerobic fitness and muscular endurance in females. *Appl Physiol Nutr Metab* 37: 1124–1131, 2012.

75. Metcalfe RS, Koumanov F, Ruffino JS, Stokes KA, Holman GD, Thompson D, et al. Physiological and molecular responses to an acute bout of reduced-exertion high-intensity interval training (REHIT). *Eur J Appl Physiol* 115: 2321–2334, 2015.

76. Miller BF, Hamilton KL. A perspective on the determination of mitochondrial biogenesis. *Am J Physiol* 302: E496-9, 2012.

77. Miller BF, Konopka AR, Hamilton KL. The rigorous study of exercise adaptations: why mRNA might not be enough. *J Appl Physiol* 121: 594–596, 2016.

78. Morgan TE, Cobb LA, Short FA, Ross R, Gunn DR. Effects of long-term exercise on human muscle mitochondria. In: *Muscle Metabolism During Exercise*. Boston, MA: Springer, 1971, p. 87–95.

79. Parker L, Trewin A, Levinger I, Shaw CS, Stepto NK. The effect of exercise-intensity on skeletal muscle stress kinase and insulin protein signaling. *PLOS ONE* 12: e0171613, 2017.

80. Parolin ML, Chesley A, Matsos MP, Spriet LL, Jones NL, Heigenhauser GJ. Regulation of skeletal muscle glycogen phosphorylase and PDH during maximal intermittent exercise. *Am J Physiol* 277: E890–E900, 1999.

81. Perry CG, Heigenhauser GJ, Bonen A, Spriet LL. High-intensity aerobic interval training increases fat and carbohydrate metabolic capacities in human skeletal muscle. *Appl Physiol Nutr Metab* 33: 1112–1123, 2008.

82. Perry CG, Lally J, Holloway GP, Heigenhauser GJ, Bonen A, Spriet LL. Repeated transient mRNA bursts precede increases in transcriptional and mitochondrial proteins during training in human skeletal muscle. *J Physiol* 588: 4795–4810, 2010.

83. Place N, Ivarsson N, Venckunas T, Neyroud D, Brazaitis M, Cheng AJ, et al. Ryanodine receptor fragmentation and sarcoplasmic reticulum Ca2+ leak after one session of high-intensity interval exercise. *Proc Natl Acad Sci U S A* 112: 15492–15497, 2015.

84. Poole DC, Burnley M, Vanhatalo A, Rossiter HB, Jones AM. Critical power: an important fatigue threshold in exercise physiology. *Med Sci Sport Exerc* 48: 2320–2334, 2016.

85. Psilander N, Wang L, Westergren J, Tonkonogi M, Sahlin K. Mitochondrial gene expression in elite cyclists: effects of high-intensity interval exercise. *Eur J Appl Physiol* 110: 597–606, 2010.

86. Raleigh JP, Giles MD, Islam H, Nelms M, Bentley RF, Jones JH, et al. Contribution of central and peripheral adaptations to changes in maximal oxygen uptake following 4 weeks of sprint interval training. *Appl Physiol Nutr Metab* 1068: 1059–1068, 2018.

87. Rodas G, Ventura JL, Cadefau JA, Cussó R, Parra J. A short training programme for the rapid improvement of both aerobic and anaerobic metabolism. *Eur J Appl Physiol* 82: 480–486, 2000.

88. Rose AJ, Kiens B, Richter EA. Ca2+-calmodulin-dependent protein kinase expression and signalling in skeletal muscle during exercise. *J Physiol* 574: 889–903, 2006.

89. Sahlin K, Broberg S, Ren JM. Formation of inosine monophosphate (IMP) in human skeletal muscle during incremental dynamic exercise. *Acta Physiol Scand* 136: 193–198, 1989.

90. Sahlin K, Katz A, Henriksson J. Redox state and lactate accumulation in human skeletal muscle during dynamic exercise. *Biochem J* 245: 551–556, 1987.

91. Sahlin K, Tonkonogi M, Söderlund K. Energy supply and muscle fatigue in humans. *Acta Physiol Scand* 162: 261–266, 1998.

92. Scalzo RL, Peltonen GL, Binns SE, Shankaran M, Giordano GR, Hartley DA, et al. Greater muscle protein synthesis and mitochondrial biogenesis in males compared with females during sprint interval training. *FASEB J* 28: 2705–2714, 2014.

93. Schantz P, Henriksson J, Jansson E. Adaptation of human skeletal muscle to endurance training of long duration. *Clin Physiol* 3: 141–151, 1983.

94. Schlittler M, Neyroud D, Tanga C, Zanou N, Kamandulis S, Skurvydas A, et al. Three weeks of sprint interval training improved high-intensity cycling performance and limited ryanodine receptor modifications in recreationally active human subjects. *Eur J Appl Physiol* 119: 1951–1958, 2019.

95. Scribbans TD, Edgett BA, Vorobej K, Mitchell AS, Joanisse SD, Matusiak JB, et al. Fibre-specific responses to endurance and low volume high intensity interval training: striking similarities in acute and chronic adaptation. *PLOS ONE* 9: e98119, 2014.

96. Shepherd SO, Cocks M, Meikle PJ, Mellett NA, Ranasinghe AM, Barker TA, et al. Lipid droplet remodelling and reduced muscle ceramides following sprint interval and moderate-intensity continuous exercise training in obese males. *Int J Obes* 41: 1745–1754, 2017.

97. Shepherd SO, Cocks M, Tipton KD, Ranasinghe AM, Barker TA, Burniston JG, et al. Sprint interval and traditional endurance training increase net intramuscular triglyceride breakdown and expression of perilipin 2 and 5. *J Physiol* 591: 657–675, 2013.

98. Skelly LE, Gillen JB, MacInnis MJ, Martin BJ, Safdar A, Akhtar M, et al. Effect of sex on the acute skeletal muscle response to sprint interval exercise. *Exp Physiol* 102: 354–365, 2017.

99. Søgaard D, Baranowski M, Larsen S, Taulo Lund M, Munk Scheuer C, Vestergaard Abildskov C, et al. Muscle-saturated bioactive lipids are increased with aging and influenced by high-intensity interval training. *Int J Mol Sci* 20: E1240, 2019.

100. Tabata I, Nishimura K, Kouzaki M, Hirai Y, Ogita F, Miyachi M, et al. Effects of moderate-intensity endurance and high-intensity intermittent training on anaerobic capacity and VO(2max). *Med Sci Sports Exerc* 28: 1327–1330, 1996.

101. Talanian JL, Galloway SD, Heigenhauser GJ, Bonen A, Spriet LL. Two weeks of high-intensity aerobic interval training increases the capacity for fat oxidation during exercise in women. *J Appl Physiol* 102: 1439–1447, 2007.

102. Thompson WR. Worldwide survey of fitness trends for 2020. *ACSM's Heal Fit J* 23: 10–18, 2019.

103. Tjonna AE, Lee SJ, Rognmo O, Stolen TO, Bye A, Haram PM, et al. Aerobic interval training versus continuous moderate exercise as a treatment for the metabolic syndrome: a pilot study. *Circulation* 118: 346–354, 2008.

104. Tobias IS, Lazauskas KK, Siu J, Costa PB, Coburn JW, Galpin AJ. Sex and fiber type independently influence AMPK, TBC1D1, and TBC1D4 at rest and during recovery from high-intensity exercise in humans. *J Appl Physiol* 128: 350–361, 2020.

105. Trewin AJ, Parker L, Shaw CS, Hiam DS, Garnham A, Levinger I, et al. Acute HIIE elicits similar changes in human skeletal muscle mitochondrial H2O2 release, respiration, and cell signaling as endurance exercise even with less work. *Am J Physiol* 315: R1003–R1016, 2018.

106. Wang L, Psilander N, Tonkonogi M, Ding S, Sahlin K. Similar expression of oxidative genes after interval and continuous exercise. *Med Sci Sport Exerc* 41: 2136–2144, 2009.

107. Wang L, Sahlin K. The effect of continuous and interval exercise on PGC-1α and PDK4 mRNA in type I and type II fibres of human skeletal muscle. *Acta Physiol* 204: 525–532, 2012.

108. Weston KS, Wisloff U, Coombes JS. High-intensity interval training in patients with lifestyle-induced cardiometabolic disease: a systematic review and meta-analysis. *Br J Sport Med* 48: 1227–1234, 2014.

109. Wilkinson SB, Phillips SM, Atherton PJ, Patel R, Yarasheski KE, Tarnopolsky MA, et al. Differential effects of resistance and endurance exercise in the fed state on signalling molecule phosphorylation and protein synthesis in human muscle. *J Physiol* 586: 3701–3717, 2008.

110. Winder WW, Wilson HA, Hardie DG, Rasmussen BB, Hutber CA, Call GB, et al. Phosphorylation of rat muscle acetyl-CoA carboxylase by AMP-activated protein kinase and protein kinase A. *J Appl Physiol* 82: 219–225, 1997.

111. Wisloff U, Stoylen A, Loennechen JP, Bruvold M, Rognmo O, Haram PM, et al. Superior cardiovascular effect of aerobic interval training versus moderate continuous training in heart failure patients: a randomized study. *Circulation* 115: 3086–3094, 2007.

112. Wojtaszewski JFPF, Nielsen P, Hansen BFF, Richter EAA, Kiens B. Isoform-specific and exercise intensity-dependent activation of 5'-AMP-activated protein kinase in human skeletal muscle. *J Physiol* 528: 221–226, 2000.

113. Wyckelsma VL, Levinger I, McKenna MJ, Formosa LE, Ryan MT, Petersen AC, et al. Preservation of skeletal muscle mitochondrial content in older adults: relationship between mitochondria, fibre type and high-intensity exercise training. *J Physiol* 595: 3345–3359, 2017.

12

REGULATION OF MUSCLE SATELLITE CELL ACTIVATION AND CYCLES CONSEQUENT TO VARIOUS FORMS OF TRAINING

Sophie Joanisse and Gianni Parise

Introduction

Skeletal muscle accounts for approximately 30–40% of total body weight in men and women and plays an indispensable role in force generation, movement, and posture maintenance, ultimately enabling physical activity. It is also a highly metabolically active tissue and serves as the largest reservoir for the storage of amino acids, which are utilized to support the health of all other organs and to maintain blood glucose levels during times of stress in addition to serving as the main source of glucose disposal. A core characteristic of skeletal muscle is its ability to adapt to stimuli. Adaptation, for the purposes of this chapter, can be broadly defined as a change in structure and function in response to a specific stimulus. For instance, resistance exercise training is characterized by an increase in skeletal muscle mass and muscle fibre size, which occurs to counter the mechanical stress of heavy loads, whereas aerobic exercise training is characterized by metabolic alterations such as increased mitochondrial content and function and improved fuel selection (greater reliance on fat oxidation), rendering the skeletal muscle more resistant to fatigue. Additionally, skeletal muscle is composed of oxidative, slow-twitch, fatigue-resistant type I fibres and glycolytic, fast-twitch type II fibres more susceptible to fatigue (50). Specific exercise stimuli can result in a differential recruitment pattern of muscle fibres leading to different fibre type–specific adaptations, thus emphasizing the importance of fibre type–specific analyses. Even though skeletal muscle can respond to a plethora of stimuli, it is important to note that this tissue is post-mitotic, meaning that myofibres are unable to undergo cell division. Although myonuclei are able to alter their transcriptional activity to support adaption to a certain extent, it is believed that muscle-specific stem cells, commonly referred to as satellite cells (SCs), play an important role in mediating some of these adaptations. The following sections will describe the effects of various forms of exercise training on SC content in skeletal muscle and how exercise training can alter the acute response of SCs to a stimulus.

Satellite Cell Biology

Muscle stem cells were first identified by Mauro in 1960 (38). These cells were termed *satellite cells* due to their anatomical location on the periphery of the muscle fibre, specifically between the basal lamina and the sarcolemma (Figure 12.1). In healthy adults, SCs are typically maintained in a state of quiescence; however, following exposure to appropriate cues such as signals released as a result of injury or muscle contraction, SCs can activate, proliferate, and terminally differentiate, fusing with existing fibres, while a subset of activated cells can revert to a quiescent state to maintain a basal pool of SCs (53). The process

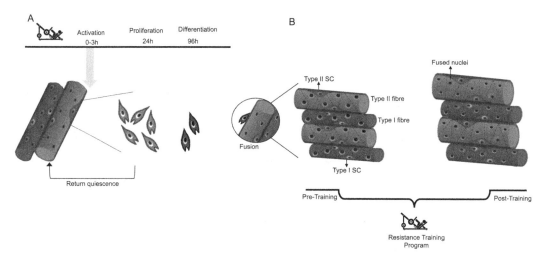

Figure 12.1 A schematic representation of (A) the acute response of SCs to a bout of resistance exercise and (B) the impact of resistance exercise training on SC content

of activation through to terminal differentiation is termed myogenesis, or the myogenic programme, and is governed by the up- and down-regulation of the paired box transcription factor Pax7 and a transcriptional network collectively referred to as the myogenic regulatory factors (MRFs) (55). Myogenic commitment of SCs is indicated by the up-regulation of myogenic factor 5 (Myf5), while activation and proliferation are indicated by the up-regulation of myoblast determination protein 1 (MyoD) (6–8, 20, 57). Following proliferation, if Pax7 remains up-regulated, cells will revert to quiescence, promoting self-renewal and replenishing the basal SC pool, whereas if Pax7 is down-regulated, with a simultaneous up-regulation of MRF4 and myogenin, SCs progress through the myogenic programme and terminally differentiate (46, 57).

SCs have been extensively studied in the context of skeletal muscle growth and regeneration using rodent models in vivo; however, extending these results to humans has proven to be challenging. In human models, SCs are often studied in an acute setting to characterize their ability to respond to a damaging stimulus like lengthening eccentric contractions or following an exercise training programme to determine their contribution to skeletal muscle adaptation. More recently researchers have also investigated whether exercise training results in an alteration in SC activation following an acute damaging stimulus in the hope of understanding how various forms of exercise may affect the acute SC response.

Satellite Cell Activation in Response to Acute Exercise

It is well accepted that SCs play an indispensable role in skeletal muscle regeneration in rodents (39, 54), which has been shown using various models of muscle damage. For example, muscle injury can be induced via mechanical insult in the form of crush, puncture, cut, or freeze injuries; injections of local anaesthetics and myotoxins; and exhaustive exercise (4, 11). Although these models are an effective way of studying SC function in rodents, the majority are not suitable to be used in humans. Therefore, a typical approach in humans utilizes a bout of acute exercise to study SC function. Using this approach, skeletal muscle biopsies are obtained using a percutaneous muscle biopsy of the vastus lateralis prior to and in the hours and days following exercise (reviewed in 60). The most commonly used model of exercise to induce structural damage in human skeletal muscle is a bout of unaccustomed eccentric exercise, where circulating levels of creatine kinase and Z-band streaming, markers of ultrastructural damage, have been reported (19, 65). The first study to report an activation of the SC pool following exercise employed an intense resistance exercise protocol consisting of several variations of eccentric contractions. The authors reported an increase in SC content up to 8 days following damage-inducing exercise (10). Dreyer et al. employed eccentric contractions to determine SC response with aging and demonstrated that 24 hours following eccentric contractions, expansion of the SC pool was relatively blunted in older compared to younger individuals (14). The information obtained from this type of model allows the researcher to determine the extent to which the SC pool is able to potentially contribute to the repair of skeletal muscle fibres and how it may be affected in different populations. The SC pool increases in the hours and days following acute eccentric exercise with a concomitant increase in the number of active or proliferating SCs at earlier time points (as early as 3 hours) during the post-exercise time course, while an increase in differentiating SCs is observed later (24–96 hours; Figure 12.1) (40). Additionally, SCs can respond in a fibre type–specific manner. Typically, the increase in type II fibre–associated SCs following unaccustomed eccentric exercise is greater than type I fibre–associated SCs. The SC response can also be evaluated following different types of "non-damaging" exercise, which allows researchers to determine the effectiveness of exercise modality to elicit an SC response and potentially contribute to exercise-induced skeletal muscle remodelling (as opposed to repair/regeneration).

Acute Response to Resistance Exercise

The involvement of SCs in skeletal muscle repair is well established and, as described earlier, damaging exercise is often used to study SC biology in humans. However, SCs are also believed to play a role in skeletal muscle hypertrophy and growth in humans (summarized in Table 12.1) (16, 28, 29, 32, 35–37, 47, 49, 66, 67) and therefore, over the last decade much research has sought to characterize the SC response to an acute bout of resistance exercise. As skeletal muscle is post-mitotic, the addition of new nuclei to support muscle growth during periods of hypertrophy, such as resistance exercise training, is mediated by SCs. Therefore, the acute activation and subsequent increase in SC content following a bout of resistance exercise has been implied to be important for mediating resistance exercise training–induced adaptations, specifically by the addition of new nuclei to support growth. In most studies involving young healthy men, an increase in SC content is reported as early as 1 hour post exercise (70) and in some cases is reported to remain elevated anywhere from 72 (3, 63) to 96 (51) hours. However, some studies using "non-damaging" resistance exercise do not report an expansion in the SC population. No appreciable increase in SC content or activity was observed 24 hours following a bout of concentric contractions; however, when matched to total work, an increase was observed following eccentric contractions (25). Eccentric, but not concentric, exercise resulted in muscle damage indirectly assessed via muscle soreness or force recovery and directly via immunostaining of Xin and tenascin C, protein markers of muscle damage and extracellular matrix deadhesion, respectively (25). Additionally, Damas et al. determined the impact of one bout of resistance exercise at three different time points during a 10-week training programme (leg press and leg extension) and only observed an increase in type I fibre–associated SCs 48 hours following the first exercise session of the 10-week training programme (12), which was the only time point associated with an increase in muscle damage, assessed via Z-line streaming (13). Although these results suggest that "damage" is required for SC activation, due to the lack of multiple time points following exercise and the lack of fibre type–specific analysis in the study by Hyldhal et al., an increase in SC content may have occurred but was simply missed (25). The acute SC response following resistance exercise rather than damage-inducing eccentric exercise is also used to determine whether differences exist between populations.

With aging, skeletal muscles become less sensitive to anabolic stimuli like feeding and resistance exercise, resulting in a progressive loss of muscle mass and strength (sarcopenia) starting as early as the fifth decade of life (24). SC dysfunction is thought to contribute to sarcopenia, and therefore researchers have examined whether a bout of resistance exercise results in a different SC response in young compared to older individuals. Although acute resistance exercise to induce activation of the SC

Table 12.1 Summary of studies examining the impact of resistance exercise training on the basal SC pool

Study	Sex	Age	Duration	fCSA	Myonuclear content	SC content
Hikida et al. (1998) (21)	M M	22.5 65	8 wks (20 sessions) 16 wks (32 sessions)	Type I + Type IIA + Type IIB + Type I + Type IIA + Type IIB +	All fibre types NC	All fibre types NC
Kadi and Thornell (2000) (29)	F	38	10 wks, 3×/wk	All fibre types +	All fibre types +	All fibre types +
Roth et al. (2001) (52)	M/F M/F	20–30 65–75	9 wks, 3×/wk	NA	NA	All fibre types +
Kadi et al. (2004) (28)	M	24	3 mts, 3×/wk	All fibre types +	All fibre types NC	All fibre types +
Petrella et al. (2006) (48)	M F M F	26.1 27.9 64.5 62.8	16 wks, 3×/wk	All fibre types + All fibre types + All fibre types + All fibre types +	All fibre types + All fibre types NC All fibre types NC All fibre types NC	All fibre types + All fibre types NC All fibre types NC All fibre types NC
Mackey et al. (2007) (36)	M F	76 74	12 wks, 3×/wk	All fibre types NC All fibre types NC	All fibre types NC All fibre types +	All fibre types + All fibre types +
Verney et al. (2008) (68)	M	73	14 wks, 3×/wk	Type I NC Type IIa NC	All fire types NC	Type I NC Type II +
Verdijk et al. (2009) (66)	M	72	12 wks, 3×/wk	Type I NC Type II +	Type I NC Type II NC	Type I NC Type II +
Mackey et al. (2011) (35)	F	44	10 wks	Type I NC Type II +	Type I NC Type II NC	Type I + Type II +
Leenders et al. (2013) (32)	M F	70 71	24 weeks	Type II + Type II +	Type II + Type II +	Type II + Type II +
Bellamy et al. (2014) (3)	M	18–35	16 wks	Type I + Type II +	All fibre types +	Type I + Type II +
Farup et al. (2014) (16)	M	23.9	12wks Ecc (Pla) (Whey) Con (Pla) (Whey)	Type I + Type II NC Type I + Type II + Type I + Type II NC Type I + Type II NC	Type I + Type II + Type I + Type II NC Type I + Type II NC Type I + Type II +	Type I NC Type II NC Type I NC Type II NC Type I + Type II + Type I + Type II +
Dammas et al. (2018) (13)	M	27	10 wks	Type I NC Type II +	Type I NC Type II NC	Type I NC Type II +
Snijders et al. (2019) (59)	M	74	12 wks (3×/wk; 2 RT, 1 AT/ wk)	Type I no change Type II no change	Type I no change Type II no change	Type I + Type II +

Abbreviations: Con, concentric; Ecc, eccentric; F, female; fCSA, fibre cross-sectional area; M, male; NC, no change; NA, data not available; mts, months; Pla, placebo; RT, resistance training; wks, weeks

pool does differ between studies, an impairment in SC pool expansion is consistently reported in older adults (69). More specifically, a complete absence (40, 43) or at least a delay (59, 63) is observed in the type II fibre–associated SC response in older compared to young adults. Since aging skeletal muscle is characterized by a reduction in the number and size of type II fibres (33), an impaired SC response associated with this fibre type is not surprising. This is a particularly poignant issue, since type II fibres are high-force-generating fibres and the loss of these fibres with age is associated with significant consequences for mobility.

Acute Response to Aerobic Exercise

Although the SC response to acute resistance exercise in humans has been extensively studied, much less is known about the SC response to aerobic exercise. To our knowledge only three studies have sought to determine the effect of aerobic exercise on the acute SC response, all employing very different exercise parameters and participant characteristics. In young healthy endurance athletes, the SC pool was increased 8 days following the completion of a 36-km run (37). Babcock et al. (2012) reported no increase in the SC pool of young healthy males 4 days following a bout of cycling at 60% of maximal workload (2). In older individuals (67 ± 7 years), there was no change in SC content following a bout of either aerobic exercise (30 mins at 55–60% HR at VO_2 peak) or high-intensity interval exercise (HIT) (10 × 60 sec cycling at 90–95% of HR at VO_2 peak). However, an increase in active SCs was observed early (24–48 hours) following HIT and later (48 hours) following aerobic exercise (43). The inconclusive results are likely due to the varying exercise protocols, age and fitness levels of participants, and the time course of biopsies. Nonetheless, it seems reasonable to conclude that SCs are involved in remodelling of tissue following aerobic exercise. However, their precise role in remodelling of tissue remains to be elucidated. For example, following resistance exercise it is generally believed that SCs donate their nuclei to existing fibres to support muscle hypertrophy. It is unclear whether SCs act to donate nuclei following aerobic exercise—a mode of exercise not typically associated with hypertrophy. It is possible that the activation of SCs from the quiescent state following aerobic exercise may be for the purposes of signalling other cells to contribute to adaptation and remodelling following aerobic activity.

There is a growing body of literature regarding the molecular responses following concurrent exercise training, defined as the combination of endurance and resistance exercise in one training session. It has been suggested that the effect of endurance exercise prior to resistance exercise may blunt some of the adaptations, such as skeletal muscle fibre hypertrophy, associated with resistance training. As SCs are associated with hypertrophy in humans, it stands to reason that the SC response to concurrent exercise may be different from that of traditional resistance exercise. To this end, an impairment in the expansion of the SC pool following a bout of concurrent exercise compared to resistance exercise alone has been reported (2). Somewhat consistent with this finding, others have reported an increase in type II fibre–associated SC content following a bout of resistance exercise alone or a resistance exercise bout followed by HIT. However, only resistance exercise alone resulted in a greater proportion of type I fibre–associated active SCs 96 hours following exercise, whereas type II fibre–associated active SCs were greater in the resistance exercise–alone group (main effect of group) (51). The differences observed with respect to SC activation between exercise interventions may be due to the inclusion of only one post-exercise time point (96 hours) and may have "missed" the increase in activation in the resistance exercise and HIT group. Additionally, the resistance exercise and HIT group had a greater proportion of type II fibre–associated active SCs at baseline compared to the resistance exercise–only group. Others still report an increase in total and active SCs following a bout of combined aerobic and resistance training (61). Reports from acute aerobic exercise studies are rare and results are varied, again likely due to inconsistencies with exercise interventions, participant characteristics, and timing of biopsies in the hours and days following the acute exercise bout. The acute response of SCs to a stimulus like damage-inducing eccentric contractions may be indicative of the muscle's ability to repair and regenerate, whereas the acute response to an exercise training session, whether it be resistance or aerobic in nature, may indicate the role SCs play in mediating adaptations associated with the respective training programmes. In any event, it is fair to say that SCs play a role in mediating plasticity of skeletal muscle, which may include repair of damage or shifting phenotypes in response to specific stimuli.

The Impact of Exercise Training on Satellite Cell Content

Exercise training results in a vast adaptation in skeletal muscle, and these adaptations are exercise specific. Aerobic exercise typically results in remodelling of skeletal muscle towards a more oxidative phenotype characterized by an increase in capillary and mitochondrial density and fatty acid oxidation, resulting in an increased VO_2 peak (18, 23). In contrast, resistance exercise training results in an increase in activation of anabolic signalling, resulting in increases in muscle protein synthesis and leading to increases in muscle mass and fibre cross-sectional area (fCSA), which are associated with a concomitant increase in myonuclear content (30, 48).

Resistance Exercise Training and Satellite Cell Content

It is widely accepted that SCs are the primary source of new nuclei for skeletal muscle fibres. The myonuclear domain theory explains that each nucleus is responsible for a set volume of sarcoplasm (Figure 12.1). When this volume grows and exceeds the transcriptional capacity of a nucleus, new myonuclei must be added to maintain the myonuclear domain (1). Several studies have reported an association between myofibre size and nuclear content, with larger fibres also having a greater number of myonuclei (15, 29, 56). Not surprisingly, an increase in muscle fCSA is also associated with an increase in SCs (summarized in Table 12.1) (3, 12, 29, 35, 49). In contrast, an increase in fCSA has also been reported without an increase in SC content (21, 48). Interestingly, previous work demonstrated that when participants were divided into groups based on the extent of muscle hypertrophy, only individuals who had the greatest increase in fCSA also had an increase in SC content (49). In addition, no differences in fCSA were observed between groups at baseline; however, the group that saw the greatest increase in fCSA did have a greater number of SCs at baseline (49). These data suggest that hypertrophy in humans is most commonly associated with an increase in SC content and the extent of hypertrophy following resistance exercise training may be related to baseline SC content.

Aerobic Exercise Training and Satellite Cell Content

Similar to the literature regarding the impact of acute aerobic exercise on SCs, the effect of aerobic exercise training on the SC pool is also sparse and inconsistent (data summarized in Table 12.2). Studies in older adults reported an expansion of the SC pool following 14 weeks of interval training (5, 68); however, an increase in fCSA was also reported in these studies, suggesting that the SC response may have been related to the relative hypertrophic stimulus of this type of exercise. While a more traditional aerobic training programme (75% VO_2 max for 40 mins) in older subjects did not result in fibre hypertrophy or affect SC content (62), a more recent study described an increase in type I fibre–associated SC content fCSA following 12 weeks of traditional aerobic exercise training in middle-aged adults (17, 42). In young adults completing 10 weeks of aerobic training, an increase in total and active SC associated with type II fibres was observed (22), but consistent with previous work, an increase in type II fCSA was also reported (31). Therefore, it is difficult to ascertain whether the expansion of the SC pool was due to an increase in fCSA or whether it occurred as a result, or in support, of skeletal muscle adaptations characteristic of aerobic training. When aerobic exercise training, whether it be moderate continuous or interval based, was not associated with increases in muscle fCSA, there was also no increase in SC content (26, 27). Although an increase in SC content was not observed, there was a greater proportion of active SCs following training (27). In further support of the importance of SCs

Table 12.2 Summary of studies examining the impact of aerobic exercise training on the basal SC pool

Study	Sex	Age	Duration	Type	fCSA	Myonuclear content	SC content
Verney et al. (2008) (68)	M	73	14 wks, 3×/wk	36 mins, 3 intervals: 2× (4 mins 75–85% HR_{max}, 1 min 80–95% HR_{max}), 2 mins recovery	Type I NC Type IIa +	All fibre types NC	Type I NC Type II +
Charifi et al. (2003) (5)	M	73	14 wks, 4×/wk	45 mins, 7 intervals: 4 min 65–75% VO_2peak, 1 min 85–95% VO_2 peak,	Type I NC Type IIa + Type IIb NC Type IIc NC	All fibre types NC	All fibre types +
Murach et al. (2016) (42)	F	56	12 wks, 3×/wk	45 mins, 65% VO_2 max	All fibre types +	NA	Type I + Type II NC
Snijders et al. (2011) (62)	M	62	6 mts, 3×/wk	40 mins, 75% VO_2 max	Type I No change Type II No change	Type I NC Type II NC	Type I NC Type II NC
Joanisse et al. (2013) (26)	F	27	6 wks, 3×/wk	20 mins, 10 intervals: 1 min, 90% HR_{max}, 1 min recovery	Type I NC Type II NC Type I/II NC	All fibre type NC	Type I NC Type II NC Type I/II +
Fry et al. (2014) (17)	M/F	47.6	12 wks, ×x/wk	45 mins, 70% $HR_{reserve}$	Type I + Type IIa + Type IIa/x NC	Type I + Type II NC	Type I + Type II NC
Joanisse et al. (2015) (27)	M/F M/F	29 21	6 wks, 3×/wk 6 wks, 4×/wk	10 mins, 3 intervals: 20s at 0.05 kg/kg body mass, 2 min recovery Group 1: 30 mins, 65% VO_2 peak Group 2: 4 mins, 8 intervals: 20s 170% VO_2 peak 10-s recovery	Type I No change Type II No change	All fibre types NC	Type I NC Type II NC
Hoedt et al. (2015) (22)	M	21	10 wks, 3×/wk	40 mins, 3×/wk: 1) continuous (70% VO_2 max) 2) 2 × 20-min intervals (80–90% VO_2 max), 5-min recovery 3) 8 × 5-min intervals (90–100% VO_2 max), 1-min recovery	NA	All fibre types NC	Type II +

Abbreviations: F, female; fCSA, fibre cross-sectional area; M, male; NC, no change; NA, data not available; mts, months; wks, weeks

in aerobic training, SC content was positively correlated to VO_2 max in individuals with a high fitness capacity (34). Although fCSA was not reported in the study, it is possible that individuals with higher VO_2 max may also have a greater fCSA, and this could account for the association between VO_2 max and SC content. However, more recently it was demonstrated that SC content is similar between individuals with high relative aerobic fitness (VO_2 peak >60 mL/kg/min) compared to average aerobic fitness (VO_2 peak = 40 mL/kg/min) (44). Additionally, SC content in endurance-trained master athletes was not different compared to either young or older healthy controls (41). Together, these data highlight that SCs respond to aerobic exercise and may have a role in mediating responses typical of this type of stimulus; however, more work is required to determine their role in non-hypertrophic adaptation.

Satellite Cells and Skeletal Muscles' Ability to Respond to Training Interventions

Skeletal muscles' impressive capacity for plasticity is contingent on aspects of metabolism and morphology to be in place for an optimal response to stimuli. One important factor for optimal plasticity in skeletal muscle is the SC pool. Rodent and human studies have highlighted the importance of SCs in muscle repair and regeneration (39, 54), and in humans, although not causative in nature, a reduction in the SC pool is associated with older age (40, 63) and various myopathies (9, 58). Earlier work demonstrated that when subjects are separated into groups (non-, moderate, and extreme responders) based on their change in muscle fCSA following resistance training, extreme-responders had greater SC content at baseline compared to other groups, and this was still the case following training. Additionally, extreme responders were the only group who were able to increase SC content with resistance exercise training (49). This work elegantly demonstrated that baseline characteristics of skeletal muscle may be related to an individual's capacity for adaptation in response to a specific stimulus. To further elaborate on this concept, a relationship between the change in SCs associated with type II fibres following resistance training and the change in quadriceps volume has been described. A positive relationship was also described between the acute response of type I fibre–associated SCs prior to the onset of training and the change in quadriceps volume (3). Together these studies highlight the importance of the contribution of SCs in the regulation of skeletal muscle hypertrophy.

Exercise Training Can Alter the Acute SC Response

It is generally thought that the acute SC response to a stimulus may provide insight into the capacity for muscle adaptation. The SC response to an acute bout of resistance exercise is affected by resistance training in young men. Damas et al. demonstrated that during a 10-week resistance training programme, only the first bout of exercise elicited an acute increase in the SC pool associated with type I fibres 48 hours following exercise, while no change was observed in type II fibre–associated SCs (12). When the acute response was determined during the third and tenth week of training, no change in SC content was observed in either fibre type. The authors attribute this to the fact that only the first bout of exercise was sufficient to induce muscle damage (12, 13). Contrary to these findings, a 16-week resistance training programme in young men resulted in an increase in type II fibre–associated SCs 24 and 72 hours following a bout of acute resistance exercise both in the trained and untrained state, with a greater activation of SCs 24 hours post resistance exercise in trained compared to untrained (45). Endurance exercise has also been shown to modulate the SC response to acute resistance exercise (12). Prior to 12 weeks of aerobic training in middle-aged women, a 29% increase in the acute type I fibre–associated SC response was observed 72 hours following an acute bout of resistance exercise (42). Following training (i.e., in the trained state) the type I fibre–associated SC response was significantly reduced 72 hours following a bout of resistance exercise (42). Here the authors hypothesize that the bout of resistance exercise may be more challenging in the untrained state and that aerobic exercise may have conditioned the muscle for more acute muscle contractions elicited by the resistance exercise bout. Additionally, the authors report an expansion of the basal SC pool following aerobic training, which may have accounted for the lack of expansion following acute resistance exercise (42). In older men 12 weeks of training (resistance twice and aerobic once weekly) resulted in expansion of the type II fibre–associated SC pool 24 and 48 hours following a bout of acute resistance exercise, an increase that was not evident prior to training (i.e., in the untrained state) (59). This finding is especially important as the impaired type II fibre–associated SC response observed in older individuals has been postulated to contribute to the age-related loss of muscle fCSA (64). These findings may have significant translational impact, as aging is associated with both a reduction in muscle mass and cardiometabolic health. Therefore, the use of training paradigms that can result in improvements in aerobic capacity and increases in fCSA are important for the maintenance of physical function throughout the lifespan, directly affecting quality of life.

Summary and Future Directions

Skeletal muscle is a highly dynamic and metabolically active tissue responsible for a variety of bodily functions. Although skeletal muscle is highly adaptable, the post-mitotic nature of skeletal muscle requires the primary muscle progenitor, SCs, to contribute new nuclei to existing muscle fibres in response to appropriate stimuli. Importantly, SCs are highly responsive to various forms of exercise and, in humans, are believed to play in important role in skeletal muscle hypertrophy following resistance exercise training and may play a role in mediating non-hypertrophic adaptations observed following aerobic training. In recent years, much research has aimed at determining optimal exercise interventions to maximize the SC response, specifically in populations where muscle mass may be compromised (i.e., aging). However, more research is required to determine the mechanisms supporting SC function and how exercise and potentially nutritional interventions may result in optimal SC function to support the maintenance of muscle health throughout the lifespan.

References

1. Allen DL, Roy RR, Edgerton VR. Myonuclear domains in muscle adaptation and disease. *Muscle Nerve* 22: 1350–1360, 1999.
2. Babcock L, Escano M, D'Lugos A, Todd K, Murach K, Luden N. Concurrent aerobic exercise interferes with the satellite cell response to acute resistance exercise. *Am J Physiol* 302: R1458–R1465, 2012.
3. Bellamy LM, Joanisse S, Grubb A, Mitchell CJ, McKay BR, Phillips SM, et al. The acute satellite cell response and skeletal muscle hypertrophy following resistance training. *PLOS ONE* 9: e109739, 2014.
4. Bodine-Fowler S. Skeletal muscle regeneration after injury: an overview. *J Voice* 8: 53–62, 1994.
5. Charifi N, Kadi F, Féasson L, Denis C. Effects of endurance training on satellite cell frequency in skeletal muscle of old men. *Muscle Nerve* 28: 87–92, 2003.
6. Cooper RN, Tajbakhsh S, Mouly V, Cossu G, Buckingham M, Butler-Browne GS. In vivo satellite cell activation via Myf5 and MyoD in regenerating mouse skeletal muscle. *J Cell Sci* 112: 2895–2901, 1999.
7. Cornelison DD, Olwin BB, Rudnicki MA, Wold BJ. MyoD(-/-) satellite cells in single-fiber culture are differentiation defective and MRF4 deficient. *Dev Biol* 224: 122–137, 2000.
8. Cornelison DD, Wold BJ. Single-cell analysis of regulatory gene expression in quiescent and activated mouse skeletal muscle satellite cells. *Dev Biol* 191: 270–283, 1997.
9. Cossu G, Mavilio F. Myogenic stem cells for the therapy of primary myopathies: wishful thinking or therapeutic perspective?. *J Clin Invest* 105: 1669–1674, 2000.
10. Crameri RM, Langberg H, Magnusson P, Jensen CH, Schrøder HD, Olesen JL, et al. Changes in satellite cells in human skeletal muscle after a single bout of high intensity exercise. *J Physiol* 558: 333–340, 2004.
11. Czerwinska AM, Streminska W, Ciemerych MA, Grabowska I. Mouse gastrocnemius muscle regeneration after mechanical or cardiotoxin injury. *Folia Histochem Cytobiol* 50: 144–153, 2012.
12. Damas F, Libardi CA, Ugrinowitsch C, Vechin FC, Lixandrão ME, Snijders T, et al. Early- and later-phases satellite cell responses and myonuclear content with resistance training in young men. *PLOS ONE* 13: e0191039, 2018.
13. Damas F, Phillips SM, Libardi CA, Vechin FC, Lixandrão ME, Jannig PR, et al. Resistance training-induced changes in integrated myofibrillar protein synthesis are related to hypertrophy only after attenuation of muscle damage. *J Physiol* 594: 5209–5222, 2016.

14. Dreyer HC, Blanco CE, Sattler FR, Schroeder ET, Wiswell RA. Satellite cell numbers in young and older men 24 hours after eccentric exercise. *Muscle Nerve* 33: 242–253, 2006.

15. Eriksson A, Kadi F, Malm C, Thornell L-E. Skeletal muscle morphology in power-lifters with and without anabolic steroids. *Histochem Cell Biol* 124: 167–175, 2005.

16. Farup J, Rahbek SK, Riis S, Vendelbo MH, Paoli F de, Vissing K. Influence of exercise contraction mode and protein supplementation on human skeletal muscle satellite cell content and muscle fiber growth. *J Appl Physiol* 117: 898–909, 2014.

17. Fry CS, Noehren B, Mula J, Ubele MF, Westgate PM, Kern PA, et al. Fibre type-specific satellite cell response to aerobic training in sedentary adults. *J Physiol* 592: 2625–2635, 2014.

18. Gibala MJ, Little JP, Macdonald MJ, Hawley JA. Physiological adaptations to low-volume, high-intensity interval training in health and disease. *J Physiol* 590: 1077–1084, 2012.

19. Gibala MJ, MacDougall JD, Tarnopolsky MA, Stauber WT, Elorriaga A. Changes in human skeletal muscle ultrastructure and force production after acute resistance exercise. *J Appl Physiol* 78: 702–708, 1995.

20. Grounds MD, Garrett KL, Lai MC, Wright WE, Beilharz MW. Identification of skeletal muscle precursor cells in vivo by use of MyoD1 and myogenin probes. *Cell Tissue Res* 267: 99–104, 1992.

21. Hikida RS, Walsh S, Barylski NA, Campos G, Hagerman FC, Staron RS. Is Hypertrophy Limited in Elderly Muscle Fibers? A comparison of elderly and young strength-trained men. *Basic Appl Myol* 8: 419–427, 1998.

22. Hoedt A, Christensen B, Nellemann B, Mikkelsen UR, Hansen M, Schjerling P, et al. Satellite cell response to erythropoietin treatment and endurance training in healthy young men. *J Physiol* 594: 727–743, 2016.

23. Hoppeler H, Howald H, Conley K, Lindstedt SL, Claassen H, Vock P, et al. Endurance training in humans: aerobic capacity and structure of skeletal muscle. *J Appl Physiol* 59: 320–327, 1985.

24. Hughes VA, Frontera WR, Wood M, Evans WJ, Dallal GE, Roubenoff R, et al. Longitudinal muscle strength changes in older adults: influence of muscle mass, physical activity, and health. *J Gerontol A Biol Sci Med Sci* 56: B209–217, 2001.

25. Hyldahl RD, Olson T, Welling T, Groscost L, Parcell AC. Satellite cell activity is differentially affected by contraction mode in human muscle following a work-matched bout of exercise. *Front Physiol* 5, 2014.

26. Joanisse S, Gillen JB, Bellamy LM, McKay BR, Tarnopolsky MA, Gibala MJ, et al. Evidence for the contribution of muscle stem cells to nonhypertrophic skeletal muscle remodeling in humans. *FASEB J* 27: 4596–4605, 2013.

27. Joanisse S, McKay BR, Nederveen JP, Scribbans TD, Gurd BJ, Gillen JB, et al. Satellite cell activity, without expansion, after nonhypertrophic stimuli. *Am J Physiol* 309: R1101–R1111, 2015.

28. Kadi F, Schjerling P, Andersen LL, Charifi N, Madsen JL, Christensen LR, et al. The effects of heavy resistance training and detraining on satellite cells in human skeletal muscles. *J Physiol* 558: 1005–1012, 2004.

29. Kadi F, Thornell LE. Concomitant increases in myonuclear and satellite cell content in female trapezius muscle following strength training. *Histochem Cell Biol* 113: 99–103, 2000.

30. Kosek DJ, Kim J-S, Petrella JK, Cross JM, Bamman MM. Efficacy of 3 days/wk resistance training on myofiber hypertrophy and myogenic mechanisms in young vs. older adults. *J Appl Physiol* 101: 531–544, 2006.

31. Larsen MS, Vissing K, Thams L, Sieljacks P, Dalgas U, Nellemann B, et al. Erythropoietin administration alone or in combination with endurance training affects neither skeletal muscle morphology nor angiogenesis in healthy young men. *Exp Physiol* 99: 1409–1420, 2014.

32. Leenders M, Verdijk LB, van der Hoeven L, van Kranenburg J, Nilwik R, van Loon LJC. Elderly men and women benefit equally from prolonged resistance-type exercise training. *J Gerontol A Biol Sci Med Sci* 68: 769–779, 2013.

33. Lexell J. Human aging, muscle mass, and fiber type composition. *J Gerontol A Biol Sci Med Sci* 50 Spec No: 11–16, 1995.

34. Macaluso F, Brooks NE, van de Vyver M, Van Tubbergh K, Niesler CU, Myburgh KH. Satellite cell count, VO(2max), and p38 MAPK in inactive to moderately active young men. *Scand J Med Sci Sports* 22: e38–44, 2012.

35. Mackey AL, Andersen LL, Frandsen U, Sjøgaard G. Strength training increases the size of the satellite cell pool in type I and II fibres of chronically painful trapezius muscle in females. *J Physiol* 589: 5503–5515, 2011.

36. Mackey AL, Esmarck B, Kadi F, Koskinen SOA, Kongsgaard M, Sylvestersen A, et al. Enhanced satellite cell proliferation with resistance training in elderly men and women. *Scand J Med Sci Sports* 17: 34–42, 2007.

37. Mackey AL, Kjaer M, Dandanell S, Mikkelsen KH, Holm L, Døssing S, et al. The influence of anti-inflammatory medication on exercise-induced myogenic precursor cell responses in humans. *J Appl Physiol* 103: 425–431, 2007.

38. Mauro A. Satellite cell of skeletal muscle fibers. *J Biophys Biochem Cytol* 9: 493–495, 1961.
39. McCarthy JJ, Mula J, Miyazaki M, Erfani R, Garrison K, Farooqui AB, et al. Effective fiber hypertrophy in satellite cell-depleted skeletal muscle. *Development* 138: 3657–3666, 2011.
40. McKay BR, Ogborn DI, Bellamy LM, Tarnopolsky MA, Parise G. Myostatin is associated with age-related human muscle stem cell dysfunction. *FASEB J* 26: 2509–2521, 2012.
41. McKendry J, Joanisse S, Baig S, Liu B, Parise G, Greig CA, et al. Superior aerobic capacity and indices of skeletal muscle morphology in chronically trained master endurance athletes compared with untrained older adults. *J. Gerontol. A Biol. Sci. Med. Sci.* Epub ahead of print: glz142, 2019.
42. Murach KA, Walton RG, Fry CS, Michaelis SL, Groshong JS, Finlin BS, et al. Cycle training modulates satellite cell and transcriptional responses to a bout of resistance exercise. *Physiol Rep* 4: e12973, 2016.
43. Nederveen JP, Joanisse S, Séguin CML, Bell KE, Baker SK, Phillips SM, et al. The effect of exercise mode on the acute response of satellite cells in old men. *Acta Physiol* 215: 177–190, 2015.
44. Nederveen JP, Joanisse S, Snijders T, Thomas ACQ, Kumbhare D, Parise G. The influence of capillarization on satellite cell pool expansion and activation following exercise-induced muscle damage in healthy young men. *J Physiol* 596: 1063–1078, 2018.
45. Nederveen JP, Snijders T, Joanisse S, Wavell CG, Mitchell CJ, Johnston LM, et al. Altered muscle satellite cell activation following 16 wk of resistance training in young men. *Am J Physiol* 312: R85–R92, 2017.
46. Olguin HC, Yang Z, Tapscott SJ, Olwin BB. Reciprocal inhibition between Pax7 and muscle regulatory factors modulates myogenic cell fate determination. *J Cell Biol* 177: 769–779, 2007.
47. Olsen S, Aagaard P, Kadi F, Tufekovic G, Verney J, Olesen JL, et al. Creatine supplementation augments the increase in satellite cell and myonuclei number in human skeletal muscle induced by strength training. *J Physiol* 573: 525–534, 2006.
48. Petrella JK, Kim J, Cross JM, Kosek DJ, Bamman MM. Efficacy of myonuclear addition may explain differential myofiber growth among resistance-trained young and older men and women. *Am J Physiol* 291: E937–E946, 2006.
49. Petrella JK, Kim J, Mayhew DL, Cross JM, Bamman MM. Potent myofiber hypertrophy during resistance training in humans is associated with satellite cell-mediated myonuclear addition: a cluster analysis. *J Appl Physiol* 104: 1736–1742, 2008.
50. Pette D, Staron RS. Myosin isoforms, muscle fiber types, and transitions. *Microsc Res Tech* 50: 500–509, 2000.
51. Pugh JK, Faulkner SH, Turner MC, Nimmo MA. Satellite cell response to concurrent resistance exercise and high-intensity interval training in sedentary, overweight/obese, middle-aged individuals. *Eur J Appl Physiol* 118: 225–238, 2018.
52. Roth SM, Martel GF, Ivey FM, Lemmer JT, Tracy BL, Metter EJ, et al. Skeletal muscle satellite cell characteristics in young and older men and women after heavy resistance strength training. *J Gerontol A Biol Sci Med Sci* 56: B240–247, 2001.
53. Rudnicki MA, Le Grand F, McKinnell I, Kuang S. The molecular regulation of muscle stem cell function. *Cold Spring Harb Symp Quant Biol* 73: 323–331, 2008.
54. Sambasivan R, Yao R, Kissenpfennig A, Van Wittenberghe L, Paldi A, Gayraud-Morel B, et al. Pax7-expressing satellite cells are indispensable for adult skeletal muscle regeneration. *Development* 138: 3647–3656, 2011.
55. Seale P, Sabourin LA, Girgis-Gabardo A, Mansouri A, Gruss P, Rudnicki MA. Pax7 is required for the specification of myogenic satellite cells. *Cell* 102: 777–786, 2000.
56. Sinha-Hikim I, Artaza J, Woodhouse L, Gonzalez-Cadavid N, Singh AB, Lee MI, et al. Testosterone-induced increase in muscle size in healthy young men is associated with muscle fiber hypertrophy. *Am J Physiol* 283: E154–164, 2002.
57. Smith CK, Janney MJ, Allen RE. Temporal expression of myogenic regulatory genes during activation, proliferation, and differentiation of rat skeletal muscle satellite cells. *J Cell Physiol* 159: 379–385, 1994.
58. Smith LR, Chambers HG, Lieber RL. Reduced satellite cell population may lead to contractures in children with cerebral palsy. *Dev Med Child Neurol* 55: 264–270, 2013.
59. Snijders T, Nederveen JP, Bell KE, Lau SW, Mazara N, Kumbhare DA, et al. Prolonged exercise training improves the acute type II muscle fibre satellite cell response in healthy older men. *J Physiol* 597: 105–119, 2019.
60. Snijders T, Nederveen JP, McKay BR, Joanisse S, Verdijk LB, van Loon LJC, et al. Satellite cells in human skeletal muscle plasticity. *Front Physiol* 6, 2015.
61. Snijders T, Verdijk LB, Beelen M, McKay BR, Parise G, Kadi F, et al. A single bout of exercise activates skeletal muscle satellite cells during subsequent overnight recovery. *Exp Physiol* 97: 762–773, 2012.
62. Snijders T, Verdijk LB, Hansen D, Dendale P, van Loon LJC. Continuous endurance-type exercise training does not modulate satellite cell content in obese type 2 diabetes patients. *Muscle Nerve* 43: 393–401, 2011.

63. Snijders T, Verdijk LB, Smeets JSJ, McKay BR, Senden JMG, Hartgens F, et al. The skeletal muscle satellite cell response to a single bout of resistance-type exercise is delayed with aging in men. *Age* 36, 2014.

64. Snijders T, Verdijk LB, van Loon LJC. The impact of sarcopenia and exercise training on skeletal muscle satellite cells. *Ageing Res Rev* 8: 328–338, 2009.

65. Stupka N, Tarnopolsky MA, Yardley NJ, Phillips SM. Cellular adaptation to repeated eccentric exercise-induced muscle damage. *J Appl Physiol* 91: 1669–1678, 2001.

66. Verdijk LB, Gleeson BG, Jonkers RAM, Meijer K, Savelberg HHCM, Dendale P, et al. Skeletal muscle hypertrophy following resistance training is accompanied by a fiber type–specific increase in satellite cell content in elderly men. *J Gerontol A Biol Sci Med Sci* 64A: 332–339, 2009.

67. Verdijk LB, Snijders T, Drost M, Delhaas T, Kadi F, van Loon LJC. Satellite cells in human skeletal muscle; from birth to old age. *Age* 36: 545–547, 2014.

68. Verney J, Kadi F, Charifi N, Féasson L, Saafi MA, Castells J, et al. Effects of combined lower body endurance and upper body resistance training on the satellite cell pool in elderly subjects. *Muscle Nerve* 38: 1147–1154, 2008.

69. Walker DK, Fry CS, Drummond MJ, Dickinson JM, Timmerman KL, Gundermann DM, et al. Pax7+ satellite cells in young and older adults following resistance exercise. *Muscle Nerve* 46: 51–59, 2012.

70. Wernbom M, Apro W, Paulsen G, Nilsen TS, Blomstrand E, Raastad T. Acute low-load resistance exercise with and without blood flow restriction increased protein signalling and number of satellite cells in human skeletal muscle. *Eur J Appl Physiol* 113: 2953–2965, 2013.

13

BIOCHEMICAL AND METABOLIC LIMITATIONS TO ATHLETIC PERFORMANCE

Brendan M. Gabriel

Background

Since the days of the ancient Olympiad (and probably beyond), it has long been known that athletic performance can be improved by exercise training and nutritional strategies. However, our knowledge of human biology has expanded within the last century to allow a thorough investigation into the myriad biochemical limitations to athletic performance. This chapter will address the known limiting biochemical factors and their associated metabolic pathways. These pathways diverge somewhat between differing athletic modalities, and exercise training specific to an athletic discipline can improve the performance or capacity of limiting metabolic pathways. However, some biochemical functionality is inherited through genetic or epigenetic means. Uncovering the biochemical and metabolic limitations to athletic performance has obvious benefits in being able to manipulate training or nutritional strategies to improve athletic performance. Additionally, elucidating these limits, and discovering their regulatory pathways can prime research into pathological conditions. Indeed, several key findings have been informed by studying highly trained athletes in addition to healthy or unhealthy subjects (15).

Historical Milestones

The study of athletic limitations has evolved from observational field studies to sophisticated mechanistic studies incorporating physiology, biochemistry, and molecular biology. Pioneering research investigating the biochemical and metabolic limitations of athletic performance has been conducted by early innovators. Much of the early research in this topic was completed by Scandinavian physiologists, often seeking to determine the metabolic limitations of endurance performance. Investigators such as August Krogh were among the first to study the metabolic limitations of athletic performance in humans. Together with Johannes Lindhard, Krogh charted changes in ventilation, blood flow, pulse rate, respiratory exchange, and alveolar CO_2 tension during the first few minutes of light or heavy exercise (31). Subsequently, Krogh performed paradigm-shifting work to uncover the regulatory mechanisms controlling capillary blood flow in resting and active skeletal muscle (28–30) for which he was awarded the Nobel Prize in Physiology or Medicine in 1920. These discoveries highlighted a crucial rate-limiting step in exercise, specifically the transport and availability of O_2 to the working muscle. Krogh and Lindhard furthered this important work by assessing how exercise performance is perturbed by ingestion of different substrates such as carbohydrates or fat (32). This work was some of the earliest to assess the effect of nutrition on athletic performance, highlighting the role of substrate metabolism in

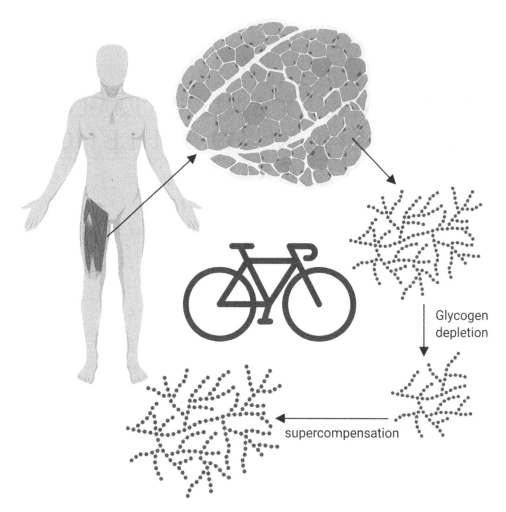

Figure 13.1 Post-exercise glycogen supercompensation as demonstrated in classic experiments by Bergström and Hultman (4, 5)

defining athletic limits. Scandinavian researchers remained at the forefront of this field in the mid-20th century, including Bergström and Hultman's seminal work demonstrating that exercise causes a rapid glycogen depletion in the working leg (4, 5). In a classical experiment, these researchers also determined that glycogen was rapidly resynthesized and restored within 24 hours after a bout of exercise. Indeed, these data suggested there was a "super-compensation" of glycogen after acute exercise, whereby the storage capacity of glycogen was transiently increased after a single bout of exercise (Figure 13.1). In another contemporaneous study, acute exercise was seen to increase the turnover and oxidation of free fatty acids. These innovative investigations into substrate utilization within a single bout of exercise encouraged researchers to explore the effects of chronic exercise training. Further work from the same decade revealed that prolonged and vigorous exercise training increases the capacity to oxidize substrates (22). This was due to an increase in the content and maximal activity of enzymes involved in these metabolic pathways, including those within mitochondria. This series of investigations was able to demonstrate the drastic remodelling of metabolic pathways within skeletal muscle in response to exercise training and went some way to explaining how highly trained athletes are able to reach the biochemical and metabolic limits of athletic performance.

Why Study the Biochemical and Metabolic Limits of Exercise?

When one assesses the biochemistry of athletic performance, it is interesting to consider an evolutionary perspective. If an Olympic games were conducted in the animal kingdom, it is almost certain that humans would specialize in endurance running events. Long limbs relative to body size and the ability to rapidly dissipate excess heat through sweating engender humans with superb endurance capabilities. This endurance capacity may have been fundamental in the evolution of humans, broadening the range of habitable environments and allowing successful persistence hunting strategies (6). Performing regular endurance activity may have also driven human evolution to some extent (44). Some researchers speculate that factors secreted from skeletal muscle during endurance exercise may drive neurological development. Additionally, the secretion of these skeletal muscle factors is associated with biochemical and metabolic changes that take place during intense exercise (51). Assessing these extreme biochemical and metabolic changes is vital to our understanding of human physiology and allows researchers to develop strategies in athletic performance, but also informs our understanding of how biochemistry responds to challenges. The biochemistry of extremes can help researchers better understand the pathology of disease and may allow improvement of disease treatment regimens. Indeed, since humans have evolved as a species capable of sustaining extreme biochemical and metabolic conditions for the duration of prolonged exercise bouts, fully understanding our own evolutionary adaptations is an important juxtaposition to research that purely assesses disease pathology.

Biochemical and Metabolic Limitations of Exercise Performance

In simplistic terms, the key biochemical and metabolic limitations of sustained, intense exercise are the ability to uptake and transport oxygen to the working muscle, the ability to sustain metabolic work without the build-up of prohibitive metabolites, and the ability to efficiently utilize readily available fuel sources (27). Outcome measurements indirectly resulting from these parameters are widely used within exercise physiology and include well-known testing procedures such as VO_2 max and blood lactate testing. Champion endurance athletes have a high innate and trained capacity to uptake, transport, and utilize oxygen, resulting in higher relative VO_2 max scores compared to moderately trained subjects. For example, elite cross-country skiers often record very high VO_2 max scores of ~90 mL·min^{-1}·kg^{-1} (48). Physiologically, cardiac output and the O_2-carrying capacity of the cardiovascular system are key rate limiters of VO_2 max at sea level (27). However, in the century since Krogh and colleagues determined oxygen utilization as a performance-limiting factor during exercise, exercise physiologists have further elucidated the complexities of oxygen delivery and utilization within this system (35, 53). Biochemically, oxygen extraction by myofibers is an important determinant of performance under some conditions, particularly, the capacity of a capillary bed within a working muscle to supply oxygen to the mitochondria of the working myofibers evenly. Endurance-trained athletes have enhanced ability to precisely match the oxygen needs of working myofibers to the delivery capacity, enhancing myofiber uptake and utilization of oxygen (15, 53).

Ultimately, oxygen bioavailability is crucial at a biochemical level, as oxygen is the final electron acceptor in the process of cellular respiration. This allows oxidative phosphorylation and generation of adenosine triphosphate (ATP) (biochemical energy), whereas a deficient matching of oxygen delivery to the working mitochondria results in reliance on anaerobic respiration. Both aerobic and anaerobic respiration result in the build-up of biochemical intermediates, which limit performance. The biochemical and metabolic limits of athletic endurance and performance can be essentially boiled down to three abilities:

- The ability to match oxygen requirement to mitochondrial respiration in a temporally and spatially specific manner
- The ability to prevent accumulation of by-products of anaerobic and aerobic respiration, which are detrimental to performance
- The ability to efficiently metabolize readily available fuel or metabolites

The Ability to Match Oxygen Requirement to Mitochondrial Respiration in a Temporally and Spatially Specific Manner

As stated, the delivery of oxygen to working mitochondria is a critical limiting factor of performance. This limitation is dictated by physiological parameters such as cardiac output, blood volume, haemoglobin mass, and capillary density (8, 27, 52). Furthermore, within the muscle, the ability of the mitochondria to extract and utilize oxygen in the most efficient manner may also determine performance capacity (15). Mitochondrial capacity has been consistently studied in exercise physiology (21). For example, it is known that citrate synthase (CS), a key enzyme in the Krebs cycle, is a rate-limiting step in oxidative metabolism (1, 13). Indeed, CS activity correlates with maximal fat oxidation in elite cross-country skiers (11). CS is localized to the mitochondrial matrix, which is encompassed by the inner mitochondrial membrane, and the area and density of this membrane are also increased in elite athletes, driven by increased cristae folding and thus density. The inner mitochondrial membrane cristae structure is the location of which a majority of the important biochemical reactions within respiration occur. In fact, cristae density (determined by electron microscopy) may be an even better predictor of oxidative capacity in athletes than CS (39). Furthermore, improved imaging techniques are constantly improving researchers' ability to study the mechanisms by which mitochondria operate in skeletal muscle, and thus determine how their biology changes in response to exercise. For example, elegant imaging techniques have been utilized to shine a light on interesting mitochondrial phenomena (17). This research challenges some aspects within the classical model of sub-sarcolemmal mitochondria and intermyofibrillar mitochondria, which are known to be heterogenous sub-populations (33). This heterogeneity is partly due to the need for subsarcolemmal mitochondria to regulate sarcolemmal membrane function, while intermyofibrillar mitochondria are regarded as the main source of ATP generation for the working muscle, due to their proximity to contracting sarcomeres (23, 34). Pioneering work demonstrates that sub-sarcolemmal and intermyofibrillar mitochondrial populations may also be part of a mitochondrial reticulum that allows conduction of biochemical energy within the myofiber (17). Within this mitochondrial reticulum, ATP synthase, which uses the proton–motive force to drive ATP production, has a higher density in the myofiber interior, whereas complexes I, II, III, and IV of the electron transport chain that generate the proton-motive force are present to a greater extent in the cell exterior. This arrangement would present an elegant method of generating proton-motive force and utilizing oxygen as the final electron acceptor in close proximity to an area to which oxygen is easily delivered. Proton-motive force could then be transferred to the interior of the myofiber, where oxygen availability may be lower, and diffusion rates slower, but where ATP is also needed for contracting sarcomeres (Figure 13.2). In other words, an area of the muscle rich with readily available oxygen has mitochondria that utilize this to create a proton gradient, whereas in an area of the muscle that has poorer oxygen delivery, mitochondria are adapted to function with less oxygen. This grid-like network provides a method of energy transfer from the perimeter to the interior of the muscle. This model is still debated to some extent and currently has only been imaged in mouse models. However, it would provide an elegant evolutionary solution to the problem of uneven oxygen distribution throughout a working myofiber.

Another aspect of the efficiency of mitochondria to utilize oxygen is how the complexes of the electron transport chain themselves are organized. The structure and formation of the electron transport chain, located on the inner mitochondrial membrane, are extremely plastic and change rapidly in response to stimuli and stress. In some cases, the members of the electron transport chain can fuse to form what are known as "super-complexes." Although this field of study is relatively new and technological challenges remain when characterizing super-complex formation, it appears that these formations may play a key role in exercise performance. For example, the formation of super-assembled complexes is increased after aerobic training (19). In this study, aerobic training promoted the redistribution of complex I from super-complex I+III$_2$ to super-complex I+III2+IV$_n$. Additionally, aerobic training preferentially favoured the re-distribution of complex III and complex IV to functional super-complex species, such

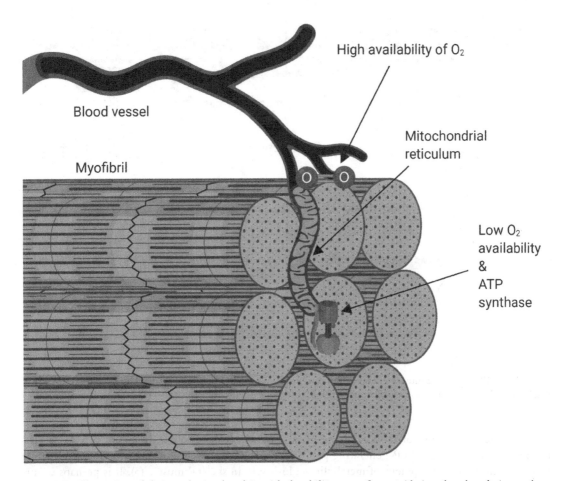

Figure 13.2 Illustration of elongated mitochondria with the ability to perform oxidative phosphorylation at the periphery of a myofiber and transfer proton gradient to areas with low O_2, hypothesized by Glancy et al. (17)

as super-complex $I+III_2+IV_n$. This shift reinforces the plasticity of the inner mitochondrial membrane and the formation of electron transport complexes. Additionally, this supports the assertion that mitochondrial function and structure are crucial components of the ability to utilize and extract oxygen during intense exercise.

The Ability to Prevent Accumulation of By-Products of Anaerobic and Aerobic Respiration, Which Are Detrimental to Performance

Preventing or managing the accumulation of by-products during exercise is a key factor in both endurance and power events. Several metabolites accumulate during intense exercise which can have deleterious effects on the ability to synthesize ATP rapidly and efficiently and thus enable skeletal muscle contractions. A famous misconception in exercise biochemistry is the historical hypothesis that lactic acid build-up contributed to fatigue. In actuality, lactic acid cannot readily form under physiological conditions (46). Although metabolic acidosis [i.e., the build-up of protons (H^+)], may contribute to fatigue by inhibiting or decreasing the efficiency of a variety of biochemical processes, the precise nature of this topic is still debated. Instead of being a waste product deleterious to exercise performance, lactate is actually a necessary metabolite in maintaining prolonged exercise performance.

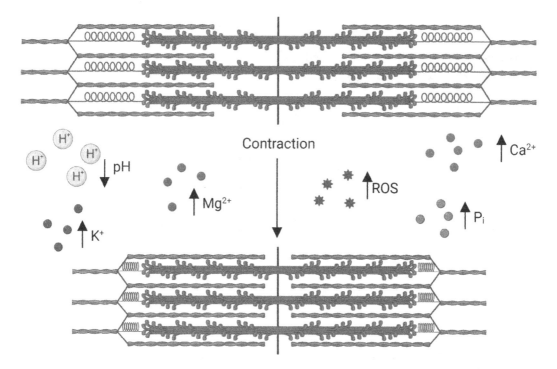

Figure 13.3 Illustration of intense exercise-induced build-up of ionic by-products, including Ca2+, H+, K+, Mg2+, and Pi (24), and reactive oxygen species (ROS) (46). Created with BioRender

For example, production of lactate during glycolysis helps to regenerate cytosolic NAD+, a critical metabolite of several ATP-generating pathways during exercise. Additionally, lactate production helps to retard the development of metabolic acidosis within skeletal muscle (3). It is perhaps unsurprising that elite endurance athletes such as marathon runners produce and can metabolize a large amount of lactate during training and competing. Interestingly, lactate may be produced in such large quantities in these athletes that lactate-metabolizing bacteria are preferentially selected for in the gut after a marathon (50). Intense exercise also results in the acute build-up of several ionic by-products, including Ca^{2+}, Cl^-, H^+, K^+, Mg^{2+}, Na^+, and P_i (24) (Figure 13.3). These ionic by-products can act to impair excitation-contraction coupling of skeletal muscle, and the ability to decrease their accumulation is a limiting factor to exercise performance.

In contracting myofibers, ATP is mainly utilized by actin–myosin cross-bridges and ion pumps. As cross-bridge cycling occurs of actin and myosin, ATP detaches from myosin after a cross-bridge power stroke. Without sufficient ATP, cross-bridges can develop rigor; thus, adequate ATP supply to these parts of the muscle fibre is imperative in maintaining optimal function. A key ion within this milieu is Ca^{2+}—a cause of fatigue involving this ion is theorized to involve insufficient sarcoplasmic reticulum pumping, resulting in unregulated increase in cytosolic free $[Ca^{2+}]$ and disruption of homeostatic Na^+ and K^+ gradients across the sarcolemma. This disruption eventually leads to an ablated action potential and the fatigue of contracting muscle fibres (2, 7). Fatigue is associated with the build-up of several other ionic by-products; for instance, Mg^{2+} in the cytosol is often bound to ATP, and a net ATP reduction is associated with an increase in the pool of free cytoplasmic $[Mg^{2+}]$ (10). Since maintaining ATP bioavailability is crucial to functioning skeletal muscle, these stores are robustly perturbed during intense exercise, and mechanisms must exist which prevent full depletion of ATP stores during intense exercise. One mechanism is via the inhibition of sarcoplasmic reticulum Ca^{2+} release in contracting myofibers. This reduces the amount of cycling cross-bridges and thus reduces ATP demand. Of course, declining sarcoplasmic reticulum Ca^{2+} release results in decreased muscle performance and is thus one limiting factor during intense exercise. Furthermore, sarcoplasmic reticulum leakage of Ca^{2+} during exercise may activate a signal transduction pathway to increase the capacity of myofibers to withstand fatigue (25). One interacting factor in Ca^{2+} metabolism during intense exercise is the sensitivity of troponin within cycling cross-bridges to local Ca^{2+} concentrations. Decreasing intracellular pH appears to inhibit troponin sensitivity to Ca^{2+}, resulting in a reduced number of cycling cross-bridges, loss of force, and thus fatigue.

Skeletal muscle pH may decline to values as low as 6.2 during intense exercise, and the magnitude of declining force during fatigue is correlated with acidosis (12). In addition to inhibiting sensitivity to Ca^{2+}, an accumulation of protons can inhibit ATPases such as the myofibril, sarcoplasmic reticulum, and Na^+–K^+ ATPases. These ATPases are essential to optimal functioning of a contracting muscle, and inhibition can contribute to reduced cross-bridge cycling, sarcoplasmic reticulum Ca^{2+} uptake and release, and surface membrane depolarization (12). Acidosis is almost certainly caused by biochemical reactions other than lactate production. For example, every time ATP is broken down to ADP and P_i, a proton is released, which can contribute to decreasing pH during intense exercise. Additionally, protons can accumulate as a result of glyceraldehyde 3-phosphate dehydrogenase reactions, which catalyze the sixth step of glycolysis, resulting in the accumulation of NADH + H^+. Thus, pathways that generate quickly available ATP without adequate mitochondrial metabolism can lead to an accumulation of protons. When the ATP demand of working muscle is met by mitochondrial oxidative phosphorylation, protons do not accumulate, as they are metabolized by working mitochondria in order to maintain the proton gradient. However, when exercise intensity exceeds mitochondrial capacity in terms of ATP demand and there is a reliance on creatine phosphate and glycolysis, excess proton accumulation occurs (46). Thus, increased mitochondrial capacity in elite endurance athletes is one method by which acidosis (i.e., the build-up of protons) is delayed and athletes can maintain a higher rate of ATP production in contracting muscle for a prolonged duration. Other mechanisms by which athletes maintain superior resistance to proton accumulation is increased buffering capacity. This buffering system consists of P_i production, HCO_3^-, creatine phosphate hydrolysis, and lactate production. These components bind or consume H^+ to help ameliorate excess proton accumulation (46), and increasing the capacity of these buffering mechanisms can increase the ability of an athlete to withstand fatigue.

Another important by-product of ATP generation during intense bouts of contracting muscle is the formation of reactive oxygen species (ROS). Multiple systems within muscle generate ROS during exercise. The most established is aerobic metabolism via the mitochondrial electron transport chain. Superoxide anions are generated as a result of incomplete reduction of oxygen at complex I and III (45). Another well-defined source of superoxide is the NADPH oxidase, which has isoforms constitutively expressed in skeletal muscle. As with most metabolites or by-products generated by metabolism of skeletal muscle during exercise, it is not entirely clear if ROS directly contributes to fatigue in a physiological setting. However, similarly to other by-products mentioned here, a series of mechanistic investigations provide evidence supporting this assertion. For example, direct exposure of intact contracting mouse muscle fibres to hydrogen peroxide reduces force during submaximal tetani (45). One mechanism by which ROS may interfere with force during skeletal muscle contraction is by promoting Ca^{2+} release from the sarcoplasmic reticulum and slowing Ca^{2+} reuptake. Endurance athletes thus have improved defences against ROS build-up during exercise in the form of scavenger molecules and enzymes which "safely" metabolize ROS.

The Ability to Efficiently Metabolize Readily Available Fuel or Metabolites

During intense or sustained exercise, the working muscle must meet energy demand by metabolizing fuel or metabolite sources to produce ATP. This includes breaking down more complex molecules suitable for storing energy such as glycogen and triglyceride. Additionally, these metabolic processes must maintain homeostasis of metabolite balances in order to preserve cellular functionality. The most obvious example of this is cellular ATP concentration, which is extremely robust, as it is vital to nearly all cellular metabolic processes. During exercise, several processes contribute to maintaining ATP concentration, which is utilized rapidly by contracting sarcomeres. Indeed, the turnover of ATP during short-duration exercise can increase by up to 1,000-fold. Even during maximally fatiguing exercise, ATP concentrations only drop a relatively small amount (e.g., in extreme cases a decrease of <30% can be detected) (3). Interestingly, the total amount of ATP stored in the muscle is very small; thus, muscle cells rely on metabolic systems to produce ATP or scavenge it from breakdown products. A major energy system in meeting the drastically increased demand for ATP during exercise is oxidative phosphorylation. Ultimately, a central part of this complex metabolic reaction is NADH breakdown to NAD^+, and the ability to maintain homeostatic balance of the $NADH/NAD^+$ ratio is another limiting factor in exercise performance. In fact, increased ratio of NAD^+ to NADH after exercise may be one way by which the transcription of genes involved in increased mitochondrial biogenesis are regulated via NAD^+-dependent sirtuin activity (18).

Fuel sources required during shorter bouts of exercise are distinct to endurance exercise. One important short-term fuel source in skeletal muscle is creatine phosphate, which provides an almost instantaneous source of ATP production and is heavily relied upon by contracting muscle during the initial ~10 seconds of intense exercise. Creatine phosphate may also play a role in energy homeostasis during longer bouts of contraction due to its role in the transfer of phosphate groups from mitochondria throughout the cytosol (46). The creatine kinase reaction consumes a proton and thus has an alkalizing effect on cellular pH levels, and improving the capacity of this system may be one of many ways exercise training is able to improve the buffering capacity of skeletal muscle and protect against acidosis.

Several other fuel sources are limiting factors in athletic performance. As demonstrated in classical experiments by Bergström and Hultman (4, 5), skeletal muscle glycogen availability during prolonged, intense exercise is a limiting metabolic factor. Glycogen is a branched polymer consisting of thousands of glucose residues and is an ideal energy storage molecule, requiring mobilization to allow its utilization during exercise. Unsurprisingly, glycogen depletion is concomitant with less readily available fuel and, hence, the onset of fatigue. Interestingly, recent studies have demonstrated that similarly to mitochondria, glycogen depots may have heterogeneity between sub-sarcolemmal and intermyofibrillar stores (41). The role of these distinct depots is not fully understood; however, intermyofibrillar pools may be preferentially depleted during exercise (40). Furthermore, sarcoplasmic reticulum Ca^{2+} release and force production are more closely associated with depletion of intermyofibrillar glycogen depots (38), although the exact mechanisms behind this are unknown.

Another source of ATP that is a limiting factor in certain types of athletic events is the availability and mobilization of lipids. Lipids are an extremely efficient storage method for biochemical energy, although as a fuel source for athletic performance, they have the downside that generation of ATP is relatively slow and consumes a large amount of O_2. Lipid catabolism is an important source of ATP generation during skeletal muscle contractions in prolonged endurance exercise. Lipids entering this process can be derived from intracellular sources such as lipid droplets within skeletal muscle, mobilized free fatty acids from adipose tissue, or lipoprotein-derived sources, whereby free fatty acids are released from lipid droplets by enzymes localized to the endothelium of the skeletal muscle capillary bed. Total lipid depots are enriched in trained endurance athletes compared to sedentary counterparts, but within this divergence, lipid droplets are also morphologically distinct from trained to sedentary (9). In another example of the benefits of assessing humans in terms of different ends of an extreme spectrum, insight regarding these lipid droplets has been garnered from experiments that evaluated patients with type 2 diabetes and endurance athletes. These investigations demonstrated that trained athletes possess predominately small lipid droplets in oxidative type I fibres within the intermyofibrillar space. In contrast, lipid droplets are larger and in the sub-sarcolemmal space in muscle of individuals with type 2 diabetes. Athletes also have higher levels of enzymes that facilitate the rapid mobilization of these lipid droplets (9). To summarize, a limiting factor to athletic performance is the ability to appropriately store and rapidly mobilize lipid and glycogen depots in order to meet the ATP demands of intense exercise.

Future Areas of Research

An important field that may become a key area of research within the study of the biochemical and metabolic limitations of exercise is the interaction between the molecular clock and metabolic processes (this topic has been reviewed in detail in 14). At first glance, the molecular clock may seem like an unlikely regulator of metabolic or biochemical limitations of exercise. However, emerging evidence suggests this may be a fundamental modulator of muscular and physiological exercise capacity. It is known that world records in nearly all sports are improved in the late afternoon or evening compared with the morning. This holds true even when accounting for temperature and other confounding factors (14). The reasons for this phenomenon are not entirely clear but may be partly related to fluctuating biochemical and metabolic perturbations within skeletal muscle. Mammalian cells possess an internal molecular clock that consists of transcriptional/translational auto-regulatory feedback loops. At a physiological level, circadian clocks drive whole-body metabolism. Molecularly, cell-autonomous circadian rhythms are produced by the activity of transcriptional activators CLOCK and BMAL1 and their target genes, which form a repressor complex that interacts with CLOCK and BMAL1 to inhibit transcriptional activity (16, 47). The feedback loop of the cell-autonomous core clock is highly regulated by several factors, including the activity of the master clock located in the hypothalamic superchiasmatic nucleus (16, 42, 47). Physical activity modulates the molecular clock in skeletal muscle, affecting both the amplitude and phase of circadian rhythms (49, 54). The skeletal muscle circadian transcriptomic response clusters around the midpoint of the active phase in mice (36). Additionally, a study of denervated skeletal muscle in rodent models demonstrates that the removal of motor neuron activation moderately dysregulates circadian transcriptional activity (37). In humans, one-legged resistance exercise altered circadian gene expression and apparently induced a phase shift of core-clock genes when compared with the contralateral control leg (55).

These data support the assertion that the core-clock machinery partly regulates the gene transcriptional response to exercise—in other words, the genes turned on in response to, or off after cessation of, intense exercise and the magnitude partly regulated by an internal cellular "clock." Additionally, genetic ablation of these molecular clocks such as *Cry1* and *Cry2* increased exercise capacity in mice and altered the exercise-induced gene signature (26), adding further weight to the evidence that the molecular clock may modulate the metabolic limits of exercise capacity. In human studies, cultured primary myotubes from endurance-trained athletes had preserved rhythmic gene expression of metabolic regulators SIRT1 and NAMPT, while myotubes derived from untrained individuals did not (20). These metabolic regulators (SIRT1 and NAMPT) are important indicators of metabolic capacity, as they are responsive to altered bioavailability of NAD^+. As detailed earlier in this chapter, the ratio of $NAD^+/NADH$ is one crucial metabolic limit of prolonged muscular function, as they are crucial metabolites in generating ATP through oxidative phosphorylation. Indeed, $NAD^+/NADH$ is hypothesized (with some evidence) to fluctuate over the course of 24 hours (43) and may be one link between the molecular clock and exercise capacity. Specifically, altering the regulation of the molecular clock can modulate the bioavailability of NAD^+ (43) and can also modify exercise performance and capacity (26).

Summary

In summary, the biochemical and metabolic limits of athletic endurance performance can essentially be boiled down to three factors:

- The ability to match oxygen requirement to mitochondrial respiration in a temporally and spatially specific manner
- The ability to prevent accumulation of by-products of anaerobic and aerobic respiration which are detrimental to performance
- The ability to efficiently metabolize readily available fuels or metabolites

Athletes have an improved ability to mobilize fuel efficiently and rapidly from readily available sources in addition to more complex storage depots such as lipid droplets. Furthermore, athletes can effectively match oxygen to areas that require this molecule as a final electron acceptor during aerobic respiration. These metabolic processes dramatically increase during exercise in order to meet a relatively huge demand for ATP. This increase in metabolism, and the process of sarcomere contraction, increases the build-up of by-products and metabolites. The ability to prevent or withstand the build-up of these by-products is also enhanced in elite athletes.

References

1. Alhindi Y, Vaanholt LM, Al-Tarrah M, Gray SR, Speakman JR, Hambly C, et al. Low citrate synthase activity is associated with glucose intolerance and lipotoxicity. *J Nutr Metab* 2019: 8594825, 2019.
2. Allen DG, Lamb GD, Westerblad H. Impaired calcium release during fatigue. *J Appl Physiol* 104: 296–305, 2008.
3. Baker JS, McCormick MC, Robergs RA. Interaction among skeletal muscle metabolic energy systems during intense exercise. *J Nutr Metab* 2010: 905612, 2010.
4. Bergstrom J, Hultman E. A study of the glycogen metabolism during exercise in man. *Scand J Clin Lab Invest* 19: 218–228, 1967.
5. Bergstrom J, Hultman E. Muscle glycogen synthesis after exercise: an enhancing factor localized to the muscle cells in man. *Nature* 210: 309–310, 1966.
6. Bramble DM, Lieberman DE. Endurance running and the evolution of Homo. *Nature* 432: 345–352, 2004.
7. Cheng AJ, Place N, Westerblad H. Molecular basis for exercise-induced fatigue: the importance of strictly controlled cellular Ca(2+) handling. *Cold Spring Harb Perspect Med* 8: a029710, 2018.
8. Costill DL, Fink WJ, Pollock ML. Muscle fiber composition and enzyme activities of elite distance runners. *Med Sci Sports* 8: 96–100, 1976.
9. Daemen S, Gemmink A, Brouwers B, Meex RCR, Huntjens PR, Schaart G, et al. Distinct lipid droplet characteristics and distribution unmask the apparent contradiction of the athlete's paradox. *Mol Metab* 17: 71–81, 2018.
10. Dahlstedt AJ, Westerblad H. Inhibition of creatine kinase reduces the rate of fatigue-induced decrease in tetanic [Ca(2+)](i) in mouse skeletal muscle. *J Physiol* 533: 639–649, 2001.
11. Dandanell S, Meinild-Lundby AK, Andersen AB, Lang PF, Oberholzer L, Keiser S, et al. Determinants of maximal whole-body fat oxidation in elite cross-country skiers: role of skeletal muscle mitochondria. *Scand J Med Sci Sports* 28: 2494–2504, 2018.
12. Fitts RH. The role of acidosis in fatigue: pro perspective. *Med Sci Sports Exerc* 48: 2335–2338, 2016.
13. Gabriel BM, Al-Tarrah M, Alhindi Y, Kilikevicius A, Venckunas T, Gray SR, et al. H55N polymorphism is associated with low citrate synthase activity which regulates lipid metabolism in mouse muscle cells. *PLOS ONE* 12: e0185789, 2017.
14. Gabriel BM, Zierath JR. Circadian rhythms and exercise - re-setting the clock in metabolic disease. *Nat Rev Endocrinol* 15: 197–206, 2019.
15. Gabriel BM, Zierath JR. The limits of exercise physiology: from performance to health. *Cell Metab* 25: 1000–1011, 2017.
16. Gerhart-Hines Z, Lazar MA. Circadian metabolism in the light of evolution. *Endocr Rev* 36: 289–304, 2015.
17. Glancy B, Hartnell LM, Malide D, Yu ZX, Combs CA, Connelly PS, et al. Mitochondrial reticulum for cellular energy distribution in muscle. *Nature* 523: 617–620, 2015.
18. Goody MF, Henry CA. A need for NAD+ in muscle development, homeostasis, and aging. *Skelet Muscle* 8: 9, 2018.
19. Greggio C, Jha P, Kulkarni SS, Lagarrigue S, Broskey NT, Boutant M, et al. Enhanced respiratory chain supercomplex formation in response to exercise in human skeletal muscle. *Cell Metab* 25: 301–311, 2017.
20. Hansen J, Timmers S, Moonen-Kornips E, Duez H, Staels B, Hesselink MK, et al. Synchronized human skeletal myotubes of lean, obese and type 2 diabetic patients maintain circadian oscillation of clock genes. *Sci Rep* 6: 35047, 2016.
21. Hawley JA, Maughan RJ, Hargreaves M. Exercise metabolism: historical perspective. *Cell Metab* 22: 12–17, 2015.
22. Holloszy JO. Biochemical adaptations in muscle. Effects of exercise on mitochondrial oxygen uptake and respiratory enzyme activity in skeletal muscle. *J Biol Chem* 242: 2278–2282, 1967.

23. Hood DA. Invited Review: contractile activity-induced mitochondrial biogenesis in skeletal muscle. *J Appl Physiol* 90: 1137–1157, 2001.

24. Hostrup M, Bangsbo J. Limitations in intense exercise performance of athletes - effect of speed endurance training on ion handling and fatigue development. *J Physiol* 595: 2897–2913, 2016.

25. Ivarsson N, Mattsson CM, Cheng AJ, Bruton JD, Ekblom B, Lanner JT, et al. SR Ca(2+) leak in skeletal muscle fibers acts as an intracellular signal to increase fatigue resistance. *J Gen Physiol* 151: 567–577, 2019.

26. Jordan SD, Kriebs A, Vaughan M, Duglan D, Fan W, Henriksson E, et al. CRY1/2 selectively repress PPARdelta and limit exercise capacity. *Cell Metab* 26: 243–255 e246, 2017.

27. Joyner MJ, Coyle EF. Endurance exercise performance: the physiology of champions. *J Physiol* 586: 35–44, 2008.

28. Krogh A. The number and distribution of capillaries in muscles with calculations of the oxygen pressure head necessary for supplying the tissue. *J Physiol* 52: 409–415, 1919.

29. Krogh A. The rate of diffusion of gases through animal tissues, with some remarks on the coefficient of invasion. *J Physiol* 52: 391–408, 1919.

30. Krogh A. The supply of oxygen to the tissues and the regulation of the capillary circulation. *J Physiol* 52: 457–474, 1919.

31. Krogh A, Lindhard J. The regulation of respiration and circulation during the initial stages of muscular work. *J Physiol* 47: 112–136, 1913.

32. Krogh A, Lindhard J. The relative value of fat and carbohydrate as sources of muscular energy: With appendices on the correlation between standard metabolism and the respiratory quotient during rest and work. *Biochem J* 14: 290–363, 1920.

33. Kuznetsov AV, Margreiter R. Heterogeneity of mitochondria and mitochondrial function within cells as another level of mitochondrial complexity. *Int J Mol Sci* 10: 1911–1929, 2009.

34. Lundby C, Jacobs RA. Adaptations of skeletal muscle mitochondria to exercise training. *Exp Physiol* 101: 17–22, 2016.

35. Lundby C, Montero D. CrossTalk opposing view: diffusion limitation of O2 from microvessels into muscle does not contribute to the limitation of VO2 max. *J Physiol* 593: 3759–3761, 2015.

36. Miller BH, McDearmon EL, Panda S, Hayes KR, Zhang J, Andrews JL, et al. Circadian and CLOCK-controlled regulation of the mouse transcriptome and cell proliferation. *Proc Natl Acad Sci U S A* 104: 3342–3347, 2007.

37. Nakao R, Yamamoto S, Horikawa K, Yasumoto Y, Nikawa T, Mukai C, et al. Atypical expression of circadian clock genes in denervated mouse skeletal muscle. *Chronobiol Int* 32: 486–496, 2015.

38. Nielsen J, Cheng AJ, Ortenblad N, Westerblad H. Subcellular distribution of glycogen and decreased tetanic Ca2+ in fatigued single intact mouse muscle fibres. *J Physiol* 592: 2003–2012, 2014.

39. Nielsen J, Gejl KD, Hey-Mogensen M, Holmberg HC, Suetta C, Krustrup P, et al. Plasticity in mitochondrial cristae density allows metabolic capacity modulation in human skeletal muscle. *J Physiol* 595: 2839–2847, 2017.

40. Ortenblad N, Nielsen J, Saltin B, Holmberg HC. Role of glycogen availability in sarcoplasmic reticulum Ca2+ kinetics in human skeletal muscle. *J Physiol* 589: 711–725, 2011.

41. Ortenblad N, Westerblad H, Nielsen J. Muscle glycogen stores and fatigue. *J Physiol* 591: 4405–4413, 2013.

42. Panda S. Circadian physiology of metabolism. *Science* 354: 1008–1015, 2016.

43. Peek CB, Affinati AH, Ramsey KM, Kuo HY, Yu W, Sena LA, et al. Circadian clock NAD+ cycle drives mitochondrial oxidative metabolism in mice. *Science* 342: 1243417, 2013.

44. Raichlen DA, Polk JD. Linking brains and brawn: exercise and the evolution of human neurobiology. *Proc Biol Sci* 280: 20122250, 2013.

45. Reid MB. Reactive oxygen species as agents of fatigue. *Med Sci Sports Exerc* 48: 2239–2246, 2016.

46. Robergs RA, Ghiasvand F, Parker D. Biochemistry of exercise-induced metabolic acidosis. *Am J Physiol* 287: R502–R516, 2004.

47. Robinson I, Reddy AB. Molecular mechanisms of the circadian clockwork in mammals. *FEBS Lett* 588: 2477–2483, 2014.

48. Sandbakk O, Holmberg HC. A reappraisal of success factors for Olympic cross-country skiing. *Int J Sports Physiol Perform* 9: 117–121, 2014.

49. Saner NJ, Bishop DJ, Bartlett JD. Is exercise a viable therapeutic intervention to mitigate mitochondrial dysfunction and insulin resistance induced by sleep loss?. *Sleep Med Rev* 37: 60–68, 2018.

50. Scheiman J, Luber JM, Chavkin TA, MacDonald T, Tung A, Pham LD, et al. Meta-omics analysis of elite athletes identifies a performance-enhancing microbe that functions via lactate metabolism. *Nat Med* 25: 1104–1109, 2019.

51. Schnyder S, Handschin C. Skeletal muscle as an endocrine organ: PGC-1alpha, myokines and exercise. *Bone* 80: 115–125, 2015.
52. Thomsen JJ, Rentsch RL, Robach P, Calbet JA, Boushel R, Rasmussen P, et al. Prolonged administration of recombinant human erythropoietin increases submaximal performance more than maximal aerobic capacity. *Eur J Appl Physiol* 101: 481–486, 2007.
53. Wagner PD. CrossTalk proposal: diffusion limitation of O2 from microvessels into muscle does contribute to the limitation of VO2 max. *J Physiol* 593: 3757–3758, 2015.
54. Wolff G, Esser KA. Scheduled exercise phase shifts the circadian clock in skeletal muscle. *Med Sci Sports Exerc* 44: 1663–1670, 2012.
55. Zambon AC, McDearmon EL, Salomonis N, Vranizan KM, Johansen KL, Adey D, et al. Time- and exercise-dependent gene regulation in human skeletal muscle. *Genome Biol* 4: R61, 2003.

14

GENETIC LIMITATIONS TO ATHLETIC PERFORMANCE

Colin N. Moran and Guan Wang

How Do We Define Athletic Performance?

Athletic performance ultimately is defined by success in winning medals and trophies. However, across sports there is no single method to achieve these goals. Some sports require power and strength, such as rugby or sprinting. Others, like cross-country skiing or marathon running, require endurance. For some, like the 100-m sprint, athletes must run in straight lines. For others, like tennis or basketball, they must twist and turn. Each of these places different demands on an athlete's physiology, and we are still only scratching the surface of the potential variety and potential for limitation.

Elite athletic performance is a complex phenomenon. In the biological context, human elite sporting performance is a phenotype, which reflects a collection of abilities required to achieve peak physiological performance. These include the ability to utilize and transport oxygen, the ability to adapt to training, and cognitive ability, to mention a few. Additionally, the lines between the necessary aspects of physiology are not easily determined. Some—in fact most—sports require a mixture of these characteristics, albeit to widely varying degrees. Whilst a 100-m sprinter will mostly benefit from strength and power, athletes playing hockey, tennis, or football would all be likely to benefit from strength, power, and endurance. Even within one sport, there is no fixed path to reach the top level of performance and achieve success. Athletes come in different shapes and sizes and excel in different aspects of their physiology (Figure 14.1) despite having the same target.

What Determines Athletic Performance?

The various aspects of physiology required in a competitive sport help define whether and how an athlete performs remarkable athletic feats. Despite the variety of paths to success, all top athletes display elite athleticism, train hard, and manage their bodies to achieve elite performance. Typically, they primarily attribute their success to hard work rather than the natural talents and attributes they were born with. Others consider the converse to be true, leading to the nature versus nurture debate. However, as David Epstein writes in *The Sports Gene: Talent, Practice and the Truth about Success*, elite athleticism is a result of both innate hardware (innate ability) and learned software (e.g., training and practice), with the greatness of athletes always characterized by both their genes and training environments (37). Neither nature nor nurture is an absolute for sports expertise. Nature and nurture are intertwined in predisposition to elite athleticism, or any complex trait. Sports geneticists seek to understand where the balance lies and how the two interact.

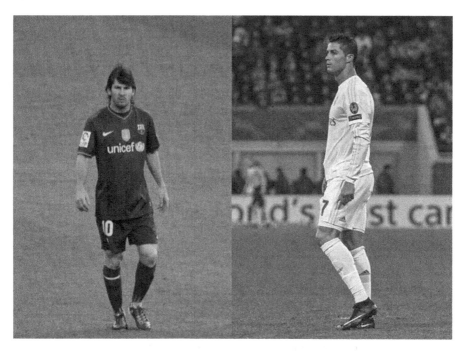

Figure 14.1 Images showing differences in physiology within one sport. Lionel Messi (1.7 m) and Cristiano Ronaldo (1.87 m), both renowned international footballers with markedly different statures

The Complexity of Nurture

Nurture plays a crucial role in developing or limiting athletic success. The characteristics of the environment in which an athlete develops and trains are only part of the equation that we (at least) perceive that we have control over: where to live, which sports to focus on, how often to train, or what nutritional advice to follow, to name a few. Socioeconomics also plays a prominent role. On one hand, low socioeconomic status may motivate athletes to perform and maintain their best condition to win competitions, to improve quality of life, and to improve social status. On the other hand, socioeconomics influences the opportunities and resources, such as facilities or equipment, which are available for the training of athletes and are also vital for discovering and shaping future Olympians.

Intensity, frequency, and type of training are important environmental components that are under an individual's control. However, the magnitude of an individual's response to training is also highly variable. In other words, we do not all respond in the same way or to the same extent. Not just because of varied training loads, durations, and patterns, but as we will explore later, this, too, is subject to genetic influence (78). Whilst individualized training according to genetic makeup would be an appealing aspect to develop, the challenge lies in decomposing the complexity of genetics (nature) that will be further illustrated in the sections that follow.

The Complexity of Nature

In the current context, nature refers to the genetic blueprints that define who we are. These blueprints are known as a genome and contain all the necessary instructions for building a human. They are the sum of all the genes in a cell or an organism. However, each one of us is unique, both in obvious ways such as hair colour or eye colour and in more complex subtle ways such as disease risks or sporting potential. Therefore, the instructions that are used to make each of us are also unique—similar because we are all humans, but different because we are all individuals—and they predispose us to be good, or not good, at different things.

Our genomes are made of four DNA letters: A, C, T, and G. The sequence of letters in the human genome was first read, or sequenced, in full during the Human Genome Project (HGP) between 1988 and 2003. The HGP was a concerted international effort across six nations outlining for the first time a complete human genetic blueprint creating a reference sequence and revealing approximately 20,500 human genes (15). A series of achievements from the HGP include characterization of 99% of the genic regions of the human genome with high accuracy (99.99%) and identification of 3.7 million human common genetic variations (although subsequently many more have been found) (15). The outcomes of the HGP had huge impacts throughout human biology and for our understanding of evolution, development, and function of human cells, medicine, and physiology. The HGP paved the way for decoding the human genetic instruction book and understanding the differences between us as individuals.

Following on the success of the HGP, the 1000 Genomes Project (2008–2015) sought to sequence multiple human genomes to understand the extent of variation. It used 2,504 individuals from ancestrally diverse populations and created a global reference for common human genetic variation (25). It catalogued a variety of different types of variation in our genomes, specifically 84.7 million single nucleotide polymorphisms (SNPs; i.e., alternative letters in the sequence) with a frequency of $\geq 1\%$ across ancestries, 3.6 million short insertions/deletions (indels; i.e., additional or missing letters in the sequence), and 60,000 structural variants (≥ 50 bp; i.e., large insertion/deletions or sections in unexpected orientations or locations) (25). Each person only carries a subset of these variants, but this library of possibilities allows each of us to be a unique individual. Typically, an individual human genome differs from the reference human genome at 4.1–5.0 million variant sites (25). These genetic variations contribute to the different physical characteristics among individuals, disease susceptibility within and among populations, and differences in almost any human trait. They predispose us to our individual sporting abilities (or lack of), making major contributions to how athletes achieve the highest performance calibre in their specialized sports (e.g., by modulating training adaptation or protecting athletes from injury).

The 1000 Genomes Project is a cornerstone of studying the functional impact of human genetic variation and disease association. The 1000 Genomes Project samples and data remain valuable open resources (12), providing information for other large genomic projects such as GEUVADIS (13) and ENCODE (10). Building on this, several nations have launched population-wide biobank projects, such as the pioneer Iceland deCODE project (founded in 1996) (6), the UK Biobank (2006–2010) (31), and the Auria Biobank in Finland (2012–ongoing) (2). These biobank projects aim to collect human genetic and clinical data on a population scale to improve disease pre-diagnoses and treatments for individuals. Significant expansions of these efforts are also already underway. For example, the 100,000 Genomes Project (England) will grow to sequence 1 million genomes through the United Kingdom's National Health Service (NHS) centres and the UK biobank, with a further plan announced for sequencing 5 million genomes in the UK within 5 years by the UK Health and Social Care Secretary Matt Hancock in October 2018 (17). Despite these biobank projects focusing on improving patient care, they also facilitate a better understanding of general populations and the interaction between an individual's unique genetic makeup and their environment, including how traits related to sporting performance are influenced positively and negatively by genetics.

Simple Versus Complex Genetic Traits

Traditionally, in high schools we are taught that genetic traits are simple and follow Mendelian rules of inheritance. This implies that there is a gene for each trait with simple alternative versions, for example, the often-used example of the eye colour gene with blue and brown versions. Some traits are relatively simple. Rare disorders such as cystic fibrosis, sickle cell anaemia, and Huntington disease are the result of changes in single genes that can cause significant disease. However, the situation is rarely so simple.

Even eye colour in reality involves differing versions of multiple genes (82). Height, a relatively simple aspect of physiology, is estimated to be determined by common variants in at least 700 genes—each with a small effect of only a few millimetres (85)—and rare variants in at least 83 genes with slightly larger effects of up to 2 centimetres (49). Other traits are also determined by multiple genes with small effects. For example, ~900 genes are involved in determining the risk of hypertension (38). In fact, the vast majority of traits are complex and the result of the combined effects of many genes.

However, genetics does not fully explain the differences in our heights or disease risks on its own. Heritability studies estimate that ~80% of the differences between us in height and ~30–50% of the differences between us in hypertension risk can be explained by heritable (genetic) factors. Consequently, the remaining 20% or 50–70%, respectively, must be explained by non-genetic factors (i.e., environmental differences between us, such as diet and lifestyle). Traits involving the interaction of multiple genetic and environmental variants are known as complex, polygenic, or multifactorial traits.

Elite sporting performance is an example of such a complex trait. A twin study investigating the heritability of elite athlete status found that 66% of the differences between us could be explained by genetic differences (35). This is consistent with the well-known quote from the renowned exercise physiologist Per-Olof Åstrand in which "anyone interested in winning Olympic gold medals must select his or her parents very carefully." However, the result means that genetics and the environment are simultaneously crucial to understanding elite sports performance, not exclusively one or the other. Whilst 66% of the differences between us can be explained by our biological inheritance from our parents, 34% cannot be explained this way and can be influenced by the choices that we make and things over which we have control. These will include, for example, training, diet, or opportunity. To understand fully the genetic determinants and limits of sporting performance, it is vital that we capture all the genetic effects, large or small, and how genes interact with the environment and choices that we make in the development of performance.

How Do We Investigate Complex Performance Traits?

Complex traits almost by definition are difficult to study. The fact that a large proportion of the differences among individuals is the result of environmental factors and choices made by individuals creates a lot of noise in experiments. In part, this problem is addressed by developing larger and larger studies. For example, recent analyses of hypertension have involved >1 million people (38). However, this approach would not be possible when studying elite athletes. Elite athletes are, by definition, rare. The problem is further compounded by the variety of paths to successful elite performance. For example, an elite 10,000-metre runner may win medals by stretching the field out from the start of the race or by bursting from the pack in a sprint finish over the final 100 metres. Each strategy relies on different aspects of physiology and therefore variation in different genes. Consequently, studies into the genetic determinants of sporting performance typically focus on measurable aspects of physiology known to be important for performance, such as $\dot{V}O_2$ max for endurance or muscle fibre type for power, rather than directly on performance itself.

Heritable Aspects of Endurance Performance

The Health, Risk factors, exercise Training And Genetics (HERITAGE) Family Study was kicked started with funding from the US government in 1992. The primary aim was to identify the role of genes in the cardiovascular and metabolic responses to regular endurance exercise (14). It was led by Professor Claude Bouchard and was a multicentre study across five institutes. It spanned 12 years and collected a range of physiological data, including but not limited to blood pressure, blood lactate, glucose, plasma lipids and lipoproteins, cardiac output, and $\dot{V}O_2$ max, in two generations of Caucasian and African American families who participated in a 20-week standardized stationary cycle ergometer programme (14). This allowed investigation of the genetic component of these traits both at baseline and in response to exercise training.

At entry to the study, participants' $\dot{V}O_2$ max scores ranged from 1.8 to 3.5 L·min⁻¹. Since the participants were family members, some more closely related than others, it was possible to see if the degree of relatedness was associated with differences in $\dot{V}O_2$ max. Approximately 51% of the differences between individuals' $\dot{V}O_2$ max scores could be explained by heritable factors (28). Following the exercise training protocol, there was, as expected, an average increase in $\dot{V}O_2$ max of ~16%. However, there were also considerable individual differences in response to training. Roughly 5% of participants had little or no improvement (i.e., <5% increase) whilst ~5% improved dramatically (i.e., >40% improvement), with every size of response in between also observed (14). This could not be accounted for by age, sex, initial fitness, or ethnicity. Importantly, there was more variance (around 2.5 times) between families than within families (i.e., two individuals were more likely to have a similar $\dot{V}O_2$ max if they were from the same family than if they were from different families), indicating a genetic component to $\dot{V}O_2$ max trainability (27). The heritability estimate reached 47% and could not be explained by baseline variables, including $\dot{V}O_2$ max. Thus, genetics is equally important to sedentary $\dot{V}O_2$ max (or $\dot{V}O_2$ max response to training) as environmental factors that are widely accepted to be important.

What Makes a Champion?

The previously mentioned study additionally suggests that the genes responsible for baseline sedentary $\dot{V}O_2$ max are different from the genes responsible for $\dot{V}O_2$ max response to training (27). Therefore, athletes with the highest $\dot{V}O_2$ max are likely to have a set of genetic variants giving them naturally high $\dot{V}O_2$ max when sedentary and have another set of genetic variants giving them a high $\dot{V}O_2$ max response to training. Additionally, of course, they must do the appropriate training and look after their diet and general health. Individuals with the best genetic profiles will not become world champion athletes if they spend their days sitting on their couch. Equally, individuals with the highest levels of performance may not be the most genetically gifted (see Figure 14.2, adapted from 78).

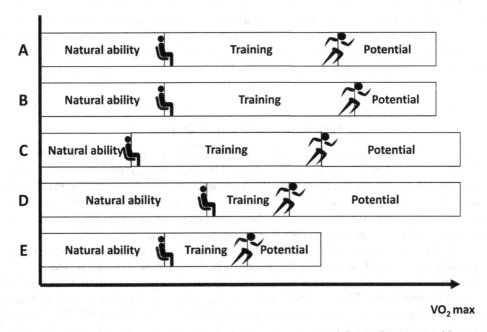

Figure 14.2 The importance of genetics in natural talent, genetics in trainability, and training. Athletes A and B have similar natural abilities (baseline genetics) and similar potential (trainability genetics), but athlete B trains harder, realizing more of their potential

Are There Really Non-Responders to Exercise?

As well as quantifying the genetic contribution to training response, the HERITAGE study suggests that some individuals' $\dot{V}O_2$ max does not respond to aerobic exercise training. Genetics is often incorrectly thought of as being both deterministic and categorical—for example, athletes have the gene for strength, or the gene for speed, whilst the rest of us do not—or that there are groups of extreme people who are responders (or non-responders) to exercise. A study by Montero and Lundby (51) reported that non-responders of $\dot{V}O_2$ max can respond given a sufficient exposure to exercise. In this study, 78 healthy young men participated in a successive 6-week endurance training programme in five groups with differing training volumes (i.e., one to five × 60 mins training sessions per week), with an average training intensity equivalent to 65% of maximal power output (Wmax) for 60 mins. The non-responders were classified given a technical error of 3.96% for Wmax based on the baseline measurements in all participants. They were then subjected to a further 6 weeks of training (identical to the first training protocols) plus two additional exercise sessions per week. The authors concluded that the non-responsiveness is diminished and eventually removed from all training groups with the increased training and demonstrated that total haemoglobin mass is a primary determinant of $\dot{V}O_2$ max. The authors pointed out that the percentage of technical error for $\dot{V}O_2$ max was not calculated due to the lack of multiple $\dot{V}O_2$ max measurements at baseline, and physiological responses in body composition changes were not measured in the study. Other criticisms that this work has received include the low Wmax error used, the failure of considering the Wmax error both at baseline and post training, and potential recruitment bias (60). Phillips et al. (60) studied $\dot{V}O_2$ max, blood pressure ,and HOMR-IR responses to 6-week high-intensity interval training (three sessions per week at workloads equivalent to ~100% or ~125% $\dot{V}O_2$ max) in 189 sedentary women and men (including 13 non-exercise participants) with impaired glucose intolerance and/or a body mass index >27 kg/m^2. They observed a comparable non-responder rate of ~15–20% for $\dot{V}O_2$ max to other large and robust exercise training studies, restating the heterogeneity of responses to exercise training (60). However, it is important to remember that complex genetics is not categorical. As clearly shown in the figures of Bouchard et al. (28), there is not a group of responders and non-responders—there is a continuum. It would be more appropriate to consider the degree of responsiveness, removing much of the conflict between the earlier studies. Those requiring extra training sessions in the Montero and Lundby study (51) could be described as being less responsive to training rather than non-responders.

Which Genes Determine $\dot{V}O_2$ max?

The HERITAGE and other studies established the magnitude of the importance of heritable factors in determining $\dot{V}O_2$ max. A best guess, based on other complex phenotypes, is that as many as 1,000 genes may be involved, each containing common genetic variants with small effects on $\dot{V}O_2$ max. However, the identity of those genes and variants remains largely unknown. Initial efforts took a candidate gene approach, which relies on existing knowledge of the underlying physiology of $\dot{V}O_2$ max and investigates variation in genes related to these physiological processes or structures.

Physiologically, $\dot{V}O_2$ max is largely determined by the capacity of the heart and oxygen transport/delivery systems (73), as well as the muscles' ability to perform aerobic respiration. However, many studies have used relatively small samples or have used differing training protocols, leading to results that are often irreproducible (73). Two of the most robustly reproduced genes associated with sporting performance are angiotensin I-converting enzyme (*ACE*) and alpha-actinin-3 (*ACTN3*), both with a link to endurance performance.

ACE is part of the renin–angiotensin system and is involved in blood pressure regulation and fluid–electrolyte balance. This gene contains a common (~40% minor allele frequency; MAF) well-studied 287-bp *Alu* insertion/deletion polymorphism in intron 16 (Ensembl Variant rs1799752). The insertion (I) allele is associated with lower levels of circulating (68) and tissue (33) ACE activity, whilst the deletion (D) allele is associated with higher levels of circulating and tissue ACE activity (61). The ACE enzyme is a dipeptidase catalysing the conversion of inactive angiotensin I to active angiotensin II. Angiotensin II is a potent vasopressor and aldosterone-stimulating peptide. Consequently, the *ACE* I/D polymorphism has the potential to alter blood pressure control and fluid electrolyte balance, depending on which version of the gene individuals carry. Control of blood flow to working muscles and fluid–electrolyte balance is crucial for sporting activity, making *ACE* I/D an excellent candidate polymorphism for sporting performance.

In 1998, the *ACE* I/D polymorphism was the first genetic variation to be associated with performance (52). Since then, the *ACE* I allele, or II homozygote, has been repeatedly associated with aerobic performance, whilst the D allele, or DD homozygote, has been repeatedly associated with strength and power performance. Some studies have failed to find these associations, although evidence from a recent meta-analysis suggests that these associations are genuine, with II homozygote individuals being 1.35 (95% confidence interval [CI] 1.17–1.55) times more likely to be endurance athletes and DD homozygote individuals being 1.21 (95% CI 1.03–1.42) times more likely to be strength athletes (46). Nonetheless, the exact molecular mechanisms by which the I/D polymorphism influences both $\dot{V}O_2$ max and strength remain elusive.

ACTN3 is perhaps the best-known sports performance gene. It is often referred to as the sprinting gene. It is a muscle structural protein primarily expressed in type II (fast) skeletal muscle fibres. There, it binds to the actin thin filaments, anchoring them at the Z discs between the sarcomeres where it is crucial for muscle function and contraction. However, it contains an unusual nonsense polymorphism at amino acid 577 (R577X; Ensembl Variant rs1815739; 56)—unusual in that it is both well tolerated and common in human populations (50). Any variant that results in the absence of a structural protein ought to have a dramatic effect on phenotype, be strongly selected against, and therefore be rare in human populations. However, the effects of this change in ACTN3 are tolerated far better than would be predicted and the underlying polymorphism far more common (~40% globally) than would be expected. This tolerance appears to be due to overlapping expression patterns and functional redundancy with the related protein ACTN2. ACTN2 can carry out the essential functions of ACTN3, meaning that ACTN3's absence is not so damaging (50). Although, given the ACTN3 R577X association with sporting performance, ACTN2 clearly cannot carry out all of ACTN3's functions equally well.

ACTN3 was first identified as an elite performance gene in 2003 in a cohort of elite Australian athletes (86). The authors compared the frequency of the RR, RX, and XX genotypes and the R and X alleles in 107 and 194 sprint and endurance athletes, respectively, to 436 controls (see Figure 14.3). They highlighted an increase in R alleles and a concomitant decrease in X alleles in sprint athletes, whilst the converse was true in endurance athletes. They suggested that the R allele was of benefit to elite sprinters, whilst the X allele was of benefit to elite endurance athletes.

Since then the R allele has been very robustly associated with sprinting ability in both elite (41) and the general population (53), despite the effect size being small, explaining ~2.3% of the variance in 40-m sprint ability of adolescent males. The X allele has also less clearly been associated with endurance ability (23, 86). However, recent work in animal models and replicated in humans has identified a plausible mechanism for the X allele to improve endurance performance through a shift towards slow myogenic programming (76). The association with endurance may become more reproducible as we understand the mechanism of action and therefore test associations in populations with the most appropriate training backgrounds.

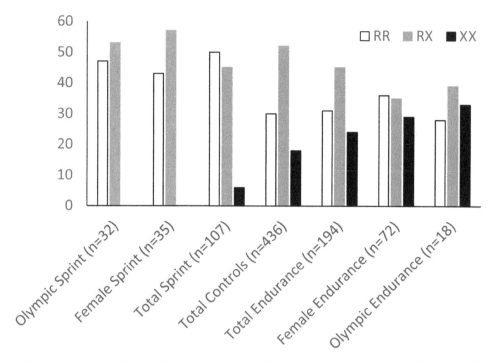

Figure 14.3 Graph showing the *ACTN3* R577X genotype frequencies in power athletes, endurance athletes, and controls

Rare Genetic Variants That Influence V̇O₂ max

ACE I/D and *ACTN3* R577X are both common genetic variants, with MAFs close to 40%. It is likely that some of the heritability of sporting performance will be the result of rarer genetic variants. These are harder to identify and study simply because they are rarer, meaning that studies to identify and investigate them need to be much larger to gather enough carriers together.

An example of a rare variant with a beneficial effect on sporting performance comes from the famous Finnish cross-country skier, Eero Mäntyranta, and his family. Mäntyranta was a phenomenal athlete who competed in four Winter Olympics (1960–1972), winning seven medals (three golds, two silver, and two bronze), as well as five World Championship medals (two gold, two silver, and one bronze; 1962 and 1966) (7, 8). He won some races by unsurpassed margins. However, he was also known to have a high haematocrit and associated high V̇O₂ max, leading to accusations of doping that he could not shake. But doping was not the source of his advantage. After his career had finished, scientists studied samples of his bone marrow and DNA to try to understand why he had such a high blood cell count (34). They were astonished to see his bone marrow producing red blood cells without any stimulation.

Normally, bone marrow produces red blood cells only when stimulated by a hormone called erythropoietin (EPO). To most sports fans, EPO is synonymous with doping. However, it is a naturally occurring hormone produced by the kidneys when oxygen levels are low. Once in the circulation, EPO binds to the EPO receptor (EPOR) on bone marrow cells, stimulating the production of new red blood cells. These red blood cells increase the oxygen-carrying capacity of the blood, counterbalancing low oxygen levels. It is only considered doping when athletes inject themselves with additional EPO to stimulate red blood cell production artificially.

The investigation of Mäntyranta's bone marrow identified a rare genetic variant (Ensembl Variant rs121917830) in his *EPOR* (34). This variant meant that the receptor constantly signalled the presence of EPO, even when there was not any there, producing a haematocrit up to 50% higher than normal.

In the general population, this variant has a MAF of <0.001%, making it incredibly rare (40). However, the study included almost 100 members of Mäntyranta's extended family and found it to be at ~30% in his close family members, giving many of them higher-than-normal haematocrit. These extra red blood cells gave Mäntyranta a significant natural advantage in endurance events. However, a permanently elevated haematocrit comes at a cost. Whilst it allows the blood to carry more oxygen, it also thickens the blood, potentially increasing the risk of heart attack and stroke. This condition is known as polycythaemia, also known as erythrocytosis (18).

Rare and Common Genetic Variants That Influence Injury Risk

Injury risk is a major concern for top athletes. Injuries can restrict training schedules or participation in major sporting events. Soft tissue injuries ranging from minor to severe, such as twisted ankles or anterior cruciate ligament (ACL) injury, are relatively common in some sports. Collagen is one of the most abundant and crucial proteins in the human body. It is a main component in the structure and support of our soft connective tissues. Collagen malfunction can manifest itself in rare genetic disorders, such as osteogenesis imperfecta, chondrodysplasias, or Ehlers-Danlos syndrome, depending on the types of collagen involved (32). However, collagen variants can also have more benign but nonetheless significant effects on athletes by influencing injury risk. Common genetic variants in the *COL5A1* gene (e.g., rs12722, T-allele MAF = 35% and rs13946 C-allele MAF = 25% estimated from 1000 Genomes Project populations) (4, 5), which encodes the type V collagen, are the most-studied genetic loci related to tendon and ligament injuries (24, 75). A recent systematic review showed that carriers of the TT genotype are 1.58 (95% CI, 1.33–1.89) times more likely to suffer soft tissue injuries such as tennis elbow, ACL rupture, and Achilles tendon pathology (45). This finding was further supported by a subsequent meta-analysis illustrating the protective role of the CC genotype of rs12722 and rs13946 to tendon–ligament injuries (57). Type V collagen molecules align themselves alongside type I collagen, regulating the diameter of these fibrils and modulating assembly of other collagen types in several tissues (26, 81). Rare mutations in *COL5A1* also associate with Ehlers-Danlos syndrome, characterized by joint hypermobility (47, 48). Links between rarer variants of *COL5A1* or other collagen genes and tissue injuries or endurance performance in athletes warranting further investigation are nevertheless interesting.

Beyond Candidate Gene Studies of $\dot{V}O_2$ max

An issue with a candidate gene approach is that it can only ever find associations in genes and processes already known to be involved. It cannot find new and unexpected relationships with $\dot{V}O_2$ max. To avoid this pitfall, variants related to any phenotype can be identified using a hypothesis-free approach known as a genome-wide association study (GWAS). GWAS tests variation at nearly all known sites in the genome and compares genotype frequencies in athletes and controls, or average phenotypic scores across genotypes in a similar manner to candidate gene studies. However, GWAS tests all known variants, regardless of whether they are from pathways known to be involved in the underlying physiology. This allows them to identify unexpected pathways involved in sporting performance.

An inherent requirement of GWAS is that they must correct for the large number of statistical tests performed. This is done by lowering the threshold at which significance is accepted from the more familiar $p < 0.05$ of many candidate gene studies to $p < 5 \times 10^{-8}$ which is known as genome-wide significance. This reduces the number of false positives but has the unfortunate consequence that GWAS need very large numbers of participants to achieve such low p-values, given that the variants mostly have small effects. Gathering a large number of high-level elite athletes is rather difficult, as only a small fraction of athletes reach the necessary performance calibre to be considered elite. GWAS are widely used in the study of complex phenotypes, although the majority of the research focuses on health conditions such as diabetes or cardiovascular disease (see the GWAS Catalog, 54). For such common conditions, large numbers of affected and unaffected individuals, often with extensive physiological measurements, are relatively easy to identify. Whilst an initial GWAS conducted in 2005 on age-related macular degeneration had only a few hundred participants (42), modern GWAS have hundreds of thousands of participants [e.g., a 5-year GWAS review (79) and a recent meta-analysis of height and body mass index in ~700,000 individuals (87)] necessary to increase power and detect variants associated with the phenotype under investigation. Typically, a GWAS will identify one genetic variant at genome-wide significance for every ~1,000 participants. This presents an additional obstacle for the study of elite sporting performance. As previously stated, elite athletes are, by definition, rare, making it difficult to achieve the necessary numbers to make this approach viable.

Consequently, GWAS with sufficient power to detect genetic variants predisposed to elite athletic performance are scarce. Some studies have used this approach to identify genes associated with elite endurance performance (20, 63). Additionally, a recent report combines GWAS and metabolic profiling in 490 endurance athletes (who also tested negative for doping) (22). However, despite their value there are also caveats to these studies, not just the relatively small number of samples analysed but also problematic categorization of elite athletes, the use of customized GWAS arrays containing a limited number of genetic variations, lack of stringent validation and replication studies, and/or multiple testing issues. Attempts are being made to unravel variants associated with elite sprint performance in three ethnic populations of world-class athletes in the hope that this may circumvent the need for a very large number of participants required for conventional GWAS. Genotype imputation and meta-analysis of the three ethnic GWAS and replication of the top findings were followed to maximize the power of GWAS to identify and verify putative common genetic variations (MAF >5%) with modest effect (effect size >2; unpublished data, Guan Wang et al). Other studies have attempted to use novel alternative approaches to focus their search for genetic variants. However, genome-wide examinations for DNA and RNA expression profiling for $\dot{V}O_2$ max response to endurance training in the HERITAGE Family Study and other cohorts yielded exciting but inconsistent molecular findings (29, 77). Again this is attributable to some inherent differences between studies such as small samples, population heterogeneity, different training programmes, and potential false-positive findings (29, 73, 77). Despite the observed inconsistencies, combining gene expression profiling with targeted genotyping showed improved explanatory power in identifying genes associated with $\dot{V}O_2$ max training response (77). Indeed, a similar approach combining genomics and transcriptomics data has produced a strong gene signature of triglyceride response to exercise training in HERITAGE white participants (72). Performing GWAS on elite performance is not straightforward. Other large-scale sequencing efforts at the DNA, RNA, and protein level and beyond (e.g., studies of epigenetic marks and DNA folding) involving recruiting participants of the highest-performance calibre, such as the ELITE (9) and the Athlome (1) projects, should shed light on our understanding of the underlying genetic mechanisms of elite human performance.

How Much Do We Understand?

This discovery journey of our understanding of elite human performance has initially been recorded in a series of annual reviews and reports—the Human Gene Map for Performance and Health-related Fitness Phenotypes (30, 59, 62, 64–66, 83) and the Advances in Exercise, Fitness and Performance Genomics (39, 44, 58, 67, 71, 74, 84) were annually published in 2001–2007 and in 2008–2015, respectively. These reviews aimed to access and summarize genetic/genomic findings associated with human performance and health, identifying existing caveats in the literature, and to explore trends for understanding the genetic basis of human performance/fitness. The authors reviewed a number of traits, including physical activity behaviour, muscle strength and power, cardiorespiratory fitness and endurance performance, body weight and adiposity, insulin and glucose metabolism, lipid and lipoprotein metabolism, and hemodynamic traits. Despite this seemingly hundreds of genes associated with the various traits (but often lacking replication), the exact casual genetic variants underlying elite athletic performance remain undetected. Small sample size, the primarily used candidate gene approach, and the failure to consider multiple testing correction in the early studies are the primary causes for inconclusive findings. Further, human genetic variation is now recognized to be individual and within-population variation being larger than between-population variation (21, 69, 70). The multifactorial nature of elite athleticism demands collaborative research studies with a versatile approach integrating the different layers of the molecular and cellular data in multiple and relevant tissues to discover and validate the results within and across populations, underpinned by concerted efforts from research communities, funding bodies and other stakeholders (e.g., government), local and global. In summary, across the whole of sports genetics, regardless of approach, only a little more than 200 genes have been associated with performance, and only 20 of those with elite performance (30). Even fewer have been robustly reproduced in multiple studies or cohorts (19).

Gene Doping

So far, we have concentrated on how natural genetic variation contributes to sporting performance. However, the knowledge gained from studying the genetics of sporting performance could ultimately be used to enhance an individual's ability to perform. Whilst "gene doping" is not currently believed to be possible, in 2003 it was added to the World Antidoping Agency (WADA) prohibited list (80). Gene doping is defined as "the non-therapeutic use of genes, genetic elements and/or cells that have the capacity to enhance athletic performance." More simply put, gene doping is gene therapy in people who have no medical need for it. Gene therapy is a medical technique that involves either transferring modified DNA into an individual or modifying the DNA of an individual to treat a medical condition. In its simplest form, this would be to provide a functional version of a missing or damaged protein.

The first clinical trial of gene therapy was conducted in 1990 (55). In the 30 years since then there have been >3,000 clinical trials of gene therapy, although very few of them have led to successful mainstream clinical applications (categorized by the four clinical trial phases during the drug development process) (11). Despite the complexities, great hope is held for the potential for gene therapy, and many trials are currently ongoing. It seems very likely that gene therapy will have more widespread success in the future, with gene doping likely following close behind. At that point, sport will have to consider its response. In fact, it is possible, perhaps likely, that some individuals have already tried gene doping.

Notably, gene doping has the potential to go beyond providing individual athletes with natural variants that they were not born with to providing them with versions of genes or amounts of protein not found naturally in the global human population—either modified proteins known to manipulate physiology in ways beneficial to performance (e.g., an always active *EPOR* variant similar to the Mäntyranta family discussed earlier) or expression of proteins at supraphysiological levels to provide performance enhancements (e.g., *IGF-1* leading to enhanced muscle growth) (43).

A significant recent advancement in the field of gene therapy is the discovery and development of the CRISPR–Cas9 system for modifying DNA. The Cas9 protein assembles with a guide RNA, enabling DNA binding and cutting much more precisely than has previously been possible in humans. This opens up possibilities for gene therapy but also for gene doping. The CRISPR–Cas9 system can create either permanent or temporary changes to the genome causing insertion, deletion, or replacement of gene(s), single-base changes, or gene suppression or activation (36). New, potentially even better, genome editing tools are also emerging, such as prime editing, CRISPR–Cas3, and EvolvR (36). Whilst gene therapy is not currently mainstream, we move ever closer to that scenario.

Despite the profound advantages of genome editing in treating and preventing genetic disease, caveats such as challenges of delivering the system to the affected tissue or target site and off-target genetic changes face the applications of genome editing tools in many research fields. Therefore, an important consideration of gene doping is the potential risk to the health of athletes. Gene doping is highly likely to be untested. If it works at all, it may include unwanted and potentially lethal side effects. Although, many of the risks are not different from more conventional doping, changes may be permanent and side effects more severe. Despite this, people are trying it. Josiah Zayner publicly attempted to modify his muscles using a CRISPR DNA kit, although he did later regret his actions (88). It is worth also considering that genetic modification with CRISPR or other tools will likely eventually succeed and become commonplace. The desire to provide one-off treatments for individuals with chronic genetic conditions drives the field forward inevitably. Sport will have to deal with it. Whilst currently morally and ethically highly questionable, the ethical viewpoint of society will likely change as treatments become possible and commonplace.

Limits of Performance

It is notable that the genetic variants most strongly linked to performance appear to have a trade-off within them. Having the right *ACTN3* R577X genotype for speed means an individual does not have the right *ACTN3* genotype for endurance and vice versa. The same is true for the *ACE* I/D polymorphism and strength- versus endurance-associated genotypes. Similarly, although Eero Mäntyranta gained a performance advantage through his rare *EPOR* variant, the variant comes at a cost to health or at least health risk. In this way there may be a genetic limit to performance. It is also important to remember that there is no such thing as a perfect genetic profile. The "best" genetic profile is only best in the environmental context in which it is measured and that environmental, even for one individual, is constantly changing. Elite athletes, who train multiple times a day whilst at their peak, do not continue with such intensive training into their retirement and may be accelerating undesirable conditions in later life if they alter their genetics.

In summary, elite athletic performance is within the constraints of both genetics and the environment, but currently only parts of the environment are within the athlete's control. Athletes should continue to train hard, frequently, with the best coaches and take care of their nutrition in an effort to achieve their potential. Meanwhile genetic research will uncover the knowledge required to best train and guide athletes to achieve their peak performance, although we have only begun to scratch the surface. This may allow athletes to bypass some unwanted limitations and stimulate achievement of their full potential. Consequently, genetic research should gain support from athletes, coaches, and other stakeholders who wish to drive performance forward. Genetics may limit an individual's performance potential, but with so many genes likely to be involved and so few of them currently identified, athletes should not consider any genetic information they have to be a hindrance to their performance; they should want to know more, as it may help them or others perform better in the future.

References

1. The Athlome Project Consortium. http://www.athlomeconsortium.org/about/.
2. Auria Biobank. https://www.auria.fi/en/index.php?lang=en.
3. Cristiano Ronaldo (The commons). https://commons.wikimedia.org/wiki/File:Cristiano_Ronaldo_ (163461623).jpeg.
4. dbSNP – rs12722. https://www.ncbi.nlm.nih.gov/snp/rs12722.
5. dbSNP – rs13946. https://www.ncbi.nlm.nih.gov/snp/rs13946.
6. deCODE genetics. www.decode.com.
7. Eero Mäntyranta. https://en.wikipedia.org/wiki/Eero_Mäntyranta.
8. Eero Mäntyranta earned his first gold medal in 1960 in Squaw Valley as a member of Finland's 4 × 10 km relay team. www.olympic.org/eero-mantyranta.
9. ELITE – Exercise at the Limit – Inherited Traits of Endurance. http://med.stanford.edu/elite.html.
10. The ENCODE Consortium. https://www.encodeproject.org/.
11. Gene Therapy Clinical Trials Worldwide, 2019. http://www.abedia.com/wiley/phases.php.
12. Genome Reference Consortium. https://www.ncbi.nlm.nih.gov/grc/human.
13. The Geuvadis Consoritum. https://www.internationalgenome.org/data-portal/data-collection/geuvadis.

14. HERITAGE - Genetics, Response to Exercise, Risk Factors. https://www.pbrc.edu/heritage/index.html.
15. The Human Genome Project. https://www.genome.gov/human-genome-project.
16. Lionel Messi (The commons). https://commons.wikimedia.org/wiki/File:Messi_Barcelona_-_Valladolid.jpg.
17. Matt Hancock announces ambition to map 5 million genomes, 2018. https://www.gov.uk/government/news/matt-hancock-announces-ambition-to-map-5-million-genomes.
18. Polycythaemia (NHS). https://www.nhs.uk/conditions/polycythaemia/.
19. Ahmetov, II, Egorova ES, Gabdrakhmanova LJ, Fedotovskaya ON. Genes and athletic performance: An update. *Med Sport Sci* 61: 41–54, 2016.
20. Ahmetov I, Kulemin N, Popov D, Naumov V, Akimov E, Bravy Y, et al. Genome-wide association study identifies three novel genetic markers associated with elite endurance performance. *Biol Sport* 32: 3–9, 2015.
21. Ahn S-M, Kim T-H, Lee S, Kim D, Ghang H, Kim D-S, et al. The first Korean genome sequence and analysis: full genome sequencing for a socio-ethnic group. *Genome Res* 19: 1622–1629, 2009.
22. Al-Khelaifi F, Diboun I, Donati F, Botrè F, Abraham D, Hingorani A, et al. Metabolic GWAS of elite athletes reveals novel genetically-influenced metabolites associated with athletic performance. *Sci Rep* 9: 19889, 2019.
23. Alfred T, Ben-Shlomo Y, Cooper R, Hardy R, Cooper C, Deary IJ, et al. ACTN3 genotype, athletic status, and life course physical capability: meta-analysis of the published literature and findings from nine studies. *Hum Mutat* 32: 1008–1018, 2011.
24. Altinisik J, Meric G, Erduran M, Ates O, Ulusal AE, Akseki D. The BstUI and DpnII variants of the COL5A1 gene are associated with tennis elbow. *Am J Sports Med* 43: 1784–1789, 2015.
25. Auton A, Brooks LD, Durbin RM, Garrison EP, Kang HM, Korbel JO, et al. A global reference for human genetic variation. *Nature* 526: 68–74, 2015.
26. Birk DE. Type V collagen: heterotypic type I/V collagen interactions in the regulation of fibril assembly. *Micron* 32: 223–237, 2001.
27. Bouchard C, An P, Rice T, Skinner JS, Wilmore JH, Gagnon J, et al. Familial aggregation of VO(2max) response to exercise training: results from the HERITAGE Family Study. *J Appl Physiol* 87: 1003–1008, 1999.
28. Bouchard C, Daw EW, Rice T, Pérusse L, Gagnon J, Province MA, et al. Familial resemblance for VO2max in the sedentary state: the HERITAGE family study. *Med Sci Sports Exerc* 30: 252–258, 1998.
29. Bouchard C, Sarzynski MA, Rice TK, Kraus WE, Church TS, Sung YJ, et al. Genomic predictors of the maximal O_2 uptake response to standardized exercise training programs. *J Appl Physiol* 110: 1160–1170, 2011.
30. Bray MS, Hagberg JM, Pérusse L, Rankinen T, Roth SM, Wolfarth B, et al. The human gene map for performance and health-related fitness phenotypes: the 2006-2007 update. *Med Sci Sports Exerc* 41: 35–73, 2009.
31. Bycroft C, Freeman C, Petkova D, Band G, Elliott LT, Sharp K, et al. The UK Biobank resource with deep phenotyping and genomic data. *Nature* 562: 203–209, 2018.
32. Chan TF, Poon A, Basu A, Addleman NR, Chen J, Phong A, et al. Natural variation in four human collagen genes across an ethnically diverse population. *Genomics* 91: 307–314, 2008.
33. Danser AH, Schalekamp MA, Bax WA, van den Brink AM, Saxena PR, Riegger GA, et al. Angiotensin-converting enzyme in the human heart. Effect of the deletion/insertion polymorphism. *Circulation* 92: 1387–1388, 1995.
34. de la Chapelle A, Träskelin AL, Juvonen E. Truncated erythropoietin receptor causes dominantly inherited benign human erythrocytosis. *Proc Natl Acad Sci U S A* 90: 4495–4499, 1993.
35. De Moor MH, Spector TD, Cherkas LF, Falchi M, Hottenga JJ, Boomsma DI, et al. Genome-wide linkage scan for athlete status in 700 British female DZ twin pairs. *Twin Res Hum Genet* 10: 812–820, 2007.
36. Doudna JA. The promise and challenge of therapeutic genome editing. *Nature* 578: 229–236, 2020.
37. Epstein D, *The Sports Gene: Talent, Practice and the Truth about Success.* Great Britain: Yellow Jersey Press, 2013, p. 338.
38. Evangelou E, Warren HR, Mosen-Ansorena D, Mifsud B, Pazoki R, Gao H, et al. Genetic analysis of over 1 million people identifies 535 new loci associated with blood pressure traits. *Nat Genet* 50: 1412–1425, 2018.
39. Hagberg JM, Rankinen T, Loos RJ, Pérusse L, Roth SM, Wolfarth B, et al. Advances in exercise, fitness, and performance genomics in 2010. *Med Sci Sports Exerc* 43: 743–752, 2011.
40. Hussein K, Percy M, McMullin MF. Clinical utility gene card for: familial erythrocytosis. *Eur J Hum Genet* 20, 2012.
41. Kikuchi N, Miyamoto-Mikami E, Murakami H, Nakamura T, Min SK, Mizuno M, et al. ACTN3 R577X genotype and athletic performance in a large cohort of Japanese athletes. *Eur J Sport Sci* 16: 694–701, 2016.
42. Klein RJ, Zeiss C, Chew EY, Tsai JY, Sackler RS, Haynes C, et al. Complement factor H polymorphism in age-related macular degeneration. *Science* 308: 385–389, 2005.
43. Lee S, Barton ER, Sweeney HL, Farrar RP. Viral expression of insulin-like growth factor-I enhances muscle hypertrophy in resistance-trained rats. *J Appl Physiol* 96: 1097–1104, 2004.

44. Loos RJ, Hagberg JM, Pérusse L, Roth SM, Sarzynski MA, Wolfarth B, et al. Advances in exercise, fitness, and performance genomics in 2014. *Med Sci Sports Exerc* 47: 1105–1112, 2015.

45. Lv ZT, Gao ST, Cheng P, Liang S, Yu SY, Yang Q, et al. Association between polymorphism rs12722 in COL5A1 and musculoskeletal soft tissue injuries: a systematic review and meta-analysis. *Oncotarget* 9: 15365–15374, 2018.

46. Ma F, Yang Y, Li X, Zhou F, Gao C, Li M, Gao L. The association of sport performance with ACE and ACTN3 genetic polymorphisms: a systematic review and meta-analysis. *PLOS ONE* 8: e54685, 2013.

47. Malfait F, De Paepe A. Molecular genetics in classic Ehlers-Danlos syndrome. *Am J Med Genet C Semin Med Genet* 139c: 17–23, 2005.

48. Malfait F, Wenstrup RJ, De Paepe A. Clinical and genetic aspects of Ehlers-Danlos syndrome, classic type. *Genet Med* 12: 597–605, 2010.

49. Marouli E, Graff M, Medina-Gomez C, Lo KS, Wood AR, Kjaer TR, et al. Rare and low-frequency coding variants alter human adult height. *Nature* 542: 186–190, 2017.

50. Mills M, Yang N, Weinberger R, Vander Woude DL, Beggs AH, Easteal S, et al. Differential expression of the actin-binding proteins, alpha-actinin-2 and -3, in different species: implications for the evolution of functional redundancy. *Hum Mol Genet* 10: 1335–1346, 2001.

51. Montero D, Lundby C. Refuting the myth of non-response to exercise training: 'non-responders' do respond to higher dose of training. *J Physiol* 595: 3377–3387, 2017.

52. Montgomery HE, Marshall R, Hemingway H, Myerson S, Clarkson P, Dollery C, et al. Human gene for physical performance. *Nature* 393: 221–222, 1998.

53. Moran CN, Yang N, Bailey ME, Tsiokanos A, Jamurtas A, MacArthur DG, et al. Association analysis of the ACTN3 R577X polymorphism and complex quantitative body composition and performance phenotypes in adolescent Greeks. *Eur J Hum Genet* 15: 88–93, 2007.

54. NHGRI-EBI. GWAS catalog - studies with available summary statistics. https://www.ebi.ac.uk/gwas/downloads/summary-statistics.

55. NIH. Results From First Human Gene Therapy Clinical Trial, 1995 https://www.genome.gov/10000521/1995-release-first-human-gene-therapy-results.

56. North KN, Yang N, Wattanasirichaigoon D, Mills M, Easteal S, Beggs AH. A common nonsense mutation results in alpha-actinin-3 deficiency in the general population. *Nat Genet* 21: 353–354, 1999.

57. Pabalan N, Tharabenjasin P, Phababpha S, Jarjanazi H. Association of COL5A1 gene polymorphisms and risk of tendon-ligament injuries among Caucasians: a meta-analysis. *Sports Med Open* 4: 46, 2018.

58. Pérusse L, Rankinen T, Hagberg JM, Loos RJ, Roth SM, Sarzynski MA, et al. Advances in exercise, fitness, and performance genomics in 2012. *Med Sci Sports Exerc* 45: 824–831, 2013.

59. Pérusse L, Rankinen T, Rauramaa R, Rivera MA, Wolfarth B, Bouchard C. The human gene map for performance and health-related fitness phenotypes: the 2002 update. *Med Sci Sports Exerc* 35: 1248–1264, 2003.

60. Phillips BE, Kelly BM, Lilja M, Ponce-González JG, Brogan RJ, Morris DL, et al. A practical and time-efficient high-intensity interval training program modifies cardio-metabolic risk factors in adults with risk factors for type II diabetes. *Front Endocrinol* 8: 229, 2017.

61. Puthucheary Z, Skipworth JR, Rawal J, Loosemore M, Van Someren K, Montgomery HE. Genetic influences in sport and physical performance. *Sports Med* 41: 845–859, 2011.

62. Rankinen T, Bray MS, Hagberg JM, Pérusse L, Roth SM, Wolfarth B, et al. The human gene map for performance and health-related fitness phenotypes: the 2005 update. *Med Sci Sports Exerc* 38: 1863–1888, 2006.

63. Rankinen T, Fuku N, Wolfarth B, Wang G, Sarzynski MA, Alexeev DG, et al. No evidence of a common DNA variant profile specific to world class endurance athletes. *PLOS ONE* 11: e0147330, 2016.

64. Rankinen T, Pérusse L, Rauramaa R, Rivera MA, Wolfarth B, Bouchard C. The human gene map for performance and health-related fitness phenotypes. *Med Sci Sports Exerc* 33: 855–867, 2001.

65. Rankinen T, Pérusse L, Rauramaa R, Rivera MA, Wolfarth B, Bouchard C. The human gene map for performance and health-related fitness phenotypes: the 2001 update. *Med Sci Sports Exerc* 34: 1219–1233, 2002.

66. Rankinen T, Pérusse L, Rauramaa R, Rivera MA, Wolfarth B, Bouchard C. The human gene map for performance and health-related fitness phenotypes: the 2003 update. *Med Sci Sports Exerc* 36: 1451–1469, 2004.

67. Rankinen T, Roth SM, Bray MS, Loos R, Pérusse L, Wolfarth B, et al. Advances in exercise, fitness, and performance genomics. *Med Sci Sports Exerc* 42: 835–846, 2010.

68. Rigat B, Hubert C, Alhenc-Gelas F, Cambien F, Corvol P, Soubrier F. An insertion/deletion polymorphism in the angiotensin I-converting enzyme gene accounting for half the variance of serum enzyme levels. *J Clin Invest* 86: 1343–1346, 1990.

69. Romualdi C, Balding D, Nasidze IS, Risch G, Robichaux M, Sherry ST, et al. Patterns of human diversity, within and among continents, inferred from biallelic DNA polymorphisms. *Genome Res* 12: 602–612, 2002.

70. Rosenberg NA, Pritchard JK, Weber JL, Cann HM, Kidd KK, Zhivotovsky LA, et al. Genetic structure of human populations. *Science* 298: 2381–2385, 2002.

71. Roth SM, Rankinen T, Hagberg JM, Loos RJ, Pérusse L, Sarzynski MA, et al. Advances in exercise, fitness, and performance genomics in 2011. *Med Sci Sports Exerc* 44: 809–817, 2012.

72. Sarzynski MA, Davidsen PK, Sung YJ, Hesselink MK, Schrauwen P, Rice TK, et al. Genomic and transcriptomic predictors of triglyceride response to regular exercise. *Br J Sports Med* 49: 1524–1531, 2015.

73. Sarzynski MA, Ghosh S, Bouchard C. Genomic and transcriptomic predictors of response levels to endurance exercise training. *J Physiol* 595: 2931–2939, 2017.

74. Sarzynski MA, Loos RJ, Lucia A, Pérusse L, Roth SM, Wolfarth B, et al. Advances in exercise, fitness, and performance genomics in 2015. *Med Sci Sports Exerc* 48: 1906–1916, 2016.

75. September AV, Cook J, Handley CJ, van der Merwe L, Schwellnus MP, Collins M. Variants within the COL5A1 gene are associated with Achilles tendinopathy in two populations. *Br J Sports Med* 43: 357–365, 2009.

76. Seto JT, Quinlan KG, Lek M, Zheng XF, Garton F, MacArthur DG, et al. ACTN3 genotype influences muscle performance through the regulation of calcineurin signaling. *J Clin Invest* 123: 4255–4263, 2013.

77. Timmons JA, Knudsen S, Rankinen T, Koch LG, Sarzynski M, Jensen T, et al. Using molecular classification to predict gains in maximal aerobic capacity following endurance exercise training in humans. *J Appl Physiol* 108: 1487–1496, 2010.

78. Tucker R, Collins M. What makes champions? A review of the relative contribution of genes and training to sporting success. *Br J Sports Med* 46: 555–561, 2012.

79. Visscher PM, Brown MA, McCarthy MI, Yang J. Five years of GWAS discovery. *Am J Hum Genet* 90: 7–24, 2012.

80. WADA. Gene Doping, 2005. https://www.wada-ama.org/sites/default/files/resources/files/PlayTrue_2005_1_Gene_Doping_EN.pdf.

81. Wenstrup RJ, Florer JB, Brunskill EW, Bell SM, Chervoneva I, Birk DE. Type V collagen controls the initiation of collagen fibril assembly. *J Biol Chem* 279: 53331–53337, 2004.

82. White D, Rabago-Smith M. Genotype-phenotype associations and human eye color. *J Hum Genet* 56: 5–7, 2011.

83. Wolfarth B, Bray MS, Hagberg JM, Pérusse L, Rauramaa R, Rivera MA, et al. The human gene map for performance and health-related fitness phenotypes: the 2004 update. *Med Sci Sports Exerc* 37: 881–903, 2005.

84. Wolfarth B, Rankinen T, Hagberg JM, Loos RJ, Pérusse L, Roth SM, et al. Advances in exercise, fitness, and performance genomics in 2013. *Med Sci Sports Exerc* 46: 851–859, 2014.

85. Wood AR, Esko T, Yang J, Vedantam S, Pers TH, Gustafsson S, et al. Defining the role of common variation in the genomic and biological architecture of adult human height. *Nat Genet* 46: 1173–1186, 2014.

86. Yang N, MacArthur DG, Gulbin JP, Hahn AG, Beggs AH, Easteal S, et al. ACTN3 genotype is associated with human elite athletic performance. *Am J Hum Genet* 73: 627–631, 2003.

87. Yengo L, Sidorenko J, Kemper KE, Zheng Z, Wood AR, Weedon MN, et al. Meta-analysis of genome-wide association studies for height and body mass index in ~700000 individuals of European ancestry. *Hum Mol Genet* 27: 3641–3649, 2018.

88. Zhang S. A biohacker regrets publicly injecting himself with CRISPR, 2018. https://www.theatlantic.com/science/archive/2018/02/biohacking-stunts-crispr/553511/.

15

THE ROLE OF EPIGENETICS IN SKELETAL MUSCLE ADAPTATIONS TO EXERCISE AND EXERCISE TRAINING

Sean L. McGee

Introduction

A landmark study in 1967 by the late John Holloszy reported that chronic endurance exercise training increased skeletal muscle metabolic enzymes and the capacity to produce adenosine triphosphate (ATP) (23). We now understand that a single bout of exercise transiently increases the expression of a subset of genes in skeletal muscle. Repeated transcriptional activation of these genes, as would occur in exercise training, leads to elevated steady-state levels of the enzymes that ultimately contribute to training adaptations in skeletal muscle (9, 16, 63). Therefore, the transcriptional response to acute exercise is thought to be an important component of the adaptive response to chronic exercise training.

Changes in the activities of intracellular signalling pathways and downstream transcriptional regulators have been observed in skeletal muscle in response to exercise and are thought to be important for coordinating gene expression responses. However, the regulation of gene transcription also involves epigenetic mechanisms. The term epigenetics broadly encompasses any mechanism that alters the expression of genes without changing DNA sequence (7). There has been considerable debate as to whether a formal definition of epigenetics should also include reference to the heritability of gene expression changes. However, some epigenetic mechanisms are dynamic, with only modest evidence of their transmissibility (7). The main epigenetic mechanisms include methylation of DNA, post-translational modifications (PTMs) to histone proteins, which are an integral component of chromatin, and control of gene expression through non-coding RNAs, including microRNA (miRNA) (22). The epigenetics field is slowly unravelling the complex interactions between these mechanisms, which together provide precise control of gene expression in changing environments. Similarly, our understanding of how epigenetic mechanisms contribute to the regulation of exercise-induced gene expression and training adaptations is slowly emerging.

The following chapter will provide a brief overview of epigenetic mechanisms before detailing our current understanding of how epigenetics influences the adaptive response to exercise and exercise training. Furthermore, this chapter will pose some unanswered questions relevant to the field that could guide future research in this area.

Epigenetics and the Control of Gene Expression

Both DNA methylation and histone modifications influence gene expression by altering chromatin structure and architecture. Chromatin is composed of repeating units of DNA wrapped around a core of histone proteins, which also form the larger chromosomes that tightly pack our genetic material into the nucleus (21). The extent of chromatin folding and the spatial relationship between DNA and histones have profound effects on transcription. Active gene transcription is generally associated with open chromatin, where DNA regions are assessable to transcriptional machinery such as the transcriptional initiation complex and RNA polymerase (21). Inactive gene regions are mostly associated with a closed chromatin structure, where transcriptional regulators cannot access gene regions (21). In contrast to these chromatin-focused mechanisms, non-coding RNA influences gene expression by regulating messenger RNA (mRNA) stability and translation.

DNA Methylation

Methylation of DNA involves the addition of a methyl group to cytosine residues within both coding and non-coding regions of DNA. Cytosine residues that are followed by guanine residues, abbreviated as CpG and referred to as CpG islands, are most frequently methylated (8). DNA methylation is generally associated with transcriptional repression through a number of different mechanisms. Methylation can prevent DNA binding of the transcriptional initiation complex and other components of the transcriptional machinery, such as transcription factors with GC-rich consensus DNA-binding sequences (61). Conversely, methylation can recruit methyl-CpG–binding proteins that have transcriptional repressive properties (32). DNA methylation is a stable modification with an extremely long half-life and was thought to predominantly occur in pluripotent cells during development (32). However, studies of identical twins have suggested that DNA methylation also occurs in terminally differentiated cells in response to environmental stimuli (29, 38, 47). Methyl groups are added to DNA by four DNA methyltransferases (DNMTs) and can be removed through the actions of ten-eleven translocation (TET) proteins, of which there are three mammalian isoforms (32). The sequence specificity of these enzymes and mechanisms regulating their activity provide precise control over DNA methylation patterns across the genome. DNA methylation is maintained through cell division through the actions of DNMTs that read and replicate existing DNA methylation marks from inherited DNA (32). However, the fidelity of DNA methylation replication is much lower than that of DNA replication (32).

Histone Modifications and Variants

DNA wraps around a core of histone proteins to form a nucleosome (48). The histone core is ordinarily organized as a central heterotetramer of histones 3 and 4, with two heterodimers of histones 2A and 2B. A length of 147 bp of DNA wraps around the histone core twice, and each nucleosome is separated by a linker of 10–60 bp of DNA (48). This repeating chromatin structure is further folded and condensed, such that access to the surrounding DNA by transcriptional regulators is compromised (48). Hence this highly compacted chromatin state is generally associated with transcriptional repression. Chromatin structure is highly dependent on histone PTMs, which affect the higher-order folding of nucleosomes (48). Such modifications include acetylation, methylation, phosphorylation, ubiquitination, and sumoylation, as well as other acylation modifications (31). These PTMs are particularly prevalent on histone lysine and arginine residues. Histone acetylation is generally associated with transcriptional activation, while methylation is associated with transcriptional repression (48). However, there are examples where acetylation can repress transcription and methylation can activate transcription. This can depend on the particular residue that is being modified or whether the residue is mono-, di-, or tri-modified. This has led to the idea that unlike the defined genetic code, there is no obvious histone code that can be assigned to a particular transcriptional or physiological outcome (48). Nonetheless, histone modifications that result in transcriptional activation cause decompaction of chromatin and often result in histone exclusion from the nucleosome, exposing DNA regulatory and gene regions to transcriptional activators (48).

The mechanisms controlling post-translational modification of histones revolve around the enzymes that regulate these particular processes. These include histone acetyltransferases and histone deacetylases, which add and remove acetylation, respectively, histone methyltransferases, demethylases, kinases, and phosphatases (48). Each family of enzymes has a number of isoforms with different substrate specificities, mechanism of activation, and regulation of sub-cellular localization, which are controlled by different intracellular signalling pathways. This ensures that only specific regions of DNA become accessible to transcriptional regulators upon activation of defined signalling pathways. These same signalling mechanisms often also regulate sequence-specific transcription factors and coactivators to provide precise control over the transcriptional response. For example, myocyte enhancer factor 2 (MEF2) transcription is acetylated by the p300 histone acetyltransferase, leading to enhanced MEF2 transcriptional activity (37). Therefore, p300 simultaneously acetylates histones and a DNA-binding transcription factor to enhance gene transcription. Adding complexity to the regulatory system are histone variants, which differ in sequence from the canonical histone proteins, but incorporate into nucleosomes regularly throughout larger chromatin fibres (17). These variants can create nucleosomes with distinct structural and regulatory features. For example, Cse4/CENP-A, a histone 3 variant, lacks a number of phosphorylation and acetylation sites that are associated with transcriptional activation (3). It is thought that the CENP-A variant retains a nucleosome in its compacted and transcriptionally repressed state (3).

The heritability of histone modifications and variants has been debated in the literature. Most histone modifications are thought to be highly dynamic, in line with the pulsatile nature of transcriptional responses. Indeed, the half-life of histone acetylation was thought to be 1–2 minutes (26); however, more recent studies suggest that some site-specific acetylation marks have a half-life of up to 30 hours (70). Nonetheless, other histone modifications are more stable, such as methylation, with a half-life of up to a number of days (68). This is sufficient to allow histone-modifying enzymes to replicate modifications from inherited histones to new histones throughout mitotic cell division. Indeed, some histone methyltransferases can recognize and amplify pre-existing histone methylation patterns (32). The influence of epigenetic inheritance on skeletal muscle phenotype will be discussed later in this chapter; however, it is likely that both histone modifications and variants play a role in retaining epigenetic information that influences transcriptional responses.

Other Epigenetic Mechanisms

A number of other epigenetic mechanisms can influence transcriptional responses without altering genome sequence. Non-coding RNA, such as miRNA, regulates gene expression by binding to untranslated regions of mRNA to either prevent its translation or promote its degradation (21). Up to 30% of the transcriptome is regulated by miRNA, which are expressed from non-coding regions of DNA (65). As such, miRNA expression is itself sensitive to canonical epigenetic mechanisms such as DNA methylation and histone modifications. Furthermore, miRNA regulation of epigenetic-modifying enzymes means that these non-coding RNAs can also feed back to control both DNA methylation and histone modifications (65). Considering this intertwined relationship, this chapter will focus on canonical epigenetic mechanisms that alter gene expression at the level of the genome, which have been implicated in the adaptive response to exercise. Readers interested in further understanding the role of miRNA and other non-coding RNA in the regulation of exercise adaptations are encouraged to read recent excellent reviews on this subject (14, 53, 54). Other novel mechanisms of transcriptional control are also regularly emerging. Indeed, the recently identified epitranscriptome—RNA modifications such as cytidine acetylation and adenosine methylation that influence mRNA stability and translation efficiency (50)—could conceivably also play a role in exercise adaptive responses. These will be critical questions for the field to address in the future.

Epigenetic Responses to Exercise and Exercise Training

Repeated, transient alterations in gene expression that over time increase protein and enzyme content are thought to contribute to the adaptive response of skeletal muscle to chronic exercise training (9, 16, 63). Although DNA methylation has traditionally been viewed as a relatively stable epigenetic mark, rapid demethylation of exercise-responsive elements of the genome has been associated with exercise-induced gene expression in skeletal muscle. In a landmark study, Juleen Zierath's laboratory revealed a global reduction in DNA methylation in response to an acute bout of exercise in humans (6). Analysis of the specific gene regions involved identified that the promoter region of peroxisome proliferator activated receptor coactivator 1 alpha (*PGC-1α*) was one region that was demethylated. PGC-1α is a coactivator of a number of transcription factors that coordinate the expression of nuclear genes involved in the structure and function of mitochondria (64) and muscle fibre type determination (33). Its expression is rapidly increased following a single acute bout of exercise (2), which is thought to be a key element of the skeletal muscle adaptive response to exercise. The reduction in *PGC-1α* promoter methylation during exercise was intensity-dependent and showed some correlation with post-exercise *PGC-1α* gene expression (6). Similar findings were also observed for the promoter regions of other exercise-responsive genes, including transcription factor A mitochondrial (*TFAM*), a transcription factor that drives expression of mitochondrial genes, and pyruvate dehydrogenase (PDH) kinase 4 (*PDK4*), a kinase that controls the oxidation of pyruvate through the PDH complex (6). Interestingly, the Zierath laboratory had also found that the *PGC-1α* promoter was predominantly methylated at non-CpG sites by DNMT3B, which was associated with skeletal muscle mitochondrial content (5). The extent to which demethylation of gene regulatory regions contributes to exercise-induced transcription in skeletal muscle remains difficult to determine, with methylation status only a moderate correlate with gene expression levels in most studies. Furthermore, the TET enzymes involved also remain elusive. However, this study and others (4) have highlighted the previously unappreciated role of dynamic changes in DNA methylation status and its relationship to transcriptional responses.

Emerging evidence suggests that histone modifications could also be an important epigenetic mechanism contributing to exercise-induced transcriptional responses in skeletal muscle. Global histone 3 acetylation at lysine 36 is increased immediately following 60 min of cycling in human skeletal muscle and is associated with the nuclear export of the class IIa histone deacetylases (HDACs) (41). This sub-family of HDACs does not possess activity against acetylated lysine, but acts as scaffolds to recruit transcriptional co-repressors and other HDAC isoforms to specific transcription factors (18), such as MEF2 (45). The phosphorylation-dependent nuclear export of the class IIa HDACs disrupts this transcriptional co-repressor complex, resulting in transcription factor–specific gene expression responses (45). The importance of disrupting this co-repressor complex for the transcriptional response to exercise has been highlighted in a recent study (19). Skeletal muscle expression of HDAC4 and HDAC5 mutants that have impaired recruitment of the co-repressor complex results in an exercise-like transcriptional response and enhanced capacity for lipid oxidation (19). Phosphorylation of the class IIa HDACs appears to be regulated by a number of kinases, including the AMP-activated protein kinase (AMPK) (44), the calcium/calmodulin-dependent protein kinase II (CaMKII), and protein kinase D (PKD) (12), in a redundant fashion (43). These studies delineate important signalling pathways by which exercise can induce specific transcriptional responses through epigenetic mechanisms.

A number of studies have also characterized histone acetylation events at specific gene promoters during exercise. Swimming exercise increased histone 3 lysine 9/14 acetylation at the glucose transporter 4 (*Glut4*) promoter in rat skeletal muscle (55), which has also been observed at the *Mef2a* and nuclear respiratory factor 1 (*Nrf-1*) promoter regions (27). This suggests that histone acetylation could be a vital component of the transcriptional response to exercise. However, in contrast, a recent study found that histone acetylation across different regions of the *Pgc-1α* gene was a poor corelate with *Pgc-1α* gene expression levels in rat skeletal muscle following swimming exercise (39). The best predictor of *Pgc-1α* gene expression was histone 3 abundance across these same gene regions, suggesting that histone exchange and exclusion could also be important for exercise responses (39). It could also be interpreted that modified histones are excluded from the nucleosome and therefore were not detected in this chromatin immunoprecipitation approach. Histone phosphorylation has also been observed in skeletal muscle during exercise. Cycling exercise increases histone 3 phosphorylation at serine 10 in both trained and untrained subjects (67). This observation has a number of important implications for understanding epigenetic regulation during exercise. Firstly, this site is a substrate for both AMPK and CaMKII (1, 51), which are exercise-responsive kinases that also inactivate the class IIa HDAC through phosphorylation-dependent nuclear export. Secondly, phosphorylation of serine 10 appears to be required to allow acetylation of lysine 14, a modification that is associated with transcriptional initiation (36). This suggests that there is highly coordinated control of epigenetic mechanisms in skeletal muscle in response to exercise, driven by a number of exercise-responsive kinases that control the stepwise progression of epigenetic-mediated transcriptional responses. Furthermore, as multiple kinases appear capable of regulating these mechanisms, it highlights the redundancy in this system and offers explanations as to why some genetic loss-of-function animal models fail to have phenotypic effects in the transcriptional response to exercise (42). While these early studies within the field have provided important insights into the potential importance of epigenetics in exercise-adaptive responses, our understanding of this regulatory system remains rudimentary at this present time. As omics approaches to address these questions become more accessible, our appreciation of the intricacies of epigenetic control of exercise-dependent transcriptional responses will increase.

It is generally well accepted that repeated bouts of acute exercise and corresponding dynamic alterations in the expression of exercise-responsive genes play an important role in skeletal muscle adaptations to exercise training. However, a key question is whether exercise training induces stable epigenetic alterations that could confer a persistent memory of muscle adaptation. A number of studies have observed hypomethylation of exercise-responsive genes in skeletal muscle following exercise training interventions (28, 35, 46), which were generally associated with gene expression patterns. Gene ontology analysis found that many of the gene regions that displayed reduced methylation following exercise training were associated with various metabolic processes and insulin signalling (46). Interestingly, many of these same pathways were also identified in ontology analysis of gene regions that displayed increased methylation after training (46). The functional significance of these findings remains unclear, but could be explained by other findings that have questioned the extent to which methylation contributes to the global control of gene expression levels in differentiated tissue (20, 69). Nitert and colleagues (46) directly addressed this question by analysing the effect of methylation on promoter reporters of a number of genes found to be hypomethylated in skeletal muscle following exercise training. These experiments showed that methylation of the promoters of the *NDUFC2, RUNX1, MEF2A,* and *THADA* genes significantly reduced reporter expression (46), providing strong evidence that hypomethylation of these gene regions enhances the transcription of these genes. The concept of an exercise training transcriptional memory has also been examined more directly in a well-controlled study where subjects completed two 3-month training periods, separated by a 9-month period of detraining (34). Following the 9-month detraining period, there was no retention of the training-induced transcriptional profile, although there were subtle differences in the transcriptional response to the second training period (34). At present no studies have rigorously assessed whether histone modifications are persistently altered following exercise training. However, given the short half-life and enzymatic reversibility of these modifications, it is difficult to envisage a scenario where persistent histone modifications contribute to maintenance of a training phenotype. On balance, these data collectively suggest that there is not a clearly defined epigenetic memory of exercise training that is retained beyond the termination of training.

As our understanding of the role of epigenetics increases, so, too, does our understanding of the role of epigenetics in exercise and exercise training responses. Both alterations in DNA methylation and histone modifications appear to operate in concert to contribute to precise regulation of the exercise-induced transcriptional response. It also appears that it is acute epigenetic alterations associated with each individual exercise bout, rather than persistent epigenetic changes, that confer the adaptive response to exercise training, although there could be a role for DNA hypomethylation in fine-tuning training-induced gene expression profiles.

Unanswered Questions

As the role of epigenetics in mediating the adaptive response to exercise and exercise training becomes more clearly defined, a number of important questions for the field remain. One such important question to definitively answer is whether exercise adaptations are transmissible to subsequent generations. Indeed, polymorphisms in enzymes involved in DNA methylation and methyl group synthesis appear to be more prevalent in elite athletes than sedentary control subjects, which is linked to the induction of myogenic genes and increased muscle cell size (59). This suggests that epigenetics could contribute to the transmission of athletic performance across generations. However, does exercise training induce persistent epigenetic alterations that can be passed onto progeny with effects on physiology? This has become a highly relevant question, which has been partially addressed in an emerging field of research examining whether exercise training in parents reverses the heritability of metabolic diseases in progeny. For example, in mothers fed a high-fat diet, exercise prevented hypermethylation of the $Pgc\text{-}1\alpha$ promoter, which was associated with increased skeletal muscle $Pgc\text{-}1\alpha$ expression and metabolic function in offspring (30). Similar studies have observed the beneficial effects of both maternal (10, 11, 56, 58) and paternal (57) exercise training on aspects of metabolism in offspring. It remains to be mechanistically determined whether these effects are conferred through epigenetics and whether specific epigenetic marks related to these phenotypes are inherited in offspring. However, assuming that they are, the effects of maternal exercise could be conferred in the preconception, perinatal, or postnatal periods. However, the beneficial effects of paternal exercise must be transmitted to offspring through sperm. Studies from independent research groups have documented DNA methylation and non-coding RNA changes in response to exercise training in human sperm (13, 25). Interestingly, both studies noted that altered DNA methylation patterns were associated with genes involved in neurological processes and neurological diseases, including schizophrenia and Parkinson's disease (13). In contrast to somatic cells, only ~15% of sperm DNA is associated with histone proteins, with the remainder associated with protamine proteins (15). The retention of histones is not random and appears to be a mechanism regulating specific sperm DNA folding and compaction patterns (15). Although histone modifications are retained on remaining sperm histones, there has been no characterization of the effects of exercise on these epigenetic marks. Additional research will be required to further characterize the role of epigenetics in how exercise training positively influences metabolic health in offspring.

Another area within the field that requires further research is the bidirectional relationship between metabolism and epigenetics. The availability of metabolic intermediates is rate limiting for both methylation and acetylation reactions (24). Methylation of both DNA and histones requires S-adenosyl-L-methionine (SAMe), a product of the methionine pathway, while acetyl-CoA, the intermediate metabolite of oxidative metabolism, is required for histone acetylation (24). The role of exercise training on the methionine pathway is unclear; however, the skeletal muscle adaptive response to exercise involves reprogramming of metabolic pathways that produce acetyl-CoA, particularly beta oxidation of fatty acids (52, 60). Indeed, epigenetic mechanisms appear to be involved in this adaptive response (19). Interestingly, increased skeletal muscle fatty acid utilization following endurance exercise training could have a profound influence on histone acetylation. This is based on observations using stable isotope fatty acid tracers, which revealed that fatty acid oxidation was the major contributor of acetyl groups for histone acetylation in cell culture (40). Indeed, acetyl-CoA produced by mitochondrial beta oxidation can enter the tricarboxylic acid (TCA) cycle and be converted to citrate before being exported to the cytosol via a citrate transporter, whereupon it can be reconverted to acetyl-CoA through the actions of ATP-citrate lyase. This occurs in the nucleus, where acetyl-CoA is then available to participate in histone acetylation (62). The raises a number of pertinent questions for the field. For example, does increased fatty acid utilization for ATP production during exercise in trained skeletal muscle mean that there is reduced acetyl-CoA available for histone acetylation? Does this contribute to the tempered transcriptional response in exercise-trained individuals? Furthermore, chromatin is able to store ~3 mM of acetyl-CoA in the form of acetylated histone proteins (66). Does exercise training enhance the capacity of skeletal muscle to use this stored acetyl-CoA for ATP or substrate regeneration if required, through its liberation from histones by histone deacetylases?

Interestingly, metabolites that are ordinarily TCA-cycle intermediates are important regulators of the TET enzymes that enzymatically remove DNA methylation. The TET enzymes require α-ketoglutarate as a co-factor for full activity (49). Although α-ketoglutarate is an integral component of the TCA cycle, it can also be synthesized in the cytosol/nuclear compartments from glutamate via transamination. Therefore, enhanced α-ketoglutarate synthesis could conceivably reduce DNA methylation. Whether this mechanism contributes to exercise-induced DNA hypomethylation remains to be determined. Furthermore, mutant isocitrate dehydrogenase enzymes, which are often observed in certain cancers, can also produce 2-hydroxyglutarate (2-HG) from α-ketoglutarate (49). The 2-HG metabolite inhibits TET function and has been associated with DNA hypermethylation and repression of gene expression (49). Whether exercise training influences any of these metabolic mechanisms regulating epigenetics remains to be determined. These studies highlight the emerging interactions between metabolism and epigenetics, which will be an important area of study in the future to further our understanding of the molecular mechanisms mediating exercise adaptations in skeletal muscle.

Concluding Remarks

Skeletal muscle adaptations to exercise training involve repeated transcriptional activation of exercise-responsive genes, which ultimately increase the protein abundance of numerous metabolic enzymes and proteins involved in muscle function. Transient regulation of epigenetic mechanisms appears to contribute to this response, including reduced DNA methylation and histone modifications that confer transcriptional activation. Our current understanding of these mechanisms is elementary at best, and future research will better define the exact epigenetic signatures that occur in response to exercise and exercise training. Whether any of these epigenetic mechanisms can be passed on to subsequent generations remains to be determined. Furthermore, the interactions between epigenetics and skeletal muscle metabolism will likely reveal important insights into how energetics during exercise and after exercise training influence adaptive responses.

References

1. Awad S, Kunhi M, Little GH, Bai Y, An W, Bers D, et al. Nuclear CaMKII enhances histone H3 phosphorylation and remodels chromatin during cardiac hypertrophy. *Nucleic Acids Res* 41: 7656–7672, 2013.
2. Baar K, Wende AR, Jones TE, Marison M, Nolte LA, Chen M, et al. Adaptations of skeletal muscle to exercise: Rapid increase in the transcriptional coactivator PGC-1. *FASEB J* 16: 1879–1886, 2002.
3. Bailey AO, Panchenko T, Sathyan KM, Petkowski JJ, Pai PJ, Bai DL, et al. Posttranslational modification of CENP-A influences the conformation of centromeric chromatin. *Proc Nat Acad Sci USA* 110: 11827–11832, 2013.
4. Bajpeyi S, Covington JD, Taylor EM, Stewart LK, Galgani JE, Henagan TM. Skeletal muscle PGC1alpha -1 nucleosome position and -260 nt DNA methylation determine exercise response and prevent ectopic lipid accumulation in men. *Endocrinology* 158: 2190–2199, 2017.
5. Barres R, Osler ME, Yan J, Rune A, Fritz T, Caidahl K, et al. Non-CpG methylation of the PGC-1alpha promoter through DNMT3B controls mitochondrial density. *Cell Metab* 10: 189–198, 2009.
6. Barres R, Yan J, Egan B, Treebak JT, Rasmussen M, Fritz T, et al. Acute exercise remodels promoter methylation in human skeletal muscle. *Cell Metab* 15: 405–411, 2012.
7. Bird A. Perceptions of epigenetics. *Nature* 447: 396–398, 2007.
8. Bird AP, Wolffe AP. Methylation-induced repression–belts, braces, and chromatin. *Cell* 99: 451–454, 1999.
9. Booth FW, Neufer PD. Exercise genomics and proteomics. In: *ACSM Advanced Exercise Physiology*, edited by Farrell PA, Joyner MJ, Caiozzo VJ. Philadelphia: Lippincott, Williams & Wilkins, 2012, p. 669–698.
10. Carter LG, Lewis KN, Wilkerson DC, Tobia CM, Ngo Tenlep SY, Shridas P, et al. Perinatal exercise improves glucose homeostasis in adult offspring. *Am J Physiol* 303: E1061–E1068, 2012.
11. Carter LG, Qi NR, De Cabo R, Pearson KJ. Maternal exercise improves insulin sensitivity in mature rat offspring. *Med Sci Sport Exerc* 45: 832–840, 2013.

12. Chang S, Bezprozvannaya S, Li S, Olson EN. An expression screen reveals modulators of class II histone deacetylase phosphorylation. *Proc Nat Acad Sci USA* 102: 8120–8125, 2005.

13. Denham J, O'Brien BJ, Harvey JT, Charchar FJ. Genome-wide sperm DNA methylation changes after 3 months of exercise training in humans. *Epigenomics* 7: 717–731, 2015.

14. Domanska-Senderowska D, Laguette MN, Jegier A, Cieszczyk P, September AV, Brzezianska-Lasota E. MicroRNA profile and adaptive response to exercise training: A review. *Int J Sports Med* 40: 227–235, 2019.

15. Donkin I, Barres R. Sperm epigenetics and influence of environmental factors. *Mol Metab* 14: 1–11, 2018.

16. Egan B, Zierath JR. Exercise metabolism and the molecular regulation of skeletal muscle adaptation. *Cell Metab* 17: 162–184, 2013.

17. Filipescu D, Szenker E, Almouzni G. Developmental roles of histone H3 variants and their chaperones. *Trends Genet* 29: 630–640, 2013.

18. Fischle W, Dequiedt F, Hendzel MJ, Guenther MG, Lazar MA, Voelter W, et al. Enzymatic activity associated with class II HDACs is dependent on a multiprotein complex containing HDAC3 and SMRT/N-CoR. *Mol Cell* 9: 45–57, 2002.

19. Gaur V, Connor T, Sanigorski A, Martin SD, Bruce CR, Henstridge DC, et al. Disruption of the class IIa HDAC corepressor complex increases energy expenditure and lipid oxidation. *Cell Rep* 16: 2802–2810, 2016.

20. Gibbs JR, van der Brug MP, Hernandez DG, Traynor BJ, Nalls MA, Lai SL, et al. Abundant quantitative trait loci exist for DNA methylation and gene expression in human brain. *PLoS Genet* 6: e1000952, 2010.

21. Goldberg AD, Allis CD, Bernstein E. Epigenetics: A landscape takes shape. *Cell* 128: 635–638, 2007.

22. Henikoff S, Greally JM. Epigenetics, cellular memory and gene regulation. *Curr Biol* 26: R644–648, 2016.

23. Holloszy JO. Biochemical adaptations in muscle. Effects of exercise on mitochondrial oxygen uptake and respiratory enzyme activity in skeletal muscle. *J Biol Chem* 242: 2278–2282, 1967.

24. Howlett KF, McGee SL. Epigenetic regulation of skeletal muscle metabolism. *Clin Sci* 130: 1051–1063, 2016.

25. Ingerslev LR, Donkin I, Fabre O, Versteyhe S, Mechta M, Pattamaprapanont P, et al. Endurance training remodels sperm-borne small RNA expression and methylation at neurological gene hotspots. *Clin Epigenetics* 10: 12, 2018.

26. Jackson V, Shires A, Chalkley R, Granner DK. Studies on highly metabolically active acetylation and phosphorylation of histones. *J Biol Chem* 250: 4856–4863, 1975.

27. Joseph JS, Ayeleso AO, Mukwevho E. Exercise increases hyper-acetylation of histones on the Cis-element of NRF-1 binding to the Mef2a promoter: Implications on type 2 diabetes. *Biochem Biophys Res Commun* 486: 83–87, 2017.

28. Kanzleiter T, Jahnert M, Schulze G, Selbig J, Hallahan N, Schwenk RW, et al. Exercise training alters DNA methylation patterns in genes related to muscle growth and differentiation in mice. *Am J Physiol* 308: E912–E920, 2015.

29. Kuratomi G, Iwamoto K, Bundo M, Kusumi I, Kato N, Iwata N, et al. Aberrant DNA methylation associated with bipolar disorder identified from discordant monozygotic twins. *Mol Psychiatry* 13: 429–441, 2008.

30. Laker RC, Lillard TS, Okutsu M, Zhang M, Hoehn KL, Connelly JJ, et al. Exercise prevents maternal high-fat diet-induced hypermethylation of the Pgc-1alpha gene and age-dependent metabolic dysfunction in the offspring. *Diabetes* 63: 1605–1611, 2014.

31. Lee JS, Smith E, Shilatifard A. The language of histone crosstalk. *Cell* 142: 682–685, 2010.

32. Li E, Zhang Y. DNA methylation in mammals. *Cold Spring Harb Perspect Biol* 6: a019133, 2014.

33. Lin J, Wu H, Tarr PT, Zhang CY, Wu Z, Boss O, et al. Transcriptional co-activator PGC-1 alpha drives the formation of slow-twitch muscle fibres. *Nature* 418: 797–801, 2002.

34. Lindholm ME, Giacomello S, Werne Solnestam B, Fischer H, Huss M, Kjellqvist S, et al. The impact of endurance training on human skeletal muscle memory, global isoform expression and novel transcripts. *PLoS Genet* 12: e1006294, 2016.

35. Lindholm ME, Marabita F, Gomez-Cabrero D, Rundqvist H, Ekstrom TJ, Tegner J, et al. An integrative analysis reveals coordinated reprogramming of the epigenome and the transcriptome in human skeletal muscle after training. *Epigenetics* 9: 1557–1569, 2014.

36. Lo WS, Trievel RC, Rojas JR, Duggan L, Hsu JY, Allis CD, et al. Phosphorylation of serine 10 in histone H3 is functionally linked in vitro and in vivo to Gcn5-mediated acetylation at lysine 14. *Mol Cell* 5: 917–926, 2000.

37. Ma K, Chan JK, Zhu G, Wu Z. Myocyte enhancer factor 2 acetylation by p300 enhances its DNA binding activity, transcriptional activity, and myogenic differentiation. *Mol Cell Biol* 25: 3575–3582, 2005.

38. Mastroeni D, McKee A, Grover A, Rogers J, Coleman PD. Epigenetic differences in cortical neurons from a pair of monozygotic twins discordant for Alzheimer's disease. *PLOS ONE* 4: e6617, 2009.

39. Masuzawa R, Konno R, Ohsawa I, Watanabe A, Kawano F. Muscle type-specific RNA polymerase II recruitment during PGC-1alpha gene transcription after acute exercise in adult rats. *J Appl Physiol* 2018.

40. McDonnell E, Crown SB, Fox DB, Kitir B, Ilkayeva OR, Olsen CA, et al. Lipids reprogram metabolism to become a major carbon source for histone acetylation. *Cell Rep* 17: 1463–1472, 2016.

41. McGee SL, Fairlie E, Garnham AP, Hargreaves M. Exercise-induced histone modifications in human skeletal muscle. *J Physiol* 587: 5951–5958, 2009.

42. McGee SL, Hargreaves M. Epigenetics and exercise. *Trend Endocrinol Metab* 30: 636–645, 2019.

43. McGee SL, Swinton C, Morrison S, Gaur V, Campbell DE, Jorgensen SB, et al. Compensatory regulation of HDAC5 in muscle maintains metabolic adaptive responses and metabolism in response to energetic stress. *FASEB J* 28: 3384–3395, 2014.

44. McGee SL, van Denderen BJ, Howlett KF, Mollica J, Schertzer JD, Kemp BE, et al. AMP-activated protein kinase regulates GLUT4 transcription by phosphorylating histone deacetylase 5. *Diabetes* 57: 860–867, 2008.

45. McKinsey TA, Zhang CL, Lu J, Olson EN. Signal-dependent nuclear export of a histone deacetylase regulates muscle differentiation. *Nature* 408: 106–111, 2000.

46. Nitert MD, Dayeh T, Volkov P, Elgzyri T, Hall E, Nilsson E, et al. Impact of an exercise intervention on DNA methylation in skeletal muscle from first-degree relatives of patients with type 2 diabetes. *Diabetes* 61: 3322–3332, 2012.

47. Oates NA, van Vliet J, Duffy DL, Kroes HY, Martin NG, Boomsma DI, et al. Increased DNA methylation at the AXIN1 gene in a monozygotic twin from a pair discordant for a caudal duplication anomaly. *Am J Hum Genet* 79: 155–162, 2006.

48. Peterson CL, Laniel MA. Histones and histone modifications. *Curr Biol* 14: R546–R551, 2004.

49. Prensner JR, Chinnaiyan AM. Metabolism unhinged: IDH mutations in cancer. *Nature Med* 17: 291–293, 2011.

50. Roundtree IA, Evans ME, Pan T, He C. Dynamic RNA modifications in gene expression regulation. *Cell* 169: 1187–1200, 2017.

51. Schaffer BE, Levin RS, Hertz NT, Maures TJ, Schoof ML, Hollstein PE, et al. Identification of AMPK phosphorylation sites reveals a network of proteins involved in cell invasion and facilitates large-scale substrate prediction. *Cell Metab* 22: 907–921, 2015.

52. Schrauwen P, van Aggel-Leijssen DP, Hul G, Wagenmakers AJ, Vidal H, Saris WH, et al. The effect of a 3-month low-intensity endurance training program on fat oxidation and acetyl-CoA carboxylase-2 expression. *Diabetes* 51: 2220–2226, 2002.

53. Silva GJJ, Bye A, El Azzouzi H, Wisloff U. MicroRNAs as important regulators of exercise adaptation. *Prog Cardiovasc Dis* 60: 130-151, 2017.

54. Sjogren RJO, Lindgren Niss MHL, Krook A. Skeletal Muscle MicroRNAs: Roles in Differentiation, Disease and Exercise. In: *Hormones, Metabolism and the Benefits of Exercise*, edited by Spiegelman B. Springer International Publishing AG: Cham: 2017, p. 67–81.

55. Smith JA, Kohn TA, Chetty AK, Ojuka EO. CaMK activation during exercise is required for histone hyperacetylation and MEF2A binding at the MEF2 site on the Glut4 gene. *Amer J Physiol* 295: E698–E704, 2008.

56. Stanford KI, Lee MY, Getchell KM, So K, Hirshman MF, Goodyear LJ. Exercise before and during pregnancy prevents the deleterious effects of maternal high-fat feeding on metabolic health of male offspring. *Diabetes* 64: 427–433, 2015.

57. Stanford KI, Rasmussen M, Baer LA, Lehnig AC, Rowland LA, White JD, et al. Paternal exercise improves glucose metabolism in adult offspring. *Diabetes* 67: 2530–2540, 2018.

58. Stanford KI, Takahashi H, So K, Alves-Wagner AB, Prince NB, Lehnig AC, et al. Maternal exercise improves glucose tolerance in female offspring. *Diabetes* 66: 2124–2136, 2017.

59. Terruzzi I, Senesi P, Montesano A, La Torre A, Alberti G, Benedini S, et al. Genetic polymorphisms of the enzymes involved in DNA methylation and synthesis in elite athletes. *Physiol Genomics* 43: 965–973, 2011.

60. Tunstall RJ, Mehan KA, Wadley GD, Collier GR, Bonen A, Hargreaves M, et al. Exercise training increases lipid metabolism gene expression in human skeletal muscle. *Amer J Physiol* 283: E66–72, 2002.

61. Watt F, Molloy PL. Cytosine methylation prevents binding to DNA of a HeLa cell transcription factor required for optimal expression of the adenovirus major late promoter. *Genes Dev* 2: 1136–1143, 1988.

62. Wellen KE, Hatzivassiliou G, Sachdeva UM, Bui TV, Cross JR, Thompson CB. ATP-citrate lyase links cellular metabolism to histone acetylation. *Science* 324: 1076–1080, 2009.

63. Williams RS, Neufer PD. Regulation of Gene Expression in Skeletal Muscle by Contractile Activity. In: *Handbook of Physiology Exercise: Regulation and Integration of Multiple Systems*, edited by Rowell LB & Shepherd JT. Bethesda, MD: American Physiological Society, 1124–1150, 1996.

64. Wu Z, Puigserver P, Andersson U, Zhang C, Adelmant G, Mootha V, et al. Mechanisms controlling mitochondrial biogenesis and respiration through the thermogenic coactivator PGC-1. *Cell* 98: 115–124, 1999.

65. Yao Q, Chen Y, Zhou X. The roles of microRNAs in epigenetic regulation. *Curr Opin Chem Biol* 51: 11–17, 2019.

66. Ye C, Tu BP. Sink into the epigenome: Histones as repositories that influence cellular metabolism. *Trends Endocrinol Metab* 29: 626–637, 2018.

67. Yu M, Stepto NK, Chibalin AV, Fryer LG, Carling D, Krook A, et al. Metabolic and mitogenic signal transduction in human skeletal muscle after intense cycling exercise. *J Physiol* 546: 327–335, 2003.

68. Zee BM, Levin RS, Xu B, LeRoy G, Wingreen NS, Garcia BA. In vivo residue-specific histone methylation dynamics. *J Biol Chem* 285: 3341–3350, 2010.

69. Zhang D, Cheng L, Badner JA, Chen C, Chen Q, Luo W, et al. Genetic control of individual differences in gene-specific methylation in human brain. *Am J Hum Genet* 86: 411–419, 2010.

70. Zheng Y, Thomas PM, Kelleher NL. Measurement of acetylation turnover at distinct lysines in human histones identifies long-lived acetylation sites. *Nature Commun* 4: 2203, 2013.

16

STATISTICAL CONSIDERATIONS AND BIOLOGICAL MECHANISMS UNDERLYING INDIVIDUAL DIFFERENCES IN ADAPTATIONS TO EXERCISE TRAINING

Jacob T. Bonafiglia, Hashim Islam, Nir Eynon,
and Brendon J. Gurd

General Introduction

Although the multifaceted benefits of exercise are consistently observed at the group level, it is becoming increasingly apparent that individuals respond differently to exercise training (68, 71, 82). A growing number of studies have identified a portion of participants as "non-responders" that do not appear to demonstrate meaningful benefit after completing exercise training (63, 71). Given issues associated with the term "non-responder" (discussed in *Concerns with labelling individuals as "non-responders"*), we will instead use the term "low responder." Interindividual variability and the purported existence of "low-responders" suggests that a "one size fits all" approach is not suitable when prescribing exercise in clinical/applied settings (21). While the existence of variability in observed physiological responses to exercise training cannot be questioned, the mechanisms explaining this variability remain unclear.

The purpose of this chapter is to discuss the evidence highlighting genetic factors and other mechanisms that appear to contribute to variability in observed responses to exercise training. Given the importance in understanding statistical concepts related to analysis of individual responses, this chapter begins by overviewing methods for defining "responders" and "low-responders," as well as estimating variability in responses to training. In closing, this chapter acknowledges two large-scale collaborative projects that are anticipated to provide valuable insight into the mechanisms underlying training responsiveness.

Defining "Responders" and "Low-Responders"

Two main observations have emerged from a growing body of literature examining individual responses to exercise training. First, despite exercise training resulting in improvements at the group level, a portion of individuals do not appear to benefit from exercise training and have thus been labelled "low-responders" (reviewed in 13). Second, despite individuals completing identical training protocols, there appears to be interindividual variability in the observed responses to exercise training (reviewed in 11). Although these two observations have gained considerable research interest and have led to discussions of utilizing exercise as personalized medicine (21), concerns have been raised regarding the statistical approaches for classifying "responders" and "low responders" (4, 13, 14, 32, 71, 78) and quantifying the existence/magnitude of interindividual response variability (3, 4, 11, 71, 78).

This section first outlines the sources of variation that are relevant to interpreting individual responses to training. We then discuss several lines of evidence that raise concerns for labelling individuals as "non-responders" and preface the rest of this chapter.

Analysing Individual Responses to Exercise Training

Sources of Variation Influencing the Observed Response to Exercise Training

There are three main sources of variation influencing an individual's observed response to exercise training. The first source of variation is an individual's true response to exercise training (*TRUE*), which describes a real change in a physiological variable that is attributable to the effect of exercise training. The second source of variation is within-subject variability (*WS*), which refers to real physiological changes associated with alterations in behavioural and/or environmental factors (e.g., changes in long-term physical activity or diet patterns) (31, 74) over the course of an exercise training intervention. Although the influence of *WS* can produce real physiological changes, it is important to emphasize that changes caused by *WS* are separate from the effects of exercise training (11). The third source of variation is the typical error of measurement (*TE*), which comprises random measurement error introduced by technical noise (e.g., equipment or experimenter error) and random day-to-day variability in biological factors (e.g., circadian rhythms, sleep patterns, diet) (35). Within the context of an individual's response to exercise training, *TE* will introduce noise into both pre- and post-training measurements. Taken together, an individual's observed response to exercise training is composed of *TRUE*, *WS*, and *TE* (11):

Individual's Observed Response

$$= \Delta TRUE \pm \Delta WS \pm \Delta TE \tag{16.1}$$

where $\Delta TRUE$ represents true changes attributable to exercise training, ΔWS represents true changes attributable to *WS* (i.e., not attributable to exercise training), and ΔTE represents the impact of *TE* in both pre- and post-training measurements.

Classifying "Responders" and "Low-Responders"

Given that $\Delta TRUE$ is one of three sources of variation comprising an individual's observed response to exercise training (Equation 16.1), it is inappropriate to assume that an individual's observed response reflects $\Delta TRUE$. Therefore, rather than using an arbitrary threshold to dichotomously classify responses based on observed responses, classification of "responders" and "low-responders" may require utilizing a statistical approach that considers the influence of ΔTE and/or ΔWS (13). Additionally, recent articles have suggested that analysing individual responses on a continuous axis is more appropriate, and potentially less erroneous, than categorically classifying responses (4, 13). For more information regarding recommended methods for identifying "responders" and "low responders," we refer the reader to several articles that describe relevant statistical approaches (4, 13, 14, 32, 78).

Analysing Interindividual Variability in Responses to Exercise Training

Sources of Variation Influencing Interindividual Variability in Responses to Exercise Training

The three main sources of variation that influence an individual's observed response (ΔTE, ΔWS, and $\Delta TRUE$; Equation 16.1) can vary between individuals and thus contribute to interindividual variability (standard deviation; SD) in observed responses to exercise training (herein referred to as SD_{EX}):

$$SD_{EX} = V\Delta TRUE \pm V\Delta WS \pm V\Delta TE \qquad (16.2)$$

where $V\Delta TRUE$ represents interindividual variability in true changes attributable to exercise training, $V\Delta WS$ represents interindividual variability in true changes attributable to behavioural/environmental factors, and $V\Delta TE$ represents interindividual variability in TE in both pre- and post-training measurements (11).

Quantifying Interindividual Variability in Responses to Exercise Training

Given that $V\Delta TRUE$ is one of three sources of variation comprising interindividual variability in observed responses (Equation 16.2), it is inappropriate to assume that variability in observed responses reflects $V\Delta TRUE$ (3). For instance, we recently reported interindividual variability in behavioural factors (e.g., diet and physical activity patterns) over the course of an exercise training intervention, which highlights the possibility that SD_{EX} is influenced by $V\Delta WS$ and that SD_{EX} is not an accurate depiction of $V\Delta TRUE$ (11). Further, recent articles have suggested that the influence of $V\Delta WS$ and/or $V\Delta TE$ are so large that the magnitude of $V\Delta TRUE$ is minimal or does not exist (3). Quantifying the existence and magnitude of $V\Delta TRUE$ is a complex issue, and we refer the reader to several articles that have outlined statistical approaches for estimating $V\Delta TRUE$ using various study designs (3, 31, 32, 74).

Concerns with Labelling Individuals as "Non-Responders"

Concurrent with the increasing popularity of examining individual responses to exercise training are growing concerns with labelling individuals as "non-responders" (16, 63). Understanding these concerns is crucial for discussing individual responses to exercise training, especially when translating findings to broader audiences, and is therefore relevant for research exploring mechanisms contributing to individual differences in adaptations to training. The four major concerns addressed in the literature are as follows:

1. *Dichotomous classification methods:* Dichotomous classification methods risk labelling individuals as "non-responders" despite these participants potentially experiencing true physiological adaptations to exercise training (13). Although conservative low-response thresholds (e.g., −2x TE) decrease the risk in misclassifying participants as "non-responders," previous work (reviewed in 13) has inappropriately classified "non-responders" using non-conservative thresholds (e.g., +2x TE thresholds). In general, we recommend analysing responses to exercise interventions on continuous axes rather than using dichotomous, and often arbitrary, cut-off points.

2. *Individual patterns of response:* Many studies have observed individual patterns of response across multiple outcomes (reviewed in 13) whereby a given individual can respond positively in one outcome but fail to respond in others. The observation that individuals respond differently across a range of outcomes suggests that it is inappropriate to label individuals as "non-responders" to exercise training. In other words, it is critical to specify the outcome (specific trait) when labelling responders (e.g., "VO_2 max low-responder") given the possibility that these individuals responded in other unmeasured outcomes (16).

3. *Intraindividual variability:* We recently found that individual VO_2 max responses were not reproducible after completing two identical training periods (26). This observation suggests that non-response is not a permanent feature, as "non-responders" may positively respond after repeatedly being exposed to the same stimulus. There is also evidence that "non-responders" can elicit a

positive response after changing the training stimulus (15) or augmenting exercise training frequency (55) or exposure (70).

4. *Public health concern:* Individuals that view themselves as "non-responders" may refrain from exercising under the belief that exercise will not provide any benefit—a concern that is heightened by the low physical activity rates observed worldwide. This public health concern may be alleviated by using alternative terminology such as "did not respond" instead of "non-responder" (63).

Investigating Mechanisms of Individual Response Variability

Given the complex statistical considerations mentioned earlier, it reasonably follows that identifying mechanisms that underlie individual response variability is also a complex task requiring the use of nuanced statistical approaches (3). The remainder of this chapter reviews studies that have explored potential mechanisms that underlie interindividual variability in observed responses. It is important to note that these studies did not use the earlier-referenced statistical approaches to determine the mechanisms underlying $V\Delta TRUE$. Nevertheless, the studies discussed throughout the remainder of this chapter highlight many possible mechanisms underlying individual response variability and point to several areas for future work.

Genetic Influence on Individual Responses to Exercise

Since the pioneer HERITAGE study demonstrated interindividual differences in observed responses to aerobic training, there has been considerable interest in exploring the role of genetics in regulating adaptations to exercise training. The focus of this section is to review the evidence from animal models and human studies supporting the notion that genetics partly explains the variability in adaptations to exercise training.

Evidence from Animal Studies

A unique advantage in animal studies is the ability to tightly control for behavioural/environmental factors (e.g., physical activity levels, diet composition) and thus minimize variability in true changes caused by these factors ($V\Delta WS$). Therefore, animal studies provide an opportunity to investigate the genetic mechanisms that may explain $V\Delta TRUE$. In this section, we briefly highlight animal models that have been used to demonstrate that genetics contributes to the magnitude of adaptations to exercise training, and we review animal studies that attempted to identify specific genetic variants associated with training responsiveness.

Inbred Strains

Inbred strains/lines are created by strict brother–sister mating for many generations (usually 20+) to produce genetically unique lines. Given the virtually isogenic nature of each inbred line (~98.6% identical genome after 20 generations of inbreeding), these animal models can interrogate the influence of genetics on variability in responses to exercise training. Specifically, variability in training responses between inbred strains, and thus between different genetic profiles, reflects variability that can be attributed to genetics.

Several studies have demonstrated variability in training responses between inbred lines, suggesting that genetic variation contributes to observed variability in training adaptations. Between-line variability in exercise responsiveness has been reported for aerobic exercise capacity, heart and muscle mass, body weight, and skeletal muscle morphological and molecular characteristics (39, 47). An interesting finding is that certain inbred lines appear to be "resistant" to exercise training, as rodents within these lines fail to improve their exercise capacity following standardized training (5, 41, 42). Importantly, the existence of between-line variability in exercise response and the demonstration of "exercise-resistant" inbred lines support the role of genetics in influencing exercise (low) response.

Selective Breeding for Low and High Responses to Exercise Training

In the late 2000s, a selective breeding rat model was developed based on changes in exercise capacity following aerobic training (42, 43). This model produced two genetically independent lines: low-response trainers (LRTs) and high response trainers (HRTs). Studies using this model have demonstrated that HRTs exhibit larger changes in exercise capacity (42, 45, 89), muscle strength (2), and parameters of whole-body metabolic function (43). Potential mechanisms underlying observed differences in whole-body exercise capacity and metabolic function responses between HRTs and LRTs include skeletal muscle morphological factors (43, 45), regulators of skeletal muscle mitochondrial biogenesis (45), and cellular characteristics of the left ventricle (89). Collectively, these findings from selectively bred rat models provide convincing, and perhaps the strongest (71), evidence that genetics contributes to the magnitude of adaptations following exercise training.

Quantitative Trait Loci Mapping for Exercise Training Responses

Quantitative trait loci (QTL) are polymorphic regions (loci) associated with variability in a given phenotype. QTL mapping involves correlating tagged genetic variants (i.e., selected variants that are meant to cover a given genomic region) with variation in a given phenotype (87). It is important to note that the goal of QTL mapping is to determine whether phenotype variability is associated with a given locus or loci rather than specific genetic variants per se. Therefore, QTL mapping is often followed with more detailed analysis (e.g., "fine-mapping") to identify specific genetic variants within a given loci that correlate with a given phenotype.

To our knowledge, few studies have conducted QTL mapping for aerobic exercise training phenotypes in animal models. Massett et al. identified a single QTL that was significantly associated with changes in aerobic exercise capacity (46). This single QTL contains *CPVL* (a carboxypeptidase gene), suggesting that this gene is associated with changes in aerobic exercise capacity following training in mice (46). However, large-scale human studies have failed to reproducibly identify significant associations between variants in *CPVL* and training responses in maximal exercise capacity (86). Given the dearth of QTL mapping studies in animal models, it is possible that future investigations using a large number of genetically diverse lines reveal more QTLs linked to variation in adaptations to exercise training.

Evidence from Human Studies

Many human studies have provided different lines of evidence supporting an association between genetics and exercise training responses. As described in the sections that follow, the bulk of these studies come from Dr Claude Bouchard and his colleagues beginning in the early 1980s and continuing today. Despite many reports demonstrating genetic associations with exercise training, several shortcomings remain that currently limit the application of genetic factors to predict the magnitude of individual responses.

Twin and Family Studies

Experiments conducted at the University of Laval (Ste-Foy, Quebec, Canada) were the first to provide evidence linking genetics to variability in observed responses to exercise training. Exercise training studies involving monozygotic twins (i.e., siblings with nearly identical genomes) found moderate-to-strong correlations in changes in skeletal muscle outcomes, body composition, and exercise performance between twin pairs (reviewed in 72). Subsequently, the HERITAGE Family Study demonstrated familial aggregation in exercise responses with heritability estimates (i.e., an estimate of the degree of variation in a given outcome that can be explained by genetics) ranging from ~14% to 51% across a number of physiological outcomes (reviewed in 72). Collectively, twin and family studies suggest that genetics partially explains the variability in observed responses to exercise training in humans.

It is important to recognize that shared behavioural/environmental factors may contribute to the aggregation of observed responses among monozygotic twins and nuclear families (74). As discussed earlier, variability in observed responses comprises both variability in responsiveness to exercise training ($V\Delta TRUE$) and variability in real physiological changes attributable to behavioural/environmental factors $(V\Delta WS)$. Therefore, it is possible that similar observed responses among twins and families reflect shared behaviour/environmental factors rather than genetic associations to $V\Delta TRUE$ (74).

Studies Examining Specific Genetic Variants: From Candidate Genes to a Genome-Wide Approach

The sequencing of the human genome provided experimental opportunities beyond twin/familial aggregation studies for investigating whether specific genetic variants underlie complex human phenotypes. Experiments investigating genetic associations to human phenotypes follow either a candidate-gene or a hypothesis-free approach (86). Candidate-gene approaches involve testing the hypothesis that predetermined, specific genetic variants are associated with a given phenotype. Conversely, hypothesis-free approaches involve genome-wide association studies (GWAS) to identify genetic associations with human phenotypes in hundreds of thousands to millions of variations across the human genome. For the remainder of this section, we will discuss genetic associations with exercise-induced changes in VO_2 max, as this is the most commonly studied outcome in exercise genomics (72). For more information on other exercise-related outcomes, we refer the reader to annual reviews completed by leaders in exercise genomics (most recent report, 73).

Early candidate-gene approaches in human training studies used QTL mapping to identify chromosomal locations associated with changes in maximal exercise capacity (19, 67). Later work explored specific genetic variants, and Williams and colleagues recently conducted a systematic review of specific variants associated with exercise-induced changes in VO_2 max (86). As reported by Williams et al. (86), variants associated with changes in VO_2 max have small/weak effect sizes, and only a few genetic variants have been successfully replicated in different cohorts (Table 16.1).

A limitation of studying single genetic variants is the inherent complexity of the adaptive response to exercise—a complexity that reflects combined contributions from multiple genetic variants (i.e., polygenic) (72, 86). Cognizant of this genetic complexity, Bouchard and colleagues re-analysed samples from the HERITAGE study using combined association scores across multiple variants (20). Specifically, they conducted a GWAS examining over 324,000 single nucleotide polymorphisms (SNPs) and identified 39 SNPs that were significantly ($p < 1.5 \times 10^{-4}$) associated with changes in VO_2 max (20). Multivariate regression analysis found that the combined effects of 21 of these SNPs accounted for ~49% of the variance in observed VO_2 max responses—an effect size that is similar to the heritability estimate (~47%) derived from the familial aggregation analysis reported in 1999 (18). Importantly, these 21 SNPs accounted for a larger amount of variance in observed VO_2 max responses compared to the strongest individual variant (only ~7% of variance explained by *ACSL1*), thus highlighting the strength of multivariate polygenic approaches. Bouchard and colleagues also created "predictor scores" based on zygosity for each of the 21 SNPs, and these scores effectively separated high and low VO_2 max responses (20). Evidently, findings from the HERITAGE Family Study suggest that genetics contributes to variability in VO_2 max response and support the notion that low and high VO_2 max responders exhibit divergent genetic profiles (82). However, these data should be looked at with caution, since many of these identified SNPs have not been replicated (86) and the statistical threshold chosen was low compared to other GWAS studies.

Table 16.1 Genetic variants identified by Williams et al. (86) that are significantly associated with changes in VO$_2$ max following exercise training and have been replicated in different samples

Gene symbol	Pathway(s)
ACE	Renin–angiotensin system; protein digestion and absorption
ACSL1	Fatty acid biosynthesis; fatty acid degradation; "metabolic pathways"; fatty acid metabolism; PPAR signalling pathway; peroxisome; ferroptosis; thermogenesis; adipocytokine signalling pathway
AMPD1	Purine metabolism; "metabolic pathways"
APOE	Cholesterol metabolism; Alzheimer disease
BIRC7/YTHDF1	Ubiquitin-mediated proteolysis; apoptosis; toxoplasmosis; pathways in cancer; small cell lung cancer
CAMTA1	N/A*
CD44	ECM-receptor interaction; hematopoietic cell lineage; shigellosis; Epstein–Barr virus infection; proteoglycans in cancer; microRNAs in cancer
CKM	Arginine and proline metabolism; "metabolic pathways"
DAAM1	Wnt signalling pathway
NDN	N/A*
RGS18	N/A*
RYR2	Calcium signalling pathway; cAMP signalling pathway; cardiac muscle contraction; adrenergic signalling in cardiomyocytes; apelin signalling pathway; circadian entrainment; insulin secretion; oxytocin signalling pathway; pancreatic secretion; hypertrophic cardiomyopathy; arrhythmogenic right ventricular cardiomyopathy; dilated cardiomyopathy
ZIC4	N/A*

Pathways were determined by performing individual searches on the Kyoto Encyclopedia of Genes and Genomes (KEGG).
* N/A refers to genes that are not involved in a known pathway

Current Perspectives and Future Directions

Despite the intriguing results discussed earlier, exercise genomics experts remain doubtful that genetic variants can be accurate predictors of individual exercise responses due to three apparent limitations:

1. Few of the variants associated with changes in VO$_2$ max are linked to the physiological mechanisms that determine VO$_2$ max (72) (Table 16.1). For instance, improvements in VO$_2$ max are primarily driven by increases in cardiac output, stroke volume, and blood volume (33); however, none of the SNPs identified in the HERITAGE analysis are functionally related to these mechanisms (38, 72). As discussed earlier, the function of some of the SNPs from HERITAGE have yet to be discovered (20), and thus it is possible that future studies discover that some SNPs are functionally linked to exercise-induced improvements in VO$_2$ max.

2. The majority of significant relationships between genetic variants and changes in VO$_2$ max are either weak or have small effect sizes. The majority of significant SNPs only explain ~1–2% of the variance in observed VO$_2$ max responses (20). Although this section has focused on changes in VO$_2$ max following training, individual genetic variants associated with other complex human traits have yielded disappointingly small effect sizes (17, 22). These disappointing results may be explained by the polygenic nature of human phenotypes whereby many genetic variants, each with small effect sizes, and/or a few rare variants with large effect sizes collectively influence a given complex trait (17, 29). In support of a polygenic explanation is the observation of a larger effect size for the regression with changes in VO$_2$ max when Bouchard et al. (20) combined 21 SNPs. Nevertheless, studying genomics alone may not provide enough mechanistic information (22),

suggesting that that multiomic approaches are required to confidently predict complex human phenotypes (17, 29).

3. Perhaps the most problematic limitation is the inability to replicate genetic associations across multiple cohorts. For instance, although ~100 genetic variants are associated with changes in VO_2 max (86), only 14 have been corroborated in some, but not all, studies (Table 16.1). It is also important to emphasize that significant associations do not necessarily confer causation, which highlights the need to follow successful replication studies with mechanistic and functional experiments to ascertain causal evidence (29). For example, a recent study suggested that the angiotensin-converting enzyme (ACE) insertion/deletion variant is associated with the ACE content in the blood, thus offering a strong biological marker that can potentially be predicted by the genotype (90).

Despite the scepticism among experts in exercise genomics (17, 38), several companies advertise the ability to predict training responsiveness based on algorithms derived from genetic associations. These "direct-to-consumer" claims have received justifiable criticism (17, 84), as future work is needed, including collaborative multiomic approaches, before commercially marketing the ability to predict training responsiveness using genetic variants (84).

Biological Mechanisms Underlying Individual Differences in Adaptations to Exercise Training

This section reviews non-genetic biological mechanisms associated with individual variability in adaptations to exercise training. The majority of this section focuses on skeletal muscle mechanisms. Therefore, it is important to preface this section by briefly describing the molecular basis of skeletal muscle adaptations to exercise training (described in the next paragraph). Additionally, given that VO_2 max is the most studied outcome in exercise genomics, the final section reviews studies that have investigated mechanisms that may be associated with individual differences in VO_2 max responses to exercise training.

The molecular basis of skeletal muscle adaptations is illustrated in Figure 16.1 and has been described in detail elsewhere (23, 28, 60). Skeletal muscle adaptations to exercise training are characterized by a series of molecular events occurring in response to individual acute exercise bouts. In brief, physical activity increases the production of contractile and/or metabolic by-products (e.g., increased myocellular

Acute Exercise

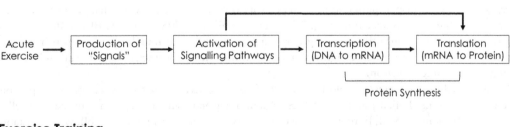

Exercise Training

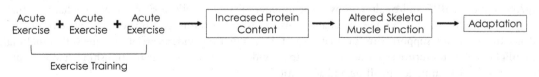

Figure 16.1 The molecular basis of skeletal muscle adaptation to exercise training

calcium, elevated AMP/ATP ratio) that act as signals to initiate skeletal muscle adaptation. These signals activate signalling pathways (e.g., AMPK, CaMK, p38 MAPK) that converge on various transcription factors and co-activators to promote transcription. Consequently, acute exercise is associated with transient bursts in mRNA that typically occur in the early post-exercise period (e.g., 1–3 hours). Over the course of repeated exercise bouts (i.e., exercise training), frequent mRNA bursts augment protein translation, thereby altering skeletal muscle protein content. Signalling pathways also promote protein translation and thus increase rates of protein synthesis. Finally, altered protein levels improve skeletal muscle function and consequently increase exercise performance and other whole-body outcomes (e.g., glucose metabolism, cardiorespiratory fitness).

Within the context of individual responses to exercise training, it is reasonable to hypothesize that variability in any of these acute molecular events (Figure 16.1) may explain the variability in responses to exercise training. Additionally, although "exercise epigenetics" is still in its infancy (37, 50) and epigenetic processes are often overlooked in depictions of the molecular basis of adaptations to exercise (Figure 16.1), we overview the evidence linking acute alterations in skeletal muscle epigenetics and adaptations following exercise training. Further, the final subsection briefly overviews studies that relate variability in adaptations to exercise training with chronic changes in skeletal muscle characteristics (i.e., measuring pre- vs. post-training changes rather than before vs. after an acute bout of exercise). As discussed throughout this section, there is an overall dearth of evidence mechanistically linking acute and chronic skeletal muscle responses to variability in adaptations to exercise training, thus highlighting the need for future investigations.

Acute Changes in Skeletal Muscle Signalling Pathways and Training Adaptations

Although there is some evidence supporting and refuting the hypothesis that acute changes in skeletal muscle signalling play a role in predicting the magnitude of adaptations to resistance training (49, 51–53, 79), we are unaware of any evidence exploring this relationship with aerobic exercise. With respect to resistance exercise, acute changes in phosphorylation of ribosomal protein S6 kinase beta-1 (p70S6K) positively correlate with subsequent muscle strength and size gains following training (49, 51, 79). Despite three separate studies reporting this relationship (49, 51, 79), a significant correlation between acute changes in phosphorylation of p70S6K and hypertrophy is not always observed (53). p70S6K is a downstream target of mammalian target of rapamycin (mTOR), which is a key regulator of protein synthesis and hypertrophic adaptations to resistance training (23). In addition to p70S6K, acute changes in the phosphorylation of eukaryotic translation initiation factor 4E-binding protein 1(4E-BP1), another downstream target of mTOR (23), also correlate with changes in muscle size following resistance training (52). Interestingly, acute changes in phosphorylation of protein kinase B (Akt), an upstream activator of mTOR, or phosphorylation of mTOR itself do not correlate with changes in muscle size or strength following resistance training (52, 79). Thus, while the p70S6K and 4E-BP1 findings suggest that acute activation of mTOR signalling may explain variability in muscle adaptations to resistance training, the inability to observe significant correlations with phosphorylation of Akt and mTOR complicates this interpretation.

An additional area of interest is exploring the role of satellite cells in mediating hypertrophic adaptations to resistance training. Bellamy and co-workers (9) found that acute alterations in the number of satellite cells in type I, but not type II, fibres positively correlate with changes in muscle size following resistance training. Collectively, these findings support the speculation that changes in skeletal muscle signalling (p70S6K and 4E-BP1) and/or alterations in the number of satellite cells represent acute mechanisms that may explain individual differences in adaptations to resistance training. However, the paucity of evidence that currently supports this speculation and the conflicting evidence related to mTOR signalling highlights a need for future replication studies to provide more insight in the relationship between acute changes in skeletal muscle signalling and adaptations to training.

As mentioned earlier, no study has directly tested the hypothesis that variability in activation of skeletal muscle signalling pathways predicts interindividual differences in adaptations to aerobic exercise training. Despite this knowledge gap, we recently reported that blood lactate responses during an acute bout of aerobic exercise strongly correlate with changes in VO_2 max following 4 weeks of aerobic training (64). Although we did not directly measure skeletal muscle signalling, it is possible that blood lactate concentrations reflect muscle lactate concentrations, intramuscular stress, and thus the activation of skeletal muscle signalling pathways (64). Therefore, our observed correlation may provide indirect evidence linking variation in skeletal muscle signalling and variation in training responses; however, future work should directly test this hypothesis.

Acute Changes in Skeletal Muscle mRNA and Training Adaptations

Although several studies have reported a temporal relationship whereby acute alterations in messenger RNA (mRNA) levels precede adaptations to training (27, 61), few studies have directly tested the hypothesis that the magnitude of acute changes in mRNA levels predict the variance in adaptations to exercise training. Granata et al. (30) found that aerobic training–induced changes in mitochondrial content positively correlate with acute changes in p53 mRNA content. While this finding supports the role of p53 in regulating mitochondrial adaptations to exercise training (75), there is conflicting evidence for whether acute mRNA responses of other key regulators of mitochondrial biogenesis, including PGC-1α, positively correlate with mitochondrial adaptations to aerobic training (12, 30). Within the context of resistance exercise, acute changes in levels of mRNA linked to modulating muscle growth appear to be largest in participants identified as "extreme responders" in skeletal muscle hypertrophy following training (7, 40). Further, Raue et al. (66) used microarray analysis to demonstrate that acute changes in over 1,700 mRNA correlated with changes in muscle strength and size following training. In summary, although there is some evidence supporting the speculation that acute changes in skeletal muscle mRNA levels underlie individual differences in training responses to exercise training, the small number of studies investigating this speculation highlights a need for future work.

In an attempt to provide more insight into the potential importance of mRNA responses to acute exercise, we recently examined the repeatability of mRNA responses to two identical bouts of acute endurance exercise (36). Our hypothesis was if the magnitude of an individual's mRNA response to acute exercise predicts the magnitude of their subsequent adaptations to training, then the degree of acute mRNA responses should be somewhat repeatable at the individual level. Acute changes of mRNA implicated in regulating skeletal muscle adaptations to aerobic training (e.g., PGC-1α, PDK4, NRF-1, VEGF-A, p53) were not repeatable, and several follow-up experiments confirmed that this lack of repeatability could not be explained by technical or measurement error (36). This apparent lack of repeatability supports the observations of non-significant relationships between acute changes in mRNA levels and adaptations to training (7, 12, 30, 40), possibly questioning the spuriousness of the earlier-mentioned significant correlations and relationships (7, 12, 30, 40, 66), and ultimately suggesting that acute changes in mRNA may not be a viable biomarker for gauging individual responsiveness to exercise training (36).

Acute Changes in Rates of Skeletal Muscle Protein Synthesis and Training Adaptations

To our knowledge, only studies using resistance exercise have directly tested the hypothesis that acute changes in rates of protein synthesis predict adaptations to training (24, 49, 52). In opposition to this hypothesis, there is some evidence that changes in the rate of myofibrillar protein synthesis in response to a single pre-training bout of resistance exercise does not correlate with hypertrophic adaptations following resistance training (49, 52). Conversely, Damas et al. (24) found that changes in the rate of myofibrillar protein synthesis following an acute bout of resistance exercise in the third week of training positively correlates with hypertrophic responses to 10 weeks of training. While it is possible that the incongruent findings between these studies are explained by differences in the time points used to characterize changes in rates of muscle protein synthesis (i.e., changes following a single bout of exercise vs. 3 weeks of training) (68), the small number of studies investigating this relationship warrants a need for further investigation. Further, future work should explore this hypothesis using aerobic exercise protocols.

Acute Epigenetic Changes in Skeletal Muscle and Training Adaptations

Epigenetics Overview

The term *epigenetics* translates to "in addition to changes in genetic sequence" and refers to chemical modifications to DNA (such as DNA methylation) that regulate the expression of genes without altering the underlying DNA sequence, which can ultimately result in downstream changes in protein expression (10). There are two main types of epigenetic modifications (37). First, DNA methylation involves the addition of methyl groups directly to the DNA sequence by DNA methyltransferases (50). DNA methylation results in decreased transcription of the targeted gene, whereas DNA demethylation (or hypomethylation), a process regulated by ten-eleven translocation enzymes (50), increases gene transcription (see 58 for details). The second epigenetic process is histone modification, which involves post-translational modifications to histones (the protein forming the nucleosome core and providing structural stability) that ultimately affect transcription by allowing or inhibiting the transcriptional machinery access to promoter regions of target genes (50). Although not often considered an epigenetic process (37), the actions of non-coding RNAs (such as micro RNA) can also influence gene expression without altering DNA sequence. Collectively, DNA (de)methylation, histone modification, and non-coding RNAs influence gene expression and may therefore play important roles in the adaptive process to exercise (37, 50, 83, 85).

Skeletal Muscle Epigenetics: Possible Mechanisms Underlying Individual Differences in Responses to Exercise Training

Although no study has directly examined both acute changes in skeletal muscle DNA methylation and training-induced phenotypes in the same participants, some findings from acute exercise studies highlight the possibility that changes in DNA methylation contribute to individual differences in exercise training responses. For instance, Barrès et al. (8) found that exercise decreased global DNA methylation as well as methylation of genes known to regulate skeletal muscle adaptations (e.g., PGC-1α, PDK4, and PPARδ/β). Importantly, Barrès et al. (8) found that DNA hypomethylation preceded increases in gene expression, suggesting that alterations in DNA methylation are functionally important for transcriptional responses to acute exercise. In support of this assertion, a recent acute exercise study found that individuals who displayed DNA hypomethylation at the PGC-1α promoter had larger increases in PGC-1α mRNA compared to individuals who displayed increases in DNA methylation at the PGC-1α promoter (6). Given the aforementioned relationship between acute changes in PGC-1α mRNA and changes in skeletal muscle oxidative capacity following training (12), these findings raise the possibility that acute changes in DNA methylation may explain interindividual differences in training responsiveness (85). However, future studies are needed to test this hypothesis.

Although many studies have reported histone modifications in skeletal muscle following acute exercise (reviewed in 37, 85), studies examining both histone modifications to acute exercise and adaptations to training in the same group of individuals are lacking. However, recent experiments in rodent skeletal muscle have found that acute exercise results in histone modifications on the PGC-1α promoter (44, 48) and, as described earlier, differences in epigenetic regulation on the PGC-1α promoter may explain variability in adaptations to training (85). The potential importance of histone modifications on mediating exercise responsiveness was also demonstrated in a histone deacetylation 3 (HDAC3) knockout model (34). Mice lacking HDAC3, a histone-modifying protein associated with transcriptional repression (50), exhibited suppressed endurance and force production as well as greater muscle fatigue (34). Despite these findings from rodent experiments, there is a need for future studies to examine the relationship between histone modifications following acute exercise and adaptations to exercise training in human participants.

Although not examining responses to acute exercise per se, studies examining baseline epigenetic characteristics have provided additional evidence supporting the notion that epigenetic processes play an important role in predicting variability in training responses. For instance, Stephens et al. (77) reported baseline differences in genome-wide DNA methylation between "low responders" and "responders" in mitochondrial function following aerobic training. Additionally, Thalacker-Mercer et al. (80) found that "moderate and extreme responders" in hypertrophy following resistance training exhibited lower baseline levels of acetylated histone H3, a histone associated with increasing transcription (50), compared to "low responders." Collectively, these findings suggest that "responders" are more "primed" to experience transcriptional responses to acute exercise and thus exhibit large adaptations to exercise training. Future studies should couple characterizing baseline epigenetic profiles with skeletal muscle responses to acute exercise in an attempt to provide a mechanistic link between baseline epigenetics and adaptations to training.

Chronic Skeletal Muscle Changes and Training Adaptations

Overview of "Chronic Skeletal Muscle Changes"

For the purpose of this section, "chronic changes" refer to pre- vs. post-training changes that reflect an accumulation of the acute molecular events occurring after each individual exercise session over the course of a training period. The findings from an elegant study by Perry and colleagues (61) can help explain this concept. Perry et al. (61) found that exercise training concomitantly increased mitochondrial content (adaptation to training) and PGC-1α protein content ("chronic change"). Importantly, the observed chronic increase in PGC-1α protein content appeared to result from acute transient bursts of PGC-1α mRNA occurring after each individual exercise training session (61). Therefore, while changes in PGC-1α protein were measured pre- vs. post-training, these chronic changes were a result of acute molecular events occurring after serial training sessions (61).

Although there is evidence suggesting that chronic skeletal muscle changes are associated with variability in a range of adaptations to exercise training, the bulk of this evidence has explored mechanisms linked to hypertrophic adaptations following resistance training (68). Therefore, the remainder of this section focuses on studies that have linked chronic skeletal muscle changes and hypertrophic adaptations to resistance training.

Chronic Skeletal Muscle Changes and Hypertrophic Adaptations to Resistance Training

Studies that have tested the hypothesis that chronic changes in skeletal muscle explain the variability in hypertrophy following resistance training have examined many different types of chronic skeletal muscle alterations (68). First, an early investigation found that chronic increases in both myonuclei and satellite cell content only occurred in "extreme responders" (62), findings not supported by a more recent study (54). Second, although one study reported that chronic increases in total RNA and rRNA content only occurred in "extreme responders" in hypertrophy (76), a later study failed to replicate this finding (54). Third, several resistance training studies have concurrently measured hypertrophy and chronic changes in androgen receptor content (1, 51, 54, 56), which is a transcription factor that alters transcription to promote skeletal muscle cell growth and protein synthesis (68). Despite recent studies failing to observe differences in chronic changes in androgen receptor content between "low" and "high" hypertrophic responders (54, 56), earlier studies reported positive correlations between chronic changes in androgen receptor content and myofiber hypertrophy (1, 51). Taken together, these studies have produced several lines of conflicting evidence, which makes it difficult to conclude whether the current literature supports or refutes the hypothesis that chronic skeletal muscle changes explain the variability in hypertrophic adaptations to resistance training. Given that these studies did not attempt to capture the molecular events following acute exercise (57), future work should couple pre- vs. post-training measures with acute exercise measures to comprehensively characterize skeletal muscle changes that may account for individual differences in adaptations to training.

Mechanisms Associated with Changes in VO_2 max Following Aerobic Training

It is widely accepted that training-induced improvements in VO_2 max are driven by chronic (i.e., pre- vs. post-training) changes in features of the oxygen transport/consumption cascade, including cardiac output, convective oxygen delivery through the cardiovascular system, and skeletal muscle oxygen uptake and consumption (33). However, few studies have examined individual responses in both changes in VO_2 max and changes in components of the oxygen transport/delivery cascade following aerobic exercise training.

To our knowledge, only studies using high intensity interval training (HIIT; including its higher intensity variant, sprint interval training [SIT]) have tested the hypothesis that individual responses in components of the oxygen transport/consumption cascade explain individual variability in VO_2 max responses. Interestingly, these studies have produced several lines of conflicting evidence. First, Daussin et al. (25) found that changes in maximal cardiac output and VO_2 max were positively correlated following 8 weeks of HIIT. Conversely, we recently demonstrated that maximal cardiac output remained unchanged in both "low" and "high" VO_2 max responders following 4 weeks of SIT (65). Second, while there is evidence that changes in VO_2 max positively correlate with changes in mitochondrial respiration following HIIT (25) and changes in arteriovenous oxygen difference (a marker of active muscle oxygen consumption) following SIT (65), other findings demonstrate that markers of skeletal muscle mitochondrial content do not positively correlate with changes in VO_2 max following SIT (12, 65). Third, changes in capillary density positively correlate with observed VO_2 max responses following HIIT (25) but not SIT (12, 65). While it is possible that the previously mentioned lines of conflicting evidence are attributable to methodological differences between studies, future large-scale studies measuring several components of the oxygen transport/consumption cascade are needed to further investigate these discrepant findings.

Future Directions: Multiomic Approaches

Many experts in the field of exercise "-omics" have emphasized the need for multiomic approaches to better understand the mechanisms underlying variability in individual responses to exercise training (17, 29). In brief, multiomic approaches involve genome-wide (-omic) analysis across multiple levels of biological information, including but not limited to genomics (DNA sequences), transcriptomics (gene expression), epigenomics (epigenetics), proteomics (protein), and metabolomics (metabolites) (22). The enthusiasm underlying multiomic approaches is rooted in the belief that synthesizing data across multiple biological levels provides more information than what can be gleaned from any single "-omic" layer alone (88). Within the context of exercise science, it is believed that combining information in a multiomic fashion can leverage current genomic, transcriptomic, epigenomic, and other "-omic" findings to better identify the mechanisms underlying variability in responses to exercise training.

Although a comprehensive multiomics study has yet to take place, a small number of studies have combined data across multiple biological layers in an attempt to identify mechanisms of training response variability (69, 81). For instance, RNA expression profiling (transcriptomic) was performed on HERITAGE samples to identify a number of transcripts that were associated with variability in observed VO_2 max responses to aerobic exercise training (reviewed in 72). This information was then used to identify a number of SNPs (genomic) that were also related to changes in VO_2 max following training; however, none of these SNPs were among the group of variants that Bouchard and colleagues later identified in their GWAS on HERITAGE samples (20). While other exercise studies have combined transcriptomics with epigenomics (DNA methylomics) (69, 81) or proteomics (69), these studies contained relatively small sample sizes. Unfortunately, large sample sizes are needed in multiomic approaches in order to achieve the statistical power necessary to detect factors associated with variance in a given phenotype (17).

One proposed solution to acquire large sample sizes is to conduct large-scale collaborative projects across multiple research sites (29). To our knowledge, two multiomic collaborative initiatives have been announced: the Molecular Transducers of Physical Activity Consortium (MoTrPAC) (59) and the Gene SMART (Skeletal Muscle Adaptive Response to Training) study (91). While the specifics of these two projects differ, they share the goal of harnessing the power of multiomics to identify mechanisms that underlie variability in adaptations to exercise training. Indeed, it is highly anticipated that these two initiatives will produce valuable insight in identifying the mechanisms underlying individual response variability to exercise training.

References

1. Ahtiainen JP, Lehti M, Hulmi JJ, Kraemer WJ, Markku A, Nyman K, et al. Recovery after heavy resistance exercise and skeletal muscle androgen receptor and insulin-like growth factor-I isoform expression in strength trained men. *J Strength Cond Res* 25: 767–777, 2011.
2. Ahtiainen JP, Lensu S, Ruotsalainen I, Schumann M, Ihalainen JK, Fachada V, et al. Physiological adaptations to resistance training in rats selectively bred for low and high response to aerobic exercise training. *Exp Physiol* 103: 1513–1523, 2018.
3. Atkinson G, Batterham AM. True and false interindividual differences in the physiological response to an intervention. *Exp Physiol* 100: 577–588, 2015.
4. Atkinson G, Williamson P, Batterham AM. Issues in the determination of "responders" and "non-responders" in physiological research. *Exp. Physiol* 104: 1215–1225, 2019.
5. Avila JJ, Kim SK, Massett MP. Differences in exercise capacity and responses to training in 24 inbred mouse strains. *Front Physiol* 8: 1–12, 2017.
6. Bajpeyi S, Covington JD, Taylor EM, Stewart LK, Galgani JE, Henagan TM. Skeletal muscle PGC1α −1 nucleosome position and −260 nt DNA methylation determine exercise response and prevent ectopic lipid accumulation in men. *Endocrinology* 158: 2190–2199, 2017.
7. Bamman MM, Petrella JK, Kim JS, Mayhew DL, Cross JM. Cluster analysis tests the importance of myogenic gene expression during myofiber hypertrophy in humans. *J Appl Physiol* 102: 2232–2239, 2007.
8. Barrès R, Yan J, Egan B, Treebak JT, Rasmussen M, Fritz T, et al. Acute exercise remodels promoter methylation in human skeletal muscle. *Cell Metab* 15: 405–411, 2012.
9. Bellamy LM, Joanisse S, Grubb A, Mitchell CJ, McKay BR, Phillips SM, et al. The acute satellite cell response and skeletal muscle hypertrophy following resistance training. *PLOS ONE* 9: e109739, 2014.
10. Bird A. Perceptions of epigenetics. *Nature* 447: 396–398, 2007.
11. Bonafiglia JT, Brennan AM, Ross R, Gurd BJ. An appraisal of the SD IR as an estimate of true individual differences in training responsiveness in parallel-arm exercise randomized controlled trials. *Physiol Rep* 7: e14163, 2019.
12. Bonafiglia JT, Edgett BA, Baechler BL, Nelms MW, Simpson CA, Quadrilatero J, et al. Acute upregulation of PGC-1α mRNA correlates with traininginduced increases in SDH activity in human skeletal muscle. *Appl Physiol Nutr Metab* 42, 2017.
13. Bonafiglia JT, Nelms MW, Preobrazenski N, LeBlanc C, Robins L, Lu S, et al. Moving beyond threshold-based dichotomous classification to improve the accuracy in classifying non-responders. *Physiol Rep* 6: e13928, 2018.

14. Bonafiglia JT, Ross R, Gurd BJ. The application of repeated testing and monoexponential regressions to classify individual cardiorespiratory fitness responses to exercise training. *Eur J Appl Physiol* 119: 889–900, 2019.

15. Bonafiglia JT, Rotundo MP, Whittall JP, Scribbans TD, Graham RB, Gurd BJ. Inter-individual variability in the adaptive responses to endurance and sprint interval training: A randomized crossover study. *PLOS ONE* 11, 2016.

16. Booth FW, Laye MJ. The future: Genes, physical activity and health. *Acta Physiol* 199: 549–556, 2010.

17. Bouchard C. Exercise genomics — a paradigm shift is needed : A commentary. *Br J Sports Med* 49: 1492–1496, 2015.

18. Bouchard C, An P, Rice T, Skinner JS, Wilmore JH, Gagnon J, et al. Familial aggregation of VO2 max response to exercise training: Results from the HERITAGE Family Study. *J Appl Physiol* 87: 1003–1008, 1999.

19. Bouchard C, Rankinen T, Chagnon YC, Rice T, Pérusse L, Gagnon J, et al. Genomic scan for maximal oxygen uptake and its response to training in the HERITAGE Family Study. *J Appl Physiol* 88: 551–559, 2000.

20. Bouchard C, Sarzynski MA, Rice TK, Kraus WE, Church TS, Sung YJ, et al. Genomic predictors of the maximal O_2 uptake response to standardized exercise training programs. *J Appl Physiol* 110: 1160–1170, 2011.

21. Buford TW, Roberts MD, Church TS. Toward exercise as personalized medicine. *Sport Med* 43: 157–165, 2013.

22. Civelek M, Lusis AJ. Systems genetics approaches to understand complex traits. *Nat Rev Genet* 15: 34–48, 2014.

23. Coffey VG, Hawley JA. The molecular bases of training adaptation. *Sport Med* 37: 737–763, 2007.

24. Damas F, Phillips SM, Libardi CA, Vechin FC, Lixandrão ME, Jannig PR, et al. Resistance training-induced changes in integrated myofibrillar protein synthesis are related to hypertrophy only after attenuation of muscle damage. *J Physiol* 594: 5209–5222, 2016.

25. Daussin FN, Zoll J, Dufour SP, Ponsot E, Lonsdorfer-Wolf E, Doutreleau S, et al. Effect of interval versus continuous training on cardiorespiratory and mitochondrial functions: Relationship to aerobic performance improvements in sedentary subjects. *Am J Physiol* 295: R264–R272, 2008.

26. Del Giudice M, Bonafiglia JT, Islam H, Preobrazenski N, Amato A, Gurd BJ. Investigating the reproducibility of maximal oxygen uptake responses to high-intensity interval training. *J Sci Med Sport* 29: 100820, 2019.

27. Egan B, O'Connor PL, Zierath JR, O'Gorman DJ. Time course analysis reveals gene-specific transcript and protein kinetics of adaptation to short-term aerobic exercise training in human skeletal muscle. *PLoS One* 8, 2013.

28. Egan B, Zierath JR. Exercise metabolism and the molecular regulation of skeletal muscle adaptation. *Cell Metab* 17: 162–184, 2013.

29. Eynon N, Voisin S, Lucia A, Wang G, Pitsiladis Y. Preface: Genomics and biology of exercise is undergoing a paradigm shift. *BMC Genomics* 18: 17–19, 2017.

30. Granata C, Jamnick NA, Bishop DJ. Training-induced changes in mitochondrial content and respiratory function in human skeletal muscle. *Sport Med* 48: 1809–1828, 2018.

31. Hecksteden A, Kraushaar J, Scharhag-Rosenberger F, Theisen D, Senn S, Meyer T. Individual response to exercise training - a statistical perspective. *J Appl Physiol* 118: 1450–1459, 2015.

32. Hecksteden A, Pitsch W, Rosenberger F, Meyer T. Repeated testing for the assessment of individual response to exercise training. *J Appl Physiol* 124: 1567–1579, 2018.

33. Hellsten Y, Nyberg M. Cardiovascular adaptations to exercise training. *Compr Physiol* 6: 1–32, 2016.

34. Hong S, Zhou W, Fang B, Lu W, Loro E, Damle M, et al. Dissociation of muscle insulin sensitivity from exercise endurance in mice by HDAC3 depletion. *Nat Med* 23: 223–234, 2017.

35. Hopkins WG. Measures of reliability in sports medicine and science. *Sports Med* 30: 1–15, 2000.

36. Islam H, Edgett BA, Bonafiglia JT, Shulman T, Ma A, Quadrilatero J, et al. Repeatability of exercise-induced changes in mRNA expression and technical considerations for qPCR analysis in human skeletal muscle. *Exp Physiol* 104: 407–420, 2019.

37. Jacques M, Hiam D, Craig J, Barrès R, Eynon N, Voisin S. Epigenetic changes in healthy human skeletal muscle following exercise– a systematic review. *Epigenetics* 14: 1–16, 2019.

38. Joyner MJ, Lundby C. Concepts about VO_2max and trainability are context dependent. *Exerc Sport Sci Rev* 46: 138–143, 2018.

39. Kilikevicius A, Venckunas T, Zelniene R, Carroll AM, Lionikaite S, Ratkevicius A, et al. Divergent physiological characteristics and responses to endurance training among inbred mouse strains. *Scand J Med Sci Sports* 23: n/a–n/a, 2012.

40. Kim J, Petrella JK, Cross JM, Bamman MM. Load-mediated downregulation of myostatin mRNA is not sufficient to promote myofiber hypertrophy in humans: A cluster analysis. *J Appl Physiol* 103: 1488–1495, 2007.

41. Koch LG, Green CL, Lee AD, Hornyak JE, Cicila GT, Britton SL. Test of the principle of initial value in rat genetic models of exercise capacity. *Am J Physiol* 288: R466–R472, 2005.

42. Koch LG, Pollott GE, Britton SL. Selectively bred rat model system for low and high response to exercise training. *Physiol Genomics* 45: 606–614, 2013.

43. Lessard SJ, Rivas DA, Alves-Wagner AB, Hirshman MF, Gallagher IJ, Constantin-Teodosiu D, et al. Resistance to aerobic exercise training causes metabolic dysfunction and reveals novel exercise-regulated signaling networks. *Diabetes* 62: 2717–2727, 2013.

44. Lochmann TL, Thomas RR, Bennett JP, Taylor SM. Epigenetic modifications of the PGC-1α promoter during exercise induced expression in mice. *PLoS One* 10: 1–16, 2015.

45. Marton O, Koltai E, Takeda M, Koch LG, Britton SL, Davies KJA, et al. Mitochondrial biogenesis-associated factors underlie the magnitude of response to aerobic endurance training in rats. *Pflugers Arch* 467: 779–88, 2015.

46. Massett MP, Avila JJ, Kim SK. Exercise capacity and response to training quantitative trait loci in a NZW X 129S1 intercross and combined cross analysis of inbred mouse strains. *PLoS One* 10: 1–19, 2015.

47. Massett MP, Berk BC. Strain-dependent differences in responses to exercise training in inbred and hybrid mice. *Am J Physiol* 288: R1006–R1013, 2005.

48. Masuzawa R, Konno R, Ohsawa I, Watanabe A, Kawano F. Muscle type-specific RNA polymerase II recruitment during PGC-1α gene transcription after acute exercise in adult rats. *J Appl Physiol* 125: 1238–1245, 2018.

49. Mayhew DL, Kim J-S, Cross JM, Ferrando AA, Bamman MM. Translational signaling responses preceding resistance training-mediated myofiber hypertrophy in young and old humans. *J Appl Physiol* 107: 1655–1662, 2009.

50. McGee SL, Walder KR. Exercise and the skeletal muscle epigenome. *Cold Spring Harb Perspect Med* 7: a029876, 2017.

51. Mitchell CJ, Churchward-Venne TA, Bellamy L, Parise G, Baker SK, Phillips SM. Muscular and systemic correlates of resistance training-induced muscle hypertrophy. *PLOS ONE* 8: 1–10, 2013.

52. Mitchell CJ, Churchward-venne TA, Parise G, Bellamy L, Baker SK, Smith K, et al. Acute post-exercise myofibrillar protein synthesis is not correlated with resistance training-induced muscle hypertrophy in young men. *PLoS One* 9: 1–7, 2014.

53. Mitchell CJ, Churchward-Venne TA, West DWD, Burd NA, Breen L, Baker SK, et al. Resistance exercise load does not determine training-mediated hypertrophic gains in young men. *J Appl Physiol* 113: 71–77, 2012.

54. Mobley CB, Haun CT, Roberson PA, Mumford PW, Kephart WC, Romero MA, et al. Biomarkers associated with low, moderate, and high vastus lateralis muscle hypertrophy following 12 weeks of resistance training. *PLoS One* 13: e0195203, 2018.

55. Montero D, Lundby C. Refuting the myth of non-response to exercise training: 'Non-responders' do respond to higher dose of training. *J Physiol* 595: 3377–3387, 2017.

56. Morton RW, Sato K, Gallaugher MPB, Oikawa SY, McNicholas PD, Fujita S, et al. Muscle androgen receptor content but not systemic hormones is associated with resistance training-induced skeletal muscle hypertrophy in healthy young men. *Front Physiol* 9: 1–11, 2018.

57. Murton AJ, Billeter R, Stephens FB, Des Etages SG, Graber F, Hill RJ, et al. Transient transcriptional events in human skeletal muscle at the outset of concentric resistance exercise training. *J Appl Physiol* 116: 113–125, 2014.

58. Nakao M. Epigenetics: Interaction of DNA methylation and chromatin. *Gene* 278: 25–31, 2001.

59. National Institutes of Health. Molecular transducers of physical activity in humans. https://commonfund.nih.gov/MolecularTransducers.

60. Perry CGR, Hawley JA. Molecular basis of exercise-induced skeletal muscle mitochondrial biogenesis: Historical advances, current knowledge, and future challenges. *Cold Spring Harb Perspect Med* 8: a029686, 2017.

61. Perry CGR, Lally J, Holloway GP, Heigenhauser GJF, Bonen A, Spriet LL. Repeated transient mRNA bursts precede increases in transcriptional and mitochondrial proteins during training in human skeletal muscle. *J Physiol* 588: 4795–4810, 2010.

62. Petrella JK, Kim J, Mayhew DL, Cross JM, Bamman MM. Potent myofiber hypertrophy during resistance training in humans is associated with satellite cell-mediated myonuclear addition: A cluster analysis. *J Appl Physiol* 104: 1736–1742, 2008.

63. Pickering C, Kiely J. Do non-responders to exercise exist—and if so, what should we do about them? *Sport Med* 49: 1–7, 2019.

64. Preobrazenski N, Bonafiglia JT, Nelms MW, Lu S, Robins L, LeBlanc C, Gurd BJ. Does blood lactate predict the chronic adaptive response to training: A comparison of traditional and talk test prescription methods. *Appl Physiol Nutr Metab* 44: 179–186, 2019.

65. Raleigh JP, Giles MD, Islam H, Nelms M, Bentley RF, Jones JH, et al. Contribution of central and peripheral adaptations to changes in maximal oxygen uptake following 4 weeks of sprint interval training. *Appl Physiol Nutr Metab* 43: 1059–1068, 2018.

66. Raue U, Trappe TA, Estrem ST, Qian H-R, Helvering LM, Smith RC, et al. Transcriptome signature of resistance exercise adaptations: Mixed muscle and fiber type specific profiles in young and old adults. *J Appl Physiol* 112: 1625–1636, 2012.

67. Rico-Sanz J, Rankinen T, Rice T, Leon AS, Skinner JS, Wilmore JH, et al. Quantitative trait loci for maximal exercise capacity phenotypes and their responses to training in the HERITAGE Family Study. *Physiol Genomics* 16: 256–260, 2004.

68. Roberts MD, Haun CT, Mobley CB, Mumford PW, Romero MA, Roberson PA, et al. Physiological differences between low versus high skeletal muscle hypertrophic responders to resistance exercise training: Current perspectives and future research directions. *Front Physiol* 9: 1–17, 2018.

69. Robinson MM, Dasari S, Konopka AR, Johnson ML, Manjunatha S, Esponda RR, et al. Enhanced protein translation underlies improved metabolic and physical adaptations to different exercise training modes in young and old humans. *Cell Metab* 25: 581–592, 2017.

70. Ross R, De Lannoy L, Stotz PJ. Separate effects of intensity and amount of exercise on interindividual cardiorespiratory fitness response. *Mayo Clin Proc* 90: 1506–1514, 2015.

71. Ross R, Goodpaster BH, Koch LG, Sarzynski MA, Kohrt WM, Johannsen NM, et al. Precision exercise medicine: Understanding exercise response variability. *Br J Sport Med* 0: 1–13, 2019.

72. Sarzynski MA, Ghosh S, Bouchard C. Genomic and transcriptomic predictors of response levels to endurance exercise training. *J Physiol* 595: 2931–2939, 2017.

73. Sarzynski MA, Loos RJF, Lucia A, Perusse L, Roth SM, Wolfarth B, et al. Advances in exercise, fitness, and performance genomics in 2015. *Med Sci Sport Exerc* 48: 1906–1916, 2016.

74. Senn S. Individual therapy: New dawn or false dawn? *Drug Inf J* 35: 1479–1494, 2001.

75. Smiles WJ, Camera DM. The guardian of the genome p53 regulates exercise-induced mitochondrial plasticity beyond organelle biogenesis. *Acta Physiol* 222: e13004, 2018.

76. Stec MJ, Kelly NA, Many GM, Windham ST, Tuggle SC, Bamman MM. Ribosome biogenesis may augment resistance training-induced myofiber hypertrophy and is required for myotube growth in vitro. *Am J Physiol* 310: E652–E661, 2016.

77. Stephens NA, Brouwers B, Eroshkin AM, Yi F, Cornnell HH, Meyer C, et al. Exercise response variations in skeletal muscle PCr recovery rate and insulin sensitivity relate to muscle epigenomic profiles in individuals with type 2 diabetes. *Diabetes Care* 41: 2245–2254, 2018.

78. Swinton PA, Hemingway BS, Saunders B, Gualano B, Dolan E. A statistical framework to interpret individual response to intervention: Paving the way for personalised nutrition and exercise prescription. *Front Nutr* 5: 41, 2018.

79. Terzis G, Georgiadis G, Stratakos G, Vogiatzis I, Kavouras S, Manta P, et al. Resistance exercise-induced increase in muscle mass correlates with p70S6 kinase phosphorylation in human subjects. *Eur J Appl Physiol* 102: 145–152, 2007.

80. Thalacker-Mercer A, Stec M, Cui X, Cross J, Windham S, Bamman M. Cluster analysis reveals differential transcript profiles associated with resistance training-induced human skeletal muscle hypertrophy. *Physiol Genomics* 45: 499–507, 2013.

81. Turner DC, Seaborne RA, Sharples AP. Comparative yranscriptome and methylome analysis in human skeletal muscle anabolism, hypertrophy and epigenetic memory. *Sci Rep* 9: 4251, 2019.

82. Vellers HL, Kleeberger SR, Lightfoot JT. Inter-individual variation in adaptations to endurance and resistance exercise training: Genetic approaches towards understanding a complex phenotype. *Mamm. Genome* 29: 48–62, 2018.

83. Voisin S, Eynon N, Yan X, Bishop DJ. Exercise training and DNA methylation in humans. *Acta Physiol* 213: 39–59, 2015.

84. Webborn N, Williams A, Mcnamee M, Bouchard C, Pitsiladis Y, Ahmetov I, et al. Direct-to-consumer genetic testing for predicting sports performance and talent identification: Consensus statement. *Br J Sports Med* 49: 1486–1491, 2015.

85. Widmann M, Nieß AM, Munz B. Physical exercise and epigenetic modifications in skeletal muscle. *Sport Med* 49: 509–523, 2019.

86. Williams CJ, Williams MG, Eynon N, Ashton KJ, Little JP, Wisloff U, et al. Genes to predict VO2max trainability: A systematic review. *BMC Genomics* 18: 831, 2017.
87. Williams EG, Auwerx J. The convergence of systems and reductionist approaches in complex trait analysis. *Cell* 162: 23–32, 2015.
88. Williams EG, Wu Y, Jha P, Dubuis S, Blattmann P, Argmann CA, et al. Systems proteomics of liver mitochondria function. *Science* 352: aad0189, 2016.
89. Wisløff U, Bye A, Stølen T, Kemi OJ, Pollott GE, Pande M, et al. Blunted cardiomyocyte remodeling response in exercise-resistant rats. *J Am Coll Cardiol* 65: 1378–1380, 2015.
90. Yan X, Dvir N, Jacques M, Cavalcante L, Papadimitriou ID, Munson F, et al. ACE I/D gene variant predicts ACE enzyme content in blood but not the ACE, UCP2, and UCP3 protein content in human skeletal muscle in the Gene SMART study. *J Appl Physiol* 125: 923–930, 2018.
91. Yan X, Eynon N, Papadimitriou ID, Kuang J, Munson F, Tirosh O, et al. The gene SMART study: Method, study design, and preliminary findings. *BMC Genomics* 18: 821, 2017.

17

EFFECTS OF HYPOXIA/BLOOD FLOW RESTRICTION ON CELLULAR ADAPTATIONS TO TRAINING

Scott J. Dankel and Jeremy P. Loenneke

Introduction

Aerobic exercise results in improvements in the body's ability to uptake and utilize oxygen, while resistance exercise results in increases in muscle size and strength. As it relates to both modes of exercise, scientists are always looking for new and innovative training methods to enhance exercise adaptations and help individuals overcome plateaus in training. Two well-studied methods involve the use of either systemic hypoxia or localized hypoxia via blood flow restricted exercise. Systemic hypoxia is commonly employed by endurance athletes looking to improve athletic performance, while blood flow restricted exercise may be more beneficial for populations that are contraindicated to exercise. The purpose of this chapter is to provide a brief background of each training method and to examine the potential efficacy and physiologic mechanisms responsible for augmenting endurance and resistance training performance.

Systemic Hypoxia

Creating a Hypoxic Environment

The process of breathing occurs so that the body can get oxygen into the tissues while disposing of the carbon dioxide that is produced from metabolism. The breathing process occurs due to the pressure difference between the atmosphere and the lungs. When the pressure in the atmosphere exceeds the pressure in the lungs, air flows into the lungs (inhalation), and when the pressure in the lungs exceeds the pressure in the atmosphere, air flows out (exhalation). As an individual ascends to altitude, the atmospheric pressure becomes progressively lower than at sea level, and this causes the partial pressure of oxygen to also be reduced. For this reason, it is difficult to consume as much oxygen, which in turn creates a hypoxic environment. The hypoxia that results from travelling to altitude is not related to any change in the fraction of oxygen in the air, because oxygen always comprises approximately 21% of atmospheric air. In order to simulate altitude and more easily assess the effects of hypoxia independent of changes in wind conditions or temperature that occur at altitude, hypobaric chambers are sometimes used. These hypobaric chambers provide the most realistic simulation of altitude because they reduce the partial pressure of oxygen by reducing the magnitude of atmospheric pressure. An alternative method of simulating altitude involves reducing the partial pressure of oxygen in the air by reducing the fraction of inspired oxygen (i.e., <21% of oxygen and typically between 12% and 16%) via a normobaric hypoxic chamber, but these methods do not always produce the same results. Nonetheless, moving to altitude, artificially reducing the atmospheric pressure, and artificially reducing the fraction of oxygen in the air are all ways by which the effects of hypoxia can be studied. While the body is exposed to conditions that initially result in tissue hypoxia, adaptations will occur to increase the delivery of oxygen to peripheral tissues. Thus, adaptations that occur when the body is exposed to hypoxia are to maintain normoxia under otherwise hypoxic conditions. We will not discuss the altitude training mask as a method of hypoxia, since it does not actually alter the partial pressure of atmospheric oxygen, but rather may serve as a respiratory training device.

Strategies for Using Hypoxia to Enhance Training Adaptations

Several different methods are employed to try and enhance training adaptations via hypoxia. These methods differ based on whether individuals are living under hypoxic conditions and/or training under hypoxic conditions. The "live high, train high" philosophy is a method in which individuals will simply live and train under hypoxia. Another method involves the "live high, train low" philosophy, by which individuals live under hypoxia but train under normoxia. The "live high, train low" philosophy is centred on the idea that individuals must live at altitude to get the benefits that are associated with the reduced partial pressure of oxygen, but they should train near sea level so their performance does not suffer from being at altitude. This theory operates under the assumption that an acute impairment in training ability will negatively affect chronic adaptations, but there is little support for this claim, particularly given that localized hypoxia (i.e., blood flow restricted exercise) enhances exercise adaptations while directly limiting acute performance. Both the "live high, train high" and "live high, train low" methods involve chronic exposure to hypoxia, being that these individuals are living in an environment with a reduced partial pressure of oxygen. Living in a hypoxic environment may be beneficial in and of itself, as many of the proposed adaptations attributed to hypoxia come in response to just being at altitude in the absence of exercise. Given the reduced availability of oxygen, the body responds by trying to enhance the delivery of oxygen to the tissues. These positive adaptations are generally lost after spending some time back at normal elevation. Of course, individuals must continue to train, or they will lose adaptations that are specific to exercise training. A completely different philosophy is the "live low, train high" strategy by which individuals only complete their training under hypoxia while living at normoxia. This strategy will not provide some of the beneficial adaptations associated with living under conditions with lower atmospheric pressure but will negate some of the negative adaptations associated with it. The premise behind training at hypoxia is that it may provide an added stress to exercise that may produce even greater benefits than exercising under normoxic conditions. While hypoxia is generally thought to improve adaptations to aerobic exercise performance, we will discuss the potential benefits for aerobic, anaerobic, and resistance exercise performance. When examining the potential adaptations that occur in response to acclimating to hypoxia, we will focus on adaptations that are not immediately reversible because the goal is generally to improve exercise performance under normoxic conditions.

Aerobic Exercise Adaptations

Positive Adaptations to Hypoxia Independent of Exercise

The primary benefit of training at altitude is thought to involve improvements in aerobic exercise performance (i.e., a timed trial). Many of the adaptations brought about by acclimation to altitude are modulated by hypoxia-inducible factor 1-alpha (HIF-1α), which is a gene transcription factor present in all nucleated cells and is up-regulated during cellular hypoxia (33). When sufficient oxygen is present, HIF-1α binds to an E3 ligase and is degraded at the proteasome (i.e., it is disposed of). When insufficient oxygen is present, as is the case in hypoxia, HIF-1α binds to DNA and alters the transcriptional activity (i.e., it increases the RNA production) of several genes, one of which regulates erythropoietin (EPO) production. EPO is a hormone produced and secreted primarily by the kidneys when the peritubular capillaries in the kidneys sense lower levels of oxygen. EPO is responsible for stimulating the formation of new red blood cells and thus improves the ability to transport oxygen. To illustrate the effectiveness of EPO for exercise performance, a synthetic form of EPO was created in 1970 to combat anaemia, but quickly became used as an ergogenic aid in various sports (often termed blood doping) and has since been banned by the World Anti-Doping Agency. As such, acclimating to altitude can serve as a legal form of blood doping by increasing endogenous EPO production, albeit to a lesser extent than that which occurs via synthetic drugs. The hypoxia-induced increase in EPO production generally takes 24–48 hours, with the subsequent increase in haemoglobin and red blood cell mass increasing after about 3 weeks of hypoxia acclimation. These adaptations are not permanent, however, and red blood cell mass and haemoglobin content return to pre-altitude levels within approximately 2 weeks of returning to areas with higher atmospheric pressure.

Other physiologic adaptations that are regulated by increased activity of HIF-1α include an up-regulation of the signalling protein, vascular endothelial growth factor (VEGF), which is responsible for the formation of new blood vessels (i.e., angiogenesis). Increased capillarization would theoretically improve one's ability to transport oxygen and nutrients, while also clearing metabolic by-products. While there is some suggestion that new blood vessels are formed as a result of hypoxic exposure (1), others have suggested that there is not an increase in blood vessels per se, but rather an increase in blood vessels per unit of muscle mass (12, 16), and this is related to a decrease in muscle mass accompanying hypoxia acclimation. With that being said, an increase in the ratio of capillaries to muscle fibre area would still enable a greater transport of oxygen and clearance of waste products. Additionally, an increase in myoglobin content may enhance the ability to carry and store oxygen within the muscle and generate adenosine triphosphate (ATP), the body's energy source.

In addition to the cardiovascular adaptations mentioned, there is an increase in minute ventilation (the amount of air moved in 1 minute), which allows the body to consume more oxygen. The increase in minute ventilation appears to occur as an additional strategy to prevent low oxygen levels in the peripheral tissues, and this is brought about by stimulation of the peripheral chemoreceptors. The peripheral chemoreceptors are located in the aortic and carotid bodies and send afferent impulses back to the central nervous system in response to changes in chemical concentrations. As it relates to hypoxia, the peripheral chemoreceptors sense reductions in arterial oxygen concentrations and send signals back to the central nervous system to increase respiration. Increased minute ventilation increases the level of alveolar oxygen, which subsequently increases the level of arterial oxygen and allows for a greater amount of oxygen to be sent to and extracted by peripheral tissues. An increase in sympathetic nerve activity results in cardiovascular adaptations (i.e., increased heart rate and blood pressure), but these will be discussed later, as they are not necessarily positive adaptations for performance. Collectively, with the adaptations to the cardiovascular system, it appears that the adaptations from acclimating to altitude would allow for more oxygen to be taken in and then transported throughout the body. These positive adaptations usually require long-term acclimation (i.e., at least 2–3 weeks) to hypoxia and are generally not acquired from brief intermittent exposure to hypoxia. This is apparent in that individuals who work (~8 hours/day) at very high altitudes but live near sea level never fully acclimate to their work conditions at altitude. Although positive adaptations appear to occur in response to acclimating to altitude, it is also important to consider potential negative adaptations that may occur.

Negative Adaptations to Hypoxia Independent of Exercise

Not all adaptations that occur with acclimation to hypoxia are positive. Some of these adaptations are also present for several weeks or longer upon return to sea level, and therefore may wash out any potential positive adaptations that would also be present. Thus, while the "live high, train low" philosophy exists because of positive adaptations associated with living at altitude, negative adaptations are less discussed. For example, a reduced stroke volume and reduced maximal heart rate persists for about 2 weeks after return to normoxia. Plasma volume is usually reduced by about 10–15% and is likely related to the increased EPO production and maintenance of plasma pH by the kidneys (30). The reduced plasma volume will limit maximal stroke volume because there is less blood flow returning to the heart that can subsequently be pumped back out (i.e., there is a reduced end diastolic volume). This reduction in maximal stroke volume will limit the increase in maximal oxygen uptake by hindering oxygen transport. The reduced stroke volume at rest is counteracted by an increase in resting heart rate to maintain cardiac output. The increased resting heart rate is brought about by an increase in sympathetic nerve activity that persists for several days after returning to normoxia, but the specific cause of this prolonged elevation in sympathetic activity is unknown. It has been hypothesized that this may be due to changes in neurohormonal levels, altered sensitivity, or resetting of control mechanisms (i.e., baroreceptors and/or chemoreceptors) (15). While the increase in resting heart rate maintains cardiac output at rest, it does not mitigate the reduction in maximal cardiac output during exercise, since maximal heart rate cannot be increased. In addition to cardiovascular adaptations, detrimental effects also appear to occur to the mitochondria, including a decrease in mitochondrial volume and gene expression of peroxisome proliferator activated receptor gamma co-activator 1 alpha (PGC1α), which is considered the master regulator of mitochondrial biogenesis (28). This is thought to occur in an attempt to reduce mitochondrial biogenesis and subsequently lower the oxygen demand to better match the reduced oxygen supply (20). In addition to a decrease in mitochondrial density, there appears to be a reduction in the efficiency of mitochondria, thought to be related to damage to the mitochondrial machinery brought about by reactive oxygen species. A decrease in mitochondrial size and efficiency would reduce one's ability to produce energy via aerobic respiration. While also listed as a potential benefit, the increase in minute ventilation may result in an increased consumption of oxygen by the respiratory musculature that could otherwise be used by the exercising skeletal musculature. Lastly, there appears to be an accumulation of lipofuscin, which is a material that accumulates in lysosomes of cells (23) and is generally used as a marker of reduced overall function typically associated with aging. Put simply, altitude appears to add wear and tear on the body similar to the ageing process.

Unlike the previously discussed positive adaptations that return to baseline levels when acclimating back to normoxia, some of the maladaptations from acclimating to hypoxia remain present (8). For example, long-term exposure to hypoxia results in an increased sympathetic nerve activity to the vasculature, and this maladaptation remains present even after all positive adaptations from hypoxia are washed away. Increased constriction of the pulmonary vasculature can result in pulmonary hypertension for up to 2 years, or in some cases can be a permanent maladaptation to altitude. This indicates that acclimation to hypoxia may not just be negligible in terms of benefitting exercise performance, but it may be detrimental for not only aerobic exercise adaptations but also for general health. These potentially negative physiologic adaptations are present for individuals temporarily residing at altitude, as well as those living at altitude. A summary of the positive and negative adaptations brought about by acclimating to hypoxic conditions independent of exercise are detailed in Figure 17.1.

Aerobic Adaptations to Training under Hypoxia

A number of potential adaptations have been observed when training under hypoxia compared to training in normoxic conditions. Some of these adaptations have been suggested to be related to a greater up-regulation of HIF-1α during training. These adaptations include an increase in mitochondrial density, increased capillarization, and improved oxygen delivery to the musculature via increased myoglobin content (16). Thus, employing the "live low, train high" strategy may augment mitochondrial adaptations to training while eliminating the negative mitochondrial adaptations associated with acclimating to hypoxia. Unlike long-term exposure to hypoxia, which may down-regulate oxidative

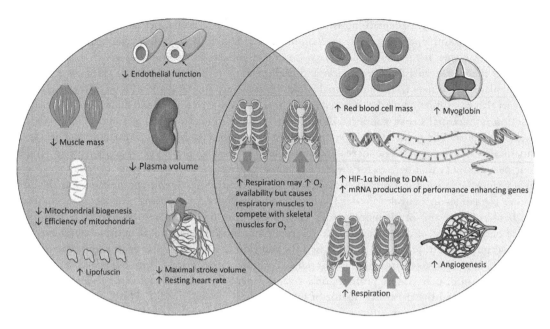

Figure 17.1 Adaptations resulting from acclimation to hypoxia independent of exercise

enzymes, acute exercise under hypoxia may up-regulate oxidative enzymes more so than training under normoxic conditions (24). While some argue that performing aerobic exercise under hypoxia results in a more intensified exercise stress, others argue that it may result in a somewhat lessened exercise stimulus, given the lower intensity of exercise that is able to be performed. This blunted ability for individuals to perform aerobic exercise is a direct result of the reduced oxygen availability. Collectively, it appears that exercising under hypoxic conditions may reduce the workload capable of being performed, but at the same time, it may augment adaptations that benefit aerobic performance when returning to normoxic conditions. For individuals with the sickle cell trait, exercising under hypoxic conditions is not recommended, as this may cause red blood cells to stick to vessel walls and one another, forming blood clots, which could be potentially fatal.

Aerobic Performance Benefits of Hypoxia

The primary goal of hypoxic training is usually to increase performance under normoxic conditions. With respect to the adaptations accompanying acclimation to altitude, it is important to consider whether these adaptations are truly contributing to improved exercise performance. An increase in laboratory measures such as red blood cell mass and even improvements in maximal oxygen uptake (VO_2 max) brought about by acclimating to hypoxia are meaningless for athletes if it does not result in improvements in actual performance measures. It is entirely plausible that an increase in VO_2 max may simply be going to fuel the respiratory muscles to support the increased minute ventilation. After all, there is no athletic event that assesses aerobic performance based on who can consume the most oxygen—these events are based on who can complete the established distance in the shortest time (i.e., a time trial).

There are numerous studies measuring actual performance outcomes to long-term acclimation to hypoxia, and the results are inconclusive (1). Nonetheless, if there is a benefit from acclimating to altitude, it appears to be extremely small in comparison to the benefits that accompany exercise itself. When examining acute exercise performed under hypoxia, the results are again somewhat inconclusive, with some studies showing beneficial effects and others showing no additive effect beyond adaptations that would occur with training under normoxic conditions (21). After considering the costs of living and training under hypoxic conditions, accompanied with the potential negative adaptations particularly to long-term exposure to hypoxia, it seems reasonable to questions its efficacy as a method for improving aerobic exercise performance. The one area that it may benefit is if individuals are planning on competing under hypoxic conditions (i.e., a competition at altitude), in which case it will likely be of benefit to acclimatize and train under hypoxic conditions (1) in adherence with the principle of specificity. With that being said, the goal of using hypoxia is usually to boost performance under normoxic conditions, and the evidence to support its efficacy is underwhelming.

Anaerobic/Resistance Exercise Adaptations

Positive Adaptations to Hypoxia Independent of Exercise

While the primary benefits of exposure to hypoxia are traditionally thought to enhance aerobic exercise adaptations, it is also believed that anaerobic exercise adaptations may be enhanced as well. The same gene transcription factor, HIF-1α, thought to improve aerobic adaptations may also play a role in improving anaerobic adaptations by up-regulating enzymes associated with glycolysis and down-regulating enzymes associated with oxidative metabolism (12). Additionally, the increase in VEGF that is present from long-term exposure to hypoxia is accompanied with an increased capillary to muscle fibre area ratio, which may improve nutrient delivery and the ability to clear metabolic by-products. Another potential adaptation exists in that long-term exposure to hypoxia increases isoforms of carbonic anhydrase, which may improve the buffer capacity of skeletal muscle to remove metabolites and limit the decrease in pH (24). Finally, long-term exposure to hypoxia has been shown to increase satellite cell concentrations (23), which may help with muscle regeneration. Satellite cells can also fuse with and add nuclei to the existing muscle fibres (termed myonuclei). These myonuclei may assist with long-term muscle growth by providing more genetic material to increase gene transcription (i.e., turn DNA to mRNA) and by increasing the number of ribosomes, which would enhance the translational capacity (i.e., turning messenger RNA [mRNA] into proteins). Despite the increase in myonuclei and theoretical benefits that it would have on increasing muscle mass, there appears to be a decrease in muscle mass with long-term exposure to hypoxia.

Negative Adaptations to Hypoxia Independent of Exercise

Similar to that of endurance exercise, some of the adaptations that occur in response to chronic hypoxia exposure may be detrimental for anaerobic and resistance exercise adaptations. The most notable detrimental adaptation appears to be the loss of muscle mass, and this is likely related to both a decrease in protein synthesis and an increase in protein breakdown. The reduction in protein synthesis is likely brought about by a decrease in mechanistic target of rapamycin complex 1 (mTORC1) signalling, which is an important regulator of muscle mass. The increase in protein breakdown is likely related to an increase in the rates of both autophagy and ubiquitination, given the up-regulation of markers that are associated with both degradation pathways (12). Additionally, there is an increase in systemic blood pressure and arterial stiffness, as well as a reduction in vascular conductance, which indicates that hypoxia may reduce endothelial function (5). Given that some evidence indicates that resistance exercise may increase arterial stiffness, this may be exacerbated by acclimating to hypoxia.

Positive Adaptations to Performing Anaerobic/Resistance Exercise under Hypoxia

Training under hypoxia is thought to be potentially beneficial largely due to the ability to enhance phosphocreatine synthesis while also improving the ability to clear metabolites (i.e., inorganic phosphate and hydrogen ions) following rest between sets or sprints. This potential adaptation would likely be related to an enhanced perfusion of muscle blood flow through nitric oxide–induced vasodilation (11). Additionally, the lack of oxygen may result in a greater accumulation of metabolites produced during resistance exercise, and this could potentially augment increases in muscle size. The benefit of metabolic accumulation could serve as a mechanism to fatigue the muscle and thus recruit more muscle fibres to generate enough force to complete the exercise. Thus, metabolites may indirectly increase muscle size by increasing the number of motor units being activated, and subsequently the number of muscle fibres being stimulated. Other mechanisms that have been proposed as to how metabolite production from training under hypoxia may regulate muscle hypertrophy include myokine production, hormone release, and reactive oxygen species production, but there is limited evidence that these mechanisms play a role with increasing muscle size in humans. Thus, it seems more likely that metabolically induced fatigue would be the mechanism responsible for any augmentations in muscle size. As for potential increases in muscle strength and power, it has been suggested that this may be due to enhanced firing rates of motor neurons or increases in spinal excitability (13). Whatever specific mechanisms are responsible for augmenting anaerobic exercise adaptations in hypoxia are unlikely to be limited by a reduced exercise capacity. This is because, unlike aerobic exercise, short bouts of anaerobic activities such as sprinting or performing maximal strength tests do not appear to be negatively affected when performed under hypoxia, since the primary energy system is the phosphocreatine system. Performing multiple sprints, however, may result in a delayed recovery as the aerobic system plays a role with recovery from exercise and restoration of phosphocreatine stores. Exercises involving a multitude of repetitions that target local muscular endurance will likely result in fewer repetitions being completed because of metabolically activated muscle afferents that inhibit voluntary muscle activation.

Anaerobic/Resistance Performance Benefits of Hypoxia

With respect to anaerobic exercise adaptations, the most promising results occur in response to acute exercise under hypoxia. The primary benefit does not appear to be an improvement in sprinting speed, but rather an improved ability to recover between short bursts of high intensity exercises such as repeated sprints (11). This particularly has utility for sports that often require numerous maximal effort sprints within a given event (e.g., American football, rugby, soccer, basketball). As for resistance exercise adaptations, the totality of evidence seems to suggest that there is no added benefit of performing resistance exercise under hypoxic compared to normoxic conditions (29). Provided resistance exercise is performed to task failure, it would be difficult to reconcile mechanistically why and how performing resistance exercise under hypoxic conditions would result in greater adaptations to muscle size and strength compared to the same exercise performed under normoxic conditions.

Future Directions

There are several considerations, with the current literature studying the effects of systemic hypoxia on exercise performance. One of the largest limitations is the sample sizes that are often used, which generally include fewer than 20 individuals per group (3). To appropriately power such studies, the sample size would need to be much larger, particularly given the small magnitude of effect that would be expected and the between-subject nature of the studies being employed. Assuming a small effect size (Cohen's d = 0.2), an alpha level of 0.05, and power of 0.8, a simple sample size estimation would recommend 394 individuals per group, and even a very optimistic moderate intervention effect (Cohen's d = 0.5) would recommend 64 individuals per group, both of which far exceed the sample sizes commonly used. Additionally, numerous studies do not include control groups continuing to exercise without being introduced to normoxia, which makes it difficult to determine if the effect of the intervention was truly due to the hypoxic stimulus or simply continued training. Even studies that do include control groups have the difficulty of trying to blind the participants to which group they are assigned to. While relocating to altitude will likely give away an individual's group assignment, even hypobaric or hypoxic normobaric chambers may create an environment that individuals can easily detect as being different. If individuals are assigned to a control group, they may observe a nocebo effect, whereby they understand that they are in the group not expected to benefit, which may have a negative psychological impact on performance. Finally, studies demonstrating an improvement in performance in response to hypoxia should seek to determine what specific physiologic mechanisms are responsible for these improvements.

Local Blood Flow Restriction

Differentiating Blood Flow Restriction with Systemic Hypoxia

Blood flow restricted exercise differs from traditional hypoxic training in that the stimulus is localized and is not applied chronically, as is the case when acclimating to systemic hypoxia. For this reason, several of the adaptations are likely to differ. For example, EPO production will only be elevated in response to systemic hypoxia, since it is the peritubular capillaries in the kidneys that secrete EPO in response to lower levels of oxygen. With blood flow restricted exercise, blood flow to the limbs may be altered, but arteries supplying blood flow to the kidneys are not directly affected. Therefore, adaptations that will occur in response to blood flow restricted exercise will either be local adaptations to the limb in which blood flow is being restricted or adaptations that result indirectly due to the pooling blood within the limbs.

Application of Blood Flow Restriction

Blood flow restriction involves the use of pneumatic cuffs (similar to that of blood pressure cuffs) placed on the most proximal part of the arms or legs. This can also be done in a more practical way by using elastic wraps or medical tourniquets to restrict blood flow. The goal of applying blood flow restriction is to reduce (not completely cut off) the arterial inflow to the muscle while also occluding venous blood flow out of the muscle. It is generally recommended to first take the individual's systolic blood pressure with the specific device/cuff that will be used during exercise on the specific limb that will be exercised (often termed arterial occlusion pressure). This then enables the pressure to be set relative to that which causes the complete cessation of arterial blood flow. As the goal is not to completely cut off arterial blood flow to the muscle, the pressure may be prescribed as a percentage of the individual's arterial occlusion pressure (40% or 80%, for example). This method helps to ensure that the pressure is not completely occlusive and provides a more homogenous stimulus across individuals. While various devices and cuffs can be used to restrict blood flow, the differences across devices and cuff sizes are likely minimal, provided the pressure is made relative to the individual and the cuff being used. There may not be a 1:1 ratio for the level of restriction being applied and the level of blood flow being reduced, but applying a relative pressure causes a similar reduction in blood flow irrespective of the cuff sizes being used (26). Figure 17.2 illustrates how blood flow restriction applied at rest and during low-intensity aerobic exercise and low-load resistance exercise may be beneficial for muscle mass. This will be discussed in the subsequent sections.

Blood Flow Restriction by Itself

The application of blood flow restriction in the absence of any exercise has been shown to be beneficial for reducing the loss of muscle mass (6) and strength (18) that may accompany periods of immobilization.

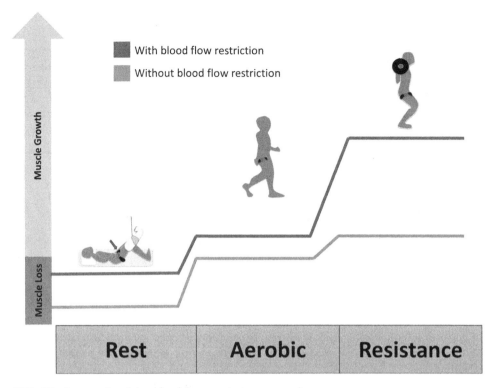

Figure 17.2   The impact of applying blood flow restriction on muscle mass

These protocols often involve repeated 5-minute inflations followed by 3-minute deflations of the pressure cuff. Since there is no muscle activity occurring from simply inflating and deflating the pressure cuff, it is difficult to determine what is causing the reductions in muscle mass and strength loss that occur with immobilization. The most widely accepted mechanism for explaining the maintenance of muscle mass is the increase in muscle swelling that occurs from inflating the pressure cuff may activate the anabolic mTORC1 and mitogen-activated protein kinase (MAPK) pathways. In other words, instead of a mechanical sensor that is sensitive to muscle contraction when exercising, there may be an osmotic sensor that is sensitive to increased fluid pressure when swelling is present, although there is little experimental evidence to directly support this. As no muscle contraction is occurring, the maintenance of muscle mass is unlikely to be explained by the accumulation of metabolites, which is often used to explain some of the adaptations that occur during exercise. It is important to mention that the application of blood flow restriction in the absence of exercise is unlikely to increase muscle size or strength above an individual's baseline levels—it simply attenuates the loss of muscle size and strength. Therefore, applying the cuff, independent of muscle contraction, is only likely to benefit individuals who must be immobilized.

One other utility of blood flow restriction in the absence of exercise involves its use to enhance acute exercise performance in what is known as ischemic pre-conditioning. This differs from traditional blood flow restriction applied at rest or during exercise, in that the pressure applied is intended to completely cut off arterial blood flow to the muscle. Ischemic pre-conditioning consists of occluding blood flow for 5-minute periods interspersed by 3-minute unoccluded or unrestricted blood flow. The repeated cessation and subsequent reperfusion of blood flow is done prior to exercise and is thought to enhance performance, but the mechanisms by which it does so are unknown. The most commonly speculated mechanism is through an increase in nitric oxide–induced vasodilation allowing for greater blood flow. This could improve performance by enabling a greater delivery of oxygen and a greater clearance of metabolic by-products, under the assumption that this magnitude of vaso-dilation would exceed that which would occur via exercise itself. Another hypothesized mechanism is via a greater activation of ATP-sensitive potassium channels, reducing energy depletion. Despite some studies showing beneficial effects of ischemic pre-conditioning, the results are far from conclusive, with numerous studies showing no additional benefit over exercise performed without ischemic preconditioning (17).

Blood Flow Restriction with Aerobic Exercise

Several studies have examined the effectiveness of different low-intensity aerobic exercise interventions with and without blood flow restriction. It appears that both cycling and walking exercises performed with blood flow restriction may be more beneficial at increasing various functional tests and VO_2 max, although the findings are not conclusive (2). Although not typically associated with aerobic exercise, increases in muscle size have been observed when aerobic exercise is performed in conjunction with blood flow restriction. This is likely due to the increased local stress being placed on the exercised musculature that more so resembles that of resistance exercise when in comparison to unrestricted aerobic exercise. The increased demand on the muscle will likely increase motor unit activation by reducing oxygen delivery to the muscle and causing an accumulation of metabolites. The accumulation of metabolites will inhibit cross-bridge cycling within activated muscle fibres and subsequently cause more muscle fibres to be recruited to maintain exercise at the same intensity relative to what would be required if blood flow were not being restricted. Since muscle fibres must be activated to grow, it is likely that a greater proportion of the muscle is being activated with blood flow restriction, and therefore, more muscle fibres are stimulated to grow. However, the increases in muscle size that accompany blood flow restricted aerobic exercise are smaller than those which are observed following resistance exercise. This may again be related to the idea that while muscle activation is increased by restricting blood flow during low-intensity aerobic exercise, it does not reach the level of activation present when performing resistance exercise. Therefore, individuals already performing resistance exercise should not expect even greater increases in muscle mass if they also perform blood flow restricted aerobic exercise. Nonetheless, this may serve as a time-efficient method to increase both muscle mass and cardiorespiratory endurance, particularly among individuals who get limited physical activity.

An important consideration is that most of these studies are examining adaptations to low-intensity aerobic exercise. The results appear to demonstrate that at any given absolute exercise intensity, the application of blood flow restriction is likely to promote greater exercise adaptations. At the same time, applying blood flow restriction is also likely to cause the individuals to perceive the exercise to be more difficult and more discomforting. The increased level of discomfort associated with restricting blood flow is thought to be related to metabolically activated afferents, which signal to the brain to increase the perception of discomfort. As such, the absolute exercise intensity that someone can achieve is likely to be reduced with blood flow restriction, and this is probably the combined result of increased discomfort, increased localized fatigue within the muscles being restricted, and decreased stroke volume and cardiac output resulting from a lower overall blood volume returning to the heart (since it is trapped within the limbs being restricted). Therefore, if the goal of exercise is to improve VO_2 max, it is probably best to perform higher intensities of exercise in the absence of blood flow restriction. However, if individuals do not enjoy performing high-intensity exercise or desire to obtain adaptations common to both aerobic and resistance exercise, blood flow restriction appears to be an alternative to traditional aerobic exercise. This mode of exercise is particularly beneficial for individuals looking to reduce the stress placed on their bones and joints or for individuals who are unable or unwilling to perform aerobic exercise at higher intensities.

Blood Flow Restriction with Anaerobic Exercise

Several studies have examined the effectiveness of applying blood flow restriction in combination with high-intensity interval training. The results of these studies suggest that there may be improvements in VO_2 max despite no difference in capillarity or mitochondrial protein content (25). This would indicate that the improved VO_2 max may be the result of increased cardiac output as opposed to local mechanisms. This may be attributed to improvements in stroke volume that are associated with the increased cardiovascular stress brought about by an augmented exercise pressor reflex occurring with blood flow restricted exercise. In other words, the increase in metabolites will increase the firing rate of metabolically activated afferent fibres, and this will signal to the brainstem to increase blood pressure in part by increasing cardiac output. Over time, this increased stress placed on the heart may augment maximal cardiac output. Another study demonstrated similar changes in various genes when sprint interval training was performed with or without blood flow restriction; however, greater improvements in VO_2 max were observed with the application of blood flow restriction (32). It seems very possible that the greater improvements in VO_2 max may be specific to performing a VO_2 max test on a cycle as opposed to a treadmill. A maximal cycling test is likely to put a greater stress on local muscle endurance when compared to that of a maximal running test, so the addition of blood flow restriction may be more beneficial for cyclists as compared to runners. It is also possible that sprinting with blood flow restriction may negatively alter running mechanics, as the range of motion is not fixed. For cycling exercise, this is unlikely to be problematic because the pedals always travel through the same set path and there is no freedom to alter it. Overall, it seems as though applying blood flow restriction may provide a slightly greater improvement in VO_2 max, but this adaptation does not seem to be corroborated by an improvement in exercise performance (i.e., a timed trial) (32).

Blood Flow Restriction with Low-Load Resistance Exercise

The most widely used application of blood flow restriction is done in conjunction with low-load resistance exercise (typically 20–30% of one-repetition maximum). While both low-load and high-load resistance training produce similar increases in muscle size if performed until volitional failure, combining blood flow restriction with low-load exercise reduces the number of repetitions required to reach task failure (10). Therefore, a repetition-matched protocol performed with blood flow restriction will produce greater muscle growth than the same protocol performed in the absence of blood flow restriction, and this is related to the level of fatigue and subsequent muscle activation achieved. If low-load exercise is performed until task failure, the increases in muscle size will be similar regardless of whether blood flow restriction is applied, but fewer repetitions will be required to reach task failure if blood flow is restricted. As it relates to the level of restriction pressure applied, it seems to be of minimal importance as it relates to changes in muscle size and strength (7), but higher pressures may provide greater adaptations to the vascular system in the form of increased capillarization (27). Higher restriction pressures will reduce the number of repetitions required to reach volitional failure but will also increase how difficult and discomforting the exercise is, so the chosen pressure should be selected accordingly.

The increases in muscle size that accompany low-load blood flow restricted exercise have been postulated to be due to numerous mechanisms, most of which are centred on the accumulation of metabolites caused by the restriction of venous outflow. The idea that blood flow restricted exercise reduces the magnitude of tension placed on the muscle (because the load is lower) has led some to hypothesize that adaptations to blood flow restricted exercise may work through an alternative mechanism. Despite this hypothesis, both low-load blood flow restricted exercise and traditional high-load exercise have been shown to result in similar changes in a wide range of gene expressions thought to regulate increases in muscle size (9). Therefore, the most likely explanation seems to be that the accumulation of metabolites results in an increase in muscle activation by inducing fatigue (31). The onset of fatigue causes more muscle fibres to be activated to make up for the loss of force production, and this results in the hypertrophic stimulus being received by a larger proportion of total muscle fibres. The actual molecular events that occur within each muscle fibre are likely the same regardless of what mode of exercise is performed—these modes of exercise just provide an alternative means to activate muscle fibres and the same mTORC1 cascade (14) that is an important regulator of muscle mass. The difference between these methods may be the way in which muscle fibres are activated (i.e., via heavy loads or via fatigue), but ultimately both activate a large proportion of muscle fibres and induce similar levels of muscle growth. In addition to metabolically induced fatigue, the reduction in oxygenated blood flow to the muscles up-regulates the gene transcription factor HIF-1α, which increases the expression of the signalling protein VEGF. The localized up-regulation of VEGF increases the formation of blood vessels, which may help to enhance nutrient (i.e., amino acid) delivery to the muscles and increase mTROC1 activation. Additionally, VEGF increases the expression of nitric oxide synthase, which is an enzyme responsible for converting L-arginine to nitric oxide. The increase in nitric oxide can stimulate the release of hepatocyte growth factor, which activates satellite cells (22). The activated satellite cells can then help with muscle regeneration, as well as increasing the number of nuclei within muscle fibres. The added myonuclei may assist with long-term muscle growth by providing more genetic material to increase gene transcription (i.e., turn DNA to mRNA) and by increasing the number of ribosomes, which would enhance the translational capacity (i.e., turning mRNA into proteins).

As it relates to strength adaptations, blood flow restricted exercise has been shown to increase strength above that of a load-matched protocol performed in the absence of blood flow restriction. This increase in strength, however, is less than that which is observed following higher-load exercise in the absence of blood flow restriction. For this reason, individuals who are looking to get stronger should lift with heavier weights if they are capable of doing so. This should not be surprising, given the principle of specificity, in that individuals who are lifting closer to their maximum strength will increase their maximum strength more so than those lifting further from their maximum strength. The mechanism as to how blood flow restriction training increases strength more so than performing the same protocol in the absence of blood flow restriction is unknown but may be related to an increased corticomotor excitability (4). In other words, the accumulation of metabolites may signal group three and four afferents to alter the motor unit recruitment pattern such that the same level of electrical activity to the primary motor cortex can generate more force. Another possibility is that changes within the muscle fibres themselves may be altered, possibly through changes in calcium kinetics. Therefore, the greater number of activated muscle fibres will cause a greater proportion of muscle fibres to undergo this adaptation.

Blood Flow Restriction with High-Load Resistance Exercise

Few studies have examined whether adding blood flow restriction to high-load exercise will produce even greater increases in muscle size and strength as compared to unrestricted high-load exercise. The results of these studies do not support a benefit of adding blood flow restriction to high-load exercise (19). As it will not require as many repetitions to reach volitional failure when performing high-load exercise, the utility of blood flow restriction with this mode of exercise is not supported. There will already be a high degree of muscle activation at the onset of exercise, and the fatiguing effects of blood flow restriction will not have a large impact on reducing the required exercise volume to achieve a high degree of muscle activation. Adding blood flow restriction will likely provide no added benefit while also increasing participant discomfort during the exercise.

Future Directions

There are several considerations to be made when examining studies pertaining to blood flow restricted exercise. First, a wide variety of arbitrary pressures are used, meaning everyone participating in a study will have the same pressure applied (i.e., 160 mmHg). This is potentially problematic, as it will likely result in a different stimulus across individuals and is also hard to replicate across studies in which laboratories use different equipment. Additionally, less is known about the best way to standardize the level of restriction being applied when using elastic wraps, since the pressure is not easily quantifiable compared to inflatable cuffs. Some suggestions have been to use a subjective feeling scale or to tighten the cuffs relative to limb circumference, but more studies are necessary to determine the best method for standardization. Furthermore, while there is some indication that the restriction pressure matters little for chronic muscle adaptations, preliminary evidence suggests that higher pressures may be necessary for producing vascular adaptations when lower loads are used. Future studies may wish to examine the importance of the applied pressure with respect to vascular adaptation. Finally, the molecular mechanisms responsible for the adaptations that occur in response to blood flow restriction are not well understood and require future research.

Take-Home Points

- Acclimating to hypoxia may result in many physiologic adaptations that are beneficial; however, there are numerous adaptations that are also detrimental for exercise performance and general health.
- There is little support for a benefit of acclimation to hypoxia for improving aerobic, anaerobic, or resistance exercise performance.
- The strongest support for a benefit of hypoxia on exercise performance appears to be an improvement in recovery during repeated sprinting, but more research is necessary to make a definitive conclusion.
- Blood flow restriction applied independent of exercise may be beneficial for slowing degeneration of muscle size and strength during periods of immobilization.
- Blood flow restriction applied during aerobic exercise appears to result in increases in muscle mass otherwise not observed when performed without blood flow restriction.
- Blood flow restriction appears to reduce the number of repetitions required to induce muscle adaptations during low-load exercise, but it is unlikely to have an additive effect when combined with high-load exercise.
- The mechanisms by which blood flow restriction increases muscle mass appear to be similar to high-load exercise, which is dependent upon achieving a high level of muscle activation and subsequently activating the mTORC1 cascade in a large proportion of muscle fibres.

References

1. Bailey DM, Davies B. Physiological implications of altitude training for endurance performance at sea level: A review. *Br J Sports Med* 31: 183–190, 1997.
2. Bennett H, Slattery F. Effects of blood flow restriction training on aerobic capacity and performance: A systematic review. *J Strength Cond Res* 33: 572–583, 2019.
3. Bonetti DL, Hopkins WG. Sea-level exercise performance following adaptation to hypoxia. *Sports Med* 39: 107–127, 2009.
4. Brandner CR, Warmington SA, Kidgell DJ. Corticomotor excitability is increased following an acute bout of blood flow restriction resistance exercise. *Front Hum Neurosci* 9: 652, 2015.
5. Calbet JA, Boushel R, Robach P, Hellsten Y, Saltin B, Lundby C. Chronic hypoxia increases arterial blood pressure and reduces adenosine and ATP induced vasodilatation in skeletal muscle in healthy humans. *Acta Physiol* 211: 574–584, 2014.
6. Clark BC, Fernhall B, Ploutz-Snyder LL. Adaptations in human neuromuscular function following prolonged unweighting: I. Skeletal muscle contractile properties and applied ischemia efficacy. *J Appl Physiol* 101: 256–263, 2006.
7. Counts BR, Dankel SJ, Barnett BE, Kim D, Mouser JG, Allen KM, et al. Influence of relative blood flow restriction pressure on muscle activation and muscle adaptation. *Muscle Nerve* 53: 438–445, 2016.
8. Dempsey JA, Morgan BJ. Humans in hypoxia: A conspiracy of maladaptation?! *Physiology (Bethesda)* 30: 304–316, 2015.

9. Ellefsen S, Hammarström D, Strand TA, Zacharoff E, Whist JE, Rauk I, et al. Blood flow-restricted strength training displays high functional and biological efficacy in women: A within-subject comparison with high-load strength training. *Am J Physiol* 309: R767–R779, 2015.

10. Fahs CA, Loenneke JP, Thiebaud RS, Rossow LM, Kim D, Abe T, et al. Muscular adaptations to fatiguing exercise with and without blood flow restriction. *Clin Physiol Funct Imaging* 35: 167–176, 2015.

11. Faiss R, Girard O, Millet GP. Advancing hypoxic training in team sports: From intermittent hypoxic training to repeated sprint training in hypoxia. *Br J Sports Med* 47: i45–i50, 2013.

12. Favier FB, Britto FA, Freyssenet DG, Bigard XA, Benoit H. HIF-1-driven skeletal muscle adaptations to chronic hypoxia: Molecular insights into muscle physiology. *Cell Mol Life Sci* 72: 4681–4696, 2015.

13. Feriche B, García-Ramos A, Morales-Artacho AJ, Padial P. Resistance training using different hypoxic training strategies: A basis for hypertrophy and muscle power development. *Sports Med Open* 3: 12, 2017.

14. Fry CS, Glynn EL, Drummond MJ, Timmerman KL, Fujita S, Abe T, et al. Blood flow restriction exercise stimulates mTORC1 signaling and muscle protein synthesis in older men. *J Appl Physiol* 108: 1199–1209, 2010.

15. Hansen J, Sander M. Sympathetic neural overactivity in healthy humans after prolonged exposure to hypobaric hypoxia. *J Physiol* 546: 921–929, 2003.

16. Hoppeler H, Vogt M, Weibel ER, Flück M. Response of skeletal muscle mitochondria to hypoxia. *Exp Physiol* 88: 109–119, 2003.

17. Horiuchi M. Ischemic preconditioning: Potential impact on exercise performance and underlying mechanisms. *J Phys Fit Sports Med* 6: 15–23, 2017.

18. Kubota A, Sakuraba K, Sawaki K, Sumide T, Tamura Y. Prevention of disuse muscular weakness by restriction of blood flow. *Med Sci Sports Exerc* 40: 529–534, 2008.

19. Laurentino G, Ugrinowitsch C, Aihara AY, Fernandes AR, Parcell AC, Ricard M, et al. Effects of strength training and vascular occlusion. *Int J Sports Med* 29: 664–667, 2008.

20. Levett DZ, Radford EJ, Menassa DA, Graber EF, Morash AJ, Hoppeler H, et al. Acclimatization of skeletal muscle mitochondria to high-altitude hypoxia during an ascent of Everest. *FASEB J* 26: 1431–1441, 2011.

21. Levine BD. Intermittent hypoxic training: Fact and fancy. *High Alt Med Biol* 3: 177–193, 2002.

22. Loenneke JP, Wilson GJ, Wilson JM. A mechanistic approach to blood flow occlusion. *Int J Sports Med* 31: 1–4, 2010.

23. Martinelli M, Winterhalder R, Cerretelli P, Howald H, Hoppeler H. Muscle lipofuscin content and satellite cell volume is increased after high altitude exposure in humans. *Experientia* 46: 672–676, 1990.

24. Millet GP, Roels B, Schmitt L, Woorons X, Richalet JP. Combining hypoxic methods for peak performance. *Sports Med* 40: 1–25, 2010.

25. Mitchell EA, Martin NRW, Turner MC, Taylor CW, Ferguson RA. The combined effect of sprint interval training and postexercise blood flow restriction on critical power, capillary growth, and mitochondrial proteins in trained cyclists. *J Appl Physiol* 126: 51–59, 2019.

26. Mouser JG, Dankel SJ, Jessee MB, Mattocks KT, Buckner SL, Counts BR, et al. A tale of three cuffs: The hemodynamics of blood flow restriction. *Eur J Appl Physiol* 117: 1493–1499, 2017.

27. Mouser JG, Mattocks KT, Buckner SL, Dankel SJ, Jessee MB, Bell ZW, et al. High-pressure blood flow restriction with very low load resistance training results in peripheral vascular adaptations similar to heavy resistance training. *Physiol Meas* 40: 35003, 2019.

28. Murray AJ. Energy metabolism and the high-altitude environment. *Exp Physiol* 101: 23–27, 2016.

29. Ramos-Campo DJ, Scott BR, Alcaraz PE, Rubio-Arias JA. The efficacy of resistance training in hypoxia to enhance strength and muscle growth: A systematic review and meta-analysis. *Eur J Sport Sci* 18: 92–103, 2018.

30. Sinex JA, Chapman RF. Hypoxic training methods for improving endurance exercise performance. *J Sport Health Sci* 4: 325–332, 2015.

31. Suga T, Okita K, Takada S, Omokawa M, Kadoguchi T, Yokota T, et al. Effect of multiple set on intramuscular metabolic stress during low-intensity resistance exercise with blood flow restriction. *Eur J Appl Physiol* 112: 3915–3920, 2012.

32. Taylor CW, Ingham SA, Ferguson RA. Acute and chronic effect of sprint interval training combined with postexercise blood-flow restriction in trained individuals. *Exp Physiol* 101: 143–154, 2016.

33. West JB. High-altitude medicine. *Am J Respir Crit Care Med* 186: 1229–1237, 2012.

SECTION III

Exercise Biochemistry/Nutrition Nexus in Physical Activity and Sport Performance

Andrea R. Josse

Nutrition can have a profound impact on physical activity, exercise, and sport performance. It provides the energy needed to perform everyday active tasks and the necessary fuel to complete a marathon, recover from a sprint, and build and maintain our musculoskeletal system. It can also offer a slight competitive edge, beyond optimal training, that may separate those on the competitive podium.

Recent research in the areas of exercise and sport nutrition has dramatically increased our understanding of how foods, nutrients, and dietary supplements are metabolized and utilized to enhance exercise performance, training, and recovery. These chapters, written by leaders in the field, focus on the importance of nutrition for physical activity, exercise, and sport and explore how nutrition, in various forms, can augment the effects of exercise and training to improve health and optimize athletic performance. This section also highlights exercise- and sport-specific nutritional strategies to improve exercise adaptations and sport performance in certain contexts and includes discussions of the biochemical underpinnings and regulatory mechanisms responsible for their effects. Concepts such as timing, dose and duration of food, nutrient and dietary supplement consumption to optimize exercise and performance outcomes are also discussed.

Specifically, this section includes important, exciting, and cutting-edge information about nutritional strategies that regulate energy balance and weight control, optimize endurance training adaptations, promote muscle protein synthesis and hypertrophy, and regulate intracellular and extracellular acid–base balance mitigating muscular fatigue. As well, new and essential information on the use of common ergogenic aids, including whey protein and leucine, caffeine, creatine, select micronutrients (zinc, iron, magnesium, and vitamin D), beetroot/dietary nitrate, beta-alanine, sodium bicarbonate, sodium citrate, and sodium and calcium lactate to facilitate improvements in physical activity, exercise, and sport performance is discussed. The final chapter in this section highlights the emerging area of sport nutrigenomics. While nutritional programmes should be tailored towards the specific needs and goals of the individual to maximize exercise adaptation, sport performance, and overall health, this newer area of research explores how one's own genetic variability may further influence this paradigm.

The fields of exercise and sport nutrition are constantly evolving, and in all these exciting areas, many unanswered questions remain and more research is needed. Thus, each chapter also highlights suggestions for future research, leaving the reader with an idea of the important issues and next steps in each respective area.

18

EXERCISE AND DIETARY INFLUENCES ON THE REGULATION OF ENERGY BALANCE AND IMPLICATIONS FOR BODY WEIGHT CONTROL

Andrea M. Brennan and Robert Ross

Introduction

It is without question that the prevalence of overweight and obesity has seen unprecedented increases over the last several decades. Typically defined by body mass index (BMI; weight [kg] over height [m^2]), the most recent Canadian data from 2014 indicate that the overall age-adjusted prevalence of obesity was 37.7% (100). These rates represent a staggering economic burden. In 2004, the direct and indirect cost associated with obesity in Canada was $4.3 billion (43) and this figure rose to $6 billion in 2006 (1). The obesity epidemic is not exclusive to North America. The World Health Organization has pointed out similar trends in rates of obesity in both developed and developing nations (70).

The adverse consequences of obesity are well-documented and ubiquitous across virtually all body systems. These include but are not limited to increases in insulin resistance, hypertension, dyslipidaemia, endothelial dysfunction, systemic inflammation, heart failure, coronary heart disease, atrial fibrillation, obstructive sleep apnoea, osteoarthritis, and certain cancers (6, 51, 72), all of which increase the risk for morbidity and mortality (28, 72). The available evidence of the wide-reaching impact of obesity and its related comorbidities is indisputable and prompts interdisciplinary efforts to mitigate its consequences.

It is largely agreed upon that one of the largest contributors to body weight change is an imbalance in the energy consumed and energy expended, wherein weight gain results from a positive energy balance and weight loss is induced by a negative energy balance. Energy here is described as kilocalories (kcal). Energy balance relies on the first law of thermodynamics in which energy cannot be created or destroyed; rather, it is transformed from one form to another (111). Thus, the storage of energy in the form of adipose and lean tissue depends on the amount of energy consumed and the amount of energy expended by the body to maintain metabolic homeostasis, sustain vital organ functions, and perform physical work as needed (92, 111). The energy balance equation provides a viable framework for studying the influence of exercise and dietary intervention on the regulation of body weight.

Energy intake refers to the energy consumed through food and fluids. It includes chemical energy derived from the digestion and absorption of carbohydrates, protein, fat, and alcohol minus faecal losses (111). Substrates derived from macronutrients can be oxidized to produce energy in the form of adenosine triphosphate (ATP) to drive biological processes or be stored as adipose tissue, glycogen, and skeletal muscle for later use.

Energy expenditure includes the energy consumed in metabolic reactions to maintain physiological homeostasis at rest and during exercise (36). Total energy expenditure is the sum of the following components:

1. *Thermic effect of food (TEF)*: The energy required to ingest, digest, absorb, and store nutrients from food and fluids we consume is the smallest component of daily energy expenditure in humans (~10%) (98). The digestion of protein requires the greatest amount of energy, followed by carbohydrates and fat (38).
2. *Resting energy expenditure (REE)*: The energy required to sustain vital homeostatic functions of our cells and organs, including body maintenance and growth, when not performing physical work. REE is reliant on many factors, including body composition (fat-free mass vs. fat mass), age, biological sex, health status, pregnancy/lactation, environment, etc. (36).
3. *Physical activity energy expenditure (PAEE)*: The energy required to perform volitional and purposeful exercise. PAEE is determined by the type, duration, and intensity of exercise and varies according to overall body weight (36, 38, 103). For example, an individual weighing 120 kg will require more energy to perform the same duration and intensity of exercise as an individual who weighs 80 kg.
4. *Non-exercise activity thermogenesis (NEAT)*: The energy required to perform activities of daily living, including household chores, gardening, sitting and standing, etc. (55).

Energy that is not used by the body for the preceding uses is stored in the forms of glycogen, lipids, and protein (98). Glycogen stores in the liver and skeletal muscle consisting of glucose molecules are relatively small and characterized by rapid turnover; thus, it is primarily used as a short-term energy resource. Conversely, lipids in the form of fatty acids can be stored in large quantities for extended periods of time and represent the largest fuel reserve to support long-term low-intensity activity and REE. In the form of triglycerides, lipids can be stored in adipose tissue depots throughout the body. Protein can either be stored in the body's muscle or broken down to amino acids and transformed to glucose for energy production (31).

Energy storage is determined by the difference between energy intake and energy expenditure. Any imbalance in the consumption and use of protein, fat, and carbohydrates can lead to changes in body composition and body weight.

This chapter will highlight the regulation of energy intake and energy expenditure and discuss the influence of lifestyle-based interventions on the energy balance equation and body weight. In particular, biochemical and physiological compensatory responses to exercise or diet-induced weight loss will be reviewed in addition to their implications for weight maintenance and weight regain. Finally, suggestions for future research aims in this area will be proposed to better delineate the genetic, metabolic, and physiological mechanistic underpinnings of behavioural factors that influence energy balance.

Regulation of Energy Balance

Metabolic Adaptation

Traditional representations of energy balance assume static models wherein energy intake minus energy expenditure equals energy storage and thus body weight. In fact, the origin of the "3500 kcal per pound" rule wherein a 3500-kilocalorie deficit by diet or exercise is required for 1 pound of weight loss is derived from this static model and is often inappropriately used to predict weight loss over time (38). Contrary to this model, energy balance is hugely dynamic and far more complex. More recently, mathematical models to predict weight change have been proposed to reflect the dynamic nature of energy balance (36).

Metabolic adaptation, or adaptive thermogenesis, is a term used to describe our body's adaptation to reductions in energy intake or a negative energy balance (38). Evolutionarily, metabolic adaptation was an important response to the body's perceived state of starvation wherein a negative energy balance was matched with a reduced energy expenditure to maintain body functions and conserve energy stores. In our current obesogenic environment that characterizes North America, this reduced energy expenditure in response to an energy deficit has contributed to weight loss that is less than predicted by a given intervention (97). Reduction in whole-body energy expenditure following reduced energy intake is partly explained by the reduction in lean and fat mass that make up a large component of REE, reductions in energy expenditure following physical activity due to a reduced cost of activity, and a decrease in TEF due to reduced energy intake (75, 78).

While the underlying mechanisms that explain metabolic adaptation are unclear, researchers have suggested reduced sympathetic nervous system activity (36, 79) and decreased leptin as potential contributors (7, 52). Compensatory responses to diet and exercise-induced changes in energy balance will be discussed in greater detail in the ensuing sections.

Regulation of Energy Intake

Energy intake is regulated in part by both homeostatic and hedonic pathways. Homeostatic regulation of eating depends on an integrated network of peripheral signals that converge on the brainstem and the hypothalamus to either stimulate or inhibit feeding (12). These actions function to maintain energy balance in an organism, which is reflected by both acute nutritional state and adiposity (67). Hedonic regulation of eating, rather, depends on the pleasure or reward-related activation of the brain's neural circuitries that respond to food cues and can ultimately promote eating in the absence of negative energy balance signals (12, 101). In this chapter, we will focus on homeostatic mechanisms of energy intake regulation in response to changes in energy balance.

Homeostatic Signals

Homeostatic regulation of ingestive behaviour involves the activity of a variety of neuropeptides that reflect both chronic energy stores and prandial state. Two types of signals from the periphery provide information to the brain related to hunger and satiety. Gut hormones, including cholecystokinin (CCK), peptide YY (PYY), glucagon-like peptide-1 (GLP-1), oxyntomodulin, and ghrelin, reflect the acute nutritional (prandial) state and either stimulate or inhibit food intake. Adiposity signals, including leptin and insulin, reflect the body's longer-term energy stores and affect energy balance. The combined influence of these hormones functions to maintain energy homeostasis (8). Table 18.1 describes these signals in greater detail.

The aforementioned episodic (CCK, GLP-1, ghrelin, PYY, oxyntomodulin) and tonic (leptin, insulin) signalling peptides are integrated in the hypothalamus to regulate energy intake. This integration and resulting downstream effects represent the brain's awareness of chronic energy stores (adiposity) and acute changes in nutrient flux (8). Receptors for these hormones are located within hypothalamic neurons, specifically in the arcuate nucleus (ARC). Leptin, PYY, and GLP-1 inhibit food intake by inhibiting neuropeptide Y (NPY)/agouti-related neuropeptide (AgRP) neurons and stimulating pro-opiomelanocortin (POMC)/cocaine- and amphetamine-regulated transcript (CART) neurons (88). Conversely, ghrelin stimulates food intake by stimulating NPY/AgRP neurons and inhibiting POMC/CART neurons (88). These neurons do not exert their effects in isolation from one another, but rather, via a coordinated response that promotes an inhibitory effect between NPY/AgRP and POMC/CART neurons (101). The hypothalamic paraventricular nucleus (PVN) is postulated to be a target for the ARC neurons, wherein PVN activation signals to higher brain centres and the sympathetic nervous system to alter energy intake (67).

In addition to the hypothalamus, the brainstem is an important regulatory region for food intake and coordinates its effects with the hypothalamus via extensive connections between the two regions. Gut hormones that are initiated in response to mechanical or chemical stimulation of the gastrointestinal tract

Table 18.1 Signals regulating energy intake

Signal	Tissue release	Features and function	Energy intake
Episodic/Short–Term Signals			
Cholecystokinin (CCK)	Small intestine	• Released 15 minutes after meal initiation in response to the presence of lipids and proteins (57) • Initiates meal termination via effects on gastric emptying (66) • Reduces meal size and duration (88)	⇓
Peptide YY (PYY)	Distal ileum and colon	• Released in response to a meal (101) • Postprandial changes in PYY are positively associated with postprandial changes in ratings of satiety (65) • Prompts meal termination (65)	⇓
Glucagon-like peptide (GLP-1)	Intestine	• Released post-prandially in response to carbohydrate, fat, and protein ingestion (65) • Inhibits gastric emptying and appetite (88, 101)	⇓
Ghrelin	Stomach	• Binds to growth hormone secretogue receptors and stimulates growth hormone and food intake (101) • Levels in the pre-prandial period are elevated and correlate with hunger scores (65) • Stimulates gastric emptying (2)	⇑
Tonic/Long-Term Signals			
Leptin	Adipose tissue	• Binds to leptin receptors in the hypothalamus and inhibits appetitive neurons while stimulating inhibitory neurons (62, 85, 87) • Serum and plasma levels reflect energy stores (adiposity) (87) • Leptin signalling becomes maladaptive under obese conditions (65)	⇓
Insulin	Pancreas	• Released in response to elevated blood glucose (65) • Enters brain and binds to receptors that inhibit appetitive neurons and stimulate inhibitory neurons (88) • Circulating insulin levels in the blood are proportional to adiposity (4)	⇓

during food ingestion can signal to the brainstem via the afferent fibres of the vagus nerve to mediate its regulatory effects (66). Second, while mesolimbic dopamine pathways (49) appear to contribute to the rewarding aspects of consuming palatable foods (73), dopamine signalling in the hypothalamus has been suggested to inhibit food intake. Finally, serotonin receptor signalling is often increased via anti-obesity drugs to suppress food intake and leptin increases serotonin turnover (13), suggesting an additional role for serotonin in the modulation of energy homeostasis.

Resting Energy Expenditure

More recently, it has been suggested that changes in REE resulting from increases or decreases in fat-free mass also play a role in regulating energy intake (9, 42). This hypothesis is supported by evidence that REE significantly determined the size of a meal, the intensity of hunger, and objectively measured total daily energy intake in both obese and lean individuals (9). This evidence suggests that energy intake related to appetite control may be regulated by fat-free mass and REE to support the physiological demand for energy.

Regulation of Energy Expenditure

Resting Energy Expenditure

Body composition explains the majority (~60–80%) of the variability in REE and is demonstrated by a linear relationship between body weight and energy expenditure at rest (36). Fat-free mass, in particular, comprises the most metabolically active tissues of the body, including skeletal muscle, liver, heart, and brain. These tissues require a higher energy cost to maintain their vital functions than tissues characterized by high fat mass (19, 76, 106). However, during weight loss interventions, the decrease in REE is greater than expected based on body weight reduction and body composition changes (9).

The remaining variability (~30%) not explained by changes in body weight or body composition may be explained by the change in activity of several anabolic pathways. Gluconeogenesis, de novo lipogenesis, and protein turnover all require varying amounts of energy, and so changes in energy intake and/ or diet composition may result in up- or down-regulation of the preceding pathways (35). Furthermore, with respect to exercise-induced weight loss interventions, improvements in energy efficiency resulting in a lesser energy cost to maintain vital functions at rest may also contribute to the decrease in REE with weight loss.

Thermic Effect of Feeding

Just as the energy cost of storing carbohydrates, lipids, and protein vary, so, too, does the cost of ingesting, digesting, and absorbing these nutrients from the diet (102). Protein requires more energy than carbohydrate, which requires more energy than fat. These discrepancies may alter energy expenditure due to the thermic effect of feeding, although precise mechanisms are not clear (36).

Non-Exercise Activity Thermogenesis

Only 15% of North Americans report meeting the national recommendations for structured exercise (150 minutes of moderate-to-vigorous intensity physical activity per week) (16). Therefore, activity performed outside of structured exercise is an important and often understated component of activity-associated energy expenditure. While it is well understood that environmental and socioeconomic access and constraints can affect NEAT (e.g., proximity to parks, occupation type, affordability, etc.), there is also evidence that biological regulation of NEAT exists to some extent (55). Kotz et al. (2002) demonstrated that the protein orexin acts on energy regulatory centres in the brain to up-regulate NEAT in mice (50). In addition, though not well defined in humans, evidence suggests that increases in thyroid hormone and leptin in animals increases NEAT (56, 71). Finally, the common sentiment that increases in exercise training results in decreases in NEAT have not been supported by the majority of existing evidence. Clearly, potential biological and metabolic regulators of NEAT require further exploration in humans and offer potentially important insights to one of the major components of total energy expenditure.

Exercise Energy Expenditure

Energy expended via structured exercise is primarily determined by changes in body weight and body composition. It is well understood that for a given duration and intensity of exercise, obese individuals will expend a greater amount of energy than those who are lean, which can be explained by differences in body mass (104). Furthermore, increased efficiency associated with exercise training also reduces the cost of performing physical work over the course of several months of intervention (103).

Regulation of Energy Storage

The widely held belief that body weight and composition simply result from kilocalories being consumed and those being expended has evolved to our current understanding of the dynamic model of energy balance regulation, wherein intake and expenditure are directly related and central/peripheral feedback signals are important contributors (36). Acknowledgement of various determinants of body weight and fat mass beyond this static model will help practitioners and researchers predict an individual's response to a weight loss intervention and setting realistic expectations.

The following factors influence energy storage and body weight:

Genetics: There is a strong consensus that genetic influences play a large role in body weight and body composition in addition to responses to intervention. Potential gene targets are beyond the scope of this chapter, but the reader is encouraged to review several comprehensive examinations on the topic (10, 60, 74). Instead, this section will focus on biological and metabolic determinants of body weight and fat distribution.

Low metabolic rate: While there is a clear and consistent relationship between metabolic rate and body size, substantial interindividual variability exists, suggesting that individuals who vary in size may also vary in metabolic rate. Indeed, the well-studied Pima Indian population is characterized by low metabolic rates even after adjusting for fat-free mass, fat mass, age, and sex (77). Additionally, over the long term, those with a low REE had a greater risk of weight gain than those with a high REE (31).

Metabolic flexibility: Equally important to energy balance is macronutrient balance, specifically, whether the intake of each macronutrient matches its oxidation. The ability of the body to adjust the flux of metabolic pathways in response to changes in macronutrient consumption is defined as metabolic flexibility (31). Metabolic flexibility can be studied using the respiratory quotient (RQ) as an indicator. The RQ represents the ratio of carbohydrate to fat oxidation, with lower fasting values (~0.80) reflecting a greater reliance on fat for fuel and conversely, higher values (~1.00) reflecting a greater reliance on carbohydrates (27, 112). Those individuals who rely more heavily on carbohydrates as the substrate for energy production are more likely to gain body weight than those who rely more heavily on fat. In the context of metabolic flexibility, those individuals who are better able to match fuel oxidation to fuel availability decrease their risk of body weight gain.

Influence of Exercise Training on Energy Balance and Body Weight

Consensus surrounding the use of exercise as an effective strategy for weight loss is controversial (17). Popular media and news outlets propagate the notion that participation in regular exercise will not result·in meaningful weight loss; however, they fail to discuss the intricacies and assumptions inherent in this conclusion.

In fact, evidence from randomized controlled trials (RCTs) has firmly established that exercise in the absence of alterations in energy intake is associated with varying reductions in body weight and total adiposity (5, 14, 21, 22, 32, 64, 68, 80, 82, 84, 90), independent of age and sex. One important issue in the discussion concerning the use of exercise for weight loss is the amount of exercise performed. Indeed, in those studies that utilize exercise prescriptions consistent with the minimum levels of national guideline recommendations, only modest weight loss is observed (~2–3 kg) (90, 96, 108). However, these physical activity guidelines are not meant to promote weight loss; rather, they aim to improve and maintain cardiovascular health. The American College of Sports Medicine (ACSM) currently recommends

225–420 min/week (41) of aerobic exercise for individuals with obesity who intend to lose weight. Indeed, when energy expenditure is matched to the energy deficit incurred through diet-induced weight loss programmes (~500–700 kcal), similar reductions in weight are observed (22, 80, 83).

While it is well understood that aerobic exercise results in greater energy expenditure than resistance exercise and thus leads to further weight loss, there is still an important role for resistance training in the study of energy balance. Resistance training alone is not likely to result in meaningful weight loss (96); however, resistance training can lead to potential gains in lean body mass. It is understood that lean mass is highly correlated with REE and so, over time, this increase may attenuate the reduction in REE due to increased muscle protein turnover (93, 107). Additionally, by maintaining lean body mass over extended periods, the age-associated increase in body weight and fat mass weakens.

Influence of Dietary Intake on Energy Balance and Body Weight

It is clear that caloric restriction results in weight loss; however, the impact of diet composition may also be influential. Traditionally, the dogma that "a calorie is a calorie" has provided the framework for obesity interventions that focus primarily on energy restriction regardless of macronutrient distribution. While thermodynamically, this may be true when focusing on oxidative phosphorylation, different effects of macronutrient consumption on energy storage patterns may influence weight and body composition beyond total caloric restriction (26, 38).

Of the three macronutrients of focus, dietary protein is particularly understood to affect levels of fat-free mass. Supplementation of dietary protein during weight loss interventions attenuates the loss of lean body mass over time (11, 54, 105). As discussed previously, lean body mass is a primary determinant of REE; thus, by supplementing the diet with protein and preserving lean body mass, energy expenditure can be maintained with weight loss and attenuate the probability of weight regain (25, 110). Higher protein diets have also been associated with reductions in appetite due to increased satiety leading to reductions in overall energy intake (29, 86).

While it is apparent that higher protein diets are useful for maintaining lean body mass and weight, the relative importance of carbohydrate and fat consumption is controversial. Proponents of low carbohydrate diets have argued that since increased carbohydrate consumption is associated with an increase in insulin (storage hormone), higher carbohydrate diets will inevitably lead to an increase in energy storage in the form of fat mass and a decrease in substrate oxidation. Over time, this may result in an overall decrease in REE (34, 58). However, experimental evidence does not support this theory. Hall et al. conducted a meta-analysis including 32 studies and 563 participants on the effects of isocaloric diets differing in carbohydrate and fat on daily energy expenditure and body fat. Contrary to popular belief, the authors found a 25 kcal/day energy expenditure gain and 16 g/day body fat loss in favour of lower fat diets (38). While these findings were statistically significant, the authors note the clinical implication of these values is extremely small and conclude that the ratio of carbohydrate to fat has little importance for body fat and energy expenditure changes.

While there is much left to learn on the impact of varying macronutrient distribution intake patterns and effects on energy balance and body weight, an important caveat to note is that long-term weight loss from any diet intervention shows little promise. Lifestyle interventions are notoriously associated with decreased adherence over time (30). In addition to mechanistic work in this area, behavioural interventions are equally as important and necessary to identify effective strategies that increase adherence and compliance in a largely obesogenic environment.

Interactions Between Diet and Exercise Interventions on Weight Loss

Multiple RCTs have been conducted to study the impact of combined exercise and diet interventions compared to diet or exercise interventions alone for weight loss. Four meta-analyses published in 1998 (64), 2005 (20), 2009 (109), and 2011 (17) demonstrate consistent evidence for a superior effect of diet and exercise combined interventions than either alone for weight loss, with one showing a 20% greater decrease in weight in the combination groups (20). However, one important caveat of studying relative effects of exercise and diet on any outcome is that typically, equivalent energy deficits are not achieved across groups. For example, interventions that are based on minutes of exercise performed will likely have varying amounts of kilocalories expended, as individuals who differ in sex and body size do not expend the same number of kilocalories for a given time period and so, whether effects on weight loss are due to a greater energy deficit in the combined group is unclear. Nevertheless, of the available evidence, it appears that dietary restriction with the addition of exercise is a more efficacious strategy for weight loss than either lifestyle intervention alone.

Potential Mechanisms

Various potential mechanisms have been suggested to mediate the effect of exercise on homeostatic eating behaviours, though literature specifically evaluating this question is scarce and represents an important knowledge gap (Figure 18.1). Animal studies suggest that exercise has positive effects on brain structure and function, including increased neurogenesis, neuroprotection, and neuroplasticity, which can affect communication between brain regions through increases or decreases in the strength of synapses and neurotransmitter receptors located there (44, 48). These effects may be mediated by exercise-induced increases in brain-derived neurotrophic factor (BDNF) expression. BDNF has been shown to play a critical role in homeostatic control of food intake as an anorexigenic factor (3). BDNF is highly expressed in the hypothalamus, as well as brain regions associated with hedonic eating such as the hippocampus and praecuneus (3, 48). Alpha-melanocyte stimulating hormone (alpha-MSH) is derived from the anorexigenic ARC neuron POMC and acts on MC4R receptors to exert its anorexigenic effects. Activation of MC4R is required for CCK-induced satiety, and BDNF has been shown to participate in activation of MC4R to mediate the effects of CCK (3). BDNF has also been shown to participate in the homeostatic control of energy intake through effects downstream of leptin signalling. Furthermore, BDNF has been observed to influence neurotransmitter turnover, as BDNF-infused rats display a dose-dependent increase in serotonin turnover in the hypothalamus (59). Increasing serotonin turnover is associated with anorectic effects. The fact that BDNF is expressed in both homeostatic and hedonic brain regions suggests its role in mediating the effect of exercise on these systems (59).

Others suggest that the effect of exercise on leptin action can explain the hedonic alterations in response. Exercise may enhance leptin sensitivity, which could explain why not all studies observe changes in leptin in response to exercise (18). It may be that similar leptin concentrations can exert their effects more potently after exercise due to increased leptin sensitivity. It is suggested that higher leptin sensitivity can alter higher brain responses such as those in reward-mediating regions to food stimuli (18, 44). Furthermore, fat mass loss associated with chronic exercise training may mediate the effect of exercise on both homeostatic and hedonic eating regulation, as it is consistently shown that individuals with overweight/obesity have greater activation in response to visual food cues in reward-associated brain regions, as well as attenuated responses of homeostatic hormones that exert anorexigenic effects (12).

In summary, both acute and chronic exercise appear to affect homeostatic and hedonic eating in the direction of reducing ingestive behaviour, though not all findings agree, especially those concerning homeostatic outcomes. Clearly, further work needs to be done to investigate the impact of chronic exercise training on homeostatic eating. Specifically, the effect of exercise mode, duration, and intensity, as well as baseline weight status and subsequent weight loss from training, needs to be elucidated.

Biochemical and Physiological Compensatory Responses to Exercise or Diet-Induced Weight Loss

In several diet and exercise-induced weight loss interventions, the expected weight loss based on kilocalorie restriction or expenditure does not match the actual weight loss that occurs from pre- to

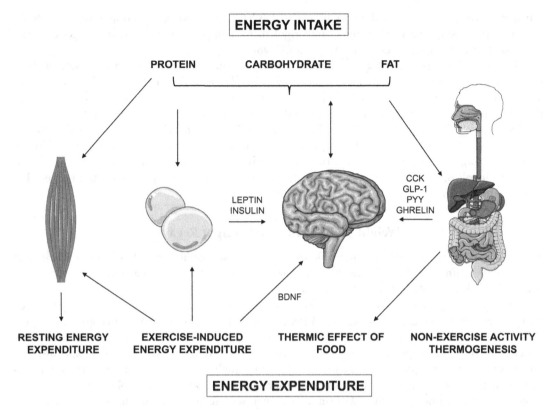

Figure 18.1 (A) Skeletal muscle, (B) adipose tissue, (C) central nervous system, and (D) gastrointestinal system. CCK, cholecystokinin; GLP-1, glucagon-like peptide-1; PYY, peptide YY; BDNF, brain-derived neurotrophic factor. Figure created with smart SERVIER MEDICAL ART (https://smart.servier.com/)

post-intervention (15, 24). For example, in our own work wherein we randomized 300 participants to four groups varying in exercise amount (kilocalories expended) and intensity, we did not observe between-group differences in weight loss (81). This is noteworthy, as the high-amount low-intensity exercise group expended double the kilocalories as the low-amount low-intensity exercise group (600 vs. 300 kilocalories for men; 360 vs. 180 kilocalories for women). While perplexing, this observation is supported by several other RCTs (14). While the exact mechanisms by which this compensation occurs is not clear, several hypotheses have been proposed.

The research group of King et al. have made several observations to explain the apparent compensatory factors that attenuate exercise-induced weight changes to defend body weight loss and maintain homeostasis (45, 47). They have noted both behavioural and metabolic responses to exercise that may compensate for changes in energy balance. Behavioural responses, those that individuals are conscious of and can control to some extent, include alterations in food intake (both quantity and macronutrient composition of the diet) and decreases in NEAT. Metabolic responses, on the other hand, are autonomic in nature, including changes in REE, energy cost of exercise, appetite regulation, and substrate oxidation, which have evolved over time to defend loss in body weight. Further, both compliance with the prescribed intervention (46) and the amount and intensity of exercise prescribed (15) may influence weight or adiposity responses to exercise differently.

One important issue in the study of compensatory responses to weight loss is the predictive model used to explore apparent discrepancies in observed and expected weight change (97). As discussed previously, the often-cited rule that a 3500-kcal deficit results in 1 lb of weight loss is regularly used as a model to describe expected weight change. It is now widely accepted that the use of such a static model is inappropriate (37). Several modern predictive models have been developed in response to include the dynamic relationships between changes in energy balance components and weight changes that may help calculate any compensation that may occur (37, 98).

A formidable gap exists in the knowledge concerning the mechanisms by which exercise alters both behavioural and metabolic compensatory responses (63). This is likely due to variability in compensatory responses between individuals. It is important to recognize that just as individuals differ in their response for a given outcome, they also differ in their propensity to compensate for changes in energy balance (45). King et al. proposes that the susceptibility of individuals to the benefits of exercise will depend on the direction and magnitude by which an individual's autonomic and volitional responses change (45, 94). Furthermore, important study design characteristics, including the magnitude of weight loss, the prescribed energy deficit, exercise dose, and participant characteristics, need to be factored into any conclusions (89).

Weight Maintenance and Weight Regain

Arguably as important as establishing viable interventions for weight loss is determining factors that affect weight maintenance. Body weight maintenance is closely linked to the components of energy balance, namely REE, NEAT, and energy intake.

In 1956, Jean Mayer published landmark observations in which he measured the relationship between energy expenditure and energy intake in 213 Bengali workers who engaged in 16 occupations varying in physical activity (61). His findings suggested that energy intake and energy expenditure are closely matched when energy expenditure is high ("regulated zone"); however, when energy expenditure is low, this balance is disrupted ("unregulated zone"). This coupling of energy intake to energy expenditure at high levels of activity has been studied in subsequent investigations. Stubbs et al. used whole-room indirect calorimetry to study six lean healthy men who reduced habitual physical activity levels from active to sedentary over 7 days. The authors observed no reduction in energy intake to match the decrease in expenditure (94).

Hand et al. extended this theory by suggesting that high levels of energy flux, the rate of conversion of energy from absorption to expenditure/storage, may be important for preventing weight gain by improving the coupling between changes in energy intake and activity (40). Perhaps maintaining high levels of activity even in cases of higher energy intake is a more practical and efficacious strategy for preventing weight gain than restricting energy intake alone. This strategy is supported by recent observations from Hagele et al. wherein 16 healthy adults participated in four energy balance protocols for 3 days each (33). Energy balance conditions included ad libitum energy intake, zero energy balance, -25% kilocalorie restriction, and +25% kilocalorie overfeeding at three different levels of energy expenditure defined by physical activity level (PAL). They observed that low energy expenditure led to decreased GLP-1 regardless of the prescribed energy balance condition and increased ghrelin in the caloric restriction and overfeeding group. The authors concluded that these two important appetite hormones responded appropriately at high levels of energy expenditure and overeating, and subsequent weight gain is more likely to occur at low levels of energy expenditure.

Another important factor to consider in the context of energy balance and body weight regulation is the maintenance of body weight after substantial weight reduction. Across both exercise and diet-based weight loss interventions, weight regain is extremely common (20, 96). Suggested mechanisms to explain the trend for regain includes increases in appetitive hormones that stimulate intake (e.g., ghrelin) in addition to decreases in inhibitory hormones that signal satiety (e.g., leptin, GLP-1) following substantial weight loss due to diet (23, 53, 95). Additionally for both diet and exercise interventions, compliance with habits developed during the intervention, including self-monitoring, may subside, leading to an increase in weight (91, 99). Finally, as discussed previously, decreases in REE with weight loss may make it more difficult to maintain body weight, as greater amounts of energy expenditure are needed to reach energy balance (69, 95). Indeed, while national physical activity guidelines recommend 150 min/week of moderate-to-vigorous physical activity for optimal health, 200–300 minutes of moderate physical activity per week is encouraged to prevent weight regain after initial losses.

Summary and Future Directions

Our understanding of energy balance, its components, and their interaction with each other in the short term has improved substantially over the past 60 years. However, remaining gaps in knowledge include understanding the long-term interaction in energy balance components in addition to precise mechanisms by which lifestyle interventions, including diet and exercise, mediate changes in energy balance and weight change. Future longitudinal studies following children and adults may provide important insights for how energy balance is regulated over the lifespan (38). Additionally, RCTs of appropriate length are necessary to determine the influence of exercise type, volume, and intensity on components of energy balance and body composition. Related to the influence of structured exercise, the impact of NEAT across the 24-hour period will be particularly insightful and offer potentially important considerations for lifestyle recommendations. Finally, assessment of the challenges that remain for adults to maintain weight loss interventions, wherein a substantial negative energy balance due to exercise or diet is prescribed, will be vitally important to subsequently devise solutions in line with our current obesogenic environment.

The individual variation in weight loss in response to lifestyle interventions is substantial (39); however, mechanisms underlying variability in responses are unknown. While compensatory behaviours such as energy intake have been shown to play a role, there may be a plethora of genetic or biochemical reasons that have yet to be discovered and interrogated. The advance of multi-omics technologies has greatly expanded our ability to examine changes in specific genes, transcription factors, metabolites, and proteins that may predict or explain phenotypic responses to an intervention. These technologies may provide insight into metabolic flexibility adaptations, alterations in energy balance, and individual exercise prescriptions that will maximize the benefits of lifestyle interventions.

Finally, an unappreciated gap in knowledge concerning exercise/diet interventions, energy balance, and body weight responses is the uncertainty of the impact of age, sex, and race. Non-white individuals have been hugely understudied despite the large percentage of the population they make up. It is possible that racial differences in genetics, biology, and physiology affect the translation of current research interventions to this population. In addition, adequately powered studies need to be conducted to determine differences in how women and men respond to a given energy balance intervention and how long-term energy balance physiology evolves across the lifespan. With the advance of technology in the last few decades, several innovative methodological opportunities have emerged that can provide a more comprehensive understanding of energy balance, body weight and composition, and the impact of lifestyle interventions.

References

1. Anis AH, Zhang W, Bansback N, Guh D, Amarsi Z, Birmingham C. Obesity and overweight in Canada: An updated cost-of-illness study. *Obesity Reviews* 11: 31–40, 2010.
2. Asakawa A, Inui A, Fujimiya M, Sakamaki R, Shinfuku N, Ueta Y, et al. Stomach regulates energy balance via acylated ghrelin and desacyl ghrelin. *Gut* 54: 18–24, 2005.
3. B Lebrun BB, Moyse E, Jean A. Brain-derived neurotrophic factor (BDNF) and food intake regulation: A minireview. *Auton Neurosci* 30: 126–127, 2006.
4. Bagdade JD, Bierman EL, Porte D, Jr. The significance of basal insulin levels in the evaluation of the insulin response to glucose in diabetic and nondiabetic subjects. *J Clin Invest* 46: 1549–1557, 1967.
5. Ballor D, Keesey RE. A meta-analysis of the factors affecting exercise-induced changes in body mass, fat mass and fat-free mass in males and females. *Int J Obes* 15(11):717–726, 1991.
6. Bastien M, Poirier P, Lemieux I, Despres JP. Overview of epidemiology and contribution of obesity to cardiovascular disease. *Prog Cardiovasc Dis* 56: 369–381, 2014.
7. Berthoud HR. The neurobiology of food intake in an obesogenic environment. *Proceedings of the Nutrition Society* 71: 478–487, 2012.

8. Blundell JE. Perspective on the central control of appetite. *Obesity (Silver Spring)* 14 Suppl 4: 160S–163S, 2006.

9. Blundell JE, Finlayson G, Gibbons C, Caudwell P, Hopkins M. The biology of appetite control: Do resting metabolic rate and fat-free mass drive energy intake? *Physiol Behav* 152: 473–478, 2015.

10. Bouchard C, Tremblay A. Genetic influences on the response of body fat and fat distribution to positive and negative energy balances in human identical twins. *J Nutr* 127: 943S–947S, 1997.

11. Bray GA, Smith SR, de Jonge L, Xie H, Rood J, Martin CK, et al. Effect of dietary protein content on weight gain, energy expenditure, and body composition during overeating: A randomized controlled trial. *JAMA* 307: 47–55, 2012.

12. Burger KS, Berner LA. A functional neuroimaging review of obesity, appetitive hormones and ingestive behavior. *Physiol Behav* 136: 121–127, 2014.

13. Calapai G, Corica F, Corsonello A, Sautebin L, Di Rosa M, Campo GM, et al. Leptin increases serotonin turnover by inhibition of brain nitric oxide synthesis. *J Clin Invest* 104: 975–982, 1999.

14. Catenacci VA, Wyatt HR. The role of physical activity in producing and maintaining weight loss. *Nat Clin Pract Endocrinol Metab* 3: 518–529, 2007.

15. Church TS, Martin CK, Thompson AM, Earnest CP, Mikus CR, Blair SN. Changes in weight, waist circumference and compensatory responses with different doses of exercise among sedentary, overweight postmenopausal women. *PLOS ONE* 4: e4515, 2009.

16. Colley RC, Garriguet D, Janssen I, Craig CL, Clarke J, Tremblay MS. Physical activity of Canadian adults: Accelerometer results from the 2007 to 2009 Canadian Health Measures Survey. *Health Rep* 22: 7–14, 2011.

17. Cook CM, Schoeller DA. Physical activity and weight control: Conflicting findings. *Curr Opin Clin Nutr Metab Care* 14: 419–424, 2011.

18. Cornier MA, Melanson EL, Salzberg AK, Bechtell JL, Tregellas JR. The effects of exercise on the neuronal response to food cues. *Physiol Behav* 105: 1028–1034, 2012.

19. Cunningham JJ. Body composition as a determinant of energy expenditure: A synthetic review and a proposed general prediction equation. *Am J Clin Nutr* 54: 963–969, 1991.

20. Curioni CC, Lourenco PM. Long-term weight loss after diet and exercise: A systematic review. *Int J Obes* 29: 1168–1174, 2005.

21. Davidson LE, Hudson R, Kilpatrick K, Kuk JL, McMillan K, Janiszewski PM, et al. Effects of exercise modality on insulin resistance and functional limitation in older adults: A randomized controlled trial. *Arch Intern Med* 169: 122–131, 2009.

22. Donnelly JE, Hill JO, Jacobsen DJ, Potteiger J, Sullivan DK, Johnson SL, et al. Effects of a 16-month randomized controlled exercise trial on body weight and composition in young, overweight men and women: The Midwest Exercise Trial. *Arch Intern Med* 163: 1343–1350, 2003.

23. Doucet E, Imbeault P, St-Pierre S, Almeras N, Mauriege P, Richard D, et al. Appetite after weight loss by energy restriction and a low-fat diet–exercise follow-up. *Int J Obes* 24: 906, 2000.

24. Drenowatz C. Reciprocal compensation to changes in dietary intake and energy expenditure within the concept of energy balance. *Adv Nutr* 6: 592–599, 2015.

25. Ebbeling CB, Swain JF, Feldman HA, Wong WW, Hachey DL, Garcia-Lago E, et al. Effects of dietary composition on energy expenditure during weight-loss maintenance. *JAMA* 307: 2627–2634, 2012.

26. Feinman RD, Fine EJ. Thermodynamics and metabolic advantage of weight loss diets. *Metab Syndr Relat Disord* 1: 209–219, 2003.

27. Flatt J, Ravussin E, Acheson KJ, Jequier E. Effects of dietary fat on postprandial substrate oxidation and on carbohydrate and fat balances. *J Clin Invest* 76: 1019–1024, 1985.

28. Flegal KM, Kit BK, Orpana H, Graubard BI. Association of all-cause mortality with overweight and obesity using standard body mass index categories: A systematic review and meta-analysis. *JAMA* 309: 71–82, 2013.

29. Foster GD, Wyatt HR, Hill JO, McGuckin BG, Brill C, Mohammed BS, et al. A randomized trial of a low-carbohydrate diet for obesity. *NEJM* 348: 2082–2090, 2003.

30. Freedhoff Y, Hall KD. Weight loss diet studies: We need help not hype. *The Lancet* 388: 849–851, 2016.

31. Galgani J, Ravussin E. Energy metabolism, fuel selection and body weight regulation. *Int J Obes* 32(Suppl 7): S109–119, 2008.

32. Garrow JS, Summerbell CD. Meta-analysis: Effect of exercise, with or without dieting, on the body composition of overweight subjects. *Eur J Clin Nutr* 49: 1–10, 1995.

33. Hägele FA, Büsing F, Nas A, Hasler M, Müller MJ, Blundell JE, et al. Appetite control is improved by acute increases in energy turnover at different levels of energy balance. *J Clin Endocrinol Metab* 104: 4481–4491, 2019.

34. Hall K. A review of the carbohydrate–insulin model of obesity. *Eur J Clin Nutr* 71: 323, 2017.

35. Hall KD. Computational model of in vivo human energy metabolism during semistarvation and refeeding. *Am J of Physiol Endocrinol and Metab* 291: E23–E37, 2006.

36. Hall KD. Modeling metabolic adaptations and energy regulation in humans. *Ann Rev Nutr* 32: 35–54, 2012.

37. Hall KD. What is the required energy deficit per unit weight loss? *Int J Obes* 32: 573, 2008.

38. Hall KD, Guo J. Obesity energetics: Body weight regulation and the effects of diet composition. *Gastroenterology* 152: 1718–1727 e1713, 2017.

39. Hammond BP, Stotz PJ, Brennan AM, Lamarche B, Day AG, Ross R. Individual variability in waist circumference and body weight in response to exercise. *MSSE* 51: 315–322, 2019.

40. Hand GA, Blair SN. Energy flux and its role in obesity and metabolic disease. *Eur Endocrinol* 10: 131, 2014.

41. Haskell WL, Lee IM, Pate RR, Powell KE, Blair SN, Franklin BA, et al. Physical activity and public health: Updated recommendation for adults from the American College of Sports Medicine and the American Heart Association. *Circulation* 116: 1081–1093, 2007.

42. Hopkins M, Finlayson G, Duarte C, Whybrow S, Ritz P, Horgan GW, et al. Modelling the associations between fat-free mass, resting metabolic rate and energy intake in the context of total energy balance. *Int J Obes* 40: 312–318, 2016.

43. Katzmarzyk PT, Janssen I. The economic costs associated with physical inactivity and obesity in Canada: An update. *Can J Appl Physiol* 29: 90–115, 2004.

44. Killgore WD, Kipman M, Schwab ZJ, Tkachenko O, Preer L, Gogel H, et al. Physical exercise and brain responses to images of high-calorie food. *Neuroreport* 24: 962–967, 2013.

45. King NA, Caudwell P, Hopkins M, Byrne NM, Colley R, Hills AP, et al. Metabolic and behavioral compensatory responses to exercise interventions: Barriers to weight loss. *Obesity* 15: 1373–1383, 2007.

46. King NA, Hopkins M, Caudwell P, Stubbs R, Blundell JE. Individual variability following 12 weeks of supervised exercise: Identification and characterization of compensation for exercise-induced weight loss. *Int J Obes* 32: 177, 2008.

47. King NA, Horner K, Hills AP, Byrne NM, Wood RE, Bryant E, et al. Exercise, appetite and weight management: understanding the compensatory responses in eating behaviour and how they contribute to variability in exercise-induced weight loss. *Br J Sports Med* 46: 315–322, 2012.

48. McFadden KL, Cornier M-A, Melanson EL, Bechtell JL, Tragellas JR. Effects of exercise on resting-state default mode and salience network activity in overweight/obese adults. *Neuroreport* 24: 866–871, 2013.

49. Klok MD, Jakobsdottir S, Drent ML. The role of leptin and ghrelin in the regulation of food intake and body weight in humans: A review. *Obes Rev* 8: 21–34, 2007.

50. Kotz CM, Teske JA, Levine JA, Wang C. Feeding and activity induced by orexin A in the lateral hypothalamus in rats. *Reg Peptides* 104: 27–32, 2002.

51. Lavie CJ, Milani RV, Ventura HO. Obesity and cardiovascular disease: Risk factor, paradox, and impact of weight loss. *JACC* 53: 1925–1932, 2009.

52. Lecoultre V, Ravussin E, Redman LM. The fall in leptin concentration is a major determinant of the metabolic adaptation induced by caloric restriction independently of the changes in leptin circadian rhythms. *J Clin Endocrinol Metab* 96: E1512–E1516, 2011.

53. Leibel RL, Rosenbaum M, Hirsch J. Changes in energy expenditure resulting from altered body weight. *NEJM* 332: 621–628, 1995.

54. Leidy HJ, Clifton PM, Astrup A, Wycherley TP, Westerterp-Plantenga MS, Luscombe-Marsh ND, et al. The role of protein in weight loss and maintenance. *Am J Clin Nutr* 101: 1320S-1329S, 2015.

55. Levine JA, Kotz CM. NEAT–non-exercise activity thermogenesis–egocentric & geocentric environmental factors vs. biological regulation. *Acta Physiologica Scandinavica* 184: 309–318, 2005.

56. Levine JA, Nygren J, Short KR, Nair KS. Effect of hyperthyroidism on spontaneous physical activity and energy expenditure in rats. *J Appl Physiol* 94: 165–170, 2003.

57. Liddle RA, Goldfine ID, Rosen MS, Taplitz RA, Williams JA. Cholecystokinin bioactivity in human plasma. Molecular forms, responses to feeding, and relationship to gallbladder contraction. *J Clin Invest* 75: 1144–1152, 1985.

58. Ludwig DS, Friedman MI. Increasing adiposity: Consequence or cause of overeating? *JAMA* 311: 2167–2168, 2014.

59. Marosi K, Mattson MP. BDNF mediates adaptive brain and body responses to energetic challenges. *Trends Endocrinol Metab* 25: 89–98, 2014.

60. Marti A, Moreno-Aliaga MJ, Hebebrand J, Martinez JA. Genes, lifestyles and obesity. *Int J Obes Relat Metab Disord* 28(Suppl 3): S29–36, 2004.

61. Mayer J, Roy P, Mitra KP. Relation between caloric intake, body weight, and physical work: Studies in an industrial male population in West Bengal. *Am J Clin Nutr* 4: 169–175, 1956.

62. Meister B. Control of food intake via leptin receptors in the hypothalamus. *Vitam Horm* 59: 265–304, 2000.

63. Melanson EL, Keadle SK, Donnelly JE, Braun B, King NA. Resistance to exercise-induced weight loss: Compensatory behavioral adaptations. *MSSE* 45: 1600, 2013.

64. Miller WC, Koceja DM, Hamilton EJ. A meta-analysis of the past 25 years of weight loss research using diet, exercise or diet plus exercise intervention. *Int J Obes Relat Metab Disord* 21: 941–947, 1997.

65. Moehlecke M, Canani LH, Silva LO, Trindade MR, Friedman R, Leitao CB. Determinants of body weight regulation in humans. *Arch Endocrinol Metab* 60: 152–162, 2016.

66. Moran TH, Kinzig KP. Gastrointestinal satiety signals II. Cholecystokinin. *Am J Physiol Gastrointest Liver Physiol* 286: G183–188, 2004.

67. Murphy KG, Dhillo WS, Bloom SR. Gut peptides in the regulation of food intake and energy homeostasis. *Endocr Rev* 27: 719–727, 2006.

68. Nordby P, Auerbach PL, Rosenkilde M, Kristiansen L, Thomasen JR, Rygaard L, et al. Endurance training per se increases metabolic health in young, moderately overweight men. *Obesity (Silver Spring)* 20: 2202–2212, 2012.

69. Ochner CN, Barrios DM, Lee CD, Pi-Sunyer FX. Biological mechanisms that promote weight regain following weight loss in obese humans. *Physiology & Behavior* 120: 106–113, 2013.

70. World Health Organization. Global strategy on diet, physical activity and health. https://www.who.int/ publications/i/item/9241592222 Website: https://www.who.int/nmh/wha/59/dpas/en/

71. Pelleymounter MA, Cullen MJ, Baker MB, Hecht R, Winters D, Boone T, et al. Effects of the obese gene product on body weight regulation in ob/ob mice. *Science* 269: 540–543, 1995.

72. Poirier P, Giles TD, Bray GA, Hong Y, Stern JS, Pi-Sunyer FX, et al. Obesity and cardiovascular disease: Pathophysiology, evaluation, and effect of weight loss. *Arterioscler Thromb Vasc Biol* 26: 968–976, 2006.

73. Pothos EN, Creese I, Hoebel BG. Restricted eating with weight loss selectively decreases extracellular dopamine in the nucleus accumbens and alters dopamine response to amphetamine, morphine, and food intake. *J Neurosci* 15: 6640–6650, 1995.

74. Ravussin E, Bogardus C. Energy balance and weight regulation: Genetics versus environment. *Br J Nutr* 83(Suppl 1): S17–20, 2000.

75. Ravussin E, Burnand B, Schutz Y, Jequier E. Energy expenditure before and during energy restriction in obese patients. *Am J Clin Nutr* 41: 753–759, 1985.

76. Ravussin E, Lillioja S, Anderson TE, Christin L, Bogardus C. Determinants of 24-hour energy expenditure in man. Methods and results using a respiratory chamber. *J Clin Inv* 78: 1568–1578, 1986.

77. Ravussin E, Lillioja S, Knowler WC, Christin L, Freymond D, Abbott WG, et al. Reduced rate of energy expenditure as a risk factor for body-weight gain. *NEJM* 318: 467–472, 1988.

78. Redman LM, Heilbronn LK, Martin CK, De Jonge L, Williamson DA, Delany JP, et al. Metabolic and behavioral compensations in response to caloric restriction: Implications for the maintenance of weight loss. *PLOS ONE* 4: e4377, 2009.

79. Rosenbaum M, Leibel RL. Adaptive thermogenesis in humans. *Int J Obes* 34: S47, 2010.

80. Ross R, Dagnone D, Jones PJ, Smith H, Paddags A, Hudson R, et al. Reduction in obesity and related comorbid conditions after diet-induced weight loss or exercise-induced weight loss in men. A randomized, controlled trial. *Ann Intern Med* 133: 92–103, 2000.

81. Ross R, Hudson R, Stotz PJ, Lam M. Effects of exercise amount and intensity on abdominal obesity and glucose tolerance in obese adults: A randomized trial. *Ann Intern Med* 162: 325–334, 2015.

82. Ross R, Janssen I. Physical activity, total and regional obesity: Dose-response considerations. *Med Sci Sports Exerc* 33: S521–527, 2001.

83. Ross R, Janssen I, Dawson J, Kungl AM, Kuk JL, Wong SL, et al. Exercise-induced reduction in obesity and insulin resistance in women: a randomized controlled trial. *Obes Res* 12: 789–798, 2004.

84. Ross RH, Stotz PJ, Lam M. Effects of exercise amount and intensity on abdominal obesity and glucose tolerance in obese adults. A randomized controlled trial. *Ann Intern Med*. Mar 3;162(5):325–34, 2015.

85. Sahu A. Evidence suggesting that galanin (GAL), melanin-concentrating hormone (MCH), neurotensin (NT), proopiomelanocortin (POMC) and neuropeptide Y (NPY) are targets of leptin signaling in the hypothalamus. *Endocrinology* 139: 795–798, 1998.

86. Samaha FF, Iqbal N, Seshadri P, Chicano KL, Daily DA, McGrory J, et al. A low-carbohydrate as compared with a low-fat diet in severe obesity. *NEJM* 348: 2074–2081, 2003.

87. Schwartz MW, Seeley RJ, Campfield LA, Burn P, Baskin DG. Identification of targets of leptin action in rat hypothalamus. *J Clin Invest* 98: 1101–1106, 1996.

88. Schwartz MW, Woods SC, Porte D Jr., Seeley RJ, Baskin DG. Central nervous system control of food intake. *Nature* 404: 661–671, 2000.

89. Silva AM, Judice PB, Carraca EV, King N, Teixeira PJ, Sardinha LB. What is the effect of diet and/or exercise interventions on behavioural compensation in non-exercise physical activity and related energy expenditure of free-living adults? A systematic review. *Br J Nutr* 119: 1327–1345, 2018.

90. Slentz CA, Duscha BD, Johnson JL, Ketchum K, Aiken LB, Samsa GP, et al. Effects of the amount of exercise on body weight, body composition, and measures of central obesity: STRRIDE–a randomized controlled study. *Arch Intern Med* 164: 31–39, 2004.

91. Soleymani T, Daniel S, Garvey WT. Weight maintenance: Challenges, tools and strategies for primary care physicians. *Obes Rev* 17: 81–93, 2016.

92. Spiegelman BM, Flier JS. Obesity and the regulation of energy balance. *Cell* 104: 531–543, 2001.

93. Strasser B, Schobersberger W. Evidence for resistance training as a treatment therapy in obesity. *J Obes* 2011.

94. Stubbs RJ, Hughes DA, Johnstone AM, Whybrow S, Horgan GW, King N, et al. Rate and extent of compensatory changes in energy intake and expenditure in response to altered exercise and diet composition in humans. *Am J Physiol Reg Int and Comp Physiol* 286: R350–R358, 2004.

95. Sumithran P, Proietto J. The defence of body weight: A physiological basis for weight regain after weight loss. *Clin Sci* 124: 231–241, 2013.

96. Swift DL, McGee JE, Earnest CP, Carlisle E, Nygard M, Johannsen NM. The effects of exercise and physical activity on weight loss and maintenance. *Prog Cardiovasc Dis* 61: 206–213, 2018.

97. Thomas DM, Bouchard C, Church T, Slentz C, Kraus WE, Redman LM, et al. Why do individuals not lose more weight from an exercise intervention at a defined dose? An energy balance analysis. *Obes Rev* 13: 835–847, 2012.

98. Thomas DM, Martin CK, Heymsfield S, Redman LM, Schoeller DA, Levine JA. A simple model predicting individual weight change in humans. *J Biol Dyn* 5: 579–599, 2011.

99. Thomas JG, Bond DS, Phelan S, Hill JO, Wing RR. Weight-loss maintenance for 10 years in the National Weight Control Registry. *Am J Prev Med* 46: 17–23, 2014.

100. Twells LK, Gregory DM, Reddigan J, Midodzi WK. Current and predicted prevalence of obesity in Canada: A trend analysis. *CMAJ* 2: E18, 2014.

101. Van Vugt DA. Brain imaging studies of appetite in the context of obesity and the menstrual cycle. *Hum Reprod Update* 16: 276–292, 2010.

102. Westerterp KR. Diet induced thermogenesis. *Nutr Metab* 1: 5, 2004.

103. Westerterp KR. Exercise, energy expenditure and energy balance, as measured with doubly labelled water. *Proc Nutr Soc* 77: 4–10, 2018.

104. Westerterp KR. Exercise, energy balance and body composition. *Eur J Clin Nutr* 72: 1246–1250, 2018.

105. Westerterp-Plantenga M, Nieuwenhuizen A, Tome D, Soenen S, Westerterp K. Dietary protein, weight loss, and weight maintenance. *Ann Rev Nutr* 29: 21–41, 2009.

106. Weyer C, Snitker S, Rising R, Bogardus C, Ravussin E. Determinants of energy expenditure and fuel utilization in man: Effects of body composition, age, sex, ethnicity and glucose tolerance in 916 subjects. *Int J Obes* 23: 715, 1999.

107. Willis LH, Slentz CA, Bateman LA, Shields AT, Piner LW, Bales CW, et al. Effects of aerobic and/or resistance training on body mass and fat mass in overweight or obese adults. *J Appl Physiol* 113: 1831–1837, 2012.

108. Wilmore JH, Després J-P, Stanforth PR, Mandel S, Rice T, Gagnon J, et al. Alterations in body weight and composition consequent to 20 wk of endurance training: The HERITAGE Family Study. *Am J Clin Nutr* 70: 346–352, 1999.

109. Wu T, Gao X, Chen M, van Dam RM. Long-term effectiveness of diet-plus-exercise interventions vs. diet-only interventions for weight loss: A meta-analysis. *Obes Rev* 10: 313–323, 2009.

110. Wycherley TP, Moran LJ, Clifton PM, Noakes M, Brinkworth GD. Effects of energy-restricted high-protein, low-fat compared with standard-protein, low-fat diets: A meta-analysis of randomized controlled trials. *Am J Clin Nutr* 96: 1281–1298, 2012.

111. Yoo S. Dynamic energy balance and obesity prevention. *J Obes Metab Syndr* 27: 203–212, 2018.

112. Zurlo F, Lillioja S, Esposito-Del Puente A, Nyomba B, Raz I, Saad M, et al. Low ratio of fat to carbohydrate oxidation as predictor of weight gain: Study of 24-h RQ. *Am J Physiol Endocrinol Metab* 259: E650–E657, 1990.

19

DIETARY MANIPULATION FOR OPTIMIZING ENDURANCE TRAINING ADAPTATIONS AND PERFORMANCE: CARBOHYDRATE VS. FAT

Jamie Whitfield and Louise M. Burke

Introduction

Over 50 years ago, pioneering work by John Holloszy demonstrated that endurance-based exercise induced an increase in skeletal muscle mitochondrial content (26). Today, this finding has been replicated by numerous labs and is considered to represent one of the hallmark adaptations to prolonged endurance training (23). The emergence of molecular biology techniques in the sport and exercise sciences has provided researchers with the tools to evaluate the effects of specific training interventions on training adaptation by elucidating many of the cellular and molecular markers that underpin exercise performance. While countless studies have sought to determine the optimal intensity, duration, or modality of exercise to induce adaptation, the role of nutrient availability in maximizing these effects has received less attention. Indeed, recognition that changes in nutrient status can alter a number of cell-signalling pathways via nutrient–gene or nutrient–protein interactions is only a recent phenomenon. As a result, there has been increased interest in how nutrient availability may promote or inhibit training adaptation and, ultimately, performance capacity. However, it remains to be determined whether it is a *surplus* or a *lack* of substrate that triggers adaptation (17). For example, if ingestion of carbohydrate during exercise allows an athlete to train harder, will the elevated work rate result in a greater training stimulus? Or should an athlete train in a fasted state, which may result in greater disturbance to cellular homeostasis and upregulation of adaptive responses? Undoubtedly, as demonstrated by our developing knowledge of the optimal model of exercise for performance benefits, the answer will lie in combining and integrating a range of these approaches to nutrient support. While other chapters in this textbook extensively detail the regulation of substrate metabolism (Chapters 1 and 2) and the cellular signalling cascades initialized by exercise (Chapters 8 and 9), this chapter seeks to address where these two fields overlap and outlines some of the existing and emerging theories regarding how endurance adaptations may be optimized through nutrition, with an emphasis on the role of carbohydrate and fat as key macronutrients.

Pathways of Energy Production

Skeletal muscle is unique amongst tissues in the body in its range of metabolic activity, with adenosine triphosphate (ATP) turnover increasing up to 100-fold over rest during maximal exercise (18, 45). To meet this increased demand, several energy pathways contribute to both substrate-level and oxidative phosphorylation to replenish the ATP store from adenosine diphosphate (ADP) and inorganic phosphate (Pi). During more prolonged exercise, the muscle relies on oxidative metabolism within the mitochondria, with substrate coming from carbohydrate and lipid stores. Specifically, skeletal muscle relies on the breakdown of endogenous stores of fuel (i.e., glycogen, the storage form of carbohydrate, and intramuscular triglycerides [IMTGs], an endogenous lipid store) as well as the uptake of blood-borne substrates (glucose and free fatty acids [FFAs]) for the production of ATP. At the onset of exercise and at higher intensities, skeletal muscle glycogen is the dominant source of substrate, while during more prolonged exercise of low to moderate intensity, there is increased reliance on plasma-derived glucose produced via liver glycogen breakdown and intracellular and extracellular lipid sources (53, 54). However, it is important to note that neither fuel source is used in isolation; rather, they display a reciprocal relationship in which an increase in utilization of one fuel source results in a concomitant decrease in the other, provided the demand for energy is constant.

During exercise, shifts in fuel utilization are driven primarily by changes in the intracellular and extracellular environments as a result of changes in exercise intensity and duration (35, 53). This ultimately results in allosteric and covalent modifications of the rate-limiting steps in both the lipid and carbohydrate metabolic pathways. While carbohydrates and FFAs are metabolized via different pathways, they share many similarities and potential sites of regulation, namely (1) mobilization and delivery of blood-borne substrate, (2) transport across the sarcolemmal membrane and into the myocyte, (3) the activity of enzymes involved in ensuing flux through the respective metabolic pathways, and finally (4) transport into the mitochondria. While the full intricacies of these relationships are beyond the scope of this chapter, an overview of these metabolic pathways and how they may be upregulated or downregulated in response to training and nutrition are presented in Figure 19.1.

Training Adaptation

In the context of exercise, it is well accepted that the cellular perturbations elicited by skeletal muscle contraction (e.g., Ca^{2+} flux, reactive oxygen species production, and changes in intracellular pH and energy status) result in the activation of a number of signalling cascades, including AMP-activated protein kinase, Ca^{2+}/calmodulin-dependent protein kinase II (CaMKII), and p38 mitogen-activated protein kinase (p38 MAPK), with putative roles in training and adaptation (37). These signalling proteins converge on downstream transcriptional activators (e.g., peroxisome proliferator-activated γ receptor coactivator, PGC-1α) and transcription factors (e.g., nuclear respiratory factors [NRF] 1 and 2) to control and regulate the expression of targeted genes. It is the cumulative response to these transient changes in gene expression that result in physiological and metabolic adaptation (46). Additionally, one consistent adaptation to exercise training is increased reliance on fat oxidation to fuel the same absolute power output, with a concomitant decrease in carbohydrate utilization resulting in a sparing of intramuscular glycogen (23). While this is generally attributed to an increase in mitochondrial content (26) and tighter metabolic control (decreasing reliance on substrate-level phosphorylation [i.e., PCr]) and better matching of energy production and oxidative supply for a given workload, the resulting reduction in concentrations of free ADP and adenosine monophosphate (AMP)—two potent allosteric activators of regulatory steps in the carbohydrate metabolic pathway—also drives the reduction in carbohydrate use.

Because the majority of scientific interest on training adaptations and training–nutrition interactions has focused on changes in fuel utilization for the same *absolute power* output, it is often forgotten that training increases the muscle's total capacity to produce power and that the ratio of substrate use at any *relative* percentage of this total appears to remain largely unchanged (24). Therefore, as training also increases the muscle's capacity for carbohydrate oxidation, mechanisms and strategies to further enhance this are of interest, since the intensity of most endurance events in high-performance sport, either sustained throughout the event or for the critical stages that determine success, are dependent on carbohydrate utilization (11, 24). Although this aspect of training/nutrient interactions is less well

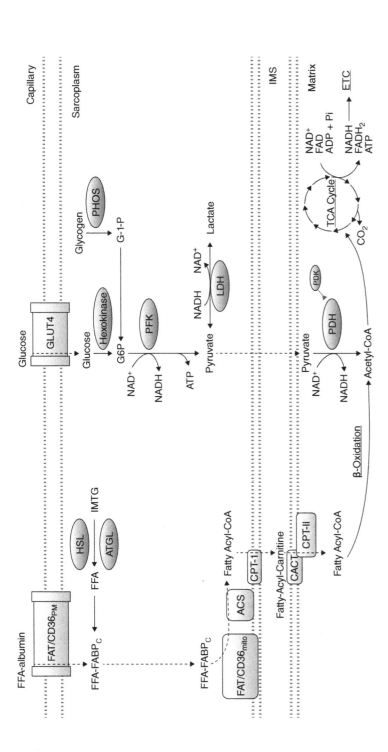

Figure 19.1 Overview of skeletal muscle metabolic pathways. During exercise, skeletal muscle relies on both exogenous and endogenous sources of lipid (plasma FFA and IMTG, respectively) and carbohydrate (plasma glucose and glycogen, respectively) for energy production via mitochondrial oxidative phosphorylation. Both pathways rely on protein-mediated transport for exogenous substrate into the cytoplasm, utilizing glucose transporter 4 (GLUT4) as well as a family of fatty acid transporters (example used above, fatty acid translocase/CD36 (FAT/CD36)). Highlighted are key regulatory enzymes in the carbohydrate metabolic pathway resulting in ATP and reducing equivalent production/consumption including glycogen phosphorylase (PHOS), hexokinase (HK), phosphofructokinase (PFK), lactate dehydrogenase (LDH), and pyruvate dehydrogenase (PDH). Lipid metabolism is more heavily regulated by transport into the mitochondria. Free fatty acids (FFA) taken up from plasma or liberated from IMTG by adipose triglyceride lipase (ATGL) and hormone sensitive lipase (HSL), are converted to fatty Acyl-CoA by Acyl-CoA synthase (ACS), and subsequently moved across the mitochondrial membranes by the carnitine palmitoyltransferase complex, consisting of carnitine palmitoyltransferase (CPT-I), carnitine acylcarnitine transferase (CACT), and CPT-II. While each of these enzymes is subject to multiple levels of allosteric and covalent regulation, the inhibitory enzyme pyruvate dehydrogenase kinase (PDK) has been included as it is heavily upregulated in response to conditions of elevated intramuscular FFA such as a low-carbohydrate, high-fat diet, or training with reduced glycogen content. Additional sites of regulation modified by these nutritional interventions include beta(3)-hydroxyacyl-CoA dehydrogenase (β-HAD), a key enzyme in the β-oxidation pathway, as well as the fatty acid transporters FAT/CD36 and CPT-I. Figure created with https://biorender.com/ (licenced version)

developed and will not be a focus of this review, it is noted that strategies that enhance fat oxidation at the expense of the carbohydrate pathways should be carefully considered in terms of the likely impairment of the performance of competitive endurance athletes.

Carbohydrate and Lipid Storage

The discovery of a significant increase in skeletal muscle glycogen stores and an associated increase in exercise capacity with 3–5 days of increased carbohydrate intake following an exhaustive bout of exercise marked an important milestone in sports nutrition (3, 4). Given the limited nature of glycogen stores within the body (~400 g in muscle and ~100 g in liver) relative to the abundance of lipids, the practice of "carbohydrate loading" or "glycogen supercompensation" has been widely utilized by athletes and practitioners in order to reduce or offset the effects of depletion on exercise capacity and performance. Modern practices, which account for the superior glycogen storage capacity of trained individuals, now consist of 24–48 hours of carbohydrate intakes of 7–12 $g \cdot kg^{-1}$ body mass·day^{-1} in concert with a taper in daily training (11). In contrast, while IMTGs represent a key fuel source during lower-intensity exercise (i.e., <65% VO_{2max}), there is no strong evidence that their intracellular concentrations limit performance (12). However, consumption of a low-carbohydrate, high-fat (LCHF) diet (68% of energy intake [EI] from fat) in the 24 hours post-exercise has been shown to increase IMTG storage when compared to a low-fat (5% of EI from fat) diet (59), demonstrating that acute "super-compensation" of intramuscular lipid stores is possible in a manner similar to glycogen. Furthermore, chronic consumption of high amounts of fat (up to 7 weeks) also acts to increase IMTG stores, potentially as a result of an overall positive fat balance, where fat intake exceeds oxidation rates and adipose tissue storage (55).

The Role of Glycogen in Cell Signalling

Recent research has suggested that glycogen plays a role beyond simply acting as a source of substrate—it can actually modulate the response to training. In an elegant study performed by Pilegaard et al. (48), subjects performed one-legged cycling to deplete glycogen content by ~50% in one leg the day prior to cycling for 2.5 hours at a low intensity (~45% VO_{2max}). In doing so, the researchers were able to minimize confounders (circulating factors, training status, etc.) and compare the effect of an acute bout on exercise performed with either low or high glycogen within the same individuals. They demonstrated greater transcription of metabolic genes, including pyruvate dehydrogenase kinase (PDK) 4 and uncoupling protein (UCP) 3, in the glycogen-depleted leg compared to its "control" glycogen-replete counterpart. This "ramped-up" training signal in response to low-glycogen conditions is underpinned by the finding that several promoters and transcription factors include carbohydrate response elements that are sensitive to glycogen levels (6). For example, the cellular metabolic energy sensor AMPK also contains a glycogen-binding domain on its β subunit, which has been proposed as a sensor of stored cellular energy (29). It has therefore been hypothesized that when the size of the glycogen granule decreases during exercise as a result of glycogenolysis, AMPK and other transcription factors with carbohydrate response elements are released and become free to associate with different target proteins. In support of this, it has been demonstrated that both the activity (65) and nuclear abundance of AMPKα2 (61), the predominant AMPK isoform in skeletal muscle, is increased under low-glycogen content conditions.

Glycogen content may also augment cellular signalling cascades indirectly. Since each gram of glycogen is bound to 3–4 grams of water (44), glycogen depletion may result in an increase in osmotic pressure within skeletal muscle (36), with a downstream increase in the activity of p38 MAPK, which is sensitive to increases in hyperosmotic-induced cellular stress (56). In the context of endurance training, this is a significant finding, as the γ subunit of p38 is required for the induction of peroxisome proliferator-activated receptor γ coactivator (PGC)-1α expression (50), the so-called master regulator of mitochondrial biogenesis, and therefore may drive subsequent mitochondrial adaptation. Consistent with these findings, manipulation of human skeletal muscle glycogen content via either nutrition or exercise increases both the phosphorylation (15, 16) and nuclear abundance (15) of p38 MAPK. It has also been demonstrated that there is a linear relationship between the exercise-induced increases in PGC-1α protein and the level of glycogen depletion following acute exercise (40). These findings can therefore be used to create a molecular framework around how manipulation of intramuscular glycogen content can augment training adaptation and performance (Figure 19.2) and set the stage for a series of studies seeking to test this theory utilizing different experimental approaches.

Nutritional Strategies to Manipulate Glycogen Status and Training Adaptation

Training Twice Per Day

The first study to truly investigate the effect of prolonged training with decreased glycogen content was performed by Hansen and colleagues (21). Much like earlier work from the same group (48), researchers employed a single leg exercise protocol in untrained males where one leg performed 2 × 1 hour bouts of leg extensions every other day separated by 2 hours, while the opposite leg performed 1 hour of exercise every day. In this manner, every second bout of exercise was performed in a glycogen-depleted state, while the contralateral control leg always undertook exercise with fully replete energy stores. Furthermore, this elegant study design permitted researchers to directly evaluate the effect of glycogen status independent of any other systematic or environmental factors, while also matching the total work performed across both legs. Following 10 weeks of a schedule involving five training bouts per week, activity of the mitochondrial enzyme beta (3)-hydroxyacyl-CoA dehydrogenase (β-HAD), a key component in the β-oxidation pathway, was increased only in the leg that undertook every second session with depleted glycogen. Furthermore, there was also a greater increase in citrate synthase (CS) activity, a marker of mitochondrial content, and improved time to exhaustion compared to the control leg (21). Studies comparing this same model (daily cycling training vs. twice per day every other day) in trained cyclists and triathletes have replicated these biochemical results; the leg that "trained low" for 50% of sessions achieved increases in markers of mitochondrial content (CS, cytochrome c oxidase [COXIV]) and increased capacity for lipid oxidation through increases in β-HAD (27, 66) and expression of the fatty acid transporter (FAT) CD36 (27). However, despite increases in the machinery required for the transport and subsequent oxidation of substrate in skeletal muscle, neither of the aforementioned studies were able to demonstrate a greater enhancement of performance associated with the 3-week training protocol (i.e., control and intervention groups saw similar performance gains).

Fasted Training

A major limitation of the twice per day training model is that it is difficult to clearly ascertain whether all training effects are due to performing the second session with reduced glycogen content. Indeed, repeated bouts of exercise in close proximity (i.e., ≤2 hours) may also alter the metabolic responses and subsequent adaptation to training. In contrast, a simpler form of "training low" can be achieved by performing exercise in the overnight fasted state. While muscle glycogen is unaltered by an overnight fast, liver glycogen is decreased and circulating FFAs, epinephrine, and cortisol are elevated (60), resulting in a change in the exogenous delivery of substrate to the working muscle. However, while results of acute exercise in the overnight fasted state have yielded equivocal increases in markers of cell signalling (AMPK activity) relative to the fed condition (1, 34), chronic (6–8 weeks) training in the glycogen-depleted state resulted in significant increases in FATs (5), β-HAD activity, and mitochondrial content (43, 51).

In order to better target both skeletal muscle and liver glycogen stores for depletion, researchers have also utilized a "sleep low" paradigm, where subjects complete a bout of exhaustive glycogen-lowering exercise on day one with restricted carbohydrate intake during recovery followed by a second bout of

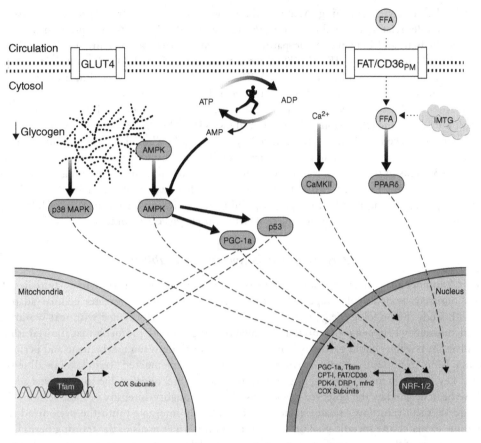

Figure 19.2 Simplified schematic outlining the putative cell signalling cascades activated through exercise with low glycogen availability. Exercise will result in an increase in energy turnover, increasing the intracellular concentration of metabolites such as calcium (Ca²⁺), AMP, and ADP, activating calcium/calmodulin-dependent protein kinase II (CaMKII) and the AMP protein kinase (AMPK). These kinases can then translocate to the nucleus in order to increase gene transcription. AMPK may also be bound to glycogen through a carbohydrate binding domain on its β-subunit. In conditions where intramuscular glycogen is decreased, AMPK is released, resulting in an increase in its activity, promoting phosphorylation of the downstream target PGC-1α as well as translocation to nucleus. PGC-1α can also translocate to the nucleus, where it autoregulates its own expression, and positively effects gene transcription through interactions with a variety of hormone receptors and transcription factors, including nuclear respiratory factors (NRF) 1 and 2. These two transcription factors promote the transcription of nuclear genes controlling the expression of cytochrome oxidase (COX) subunits. Additionally, NRF-1 also induces the expression of mitochondrial transcription factor A (Tfam), which is imported into the mitochondria in order to regulate the expression of mitochondrial (mt) DNA. AMPK can also increase the activity and alter the cellular localization of the tumor suppressor protein p53. Upon redistribution to the nucleus, both p53 and PGC-1α can coactivate Tfam to increase the expression of proteins that form subunits of the electron transport chain respiratory complexes. A decrease in glycogen content can induce cellular stress and increase the activity of p38 mitogen-activated protein kinase (p38 MAPK), promoting its translocation to the nucleus where it induces the expression of PGC-1α. Finally, exercise in a low glycogen state elevates circulating catecholamines increasing lipolysis and the breakdown of intramuscular triglycerides (IMTG). This increases the release of free fatty acids within muscle, activating the nuclear transcription factor peroxisome proliferator-activated receptor delta (PPARδ), which controls the expression of key metabolic regulatory genes including fatty acid transporters (FAT/CD36 and CPT-I), and negative regulators of carbohydrate metabolism (PDK4). Figure created with https://biorender.com/ (licenced version)

exercise on the subsequent morning. Acute exercise studies have demonstrated greater increases in the "sleep low" model relative to a fed control in the messenger RNA (mRNA) expression of regulators of the carbohydrate and lipid metabolic pathways, including pyruvate dehydrogenase kinase (PDK) 4 (2, 32, 48, 52), hexokinase (HK) II (48), glucose transporter (GLUT) 4 (61), and lipid transporters FAT/CD36 and fatty acid binding protein (FABP) 3 (32). Additionally, signalling cascades linked to training adaptation were also upregulated, with "sleep low" protocols increasing phosphorylation of p38 MAPK (15) and p53 (2), AMPK activity and downstream signalling (32, 61, 65), AMPKα2 nuclear localization (61), and the expression of PGC-1α and COXIV (32, 52). Perhaps as a result of the greater perturbation to intracellular homeostasis induced by the "sleep low" model, chronic studies employing this paradigm have demonstrated an improvement in both running (38) and cycling (39) performance following 1–3 weeks of training, at least in sub-elite athletes, whereas merely training in the overnight fasted state ("train low") yielded similar results to the carbohydrate-fed controls (43, 51). Collectively, these findings suggest that in order to augment training adaptation and maximize the cellular response to exercise, it is critically important to deplete skeletal muscle glycogen content.

Periodized Carbohydrate Availability

There are a number of explanations for the failure of early studies involving "train low" strategies (27, 66) to find consistent evidence of a superior performance outcome despite greater cellular adaptations. Issues with study methodology (e.g., the difficulty of measuring performance with real-world significance; inconsistency between protocols that clamped training loads vs. protocols that allowed athletes to train as hard as possible) could partly explain this "disconnect" between mechanistic and performance outcomes. More importantly, however, since these protocols implemented "train low" in all sessions or all of the key (high-intensity) sessions in the training programme, benefits due to enhanced adaptation may have been negated by the observed reductions (7–8%) in quality/intensity of these sessions (27, 66). This suggests that "train low" strategies need to be carefully integrated into the periodized training programme to match the specific goal of the session and the larger goals of the training period.

The evolution of the "sleep low" strategy in which the delay in restoration of glycogen during post-exercise recovery is able to upregulate markers of mitochondrial biogenesis and lipid oxidation offers a number of practical advantages for athletes. First, it can be implemented after the completion of a high-intensity training session that is optimally supported by strategies to achieve high carbohydrate availability, without interfering with the quality of performance goals of that session. Second, it sets up conditions for the next training bout to be undertaken with low glycogen content (preferably, a moderate-intensity session), thus allowing the athlete, coach, and sports scientist to work together to develop intuitive sequences of training and nutrition strategies that amplify the different requirements and goals of each session. Indeed, as identified previously, superior training adaptation and performance outcomes have recently been reported when three cycles of this sequence were introduced into the weekly training programmes of sub-elite athletes over both a 3-week (38) and 1-week (39) period of observation. In these studies, benefits were seen with this periodized approach to carbohydrate availability, which were not observed in another group who undertook similar training with a similar but evenly distributed carbohydrate intake. These studies provide encouraging evidence that a range of "train high" and "train low" strategies could be individually integrated into the athlete's training programme to amplify the desired adaptation and performance outcomes. Such an approach has been described in case studies of the preparation of elite endurance athletes (62), and a recent review of the terminology and intention of the various types of manipulation of carbohydrate availability has been prepared to better identify the suitability of different strategies (10).

It is of some interest that studies involving elite athletes show that they may be less responsive to periodization of carbohydrate availability than their sub-elite counterparts. An investigation of a 3-week programme of intensified training in world-class race walkers failed to detect any difference in the immediate performance benefits achieved by the group who consumed a periodized carbohydrate diet and another group who consumed the same total carbohydrate intake but evenly spread to promote high carbohydrate availability for all training sessions (13). Another study of elite endurance athletes reported no benefits to training adaptation or performance gains from the integration of a within-day sequence of a high-quality "train high"/"sleep (recover) low"/moderate-intensity "train low" protocol 3 days a week compared with a diet providing more consistent carbohydrate availability (19). It is therefore uncertain whether the observed lack of additional benefits is systematically related to the calibre of the athlete. For example, it is possible that a reduced ceiling for improvements makes differences harder to detect (e.g., athletes are already world-class and therefore performance improvements are likely to be small). Elite athletes may also maintain an ability to undertake intensified training where the stimulus already maximizes the adaptive response (30) and depletes carbohydrate stores even in the face of high-carbohydrate intakes around training, such that the actual differential between a diet with high or periodized carbohydrate availability is reduced (13). Further investigation is therefore merited.

Low-Carbohydrate, High-Fat Diets

While restriction of carbohydrate provision represents one way of modulating energy provision and adaptation, it has also been promoted as a strategy to maximize sports performance (42, 64). Indeed, the short-term consumption of a LCHF diet can result in a similar metabolic adaptation to training in terms of increased rates of fat oxidation and glycogen sparing (9, 14, 47), and as a result, this has become a popular strategy explored both in the literature and in the practical setting by athletes (7, 8).

Unfortunately, a growing body of evidence has shown negative effects of a short-term (5–7 days) LCHF diet on exercise performance. Several studies have demonstrated a decrease in metabolic flexibility across a range of sub-maximal intensities as shown by impaired ability to utilize glycogen (9, 14, 20, 31), which has been attributed to decreased glycogenolysis (63). Furthermore, a consistent side effect of a LCHF diet is a decrease in total resting muscle glycogen levels (59), which in and of itself can result in a decrease in glycogen utilization (22). While this may be beneficial for signalling, as outlined earlier, work by Stellingwerff et al. demonstrated that even when a carbohydrate restoration period was employed to maintain resting glycogen, the activation of pyruvate dehydrogenase (PDH) was lower during cycling at 70% $VO_{2\,peak}$ despite similar increases in allosteric activators of the enzyme (63). As PDH represents the rate-limiting step for entry of carbohydrate-derived substrate into the mitochondria and the subsequent production of reducing equivalents by the tricarboxylic acid (TCA) cycle and ATP by the electron transport chain (ETC) (58), this has profound implications for overall energy production during endurance exercise. Furthermore, these authors also showed a decrease in muscle glycogenolysis in the LCHF condition, along with impaired capacity to exercise in a simulated sprint at 150% of peak power output, which has real-world implications for the ability to produce power in race-deciding situations (63).

Recent investigations have also looked at the effects of longer (3-week) LCHF interventions in world-class athletes. In the study by Burke and co-workers in elite race-walkers (13), the effect of a LCHF diet (<50 g carbohydrate per day, 78% of EI as fat) was compared with a high (8.6 g·kg⁻¹ BM carbohydrate) or periodized carbohydrate diet, where macronutrient intake was identical but periodized within or between days to alternate between low and high carbohydrate availability. While all three groups displayed similar improvements in VO_{2peak} over the 3 weeks of intensified training, only the high and periodized carbohydrate groups improved their 10,000 m race times. In contrast, there was no difference in the LCHF race performance; this was attributed, at least in part, to an observed decrease in exercise economy such that walking at race pace occurred at a higher absolute oxygen cost, negating the increase in their VO_{2peak} and preventing them from capitalizing on their training-based improvements in aerobic capacity.

While these results strongly suggest a LCHF diet is not beneficial for performance of endurance exercise undertaken at high relative intensities, one outstanding question is whether the impairments are driven by low carbohydrate or rather by the increase in fat, as both variables are manipulated simultaneously. To answer this question, Leckey et al. (33) compared the metabolic responses to exercise in trained cyclists consuming a 5-day high-carbohydrate diet, followed by either a 5-day high-fat (>65% EI) or high-protein (>65%) diet during which the carbohydrate was clamped at <20% EI. They demonstrated that high dietary fat, rather than low carbohydrate, contributed to impairments in mitochondrial respiration, despite no changes in mitochondrial protein content. Interestingly, this impairment in mitochondrial respiration was reversed with 1 day of carbohydrate restoration, suggesting transient modifications to the mitochondria or the electron transport chain proteins themselves. These biochemical findings are supported by work performed by Skovbro et al. (57) utilizing a longer (16-day) LCHF diet with a similar macronutrient breakdown (~55–60% fat, 25–30% carbohydrate, 10–15% protein). They demonstrated impaired ADP-driven mitochondrial respiration in the LCHF condition post-exercise compared to baseline (57). Critically, these experiments utilized substrates that would circumvent PDH from entering the TCA cycle and were performed with saturating ADP, which should promote flux through other rate-limiting enzymes (i.e., NADH and $FADH_2$ producing steps within the TCA cycle). Therefore, it appears that in addition to impairing flux through PDH, the LCHF diet may induce an intrinsic change in mitochondrial function either within the TCA cycle or within the electron transport chain itself.

Emerging Topics and Future Directions

Research in the last decade has demonstrated that glycogen may mediate some of the adaptive response to training. As a result, dietary guidelines for athletic performance have moved away from a one-size-fits-all approach of completing all sessions and competition in a carbohydrate-loaded state to one that promotes manipulation of carbohydrate availability on a day-to-day, meal-by-meal basis according to the intensity, duration, and goals of each individual session. Furthermore, while there is now a wealth of research focusing on manipulation of nutrient intake and the resulting impact on performance, more recently there has been a growing interest in whether a specific "glycogen threshold" that intracellular contents must fall below exists, in order to augment the exercise-induced signalling responses and accumulation of mRNA of targeted genes (28). Well-designed studies are therefore required both to determine the acute effects of exercise on cell signalling at a variety of glycogen levels and to determine what effects this has chronically in adaptation and, ultimately, performance. Additionally, research has demonstrated that provision of carbohydrate between training sessions attenuates the oxidative adaptation to training in a glycogen-depleted state (41, 49). For both athletic populations and practitioners, it would be useful to determine whether there is a minimum time frame for restriction, and therefore more research in this area is warranted. Finally, it remains unclear why increases in cell signalling, as a result of nutritional interventions such as training in an overnight fasted condition, do not translate into improvements in performance. To date much of the research has focused on relatively few pathways (i.e., AMPK); therefore, technological advances and increased access to "-omics"-based techniques may elucidate novel targets and pathways that are key to adaptation (25).

References

1. Akerstrom TCA, Birk JB, Klein DK, Erikstrup C, Plomgaard P, Pedersen BK, Wojtaszewski JFP. Oral glucose ingestion attenuates exercise-induced activation of 5′-AMP-activated protein kinase in human skeletal muscle. *Biochem Biophys Res Commun* 342: 949–955, 2006.
2. Bartlett JD, Louhelainen J, Iqbal Z, Cochran AJ, Gibala MJ, Gregson W, et al. Reduced carbohydrate availability enhances exercise-induced p53 signaling in human skeletal muscle: Implications for mitochondrial biogenesis. *Am J Physiol - Regul Integr Comp Physiol* 304: 450–458, 2013.
3. Bergström J, Hermansen L. Diet, muscle glycogen and physical performance. *Acta Physiol Scand* 71: 140–150, 1967.
4. Bergström J, Hultman E. Muscle glycogen synthesis after exercise: An enhancing factor localized to the muscle cells in man. *Nature* 210: 309–310, 1966.

5. De Bock K, Derave W, Eijnde BO, Hesselink MK, Koninckx E, Rose AJ, et al. Effect of training in the fasted state on metabolic responses during exercise with carbohydrate intake. *J Appl Physiol* 104: 1045–1055, 2008.

6. Boraston AB, Bolam DN, Gilbert HJ, Davies GJ. Carbohydrate-binding modules: Fine-tuning polysaccharide recognition. *Biochem J* 382: 769–781, 2004.

7. Burke LM. Re-examining high-fat diets for sports performance: Did we call the 'nail in the coffin' too sSoon? *Sport Med* 45: 33–49, 2015.

8. Burke LM. Ketogenic low CHO, high fat diet: The future of elite endurance sport? *J. Physiol* 2020. doi: https://doi.org/10.1113/JP278928.

9. Burke LM, Angus DJ, Cox GR, Cummings NK, Febbraio MA, Gawthorn K, et al. Effect of fat adaptation and carbohydrate restoration on metabolism and performance during prolonged cycling. *J Appl Physiol* 89: 2413–2421, 2000.

10. Burke LM, Hawley JA, Jeukendrup A, Morton JP, Stellingwerff T, Maughan RJ. Toward a common understanding of diet-exercise strategies to manipulate fuel availability for training and competition preparation in endurance sport. *Int J Sport Nutr Exerc Metab* 28: 451–463, 2018.

11. Burke LM, Jones AM, Jeukendrup AE, Mooses M. Contemporary nutrition strategies to optimize performance in distance runners and race walkers. *Int J Sport Nutr Exerc Metab* 29: 117–129, 2019.

12. Burke LM, Kiens B, Ivy JL. Carbohydrates and fat for training and recovery. *J Sports Sci* 22: 15–30, 2004.

13. Burke LM, Ross ML, Garvican-Lewis LA, Welvaert M, Heikura IA, Forbes SG, et al. Low carbohydrate, high fat diet impairs exercise economy and negates the performance benefit from intensified training in elite race walkers. *J Physiol* 595: 2785–2807, 2017.

14. Carey AL, Staudacher HM, Cummings NK, Stepto NK, Nikolopoulos V, Burke LM, et al. Effects of fat adaptation and carbohydrate restoration on prolonged endurance exercise. *J Appl Physiol* 91: 115–122, 2001.

15. Chan MHS, McGee SL, Watt MJ, Hargreaves M, Febbraio MA. Altering dietary nutrient intake that reduces glycogen content leads to phosphorylation of nuclear p38 MAP kinase in human skeletal muscle: Association with IL-6 gene transcription during contraction. *FASEB J* 18: 1785–1787, 2004.

16. Cochran AJR, Little JP, Tarnopolsky MA, Gibala MJ. Carbohydrate feeding during recovery alters the skeletal muscle metabolic response to repeated sessions of high-intensity interval exercise in humans. *J Appl Physiol* 108: 628–636, 2010.

17. Coyle EF. Physical activity as a metabolic stressor. *Am J Clin Nutr* 72: 512S–520S, 2000.

18. Gaitanos GC, Williams C, Boobis LH, Brooks S. Human muscle metabolism during intermittent maximal exercise. *J Appl Physiol* 75: 712–719, 1993.

19. Gejl KD, Thams LB, Hansen M, Rokkedal-Lausch T, Plomgaard P, Nybo L, et al. No superior adaptations to carbohydrate periodization in elite endurance athletes. *Med Sci Sports Exerc* 49: 2486–2497, 2017.

20. Goedecke JH, Christie C, Wilson G, Dennis SC, Noakes TD, Hopkins WG, et al. Metabolic adaptations to a high-fat diet in endurance cyclists. *Metabolism* 48: 1509–1517, 1999.

21. Hansen AK, Fischer CP, Plomgaard P, Andersen JL, Saltin B, Pedersen BK. Skeletal muscle adaptation: Training twice every second day vs. training once daily. *J Appl Physiol* 98: 93–99, 2005.

22. Hargreaves M, Hawley JA, Jeukendrup A. Pre-exercise carbohydrate and fat ingestion: Effects on metabolism and performance. *J Sports Sci* 22: 31–38, 2004.

23. Hawley JA. Adaptations of skeletal muscle to prolonged, intense endurance training. *Clin Exp Pharmacol Physiol* 29: 218–222, 2002.

24. Hawley JA, Leckey JJ. Carbohydrate dependence during prolonged, intense endurance exercise. *Sport Med* 45: 5–12, 2015.

25. Hoffman NJ. Omics and exercise: Global approaches for mapping exercise biological networks. *Cold Spring Harb Perspect Med* 7: a029884, 2017.

26. Holloszy JO. Biochemical adaptations in muscle. Effects of exercise on mitochondrial oxygen uptake and respiratory enzyme activity in skeletal muscle. *J Biol Chem* 242: 2278–2282, 1967.

27. Hulston CJ, Venables MC, Mann CH, Martin C, Philp A, Baar K, et al. Training with low muscle glycogen enhances fat metabolism in well-trained cyclists. *Med Sci Sports Exerc* 42: 2046–2055, 2010.

28. Impey SG, Hearris MA, Hammond KM, Bartlett JD, Louis J, Close GL, et al. Fuel for the work required: A theoretical framework for carbohydrate periodization and the glycogen threshold hypothesis. *Sport Med* 48: 1031–1048, 2018.

29. Janzen NR, Whitfield J, Hoffman NJ. Interactive roles for AMPK and glycogen from cellular energy sensing to exercise metabolism. *Int J Mol Sci* 19: 3344, 2018.

30. Jensen L, Gejl KD, Ørtenblad N, Nielsen JL, Bech RD, Nygaard T, et al. Carbohydrate restricted recovery from long term endurance exercise does not affect gene responses involved in mitochondrial biogenesis in highly trained athletes. *Physiol Rep* 3: e12184, 2015.

31. Lambert E V, Speechly DP, Dennis SC, Noakes TD. Enhanced endurance in trained cyclists during moderate intensity exercise following 2 weeks adaptation to a high fat diet. *Eur J Appl Physiol Occup Physiol* 69: 287–293, 1994.

32. Lane SC, Camera DM, Lassiter DG, Areta JL, Bird SR, Yeo WK, et al. Effects of sleeping with reduced carbohydrate availability on acute training responses. *J Appl Physiol* 119: 643–655, 2015.

33. Leckey JJ, Hoffman NJ, Parr EB, Devlin BL, Trewin AJ, Stepto NK, et al. High dietary fat intake increases fat oxidation and reduces skeletal muscle mitochondrial respiration in trained humans. *FASEB J* 32: 2979–2991, 2018.

34. Lee-Young RS, Palmer MJ, Linden KC, LePlastrier K, Canny BJ, Hargreaves M, et al. Carbohydrate ingestion does not alter skeletal muscle AMPK signaling during exercise in humans. *Am J Physiol - Endocrinol Metab* 291: 566–573, 2006.

35. van Loon LJC, Greenhaff PL, Constantin-Teodosiu D, Saris WHM, Wagenmakers AJM. The effects of increasing exercise intensity on muscle fuel utilisation in humans. *J Physiol* 536: 295–304, 2001.

36. Low SY, Rennie MJ, Taylor PM. Modulation of glycogen synthesis in rat skeletal muscle by changes in cell volume. *J Physiol* 495: 299–303, 1996.

37. Mahoney DJ, Parise G, Melov S, Safdar A, Tarnopolsky MA. Analysis of global mRNA expression in human skeletal muscle during recovery from endurance exercise. *FASEB J* 19: 1498–1500, 2005.

38. Marquet LA, Brisswalter J, Louis J, Tiollier E, Burke LM, Hawley JA, et al. Enhanced endurance performance by periodization of carbohydrate intake: "Sleep Low" strategy. *Med Sci Sports Exerc* 48: 663–672, 2016.

39. Marquet LA, Hausswirth C, Molle O, Hawley JA, Burke LM, Tiollier E, et al. Periodization of carbohydrate intake: Short-term effect on performance. *Nutrients* 8: 755, 2016.

40. Mathai AS, Bonen A, Benton CR, Robinson DL, Graham TE. Rapid exercise-induced changes in PGC-1α mRNA and protein in human skeletal muscle. *J Appl Physiol* 105: 1098–1105, 2008.

41. Morton JP, Croft L, Bartlett JD, MacLaren DPM, Reilly T, Evans L, et al. Reduced carbohydrate availability does not modulate training-induced heat shock protein adaptations but does upregulate oxidative enzyme activity in human skeletal muscle. *J Appl Physiol* 106: 1513–1521, 2009.

42. Noakes T, Volek JS, Phinney SD. Low-carbohydrate diets for athletes: What evidence? *Br J Sports Med* 48: 1077–1078, 2014.

43. Nybo L, Pedersen K, Christensen B, Aagaard P, Brandt N, Kiens B. Impact of carbohydrate supplementation during endurance training on glycogen storage and performance. *Acta Physiol* 197: 117–127, 2009.

44. Olsson K - E, Saltin B. Variation in total body water with muscle glycogen changes in man. *Acta Physiol Scand* 80: 11–18, 1970.

45. Parolin ML, Chesley A, Matsos MP, Spriet LL, Jones NL, Heigenhauser GJ. Regulation of skeletal muscle glycogen phosphorylase and PDH during maximal intermittent exercise. *Am J Physiol* 277: E890–E900, 1999.

46. Perry CGR, Lally J, Holloway GP, Heigenhauser GJF, Bonen A, Spriet LL. Repeated transient mRNA bursts precede increases in transcriptional and mitochondrial proteins during training in human skeletal muscle. *J Physiol* 588: 4795–4810, 2010.

47. Phinney SD, Bistrian BR, Evans WJ, Gervino E, Blackburn GL. The human metabolic response to chronic ketosis without caloric restriction: Preservation of submaximal exercise capability with reduced carbohydrate oxidation. *Metabolism* 32: 769–776, 1983.

48. Pilegaard H, Keller C, Steensberg A, Helge JW, Pedersen BK, Saltin B, et al. Influence of pre-exercise muscle glycogen content on exercise-induced transcriptional regulation of metabolic genes. *J Physiol* 541: 261–271, 2002.

49. Pilegaard H, Osada T, Andersen LT, Helge JW, Saltin B, Neufer PD. Substrate availability and transcriptional regulation of metabolic genes in human skeletal muscle during recovery from exercise. *Metabolism* 54: 1048–1055, 2005.

50. Pogozelski AR, Geng T, Li P, Yin X, Lira VA, Zhang M, et al. p38γ mitogen-activated protein kinase is a key regulator in skeletal muscle metabolic adaptation in mice. *PLOS ONE* 4: e7934, 2009.

51. Van Proeyen K, Szlufcik K, Nielens H, Ramaekers M, Hespel P. Beneficial metabolic adaptations due to endurance exercise training in the fasted state. *J Appl Physiol* 110: 236–245, 2011.

52. Psilander N, Frank P, Flockhart M, Sahlin K. Exercise with low glycogen increases PGC-1α gene expression in human skeletal muscle. *Eur J Appl Physiol* 113: 951–963, 2013.

53. Romijn J, Gastaldelli A, Horowitz J, Endert E, Wolfe R. Regulation of endogenous fat and carbohydrate metabolism in relation to exercise intensity and duration. *Am J Physiol* 265: 380–391, 1993.

54. Rose AJ, Richter EA. Skeletal muscle glucose uptake during exercise: How is it regulated? *Physiology* 20: 260–270, 2005.

55. Schrauwen-Hinderling VB, Hesselink MKC, Schrauwen P, Kooi ME. Intramyocellular lipid content in human skeletal muscle. *Obesity* 14: 357–367, 2006.

56. Sheikh-Hamad D, Gustin MC. MAP kinases and the adaptive response to hypertonicity: Functional preservation from yeast to mammals. *Am J Physiol - Ren Physiol* 287: F1102–F1110, 2004.

57. Skovbro M, Boushel R, Hansen CN, Helge JW, Dela F. High-fat feeding inhibits exercise-induced increase in mitochondrial respiratory flux in skeletal muscle. *J Appl Physiol* 110: 1607–1614, 2011.

58. Spriet LL, Heigenhauser GJF. Regulation of pyruvate dehydrogenase (PDH) activity in human skeletal muscle during exercise. *Exerc Sport Sci Rev* 30: 91–95, 2002.

59. Starling RD, Trappe TA, Parcell AC, Kerr CG, Fink WJ, Costill DL. Effects of diet on muscle triglyceride and endurance performance. *J Appl Physiol* 82: 1185–1189, 1997.

60. Steensberg A, Van Hall G, Keller C, Osada T, Schjerling P, Pedersen BK, et al. Muscle glycogen content and glucose uptake during exercise in humans: Influence of prior exercise and dietary manipulation. *J Physiol* 541: 273–281, 2002.

61. Steinberg GR, Watt MJ, McGee SL, Chan S, Hargreaves M, Febbraio MA, et al. Reduced glycogen availability is associated with increased AMPKα2 activity, nuclear AMPKα2 protein abundance, and GLUT4 mRNA expression in contracting human skeletal muscle. *Appl Physiol Nutr Metab* 31: 302–312, 2006.

62. Stellingwerff T. Contemporary nutrition approaches to optimize elite marathon performance. *Int J Sports Physiol Perform* 8: 573–578, 2013.

63. Stellingwerff T, Spriet LL, Watt MJ, Kimber NE, Hargreaves M, Hawley JA, et al. Decreased PDH activation and glycogenolysis during exercise following fat adaptation with carbohydrate restoration. *Am J Physiol Metab* 290: E380–E388, 2006.

64. Volek JS, Noakes T, Phinney SD. Rethinking fat as a fuel for endurance exercise. *Eur J Sport Sci* 15: 13–20, 2015.

65. Wojtaszewski JFP, MacDonald C, Nielsen JN, Hellsten Y, Hardie DG, Kemp BE, et al. Regulation of 5'AMP-activated protein kinase activity and substrate utilization in exercising human skeletal muscle. *Am J Physiol Metab* 284: E813–E822, 2003.

66. Yeo WK, Paton CD, Garnham AP, Burke LM, Carey AL, Hawley JA. Skeletal muscle adaptation and performance responses to once a day versus twice every second day endurance training regimens. *J Appl Physiol* 105: 1462–1470, 2008.

20

DIETARY INFLUENCE ON MUSCLE PROTEIN SYNTHESIS AND HYPERTROPHY

James McKendry and Stuart M. Phillips

Glossary of terms

4E-BP1	Eukaryotic translation initiation factor 4E-binding protein 1
AA	Amino acids
AMP	Adenosine monophosphate
AMPK	Adenosine monophosphate-activated protein kinase
ATP	Adenosine triphosphate
BCAA	Branched chain amino acid
Ca2+	Calcium
CaM	Calmodulin
DGKζ	Diacylglycerol kinase ζ
EAA	Essential amino acid
eEF2k	Eukaryotic elongation factor 2 kinase
eIF4E	Eukaryotic initiation factor 4E
ER	Endoplasmic reticulum
ERK	Extra-cellular regulated pathway
FAK	Focal adhesion kinase
FKBP12	FK506-binding protein
GATOR 1	Gap Activity TOward Rags 1
GATOR 2	Gap Activity TOward Rags 2
GDP	Guanosine diphosphate
GTP	Guanosine triphosphate
GTPase	Guanosine triphosphatase
HMB	β-hydroxy-β-methylbutyrate
IGF-1	Insulin-like growth factor 1
LAT-1	L-Type amino acid transporter 1
LeuRS	Leucyl-tRNA synthetase
MAPK	Mitogen-activated protein kinase
MPB	Muscle protein breakdown
MPS	Muscle protein synthesis
mRNA	Messenger ribonucleic acid
mTORC1	Mechanistic target of rapamycin complex 1

mTORC2	Mechanistic target of rapamycin complex 2
n-3PUFA	Long chain n-3 polyunsaturated fatty acids
NBAL	Muscle net protein balance
NEAA	Non-essential amino acid
p70S6K1	Ribosomal protein S6 kinase 1
PA	Phosphatidic acid
PI3-K	Phosphoinositide 3-kinase
PKB or Akt	Protein kinase B
Raptor	regulatory-associated protein of mTOR
RDA	Recommended dietary allowance
RE	Resistance exercise
RET	Resistance exercise training
REDD1	Regulated in DNA damage and development 1
Rheb	Ras homolog enriched in brain
RNA	Ribonucleic acid
RPS6	Ribosomal protein S6
Thr	Threonine
TOR1	Target of rapamycin 1
TOR2	Target of rapamycin 2
tRNA	Transfer ribonucleic acid
TSC1/2	Tuberous sclerosis 1/2
v-ATPase	Vacuolar H+–adenosine triphosphatase ATPase
VPS34	Human vacuolar protein sorting 34

General Introduction

Skeletal muscle constitutes ~40% of total body mass and plays a critical role in a multitude of mechanical and metabolic functions. Specifically, muscle serves as the principal site for amino acid (AA) storage, contributes (due to its mass) to basal metabolism, and enables locomotion and athletic performance by way of contractile activity (41). Moreover, skeletal muscle mass is, in certain situations, related to all-cause mortality (99). The size and quality of skeletal muscle decline with advancing age, which increases the risk of disease development and mobility impairment (22). Accordingly, the development, and conservation, of skeletal muscle throughout the lifespan with appropriate lifestyle habits should be a principal focus for individuals looking to maximize athletic performance and enhance quality of life with age. Skeletal muscle is a highly plastic tissue, the malleability of which involves the sensing of internal and external signals and orchestrating an appropriate adaptive response. Significant progress has been made in the field of skeletal muscle protein metabolism. As such, skeletal muscle turnover is regulated by two intricately controlled processes, muscle protein synthesis (MPS) and muscle protein breakdown (MPB) (88). The balance between these two processes determines whether skeletal muscle is built (hypertrophy) or lost (atrophy). Importantly, MPS, and to some extent MPB, can be modified by a number of physiological and environmental stimuli.

Nutrition, in particular protein, is a crucial determinant in skeletal muscle mass regulation. For the purpose of this chapter, we will focus predominantly on the influence of protein nutrition to modulate MPS, though other macronutrients and nutraceuticals will be discussed. We will examine the molecular mechanisms that dictate skeletal muscle mass, and crucially how they can be modified by nutrition. First, we will highlight seminal studies regarding nutritional influences on muscle mass regulation. Thereafter, we describe the current understanding and propose an optimal strategy for maximizing MPS and lastly where the future of this fascinating area of research may be heading.

Regulation of Skeletal Muscle Mass: Protein Turnover

The regulation of skeletal muscle mass has been the subject of concentrated scientific attention for ~40 years. Much of what is known about how humans regulate skeletal muscle mass can be attributed to the development, and utilization, of stable isotopically labelled tracers [for extensive reviews see (64, 109)]. Skeletal muscle mass is determined by the balance of MPS and MPB. Both are dynamic in nature and continuously fluctuate in order to synthesize new muscle proteins (MPS) and facilitate the removal of damaged (i.e., through oxidation or mechanical damage) or dysfunctional (i.e., through misfolding) proteins (MPB). Put simply, in situations where MPS exceeds MPB, the muscle net protein balance (NBAL = MPS – MPB) is positive and a small amount of new muscle protein is added to skeletal muscle, increasing the total protein pool size. On the other hand, when MPB exceeds MPS, the result is a negative muscle NBAL and protein is lost from skeletal muscle. The relative rates of these processes are slow, at least by comparison to other tissues, and skeletal muscle protein turnover occurs at a rate of ~1.5% each day (108). During periods of fasting, MPS is reduced and skeletal muscle remains in a state of negative NBAL. In response to feeding there is a transient increase in MPS and a small suppression of MPB, both lasting a few hours (dependent on meal size and other factors). Thus, muscle protein turnover exhibits a fluctuating pattern in response to feeding and fasting throughout the day, and in healthy adults the total muscle protein pool remains relatively constant.

Protein feeding is one nutritional strategy that has been shown to modulate MPS (Figure 20.1). The late Professor Mike Rennie and colleagues carried out the first human investigation utilizing stable isotope methodology and demonstrated the rate of incorporation of ^{13}C-leucine into skeletal muscle was increased following protein feeding when compared with fasting (77, 89). Numerous studies have since been undertaken to investigate the impact of activity (79), inactivity (12, 14, 73), ageing (15), and feeding (5, 81) on the regulation of skeletal muscle mass. As a result, it is now widely accepted that resistance exercise (RE) is a potent stimulator of MPS (12, 70). In response to RE performed in a fasted state, despite an increase in MPS, muscle NBAL is reduced (i.e., less negative) but remains negative

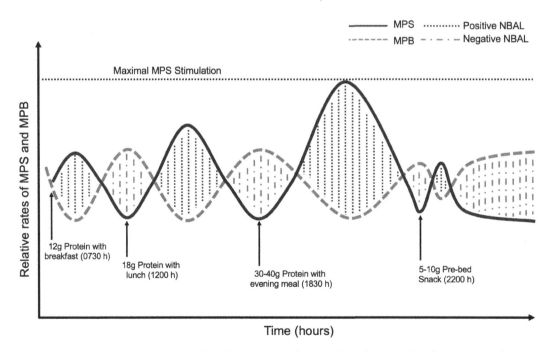

Figure 20.1 Schematic representation of muscle protein synthesis and muscle protein breakdown throughout a typical daily protein feeding pattern [redrawn with permission from (84)]

as MPB also increases (88). For muscle NBAL to become positive, RE should be followed by protein ingestion leading to elevated blood AAs (hyperaminoacidemia) to stimulate MPS (113). Eventually, persistent practice of RE and protein ingestion leads to skeletal muscle hypertrophy (23, 82), emphasizing the central role that protein nutrition plays in regulating MPS. Conversely, methodological difficulties of assessing MPB in humans (105) make it far less thoroughly explored. MPB remains largely unchanged during most situations, excluding those of extreme stress (i.e., cancer cachexia, burn injury), and the role of MPB appears permissive for skeletal muscle mass regulation during most circumstances. Nevertheless, the small fluctuations in MPB facilitate the removal of damaged proteins and this contributes AAs for the synthesis of new functional proteins (27). Interestingly, the efficiency of this process is high, and so AAs released into the free pool due to MPB are efficiently reutilized (>80%) for MPS. Therefore, while MPB is undoubtedly important, the changes in MPS, and the focus of this chapter, will be the factors that affect MPS as it is in response to nutritional influences.

Molecular Mechanisms Underpinning Muscle Protein Synthesis

The process that leads from a mechanical stimulus of contraction to MPS is extraordinarily complex and well-orchestrated. Molecular exercise physiologists have made substantial progress determining how signals are sensed, transduced, and ultimately result in MPS being stimulated to promote an adaptive response. The ribosome is an essential RNA-containing-protein complex which directly facilitates the translation of messenger RNA (mRNA) to a polypeptide AA chain. First, translational efficiency specifically refers to the protein synthesis rate per ribosome/unit of mRNA. Typically, acute increases in the rates of protein synthesis are attributed to the activation of pre-existing translational machinery and thus increased efficiency (24), whereas translational capacity is determined by the total amount of translational machinery per unit of tissue (including ribosomal subunits 40s and 60s, tRNAs, and translation factors). Much of the current understanding surrounding translational control of MPS is linked to the identification and examination of a key signalling protein, mechanistic target of rapamycin complex 1 (mTORC1), which serves as a central integration point for a number of physiological stimuli.

mTORC1: A Central Integration Point

The quest to unravel the complex control of important biological processes has been at the forefront of scientific research for many years. Following the discovery of rapamycin, in 1964 (93), a series of seminal studies utilized a genetic screen to identify genetic mutants (55) and determined that peptidyl-prolyl-isomerase FKBP12 was the cellular receptor for rapamycin (92). Furthermore, two targets of rapamycin (TOR) genes (TOR1 and TOR2) that encoded for two large kinases that resembled phosphoinositide 3-kinase (PI3-K) were identified (67), successfully pinpointing the biochemical mechanism of action. These significant breakthroughs paved the way for a plethora of research studies focused on TOR, and it is now understood that mTOR is an evolutionarily conserved serine/threonine kinase present in two structurally distinct protein complexes (i.e., mTORC1 and mTORC2). Both complexes play pivotal roles as integration hubs of numerous physiological stimuli. However, attention will be directed towards mTORC1-dependent mechanisms, as the role of this protein complex is the better characterized of the two protein complexes (68).

mTORC1: Activation

mTORC1 integrates several upstream signals, importantly AAs, growth factors, and mechanical stress. Typically, mTORC1 resides in the cell cytoplasm and plays a fundamental role in cell signalling and membrane trafficking (68). In order to become phosphorylated or "activated" mTORC1, two conditions must be met. First, translocation of mTORC1 to the lysosome (91), and second the interaction with the small guanosine triphosphatase (GTPase) Ras homolog enriched in brain (Rheb), while Rheb is in a

GTP-bound state. Rheb-mediated activation of mTORC1 is dictated by an upstream GTPase-activating protein, tuberous sclerosis complex 2 (TSC2) (4). TSC2 is particularly important, as its phosphorylation, predominantly by protein kinase b (PKB or Akt) and/or the mitogen-activated protein kinase (MAPK)/ extracellular signal-regulated kinase (ERK) pathway, initiates the translocation of TSC2 from the lysosomal membrane, which prevents the inhibitory effect on mTORC1 complexing with the lysosome. Inhibition of mTORC1 activity occurs when TSC2 binds to GTP and hydrolyzes it to form GDP, thus raising the ratio of GDP-Rheb to GTP-Rheb and subsequently quenches mTORC1 kinase activity (58). Recently, significant strides have been made towards unravelling the mechanisms through which mechanical stress and, crucially for this chapter, AAs influence mTORC1 kinase activity.

Mechanical stress, or skeletal muscle contraction, has repeatedly been shown to induce increases in mTORC1 activity and its downstream effectors. Yet identifying specific mechano-sensitive proteins has proved challenging. Nevertheless, candidates for mechanically induced mTORC1 activators have been put forward. The IGF-1 and ERK pathways have previously been implicated in the mechano-stimulation of mTORC1 activity, although controversial (47), and phosphatidic acid (PA), a glycerophospholipid, has been shown to directly bind to the FRB-domain of mTORC1 to augment its kinase activity (94). Another theory, possibly not at the mutual exclusion of the PA mechanism, is that focal adhesion kinase (FAK), an integrin protein located within the costameres of skeletal muscle, has been shown in numerous models to exhibit mechanically sensitive attributes (39, 48). Purportedly, FAK acts through TSC2-dependent abrogation of mTORC1 (20). Here, we briefly mention some purported mechanosensitive mTORC1 pathways, which are discussed in greater detail in Chapters 6, 8, and 10. Despite considerable efforts to decipher elusive mechano-sensitive proteins responsible for mTORC1 activity and subsequent increased MPS, this avenue of research remains in its infancy, but will no doubt yield new information with future investigations.

AAs are fundamental in driving increased MPS via mTORC1 activity, though, again, determining the mechanisms through which AAs drive increased rates of MPS has been somewhat elusive. Increased circulating concentrations of AAs following digestion and absorption of protein are transported into skeletal muscle. The L-type amino acid transporter 1 (LAT1) plays a vital role in transporting AAs, mainly the branched-chain amino acid (BCAA) leucine, into skeletal muscle (57). Once inside the muscle, AAs influence mTORC1 activity via conversion of the Rag GTPases (Rag A/B and Rag C/D) to a nucleotide-bound state and association with the Ragulator complex, which subsequently binds directly to Raptor and facilitates the recruitment of mTORC1 to the lysosomal surface, increasing mTORC1 kinase activity. Conversely, the absence of AAs results in mTORC1 dissociating from the lysosomal membrane, preventing the essential interactions with co-activators (69). AAs also augment mTORC1 activity via human vacuolar protein sorting 34 (VPS34) and a calcium (Ca^{2+})/calmodulin (CaM)−dependent interaction (51). Building on these important discoveries, mTORC1 has been shown to "sense" AAs through two distinct mechanisms: vacuolar H^+−adenosine triphosphatase ATPase (v-ATPase) (117) and GATOR 1−, GATOR 2−, and Sestrin2-mediated regulation (11, 25), both of which act via Rag GTPases and the Ragulator complex. Leucyl-tRNA synthetase (LeuRS) has been proposed as another candidate contributing to the AA sensing mechanism (61), though much work is still required to fully elucidate the AA-mediated mTORC1 activity.

The main focus of this chapter is the activation of anabolism by mTORC1; however, it is important to acknowledge that a number of signals may reduce mTORC1 activity. mTORC1 kinase activity is negatively regulated by intracellular and extracellular stressors that oppose growth-stimulating effects. These signals are primarily induced by exercise of significant intensity and duration. For example, energy stress and hypoxia can reduce adenosine triphosphate (ATP) concentrations to a small degree, but importantly increase the adenosine monophosphate (AMP) to ATP ratio. The result of the increased AMP/ATP ratio is an activation of SIRT1 and induction of endoplasmic reticulum (ER) stress (42). Following this, the phosphorylation of AMP-activated protein kinase (AMPK) and regulated in DNA damage and development 1 (REDD1) serve to phosphorylate and activate TSC2 attenuating mTORC1 activity (16, 52, 59). Thus, theoretically, energy stress and hypoxia may exert an inhibitory effect on mTORC1 and acute MPS responses to exercise (28), potentially hampering long-term muscle adaptations (56), though evidence to support an interference effect of this nature is lacking (42).

Downstream Signaling Targets of mTORC1

Activation of mTORC1 initiates a cascade of downstream signalling events that ultimately culminate in an increase in MPS (Figure 20.2). Ribosomal protein S6 kinase 1 (p70S6K1) and eukaryotic translation initiation factor 4E-binding protein 1 (4E-BP1) are currently the two best characterized downstream targets of mTORC1, both of which are paramount in the initiation and elongation in protein translation (68). A seminal study by Baar and Esser demonstrated that phosphorylation of p70S6K1 at 6 hours post-exercise was correlated with the extent of muscle hypertrophy over 6 weeks of electrically stimulated resistance exercise training (RET) (9). The phosphorylation of p70S6K1 and 4E-BP1 occurs rapidly and remains elevated for a number of hours following RE (35). Once phosphorylated by mTORC1 at Thr389, p70S6K1 phosphorylates further downstream effectors, including eukaryotic elongation factor 2 kinase (eEF2k) and ribosomal protein S6 (RPS6), which facilitate translational elongation (46) and ribosomal biogenesis (24), whereas 4E-BP1 is phosphorylated by mTORC1 at Thr37/46, causing dissociation from eukaryotic initiation factor 4E (eIF4E) complex and facilitates translation initiation (43). Thus, phosphorylation of p70S6K1 and 4E-BP1 regulate MPS through increased translational efficiency and signalling increases in translational capacity. p70S6K1 and 4E-BP1 are frequently used as proxy indicators of mTORC1 activity. However, acute increases in the phosphorylation status of intramuscular signalling proteins in humans are not always related to the degree of muscle hypertrophy over time (78, 79). Regardless, phosphorylation and activation of downstream targets of mTORC1 have provided important mechanistic insight into the molecular events that dictate the MPS response to various environmental stressors [i.e., RE (37) and AA provision (34)]. Thus, intramuscular signalling targets should continue to be incorporated within research to enhance our understanding of the molecular control surrounding MPS and muscle hypertrophy.

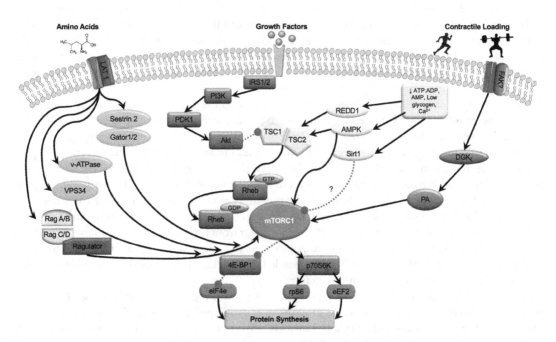

Figure 20.2 A schematic overview of the cellular signalling pathways regulating skeletal muscle protein synthesis in response to AAs, growth factors, and muscular contraction from endurance and resistance exercise

Skeletal Muscle Hypertrophy

Skeletal muscle hypertrophy specifically refers to the increase in size, through the addition of protein, of existing muscle fibres and thus whole muscle, without an increase in the fibre number. Hypertrophy is the consequence of cumulative periods of MPS exceeding MPB, leading to a positive muscle NBAL over time and thus net protein accretion. Exercise is the foundation, and nutrition plays a role in regulating skeletal muscle mass, and they act synergistically to promote increased MPS and muscle hypertrophy (113). RET has been repeatedly shown to elicit skeletal muscle hypertrophy, as demonstrated by a ~5–10% increase of muscle cross-sectional area following 10 weeks of RET (31), which is augmented to a mild degree with appropriate nutritional strategies such as increased protein consumption (23, 82). Increasing the abundance of muscle tissue provides significant athletic advantages and confers important protective benefits against disease development during periods of disuse and reduced physical activity with advancing age.

Dietary Components Influencing MPS

Since the early stable isotopic tracer studies (89), a considerable body of knowledge has accumulated examining nutritional influences on MPS, and protein nutrition is the most comprehensively studied. Dietary protein comprises a varying portion of daily macronutrient intake (usually 15–20% of total energy intake) and is essential for muscle function and growth. Following protein ingestion, the ensuing hyperaminoacidemia leads to an influx of AAs into muscle cells and a stimulation of MPS, the magnitude and duration of which can be influenced by a variety of factors (i.e., the dose, AA composition, source, distribution, and co-ingestion with other macronutrients).

Protein Dose – Individual Dose and Total Protein Intake

The amount of protein consumed is an important consideration for individuals looking to maintain or increase skeletal muscle mass. One might assume that MPS and muscle hypertrophy increase linearly with increasing protein intake; however, the process of MPS and hypertrophy appear to be dose-saturable. Moore and colleagues fed differing doses of protein following RE and showed that the magnitude of MPS increased in response to greater doses of egg protein up to a dose of 20 g, with no further rise in MPS even when the protein dose was doubled to 40 g (81). This suggests an upper limit exists for protein intake that the muscle could utilize and direct towards MPS in a single bolus. In further support of a ceiling response, 40 g of whey was no more effective than 20 g at stimulating MPS following RE (113). Therefore, on an individual protein feeding occasion, it appears that ~20 g of high-quality protein is sufficient to maximally stimulate MPS, which, in an 80-kg individual, equates to ~0.25 g/kg body mass, and doses above this amount lead to increased AA oxidation and urea production (113). More recently, following whole-body RE the consumption of 40 g compared with 20 g of whey protein conferred little additional benefit in augmenting MPS (~18%) (71). Thus, in most cases in young healthy individuals 20 g of high-quality protein is sufficient to maximize the MPS response. However, it has been shown that higher per-meal doses of protein (~0.4 g/kg) are required in older individuals to maximally stimulate MPS (80). It is also clear from the aforementioned studies that a high degree of interindividual variability in the responsiveness to a single dose of protein exists. Therefore, on a per meal/protein feeding basis, it is recommended that ~0.4 g/kg body mass be consumed in order to ensure that a maximal MPS response is attained.

Aside from physical activity, total daily protein intake is still regarded as the most significant contributor to muscle mass maintenance, or growth, over prolonged periods (101). Current guidelines suggest that the recommended dietary allowance (RDA) of protein for a healthy, non-diseased adult (>18 years) is equivalent to 0.8 g/kg/d (40). However, this represents the minimum amount required to maintain nitrogen balance (115), and not surprisingly up to ~35% of individuals in the United States consume less than the RDA (3). Existing protein intake recommendations are far from optimal when considering those individuals that adopt a highly active lifestyle or older individuals that display reduced physical activity and often experience situations of compromised mobility (21). Thus, an increased total protein intake to support muscle remodelling with exercise (62) or prevent losses with ageing is an advantageous strategy (63). A recent meta-analysis conducted by Morton and colleagues identified that a protein intake up to ~1.6 g/kg/d elicited significantly greater gains in muscle mass when combined with RET, and above this intake induced no further gains in muscle mass (82). Furthermore, consumption of a higher-protein diet (~1.2–1.6 g protein·kg^{-1} body mass·day^{-1}) is recommended for older individuals that may experience compromised sensitivity to protein feeding (87). Therefore, a total daily protein intake equivalent to two times the RDA appears favourable for skeletal muscle protein accretion, and beyond this amount of protein intake the benefits were inconsequential.

Essential and Non-essential Amino Acids

Broadly, AAs can be sub-divided into two distinct categories: those that cannot be endogenously synthesized *de novo* or nutritionally essential (or indispensable) AAs (EAA) and those that can be synthesized endogenously in adequate amounts or nutritionally non-essential (or dispensable) AAs (NEAA) (116). Stimulation of MPS in skeletal muscle is dictated by EAAs (97, 98, 103), whereas the impact of NEAAs on MPS was shown to be trivial (104). Thus, protein sources with a greater EAAs content are far superior (i.e., of greater quality) in terms of their capacity to stimulate MPS. Specifically, the BCAA leucine is the primary EAA that directly stimulates MPS (8, 30). The potency of leucine in stimulating the mTORC1 pathway and upregulating MPS has been consistently shown when compared with other AAs (38) and appears to saturate at ~ 3 g per meal serving (26). Rapidly digestible protein sources containing a high leucine content (i.e., milk proteins) are superior at stimulating MPS when compared with isonitrogenous and isoenergetic quantities of soy protein (112). Interestingly, however, it has been shown that leucine supplementation alone was not able increase skeletal muscle mass throughout an extended supplementation period in both rats and older humans (72, 107). This may suggest that when a single EAA (e.g., leucine) is provided in a sufficient quantity, additional leucine appears to confer no further benefit in stimulating MPS (44). Despite the fundamental role of leucine in stimulating MPS, the duration of the response eventually becomes limited due to the lowered availability of other EAAs (101). When sufficient leucine is provided in the presence of other EAAs the MPS response in skeletal muscle is enhanced and prolonged (7, 33, 83). Taken together, this suggests leucine as fundamental in "triggering" the MPS response (13), yet a full complement of EAAs may be required to maximize (i.e., sustain) the MPS response.

Protein Source

Current recommendations for protein intake suggest that consuming "high-quality" protein foods is key in ensuring sufficient provision of AAs for muscle maintenance or growth. For those looking to increase/maintain skeletal muscle mass, the incorporation of dietary protein sources that contain sufficient amounts of EAAs to stimulate MPS is of primary importance. Ingestion of milk-based protein has been shown to be superior when compared with ingestion of isonitrogenous soy protein beverage at stimulating MPS (112). Tang and colleagues demonstrated that whey and soy protein were both superior in stimulation of MPS when compared with casein protein both at rest and following RE (102), which holds true in older individuals (19). This is because the matrix in which protein is consumed and the specific method of preparation are factors that can significantly modify the digestibility of proteins and the postprandial rate of appearance of EAAs for MPS (29, 49). Moreover, the provision of a low dose of total protein can elicit the same maximal MPS response as a high protein dose when supplemented with additional leucine (26). Thus, the ability of a protein source to stimulate MPS is dictated by the quantity and availability of the EAAs, in particular, leucine. Crucially, the protein food source should match the requirement of the consumer (17); hence to maximally stimulate MPS post-ingestion, the protein source should be rapidly digestible and contain sufficient EAAs (specifically leucine).

Protein Distribution

In many cultures, dietary protein is commonly consumed in an uneven pattern throughout the day. Specifically, increasing amounts of protein are eaten with each subsequent meal (i.e., breakfast < lunch < dinner), and the amount of protein required to maximally stimulate MPS may only be consumed with one meal, usually in the evening (dinner) meal (85). The transient elevation in MPS following protein ingestion returns to basal after a few (~2–3) hours, and importantly, this occurs despite the continued availability of AAs in the circulation (6). Therefore, the development of protein feeding strategies that maximally stimulate the muscle building response repeatedly throughout the day may be of significant interest for those looking to maximize increases in, or retention of, skeletal muscle mass. More evenly distributing protein intake throughout the day could, theoretically, maximize the cumulative daily NBAL (Figure 20.3) (2). Currently, no guidelines exist that promote an evenly distributed protein intake for the enhancement of MPS for muscle mass growth/maintenance. However, Areta and colleagues showed that four meals at 20 g per meal of whey protein was superior in stimulating MPS over a 12-hour period when compared with two larger meals (2 × 40 g) or eight smaller (8 × 10 g) evenly distributed meals (2). In addition, a moderate amount of protein (~30 g) with each meal stimulated 24-hour MPS to a greater extent when compared with a distribution skewed towards the evening meal (73). Conversely, others suggest total protein intake and not meal-to-meal distribution has a greater influence on the 24-hour MPS response and that the impact of distribution pattern was negligible (63). Taken together, if a sufficient daily protein intake cannot be achieved, distributing protein intake throughout the day may offer a feasible solution to potentiate daily MPS.

Pre-sleep protein ingestion offers another timing-based feeding strategy that may be utilized to enhance MPS. Typically, during an overnight fast, MPB exceeds MPS, in all likelihood, for a period

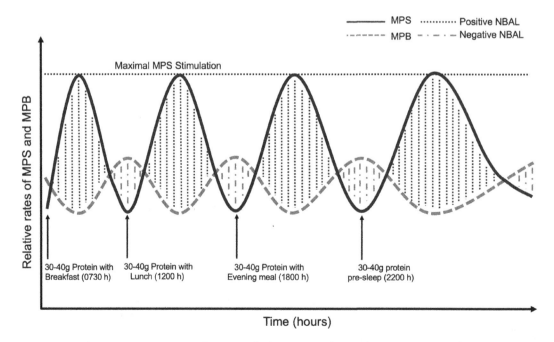

Figure 20.3 Schematic representation of a protein feeding pattern designed to maximize muscle protein synthesis and the muscle NBAL, subsequently facilitating skeletal muscle hypertrophy

of ~8 hours. Therefore, protein consumption in relatively close temporal proximity prior to sleep may help to mitigate some of the protein losses that occur overnight. The ingestion of a slower-digesting protein source (i.e., casein) prior to sleep may offer a useful strategy to provide EAAs over a prolonged time period to prevent a decline in MPS and enhance overall NBAL (106); however, thus far, there have been no comparisons between slow- and fast-digesting proteins to allow a conclusion to be made. Pre-sleep protein ingestion has been shown to significantly augment the overnight MPS response and whole-body protein balance (66, 90). As such, it appears the protein distribution, and in particular, pre-sleep protein ingestion, may play an important role in determining daily MPS response and total NBAL.

Carbohydrate and Other Nutraceutical Compounds

Protein ingestion is not the only nutritional strategy that has been investigated to influence MPS. Co-ingestion of carbohydrate with protein has been proposed as an approach to enhance MPS (45, 65, 100). Carbohydrate ingestion increases circulating insulin concentrations; however, in humans, the impact of elevated insulin concentrations on MPS appears permissive rather than stimulatory (1). Primarily, the role of insulin, rather than being stimulatory for MPS, is in suppressing MPB, independent of elevated circulating AAs (1). Greenhaff and colleagues showed that insulin influences muscle NBAL by suppressing MPB up to a moderate insulin concentration (50). Yet no further suppression occurs with greater circulating insulin concentrations. In further support of this premise, the addition of 50 g of carbohydrate to 25 g of whey protein was no more effective than protein alone at stimulating MPS (100). Thus, so long as sufficient protein is ingested, the addition of carbohydrate to protein feeding confers no significant benefit when aiming to increase MPS.

The pursuit to identify nutritional compounds capable of enhancing MPS has uncovered a plethora of candidates [for an extensive review see (32)]. Not surprisingly, β-hydroxy-β-methylbutyrate (HMB) a metabolite of leucine, has been shown to augment MPS to the same extent as leucine (110). Expectedly, HMB upregulates the mTORC1 pathway, and the increase in MPS has been shown to be equivalent to that typically seen with leucine alone or the ingestion of mixed meal. Interestingly, HMB ingestion also led to a suppression of MPB, the importance of which has yet to be determined. Previously, it has been shown that supplementation with HMB led to increased acute MPS and increased muscle mass (10). However, when compared with leucine, supplementation with HMB during 12 weeks of progressive RE resulted in equivalent increases in fat- and bone-free mass, muscle morphological alterations, and strength (60). Thus, leucine and its metabolite HMB, in combination with sufficient AAs and RE, provide sufficient substrate to increase MPS and muscle mass.

Fish oil supplementation, and specifically long-chain n-3 polyunsaturated fatty acids (n-3 PUFA), has recently garnered interest regarding its ability to promote muscle anabolism. Smith and colleagues demonstrated that, regardless of age, 8 weeks of supplementation with n-3 PUFA augmented the acute MPS response to a hyperinsulinemic-euglycemic clamp when compared with corn oil (95, 96). However, when combined with adequate protein nutrition, the addition of n-3 PUFA supplementation does not further potentiate the acute MPS response (75). Purportedly, n-3 PUFA supplementation enhances skeletal muscle anabolism via alterations in cell membrane composition, thus sensitizing skeletal muscle to anabolic stimuli. In healthy uncompromised persons, however, n-3 PUFA are unlikely to confer an additional benefit in terms of MPS, yet in older or immobilized individuals, the benefits of n-3 PUFA supplementation may lie in rescuing deficits in MPS.

Phosphatidic acid, ursolic acid, vitamin D, creatine, and dietary nitrates, to name a few, have been investigated with regard to their influence on MPS. Many have shown beneficial effects in cells or animal models, yet the findings in humans appear equivocal (32). The impact of protein supplementation up to 1.6 g protein·kg^{-1} body mass·day^{-1} exerts a small, but significant, effect on gains in fat- and bone-free mass (82). Importantly, whether HMB or any of the aforementioned nutritional compounds would confer any significant benefit on MPS when sufficient AAs are present seems unlikely. However, many of these compounds may exert important functions outside of elevating MPS. Thus, if a single or a combination of nutraceutical compounds were incorporated into a structured supplementation regimen, there would likely be little to no additional benefit for muscle protein accretion beyond that of sufficient protein intake.

Exercise Interaction and Training

RE is the most potent stimulus for skeletal muscle hypertrophy. The interaction between exercise and nutrition is a major determinant of long-term skeletal muscle adaptation. Biolo and colleagues demonstrated that following RE, increased MPS is accompanied by a prolonged elevation in MPB and a diminished but still negative muscle NBAL (12). The preceding RE bout enhances skeletal muscle sensitivity to nutritional influences, essentially "priming" the muscle to be more sensitive to the hyperaminoacidemia. This sensitizing effect of RE appears to persist for up to ~48 hours (18, 88). The provision of EAAs post-exercise provides the necessary substrate to increase MPS, and prior exercise enables skeletal muscle to utilize a greater amount of the EAAs for MPS (86). Typically, with RE or protein nutrition MPS increases ~50%. However, the combination elicits an additive effect, increasing MPS by ~100–150% (36, 76, 81).

RE is often employed as the principal strategy to increase MPS and muscle hypertrophy. However, aerobic exercise has been shown to acutely increase MPS (53) and induce, at least in some populations, muscle fibre hypertrophy (54). Furthermore, with continued exercise training, the acute MPS response becomes refined in a mode-specific manner. In response to a single bout of RE, an untrained individual would experience an increase in both myofibrillar and mitochondrial protein synthetic rates (111). However, following 10 weeks of RET, exposure to a RE bout only elicited an increase in myofibrillar protein synthesis (111). Conversely, exposure to an acute endurance exercise stimulus provoked an increase in only mitochondrial synthetic rates, regardless of training status (111). Nevertheless, acute changes in MPS in specific protein sub-fractions may not translate to chronic adaptations, and caution with interpretation is warranted. Taken together, this briefly highlights the importance of exercise in maximizing MPS and sheds light on how exercise can modulate the acute MPS response following chronic training of divergent modalities.

Future Directions

Research focused on nutritional influences on skeletal muscle protein metabolism remains an exciting field of study; however, many questions remain unanswered or understudied, some of which have been well summarized (114). Future studies should endeavour to investigate whether plant-based (i.e., pea) sources can stimulate MPS to a similar extent as animal-derived sources and further elucidate the molecular control of AA and mechano-sensitive mechanisms underpinning MPS. Furthermore, with recent advances in isotopic tracers (i.e., D_2O) and the expansion of the -omics field (i.e., proteomics, transcriptomics, and metabolomics), examination of entire biological networks regulating MPS will be uncovered, alongside synthetic rates and the total abundance of individual proteins in response to a variety of interventions.

Summary and Take-Home Messages

Skeletal muscle is critical for a variety of important bodily functions. Muscle mass is determined by the balance between MPS and MPB. Fluctuations predominantly in MPS dictate the muscle NBAL, as MPB remains largely constant. RE and protein nutrition, through activation of the mTORC1 pathway, act independently and synergistically to stimulate increased MPS. Critically, positive muscle NBAL can only be achieved when both RE and protein feeding are combined. Importantly, protein feeding regimens can be manipulated (i.e., dose, quality, distribution, etc.) to modify acute MPS at rest and following exercise training. However, the investigation of other nutritional strategies has also yielded important discoveries in the field of muscle protein metabolism. Nevertheless, persistent practice of RE and protein feeding remains the most effective strategy to promote acute increases in MPS and drive the addition of newly synthesized protein to skeletal muscle over time (i.e., hypertrophy). Therefore, we have provided some practical guidelines that can be incorporated to facilitate the enhancement of MPS and subsequent muscle hypertrophy.

Ingested protein dose:

1. Consume ~0.4 g/kg of protein at each meal, either at rest or following a bout of exercise.
2. A total daily protein intake of ~1.6 g/kg/d may augment muscle protein accretion.

Protein quality:

1. Consume higher-quality protein sources and those with a high EAA content, in particular leucine. However, a full complement of EAAs is necessary to sustain the MPS response.
2. Supplementing a lower dose of protein with additional leucine may be a useful strategy in lieu of a sufficient bolus.

Protein distribution:

1. Evenly space protein-containing meals (every ~3–5 hours) to maximize the cumulative MPS response during the course of the day.
2. Ingestion of protein prior to sleep may mitigate the reductions in MPS during an overnight fast.

Co-ingestion with other macronutrients:

1. Carbohydrate or other supplements likely provide no additional benefit when combined with RE so long as sufficient EAAs are present.

References

1. Abdulla H, Smith K, Atherton PJ, Idris I. Role of insulin in the regulation of human skeletal muscle protein synthesis and breakdown: A systematic review and meta-analysis. *Diabetologia* 59: 44–55, 2016.
2. Areta JL, Burke LM, Ross ML, Camera DM, West DWD, Broad EM, et al. Timing and distribution of protein ingestion during prolonged recovery from resistance exercise alters myofibrillar protein synthesis. *J Physiol* 591: 2319–2331, 2013.
3. US. Department of Agriculture. Nutrient intakes from food and beverages: mean amounts consumed per individual, by gender and age, What We Eat in America, NHANES 2013-2014.
4. Aspuria P-J, Tamanoi F. The Rheb family of GTP-binding proteins. *Cell Signal* 16: 1105–1112, 2004.
5. Atherton PJ, Etheridge T, Watt PW, Wilkinson D, Selby A, Rankin D, et al. Muscle full effect after oral protein: Time-dependent concordance and discordance between human muscle protein synthesis and mTORC1 signaling. *Am J Clin Nutr* 92: 1080–1088, 2010.
6. Atherton PJ, Etheridge T, Watt PW, Wilkinson D, Selby A, Rankin D, et al. Muscle full effect after oral protein: Time-dependent concordance and discordance between human muscle protein synthesis and mTORC1 signaling. *Am J Clin Nutr* 92: 1080–1088, 2010.
7. Atherton PJ, Kumar V, Selby AL, Rankin D, Hildebrandt W, Phillips BE, et al. Enriching a protein drink with leucine augments muscle protein synthesis after resistance exercise in young and older men. *Clin Nutr* 36: 888–895, 2017.
8. Atherton PJ, Smith K, Etheridge T, Rankin D, Rennie MJ. Distinct anabolic signalling responses to amino acids in C2C12 skeletal muscle cells. *Amino Acids* 38: 1533–1539, 2010.
9. Baar K, Esser K. Phosphorylation of p70(S6k) correlates with increased skeletal muscle mass following resistance exercise. *Am J Physiol* 276: C120–127, 1999.
10. Baier S, Johannsen D, Abumrad N, Rathmacher JA, Nissen S, Flakoll P. Year-long changes in protein metabolism in elderly men and women supplemented with a nutrition cocktail of beta-hydroxy-beta-methylbutyrate (HMB), L-arginine, and L-lysine. *J Parenter Enteral Nutr* 33: 71–82, 2009.

11. Bar-Peled L, Chantranupong L, Cherniack AD, Chen WW, Ottina KA, Grabiner BC, et al. A tumor suppressor complex with GAP activity for the rag GTPases that signal amino acid sufficiency to mTORC1. *Science* 340: 1100–1106, 2013.

12. Biolo G, Maggi SP, Williams BD, Tipton KD, Wolfe RR. Increased rates of muscle protein turnover and amino acid transport after resistance exercise in humans. *Am J Physiol* 268: E514–E520, 1995.

13. Breen L, Churchward-Venne TA. Leucine: A nutrient 'trigger' for muscle anabolism, but what more? *J Physiol* 590: 2065–2066, 2012.

14. Breen L, Stokes KA, Churchward-Venne TA, Moore DR, Baker SK, Smith K, et al. Two weeks of reduced activity decreases leg lean mass and induces "anabolic resistance" of myofibrillar protein synthesis in healthy elderly. *J Clin Endocrinol Metab* 98: 2604–2612, 2013.

15. Brook MS, Wilkinson DJ, Mitchell WK, Lund JN, Phillips BE, Szewczyk NJ, et al. Synchronous deficits in cumulative muscle protein synthesis and ribosomal biogenesis underlie age-related anabolic resistance to exercise in humans. *J Physiol-Lond* 594: 7399–7417, 2016.

16. Brugarolas J, Lei K, Hurley RL, Manning BD, Reiling JH, Hafen E, et al. Regulation of mTOR function in response to hypoxia by REDD1 and the TSC1/TSC2 tumor suppressor complex. *Genes Dev* 18: 2893–2904, 2004.

17. Burd NA, McKenna CF, Salvador AF, Paulussen KJM, Moore DR. Dietary protein quantity, quality, and exercise are key to healthy living: A muscle-centric perspective across the lifespan. *Front Nutr* 6, 2019.

18. Burd NA, West DWD, Moore DR, Atherton PJ, Staples AW, Prior T, et al. Enhanced amino acid sensitivity of myofibrillar protein synthesis persists for up to 24 h after resistance exercise in young men. *J Nutr* 141: 568–573, 2011.

19. Burd NA, Yang Y, Moore DR, Tang JE, Tarnopolsky MA, Phillips SM. Greater stimulation of myofibrillar protein synthesis with ingestion of whey protein isolate v. micellar casein at rest and after resistance exercise in elderly men. *Br J Nutr* 108: 958–962, 2012.

20. Camera DM, Smiles WJ, Hawley JA. Exercise-induced skeletal muscle signaling pathways and human athletic performance. *Free Radic Biol Med* 98: 131–143, 2016.

21. Campbell WW, Trappe TA, Wolfe RR, Evans WJ. The recommended dietary allowance for protein may not be adequate for older people to maintain skeletal muscle. *J Gerontol Ser A* 56: M373–M380, 2001.

22. Cao L, Morley JE. Sarcopenia is recognized as an independent condition by an international classification of disease, tenth revision, clinical modification (ICD-10-CM) code. *J Am Med Dir Assoc* 17: 675–677, 2016.

23. Cermak NM, Res PT, de Groot LC, Saris WH, van Loon LJ. Protein supplementation augments the adaptive response of skeletal muscle to resistance-type exercise training: A meta-analysis. *Am J Clin Nutr* 96: 1454–1464, 2012.

24. Chaillou T, Kirby TJ, McCarthy JJ. Ribosome biogenesis: Emerging evidence for a central role in the regulation of skeletal muscle mass. *J Cell Physiol* 229: 1584–1594, 2014.

25. Chantranupong L, Wolfson RL, Orozco JM, Saxton RA, Scaria SM, Bar-Peled L, et al. The Sestrins Interact with GATOR2 to Negatively Regulate the Amino-Acid-Sensing Pathway Upstream of mTORC1. *Cell Rep* 9: 1–8, 2014.

26. Churchward-Venne TA, Breen L, Di Donato DM, Hector AJ, Mitchell CJ, Moore DR, et al. Leucine supplementation of a low-protein mixed macronutrient beverage enhances myofibrillar protein synthesis in young men: A double-blind, randomized trial. *Am J Clin Nutr* 99: 276–286, 2014.

27. Churchward-Venne TA, Burd NA, Phillips SM. Nutritional regulation of muscle protein synthesis with resistance exercise: Atrategies to enhance anabolism. *Nutr Metab* 9: 40, 2012.

28. Coffey VG, Jemiolo B, Edge J, Garnham AP, Trappe SW, Hawley JA. Effect of consecutive repeated sprint and resistance exercise bouts on acute adaptive responses in human skeletal muscle. *Am J Physiol-Regul Integr Comp Physiol* 297: R1441–R1451, 2009.

29. Conley TB, Apolzan JW, Leidy HJ, Greaves KA, Lim E, Campbell WW. Effect of food form on postprandial plasma amino acid concentrations in older adults. *Br J Nutr* 106: 203–207, 2011.

30. Crozier SJ, Kimball SR, Emmert SW, Anthony JC, Jefferson LS. Oral leucine administration stimulates protein synthesis in rat skeletal muscle. *J Nutr* 135: 376–382, 2005.

31. Damas F, Libardi CA, Ugrinowitsch C. The development of skeletal muscle hypertrophy through resistance training: The role of muscle damage and muscle protein synthesis. *Eur J Appl Physiol* 118: 485–500, 2018.

32. Deane CS, Wilkinson DJ, Phillips BE, Smith K, Etheridge T, Atherton PJ. "Nutraceuticals" in relation to human skeletal muscle and exercise. *Am J Physiol Endocrinol Metab* 312: E282–E299, 2017.

33. Devries MC, McGlory C, Bolster DR, Kamil A, Rahn M, Harkness L, et al. Leucine, not total protein, content of a supplement is the primary determinant of muscle protein anabolic responses in healthy older women. *J Nutr* 148: 1088–1095, 2018.

34. Dickinson JM, Fry CS, Drummond MJ, Gundermann DM, Walker DK, Glynn EL, et al. Mammalian target of rapamycin complex 1 activation is required for the stimulation of human skeletal muscle protein synthesis by essential amino acids. *J Nutr* 141: 856–862, 2011.

35. Dreyer HC, Fujita S, Cadenas JG, Chinkes DL, Volpi E, Rasmussen BB. Resistance exercise increases AMPK activity and reduces 4E-BP1 phosphorylation and protein synthesis in human skeletal muscle. *J Physiol* 576: 613–624, 2006.

36. Drummond MJ, Dreyer HC, Fry CS, Glynn EL, Rasmussen BB. Nutritional and contractile regulation of human skeletal muscle protein synthesis and mTORC1 signaling. *J Appl Physiol Bethesda Md 1985* 106: 1374–1384, 2009.

37. Drummond MJ, Fry CS, Glynn EL, Dreyer HC, Dhanani S, Timmerman KL, et al. Rapamycin administration in humans blocks the contraction-induced increase in skeletal muscle protein synthesis. *J Physiol* 587: 1535–1546, 2009.

38. Drummond MJ, Rasmussen BB. Leucine-Enriched Nutrients and the Regulation of mTOR Signalling and Human Skeletal Muscle Protein Synthesis. *Curr Opin Clin Nutr Metab Care* 11: 222–226, 2008.

39. Flück M, Carson JA, Gordon SE, Ziemiecki A, Booth FW. Focal adhesion proteins FAK and paxillin increase in hypertrophied skeletal muscle. *Am J Physiol-Cell Physiol* 277: C152–C162, 1999.

40. Food and Nutrition Board IOM. *Dietary reference intakes for energy, carbohydrate, fiber, fat, fatty acids, cholesterol, protein, and amino acids (macronutrients)*. National Academy Press Washington, DC, 2005.

41. Frontera WR, Ochala J. Skeletal muscle: A brief review of structure and function. *Calcif Tissue Int* 96: 183–195, 2015.

42. Fyfe JJ, Bishop DJ, Stepto NK. Interference between concurrent resistance and endurance exercise: Molecular bases and the role of individual training variables. *Sports Med* 44: 743–762, 2014.

43. Gingras AC, Gygi SP, Raught B, Polakiewicz RD, Abraham RT, Hoekstra MF, et al. Regulation of 4E-BP1 phosphorylation: A novel two-step mechanism. *Genes Dev* 13: 1422–1437, 1999.

44. Glynn EL, Fry CS, Drummond MJ, Timmerman KL, Dhanani S, Volpi E, et al. Excess leucine intake enhances muscle anabolic signaling but not net protein anabolism in young men and women. *J Nutr* 140: 1970–1976, 2010.

45. Glynn EL, Fry CS, Timmerman KL, Drummond MJ, Volpi E, Rasmussen BB. Addition of carbohydrate or alanine to an essential amino acid mixture does not enhance human skeletal muscle protein anabolism. *J Nutr* 143: 307–314, 2013.

46. Goodman CA. The role of mTORC1 in mechanically-induced increases in translation and skeletal muscle mass. *J. Appl. Physiol. Bethesda Md 1985* 127(2):581–590, 2019.

47. Goodman CA, Nilius B, Gudermann T, Jahn R, Lill R, Offermanns S, et al. The role of mTORC1 in regulating protein synthesis and skeletal muscle mass in response to various mechanical stimuli. *Rev. Physiol. Biochem. Pharmacol.* 166 (2014). doi: 10.1007/112_2013_17.

48. Gordon SE, Flück M, Booth FW. Selected contribution: Skeletal muscle focal adhesion kinase, paxillin, and serum response factor are loading dependent. *J Appl Physiol* 90: 1174–1183, 2001.

49. Gorissen SHM, Rémond D, van Loon LJC. The muscle protein synthetic response to food ingestion. *Meat Sci* 109: 96–100, 2015.

50. Greenhaff PL, Karagounis LG, Peirce N, Simpson EJ, Hazell M, Layfield R, et al. Disassociation between the effects of amino acids and insulin on signaling, ubiquitin ligases, and protein turnover in human muscle. *Am J Physiol-Endocrinol Metab* 295: E595–E604, 2008.

51. Gulati P, Gaspers LD, Dann SG, Joaquin M, Nobukuni T, Natt F, et al. Amino acids activate mTOR complex 1 via Ca2+/CaM signaling to hVps34. *Cell Metab* 7: 456–465, 2008.

52. Gwinn DM, Shackelford DB, Egan DF, Mihaylova MM, Mery A, Vasquez DS, et al. AMPK phosphorylation of raptor mediates a metabolic checkpoint. *Mol Cell* 30: 214–226, 2008.

53. Harber MP, Konopka AR, Jemiolo B, Trappe SW, Trappe TA, Reidy PT. Muscle protein synthesis and gene expression during recovery from aerobic exercise in the fasted and fed states. *Am J Physiol-Regul Integr Comp Physiol* 299: R1254–R1262, 2010.

54. Harber MP, Konopka AR, Undem MK, Hinkley JM, Minchev K, Kaminsky LA, et al. Aerobic exercise training induces skeletal muscle hypertrophy and age-dependent adaptations in myofiber function in young and older men. *J Appl Physiol* 113: 1495–1504, 2012.

55. Heitman J, Movva NR, Hall MN. Targets for cell cycle arrest by the immunosuppressant rapamycin in yeast. *Science* 253: 905–909, 1991.

56. Hickson RC. Interference of strength development by simultaneously training for strength and endurance. *Eur J Appl Physiol* 45: 255–263, 1980.

57. Hodson N, Brown T, Joanisse S, Aguirre N, West DWD, Moore DR, et al. Characterisation of L-Type amino acid transporter 1 (LAT1) expression in human skeletal muscle by immunofluorescent microscopy. *Nutrients* 10, 2017.

58. Inoki K, Li Y, Xu T, Guan K-L. Rheb GTPase is a direct target of TSC2 GAP activity and regulates mTOR signaling. *Genes Dev* 17: 1829–1834, 2003.

59. Inoki K, Zhu T, Guan K-L. TSC2 mediates cellular energy response to control cell growth and survival. *Cell* 115: 577–590, 2003.

60. Jakubowski JS, Wong EPT, Nunes EA, Noguchi KS, Vandeweerd JK, Murphy KT, et al. Equivalent hypertrophy and strength gains in β-hydroxy-β-methylbutyrate- or leucine-supplemented men. *Med Sci Sports Exerc* 51: 65–74, 2019.

61. Jewell JL, Russell RC, Guan K-L. Amino acid signalling upstream of mTOR. *Nat Rev Mol Cell Biol* 14: 133–139, 2013.

62. Kato H, Suzuki K, Bannai M, Moore DR. Protein requirements are elevated in endurance athletes after exercise as determined by the indicator amino acid oxidation method. *Plos One* 11: e0157406, 2016.

63. Kim I-Y, Schutzler S, Schrader A, Spencer H, Kortebein P, Deutz NEP, et al. Quantity of dietary protein intake, but not pattern of intake, affects net protein balance primarily through differences in protein synthesis in older adults. *Am J Physiol-Endocrinol Metab* 308: E21–E28, 2014.

64. Kim IY, Suh SH, Lee IK, Wolfe RR. Applications of stable, nonradioactive isotope tracers in in vivo human metabolic research. *Exp Mol Med* 48: e203, 2016.

65. Koopman R, Beelen M, Stellingwerff T, Pennings B, Saris WHM, Kies AK, et al. Coingestion of carbohydrate with protein does not further augment postexercise muscle protein synthesis. *Am J Physiol Endocrinol Metab* 293: E833–E842, 2007.

66. Kouw IW, Holwerda AM, Trommelen J, Kramer IF, Bastiaanse J, Halson SL, et al. Protein ingestion before sleep increases overnight muscle protein synthesis rates in healthy older men: A randomized controlled trial. *J Nutr* 147: 2252–2261, 2017.

67. Kunz J, Henriquez R, Schneider U, Deuter-Reinhard M, Movva NR, Hall MN. Target of rapamycin in yeast, TOR2, is an essential phosphatidylinositol kinase homolog required for G1 progression. *Cell* 73: 585–596, 1993.

68. Laplante M, Sabatini DM. mTOR signaling at a glance. *J Cell Sci* 122: 3589–3594, 2009.

69. Long X, Ortiz-Vega S, Lin Y, Avruch J. Rheb binding to mammalian target of rapamycin (mTOR) is regulated by amino acid sufficiency. *J Biol Chem* 280: 23433–23436, 2005.

70. MacDougall JD, Tarnopolsky MA, Chesley A, Atkinson SA. Changes in muscle protein synthesis following heavy resistance exercise in humans: A pilot study. *Acta Physiol Scand* 146: 403–404, 1992.

71. Macnaughton LS, Wardle SL, Witard OC, McGlory C, Hamilton DL, Jeromson S, et al. The response of muscle protein synthesis following whole-body resistance exercise is greater following 40 g than 20 g of ingested whey protein. *Physiol Rep* 4, 2016.

72. Magne H, Savary-Auzeloux I, Migné C, Peyron M-A, Combaret L, Rémond D, et al. Contrarily to whey and high protein diets, dietary free leucine supplementation cannot reverse the lack of recovery of muscle mass after prolonged immobilization during ageing. *J Physiol* 590: 2035–2049, 2012.

73. Mamerow MM, Mettler JA, English KL, Casperson SL, Arentson-Lantz E, Sheffield-Moore M, et al. Dietary protein distribution positively influences 24-h muscle protein synthesis in healthy adults. *J Nutr* 144: 876–880, 2014.

74. McGlory C, von Allmen MT, Stokes T, Morton RW, Hector AJ, Lago BA, et al. Failed recovery of glycemic control and myofibrillar protein synthesis with 2 wk of physical inactivity in overweight, prediabetic older adults.

75. McGlory C, Wardle SL, Macnaughton LS, Witard OC, Scott F, Dick J, et al. Fish oil supplementation suppresses resistance exercise and feeding-induced increases in anabolic signaling without affecting myofibrillar protein synthesis in young men. *Physiol. Rep.* (March 1, 2016). doi: 10.14814/phy2.12715.

76. McKendry J, Pérez-López A, McLeod M, Luo D, Dent JR, Smeuninx B, et al. Short inter-set rest blunts resistance exercise-induced increases in myofibrillar protein synthesis and intracellular signalling in young males. *Exp Physiol* 101: 866–882, 2016.

77. Millward DJ, Halliday D, Hundal H, Taylor P, Atherton P, Greenhaff P, et al. Michael John Rennie, MSc, PhD, FRSE, FHEA, 1946-2017: An appreciation of his work on protein metabolism in human muscle. *Am J Clin Nutr* 106: 1–9, 2017.

78. Mitchell CJ, Churchward-Venne TA, Bellamy L, Parise G, Baker SK, Phillips SM. Muscular and systemic correlates of resistance training-induced muscle hypertrophy. *PLOS ONE* 8: e78636, 2013.

79. Mitchell CJ, Churchward-Venne TA, Parise G, Bellamy L, Baker SK, Smith K, et al. Acute post-exercise myofibrillar protein synthesis is not correlated with resistance training-induced muscle hypertrophy in young men. *Plos One* 9: e89431, 2014.

80. Moore DR, Churchward-Venne TA, Witard O, Breen L, Burd NA, Tipton KD, et al. Protein ingestion to stimulate myofibrillar protein synthesis requires greater relative protein intakes in healthy older versus younger men. *J Gerontol Ser A* 70: 57–62, 2015.

81. Moore DR, Robinson MJ, Fry JL, Tang JE, Glover EI, Wilkinson SB, et al. Ingested protein dose response of muscle and albumin protein synthesis after resistance exercise in young men. *Am J Clin Nutr* 89: 161–168, 2009.

82. Morton RW, Murphy KT, McKellar SR, Schoenfeld BJ, Henselmans M, Helms E, et al. A systematic review, meta-analysis and meta-regression of the effect of protein supplementation on resistance training-induced gains in muscle mass and strength in healthy adults. *Br J Sports Med* 52: 376–384, 2018.

83. Murphy CH, Saddler NI, Devries MC, McGlory C, Baker SK, Phillips SM. Leucine supplementation enhances integrative myofibrillar protein synthesis in free-living older men consuming lower- and higher-protein diets: A parallel-group crossover study. *Am J Clin Nutr* 104: 1594–1606, 2016.

84. Oikawa SY, Holloway TM, Phillips SM. The impact of step reduction on muscle health in aging: Protein and exercise as countermeasures. *Front Nutr* 6: 75, 2019.

85. Paddon-Jones D, Campbell WW, Jacques PF, Kritchevsky SB, Moore LL, Rodriguez NR, et al. Protein and healthy aging. *Am J Clin Nutr* 101: 1339S–1345S, 2015.

86. Pennings B, Koopman R, Beelen M, Senden JMG, Saris WHM, van Loon LJC. Exercising before protein intake allows for greater use of dietary protein-derived amino acids for de novo muscle protein synthesis in both young and elderly men. *Am J Clin Nutr* 93: 322–331, 2011.

87. Phillips SM, Chevalier S, Leidy HJ. Protein "requirements" beyond the RDA: Implications for optimizing health. *Appl Physiol Nutr Metab Physiol Appl Nutr Metab* 41: 565–572, 2016.

88. Phillips SM, Tipton KD, Aarsland A, Wolf SE, Wolfe RR. Mixed muscle protein synthesis and breakdown after resistance exercise in humans. *Am J Physiol* 273: E99–E107, 1997.

89. Rennie MJ, Edwards RH, Halliday D, Matthews DE, Wolman SL, Millward DJ. Muscle protein synthesis measured by stable isotope techniques in man: The effects of feeding and fasting. *Clin Sci* 63: 519–523, 1982.

90. Res PT, Groen B, Pennings B, Beelen M, Wallis GA, Gijsen AP, et al. Protein ingestion before sleep improves postexercise overnight recovery. *Med Sci Sports Exerc* 44: 1560–1569, 2012.

91. Sancak Y, Bar-Peled L, Zoncu R, Markhard AL, Nada S, Sabatini DM. Ragulator-rag complex targets mTORC1 to the lysosomal surface and is necessary for its activation by amino acids. *Cell* 141: 290–303, 2010.

92. Schreiber SL. Chemistry and biology of the immunophilins and their immunosuppressive ligands. *Science* 251: 283–287, 1991.

93. Sehgal SN, Baker H, Vézina C. Rapamycin (Ay-22,989), a new antifungal antibiotic. *J Antibiot (Tokyo)* 28: 727–732, 1975.

94. Shad BJ, Smeuninx B, Atherton PJ, Breen L. The mechanistic and ergogenic effects of phosphatidic acid in skeletal muscle. *Appl Physiol Nutr Metab Physiol Appl Nutr Metab* 40: 1233–1241, 2015.

95. Smith GI, Atherton P, Reeds DN, Mohammed BS, Rankin D, Rennie MJ, et al. Dietary omega-3 fatty acid supplementation increases the rate of muscle protein synthesis in older adults: A randomized controlled trial. *Am J Clin Nutr* 93: 402–412, 2011.

96. Smith GI, Atherton P, Reeds DN, Mohammed BS, Rankin D, Rennie MJ, et al. Omega-3 polyunsaturated fatty acids augment the muscle protein anabolic response to hyperinsulinaemia-hyperaminoacidaemia in healthy young and middle-aged men and women. *Clin Sci Lond Engl 1979* 121: 267–278, 2011.

97. Smith K, Barua JM, Watt PW, Scrimgeour CM, Rennie MJ. Flooding with L-[1-13C]leucine stimulates human muscle protein incorporation of continuously infused L-[1-13C]valine. *Am J Physiol-Endocrinol Metab* 262: E372–E376, 1992.

98. Smith K, Reynolds N, Downie S, Patel A, Rennie MJ. Effects of flooding amino acids on incorporation of labeled amino acids into human muscle protein. *Am J Physiol-Endocrinol Metab* 275: E73–E78, 1998.

99. Srikanthan P, Karlamangla AS. Muscle mass index as a predictor of longevity in older adults. *Am J Med* 127: 547–553, 2014.

100. Staples AW, Burd NA, West DWD, Currie KD, Atherton PJ, Moore DR, et al. Carbohydrate does not augment exercise-induced protein accretion versus protein alone. *Med Sci Sports Exerc* 43: 1154–1161, 2011.

101. Stokes T, Hector AJ, Morton RW, McGlory C, Phillips SM. Recent perspectives regarding the role of dietary protein for the promotion of muscle hypertrophy with resistance exercise training. *Nutrients* 10, 2018.

102. Tang JE, Moore DR, Kujbida GW, Tarnopolsky MA, Phillips SM. Ingestion of whey hydrolysate, casein, or soy protein isolate: Effects on mixed muscle protein synthesis at rest and following resistance exercise in young men. *J Appl Physiol* 107: 987–992, 2009.

103. Tipton KD, Ferrando AA, Phillips SM, Doyle D, Wolfe RR. Postexercise net protein synthesis in human muscle from orally administered amino acids. *Am J Physiol-Endocrinol Metab* 276: E628–E634, 1999.

104. Tipton KD, Gurkin BE, Matin S, Wolfe RR. Nonessential amino acids are not necessary to stimulate net muscle protein synthesis in healthy volunteers. *J Nutr Biochem* 10: 89–95, 1999.

105. Tipton KD, Hamilton DL, Gallagher IJ. Assessing the role of muscle protein breakdown in response to nutrition and exercise in humans. *Sports Med* 48: 53–64, 2018.

106. Trommelen J, Van Loon LJC. Pre-sleep protein ingestion to improve the skeletal muscle adaptive response to exercise training. *Nutrients* 8: 763, 2016.

107. Verhoeven S, Vanschoonbeek K, Verdijk LB, Koopman R, Wodzig WK, Dendale P, et al. Long-term leucine supplementation does not increase muscle mass or strength in healthy elderly men. *Am J Clin Nutr* 89: 1468–1475, 2009.

108. Welle S, Thornton C, Statt M, McHenry B. Postprandial myofibrillar and whole body protein synthesis in young and old human subjects. *Am J Physiol* 267: E599–E604, 1994.

109. Wilkinson DJ. Historical and contemporary stable isotope tracer approaches to studying mammalian protein metabolism. *Mass Spectrom Rev* 37: 57–80, 2018.

110. Wilkinson DJ, Hossain T, Hill DS, Phillips BE, Crossland H, Williams J, et al. Effects of leucine and its metabolite β-hydroxy-β-methylbutyrate on human skeletal muscle protein metabolism. *J. Physiol.*591(11):2911–23 (July 27, 2017).

111. Wilkinson SB, Phillips SM, Atherton PJ, Patel R, Yarasheski KE, Tarnopolsky MA, et al. Differential effects of resistance and endurance exercise in the fed state on signalling molecule phosphorylation and protein synthesis in human muscle. *J Physiol* 586: 3701–3717, 2008.

112. Wilkinson SB, Tarnopolsky MA, Macdonald MJ, Macdonald JR, Armstrong D, Phillips SM. Consumption of fluid skim milk promotes greater muscle protein accretion after resistance exercise than does consumption of an isonitrogenous and isoenergetic soy-protein beverage. *Am J Clin Nutr* 85: 1031–1040, 2007.

113. Witard OC, Jackman SR, Breen L, Smith K, Selby A, Tipton KD. Myofibrillar muscle protein synthesis rates subsequent to a meal in response to increasing doses of whey protein at rest and after resistance exercise. *Am J Clin Nutr* 99: 86–95, 2014.

114. Witard OC, Wardle SL, Macnaughton LS, Hodgson AB, Tipton KD. Protein considerations for optimising skeletal muscle mass in healthy young and older adults. *Nutrients* 8, 2016.

115. Wolfe RR, Miller SL. The recommended dietary allowance of protein: A misunderstood concept. *JAMA* 299: 2891–2893, 2008.

116. Wu G. Amino acids: Metabolism, functions, and nutrition. *Amino Acids* 37: 1–17, 2009.

117. Zoncu R, Bar-Peled L, Efeyan A, Wang S, Sancak Y, Sabatini DM. mTORC1 senses lysosomal amino acids through an inside-out mechanism that requires the vacuolar H(+)-ATPase. *Science* 334: 678–683, 2011.

21

MICRONUTRIENTS AND NUTRACEUTICALS: EFFECTS ON EXERCISE PERFORMANCE

Stella L. Volpe and Quentin Nichols

Introduction

Exercise performance is based on a number of aspects; however, training and nutrition are two factors that can significantly influence a person's performance. An individual's dietary intake can lead to better performance. Although macronutrient intake is important as energy sources for athletes, micronutrients, as well as other compounds within foods, can also influence exercise performance. The goal of this chapter is to evaluate some micronutrients, specifically, magnesium, iron, zinc, and vitamin D, as well as food-based supplements and nutritional supplements on exercise performance.

Magnesium

Magnesium is the fourth most abundant mineral and the second most abundant intracellular divalent cation in the body and is involved in more than 300 metabolic reactions in the body. Magnesium is involved in reactions of protein synthesis, cellular energy production, and cell growth and reproduction, to name a few. Furthermore, magnesium helps maintain normal heart rhythm (cardiac excitability), vasomotor tone, blood pressure, immune system, bone integrity, and blood glucose concentrations. Because of magnesium's role in energy production and storage and normal muscle function, it has been studied as an ergogenic aid (performance enhancing) for athletes (66, 67). Good food sources of magnesium are listed in Table 21.1.

Several studies have been published with respect to magnesium intake of athletes. Raizel and colleagues (51) researched the dietary intakes of 19 male Brazilian professional soccer players. They reported that although their energy intake was adequate, their dietary magnesium intake was below national recommendations. In a study conducted in Canadian Paralympic athletes representing nine different sports, Madden et al. (39) similarly reported that they consumed adequate energy but were below the requirements for magnesium intake.

Silva and Silva (60) evaluated the body composition and dietary intake of children and adolescent male Portuguese rink hockey players. They reported that these athletes consumed below their energy requirements and consumed below the requirements for magnesium. Serairi Beji (59) researched the dietary intake of children and adolescent male Tunisian weightlifters. They reported adequate dietary intake, but magnesium intake was below recommendations.

Heffernan et al. (22) conducted a systematic review of minerals on exercise performance. They searched six databases (MEDLINE, Embase, CINHAL, SportDISCUS, Web of Science, and clinicaltrials.gov). They included 128 studies on various micronutrients, including calcium, magnesium, phosphate, zinc,

Table 21.1 Food sources of magnesium

Food	Magnesium content (mg)
1 ounce of dry roasted almonds	80
½ cup of boiled spinach	78
1 cup of plain or vanilla soymilk	61
1 medium banana	32
3 ounces of Atlantic, farm-raised salmon	26
1 cup of milk	24–27
1 slice of whole wheat bread	23
½ cup of avocado	22
3 ounces of roasted chicken breast	22
½ cup of cooked broccoli	12

Adapted from: https://fdc.nal.usda.gov/

sodium, boron, selenium, chromium, and multimineral articles. They reported that there was little evidence for the use of mineral supplementation to improve biological markers of exercise performance. Only iron and magnesium showed some merit to enhancing exercise performance.

In a meta-analysis and systematic review, Wang and colleagues (73) examined the effect of magnesium supplementation on numerous fitness variables. These variables included leg strength, knee extension strength, peak torque, muscle power, muscle work, hand grip strength, bench press, resistance exercise, lean mass, muscle strength, walking speed, muscle mass, repeated chair stands, and timed get-up-and-go. They searched the Medline database and other sources for randomized clinical trials through July 2017. Wang et al. (73) included 14 randomized clinical trials, where they identified three different population groups: athletes or physically active individuals (215 participants, mean = 24.9 years of age); untrained healthy individuals (95 participants, mean = 40.2 years of age); and older individuals or those with alcoholism (232 participants, mean = 62.7 years of age). They reported that magnesium supplementation did not lead to an ergogenic effect in athletes and physically active individuals on fitness variables who had normal magnesium status. They did report, however, that there were beneficial effects of magnesium supplementation in older individuals and those with alcoholism. More research needs to be conducted on magnesium supplementation in athletes who are magnesium deficient.

Magnesium is involved in metabolic processes that would likely be the mechanisms affecting exercise performance. For example, magnesium is involved in adenosine triphosphatase (ATPase) function, tyrosine kinase activity, lipid metabolism, protein synthesis, energy metabolism, and muscle contraction. Magnesium regulates cellular glucose metabolism because of its role as part of the activated magnesium–adenosine triphosphate (Mg-ATP) complex required for all rate-limiting enzymes of glycolysis. Magnesium is involved in all phosphorylation processes, and all reactions include utilization and transfer of ATP (7, 31, 56, 62, 67, 75).

Iron

Iron is one of the most abundant metals on earth; however, iron deficiency is the most common nutritional deficiency in the world. According to the World Health Organization, about 24.8% of the entire population has iron deficiency anaemia. Preschool-age children (47.4%), pregnant women (41.8%), and non-pregnant women (30.2%) have the highest rates of iron-deficiency anaemia (76). Good food sources of iron are listed in Table 21.2.

Iron is involved in a number of metabolic reactions in the body, including those involved with oxygen transport in red blood cells and tissues, ATP generation, prevention of lipid peroxidation, and storage and transport. One of the main functions of iron is its involvement in the synthesis of haem into

Table 21.2 Food sources of iron

Food	Iron content (mg)
1 serving of breakfast cereal (fortified with 100% of the daily value for iron)	18
1 cup of canned of white beans	8
3 ounces of dark chocolate (45–69% cacao solids)	7
½ cup of boiled lentils	3
½ cup of boiled spinach	3
3 ounces of canned (in oil) Atlantic sardines	2
½ cup of chickpeas	2
½ cup of canned, stewed tomatoes	2
1 medium baked potato (with the skin)	2
½ cup of boiled green peas	1

Adapted from: https://fdc.nal.usda.gov/

haemoglobin, which is a protein found in red blood cells. The main function of haemoglobin is the transport of oxygen from the lungs to the tissues.

A major regulator of iron homeostasis is hepcidin, which is a hormone synthesized in the liver [77]. Hepcidin plays a primary role in iron regulation by binding to the iron export protein ferroportin 1 (FPN1), thus inhibiting iron transport. Ferroportin 1 is located on the basolateral surface of the intestinal enterocytes and the plasma membrane of macrophages. By inhibiting ferroportin, hepcidin precludes iron from being exported, and thus, iron is sequestered in the cells. Hepcidin therefore decreases dietary iron absorption and decreases iron release from macrophages [5, 19, 54].

Although exercise has been well-established to be excellent for overall health, it is a stressor, resulting in acute inflammation. Hepcidin concentrations increase under conditions such as inflammation. Thus, there is something termed "exercise-induced hepcidin elevation," which could lead to increased risk of iron-deficiency anaemia in athletes [18].

Goto et al. [18] compared the effects of resistance and endurance exercise on hepcidin and iron concentrations in ten men. Both exercise sessions were 60 minutes in duration. They collected blood samples before exercise and immediately post-exercise, as well as 1, 2, 3, and 6 hours post-exercise. Plasma hepcidin concentrations were significantly increased post-exercise ($p < 0.001$); the percentage increases were greater after resistance training compared to endurance training ($463 \pm 125\%$ vs. $137 \pm 27\%$, respectively [$p = 0.03$]). They also reported that serum iron concentrations were significantly increased immediately post-exercise ($p < 0.001$), with no significant differences between resistance and endurance exercise. Although one might have postulated a greater increase in hepcidin concentrations after endurance exercise, it appears that resistance training may impose a greater increase in hepcidin concentrations. Thus, athletes who resistance train should be educated on consuming foods high in iron.

Zügel et al. [77] assessed hepcidin concentrations and iron status during a 4-week training camp of junior world elite rowers. They reported a significant increase in serum hepcidin concentrations during the first week of training (23.24 ± 2.43 ng/mL) compared to the start of training (11.47 ± 3.92 ng/mL) ($p = 0.02$). After about 2 weeks of training, hepcidin concentrations returned to baseline values (09.51 ± 3.59 ng/mL). Serum ferritin concentrations followed the similar patterns at baseline and day seven as serum hepcidin concentrations. The researchers reported that because hepcidin and ferritin are acute-phase proteins, they "are sensitive to initial increases in training load" [77]. The authors also reported that these alterations were short-term and did not affect erythropoiesis.

Iron is also involved in thyroid hormone production. Thyroid hormones are involved in nearly every process in the body, including energy metabolism and thermoregulation. Specifically, iron-deficiency anaemia can negatively affect thyroid peroxidase (TPO) activity. Thyroid peroxidase is a haem-containing enzyme. If TPO activity is impaired, thyroid-stimulating hormone (TSH) activity will be increased and thyroxine (T4) and triiodothyronine (T3) activity will be decreased (37). Therefore, iron-deficiency anaemia may lead to a decreased resting metabolic rate (RMR) and impaired thermo-regulation, especially under cold conditions (9, 53).

In a case study, Harris Rosenzweig and Volpe (21) evaluated the effect of iron supplementation on thyroid hormone concentrations and RMR in female college athletes. Two female athletes who had iron-deficiency anaemia and were 18 and 21 years of age were supplemented with 23 mg/day of elemental iron for 16 weeks. Iron-deficiency anaemia was clinically corrected in both women, with increases in haemoglobin and serum ferritin concentrations. However, RMR and thyroid hormone concentrations were oppositely affected in each participant. Due to the fact that this was a case study, no statistical changes could be evaluated.

Because iron is involved in many metabolic reactions in the body, poor iron status has been associated with increased risk of various morbidities. Kortas et al. (36) examined the relationship between iron metabolism and exerkines in older women before and after Nordic walking training. Exerkines are compounds released by the skeletal muscle, fat, liver, brain, and kidneys after exercise. Examples of exerkines include myostatin, adiponectin, and osteocalcin, which may all positively affect metabolism. Kortas et al. (36) recruited 36 post-menopausal women (66 ± 5 years of age) and randomly assigned them to a Nordic walking group or a control group. Those in the intervention group walked 3 days per week for 12 weeks. They reported that serum ferritin concentrations were inversely correlated with changes in myostatin, adiponectin, osteocalcin, and serum iron concentrations after the 12-week walking program ($p < 0.05$). Their results provide evidence that iron effects exerkine concentrations as a result of walking in older post-menopausal women.

Zinc

Zinc, an essential trace mineral, is involved in more than 300 metabolic reactions in the body; it is needed for the catalytic activity of more than 100 enzymes (17, 29, 55). Zinc is integral for immune function, wound healing, protein and DNA synthesis, and cell division (15, 17, 49, 61). Zinc is required for normal growth and development, as well as for proper sense of taste (17, 25). Good food sources of zinc are listed in Table 21.3.

Like iron, zinc is involved in the conversion of T4 to the more active T3, and thus, zinc affects energy metabolism and exercise performance (68). Maxwell and Volpe (42) evaluated the effects of zinc supplementation on plasma zinc, serum ferritin, thyroid hormone concentrations, and RMR in two physically active women who were zinc deficient. They supplemented them with 26.4 mg/dL of

Table 21.3 Food sources of zinc

Food	Zinc content (mg)
3 ounces of oysters, breaded and fried	74
3 ounces of braised chuck roast	7
½ cup of canned vegetarian baked beans	2.9
2 ounces of baked dark meat chicken	2.4
1 ounce of dried pumpkin seeds	2.2
8 ounces of low-fat fruit yogurt	1.7
½ cup of chickpeas	1.3
1 cup of milk	1
1 ounce of dry roasted almonds	0.9
1 ounce of cheddar cheese	0.9

Adapted from: https://fdc.nal.usda.gov/

zinc (as zinc gluconate) for 4 months. After 4 months of zinc supplementation, zinc deficiency was clinically corrected in both women; total T3 concentrations increased in one participant, while all thyroid hormone concentrations increased in the other. RMR increased in both participants at the end of the 4-month supplementation period. Statistical analyses could not be conducted because this was a case study; nonetheless, zinc supplementation appeared to be directly responsible for the increase in plasma zinc concentrations. In addition, zinc supplementation likely resulted in the increase in T3 concentrations and RMR.

Although serum zinc concentration is often measured as a marker of zinc status, it is not a good indicator of dietary zinc intake. Serum zinc concentrations can be influenced by age, sex, and/or timing of the blood draw (23, 24). In addition, zinc homeostasis is tightly regulated by the family of proteins called metallothioneins. Although other markers of zinc have been explored, stable isotopes of zinc can provide a clear picture of the zinc kinetics and can identify the movement of zinc within the body.

Volpe et al. (72) assessed the influence of acute exhaustive exercise versus rest on short-term zinc kinetics in 12 healthy, sedentary men, 25 to 35 years of age. In this cross-over design study, where each participant was his own control, the stable isotope, ^{70}Zinc (^{70}Zn) was infused 10 minutes post-exercise or at rest. Plasma zinc concentrations were measured at baseline and 2, 5, 10, 15, 30, 45, 60, 75, 90, and 120 minutes post-exercise or rest. Haematocrit was also assessed prior to and post-exercise to assess changes in plasma volume that occurred during exercise. Volpe et al. (72) reported significant decreases in plasma zinc concentrations ($p < 0.05$) after exercise, with a mean nadir of $13.9 \pm 4.1\%$ 70 minutes after exercise. With respect to ^{70}Zn, they reported significant increases in the size of the rapidly exchangeable plasma zinc pool (Qa; from 3.1 [0.2] to 3.6 [0.2] mg; $p < 0.05$) and the liver zinc pool (Qb; from 10.2 [0.6] to 11.4 [0.8] mg; $p = 0.12$). The results of this zinc kinetics study indicate that exercise causes a shift of plasma zinc into the interstitial fluid and liver post-exercise. These kinetic changes mirror the acute stress response of exercise. More research in zinc kinetics with exercise will help to elucidate if the acute changes in zinc persist longer after exercise.

Vitamin D

Vitamin D is both a fat-soluble vitamin and a hormone because it is activated in one part of the body but has its effects on another part of the body. Vitamin D is acquired from both the sun and food. Just 10–15 minutes of exposure to ultraviolet B (UVB) light (the sun) can provide 10,000–40,000 International Units (IU) via conversion on the skin, compared to 3 ounces of salmon, a vitamin D–rich food, which provides 530 IU (59, 61, 62). Figure 21.1 demonstrates the conversion of vitamin D from skin and food sources. Briefly, pre-vitamin D_3 is synthesized non-enzymatically in the skin from 7-dehydrocholesterol during exposure to the ultraviolet rays in sunlight. Pre-vitamin D_3 undergoes a temperature-dependent rearrangement to form vitamin D_3 (cholecalciferol). Vitamin D_3 (cholecalciferol) then travels to the liver where the first hydroxylation (addition of an OH group) occurs on the 25th position of vitamin D_3. This then becomes 25-hydroxyvitamin D, also known as calcidiol. Calcidiol then travels to the kidneys, where the second hydroxylation of vitamin D occurs, forming 1,25-dihydroxyvitamin D_3, also known as calcitriol. Calcitriol is the most active form of vitamin D and, along with parathyroid hormone (PTH), works to maintain calcium homeostasis, among many other functions in the body. Despite the fact that calcitriol is the most active form of vitamin D, calcidiol is used to measure vitamin D status because it has a longer half-life than calcitriol. Some other functions of vitamin D include modulation of bone metabolism, regulation of cell proliferation and differentiation, de novo protein synthesis, and improved muscle function (69–71).

Because of vitamin D's role in bone metabolism, a number of studies have been published in this area. One such study was published by Armstrong et al. (4), who evaluated the gene–environment interaction in 51 Royal Marines in the United Kingdom who developed a stress fracture during training. They were compared to 141 uninjured controls. They performed genotyping for the vitamin D receptor (VDR) FokI polymorphism in all participants. They reported that baseline serum calcidiol concentrations

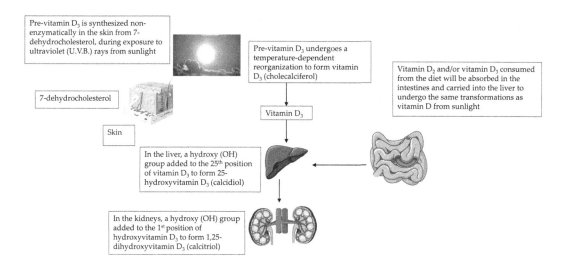

Figure 21.1: Vitamin D metabolism. *Art from:* https://smart.servier.com/

interacted with the VDR FokI polymorphism. That is, the higher the calcidiol concentrations, the lower the stress fracture risk ($p = 0.01$). Armstrong et al. (4) concluded, "This further supports the role of low serum vitamin D concentrations in causing stress fractures, and hence prophylactic vitamin D supplementation as an injury risk mitigation strategy."

Vitamin D not only affects bone but also can influence endurance capacity. Marley et al. (40) conducted a dose-response, cross-over, placebo-controlled trial in 27 recreational male combat athletes (age: 24±4 years; height: 176±6 cm; body weight: 77±14 kg). Participants were assigned to one of three levels of vitamin D supplementation: 50,000 IU, 80,000 IU, or 110,000 IU, after which they completed a 6-week placebo period followed by a 6-week supplementation period. The researchers reported that vitamin D supplementation increased endurance in recreational combat athletes; however, there were no increased benefits for doses higher than 50,000 IU.

In addition to affecting aerobic capacity, vitamin D might improve anaerobic performance. Ramezani et al. (52) conducted a double-blind, randomized controlled trial on the effect of vitamin D_3 supplementation on both anaerobic and aerobic performance in 46 active men. Participants were randomly assigned to a vitamin D_3 supplement (2,000 IU/day) or a placebo for 12 weeks. They reported an improvement in aerobic capacity, anaerobic performance, and vitamin D status following vitamin D_3 supplementation. The results from the aforementioned studies indicate that vitamin D affects bone, as well as aerobic and anaerobic capacity. Vitamin D's effects on aerobic and anaerobic capacity are likely associated with its role in muscle function. As previously stated, vitamin D concentrations are related to the presence of VDRs in nearly all human cells. Expression of transcription factors augmenting muscle cell proliferation and differentiation is caused by an interaction of skeletal muscle to vitamin D (74).

Whey Protein

In general, athletes and physically active populations require more protein than the average population (30). The current Recommended Dietary Allowance (RDA) for protein in the United States of America is 0.8 g protein/kg body mass per day, with a range of 10–35% of total energy intake (28). This amount has been appropriately deemed for healthy individuals to meet their daily nutritional requirements and is likely sufficient for many physically active individuals (63). In 2017, Jäger et al. (30) published the International Society of Sports Nutrition's position stand on protein and exercise for athletes and active populations. They stated that an adequate amount of protein for active individuals to build and maintain lean body mass is 1.4–2.0 g protein/kg body weight/day (30), which does not exceed the upper range of 35% established by the United States of America's RDA (28). Schoenfeld and Aragon (58) stated that to maximize anabolism, athletes should consume 0.4–0.55 g protein/kg/meal across four meals to reach 1.6–2.2 g protein/kg/day. The amount of protein required for athletes generally coincides with how novice they are to a sport. The more novice athlete will likely require more protein per kg of body weight, compared to a more experienced athlete.

Maintaining muscle mass for athletic performance hinges on resistance training and proper consumption of protein for muscle protein synthesis and maintaining a net protein balance (13, 30, 44). If any athlete or exerciser does not consume their required amount of protein, they will be at risk of creating a negative nitrogen balance, leading to protein breakdown and impaired recovery.

Whey protein (which is also found naturally in milk) has been shown to be a potent stimulator of muscle protein synthesis, otherwise known as myofibrillar protein synthesis (MPS), likely due to the high amount of the amino acid leucine, which is one of the three branched-chain amino acids (BCAAs) (valine and isoleucine are the other two) (46). Leucine has been shown to stimulate the mammalian target of rapamycin (mTOR), leading to MPS (1, 2, 10, 40) (Figure 21.2).

Areta et al. (3) examined how different amounts of whey protein distributed throughout a 12-hour recovery period following resistance exercise influenced MPS. Twenty-four healthy trained men were assigned to one of three groups (8 men per group), with each group receiving a total of 80 grams of whey protein. The groups were as follows: [1] 8 × 10 grams of whey protein every 1.5 hours; [2] 4 × 20 grams of whey protein every 3 hours; and [3] 2 × 40 grams of whey protein every 6 hours. The researchers took muscle biopsies from the participants at the following intervals: at rest and after 1, 4, 6, 7, and 12 hours post-exercise. Although all three regimens led to significant increases in MPS compared to rest, those who consumed 4 × 20 grams of whey protein resulted in the greatest stimulus of MPS compared to the other two regimens.

Li and Liu (38) conducted a meta-analysis to examine the effect of whey protein supplementation combined with resistance training on muscle mass and muscle strength. They used data from

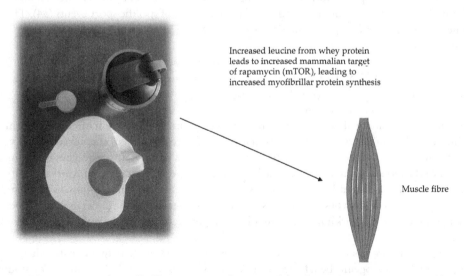

Increased leucine from whey protein leads to increased mammalian target of rapamycin (mTOR), leading to increased myofibrillar protein synthesis

Muscle fibre

Figure 21.2 Whey protein and myofibrillar protein synthesis. Art from: https://smart.servier.com/. Photo taken by S.L. Volpe

21 randomized controlled trials, with 837 participants. Compared to control groups who resistance-trained, those who combined whey protein supplementation with resistance training had significantly greater lean body mass and muscular strength, with significantly lower fat mass in healthy individuals <40 years of age.

Does whey protein improve muscle mass in older adults? Skeletal muscle mass begins to decline after about the age of 40. This loss of muscle mass is known as sarcopenia and can lead to physical disability, poor quality of life, and death (46). Nabuco et al. (45) assessed the effects of consuming whey protein immediately pre- or post-resistance training on skeletal muscle mass, muscular strength, and functional capacity in 70 already conditioned older women living in Brazil. Participants were randomly assigned to one of three groups: whey protein pre-resistance training + placebo post-resistance training ($n = 24$), placebo pre-resistance training + whey protein post-resistance training ($n = 23$), and placebo pre- and post-resistance training ($n = 23$). The resistance training program was conducted for 12 weeks, and all participants consumed 35 grams of either whey protein or a placebo. Both whey protein groups had significantly greater ($p < 0.05$) skeletal muscle mass, muscular strength, and functional capacity compared to the placebo group, regardless of timing of whey protein supplementation. In this case, whey protein supplementation was effective at improving muscle mass in older individuals.

Whey protein supplementation is an effective nutritional supplement with respect to increases in muscle mass. Although not all researchers have shown improvements in muscle mass in older adults, some researchers have shown a beneficial effect, which can help stave off the loss of muscle due to sarcopenia.

Beetroot

Beet really is "beetroot" since it is the root of the plant. It was formally known as "*Beta vulgaris*" and gets it colour from betanin, which has been suggested to prevent oxidative stress. Beetroot, as well as arugula and watermelon, provide high sources of dietary nitrate. Dietary nitrate can improve exercise performance because of an increased production of nitric oxide (32). The International Olympic Committee recommends beetroot/dietary nitrate supplementation as having enough evidence to use it in sport-specific scenarios (41). The Australian Institute of Sport also suggests that beetroot/dietary nitrate supplementation qualify as having strong sport-specific evidence to recommend its use (6). The International Society of Sports Nutrition stated in their review of the current evidence on supplementation that nitrates show an ergogenic benefit within the context of specific sport events (34). The general recommendation for nitrate supplementation is 300–600 mg (34).

Dietary nitrate's ergogenic properties result from its formation into nitric oxide (32, 33). Nitric oxide, when elevated, can improve blood flow and thus increase mitochondrial respiration during exercise (15, 32, 33) (Figure 21.3). Increasing blood flow to working muscles can also improve the recovery process in athletes and exercisers (11, 16, 32). Nitrates are naturally found in the diet from vegetables (e.g., arugula, beets, watermelon) (14, 65).

Beetroot juice has emerged as the main source of dietary nitrate supplementation due to its high content of nitrate (NO_3^-) (11, 15, 16, 32, 65). When beetroots are consumed, the nitrate mixes with bacteria in the mouth, which reduces nitrate to nitrite (15, 16). When the nitrite reaches the stomach, it is absorbed into the bloodstream, and when the body is in a low oxygen state, it converts into nitric oxide (15, 16). Nitric oxide aids in dilating blood vessels due to its effect on smooth muscle fibres and results in increased blood flow to working muscles, allowing for aerobic energy metabolism to occur (15). Improving blood flow to working muscle in a low oxygen state can produce performance-enhancing benefits.

McMahon et al. (43) conducted a systemic review and meta-analysis to evaluate whether dietary nitrate provided an ergogenic benefit for endurance exercise. The authors analysed 76 studies with various exercise testing protocols such as time to exhaustion, graded exercise testing, and time trials (43).

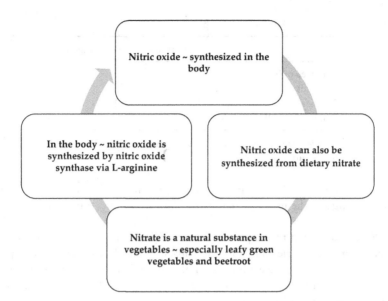

Figure 21.3 Nitric oxide production from foods

They concluded that dietary nitrate benefited time to exhaustion most consistently. They also reported that there was no consistent dosing strategy, and thus, it is difficult to provide dosing guidelines (43).

Campos et al. (11) also conducted a systematic review and meta-analysis to examine nitrate supplementation and its ergogenic effects in non-trained versus trained populations. They included 43 trials of non-trained and 63 trials of trained individuals, with the majority being cyclists. The amount of beetroot used ranged from 70 to 500 mL, 40 minutes to 24 hours prior to exercise. Nitrate supplementation provided some benefit to non-trained individuals participating in endurance exercise until fatigue. Dietary nitrate supplementation did not, however, demonstrate any benefit for the trained population in various testing protocols. Campos et al. (11) concluded that dietary nitrate supplementation benefits non-trained populations in an aerobic setting of longer duration. However, the lack of an ergogenic effect in the trained population may have resulted from the range of supplement doses and timing, both of which need to be better established to maximize performance benefits (11).

Dominguez et al. (15) reviewed the effects of beetroot juice in high-intensity exercise. They reviewed nine studies with a total of 120 individuals (107 men and 13 women). In five of the studies, beetroot juice was administered between 120 minutes and 180 minutes before exercise. Beetroot supplementation was also administered 5–7 days before physical activity in four remaining studies. They reported that acute or long-term beetroot juice supplementation showed benefits for higher-intensity exercise (15).

Beetroot juice has demonstrated ergogenic effects in endurance and high-intensity exercise. Nonetheless, there is a lack of standard consensus on dosing and timing of consumption of beetroot juice (48). Furthermore, more research needs to be conducted in women and older populations.

β-Alanine

β-alanine is a beta amino acid, which means that the amino group is at the β-position from the carboxylate group. β-Alanine is produced in the liver and can be obtained from various protein sources (64) (Table 21.4). Exogenous β-alanine supplementation has been shown to increase the concentration of carnosine in the muscle, increasing the duration of intracellular buffering capacity (27). Improving intracellular buffering capacity can potentially increase the ability to sustain higher-intensity activities

Table 21.4 Food sources of β-alanine

Food	β-alanine content (grams)
3 ounces of beef	2–3
5 ounces of chicken breast	2
3 ounces of turkey breast	<2
3 ounces of yellowtail fish	1

Adapted from: https://www.livestrong.com/article/338184-food-sources-of-beta-alanine/

for a longer period of time, thus improving exercise performance (26). Additional information on the biochemistry of buffering and the use of β-alanine for improved exercise performance can be found in Chapter 22.

Harris et al. (20) demonstrated that supplementation of β-alanine increased muscle carnosine concentration, which improves muscle pH buffering capacity. The International Olympic Committee states that β-alanine was shown to have a high level of evidence to recommend its use in performance scenarios (41). The Australian Institute of Sport classifies β-alanine as having a strong level of evidence to support or enhance athletic performance (6).

Quesnele et al. (50) conducted a systematic review of 19 studies on β-alanine and its effects on performance. They reported that doses between 3 and 6 grams were beneficial for aerobic and anaerobic performance; however, while β-alanine may improve performance, there is not enough evidence showing its safety and potential side effects (50). Saunders et al. (57) also conducted a systematic review and meta-analysis to evaluate the effect of β-alanine on exercise capacity and performance. The authors concluded that β-alanine has the greatest ergogenic benefit on exercise that lasts from 30 seconds to 10 minutes and has more benefits in non-trained versus trained populations (57).

The International Society of Sports Nutrition's position stand on β-alanine stated that doses of 4–6 grams/day improves carnosine content within the muscle (64). The International Society of Sports Nutrition noted that β-alanine, when use in the proper doses within healthy populations, shows no side effects (64). The position stand mentioned that there were some reports of paraesthesia and recommended that doses be lowered to 1.6 grams or less. In exercise events lasting 1–4 minutes, β-alanine should be dosed at 4–6 grams for a minimum of 2–4 weeks (64).

More research on β-alanine is required to evaluate its effects in highly trained athletes and contextual use in sport-specific scenarios (10, 35), as well as in longer-duration activities (41). In addition, research on β-alanine supplementation in female athletes and older populations needs to be conducted (10, 35).

Summary and Future Directions

Research on magnesium, iron, zinc, and vitamin D, as well as food-based supplements (whey protein, beetroot) and nutritional supplements (β-alanine) have been presented in this chapter. Research outcomes with some of the aforementioned micronutrients or food-based supplements are more definitive than others. For example, the effects of whey protein on lean body mass and the effects of beetroot juice on increasing nitric oxide, and hence, exercise performance, have been shown consistently throughout the literature. Less definitive results have been reported for magnesium, iron, zinc, vitamin D, and β-alanine. More research on these substances is required. The research that needs to be conducted are double-blind, placebo-controlled, and longer-term studies. In addition, overall, more research is required in female athletes, because the majority of research has been conducted in male athletes. Furthermore, research in older athletes is also required. Research needs to be conducted among different types of athletes. Finally, more research is required using more consistent doses of the aforementioned nutrients and food-based supplements. These types of studies can provide a stronger understanding of how micronutrients and food-based supplements can affect exercise performance and overall health.

References

1. Antonio J, Ellerbroek A, Evans C, Silver T, Peacock CA. High protein consumption in trained women: Bad to the bone? *J Int Society Sports Nutr* 15(1): 6–10, 2018.
2. Antonio J, Ellerbroek A, Silver T, Vargas L, Tamayo A, Buehn R, et al. A high protein diet has no harmful effects: A one-year crossover study in resistance-trained males. *J Nutr Metabol* 0–4, 2016.
3. Areta JL, Burke LM, Ross ML, Camera DM, West DW, Broad EM, et al. Timing and distribution of protein ingestion during prolonged recovery from resistance exercise alters myofibrillar protein synthesis. *J Physiol* 591(9): 2319–2331, 2013.
4. Armstrong RA, Davey T, Allsopp AJ, Lanham-New SA, Oduoza U, Cooper JA, et al. Low serum 25-hydroxyvitamin D status in the pathogenesis of stress fractures in military personnel: An evidenced link to support injury risk management. *PLOS ONE* 15(3): e0229638. eCollection 2020.
5. Ashby DR, Gale DP, Busbridge M, Murphy KG, Duncan ND, Cairns TD, et al. Plasma hepcidin levels are elevated but responsive to erythropoietin therapy in renal disease. *Kidney Int* 75(9): 976–981, 2009.
6. Australian Institute of Sport. *The Australian Institute of Sport (AIS)* Sports Supplement Framework. March 2019. https://www.ais.gov.au/nutrition/supplements, retrieved August 29, 2020.
7. Barbagallo M, Dominguez LJ. Magnesium metabolism in type 2 diabetes mellitus, metabolic syndrome and insulin resistance. *Arch Biochem Biophys* 458(1): 40–47, 2007.
8. Bond P. Regulation of mTORC1 by growth factors, energy status, amino acids and mechanical stimuli at a glance. *J Int Society of Sports Nutr* 13(1): 1–11, 2016.
9. Brigham D, Beard J. Iron and thermoregulation: A review. *Crit Rev Food Sci Nutr* 36(8): 747–763, 1996.
10. Brisola GMP and Zagatto AM. Ergogenic effects of B-Alanine supplementation on different sports modalities: Strong evidence or only incipient findings? *J of Strength Condition Res* 33(1): 253–282, 2019.
11. Campos HO, Drummond LR, Rodrigues QT, Machado FSM, Pires W, Wanner SP, et al. Nitrate supplementation improves physical performance specifically in non-athletes during prolonged open-ended tests: A systematic review and meta-analysis. *British J Nutr* 119(6): 636–657, 2018.
12. Casonato M, Jeferson R, Jacinto L, Bendito D, Rubens O, Antonio J, et al. Effects of beta-alanine supplementation on muscle function during recovery from resistance exercise in young adults. *Amino Acids* 2019.
13. Churchward-Venne TA, Burd NA, Phillips SM. Nutritional regulation of muscle protein synthesis with resistance exercise: Strategies to enhance anabolism. *Nutr Metabol* 9(1): 1, 2012.
14. Devries MC, and Phillips SM. Supplemental protein in support of muscle mass and health: Advantage whey. *J Food Science* 80(S1): A8–A15, 2015.
15. Domínguez R, Maté-Muñoz JL, Cuenca E, García-Fernández P, Mata-Ordoñez F, Lozano-Estevan MC, et al. Effects of beetroot juice supplementation on intermittent high-intensity exercise efforts. *J Int Society Sports Nutr* 15: 2, 2018.
16. Domínguez R, Cuenca E, Maté-Muñoz JL, García-Fernández P, Serra-Paya N, Estevan MCL, et al. Effects of beetroot juice supplementation on cardiorespiratory endurance in athletes. A systematic review. *Nutrients* 9(1): 1–18, 2017.
17. Frassinetti S, Bronzetti G, Caltavuturo L, Cini M, Croce CD. The role of zinc in life: A review. *J Environ Pathol Toxicol Oncol* 25(3): 597–610, 2006.
18. Goto K, Kojima C, Kasai N, Sumi D, Hayashi N, Hwang H. Resistance exercise causes greater serum hepcidin elevation than endurance (cycling) exercise. *PLoS One* 15(2): e0228766, 2020.
19. Gulec S, Anderson GJ, Collins JF. Mechanistic and regulatory aspects of intestinal iron absorption. *Am J Physiol: Gastrointest Liver Physiol* 307(4): G397–G409, 2014.
20. Harris RC, Tallon MJ, Dunnett M, Boobis L, Coakley J, Kim HJ, et al. The absorption of orally supplied β-alanine and its effect on muscle carnosine synthesis in human vastus lateralis. *Amino Acids* 30(3 SPEC. ISS.): 279–289, 2006.
21. Harris Rosenzweig P, Volpe SL. Effect of iron supplementation on thyroid hormone levels and resting metabolic rate in two college female athletes: A case study. *Int J Sport Nutr Exerc Metab* 10(4): 434–443, 2000.
22. Heffernan SM, Horner K, De Vito G, Conway GE. The role of mineral and trace element supplementation in exercise and athletic performance: A systematic review. *Nutrients* 11(3): 696, 2019.
23. Hennigar SR, Kelley AM, McClung JP. Metallothionein and zinc transporter expression in circulating human blood cells as biomarkers of zinc status: A systematic review. *Adv Nutr* 7: 735–746, 2016.
24. Hennigar SR, Lieberman HR, Fulgoni III VL, McClung JP. Serum zinc concentrations in the US population are related to sex, age, and time of blood draw but not dietary or supplemental zinc. *J Nutr* 148(8): 1341–1351, 2018.
25. Heyneman CA. Zinc deficiency and taste disorders. *Ann Pharmacother* 30: 186–187, 1996.
26. Hobson RM, Saunders B, Ball G, Harris RC, Sale C. Effects of β-alanine supplementation on exercise performance: A meta-analysis. *Amino Acids* 43(1): 25–37, 2012.

27. Hoffman JR, Varanoske A, Stout JR. Effects of β-Alanine supplementation on carnosine elevation and physiological performance. In *Advances in Food and Nutrition Research* 84:183–206, 2018.

28. Institute of Medicine. *Dietary Reference Intakes for Energy, Carbohydrate, Fiber, Fat, Fatty Acids, Cholesterol, Protein, and Amino Acids.* Washington, DC: National Academies Press, 2005.

29. Institute of Medicine, Food and Nutrition Board. *Dietary Reference Intakes for Vitamin A, Vitamin K, Arsenic, Boron, Chromium, Copper, Iodine, Iron, Manganese, Molybdenum, Nickel, Silicon, Vanadium, and Zinc.* Washington, DC: National Academy Press, 2001.

30. Jäger R, Kerksick CM, Campbell BI, Cribb PJ, Wells SD, Skwiat TM, et al. International society of sports nutrition position stand: Protein and exercise. *J Int Society Sports Nutr* 14(1): 1–25, 2017.

31. Jahnen-Dechent W, Ketteler M. Magnesium basics. *Clin Kidney J* 5(Suppl 1): i3–i14, 2012.

32. Jones AM, Thompson C, Wylie LJ, Vanhatalo A. Dietary nitrate and physical performance. *Annual Rev Nutr* 38(1): 303–328, 2018.

33. Jones AM. Dietary nitrate supplementation and exercise performance. *Sports Med* 44(Suppl. 1) S35–45, 2014.

34. Kerksick CM, Wilborn CD, Roberts MD, Smith-Ryan A, Kleiner SM, Jäger R, et al. ISSN exercise & sports nutrition review update: Research & recommendations. *J Int Society Sports Nutr* 15(1): 1–57, 2018.

35. Kimball SR. Integration of signals generated by nutrients, hormones, and exercise in skeletal muscle. *Am J Clin Nutr* 99(1): 237–242, 2014.

36. Kortas J, Ziemann E, Juszczak D, Micielska K, Kozłowska M, Prusik K, et al. Iron status in elderly women impacts myostatin, adiponectin and osteocalcin levels induced by Nordic walking training. *Nutrients* 12(4):1129, 2020.

37. Larson-Meyer DE, Gostas DE. Thyroid function and nutrient status in the athlete. *Curr Sports Med Rep* 19(2): 84–94, 2020.

38. Li M, Liu F. Effect of whey protein supplementation during resistance training sessions on body mass and muscular strength: a meta-analysis. *Food Funct* 10(5): 2766–2773, 2019.

39. Madden RF, Shearer J, Parnell JA. Evaluation of dietary intakes and supplement use in Paralympic athletes. *Nutrients* 9(11): 1266, 2017.

40. Marley A, Grant MC, Babraj J. Weekly vitamin D$_3$ supplementation improves aerobic performance in combat sport athletes. *Eur J Sport Sci* 18: 1–19, 2020.

41. Maughan RJ, Burke LM, Dvorak J, Larson-Meyer DE, Peeling P, Phillips SM, et al. IOC consensus statement: Dietary supplements and the high-performance athlete. *J Int Society Sports Nutr* 28(2): 104–125, 2018.

42. Maxwell C, Volpe SL. Effect of zinc supplementation on thyroid hormone function. A case study of two college females. *Ann Nutr Metab* 51(2): 188–194, 2007.

43. McMahon NF, Leveritt MD, Pavey TG. The effect of dietary nitrate supplementation on endurance exercise performance in healthy adults: A systematic review and meta-analysis. *Sports Med* 47(4): 735–756, 2017.

44. Murphy CH, Hector AJ, Phillips SM. Considerations for protein intake in managing weight loss in athletes. *Eur J Sport Sci* 15(1): 21–28, 2015.

45. Nabuco HCG, Tomeleri CM, Sugihara Junior P, Fernandes RR, Cavalcante EF, Antunes M, et al. Effects of whey protein supplementation pre- or post-resistance training on muscle mass, muscular strength, and functional capacity in pre-conditioned older women: A randomized clinical trial. *Nutrients* 10(5): 56, 2018.

46. Naseeb MA, Volpe SL. Protein and exercise in the prevention of sarcopenia and aging. *Nutr Res* 40: 1–20, 2017.

47. Nassis GP, Sporer B, Stathis CG. β-Alanine efficacy for sports performance improvement: From science to practice. *British J Sports Med* 51(8): 626–627, 2017.

48. Poortmans JR, Gualano B, Carpentier A. Nitrate supplementation and human exercise performance: Too much of a good thing? *Curr Opin Clin Nutr Metabolic Care* 18(6): 599–604, 2015.

49. Prasad AS. Zinc: An overview. *Nutrition* 11: 93–99, 1995.

50. Quesnele JJ, Laframboise MA, Wong JJ, Kim P, Wells GD. The effects of beta-alanine supplementation on performance: A systematic review of the literature. *J Int Society Sports Nutr* 24(1): 14–27, 2014.

51. Raizel R, da Mata Godois A, Coqueiro AY, Voltarelli FA, Fett CA, Tirapegui J, et al. Pre-season dietary intake of professional soccer players. *Nutr Health* 23(4): 215–222, 2017.

52. Ramezani Ahmadi A, Mohammadshahi M, Alizadeh A, Ahmadi Angali K, Jahanshahi A. Effects of vitamin D3 supplementation for 12 weeks on serum levels of anabolic hormones, anaerobic power, and aerobic performance in active male subjects: A randomized, double-blind, placebo-controlled trial. *Eur J Sport Sci* 18: 1–13, 2020.

53. Rosenzweig PH, Volpe SL. Iron, thermoregulation, and metabolic rate. *Crit Rev Food Sci Nutr* 39(2): 131–148, 1999.

54. Rossi E. Hepcidin-The iron regulatory hormone. *Clin Biochem Rev* 25(3): 47–49, 2005.

55. Sandstead HH. Understanding zinc: Recent observations and interpretations. *J Lab Clin Med* 124: 322–327, 1994.

56. Saris NE, Mervaala E, Karppanen H, Khawaja JA, Lewenstam A. Magnesium. An update on physiological, clinical and analytical aspects. *Clin Chim Acta* 294(1–2): 1, 2000.

57. Saunders B, Elliott-Sale K, Artioli GG, Swinton PA, Dolan E, Roschel H, et al. β-Alanine supplementation to improve exercise capacity and performance: A systematic review and meta-Analysis. *British J Sports Med* 0: 1–14, 2017.

58. Schoenfeld BJ, Aragon AA. How much protein can the body use in a single meal for muscle-building? Implications for daily protein distribution. *J Int Soc Sports Nutr* 15: 10, 2018.

59. Serairi Beji R, Megdiche Ksouri W, Ben Ali R, Saidi O, Ksouri R, Jameleddine S. Evaluation of nutritional status and body composition of young Tunisian weightlifters. *Tunis Med* 94(2): 112–117, 2016.

60. Silva MG, Silva HH. Comparison of body composition and nutrients' deficiencies between Portuguese rink-hockey players. *Eur J Pediatr* 176(1): 41–50, 2017.

61. Solomons NW. Mild human zinc deficiency produces an imbalance between cell-mediated and humoral immunity. *Nutr Rev* 56: 27–28, 1998.

62. Swaminathan R. Magnesium metabolism and its disorders. *Clin Biochemist Rev* 24(2): 47–66, 2003.

63. Tipton KD. Efficacy and consequences of very-high-protein diets for athletes and exercisers. *Proceedings Nutr Society* 70(2): 205–214, 2011.

64. Trexler ET, Smith-Ryan AE, Stout JR, Hoffman JR, Wilborn CD, Sale C, et al. International society of sports nutrition position stand: Beta-alanine. *J Int Society Sports Nutr* 12(1): 1–14: 2015.

65. Vanam De Walle, GP, Vukovich MD. The effect of nitrate supplementation on exercise tolerance and performance: A systematic review and meta-analysis. *J Strength Condition Res* 32(6): 1796–1808, 2018.

66. Volpe SL. Magnesium and the athlete. *Curr Sports Med Reports* 14(4): 279–283, 2015.

67. Volpe SL. Magnesium in disease prevention and overall health. *Adv Nutr* 4(3): 378S–383S, 2013.

68. Volpe SL. Minerals as ergogenic aids. *Curr Sports Med Rep* 7(4): 224–229, 2008.

69. Volpe SL. Vitamin D, adiposity, and exercise performance. *ACSM's Health Fit J* 19(5): 40–41, 2015.

70. Volpe SL. Vitamin D and health: Do we need more than the current DRI?: Part 2. *ACSM's Health Fit J* 13(1): 33–34, 2009.

71. Volpe SL. Vitamin D and health: Do we need more than the current DRI?: Part 1. *ACSM's Health Fit J* 12(5): 34–36, 2008.

72. Volpe SL, Lowe NM, Woodhouse LR, King JC. Effect of maximal exercise on the short-term kinetics of zinc metabolism in sedentary men. *Br J Sports Med* 41(3): 156–161, 2007.

73. Wang R, Chen C, Liu W, Zhou T, Xun P, He K, et al. The effect of magnesium supplementation on muscle fitness: A meta-analysis and systematic review. *Magnes Res* 30(4): 120–132, 2017.

74. Wiciński M, Adamkiewicz D, Adamkiewicz M, Śniegocki M, Podhorecka M, Szychta P, et al. Impact of vitamin D on physical efficiency and exercise performance - A review. *Nutrients* 11(11):2826, 2019.

75. Wolf FI, Cittadini A. Magnesium in cell proliferation and differentiation. *Front Biosci* 4: D607–D617, 1999.

76. World Health Organization. https://www.who.int/vmnis/anaemia/prevalence/summary/anaemia_data_status_t2/en/

77. Zügel M, Treff G, Steinacker JM, Mayer B, Winkert K, Schumann U. Increased hepcidin levels during a period of high training load do not alter iron status in male elite junior rowers. *Front Physiol* 10: 1577, 2020.

22

BIOCHEMISTRY OF BUFFERING CAPACITY AND INGESTION OF BUFFERS IN EXERCISE AND ATHLETIC PERFORMANCE

Bryan Saunders, Guilherme G. Artioli, Eimear Dolan, Rebecca L. Jones, Joseph Matthews, and Craig Sale

Introduction

Muscle fatigue is the loss in force or power production in response to muscle contraction (61). During exercise, this results in the inability to sustain exercise at a given intensity. It is widely accepted that exercise-induced muscle fatigue is a complex, multifactorial phenomenon caused by several mechanisms that can vary according to exercise type, intensity, and duration. Both central (i.e., arising in the central nervous system) and peripheral (i.e., arising in skeletal muscle or the neuromuscular junction) events have been implicated in fatigue development (61).

Contracting the muscle at a high rate significantly increases the demand for adenosine-5'-triphosphate (ATP) turnover in order to meet the increased energy demand and maintain the rate of muscle contraction. Resynthesis of ATP is supported by the hydrolysis of phosphorylcreatine, glycolysis, and oxidative phosphorylation in mitochondria, provided sufficient oxygen is available. During high-intensity exercise, however, the rate of ATP hydrolysis can exceed the rate of ATP resynthesis provided by aerobic means, meaning that the shortfall in ATP must be met by the hydrolysis of phosphorylcreatine and anaerobic glycolysis (53). Meeting these energy demands comes at a cost, with anaerobic glycolysis being the primary metabolic process responsible for hydrogen cation (H^+) production in skeletal muscle and thus a reduction in the intramuscular pH, which is suggested to disrupt muscle energetics and muscle contraction (118). Specifically, intramuscular acidosis can inhibit the activity of key enzymes of energy metabolism, in particular phosphofructokinase, a key regulator of glycolysis (120), and can inhibit the resynthesis of phosphorylcreatine (97). Acidosis can also disrupt skeletal muscle contractility by reducing the sensitivity of the calcium-binding site of troponin to the Ca^{2+} ions (30, 118), and can directly interfere with actomyosin interactions by inhibiting the transition from the low- to the high-force state of the actin–myosin cross-bridge (25, 119). Since acidosis rapidly builds up during high-intensity exercise, it is assumed that it plays a major causative role in peripheral fatigue during this type of exercise (64).

Any strategy capable of delaying the increase in intramuscular H^+ concentration that accompanies high-intensity exercise has the potential to delay the onset of fatigue and is thus potentially ergogenic. The regulation of acid–base balance in the body is supported by several physiological mechanisms, including the actions of chemical and metabolic buffers that can alter the H^+ concentration in seconds, pulmonary ventilation that can excrete H^+ over the course of minutes, and the action of the kidneys that can excrete H^+ over the longer term. We will focus on the chemical and metabolic buffers in the intracellular (i.e., muscle) and extracellular (i.e., blood) environments that support the control of intramuscular pH during exercise. In the following sections, we will focus on nutritional interventions that might have the potential to increase intracellular or extracellular buffering capacity, which could delay H^+ accumulation and fatigue.

Biochemistry of pH, Fatigue, and Intracellular/Extracellular Buffering

Fundamental Concepts

Hydrogen is the simplest element in nature, formed by a single positively charged proton and a single negatively charged electron. Single hydrogen atoms are, however, not common on earth, since they naturally combine with other elements to form molecules, such as the diatomic gas form of hydrogen (H_2) or water (H_2O). Water is essential for virtually all known forms of life, since all biochemical reactions require an aqueous medium to occur. Due to its molecular arrangement, in particular the hydrogen side of the molecule being positively charged and the oxygen side of the molecule being negatively charged, water becomes a polar molecule, with a high dielectric constant and it easily forms hydrogen bonds. These characteristics make water an excellent solvent, as the electric charges interact with numerous elements and molecules.

Water causes polar molecules to dissociate into ions, which are then dissolved to form a solution. In pure water, the only ions present are H^+ and OH^-, both in equal concentrations. Since the concentration of positively and negatively charged ions is equal, pure water is neutral. Secondly, their concentrations are remarkably low. Thirdly, water neutrality is seen only when the concentration of both H^+ and OH^- is 10^{-7} M. Finally, the product of H^+ and OH^- concentration in pure water is 10^{-14}.

Since the concentration of ions in pure water is very low, it is convenient to use negative log; this avoids working with several decimal places. By calculating the negative log of the concentration of H^+ in pure water, we obtain pH, where "p" stands for the negative log of the hydrogen cation concentration in water. pH, therefore, is a measure of the hydrogen cation concentration in an aqueous solution, being expressed in a negative logarithmic scale. The pH of pure water is calculated to be 7. Because H^+ concentration is equal to the concentration of OH^-, pOH is also 7. For that reason, 7 is the pH value that represents neutrality of an aqueous solution. When H^+ concentration increases, the solution becomes acidic, its pH decreases and its OH^- concentration decreases because of Le Chatelier's principle. Conversely, when OH^- concentration increases, the solution becomes alkaline (i.e., pH increases) and its H^+ concentration decreases.

According to the Brønsted-Lowry definition of acids and bases, the term acid refers to a substance that can donate protons (i.e., H^+), whilst the term base refers to a substance that is able to accept protons. Acids and bases tend to ionize in water, although the level of ionization depends upon the pH of the solution and the dissociation constant of the acid (Ka) or the base (Kb). Strong acids and bases completely dissociate in aqueous solutions, whereas weak acids and bases only partially dissociate. The dissociation of an acid (HA) can be expressed in the following simplified reaction:

$$HA \leftrightarrow H^+ + A^-$$

To identify the strength of the acid or, in other words, its ability to dissociate and donate protons, it is necessary to calculate the dissociation constant of the acid (Ka) using the formula:

$$K_d = \frac{[H^+] \times [A^-]}{[HA]}$$

Table 22.1 Dissociation constant (Ka) and its negative log (pKa) of a few organic weak acids

Acid	Ka	pKa
Pyruvic Acid	3.98×10^{-3}	2.4
Citric Acid	7.94×10^{-4}	3.1
Formic Acid	1.78×10^{-4}	3.75
Imidazole	1.26×10^{-7}	6.9

Since stronger acids tend to dissociate more than the weaker ones, the stronger the acid, the higher its Ka value. Likewise, the weaker the acid, the lower its Ka value. Because the Ka values can differ by several orders of magnitude between weak and strong acids, it is convenient to work with their negative logarithms, thereby obtaining the pKa of an acid. Hence, the pKa of an acid represents the negative log of its dissociation constant, as exemplified in Table 22.1.

From the dissociation equation, one can calculate their log on both sides of the equation, as follows:

$$K_a = \frac{[H^+] \times [A^-]}{[HA]}$$

$$\log K_a = \log\left(\frac{[H^+] \times [A^-]}{[HA]}\right)$$

By splitting the log terms, we obtain:

$$\log K_a = \log[H^+] + \log\left(\frac{[A^-]}{[HA]}\right)$$

If all terms are multiplied by -1, this gives us:

$$-\log K_a = -\log[H^+] - \log\left(\frac{[A^-]}{[HA]}\right)$$

Replacing the negative logs with their respective "p" terms, we obtain:

$$pK_a = pH - \log\left(\frac{[A^-]}{[HA]}\right)$$

Or:

$$pH = pK_a + \log\left(\frac{[A^-]}{[HA]}\right)$$

This is the Henderson-Hasselbalch equation, and it is important since it relates pH, pKa, and the percentage of dissociation of an acid (or a base). From this equation, for example, we can see that an acid is 50% in its undissociated form and 50% in its dissociated form when the pH of the medium is equal to its pKa. Thus, the pKa of an acid can also be interpreted as the pH of the solution at which this acid will be 50% dissociated and 50% undissociated.

Physiological pH Buffering Systems

Since H^+ and OH^- ions are highly reactive, any shift in pH neutrality, either to the acid or the alkali side, can have a profound impact on key physiological processes, such as enzyme activity and protein structure and function. Most cells and physiological systems operate with their pH tightly regulated and close to neutrality. Such a fine-tuning of pH is achieved thanks to several buffering systems that prevent abrupt changes in pH, as would occur when small amounts of acid or alkali are added to an aqueous solution with no buffering systems (Figure 22.1A). In a buffered system, the addition of acid will not cause such a sudden drop in pH, at least within certain pH limits (Figure 22.1B).

In most animals, both intracellular and extracellular pH are tightly regulated, although the physiological pH range varies slightly between blood and the intracellular medium. In blood, the pH is slightly alkaline (~7.4), whereas in the intracellular medium, pH is typically close to neutrality (~7.0), although this may vary within cellular compartments or between cell types. As such, the buffering systems operating within the blood are different from those operating inside cells. In blood, the most important buffering system is bicarbonate (HCO_3^-), which works in equilibrium with carbonic acid (H_2CO_3), as depicted in the simplified reaction shown here.

$$HCO_3^- + H^+ \leftrightarrow H_2CO_3 \leftrightarrow CO_2 + H_2O$$

When there is an increase in H^+ concentration in blood (i.e., acidosis), the reaction is shifted to the right, meaning that the neutralization of H^+ by HCO_3^- increases, thereby increasing the formation of CO_2 and reducing HCO_3^- concentration. The resulting CO_2 then stimulates an increase in ventilation, through which CO_2 is eliminated. This condition is known as metabolic acidosis and occurs during high-intensity exercise. Alternatively, when there is an increase in CO_2 concentration, the reaction $H_2CO_3 \leftrightarrow CO_2 + H_2O$ is shifted to the right, thereby reducing the concentration of H_2CO_3 in relation to the HCO_3^-. This condition is known as respiratory alkalosis, and it is easily observable when an individual hyperventilates. Another way to induce blood alkalosis is through an increase in HCO_3^- concentration, a condition known as metabolic alkalosis and inducible via the ingestion of nutritional supplements, as discussed in this chapter.

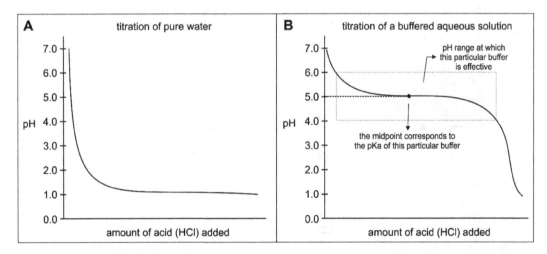

Figure 22.1 Schematic representation of titration curves of pure water (A) and a buffered aqueous solution (B). In pure water, where there is no buffering system, the addition of small amounts of acid results in a large reduction in pH, whilst in a buffered system, there is a zone where the addition of large amounts of acid does not result in a reduced pH. The zone of effectiveness refers to the pH range around the pKa of that particular buffer, thereby varying according to the buffering agent

Inside cells, the equilibrium between the protonated and non-protonated forms of dihydrogen phosphate ($H_2PO_4^-$) is one system that can prevent changes in intracellular pH when the acid or alkali load increases. Another important buffer operating inside cells is the protein system. This system relies on the ability of the amino acid residues to ionize and accept or donate H^+ within the physiological pH range. Because all amino acids have an acid group ($COOH \leftrightarrow COO^-$) and a base group ($NH_2 \leftrightarrow NH_3^+$) that have very low and high pKa's (~2 and ~10), they cannot effectively buffer pH changes within the physiological pH range; therefore, the buffering activity of an amino acid is dependent upon two characteristics of its side chain: (1) whether it is ionizable and (2) whether its pKa is close to the physiological pH. As shown in Table 22.2, histidine is the sole amino acid that can effectively work as a pH buffer in the intracellular medium where pH is close to neutrality. The pKa of amino acids can change when they bind to and interact with other amino acids. Carnosine, a dipeptide formed by histidine and beta-alanine, is a good example, as the pKa of histidine changes from 6.0 to 6.9 when it is bound with beta-alanine. This has important implications for pH regulation during exercise.

The body has several intracellular and extracellular physiological buffers that can accept or release H^+ to prevent pH changes. This is particularly important during high-intensity exercise, which causes an accumulation of H^+ that can lead to fatigue and negatively affect performance. In muscle, physicochemical buffers such as organic and inorganic phosphates, bicarbonate anions, and histidine containing dipeptides (e.g., carnosine) are the primary mediators of pH homeostasis, while H^+ are also actively and passively transported out of the muscle into the blood mediated by transport systems. Therefore, a nutritional intervention designed to increase buffering capacity may be of benefit to exercise performance. The following sections will detail the available evidence on nutritional supplements that have the potential to increase intracellular or extracellular buffering capacity.

Table 22.2 The pKa of ionizable groups of the amino acids

Amino acid	pKa of COOH	pKa of NH₂	pKa of side chain
Alanine	2.34	9.69	–
Arginine	2.17	9.04	12.48
Asparagine	2.02	8.80	–
Aspartic acid	1.88	9.60	3.65
Cysteine	1.96	10.28	8.18
Glutamic acid	2.19	9.67	4.25
Glutamine	2.17	9.13	–
Glycine	2.34	9.60	–
Histidine	1.82	9.17	6.00
Hydroxyproline	1.82	9.65	–
Isoleucine	2.36	9.60	–
Leucine	2.36	9.60	–
Lysine	2.18	8.95	10.53
Methionine	2.28	9.21	–
Phenylalanine	1.83	9.13	–
Proline	1.99	10.60	–
Serine	2.21	9.15	–
Threonine	2.09	9.10	–
Tryptophan	2.83	9.39	–
Tyrosine	2.20	9.11	10.07
Valine	2.32	9.62	–

Source: (15)

Beta-alanine Supplementation

Carnosine (comprising beta-alanine and L-histidine) is abundant in skeletal muscle and is purported to have many therapeutic (3) and ergogenic (99) properties. Potential mechanisms through which these influences occur include the reduction of reactive oxygen or nitrogen species (13), anti-glycation (51), and the regulation of calcium transients and sensitivity (35). While it is possible that some, or all, of these functions contribute toward carnosine's ergogenic and therapeutic properties, the strongest line of evidence supports an important role for carnosine as an intracellular physicochemical buffer (28). This action is possible because the pKa of carnosine (and more specifically of its imidazole ring; 6.83) (7) renders it ideally placed to act as a pH buffer across the pH transit range of the intramuscular environment, which has been reported to reduce from approximately 7.1 at rest to between 6.5 and 6.1 following exhaustive high-intensity exercise (88, 98).

The contribution of carnosine toward intracellular buffering capacity is dependent upon its content and, as such, it is desirable for individuals with a high requirement for intracellular buffering (e.g., athletes who regularly undertake high-intensity exercise) to augment their supply (Figure 22.2). Beta-alanine is the rate-limiting amino acid for carnosine synthesis (45), and supplementation with this amino acid increases carnosine content (104) and is ergogenic in certain situations (102). These properties have led to its application as one of the most widely used sports supplements available today and justifies its inclusion as one of five effective sport supplements indicated for use by various international organizations, including the International Olympic Committee (68).

Supplementation Strategies

The first study to demonstrate that beta-alanine supplementation could increase muscle carnosine content reported that beta-alanine ingestion of 3.2–5.2 g·day^{-1} (mean) for 4 weeks (equating to 89.6–145.6 g total beta-alanine) led to muscle carnosine increases of approximately 40–65% (45). Further independent studies have since confirmed these findings across a range of doses (1.6–6.4 g·day^{-1}), durations (2–24 weeks), and analysis techniques (HPLC and ^{1}H-MRS) (4, 9, 12, 49, 104).

It seems that the main determinant of carnosine content in response to supplementation is the total amount ingested. Church et al. (19) reported equivalent increases in muscle carnosine when 168 g

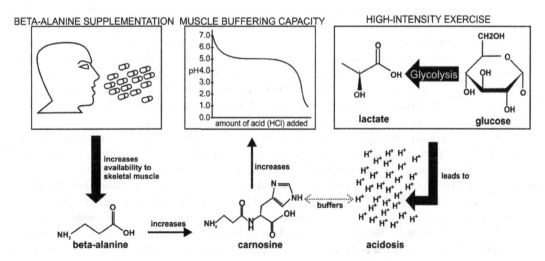

Figure 22.2 Overview of beta-alanine supplementation to increase muscle buffering capacity during high-intensity exercise

of beta-alanine was ingested, either as 12 g·day^{-1} for 2 weeks or as 6 g·day^{-1} for 4 weeks. Similarly, Stellingwerff et al. (116) reported a 2-fold greater increase in muscle carnosine content when participants ingested 3.2 as opposed to 1.6 g·day^{-1} for 4 weeks. The upper limit of carnosine content attainable via beta-alanine supplementation is currently unknown. The longest trial conducted to date supplemented 6.4 g·day^{-1} beta-alanine for 24 weeks, with muscle carnosine content measurements taken every 4 weeks throughout the investigation (104). The greatest increases were shown in the first 4–8 weeks of supplementation, although muscle carnosine content continued to increase throughout the 24 weeks, with some individuals continuing to show increases at the final 24-week collection point, demonstrating that they may not yet have reached saturation.

Effects on Exercise Performance

Hill and colleagues (49) first showed that a beta-alanine–induced increase in muscle carnosine could improve high-intensity exercise capacity. Since then, numerous studies have investigated the influence of beta-alanine supplementation on a wide range of exercise tests and performance parameters. Meta-analytical data showed a significant main effect of beta-alanine supplementation on exercise outcomes (0.18; 95% confidence interval [CI] 0.08–0.28) (102). Importantly, the authors also conducted a meta-regression to identify whether different factors—including exercise duration; type (capacity-based tests conducted to exhaustion or performance-based tests that used a set task); mode (whole body or isolated limb); and mode 2 (intermittent or continuous)—influenced this main effect. In line with an important role of muscle carnosine in delaying fatigue due to increased intracellular buffering capacity, the meta-regression indicated that beta-alanine supplementation exerted its greatest influence in capacity-based tests lasting 30 seconds to 10 minutes. In contrast, shorter (0–30 seconds) and longer (>10 minutes) tests were unlikely to be improved by beta-alanine supplementation, probably because pH changes have a smaller contribution to fatigue in very short, or more prolonged, exercise tests. The effect of beta-alanine was smaller for trained compared to non-trained individuals, although Painelli et al. (87) directly compared the efficacy of beta-alanine supplementation on training status comparing a trained and non-trained population and showed it to be equally effective in both groups. Importantly, any small gains may translate into worthwhile improvements in applied settings (i.e., competition) for competitive athletes.

The influence of beta-alanine supplementation on performance in intermittent tasks such as repeated sprint ability and resistance exercise has been widely studied; acidosis is likely to contribute, at least in part, to performance in these activities (115, 122). Theoretically, it makes sense that beta-alanine supplementation would be most efficacious toward the latter stages of repeated, intense efforts, when acidosis may negatively affect continued ATP regeneration and directly hinder muscle contractile properties (37). Repeated sprint ability is important for a wide range of intermittent team sports, such as football, hockey, rugby, and basketball. Longer-duration repeated efforts, such as repeated upper- (123) and lower- (87) body Wingates or YoYo performance (108) are more amenable to beta-alanine supplementation than are shorter-duration repeated efforts (32, 52, 105, 106, 121).

The effects of beta-alanine supplementation on strength and resistance-based exercise outcomes are equivocal. Hoffman et al. (52) showed improved repeated isotonic endurance performance with beta-alanine, although no such effect on similar exercise outcomes has been shown by others (5, 6). Mixed results have also been reported on the effects of beta-alanine on isometric hold endurance, with studies showing an improvement (6, 100) or no influence (27, 55). Such isometric holds result in reduced blood flow to the muscle and generate a hypoxic environment, increasing reliance upon anaerobic metabolism. The muscle essentially functions as a closed unit during these holds, meaning that the ability to remove H$^+$ is also limited, further exacerbating the ability of the muscle to regulate pH. Insufficient evidence is currently available to make a clear conclusion on the influence of beta-alanine supplementation on strength and resistance exercise outcomes.

The evidence described here is based upon isolated beta-alanine supplementation protocols for acute exercise, but perhaps of equal importance to the athlete is the potential for an enhanced ability to perform high-intensity exercise to contribute to a higher training intensity, which would augment training adaptations. A number of studies have investigated the influence of beta-alanine supplementation alongside a high-intensity interval training (HIIT) programme, and the majority of these showed no added effect of beta-alanine supplementation with training when compared to training alone (20, 113, 126). An important point to consider here, however, is that beta-alanine supplementation typically takes at least 2–3 weeks to show measurable muscle carnosine increases (116), and the aforementioned investigations lasted 6 weeks, meaning that these would have been less likely to show benefits of beta-alanine supplementation from the outset. Supporting this, Smith et al. (114) reported comparable exercise improvements following HIIT with beta-alanine and placebo for the first 3 weeks of the training protocol, but superior influences in the beta-alanine group after 6 weeks. Similarly, Bellinger and Minihan (8) pre-supplemented a group of cyclists with 6.4 g·day^{-1} of beta-alanine for 4 weeks prior to a 5-week sprint training programme and showed a beneficial influence of supplementation and training. Thus, beta-alanine supplementation could well have the capacity to improve exercise training outcomes, but supplementation prior to the implementation of the training programme is obviously required to ensure these benefits are achieved.

Side Effects

The longest supplementation study to date showed that 24 weeks of supplementation at 6.4 g·day^{-1} did not change clinical markers of health in healthy individuals (103). The available evidence indicates that beta-alanine supplementation (within the doses and durations that have been scientifically investigated) is safe (29). The primary side effect experienced is paraesthesia, which has been described as an uncomfortable prickly sensation on the skin. Paraesthesia most likely occurs due to the binding of beta-alanine to the peripheral neuronal receptor MrgprD (66). Although many individuals consider it an unpleasant sensation, there is no evidence to indicate that it is harmful. The occurrence and intensity of paraesthesia are dose-related and closely relate to the time and peak of blood beta-alanine concentration (45). Accordingly, strategies to slow the time or extent of peak blood beta-alanine, such as splitting the desired dose throughout the day (45) or using a slow-release capsule (26), have been reported to effectively reduce the occurrence or intensity of paraesthesia symptoms.

Animal studies show that beta-alanine supplementation may reduce intracellular taurine content, because the increase in beta-alanine availability increases competition for their shared transporter, TauT. Despite this, 24 weeks of 6.4 g·day^{-1} beta-alanine did not affect the taurine pool in muscle (103). A recent systematic risk assessment of beta-alanine supplementation meta-analysed all available data and showed no effect of beta-alanine supplementation on muscle taurine content in humans (29). The discrepant findings between humans and animals likely relates to the very large difference in dosing protocols used, with animal studies typically employing doses that are 38- to 56-fold larger than those used in human studies. Another theoretical concern of beta-alanine supplementation that has been raised is that it may reduce intracellular free histidine content (12), given that histidine is also required to synthesize carnosine. But the same meta-analysis of human data indicates that this is not the case and that beta-alanine supplementation (within doses investigated) does not reduce free histidine content. As such, the available evidence indicates that beta-alanine supplementation is a safe ergogenic aid.

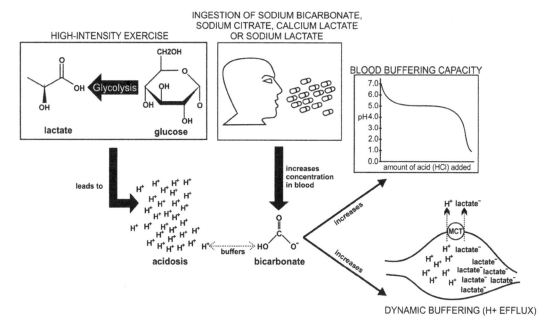

Figure 22.3 Overview of supplementation with extracellular buffers (sodium bicarbonate, sodium citrate, calcium lactate, and sodium lactate) to increase extracellular buffering capacity during high-intensity exercise

Sodium Bicarbonate Supplementation

Normal resting blood bicarbonate concentrations range between 23 and 27 mmol·L^{-1} (67). Sodium bicarbonate is a buffering agent capable of inducing alkalosis via increases in blood pH and bicarbonate (21, 60). This aids in the maintenance of muscle acid–base balance during exercise, increasing the efflux of H$^+$ from the contracting muscle (59), forming carbonic acid, and allowing further buffering by the respiratory system (Figure 22.3). Sodium bicarbonate is another supplement included as one of the five sport supplements that have sufficient evidence to support their use by the International Olympic Committee (68).

Supplementation Strategies

Available evidence suggests that to gain a potential or almost certain improvement in exercise performance, an increase in blood bicarbonate concentration in excess of +5 and +6 mmol·L^{-1} from baseline is required (17). Acute ingestion of 0.3 g·kg^{-1} body mass (BM), the most commonly ingested dose, is sufficient in increasing absolute blood bicarbonate concentrations to these levels (40, 56, 72). Doses above 0.3 g·kg^{-1}BM have demonstrated no additional performance benefits despite greater increases in bicarbonate (72), while a 0.1 g·kg^{-1}BM dose is insufficient in raising circulating blood bicarbonate concentrations >6 mmol·L^{-1} (56) and appears not to improve exercise outcomes (72). Individual variability in blood bicarbonate responses following 0.2 g·kg^{-1}BM (56) could explain why the exercise benefits with this dose are contrasting (21, 60, 72, 96). The maximal absolute increases in circulating bicarbonate following ingestion of 0.2 and 0.3 g·kg^{-1}BM are reported as being similar (44) and have comparable exercise effects. This suggests that it is useful to time supplement ingestion so that exercise coincides with peak alkalosis in order to optimize sodium bicarbonate supplementation at lower doses. Further work is necessary to clarify these claims.

It appears logical to suggest that the greatest ergogenic effect following sodium bicarbonate ingestion would occur at peak alkalosis. The most commonly employed ingestion strategy is to consume sodium bicarbonate at a standardized time point, 60–180 minutes prior to exercise (33, 92, 94, 112), albeit these data have been challenged (18, 44, 56, 111). Consumption of 0.3 g·kg⁻¹BM of sodium bicarbonate results in peak blood bicarbonate concentration between 10 (75) and 180 minutes (56) following ingestion. Therefore, rather than following generalized approaches, individualized sodium bicarbonate ingestion strategies designed to align peak alkalosis with the onset of exercise performance may be more effective. Individualized strategies have demonstrated high repeatability for time-to-peak blood bicarbonate and pH responses (43). Individuals adopting this approach, however, are required to have prior knowledge of blood bicarbonate responses together with the flexibility to manipulate the time frame leading up to performance. This may be difficult for athletes engaged in repeated events throughout the day or those that have strict schedules. More recent data suggest, however, that individualizing supplementation to a solitary peak time point is unnecessary and that there is a long-lasting ergogenic window of opportunity with sodium bicarbonate lasting approximately 3 hours from 60 minutes post-ingestion (23). Those with a short time frame to supplement prior to exercise should consider ingesting a lower dose, since 0.1–0.3 g·kg⁻¹BM showed similar blood bicarbonate responses in the initial 30 minutes post-ingestion (56). Serial sodium bicarbonate ingestion across several days is also a purported method by which to maintain chronically elevated blood bicarbonate levels (71). This serial dosing strategy can lead to exercise improvements (34, 82), although not all studies show this strategy to be effective (58). Individuals should experiment with different supplementation strategies to determine which one works best for them, although 0.3 g·kg⁻¹BM ingested 60–180 minutes before exercise appears to be beneficial under most circumstances.

Effects on Exercise Performance

To gain an ergogenic effect following sodium bicarbonate ingestion, both the duration and the intensity of the exercise should be considered. Sodium bicarbonate increases buffering capacity; therefore, performance benefits are only likely to be reported when exercise is limited by increases in H^+ accumulation. High-intensity exercise of short duration, such as those lasting 10–30 seconds, have demonstrated no improvements following sodium bicarbonate ingestion (73), while most studies report no improvements during endurance exercise (39, 81, 117). A 1- to 10-minute exercise duration is the most likely to be improved by sodium bicarbonate (40, 72, 73), although exercise intensity likely also plays an important role (48). Repeated sprint exercise, common during team sports, has been shown to be limited by H^+ buffering capacity (93). Intermittent protocols such as these (i.e., repeated sprint exercise) do appear particularly susceptible to improvements with sodium bicarbonate supplementation (10, 11, 63, 75). Similar to beta-alanine, the ergogenic effects of sodium bicarbonate appear reduced in trained individuals (90), but its application in a competitive setting may lead to worthwhile changes in performance.

The effect of sodium bicarbonate between individuals appears variable, with some individuals improving performance while others do not, despite similar increases in blood variables (107). Within-individual blood responses following ingestion of sodium bicarbonate appear consistent, although consistency of the ergogenic effect on exercise performance is disputed (40, 42). This, however, may be due to the contrasting nature of the populations employed; inconsistent exercise results have been shown with non-trained (40), but not trained (42), individuals. There is the possibility that inconsistent exercise results are due to variable blood responses between individuals, particularly in response to ingestion at a standardized time point prior to exercise, since not all individuals may have experienced sufficient alkalosis to influence performance. This has led to studies employing time-to-peak bicarbonate protocols to coincide exercise with the greatest changes in circulating bicarbonate. The only two studies to date that have employed this tactic have shown positive results (44, 75), although further work is necessary to elucidate whether this approach elicits greater and more consistent gains for exercise performance and capacity.

Most sodium bicarbonate research has focused upon acute ingestion to improve exercise performance, although a few studies have explored the influence of serial ingestion in conjunction with high-intensity interval training with conflicting results. Evidence has shown greater beneficial effects of combined training with supplementation than training alone on aerobic and anaerobic measures (36, 57, 127), although not all agree (31). There is a growing body of evidence that sodium bicarbonate may be effective for exercise performed in extreme environments, such as hypoxia (24, 41, 106) and the heat (80). These extreme environmental conditions result in greater-than-normal lactate and H^+ accumulation and are thus likely to be extremely susceptible to increased buffering capacity, suggesting a further avenue for research.

Side Effects

Upon entering the stomach, the bicarbonate neutralizes large quantities of the H^+ present within the stomach's gastric juices producing carbon dioxide, which can cause abdominal pain, flatulence, nausea, diarrhoea, and vomiting (14). The intensity and duration of these symptoms are intrinsically linked to the dose ingested, with greater discomfort experienced with increasing doses (72). It is important to determine the impact these side effects may have, since they have the potential to influence an individual's performance and potentially the overall outcome of the investigation. Saunders et al. (107) only showed improvements in high-intensity cycling capacity when individuals suffering from gastrointestinal (GI) distress were removed from the analysis. Several strategies have been developed to avoid these side effects, including split-dose strategies (101, 107), multiday consumption (71, 79), or carbohydrate ingestion alongside supplementation (17). Strategies that minimize bicarbonate losses in the stomach have been suggested to be a viable method to minimize side effects (22); this may include delayed-release (50) or enteric-coated (14) capsules, although research on this topic is currently underexplored. It is also important to note that frequent or chronic sodium bicarbonate supplementation will lead to a chronically increased sodium load for the body, which could affect kidney function, although no study has determined this directly.

Sodium Citrate

Research into the use of sodium citrate as an ergogenic aid began over 30 years ago (89). It acts as an alkalizing agent, since the utilization of protons during the oxidation of citrate indirectly generates bicarbonate, leading to an increased buffering capacity in a similar manner to sodium bicarbonate (64). Following initial positive findings, subsequent studies suggested sodium citrate had low efficacy, and it received less attention than comparable buffering agents such as sodium bicarbonate. There has been a resurgence in its popularity due to a series of recent findings and the possibility that sodium citrate carries a lower incidence of GI-related side effects than sodium bicarbonate (124).

Supplementation Strategies

Sodium citrate is supplemented in powder or capsule form and ingested acutely prior to exercise. Two key factors that may alter its efficacy are the timing and relative dose of supplementation, which should be structured to elicit the greatest alkalotic effect at the onset of exercise. Ingestion consistently leads to an increase in plasma bicarbonate, with several studies showing an increase in excess of the theoretical potential (≥ 5 mmol·L^{-1}) and certain (≥ 6 mmol·L^{-1}) ergogenic thresholds (46). McNaughton (74) first showed a dose-response to sodium citrate supplementation for intakes ranging from 0.1 to 0.5 g·kg^{-1}BM; 90 minutes post-ingestion, exercise performance, blood pH, and bicarbonate were greatest with the highest 0.5 g·kg⁻¹BM dose. The two lowest doses, 0.1 and 0.2 g·kg⁻¹BM, did not result in an ergogenic effect. As a consequence of these data, most studies have adopted 0.3 g·kg⁻¹BM or 0.5 g·kg⁻¹BM as the experimental treatment dose (70, 83, 84, 110).

Urwin and colleagues (124) investigated the time course of blood response following higher doses of sodium citrate, although results confirmed 0.5 g·kg⁻¹BM as the most effective; 0.7 g·kg⁻¹BM and 0.9 g·kg⁻¹BM led to worse side effects without further changes in blood pH or bicarbonate. Their results did, however, suggest that the standardized ingestion time used in most studies (i.e., 90 minutes pre-exercise) may be sub-optimal. Blood alkalosis peaked between 180 and 215 minutes post-ingestion, suggesting that sodium citrate should be taken a minimum of 180 minutes pre-exercise. This recent evidence may explain some of the equivocal findings in the research (86), since the greatest chance of an improvement in exercise performance is likely to come from supplementation strategies that maximize increases in blood pH and bicarbonate prior to exercise.

Effects on Exercise Performance

Parry-Billings and MacLaren (89) showed that sodium citrate had no effect on anaerobic power and capacity, with McNaughton (74) being the first to show a beneficial effect of sodium citrate supplementation on total work and peak power output during a maximal 1-minute cycle ergometer sprint. The degree of performance enhancement increased with each ascending dose and increase in blood alkalosis (74). A subsequent study supported the use of sodium citrate supplementation to enhance performance for maximal tasks lasting from 2 to 4 minutes, but not for tasks ≤30 seconds in duration (70), consistent with its role as an extracellular pH buffer. Despite these favourable results, meta-analytical data of sodium citrate supplementation showed evidence to be equivocal (16). Pooled data from 13 studies showed an unclear effect on performance (0.0 ± 1.3% change in mean power), which was not modified by sex, athletic status, or the supplement dose. The lack of effect occurred despite a similar temporal response of blood pH and bicarbonate to that of sodium bicarbonate supplementation. When standardized to an equimolar dose, sodium citrate appears less effective than sodium bicarbonate at improving exercise performance: 1% vs. 6.3% improvement in high-intensity running to exhaustion (125).

These findings question the efficacy and mechanism of action of sodium citrate. A possible explanation is that an inhibitory effect of increased intracellular citrate counteracts the increase in extracellular buffering capacity (62). Citrate can allosterically inhibit the rate-limiting glycolytic enzyme, phosphofructokinase, and thus reduce adenosine triphosphate production. A further issue could be the timing of ingestion, since most studies included in the meta-analysis supplemented sodium citrate 90 to 120 minutes prior to exercise (16). As discussed, this may be a sub-optimal strategy as it does not allow for peak blood alkalosis and coincides with greater side effects (124). Thus, improvements in exercise performance may be more apparent with a longer period between sodium citrate ingestion and the start of the task, but this remains to be experimentally confirmed.

Side Effects

There is a perceived lower risk of GI discomfort compared to sodium bicarbonate (91, 95), although side effects still occur with sodium citrate. The most common symptoms include stomach cramps, bloating, nausea, vomiting, urge to defecate, diarrhoea, thirst, and headache (84, 109, 110); essentially the same side effects as sodium bicarbonate. Early studies reported no side effects from sodium citrate doses ranging from 0.1 to 0.5 g·kg⁻¹BM (62, 74, 89), although these investigations failed to adequately record the incidence and severity of side effects, meaning that mild symptoms went unnoticed. Later studies reported side effects with doses of 0.5 g·kg⁻¹BM (83, 84, 110), but GI distress was not experienced by volunteers in all studies (125). Symptom prevalence and severity increase in a dose-dependent manner for intakes of 0.5, 0.7, and 0.9 g·kg⁻¹BM (124). Key moderators of these effects appear to be the volume of fluid supplied with the supplement and the time permitted to consume the fluid; concentrated solutions with a higher osmolality are more likely to result in GI distress (65). Higher doses potentiate these symptoms (124), and lower or staggered doses may reduce symptom prevalence and/or severity (74). Side effects may also have an ergolytic effect on exercise, particularly if sodium citrate is ingested 60–90 minutes pre-exercise, which means that individuals would perform exercise at the moment of the highest risk of GI distress and without reaching peak blood alkalosis (124).

Sodium and Calcium Lactate

Lactate supplementation has been purported as a strategy for increasing extracellular buffering capacity. Following ingestion of sodium or calcium lactate, the lactate is absorbed in the intestine, preferentially in the jejunum (47), entering the bloodstream and increasing blood lactate concentration. The lactate can subsequently be oxidized or used as a metabolic substrate in gluconeogenesis (69, 76), processes that consume H^+, subsequently altering acid–base balance. The increased lactate can also be taken up by the tissue for oxidation (54) or by hepatocytes for conversion into glucose (1). The transport of lactate into tissues is facilitated by the monocarboxylate transporters 1 and 4, which co-transport with H^+ in a 1:1 ratio (59), thereby resulting in a net loss of H^+ in blood, increasing blood pH, and sparing blood bicarbonate, which may be useful during high-intensity exercise.

Supplementation Strategies

Lactate is commonly provided in doses between 120 and 300 mg·kg⁻¹BM; one study employed a dose as low as ~14 mg·kg⁻¹BM (81), although they showed no changes in blood variables, suggesting that this low dose is incapable of increasing buffering capacity, and increases in circulating bicarbonate and blood pH were modest at best. Mean bicarbonate increases of approximately +3 mmol·L⁻¹ have been shown after ingesting 250 ml of an 80% polylactate solution (38) and 120 mg·kg⁻¹BM in gelatine capsules (78); this is approximately half the increase usually shown with a 0.3 g·kg⁻¹BM dose of sodium bicarbonate (46). De Salles Painelli et al. (85) aimed to determine the optimal lactate dose and timing for peak increases in blood pH and bicarbonate using a low (150 mg·kg⁻¹BM) and high (300 mg·kg⁻¹BM) dose of calcium lactate. Both doses only resulted in increased bicarbonate concentrations of around +2 mmol·L⁻¹, with similarly small increases in pH, and peak values occurred 60–90 minutes following supplement ingestion. Morris et al. (77) showed increases of approximately +2.5 mmol·L⁻¹ 70 minutes post-ingestion of 120 and 300 mg·kg⁻¹BM. Five days of calcium lactate supplementation at 500 mg·kg⁻¹·day⁻¹ did not result in blood alkalosis, suggesting that a chronic supplementation strategy is inefficient for increasing buffering capacity (82). Acute lactate doses of between 120 and 300 mg·kg⁻¹BM 60–90 minutes prior to exercise appear most likely to increase buffering capacity, albeit more modestly than sodium bicarbonate or sodium citrate.

Effects on Exercise Performance

Morris et al. (78) showed a 17% improvement in exercise tolerance during a high-intensity cycling capacity test to exhaustion at 100% of maximal power output with 120 mg·kg⁻¹BM calcium lactate; the same group showed improvements (+14 and +26%) in the same high-intensity exercise test following two doses of 120 and 300 mg·kg⁻¹BM of calcium lactate (77). These impressive gains are not consistent within the literature, with further studies failing to show any efficacy of this supplement (81, 82). Methodological differences may explain the lack of an effect of lactate on performance in these studies, such as a very low dose unlikely to increase buffering capacity (81) and chronic supplementation which resulted in no increases in circulating bicarbonate (82). However, performance during the three-bout upper-body Wingate test was not improved with either 150 or 300 mg·kg⁻¹BM of acute calcium lactate ingestion (85). Since this exercise test is susceptible to changes in buffering capacity with sodium bicarbonate and beta-alanine (2, 123), these findings cast doubt on the efficacy of lactate as an ergogenic aid. One study compared the efficacy of sodium lactate with sodium bicarbonate and sodium citrate in male endurance runners. A 400 mg·kg⁻¹BM dose of sodium lactate 90 minutes prior to a run to exhaustion (at maximum effort to elicit fatigue in 1–2 minutes) improved performance by 1.7%, which was higher than the improvement shown with sodium citrate (0.5%) although lower than that with sodium bicarbonate (2.7%) (125).

Side Effects

Only two studies have reported any side effects with acute lactate supplementation, with volunteers experiencing similar levels of belching and flatulence following 150 and 300 mg·kg⁻¹BM of calcium lactate (85) and very low levels of sickness and stomach ache with 400 mg·kg⁻¹BM (125). The associated side effects with lactate supplementation appear to be minor and unlikely to harm exercise performance.

Outstanding Questions and Directions for Future Research

- The greatest possible increases in muscle carnosine with beta-alanine supplementation are currently unknown and are worth determining to see if concomitant changes in exercise capacity and performance can also be maximized.
- The effects of beta-alanine for resistance and strength-based exercise is unclear. Further research using intensive protocols, those commonly used in real-life situations, are required to clarify its potential as an ergogenic aid for resistance athletes.
- The efficacy of sodium citrate and sodium/calcium lactate for exercise performance relative to sodium bicarbonate (considered the most effective of these extracellular buffers) needs to be further investigated. This will allow determination of whether supplementation with these alternative products is useful.
- The optimal timing of sodium bicarbonate (and sodium citrate) to induce the greatest alkalosis and minimal side effects at the moment exercise begins is currently suggested, but not strongly demonstrated. Studies should determine whether these claims are substantiated.
- Alternative supplementation strategies to reduce side effects with extracellular buffers warrant future investigation. This may include gastro-resistant capsules, split-dose strategies, and lower doses with adapted timing of ingestion.
- More work is necessary to determine if any of these buffering supplements are more effective for exercise performed in extreme environmental conditions that result in greater-than-normal H⁺ accumulation, such as hypoxia or heat.

Summary and Conclusions

Intense exercise challenges skeletal muscle homeostasis, partly through the production of lactic acid that occurs when the rate of glycolysis outstrips the rate of pyruvate oxidation. The resultant increase in H⁺ within the skeletal muscle contributes to fatigue, particularly in those high-intensity events lasting between 1 and 10 minutes. The action of buffers in the skeletal muscle can help to protect against the rate of H⁺ accumulation. Over time, however, H⁺ will still accumulate, and must be transported out of the muscle and into the blood, resulting in reduced blood pH. One possible means to delay the onset of fatigue during this type of exercise is to increase the intracellular and/or extracellular buffering capacity. Several dietary supplements have some potential to achieve this, with the most promising being chronic supplementation with beta-alanine (to increase intramuscular buffering via an increase in muscle carnosine content) and acute supplementation with sodium bicarbonate (to increase extracellular buffering via an increase in circulating bicarbonate). Both supplements have been listed by the International Olympic Committee as sport supplements where there is sufficient evidence to substantiate their recommendation for use to improve exercise performance (68).

References

1. Adeva-Andany MM, Perez-Felpete N, Fernandez-Fernandez C, Donapetry-Garcia C, Pazos-Garcia C. Liver glucose metabolism in humans. *Biosci Rep* 36: 2016.
2. Artioli GG, Gualano B, Coelho DF, Benatti FB, Galley AW, Lancha AH. Does sodium-bicarbonate ingestion improve simulated judo performance? *Int J Sport Nutr Exerc Metab* 17: 206–217, 2007.
3. Artioli GG, Sale C, Jones RL. Carnosine in health and disease. *Eur J Sport Sci* 1–10, 2018.
4. Baguet A, Bourgois J, Vanhee L, Achten E, Derave W. Important role of muscle carnosine in rowing performance. *J Appl Physiol (1985)* 109: 1096–1101, 2010.
5. Bailey CH, Signorile JF, Perry AC, Jacobs KA, Myers ND. Beta-alanine does not enhance the effects of resistance training in older adults. *J Diet Suppl* 15: 860–870, 2018.
6. Bassinello D, de Salles Painelli V, Dolan E, Lixandrao M, Cajueiro M, de Capitani M, et al. Beta-alanine supplementation improves isometric, but not isotonic or isokinetic strength endurance in recreationally strength-trained young men. *Amino Acids* 51(1):27–37, 2018.
7. Bate-Smith EC. The buffering of muscle in rigor; protein, phosphate and carnosine. *J Physiol* 92: 336–343, 1938.
8. Bellinger PM, Minahan CL. Additive benefits of beta-alanine supplementation and sprint-interval training. *Med Sci Sports Exerc* 48: 2417–2425, 2016.
9. Bex T, Chung W, Baguet A, Stegen S, Stautemas J, Achten E, et al. Muscle carnosine loading by beta-alanine supplementation is more pronounced in trained vs. untrained muscles. *J Appl Physiol* 116: 204–209, 2014.
10. Bishop D, Claudius B. Effects of induced metabolic alkalosis on prolonged intermittent-sprint performance. *Med Sci Sports Exerc* 37: 759–767, 2005.
11. Bishop D, Edge J, Davis C, Goodman C. Induced metabolic alkalosis affects muscle metabolism and repeated-sprint ability. *Med Sci Sports Exerc* 36: 807–813, 2004.
12. Blancquaert L, Everaert I, Missinne M, Baguet A, Stegen S, Volkaert A, et al. Effects of histidine and beta-alanine supplementation on human muscle carnosine storage. *Med Sci Sports Exerc* 49: 602–609, 2017.
13. Boldyrev AA, Stvolinsky SL, Fedorova TN, Suslina ZA. Carnosine as a natural antioxidant and geroprotector: From molecular mechanisms to clinical trials. *Rejuvenation Res* 13: 156–158, 2010.
14. Breitkreutz J, Gan TG, Schneider B, Kalisch P. Enteric-coated solid dosage forms containing sodium bicarbonate as a drug substance: An exception from the rule? *J Pharm Pharmacol* 59: 59–65, 2007.
15. Butterworth PJ. *Lehninger: principles of biochemistry* (4th edn) D. L. Nelson and M. C. Cox, W. H. Freeman & Co., New York, 1119pp (plus 17 pp glossary), ISBN 0-7167-4339-6 (2004). *Cell Biochemistry and Function* 23: 293–294, 2005.
16. Carr AJ, Hopkins WG, Gore CJ. Effects of acute alkalosis and acidosis on performance: A meta-analysis. *Sports Med* 41: 801–814, 2011.
17. Carr AJ, Slater GJ, Gore CJ, Dawson B, Burke LM. Effect of sodium bicarbonate on [HCO3-], pH, and gastrointestinal symptoms. *Int J Sport Nutr Exerc Metab* 21: 189–194, 2011.
18. Carr AJ, Slater GJ, Gore CJ, Dawson B, Burke LM. Reliability and effect of sodium bicarbonate: Buffering and 2000-m rowing performance. *Int J Sports Physiol Perform* 7: 152–160, 2012.
19. Church DD, Hoffman JR, Varanoske AN, Wang R, Baker KM, La Monica MB, et al. Comparison of two beta-alanine dosing protocols on muscle carnosine elevations. *J Am Coll Nutr* 36(8):608–616, 2017.
20. Cochran AJ, Percival ME, Thompson S, Gillen JB, MacInnis MJ, Potter MA, et al. Beta-alanine supplementation does not augment the skeletal muscle adaptive response to 6 weeks of sprint interval training. *Int J Sport Nutr Exerc Metab* 25: 541–549, 2015.
21. Costill DL, Verstappen F, Kuipers H, Janssen E, Fink W. Acid-base balance during repeated bouts of exercise: Influence of HCO3. *Int J Sports Med* 5: 228–231, 1984.
22. de Oliveira LF, Saunders B, Artioli GG. Is bypassing the stomach a means to optimize sodium bicarbonate supplementation? A case study with a postbariatric surgery individual. *Int J Sport Nutr Exerc Metab* 28: 660–663, 2018.
23. de Oliveira LF, Saunders B, Yamaguchi G, Swinton P, Artioli GG. Is individualization of sodium bicarbonate ingestion based on time to peak necessary? *Med Sci Sports Exerc* 52(8):1801–1808, 2020.

24. Deb SK, Gough LA, Sparks SA, McNaughton LR. Determinants of curvature constant (W') of the power duration relationship under normoxia and hypoxia: The effect of pre-exercise alkalosis. *Eur J Appl Physiol* 117: 901–912, 2017.

25. Debold EP, Fitts RH, Sundberg CW, Nosek TM. Muscle fatigue from the perspective of a single crossbridge. *Med Sci Sports Exerc* 48: 2270–2280, 2016.

26. Decombaz J, Beaumont M, Vuichoud J, Bouisset F, Stellingwerff T. Effect of slow-release beta-alanine tablets on absorption kinetics and paresthesia. *Amino Acids* 43: 67–76, 2012.

27. Derave W, Oezdemir MS, Harris RC, Pottier A, Reyngoudt H, Koppo K, et al. Beta-alanine supplementation augments muscle carnosine content and attenuates fatigue during repeated isokinetic contraction bouts in trained sprinters. *J Appl Physiol* 103: 1736–1743, 2007.

28. Dolan E, Saunders B, Harris RC, Bicudo J, Bishop DJ, Sale C, et al. Comparative physiology investigations support a role for histidine-containing dipeptides in intracellular acid-base regulation of skeletal muscle. *Comp Biochem Physiol A Mol Integr Physiol* 234: 77–86, 2019.

29. Dolan E, Swinton PA, Painelli VS, Stephens Hemingway B, Mazzolani B, Infante Smaira F, et al. A systematic risk assessment and meta-analysis on the use of oral beta-alanine supplementation. *Adv Nutr* 10(3):452–463, 2019.

30. Donaldson SK, Hermansen L, Bolles L. Differential, direct effects of H+ on Ca2+ -activated force of skinned fibers from the soleus, cardiac and adductor magnus muscles of rabbits. *Pflugers Arch* 376: 55–65, 1978.

31. Driller MW, Gregory JR, Williams AD, Fell JW. The effects of chronic sodium bicarbonate ingestion and interval training in highly trained rowers. *Int J Sport Nutr Exerc Metab* 23: 40–47, 2013.

32. Ducker KJ, Dawson B, Wallman KE. Effect of beta alanine and sodium bicarbonate supplementation on repeated-sprint performance. *J Strength Cond Res* 27: 3450–3460, 2013.

33. Duncan MJ, Weldon A, Price MJ. The effect of sodium bicarbonate ingestion on back squat and bench press exercise to failure. *J Strength Cond Res* 28: 1358–1366, 2014.

34. Durkalec-Michalski K, Zawieja EE, Podgorski T, Loniewski I, Zawieja BE, Warzybok M, et al. The effect of chronic progressive-dose sodium bicarbonate ingestion on CrossFit-like performance: A double-blind, randomized cross-over trial. *PLOS ONE* 13: e0197480, 2018.

35. Dutka TL, Lamb GD. Effect of carnosine on excitation-contraction coupling in mechanically-skinned rat skeletal muscle. *J Muscle Res Cell Motil* 25: 203–213, 2004.

36. Edge J, Bishop D, Goodman C. Effects of chronic NaHCO3 ingestion during interval training on changes to muscle buffer capacity, metabolism, and short-term endurance performance. *J Appl Physiol (1985)* 101: 918–925, 2006.

37. Fabiato A, Fabiato F. Effects of pH on the myofilaments and the sarcoplasmic reticulum of skinned cells from cardiace and skeletal muscles. *J Physiol* 276: 233–255, 1978.

38. Fahey TD, Larsen JD, Brooks GA, Colvin W, Henderson S, Lary D. The effects of ingesting polylactate or glucose polymer drinks during prolonged exercise. *Int J Sport Nutr* 1: 249–256, 1991.

39. Freis T, Hecksteden A, Such U, Meyer T. Effect of sodium bicarbonate on prolonged running performance: A randomized, double-blind, cross-over study. *PLOS ONE* 12: e0182158, 2017.

40. Froio de Araujo Dias G, da Eira Silva V, Painelli VS, Sale C, Giannini Artioli G, Gualano B, et al. (In) consistencies in responses to sodium bicarbonate supplementation: A randomised, repeated measures, counterbalanced and double-blind study. *PloS One* 10: e0143086, 2015.

41. Gough LA, Deb SK, Brown D, Sparks SA, McNaughton LR. The effects of sodium bicarbonate ingestion on cycling performance and acid base balance recovery in acute normobaric hypoxia. *J Sports Sci* 37: 1464–1471, 2019.

42. Gough LA, Deb SK, Sparks A, McNaughton LR. The reproducibility of 4-km time trial (TT) performance following individualised sodium bicarbonate supplementation: A randomised controlled trial in trained cyclists. *Sports Med Open* 3: 34, 2017.

43. Gough LA, Deb SK, Sparks AS, McNaughton LR. The reproducibility of blood acid base responses in male collegiate athletes following individualised doses of sodium bicarbonate: A randomised controlled crossover study. *Sports Med* 47: 2117–2127, 2017.

44. Gough LA, Deb SK, Sparks SA, McNaughton LR. Sodium bicarbonate improves 4 km time trial cycling performance when individualised to time to peak blood bicarbonate in trained male cyclists. *J Sports Sci* 1–8, 2017.

45. Harris RC, Tallon MJ, Dunnett M, Boobis L, Coakley J, Kim HJ, et al. The absorption of orally supplied beta-alanine and its effect on muscle carnosine synthesis in human vastus lateralis. *Amino Acids* 30: 279–289, 2006.

46. Heibel AB, Perim PHL, Oliveira LF, McNaughton LR, Saunders B. Time to optimize supplementation: Modifying factors influencing the individual responses to extracellular buffering agents. *Front Nutr* 5: 35, 2018.

47. Heller MD, Kern F Jr. Absorption of lactic acid from an isolated intestinal segment in the intact rat. *Proc Soc Exp Biol Med* 127: 1103–1106, 1968.

48. Higgins MF, James RS, Price MJ. The effects of sodium bicarbonate (NaHCO3) ingestion on high intensity cycling capacity. *J Sport Sci* 31: 972–981, 2013.

49. Hill CA, Harris RC, Kim HJ, Harris BD, Sale C, Boobis LH, et al. Influence of beta-alanine supplementation on skeletal muscle carnosine concentrations and high intensity cycling capacity. *Amino Acids* 32: 225–233, 2007.

50. Hilton NP, Leach NK, Sparks SA, Gough LA, Craig MM, Deb SK, et al. A novel ingestion strategy for sodium bicarbonate supplementation in a delayed-release form: A randomised crossover study in trained males. *Sports Med Open* 5: 4, 2019.

51. Hipkiss AR, Brownson C. A possible new role for the anti-ageing peptide carnosine. *Cell Mol Life Sci* 57: 747–753, 2000.

52. Hoffman JR, Ratamess NA, Faigenbaum AD, Ross R, Kang J, Stout JR, et al. Short-duration beta-alanine supplementation increases training volume and reduces subjective feelings of fatigue in college football players. *Nutr Res* 28: 31–35, 2008.

53. Hultman E, Sjoholm H. Energy metabolism and contraction force of human skeletal muscle in situ during electrical stimulation. *J Physiol* 345: 525–532, 1983.

54. Jacobs RA, Meinild AK, Nordsborg NB, Lundby C. Lactate oxidation in human skeletal muscle mitochondria. *Am J Physiol Endocrinol Metab* 304: E686–E694, 2013.

55. Jones RL, Barnett CT, Davidson J, Maritza B, Fraser WD, Harris R, et al. Beta-alanine supplementation improves in-vivo fresh and fatigued skeletal muscle relaxation speed. *Eur J Appl Physiol* 117: 867–879, 2017.

56. Jones RL, Stellingwerff T, Artioli GG, Saunders B, Cooper S, Sale C. Dose-response of sodium bicarbonate ingestion highlights individuality in time course of blood analyte responses. *Int J Sport Nutr Exerc Metab* 26: 445–453, 2016.

57. Jourkesh M, Ahmaidi S, Bita Mehdipoor K, Sadri I, Ojagi A. Effects of six weeks sodium bicarbonate supplementation and high-intensity interval training on endurance performance and body composition. *Ann Biol Res* 2: 403–413, 2011.

58. Joyce S, Minahan C, Anderson M, Osborne M. Acute and chronic loading of sodium bicarbonate in highly trained swimmers. *Eur J Appl Physiol* 112: 461–469, 2012.

59. Juel C. Lactate-proton cotransport in skeletal muscle. *Physiol Rev* 77: 321–358, 1997.

60. Katz A, Costill DL, King DS, Hargreaves M, Fink WJ. Maximal exercise tolerance after induced alkalosis. *Int J Sports Med* 5: 107–110, 1984.

61. Kent-Braun JA, Fitts RH, Christie A. Skeletal muscle fatigue. *Compr Physiol* 2: 997–1044, 2012.

62. Kowalchuk JM, Maltais SA, Yamaji K, Hughson RL. The effect of citrate loading on exercise performance, acid-base balance and metabolism. *Eur J Appl Physiol Occup Physiol* 58: 858–864, 1989.

63. Krustrup P, Ermidis G, Mohr M. Sodium bicarbonate intake improves high-intensity intermittent exercise performance in trained young men. *J Int Soc Sports Nutr* 12: 2015.

64. Lancha Junior AH, Painelli VS, Saunders B, Artioli GG. Nutritional strategies to modulate intracellular and extracellular buffering capacity during high-intensity exercise. *Sports Med* 45(Suppl 1): S71–S81, 2015.

65. Linderman JK, Gosselink KL. The effects of sodium bicarbonate ingestion on exercise performance. *Sports Med* 18: 75–80, 1994.

66. Liu Q, Sikand P, Ma C, Tang Z, Han L, Li Z, et al. Mechanisms of itch evoked by beta-alanine. *J Neurosci* 32: 14532–14537, 2012.

67. Matson LG, Tran ZV. Effects of sodium bicarbonate ingestion on anaerobic performance: A meta-analytic review. *Int J Sport Nutr* 3: 2–28, 1993.

68. Maughan RJ, Burke LM, Dvorak J, Larson-Meyer DE, Peeling P, Phillips SM, et al. IOC consensus statement: Dietary supplements and the high-performance athlete. *Br J Sports Med* 52: 439–455, 2018.

69. Mazzeo RS, Brooks GA, Schoeller DA, Budinger TF. Disposal of blood [1-13C]lactate in humans during rest and exercise. *J Appl Physiol (1985)* 60: 232–241, 1986.

70. McNaughton L, Cedaro R. Sodium citrate ingestion and its effects on maximal anaerobic exercise of different durations. *Eur J Appl Physiol Occup Physiol* 64: 36–41, 1992.

71. McNaughton L, Thompson D. Acute versus chronic sodium bicarbonate ingestion and anaerobic work and power output. *J Sports Med Phys Fitness* 41: 456–462, 2001.

72. McNaughton LR. Bicarbonate ingestion: Effects of dosage on 60 s cycle ergometry. *J Sport Sci* 10: 415–423, 1992.

73. McNaughton LR. Sodium bicarbonate ingestion and its effects on anaerobic exercise of various durations. *J Sports Sci* 10: 425–435, 1992.

74. McNaughton LR. Sodium citrate and anaerobic performance: Implications of dosage. *Eur J Appl Physiol Occup Physiol* 61: 392–397, 1990.

75. Miller P, Robinson AL, Sparks SA, Bridge CA, Bentley DJ, McNaughton LR. The effects of novel ingestion of sodium bicarbonate on repeated sprint ability. *J Strength Cond Res* 30: 561–568, 2016.

76. Morris D. Effects of oral lactate consumption on metabolism and exercise performance. *Curr Sports Med Rep* 11: 185–188, 2012.

77. Morris D, Beloni R, Wofford H. Metabolic and exercise performance responses to two different oral doses of calcium lactate. *Med Sci Sport Exer* 48: 250–250, 2016.

78. Morris DM, Shafer RS, Fairbrother KR, Woodall MW. Effects of lactate consumption on blood bicarbonate levels and performance during high-intensity exercise. *Int J Sport Nutr Exerc Metab* 21: 311–317, 2011.

79. Mueller SM, Gehrig SM, Frese S, Wagner CA, Boutellier U, Toigo M. Multiday acute sodium bicarbonate intake improves endurance capacity and reduces acidosis in men. *J Int Soc Sports Nutr* 10: 16, 2013.

80. Mundel T. Sodium bicarbonate ingestion improves repeated high-intensity cycling performance in the heat. *Temperature* 5: 343–347, 2018.

81. Northgraves MJ, Peart DJ, Jordan CA, Vince RV. Effect of lactate supplementation and sodium bicarbonate on 40-km cycling time trial performance. *J Strength Cond Res* 28: 273–280, 2014.

82. Oliveira LF, de Salles Painelli V, Nemezio K, Goncalves LS, Yamaguchi G, Saunders B, et al. Chronic lactate supplementation does not improve blood buffering capacity and repeated high-intensity exercise. *Scand J Med Sci Sports* 27: 1231–1239, 2017.

83. Oopik V, Saaremets I, Medijainen L, Karelson K, Janson T, Timpmann S. Effects of sodium citrate ingestion before exercise on endurance performance in well trained college runners. *Br J Sports Med* 37: 485–489, 2003.

84. Oopik V, Saaremets I, Timpmann S, Medijainen L, Karelson K. Effects of acute ingestion of sodium citrate on metabolism and 5-km running performance: A field study. *Can J Appl Physiol* 29: 691–703, 2004.

85. Painelli VS, da Silva RP, de Oliveira OM Jr., de Oliveira LF, Benatti FB, Rabelo T, et al. The effects of two different doses of calcium lactate on blood pH, bicarbonate, and repeated high-intensity exercise performance. *Int J Sport Nutr Exerc Metab* 24: 286–295, 2014.

86. Painelli VS, Lancha Junior AH. Thirty years of investigation on the ergogenic effects of sodium citrate: Is it time for a fresh start? *Br J Sports Med* 2016.

87. Painelli VS, Saunders B, Sale C, Harris RC, Solis MY, Roschel H, et al. Influence of training status on high-intensity intermittent performance in response to beta-alanine supplementation. *Amino Acids* 46: 1207–1215, 2014.

88. Pan JW, Hamm JR, Hetherington HP, Rothman DL, Shulman RG. Correlation of lactate and pH in human skeletal muscle after exercise by 1H NMR. *Magn Reson Med* 20: 57–65, 1991.

89. Parry-Billings M, MacLaren DP. The effect of sodium bicarbonate and sodium citrate ingestion on anaerobic power during intermittent exercise. *Eur J Appl Physiol Occup Physiol* 55: 524–529, 1986.

90. Peart DJ, Siegler JC, Vince RV. Practical recommendations for coaches and athletes: A meta-analysis of sodium bicarbonate use for athletic performance. *J Strength Cond Res* 26: 1975–1983, 2012.

91. Peeling P, Binnie MJ, Goods PSR, Sim M, Burke LM. Evidence-based supplements for the enhancement of athletic performance. *Int J Sport Nutr Exerc Metab* 28: 178–187, 2018.

92. Price MJ, Singh M. Time course of blood bicarbonate and pH three hours after sodium bicarbonate ingestion. *Int J Sports Physiol Perform* 3: 240–242, 2008.

93. Rampinini E, Sassi A, Morelli A, Mazzoni S, Fanchini M, Coutts AJ. Repeated-sprint ability in professional and amateur soccer players. *Appl Physiol Nutr Metab* 34: 1048–1054, 2009.

94. Renfree A. The time course for changes in plasma [h+] after sodium bicarbonate ingestion. *Int J Sports Physiol Perform* 2: 323–326, 2007.

95. Requena B, Zabala M, Padial P, Feriche B. Sodium bicarbonate and sodium citrate: Ergogenic aids? *J Strength Cond Res* 19: 213–224, 2005.

96. Roberges R, Hutchinson K, Hendee S, Madden S, Siegler J. Influence of pre-exercise acidosis and alkalosis on the kinetics of acid-base recovery following intense exercise. *Int J Sport Nutr Exerc Metab* 15: 59–74, 2005.

97. Sahlin K, Harris RC, Hultman E. Creatine kinase equilibrium and lactate content compared with muscle pH in tissue samples obtained after isometric exercise. *Biochem J* 152: 173–180, 1975.

98. Sahlin K, Harris RC, Nylind B, Hultman E. Lactate content and Ph in muscle samples obtained after dynamic exercise. *Pflug Arch Eur J Phy* 367: 143–149, 1976.

99. Sale C, Artioli GG, Gualano B, Saunders B, Hobson RM, Harris RC. Carnosine: from exercise performance to health. *Amino Acids* 44: 1477–1491, 2013.

100. Sale C, Hill CA, Ponte J, Harris RC. Beta-alanine supplementation improves isometric endurance of the knee extensor muscles. *J Int Soc Sports Nutr* 9: 26, 2012.

101. Sale C, Saunders B, Hudson S, Wise JA, Harris RC, Sunderland CD. Effect of beta-alanine plus sodium bicarbonate on high-intensity cycling capacity. *Med Sci Sport Exer* 43: 1972–1978, 2011.

102. Saunders B, Elliott-Sale K, Artioli GG, Swinton PA, Dolan E, Roschel H, et al. Beta-alanine supplementation to improve exercise capacity and performance: A systematic review and meta-analysis. *Br J Sports Med* 51: 658–669, 2017.

103. Saunders B, Franchi M, Oliveira LF, Silva VE, Silva RP, Painelli VS, et al. 24-Wk β-alanine ingestion does not affect muscle taurine or clinical blood parameters. *Eur J Nutr* 59: 57–65, 2020.

104. Saunders B, Painelli VS, De Oliveira LF, Eira Silva V, Silva RP, Riani L, et al. Twenty-four weeks of beta-alanine supplementation on carnosine content, related genes, and exercise. *Med Sci Sports Exerc* 49: 896–906, 2017.

105. Saunders B, Sale C, Harris RC, Sunderland C. Effect of beta-alanine supplementation on repeated sprint performance during the Loughborough Intermittent Shuttle Test. *Amino Acids* 43: 39–47, 2012.

106. Saunders B, Sale C, Harris RC, Sunderland C. Effect of sodium bicarbonate and beta-alanine on repeated sprints during intermittent exercise performed in hypoxia. *Int J Sport Nutr Exerc Metab* 24: 196–205, 2014.

107. Saunders B, Sale C, Harris RC, Sunderland C. Sodium bicarbonate and high-intensity-cycling capacity: Variability in responses. *Int J Sports Physiol Perform* 9: 627–632, 2014.

108. Saunders B, Sunderland C, Harris RC, Sale C. Beta-alanine supplementation improves YoYo intermittent recovery test performance. *J Int Soc Sports Nutr* 9: 39, 2012.

109. Schabort EJ, Wilson G, Noakes TD. Dose-related elevations in venous pH with citrate ingestion do not alter 40-km cycling time-trial performance. *Eur J Appl Physiol* 83: 320–327, 2000.

110. Shave R, Whyte G, Siemann A, Doggart L. The effects of sodium citrate ingestion on 3,000-meter time-trial performance. *J Strength Cond Res* 15: 230–234, 2001.

111. Siegler JC, Marshall PWM, Bray J, Towlson C. Sodium bicarbonate supplementation and ingestion timing: Does it matter? *J Strength Cond Res* 26: 1953–1958, 2012.

112. Siegler JC, Midgley AW, Polman RC, Lever R. Effects of various sodium bicarbonate loading protocols on the time-dependent extracellular buffering profile. *J Strength Cond Res* 24: 2551–2557, 2010.

113. Smith AE, Moon JR, Kendall KL, Graef JL, Lockwood CM, Walter AA, et al. The effects of beta-alanine supplementation and high-intensity interval training on neuromuscular fatigue and muscle function. *Eur J Appl Physiol* 105: 357–363, 2009.

114. Smith AE, Walter AA, Graef JL, Kendall KL, Moon JR, Lockwood CM, et al. Effects of beta-alanine supplementation and high-intensity interval training on endurance performance and body composition in men; a double-blind trial. *J Int Soc Sports Nutr* 6: 5, 2009.

115. Spencer M, Bishop D, Dawson B, Goodman C. Physiological and metabolic responses of repeated-sprint activities: Specific to field-based team sports. *Sports Med* 35: 1025–1044, 2005.

116. Stellingwerff T, Anwander H, Egger A, Buehler T, Kreis R, Decombaz J, et al. Effect of two beta-alanine dosing protocols on muscle carnosine synthesis and washout. *Amino Acids* 42: 2461–2472, 2012.

117. Stephens TJ, McKenna MJ, Canny BJ, Snow RJ, McConell GK. Effect of sodium bicarbonate on muscle metabolism during intense endurance cycling. *Med Sci Sports Exerc* 34: 614–621, 2002.

118. Sundberg CW, Fitts RH. Bioenergetic basis of skeletal muscle fatigue. *Curr Opin Physiol* 10: 118–127, 2019.

119. Sundberg CW, Hunter SK, Trappe SW, Smith CS, Fitts RH. Effects of elevated H(+) and Pi on the contractile mechanics of skeletal muscle fibres from young and old men: Implications for muscle fatigue in humans. *J Physiol* 596: 3993–4015, 2018.

120. Sutton JR, Jones NL, Toews CJ. Effect of PH on muscle glycolysis during exercise. *Clin Sci (Lond)* 61: 331–338, 1981.

121. Sweeney KM, Wright GA, Glenn Brice A, Doberstein ST. The effect of beta-alanine supplementation on power performance during repeated sprint activity. *J Strength Cond Res* 24: 79–87, 2010.

122. Tesch PA, Colliander EB, Kaiser P. Muscle metabolism during intense, heavy-resistance exercise. *Eur J Appl Physiol Occup Physiol* 55: 362–366, 1986.

123. Tobias G, Benatti FB, Painelli VS, Roschel H, Gualano B, Sale C, et al. Additive effects of beta-alanine and sodium bicarbonate on upper-body intermittent performance. *Amino Acids* 45: 309–317, 2013.

124. Urwin CS, Dwyer DB, Carr AJ. Induced alkalosis and gastrointestinal symptoms after sodium citrate ingestion: A dose-response investigation. *Int J Sport Nutr Exerc Metab* 26: 542–548, 2016.

125. Van Montfoort MC, Van Dieren L, Hopkins WG, Shearman JP. Effects of ingestion of bicarbonate, citrate, lactate, and chloride on sprint running. *Med Sci Sports Exerc* 36: 1239–1243, 2004.

126. Walter AA, Smith AE, Kendall KL, Stout JR, Cramer JT. Six weeks of high-intensity interval training with and without beta-alanine supplementation for improving cardiovascular fitness in women. *J Strength Cond Res* 24: 1199–1207, 2010.

127. Wang J, Qiu J, Yi L, Hou Z, Benardot D, Cao W. Effect of sodium bicarbonate ingestion during 6 weeks of HIIT on anaerobic performance of college students. *J Int Soc Sports Nutr* 16: 18, 2019.

23

CREATINE AUGMENTATION FOR MUSCLE AND BONE RESPONSES TO EXERCISE

Philip D. Chilibeck

Introduction

Creatine monohydrate (Cr) (Figure 23.1) is a nitrogenous organic acid that is found mainly in skeletal muscle (i.e., 95% of body stores), with smaller amounts found in other tissues, such as bone (65). It is synthesized endogenously (1–2 g per day) from three amino acids (arginine, glycine, and methionine) in the liver and kidneys (65) and can be obtained exogenously from the diet from beef, pork, fish (13), and poultry (35). Supplementation with Cr increases muscle creatine stores (2) and improves high-intensity exercise performance (23), and therefore there is great interest in using Cr as a supplement to improve muscular performance for athletes (13) and clinical populations, such as older adults (11). This chapter provides a review of the mechanisms by which Cr supplementation can augment muscular and skeletal responses to exercise.

Enhancement of Muscle Energy Supply with Creatine Supplementation

Creatine combines with inorganic phosphate to form phosphorylcreatine (PCr) in tissues such as muscle. When adenosine triphosphate (ATP) is broken down to provide energy for muscular contraction, it can very quickly be resynthesized by the reaction: adenosine diphosphate (ADP) + PCr → ATP + Cr; therefore, increasing PCr stores through Cr supplementation can buffer ATP levels, allowing for greater duration of high-intensity exercise (12, 65). Energy from the breakdown of ATP is important at several sites in muscle during contraction and relaxation, including the formation of actin–myosin cross-bridges, pumping of calcium into the sarcoplasmic reticulum, and pumping of sodium out and potassium into the muscle across the sarcolemma (54). Creatine can act as a shuttle for high-energy phosphate from the breakdown of ATP produced in the mitochondria to these sites of energy utilization to allow for quick re-phosphorylation of ADP to ATP (54) (Figure 23.2). Increasing Cr concentrations through supplementation with Cr can potentially enhance this shuttle system allowing for increased re-synthesis of ATP during exercise and recovery from exercise. Acute or chronic Cr supplementation can increase force output during repeated contractions, and therefore actin–myosin cross-bridge formation is most likely enhanced (12, 23). There is also evidence Cr supplementation (over 4–5 days) can enhance muscle relaxation after either electrically stimulated or voluntary contractions, therefore potentially enhancing ATP-mediated uptake of calcium into the sarcoplasmic reticulum (29, 61). Whether Cr supplementation can enhance sodium–potassium exchange across the sarcolemma has yet to be determined.

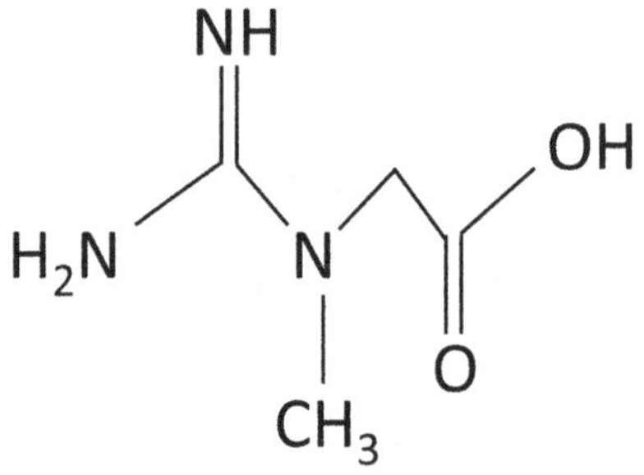

Figure 23.1   Chemical structure of creatine

Phosphorylcreatine is continuously broken down to drive re-synthesis of ATP during high-intensity exercise; therefore, sustaining high intensities of exercise is largely dependent on the amount of PCr stored in muscle (23). Exercise intensity needs to be reduced when PCr stores become depleted (65). Creatine supplementation drives the reverse of the creatine kinase reaction: $Cr + ATP \rightarrow PCr + ADP$, so that recovery of PCr after intense exercise is enhanced by supplementation with Cr (22, 56). Creatine supplementation therefore has great potential for improving repeated bouts of intense exercise (23) that are separated by short durations of recovery (i.e., characteristic of many sports such as American football).

Glycogen, the main storage form of carbohydrate in muscle, is important as a fuel source for exercise that ranges from high-intensity (i.e., anaerobic glycolysis) to sustained, low-intensity efforts (i.e., aerobic

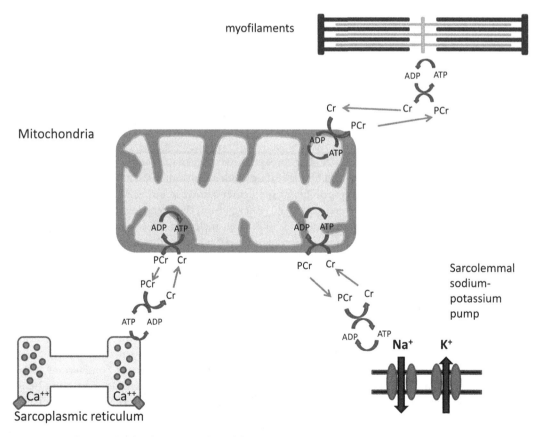

Figure 23.2   The creatine shuttle system (adapted from 54)

glycolysis). Significant glycogen depletion occurs during exercise ranging from resistance training (26) to long-distance cycling or running (48). When Cr is supplemented along with carbohydrate after glycogen-depleting exercise, there is an enhancement of glycogen re-synthesis post-exercise (48, 49). Creatine supplementation by itself (i.e., without carbohydrate supplementation) may also be effective, as rats that were supplemented with Cr for 5 days had better sparing of muscle glycogen after exhaustive intermittent swimming than rats not supplemented with Cr (50). Creatine supplementation may upregulate the expression (i.e., mRNA) and content of glucose transport proteins (GLUT-4) in muscle (17, 45) or increase the translocation of GLUT-4 to the muscle membrane (25). This may allow enhancement of glucose uptake into muscle for glycogen re-synthesis. Creatine supplementation also upregulates the expression of genes encoding for proteins involved in glycogen synthesis and downregulates the expression of genes encoding for proteins involved in glycogen breakdown (51). Supplementing with Cr facilitates the enhancement of substrates (whether PCr or glycogen) for energy during exercise or enhancement of recovery (i.e., between sets of resistance training). It may allow one to train at higher volumes of exercise (12), leading to greater adaptation during resistance training sessions.

Enhancement of Muscle Protein Synthesis with Creatine Supplementation

Supplementation with Cr may enhance pathways involved in muscle protein synthesis. Early studies by Ingwall (31, 32) showed that myofibrillar (i.e., myosin and actin) protein synthesis was increased when Cr was added to cell cultures from breast muscle of chick embryos. Creatine supplementation for 10 days in young adults upregulates proteins involved in cell swelling and detection of osmolarity, which is thought to enhance signalling for protein synthesis (51). Creatine supplementation for 5–9 days with or without an acute session of resistance training was not effective for increasing myofibrillar or sarcoplasmic protein synthesis in men or women (39, 46); however, 5 days of Cr supplementation induced an increase in myosin heavy chain IIa mRNA immediately after an acute exercise session (17), indicating that transcription is activated in this short time span. A longer duration of Cr supplementation (i.e., 12 weeks) combined with resistance training enhanced expression of myosin heavy chain type I, IIa, and IIx mRNA and myosin heavy chain I and IIx protein levels in young men (63).

The initial steps in protein synthesis involve increased expression of "myogenic regulatory factors" (transcription factors) that are involved in proliferation and differentiation of satellite cells, which are located just outside the muscle membrane; these cells can be incorporated into muscle fibres as new myonuclei, increasing capacity for protein synthesis (69). A number of myogenic regulatory factors affect satellite cell proliferation and differentiation at different time points. Myogenic factor 5 (Myf5) is involved in satellite cell activation and proliferation; myoblast determination protein 1 (MyoD) is involved in migration of satellite cells to the muscle fibre membrane and differentiation of satellite cells; myogenin is involved with fusion of satellite cells to the muscle fibre membrane; and lastly, myogenic regulatory factor 4 (Mrf4) is involved in maturation of the newly repaired muscle fibre (69). Opposite to the actions of myogenic regulatory factors, myostatin is a "myokine" produced by muscle that inhibits satellite cell activation (69). Production of insulin-like growth factor-1 (IGF-1) by muscle may be involved in expression of the myogenic regulatory factors and possibly inhibition of myostatin (68). Supplementation with Cr may affect expression of IGF-1, the myogenic regulatory factors, and myostatin. Murine (i.e., rats or mice) cell culture incubated with Cr had increased expression of mRNA encoding for IGF-1 and upregulation of myogenic regulatory factors in their expected sequence (i.e., Myf5 early time course, MyoD and myogenin intermediate, and Mrf4 late time course) (40). In young males and females, Cr supplementation during 8 weeks of resistance training increased muscle-specific IGF-1 levels (5). In young adults who were supplemented with Cr during 2 weeks of leg immobilization followed by 10 weeks of knee extension resistance training, Mrf4 levels were increased and correlated with increased muscle fibre area, whereas myogenin levels were decreased after the knee extension intervention (28). This might make sense considering the sequence of myogenic regulatory factor expression: Myogenin is expressed earlier in the process of satellite cell proliferation and differentiation, whereas

Mrf4 is expressed much later; therefore, myogenin might have already played its role well before the end of the 10 weeks of training and therefore was decreasing when assessed. Slightly contrasting these results, supplementation of Cr in young men during 12 weeks of resistance training increased mRNA and protein levels of myogenin and Mrf4 with no effect on Myf5 and MyoD (64). Again, these results may correspond to the sequence of myogenic regulatory factor expression, as Myf5 and MyoD are expressed earlier and myogenin and Mrf4 later in the process of satellite cell proliferation/differentiation (69). There is less work regarding the effects of Cr supplementation on myostatin levels. Creatine supplementation decreased mRNA coding for myostatin in pigs (67) and decreased serum levels of myostatin during 8 weeks of resistance training in young men (53); this may or may not reflect muscle levels of myostatin. The only study to assess expression of myostatin from muscle samples (i.e., mRNA) found no effect when Cr was supplemented 5 days before an acute resistance training session (17). The increased expression of myogenic regulatory factors or possible inhibition of myostatin with Cr supplementation may allow increased satellite cell activation, proliferation, and differentiation during resistance training. In a compensatory overload model in rats, where the synergist muscles of the gastrocnemius and soleus were removed to overload the plantaris, the mitotic activity of satellite cells was increased by Cr supplementation (15). Importantly in this study, Cr supplementation had no effect on the opposite (control) non-overloaded limb, implying that overload of muscle is necessary for realizing a beneficial effect from Cr. In a human study, 8 weeks of Cr supplementation during resistance training of young men resulted in faster increase in satellite number, myonuclei per muscle fibre area, and muscle fibre area (44). This response may be attenuated with ageing. In older men (73 years old) 7 weeks of Cr supplementation had no effect on satellite cell activation following an acute resistance training session (57).

Translation of mRNA on ribosomes is a key process for protein synthesis. The capacity for translation and the activation of translation are often assessed by the amount and phosphorylation state of the phosphatidylinositol 3-kinase (PI3K)–protein kinase B (Akt)–mammalian target of rapamycin (mTOR)–ribosomal protein S6 kinase beta-1 (S6K) (eukaryotic translation initiation factor 4E-binding protein 1 [4E-BP1]–eukaryotic initiation factor 4E [eIF4E]) pathway (in this last step, phosphorylation of 4E-BP1 removes its inhibition of eIF4E, which allows initiation of translation). This pathway is activated in murine cell culture with Cr supplementation (19) and also in an animal model (20). In the animal model, rats were resistance trained for 8 weeks by having them wear weights attached to their tails while performing a climbing task. Creatine supplementation upregulated muscle-specific IGF-1, IGF-1 receptors on the muscle membrane, had no effect on PI3K, increased phosphorylation (i.e., activation) of Akt, had no effect on mTOR or phosphorylation (i.e., activation) of mTOR, and had no effect on S6K (20). It was implied that Cr supplementation positively affected IGF-1, which in turn activated components of the pathway leading to increased translation. Studies in humans show that Cr supplementation for 5 days increased resting muscle IGF-1 and IGF-2 mRNA and enhanced the phosphorylation of 4E-BP1 (which removes inhibition of translation initiation) 24 hours post-exercise (17, 18).

Effect of Creatine Supplementation on Muscle Protein Degradation

Signalling pathways for protein degradation have not been studied as extensively as pathways for protein synthesis in studies of Cr supplementation. Supplementation with Cr for 5 days had no effect on muscle mRNA levels for atrophy F-box (MAFbx), a component of the ubiquitin/proteasome pathway, after an acute resistance training session (17). Eight to nine days of Cr supplementation was, however, effective in males (but not females) for reducing leucine oxidation and rate of appearance of leucine in the blood (both markers of protein degradation) (46). Urinary 3-methyl histidine can be used as a general marker of whole-body protein degradation. When Cr is given as a supplement, this marker decreases during 5–12 weeks of resistance training in young men and women (14), and older men (i.e., >55 years old) (6), but not older women (33).

Creatine is a potent antioxidant (36, 55), and in this role, it may prevent protein degradation, especially with ageing. During ageing, mitochondrial respiratory chain defects may cause increased

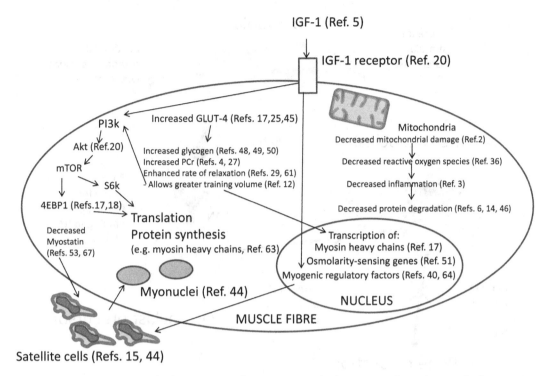

Figure 23.3 Mechanisms by which creatine supplementation can lead to increased muscle mass. References are indicated in brackets to support different mechanisms

production of reactive oxygen species, which lead to damaged cell membranes and inflammation (34). Damage to muscle membranes and inflammation may lead to increased muscle protein breakdown and loss of muscle mass (34). When Cr is added to oxidatively-damaged mouse myoblasts, there is a reduction in mitochondrial damage (2). There has been limited assessment in humans; however, 12 weeks of supplementation with Cr during exercise training reduces inflammation in older adults (3).

Figure 23.3 provides a summary of the potential effects of Cr supplementation for increasing muscle protein synthesis or decreasing muscle protein degradation.

Effects of Creatine on Bone

Bone turns over in a cycle of formation and resorption so that blood calcium levels are maintained to support excitable tissues and to repair micro-damage to bone. Bone is therefore a metabolically active tissue with cells that are activated to induce bone formation (osteoblasts) and cells that are activated to resorb bone (osteoclasts). An increased activation of osteoblasts or a decreased activation of osteoclasts will result in a greater amount of bone deposited and higher bone strength. Bone contains creatine kinase, the enzyme for breakdown of PCr; therefore, bone relies on high-energy phosphates as an energy source (62). Osteoblasts require large amounts of energy when active (30), and stimulation of bone formation results in elevated creatine kinase activity (8, 58). When Cr was added to low serum cell culture medium, it stimulated the metabolic activity, differentiation, and mineralization of osteoblast-like cells (21). Osteoblasts form bone by first depositing type I collagen, followed by deposition of minerals (i.e., calcium and phosphate). Supplementation of Cr for 5 days in humans increases mRNA for type I collagen, although this was assessed in muscle tissue (17). Supplementation of Cr in ovariectomized rats (used as a model of postmenopausal osteoporosis) or male mice increased mineralization as assessed by phosphate levels or phosphate/carbonate levels in bone (16, 42); this is associated with reduced fracture risk in humans (41).

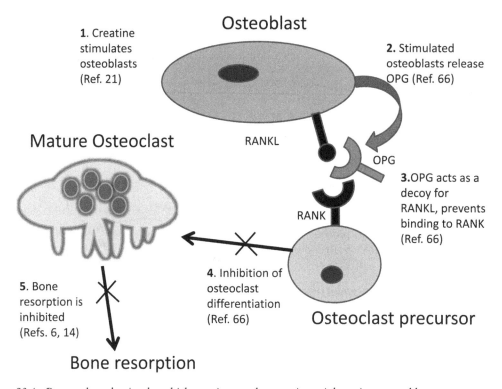

Figure 23.4 Proposed mechanism by which creatine supplementation might activate osteoblasts to secrete osteoprotegerin (OPG). Osteoprotegerin acts as a decoy for receptor activator for the nuclear factor-kappaB ligand (RANKL), preventing its binding with RANK on osteoclast precursor cells. This prevents osteoclast differentiation and reduces bone resorption

Osteoblast-induced bone formation is linked to osteoclast-induced bone resorption in the bone remodelling cycle through binding of receptors on osteoblasts to osteoclast precursor cells (66). Osteoblasts contain receptor activator for the nuclear factor-kappaB ligand (RANKL), which binds to RANK on osteoclast precursor cells, resulting in differentiation of these cells into mature osteoclasts (66). When osteoblasts are stimulated, they release a protein called osteoprotegerin which acts as a decoy for RANKL, preventing its binding with RANK. This prevents differentiation of osteoclasts. In this manner, stimulation of osteoblasts by Cr (21) may inhibit osteoclasts and bone resorption (66) (Figure 23.4). Bone resorption can be assessed by breakdown products of type I collagen in the urine (i.e., cross-linked N-telopeptides of type I collagen, NTx). Twelve to sixteen weeks of Cr supplementation decreased this marker of bone resorption in boys with muscular dystrophy (38, 59), and 5–10 weeks of Cr supplementation during resistance training programmes decreased NTx in older males (55–77 years old) (6) and young males and females (14). Other studies, however, have found that Cr supplementation over periods of 14–26 weeks failed to affect markers of bone formation or resorption during resistance training in older males or females (4, 24, 60). Also, there is evidence that the creatine kinase enzyme may be important for support of osteoclasts, the cells involved in bone resorption. When creatine kinase was suppressed in vitro, bone resorption was decreased, and mice with knockout of the creatine kinase gene were protected against bone loss after ovariectomy (7).

As with studies of the effect of Cr supplementation on bone cells, studies of Cr supplementation and effects on bone tissue are mixed in their results. The most comprehensive study found that Cr supplementation during 12 weeks of downhill treadmill run training (which produces a marked osteogenic response in bone) in ovariectomized rats failed to increase bone mineral density (43). The Cr supplementation also had no beneficial effects on bone histomorphometric properties (i.e., trabecular architecture), osteoblast or osteoclast activity, or femoral bone strength assessed directly in a bending test above the effects of exercise training alone (43). In contrast, young male rats supplemented with Cr for 8 weeks (but without exercise training) had increases in bone mineral density and femoral bone strength assessed in bending tests (1); therefore, there may be age- or sex-related differences for how bone responds to Cr supplementation.

Studies of the effect of Cr supplementation on bone mineral properties of humans are also mixed. Twelve to twenty-four months of Cr supplementation (without exercise training) had no effect on bone mineral density in older women (37, 52), although these studies involved relatively low doses of Cr (i.e., 1–3 g/d) which is about two to five times lower than typical dosing regimens. It has been argued that Cr supplementation without exercise training may not be effective for affecting bone mineral density because the increase in muscle mass with Cr and training may be necessary to provide an adequate osteogenic stimulus to bone through muscle pull on the tendons attached to bone (10). For example, Cr supplementation during 12 weeks of resistance training in older men increased bone mineral content of the arms, and this was correlated with the increase in muscle mass of the arms (10). Although most studies have shown no effect of Cr supplementation during resistance training on bone mineral density, these studies were of relatively short duration (i.e., 6 months or less) (24, 47, 60). These short durations may not permit sufficient time for full turnover of bone. The study with the longest duration of Cr supplementation during resistance training (i.e., 12 months) showed a benefit of Cr for maintaining femoral neck bone mineral density and for improving geometric properties at the hip in postmenopausal women compared to placebo (9).

Summary and Areas for Future Research

Supplementation with Cr enhances high-intensity exercise performance and increases strength and muscle mass during resistance training programmes (12, 13). Future research should clarify the effect of Cr on timing of myogenic regulatory factor expression in humans and clarify what aspect of pathways involved in translation initiation and protein degradation are affected by Cr supplementation. Myostatin is a myokine which inhibits satellite cell activation; however, there are limited studies of the effect of Cr on this myokine (17, 53, 67). Studies of the effect of Cr on the myogenic regulatory factors, myostatin, and signalling pathways are especially important in clinical populations such as older adults who may have an anabolic resistance to strength training or supplementation of Cr (57); therefore, this is an attractive area for future research.

Supplementation with Cr improves energy status in muscle by increasing PCr levels. This has benefits for enhancing energy provision to the myofilaments (23) and most likely the sarcoplasmic reticulum (based on findings that Cr supplementation shortens relaxation time after contraction) (29, 61). No studies have yet assessed whether Cr supplementation can improve function of the sodium–potassium pump in the sarcolemma, which is important for recovery of muscle after exercise.

Creatine supplementation may have benefits for bone; however, important pathways involving interaction between bone-forming cells (osteoblasts) and bone-resorbing cells (osteoclasts) such as the RANKL–RANK–osteoprotegerin pathway have not been evaluated with Cr supplementation. Bone responsiveness to Cr may be different in younger and older individuals, as evidenced by greater responsiveness in young versus older animal models (1, 43). This difference needs to be evaluated in humans to determine the best time during the lifespan to supplement Cr to improve bone health.

References

1. Antolic A, Roy BD, Tarnopolsky MA, Zernicke RF, Wohl GR, Shaughnessy SG, et al. Creatine monohydrate increases bone mineral density in young sprague-dawley rats. *Med Sci Sports Exerc* 39: 816–820, 2007.
2. Barbieri E, Guescini M, Calcabrini C, Vallorani L, Diaz AR, Fimognari C, et al. Creatine prevents the structural and functional damage to mitochondria in myogenic, oxidatively stressed C2C12 cells and restores their differentiation capacity. *Oxid Med Cell Longev* 2016: 5152029, 2016.

3. Bell KE, Snijders T, Zulyniak MA, Kumbhare D, Parise G, Chabowski A, et al. A multi-ingredient nutritional supplement enhances exercise training-related reductions in markers of systemicinflammation in healthy older men. *Appl Physiol Nutr Metab* 43: 299–302, 2018.

4. Brose A, Parise G, Tarnopolsky MA. Creatine supplementation enhances isometric strength and body composition improvements following strength exercise training in older adults. *J Gerontol A Biol Sci Med Sci* 58: 11–19, 2003.

5. Burke DG, Candow DG, Chilibeck PD, MacNeil LG, Roy BD, Tarnopolsky MA, et al. Effect of creatine supplementation and resistance-exercise training on muscle insulin-like growth factor in young adults. *Int J Sport Nutr Exerc Metab* 18: 389–398, 2008.

6. Candow DG, Little JP, Chilibeck PD, Abeysekara S, Zello GA, Kazachkov M, et al. Low-dose creatine combined with protein during resistance training in older men. *Med Sci Sports Exerc* 2008 Sep; 40(9): 1645–1652. doi: 10.1249/MSS.0b013e318176b310.

7. Chang EJ, Ha J, Oerlemans F, Lee YJ, Lee SW, Ryu J, et al. Brain-type creatine kinase has a crucial role in osteoclast-mediated bone resorption. *Nat Med* 14: 966–972, 2008.

8. Ch'ng JL, Ibrahim B. Transcriptional and posttranscriptional mechanisms modulate creatine kinase expression during differentiation of osteoblastic cells. *J Biol Chem* 269: 2336–2341, 1994.

9. Chilibeck PD, Candow DG, Landeryou T, Kaviani M, Paus-Jenssen L. Effects of creatine and resistance training on bone health in postmenopausal women. *Med Sci Sports Exerc* 47: 1587–1595, 2015.

10. Chilibeck PD, Chrusch MJ, Chad KE, Shawn Davison K, Burke DG. Creatine monohydrate and resistance training increase bone mineral content and density in older men. *J Nutr Health Aging* 9: 352–355, 2005.

11. Chilibeck PD, Kaviani M, Candow DG, Zello GA. Effect of creatine supplementation during resistance training on lean tissue mass and muscular strength in older adults: A meta-analysis. *Open Access J Sports Med* 8: 213–226, 2017.

12. Chrusch MJ, Chilibeck PD, Chad KE, Davison KS, Burke DG. Creatine supplementation combined with resistance training in older men. *Med Sci Sports Exerc* 33: 2111–2117, 2001.

13. Clark JF. Creatine: A review of its nutritional applications in sport. *Nutrition* 14: 322–324, 1998.

14. Cornish SM, Candow DG, Jantz NT, Chilibeck PD, Little JP, Forbes S, et al. Conjugated linoleic acid combined with creatine monohydrate and whey protein supplementation during strength training. *Int J Sport Nutr Exerc Metab* 19: 79–96, 2009.

15. Dangott B, Schultz E, Mozdziak PE. Dietary creatine monohydrate supplementation increases satellite cell mitotic activity during compensatory hypertrophy. *Int J Sports Med* 21: 13–16, 2000.

16. de Souza RA, Xavier M, da Silva FF, de Souza MT, Tosato MG, Martin AA, et al. Influence of creatine supplementation on bone quality in the ovariectomized rat model: An FT-Raman spectroscopy study. *Lasers Med Sci* 27: 487–495, 2012.

17. Deldicque L, Atherton P, Patel R, Theisen D, Nielens H, Rennie MJ, et al. Effects of resistance exercise with and without creatine supplementation on gene expression and cell signaling in human skeletal muscle. *J Appl Physiol* 104: 371–378, 2008.

18. Deldicque L, Louis M, Theisen D, Nielens H, Dehoux M, Thissen JP, et al. Increased IGF mRNA in human skeletal muscle after creatine supplementation. *Med Sci Sports Exerc* 37: 731–736, 2005.

19. Deldicque L, Theisen D, Bertrand L, Hespel P, Hue L, Francaux M. Creatine enhances differentiation of myogenic C2C12 cells by activating both p38 and Akt/PKB pathways. *Am J Physiol Cell Physiol* 293: C1263–C1271, 2007.

20. Ferretti R, Moura EG, Dos Santos VC, Caldeira EJ, Conte M, Matsumura CY, et al. High-fat diet suppresses the positive effect of creatine supplementation on skeletal muscle function by reducing protein expression of IGF-PI3K-AKT-mTOR pathway. *PLoS One* 13: e0199728, 2018.

21. Gerber I, Ap Gwynn I, Alini M, Wallimann T. Stimulatory effects of creatine on metabolic activity, differentiation and mineralization of primary osteoblast-like cells in monolayer and micromass cell cultures. *Eur Cells Mater* 10: 8–22, 2005.

22. Greenhaff PL, Bodin K, Soderlund K, Hultman E. Effect of oral creatine supplementation on skeletal muscle phosphocreatine resynthesis. *Am J Physiol* 266(5 Pt 1): E725–E730, 1994.

23. Greenhaff PL, Casey A, Short AH, Harris R, Soderlund K, Hultman E. Influence of oral creatine supplementation of muscle torque during repeated bouts of maximal voluntary exercise in man. *Clin Sci (Lond)* 84: 565–571, 1993.

24. Gualano B, Macedo AR, Alves CR, Roschel H, Benatti FB, Takayama L, et al. Creatine supplementation and resistance training in vulnerable older women: A randomized double-blind placebo-controlled clinical trial. *Exp Gerontol* 53: 7–15, 2014.

25. Gualano B, DE Salles Painneli V, Roschel H, Artioli GG, Neves M Jr, De Sá Pinto AL, et al. Creatine in type 2 diabetes: A randomized, double-blind, placebo-controlled trial. *Med Sci Sports Exerc* 43: 770–778, 2011.

26. Haff GG, Koch AJ, Potteiger JA, Kuphal KE, Magee LM, Green SB, et al. Carbohydrate supplementation attenuates muscle glycogen loss during acute bouts of resistance exercise. *Int J Sport Nutr Exerc Metab* 10: 326–339, 2000.

27. Harris RC, Söderlund K, Hultman E. Elevation of creatine in resting and exercised muscle of normal subjects by creatine supplementation. *Clin Sci (Lond)* 83: 367–374, 1992.

28. Hespel P, Op't Eijnde B, Van Leemputte M, Ursø B, Greenhaff PL, Labarque V, et al. Oral creatine supplementation facilitates the rehabilitation of disuse atrophy and alters the expression of muscle myogenic factors in humans. *J Physiol* 536(Pt 2): 625–633, 2001.

29. Hespel P, Op't Eijnde B, Van Leemputte M. Opposite actions of caffeine and creatine on muscle relaxation time in humans. *J Appl Physiol* 92: 513–518, 2002.

30. Heyden G, From SH. Enzyme histochemistry and its application in comparative studies of adenosinetriphosphatase (ATPase) and some oxidative enzymes in bone, cartilage and tooth germs. *Odontol Revy* 21: 129–142, 1970.

31. Ingwall JS, Morales MF, Stockdale FE. Creatine and the control of myosin synthesis in differentiating skeletal muscle. *Proc Natl Acad Sci USA* 69: 2250–2253, 1972.

32. Ingwall JS, Weiner CD, Morales MF, Davis E, Stockdale FE. Specificity of creatine in the control of muscle protein synthesis. *J Cell Biol* 62: 145–151, 1974.

33. Johannsmeyer S, Candow DG, Brahms CM, Michel D, Zello GA. Effect of creatine supplementation and drop-set resistance training in untrained aging adults. *Exp Gerontol* 83: 112–119, 2016.

34. Johnston AP, De Lisio M, Parise G. Resistance training, sarcopenia, and the mitochondrial theory of aging. *Appl Physiol Nutr Metab* 33: 191–199, 2008.

35. Jung S, Bae YS, Kim HJ, Jayasena DD, Lee JH, Park HB, et al. Carnosine, anserine, creatine, and inosine 5'-monophosphate contents in breast and thigh meats from 5 lines of Korean native chicken. *Poult Sci* 92: 3275–3282, 2013.

36. Lawler JM, Barnes WS, Wu G, Song W, Demaree S. Direct antioxidant properties of creatine. *Biochem Biophys Res Commun* 290: 47–52, 2002.

37. Lobo DM, Tritto AC, da Silva LR, de Oliveira PB, Benatti FB, Roschel H, et al. Effects of long-term low-dose dietary creatine supplementation in older women. *Exp Gerontol* 70: 97–104, 2015.

38. Louis M, Lebacq J, Poortmans JR, Belpaire-Dethiou MC, Devogelaer JP, Van Hecke P, et al. Beneficial effects of creatine supplementation in dystrophic patients. *Muscle Nerve* 27: 604–610, 2003

39. Louis M, Poortmans JR, Francaux M, Berré J, Boisseau N, Brassine E, et al. No effect of creatine supplementation on human myofibrillar and sarcoplasmic protein synthesis after resistance exercise. *Am J Physiol Endocrinol Metab* 285(5): E1089–E1094, 2003.

40. Louis M, Van Beneden R, Dehoux M, Thissen JP, Francaux M. Creatine increases IGF-I and myogenic regulatory factor mRNA in C(2)C(12) cells. *FEBS Lett* 557: 243–247, 2004.

41. McCreadie BR, Morris MD, Chen TC, Sudhaker Rao D, Finney WF, Widjaja E, et al. Bone tissue compositional differences in women with and without osteoporotic fracture. *Bone* 39: 1190–1195, 2006.

42. Mirandaa H, De Souzaa RA, Tosatoc MG, Simaob R, Oliveiraa MX, De Limaa FM, et al. Effect of different doses of creatine on the bone in thirty days of supplementation in mice. *Spectroscopy* 25: 225–233, 2011.

43. Murai IH, Roschel H, Pabis LV, Takayama L, de Oliveira RB, Dos Santos Pereira RT, et al. Exercise training, creatine supplementation, and bone health in ovariectomized rats. *Osteoporos Int* 26: 1395–1404, 2015.

44. Olsen S, Aagaard P, Kadi F, Tufekovic G, Verney J, Olesen JL, et al. Creatine supplementation augments the increase in satellite cell and myonuclei number in human skeletal muscle induced by strength training. *J Physiol* 573(Pt 2): 525–534, 2006.

45. Op 't Eijnde B, Ursø B, Richter EA, Greenhaff PL, Hespel P. Effect of oral creatine supplementation on human muscle GLUT4 protein content after immobilization. *Diabetes* 50: 18–23, 2001.

46. Parise G, Mihic S, MacLennan D, Yarasheski KE, Tarnopolsky MA. Effects of acute creatine monohydrate supplementation on leucine kinetics and mixed-muscle protein synthesis. *J Appl Physiol* 91: 1041–1047, 2001.

47. Pinto CL, Botelho PB, Carneiro JA, Mota JF. Impact of creatine supplementation in combination with resistance training on lean mass in the elderly. *J Cachexia Sarcopenia Muscle* 7: 413–421, 2016.

48. Roberts PA, Fox J, Peirce N, Jones SW, Casey A, Greenhaff PL. Creatine ingestion augments dietary carbohydrate mediated muscle glycogen supercompensation during the initial 24 h of recovery following prolonged exhaustive exercise in humans. *Amino Acids* 48: 1831–1842, 2016.

49. Robinson TM, Sewell DA, Hultman E, Greenhaff PL. Role of submaximal exercise in promoting creatine and glycogen accumulation in human skeletal muscle. *J Appl Physiol* 87: 598–604, 1999.

50. Roschel H, Gualano B, Marquezi M, Costa A, Lancha AH Jr. Creatine supplementation spares muscle glycogen during high intensity intermittent exercise in rats. *J Int Soc Sports Nutr* 7(1): 6, 2010.

51. Safdar A, Yardley NJ, Snow R, Melov S, Tarnopolsky MA. Global and targeted gene expression and protein content in skeletal muscle of young men following short-term creatine monohydrate supplementation. *Physiol Genomics* 32: 219–228, 2008.

52. Sales LP, Pinto AJ, Rodrigues SF, Alvarenga JC, Gonçalves N, et al. Creatine supplementation (3 g/day) and bone health in older women: A 2-year, randomized, placebo-controlled trial. *J Gerontol A Biol Sci Med Sci* 75: 931–938, 2020.

53. Saremi A, Gharakhanloo R, Sharghi S, Gharaati MR, Larijani B, Omidfar K. Effects of oral creatine and resistance training on serum myostatin and GASP-1. *Mol Cell Endocrinol* 317: 25–30, 2010.

54. Schlattner U, Klaus A, Ramirez Rios S, Guzun R, Kay L, Tokarska-Schlattner M. Cellular compartmentation of energy metabolism: Creatine kinase microcompartments and recruitment of B-type creatine kinase to specific subcellular sites. *Amino Acids* 48: 1751–1774, 2016.

55. Sestili P, Martinelli C, Colombo E, Barbieri E, Potenza L, Sartini S, et al. Creatine as an antioxidant. *Amino Acids* 40: 1385–1396, 2011.

56. Smith SA, Montain SJ, Matott RP, Zientara GP, Jolesz FA, Fielding RA. Creatine supplementation and age influence muscle metabolism during exercise. *J Appl Physiol* 85: 1349–1356, 1998.

57. Snijders T, Bell KE, Nederveen JP, Saddler NI, Mazara N, Kumbhare DA, et al. Ingestion of a multi-ingredient supplement does not alter exercise-induced satellite cell responses in older men. *J Nutr* 148: 891–899, 2018.

58. Somjen D, Kaye AM. Stimulation by insulin-like growth factor-I of creatine kinase activity in skeletal-derived cells and tissues of male and female rats. *J Endocrinol* 143: 251–259, 1994.

59. Tarnopolsky MA, Mahoney DJ, Vajsar J, Rodriguez C, Doherty TJ, Roy BD, et al. Creatine monohydrate enhances strength and body composition in Duchenne muscular dystrophy. *Neurology* 62: 1771–1777, 2004.

60. Tarnopolsky M, Zimmer A, Paikin J, Safdar A, Aboud A, Pearce E, et al. Creatine monohydrate and conjugated linoleic acid improve strength and body composition following resistance exercise in older adults. *PLOS ONE* 2: e991, 2007.

61. van Leemputte M, Vandenberghe K, Hespel P. Shortening of muscle relaxation time after creatine loading. *J Appl Physiol* 86: 840–844, 1999.

62. Wallimann T, Hemmer W. Creatine kinase in non-muscle tissues and cells. *Mol Cell Biochem* 133–134: 193–220, 1994.

63. Willoughby DS, Rosene J. Effects of oral creatine and resistance training on myosin heavy chain expression. *Med Sci Sports Exerc* 33: 1674–1681, 2001.

64. Willoughby DS, Rosene JM. Effects of oral creatine and resistance training on myogenic regulatory factor expression. *Med Sci Sports Exerc* 35: 923–929, 2003.

65. Wyss M, Kaddurah-Daouk R. Creatine and creatinine metabolism. *Physiol Rev* 80: 1107–1213, 2000.

66. Yasuda H, Shima N, Nakagawa N, Mochizuki SI, Yano K, Fujise N, et al. Identity of osteoclastogenesis inhibitory factor (OCIF) and osteoprotegerin (OPG): A mechanism by which OPG/OCIF inhibits osteoclastogenesis in vitro. *Endocrinology* 139: 1329–1337, 1998.

67. Young JF, Bertram HC, Theil PK, Petersen AG, Poulsen KA, Rasmussen M, et al. In vitro and in vivo studies of creatine monohydrate supplementation to duroc and landrace pigs. *Meat Sci* 76: 342–351, 2007.

68. Yu M, Wang H, Xu Y, Yu D, Li D, Liu X, et al. Insulin-like growth factor-1 (IGF-1) promotes myoblast proliferation and skeletal muscle growth of embryonic chickens via the PI3K/Akt signalling pathway. *Cell Biol Int* 39: 910–922, 2015.

69. Zanou N, Gailly P. Skeletal muscle hypertrophy and regeneration: interplay between the myogenic regulatory factors (MRFs) and insulin-like growth factors (IGFs) pathways. *Cell Mol Life Sci* 70: 4117–4130, 2013.

24

BIOCHEMISTRY OF CAFFEINE'S INFLUENCE ON EXERCISE PERFORMANCE

Jane Shearer, Robyn F. Madden, and Jill A. Parnell

Introduction

Caffeine is the most commonly consumed central nervous system stimulant worldwide. It is also frequently used as an ergogenic aid to enhance sports performance in a wide range of exercise modalities, including sprint, power, and endurance activities. For this reason, there has been intense interest in understanding the timing, dose, biochemistry, and mechanisms of caffeine's action related to sports performance. Caffeine use has been extensively studied in exercise, with one of the first scientific reports appearing as early as 1907 (78). This work concluded that "caffeine produces an increase in the capacity for muscular work, this increase not being due to the various psychical factors" (78). Since that time, thousands of studies, reviews, and recommendations examining all aspects of caffeine in sport have been conducted (33, 72, 73, 97). This chapter will review current evidence for the use of caffeine as an ergogenic aid, as well as the biochemical mechanisms mediating these effects.

Sources of Caffeine

Caffeine can be found as an alkaloid (pill, powder), but is also naturally occurring in the nuts, beans, leaves, and berries of various plants (61), such as the kola nut, guarana seed, and yerba mate. However, caffeine is most notably recognized as a derivative of tea and coffee—typically the second and third most abundantly consumed beverages in adults worldwide after water. Over the past decade, the number of caffeine-containing foods and beverages available to consumers has increased exponentially. Among children and adolescents, caffeine-containing energy drinks have become popular, with an estimated 74% of youth in North America consuming these products and 16% consuming more than two within a day (75). These statistics are highly concerning, as the low body mass of children can expose them to significant amounts of the drug (39, 40). Aside from naturally caffeinated beverages, the alkaloid form can be an additive to various foods and drinks, including chocolate, gums, candy, and alcohol. Furthermore, caffeine has pharmaceutical properties and can be found in analgesics, cold and sinus preparations, and appetite suppressants (46). Within sport, the majority of studies have examined alkaloid caffeine, although a greater number are now starting to examine alternative forms, including mouthwashes, candy (e.g., jellybeans), energy drinks, gum, and coffee.

Caffeine Consumption

Caffeine is consumed both as part of the diet and for ergogenic purposes; thus, it is often difficult to determine the intent of caffeine consumption in athlete populations. In the general population, upwards of 90% of adults consume caffeine on a daily basis (7). Specific consumption varies by region, but it is estimated that in North America, caffeine-consuming adults ingest an average of 300 mg per day, while adolescents consume 100 mg per day (82). Caffeine consumption is not recommended for children, and limits of 2.5 mg/kg body weight per day have been established for adolescents 13 years of age and older (101). Although deemed a drug, caffeine is socially accepted and frequently sought after by specific populations, including athletes, truck drivers (38), military personnel (63), and shift workers (e.g., nurses) (8), to combat fatigue and enhance performance. Caffeine use tends to be greatest in occupations with high physical demands, long commutes, tedious demands, overtime, and multiple jobs (32, 86).

Use of caffeine by athletes for performance enhancement varies by sport, but is most predominant in endurance activities (9, 49, 96). Analysis of caffeine concentrations in urine from samples obtained directly following national and international competitions from 2004 to 2008 showed that 74% of samples contained caffeine (14). This suggests that athletes consumed caffeine close to competition time, although this study was unable to determine whether caffeine was consumed as part of the diet or for performance enhancement. Only 0.6% of samples had urinary caffeine concentrations that met the threshold for "doping" at 12 $\mu g \cdot mL^{-1}$ under former World Anti-Doping Agency (WADA) rules (14). This level of caffeine is extremely high and far above what is generally accepted to be ergogenic. Of note, caffeine was removed from the WADA list in 2004 and is now a monitored substance. Part of the difficulty in monitoring caffeine was dietary consumption, individual differences in metabolism, and timing of the sport. For example, post-performance levels of urinary caffeine would be drastically different if administered prior to a 100 m run (10 seconds) versus a marathon event (2 hours).

A survey of elite athletes revealed that the majority of consumed caffeine was in the form of coffee, but that levels were generally insufficient to elicit performance enhancement (94). Of the 14 different sports examined, the highest levels of caffeine were found in triathlon, cycling, and rowing, while the lowest levels were noted for tennis and gymnastics. These findings align with athletes' perception that while caffeine is beneficial for endurance and speed, it negatively affects calmness (16). Although used by the majority of athletes, most individuals are unable to identify the amount of caffeine they would need to consume to improve performance (16). Intriguingly, older athletes tend to have higher levels of urinary caffeine compared to younger athletes, despite ergogenic benefits being found in both populations (89). Caffeine use is also prevalent among Paralympians (58, 60), although detailed examinations of levels during or after competition are lacking.

Future work is needed to determine where athletes obtain their information regarding caffeine and their level of knowledge on how their bodies react to administration (81). This is of interest, as caffeine consumption, as well as the ergogenic impacts of caffeine in sport, are genetically determined (37, 83). Additional information on the influence of genetics on caffeine can be found in Chapter 25.

Caffeine Pharmacokinetics

Absorption

Caffeine is readily absorbed and can be administered through a number of routes, including skin, membranes of the nasal and buccal cavity, and the gastrointestinal tract. Ergogenic benefits have also been reported for both caffeine mouthwashes and gums (5, 22, 48, 57). This suggests that caffeine can modulate performance benefits without being ingested, but rather via the oral cavity alone. Comparison of caffeine administered by instant coffee or as a gum shows the latter to have 18% lower absorption but results in equivalent plasma concentrations over 2 hours (80). As such, the maximum safe caffeine dose of 400 mg/day should be applicable irrespective of delivery method (91, 101).

When ingested orally, caffeine is absorbed within the small intestine of the gastrointestinal tract within 30–45 minutes (2) and then is rapidly distributed throughout the body (23). Absorption is fastest when caffeine is administered in alkaloid (capsule) form and slightly delayed when consumed as a beverage (tea or coffee) or combined with food. Both coffee and caffeine stimulate gastric acid secretions and can be stomach irritants in some individuals; determining the factors involved here is an area of ongoing interest (54, 68). Once absorbed, caffeine is rapidly distributed throughout the body and as a result it is "seen" by all physiological organ systems.

Metabolism and Excretion

Caffeine is a trimethylxanthine (1,3,7-trimethylxanthine) that is rapidly and primarily metabolized by the liver into its three related dimethylxanthines (theophylline (11%, 1,3-dimethylxanthine), theobromine (4%, 1,7-dimethylxanthine), and paraxanthine (80%, 1,7-dimethylxanthine) through a series of demethylation steps (Figure 24.1).

Over 95% of caffeine is metabolized by the CYP1A2 enzyme with <2% of ingested caffeine excreted in urine (36). Consequently, caffeine metabolism is largely genetically determined by single nucleotide polymorphisms on the *CYP1A2* gene (70). As a result, caffeine metabolism is highly variable between individuals (44, 74). Individuals are classified as either slow or fast metabolizers, with an almost equal distribution within the population. Such variation represents a major source of individuality in the pharmacokinetics of caffeine, which has a half-life generally ranging between 4 and 6 hours (93).

Caffeine metabolism is not altered by the route of administration but can be negatively affected by the presence of disease or environmental factors. For example, barbiturates and nicotine are known to induce the CYP1A2 enzyme and result in enhanced metabolism of caffeine (50). Likewise, caffeine may act as a competitive inhibitor and slow drug metabolism if significant amounts are ingested. Upon metabolism, each of the three primary caffeine metabolites are also metabolically active. Paraxanthine, comprising the majority of caffeine breakdown, is wake promoting (20). Theophylline is not ergogenic, but has been used as a bronchodilator in asthma and is an immune mediator (79). Lastly, theobromine has vasodilatory properties and can be used as a cardiac inducer, but levels resulting from caffeine consumption are very minor and are thought to have little physiological impact.

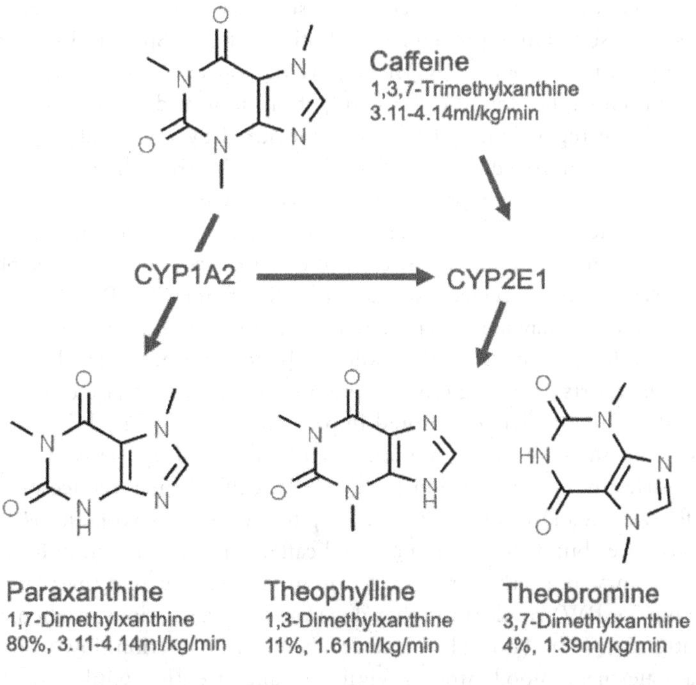

Figure 24.1 Metabolism of caffeine and its resulting metabolites. Chemical structures, metabolites, chemical name and approximate metabolite percentage are shown (53, 91). *Figures are taken from ChemSpider with permission (4).*

Exercise Performance

Caffeine is one of the few permitted ergogenic aids with established performance benefits (30). It is proposed to increase energy availability, concentration, and physical and cognitive performance, as well as decrease mental fatigue (28). Consequently, the International Olympic Committee (IOC) consensus statement on dietary supplement use in high-performance athletes concluded caffeine could exert performance benefits in endurance-based sports, as well as shorter supramaximal and/or sprint repeats primarily via its actions as a stimulant (62).

Initially, caffeine was studied for its ability to improve endurance performance, and it is in this realm where it is likely to be most effective. Endurance athletes report the highest prevalence of caffeine use (14); therefore, it may not be that caffeine consumption provides an edge over the competition, but rather prevents athletes from being disadvantaged (84). Southward et al. (84) combined the results from a suite of studies designed to evaluate the impact of caffeine on endurance performance and found that time-trial completion was improved by 2% and power output by 3%. To put this into context, in many Olympic sports, a 1% improvement in performance would make the difference between winning gold versus silver (10). Caffeine has also been found to improve performance in intermittent sports such as volleyball (15). Low (3 mg/kg body weight [BW]) and moderate (3–6 mg/kg BW) doses of supplemental caffeine in athletes have been shown to mitigate fatigue whilst enhancing performance. This difference in effective dose likely depends on genetics and the measurement of performance in relation to consumption. While the majority of studies are blinded to placebo or caffeine treatment, it is important to note that there may also be a placebo effect when it comes to performance enhancement. At least one study found faster running times when participants were told they were consuming caffeine when they were administered a placebo or caffeine as compared to when they were told they were consuming a placebo. In this case, however, the test was 1,000 m, which is a relatively short distance (41).

Performance benefits of caffeine ingestion on anaerobic exercise and muscle strength and power are emerging; however, the results are less robust. Generally, there is support for increased maximal strength, muscular endurance, and power (34). A meta-analysis evaluating caffeine consumption on a Wingate test, a 30-second cycling test designed to measure anaerobic performance and power output, found caffeine ingestion resulted in improvements in both outcomes. Specifically, average power output increased by 3% and peak power output by 4% (33). With respect to muscle strength and power, the combined results from ten studies found caffeine ingestion improved strength, the maximum weight a person could lift for one repetition, and power as measured by a vertical jump. A more in-depth analysis noted that caffeine improved upper but not lower body strength (35) in that particular set of studies. Conversely, in a 2019 study comparing the effects of caffeine ingestion on upper and lower body Wingate anaerobic test performance, peak power was increased in both the upper and lower body; however, mean power and fatigue were not statistically affected by caffeine. Remarkably, only the upper body test found a lower rate of perceived exhaustion with caffeine (21). Reasons for this discrepancy are not well understood, but it may mean that there is greater room for improvement in upper vs. lower body power activities (100). Caffeine also likely affects physicality (speed, number, and force of hits), a key component of many sports including football and hockey. A recent analysis of skills and physicality with and without caffeine demonstrated limited impact on sport-specific skills but enhanced physicality (59). Therefore, caffeine may affect the number and severity of injuries sustained in sport, as well as recovery from injuries such as concussion (99). Finally, caffeine may reduce delayed-onset muscle soreness, the pain felt within a few hours and lasting up to 3 days post-workout (34).

Adenosine receptors are abundant in the brain, and caffeine is well known to have psychoactive and cognitive benefits that may affect the performance of all athletes beyond the physiological. Caffeine consumption (3–6 mg/kg BW) results in higher dopamine concentrations, particularly in those brain areas linked with attention (65). Through this neurochemical interaction, low to moderate intakes of caffeine can increase alertness, mood, arousal, vigilance, and attention while reducing reaction time. Currently, caffeine's effects on higher cognitive functions like problem-solving and decision-making are somewhat unclear and may even be negative for some individuals (64). Specifically, the cognitive benefits of caffeine appear to be enhanced when the athlete is sleep deprived. For example, in a double-blind trial with elite rugby players, administration of caffeine at doses of 1 mg/kg BW and 5 mg/kg BW negated the impacts of sleep deprivation on performance (12). Interestingly, there is also an effect of circadian rhythm on performance, with optimal performance often demonstrated in the afternoon. Although controversial, there is limited evidence that caffeine intake prior to morning competitions may help to off-set morning performance decrement (71).

While the benefits of caffeine on performance have been extensively studied, the majority of the studies have used young, healthy males with only approximately 13% of studies including females until now (66). The available evidence suggests there are differences between the sexes. A systematic review exploring the effect of sex on caffeine supplementation found that improvements in endurance performance and reductions in fatigue were similar in magnitude between sexes; however, improvements in anaerobic performance were found to be greater in males in over 50% of the studies. When caffeine was provided males saw greater improvements in weight lifted, power generated, and sprint times than females. In the majority of these studies, the doses were the same; however, as they were based on body weight, males often were provided with greater absolute amounts (66). Differences in subjective and physiological responses to caffeine between males and females are also found in non-athletic populations (92). It should be noted that studies in females require a higher level of control, as the menstrual cycle can affect maximal endurance performance and oral contraceptives may affect caffeine metabolism (77).

Limitations to the evidence surrounding performance benefits should be noted. Age, sex, genetics, menstrual cycle (51), and drug use, among other factors, can affect caffeine metabolism, and there is likely a high level of interindividual variability even within similar groups. Consequently, it is difficult to generalize and determine the benefit or harm of caffeine ingestion on the performance of all athletes.

Dose, Timing, and Administration

As previously mentioned, athletes can ingest caffeine in multiple forms, including beverages, capsules, powders, gums, and gels. Performance benefits have been reported with doses as little as 1–2 mg/kg BW; however, they typically range from 3 mg/kg BW to 6 mg/kg BW to elicit an ergogenic effect (42, 84, 85). Higher doses do not necessarily confer any additional benefit and put the athlete at risk for adverse reactions. In addition to the dose, athletes must carefully consider the timing of caffeine ingestion, as the effects are not immediate. To optimize ergogenic effects, it is recommended that caffeine be consumed ~60 minutes prior to exercise, as this is when concentrations usually peak (62). Notably, although research often focuses on pure caffeine ingestion to study the effects on performance, athletes are likely to be consuming caffeine in the form of energy drinks, caffeinated beverages (coffee, tea, etc.), candy (bars, gum), or dietary supplements. These products are either naturally multi-ingredient or specifically formulated with a cocktail of conceivably ergogenic ingredients, including carbohydrates, antioxidants, taurine, vitamins, herbs, etc. Co-ingestion adds complexity, as it is not possible to determine if the effects are solely due to caffeine, other ingredients, or a combination of factors. Evidence already exists that co-ingestion of caffeine and a carbohydrate source can maximize performance effectiveness (11, 62).

Many caffeinated supplements such as sport gels, drinks, and gummies are designed to be consumed prior to exercise; however, less information is available on the effects of caffeine intake during exercise (where there is time for absorption to occur). One study assessed the effects of a caffeine/carbohydrate-electrolyte solution intake after 80 minutes of cycling on cycling performance greater than 2 hours and found improvements (87). Based on this study, the IOC supported a recommendation of <3 mg/kg BM, ~200 mg during exercise when consumed with a carbohydrate source (62).

The potential of mouth rinses to improve performance is intriguing, as it could help those who experience exercise-induced gastrointestinal symptoms if they drink or eat while exercising. A caffeine mouth rinse, either with or without carbohydrates, can improve time to exhaustion (27). Furthermore, high-intensity interval training (HIIT) when carbohydrate restricted (45) or in the fed state (17) was also improved with a caffeine/carbohydrate mouth rinse.

Negative Side Effects

The current body of evidence suggests that caffeine ingestion, especially in doses exceeding 6 mg/kg BW, might result in several negative side effects such as insomnia, headaches, nervousness, gastrointestinal problems, and muscle soreness, among others (3). While caffeine could increase physical performance directly, there may be negative implications for certain aspects of mental performance. For example, competition is typically a time of heightened anxiety, and the consumption of caffeine may exaggerate this response (98). For this reason, it is important for athletes to "practice" with caffeine during training to gauge their individual responses and how this could potentially affect performance. Although studies show improvements in performance on average with caffeine consumption, the variation of responses can be large, with many studies reporting some participants' performance decreased (84). Indeed, it has been suggested that the current guidelines for caffeine timing and dosing in sport need to be personalized to each athlete (72).

Other potential considerations exist related to muscle damage, habituation, withdrawal, and sleep disturbances. Caffeine consumption has been shown to increase workload and physical exertion, which may result in greater muscle damage. Increased muscle damage would have implications for recovery time or for those participating in multiday sporting events. Another factor that may influence responsiveness to caffeine supplementation is habituation. Individuals become more tolerant to caffeine, and this is mediated in part by an up-regulation of adenosine receptors (13, 24). Questions have also been raised as to whether the impact of caffeine is less in regular consumers compared to naïve users. Data on the influence of habitation are mixed, with some reports showing no impact while others reporting low users experience a greater ergogenic impact. As mentioned, caffeine is distributed throughout the body and affects all systems. It appears that individuals can habituate to some impacts of caffeine (e.g., blood pressure), but not to others (95). Having said this, habituation can likely be overcome by increasing doses of caffeine.

Associated with the reliance and recurrent consumption of caffeine is the potential for increased tolerance and, if consumption ceases, withdrawal symptoms. Withdrawal symptoms may include headache, disrupted sleep or insomnia, fatigue, irritability, mental fog, muscle tremor, dysphoria, nausea, and anxiety, among others (18). Depending on tolerance and genetic predispositions of an individual (76), higher doses may exasperate these discomforts, as the severity of withdrawal symptoms increases in tandem with daily amounts (43). Caffeine is also known to disrupt sleep in some users, although this impact varies considerably between individuals and is likely due to genetically determined slow or fast metabolism of the drug (52). A recent study by Ali and colleagues examined the impact of caffeine consumption on 800-m run performance and its subsequent influence on sleep (1). Results showed caffeine to significantly impair sleep efficiency, actual wake time, the number of awakenings, calm sleep, ease of falling asleep, and feeling refreshed after waking. Furthermore, the effects of caffeine on sleep disturbances may be prolonged, with one study finding 400 mg of caffeine negatively affecting sleep quality and duration when ingested 6 hours prior to bedtime (19).

Mechanisms of Action

The mechanisms by which caffeine exerts its ergogenic impact has been a topic of considerable debate. This is likely because caffeine affects so many different systems and signalling pathways in the body due to widespread and diverse adenosine receptor distribution. Here we outline the effects of caffeine on whole-body exercise, as well as its known impacts on skeletal muscle pertinent to exercise. A summary of systems affected by caffeine when consumed as a supplement for performance enhancement is shown in Figure 24.2.

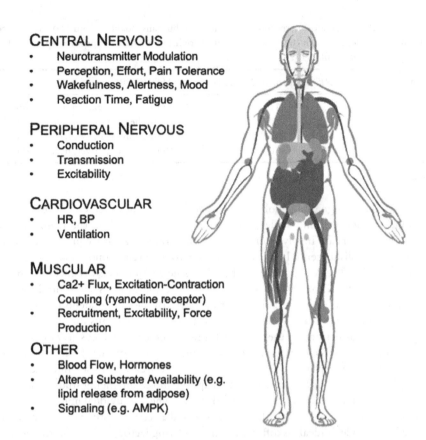

CENTRAL NERVOUS
- Neurotransmitter Modulation
- Perception, Effort, Pain Tolerance
- Wakefulness, Alertness, Mood
- Reaction Time, Fatigue

PERIPHERAL NERVOUS
- Conduction
- Transmission
- Excitability

CARDIOVASCULAR
- HR, BP
- Ventilation

MUSCULAR
- Ca2+ Flux, Excitation-Contraction Coupling (ryanodine receptor)
- Recruitment, Excitability, Force Production

OTHER
- Blood Flow, Hormones
- Altered Substrate Availability (e.g. lipid release from adipose)
- Signaling (e.g. AMPK)

Figure 24.2   The impacts of caffeine are diverse and widespread throughout the body. Potential mechanisms by which caffeine exerts ergogenic benefit are listed. Adenosine receptor expression (ADORA2A) is widespread throughout the body as shown in this diagram from the *Human Protein Atlas (102)*

A meta-analysis found no effects of caffeine on heart rate, oxygen uptake, and respiratory exchange ratio during submaximal exercise (29). Conversely, caffeine did reduce the rating of perceived exertion and increased minute ventilation (29). In the sections that follow, we outline the various proposed mechanisms by which caffeine is likely to exert benefit to athletic performance and briefly summarize the evidence for each.

Adenosine Receptor Antagonism

As previously mentioned, caffeine is a non-specific adenosine receptor antagonist. Adenosine receptors are a group of G protein–coupled receptors that mediate the physiological actions of adenosine. There are four main subtypes of adenosine receptors (A_1, A_{2A}, A_{2B}, and A_3) classified by their differential coupling to adenylyl cyclase that regulate cyclic AMP (cAMP) levels (26, 69). Receptors are distributed throughout the body, with different tissues expressing specific subtypes. Adenosine A_1 and A_3 receptors are coupled to $G_{i/o}$ proteins, while adenosine A_{2A} and A_{2B} receptors act upon $G_{s/olf}$ proteins (25, 69). Binding of adenosine to its receptors results in changes in cAMP levels that initiate a host of cell responses, including ion channels and enzymes. Caffeine has a similar structure to adenosine and therefore binds to the same receptors, essentially blocking the normal effects of adenosine (antagonist). However, caffeine has different affinities for each type of adenosine receptor, explaining why caffeine can produce distinct impacts on tissues depending on the type and level of adenosine receptors present (Table 24.1).

Table 24.1 Affinity of different adenosine receptors to caffeine in humans, adapted from (24). Affinity constant (K_D, μM) and primary tissues in which the receptor is found are listed. Caffeine expression (protein) levels were derived from the *Human Protein Atlas* (102)

Adenosine receptor	Affinity constant (K_D, μM)	Main tissues
A1	12	Brain, nerve, heart, muscle, endocrine
A2A	2.4	Brain, heart, lungs, spleen, blood, GI tract
A2B	13	Brain, bone marrow, lymphoid tissues
A3	80	Brain, GI tract, liver, heart, endocrine, blood

GI, gastrointestinal tract

Adenosine is a ubiquitous signalling molecule, which typically increases during exercise. A_1, A_{2A}, and A_{2B} are found in endothelium, while only A_{2A} and A_{2B} are found on the membrane of skeletal muscle (56). These receptors are involved in numerous important regulatory processes, including glucose uptake, lipid metabolism, central and peripheral nervous system stimulation, and cardiovascular and respiratory responses (29). Antagonism of the adenosine receptors also reduces the perception of the effort required to perform (6, 28). This is because adenosine inhibits the central nervous system by suppressing neurotransmitters and neuronal-firing rates. By blocking adenosine, caffeine has the opposite effect, increasing neurotransmitter release and firing of motor units (6).

Caffeine is proposed to directly affect the contractile properties of skeletal muscle (88). Mechanistically, it is thought that caffeine acts as an antagonist of adenosine receptors on the skeletal muscle membrane and/or binds to ryanodine receptors. The end result is a greater release of Ca^{2+} into the intramuscular space, which modifies muscle performance (88). Perhaps the most convincing studies showing caffeine enhances muscle contraction are derived from animal studies where individual muscles from rodents are isolated and tested (55). Here, muscles are placed in a bath and electrically stimulated to contract with or without caffeine. This model is ideal, as differences in circulating factors and the central nervous system are negated. Likewise, there is also ergogenic benefit for individuals with a spinal cord injury undergoing functional electrical stimulation of their paralyzed limbs to the point of fatigue. Here, caffeine improved performance showing that the drug acts, at least in part, by a direct action on the muscle (67).

It has been suggested that caffeine affects performance via inhibition of carbohydrate oxidation and increased fat oxidation (47). While caffeine certainly mobilizes fatty acids from adipose tissue, rarely have measures of the respiratory exchange ratio indicated an increase in fat oxidation during exercise (31). However, changes may be small and there is likely a genetic influence. Likewise, caffeine ingestion pre-exercise increases blood lactate and glucose levels. The mechanism is unclear; however, it has been proposed that caffeine may antagonize adenosine-facilitated intracellular glucose transport (29).

Future Directions

Caffeine has been studied extensively, as has its role in physical performance; however, many unanswered questions remain. As noted previously, there is ambiguity regarding the influence of training status on performance enhancement with caffeine supplementation e.g., trained vs. untrained or recreational vs. professional athletes. Additional research is also required to determine if habitual usage can affect performance. If yes, should abstinence for a period of time prior to competition be practised, or should the dose be modified and, if so, by how much? Additionally, the majority of the studies have investigated the impact of caffeine on acute performance e.g., time-to-exhaustion; therefore, much less is known regarding the impact of caffeine on long-term training adaptations. Moreover, the impact of biological sex, age, and circadian rhythm also requires further investigation. Finally, while a dose of 6 mg/kg BW has widely been found effective in endurance athletes, less is known regarding optimal dosing and effectiveness in anaerobic exercise or for muscle hypertrophy, especially in females. With respect to dosing, the understanding of the potential usefulness of caffeine ingestion during ultra-endurance events, including dose and timing, could also be enhanced.

Conclusions

In summary, caffeine consumption has the potential to improve all aspects of physical performance, including aerobic and anaerobic competitions, as well as alertness and mental fatigue. Caution is required to ensure athletes are aware of their individual reactions and appropriate dosage and timing. It is also important to emphasize that caffeine is not a food or nutritional supplement, but a drug that can have serious consequences. Although relatively safe in healthy adults, caffeine can be harmful for vulnerable populations and some athletes. Even at recommended doses, caffeine can exacerbate underlying health conditions, including asthma, cardiac arrhythmias, and mental illness. All considered, it is important that coaches and athletes alike be educated about caffeine consumption and test its ergogenic impacts on an individual level.

References

1. Ali A, O'Donnell J, Starck C, Rutherfurd-Markwick K. The effect of caffeine Ingestion during evening exercise on subsequent sleep quality in females. *Int J Sports Med* 36: 433–439, 2015.
2. Astorino TA, Roberson DW. Efficacy of acute caffeine ingestion for short term high intensity exercise performance: a systematic review. *J Strength Cond Res* 24: 257–265, 2010.
3. Astorino TA, Rohmann RL, Firth K. Effect of caffeine ingestion on one-repetition maximum muscular strength. *Eur J Appl Physiol* 102: 127–132, 2008.
4. Ayers M. ChemSpider: the free chemical database2012312 *ChemSpider: the free chemical database.* URL: www.chemspider.com: Royal Society of Chemistry Last visited April 2012. Gratis. *Ref Rev* 26: 45–46, 2012.
5. Beaven CM, Maulder P, Pooley A, Kilduff L, Cook C. Effects of caffeine and carbohydrate mouth rinses on repeated sprint performance. *Appl Physiol Nutr Metab* 38: 633–637, 2013.
6. Bowtell JL, Mohr M, Fulford J, Jackman SR, Ermidis G, Krustrup P, et al. Improved exercise tolerance with caffeine is associated with modulation of both peripheral and central neural processes in human participants. *Front Nutr* 5: 2018.
7. Burke LM. Caffeine and sports performance. *Appl Physiol Nutr Metab* 33: 1319–1334, 2008.
8. Centofanti S, Banks S, Colella A, Dingle C, Devine L, Galindo H, et al. Coping with shift work-related circadian disruption: a mixed-methods case study on napping and caffeine use in Australian nurses and midwives. *Chronobiol Int* 35: 853–864, 2018.
9. Chester N, Wojek N. Caffeine consumption amongst British athletes following changes to the 2004 WADA prohibited list. *Int J Sports Med* 29: 524–528, 2008.
10. Christensen PM, Shirai Y, Ritz C, Nordsborg NB. Caffeine and bicarbonate for speed. A meta-analysis of legal supplements potential for improving intense endurance exercise performance. *Front Physiol* 8: 2017.
11. Cole M, Hopker JG, Wiles JD, Coleman DA. The effects of acute carbohydrate and caffeine feeding strategies on cycling efficiency. *J Sports Sci* 36: 817–823, 2018.
12. Cook CJ, Crewther BT, Kilduff LP, Drawer S, Gaviglio CM. Skill execution and sleep deprivation: effects of acute caffeine or creatine supplementation - a randomized placebo-controlled trial. *J Int Soc Sports Nutr* 8: 2011.
13. Daly JW, Fredholm BB. Caffeine—an atypical drug of dependence. *Drug Alcohol Depend* 51: 199–206, 1998.
14. Del Coso J, Muñoz G, Muñoz-Guerra J. Prevalence of caffeine use in elite athletes following its removal from the world anti-doping agency list of banned substances. *Appl Physiol Nutr Metab* 36: 555–561, 2011.
15. Del Coso J, Pérez-López A, Abian-Vicen J, Salinero JJ, Lara B, Valadés D. Enhancing physical performance in male volleyball players with a caffeine-containing energy drink. *Int J Sports Physiol Perform* 9: 1013–1018, 2014.
16. Desbrow B, Leveritt M. Well-trained endurance athletes' knowledge, insight, and experience of caffeine use. *Int J Sport Nutr Exerc Metab* 17: 328–39, 2007.
17. Devenney S, Mangan S, Shortall M, Collins K. Effects of carbohydrate mouth rinse and caffeine on high-intensity interval running in a fed state. *Appl Physiol Nutr Metab* 43:517–521, 2018.
18. Dews PB, O'Brien CP, Bergman J. Caffeine: behavioral effects of withdrawal and related issues. *Food Chem Toxicol* 40: 1257–1261, 2002.

19. Drake C, Roehrs T, Shambroom J, Roth T. Caffeine effects on sleep taken 0, 3, or 6 hours before going to bed. *J Clin Sleep Med* 9: 1195–1200, 2013.

20. Dulloo AG, Seydoux J, Girardier L. Paraxanthine (metabolite of caffeine) mimics caffeine's interaction with sympathetic control of thermogenesis. *Am J Physiol* 267: E801–E804, 1994.

21. Duncan MJ, Eyre E, Grgic J, Tallis J. The effect of acute caffeine ingestion on upper and lower body anaerobic exercise performance. *Eur J Sport Sci* 19: 1359–1366, 2019.

22. Evans M, Tierney P, Gray N, Hawe G, Macken M, Egan B. Acute ingestion of caffeinated chewing gum improves repeated sprint performance of team sport athletes with low habitual caffeine consumption. *Int J Sport Nutr Exerc Metab* 28: 221–227, 2018.

23. Fisone G, Borgkvist A, Usiello A. Caffeine as a psychomotor stimulant: mechanism of action. *Cell Mol Life Sci* 61: 857–872, 2004.

24. Fredholm BB, Bättig K, Holmén J, Nehlig A, Zvartau EE. Actions of caffeine in the brain with special reference to factors that contribute to its widespread use. *Pharmacol Rev* 51: 83–133, 1999.

25. Fredholm BB, Hökfelt T, Milligan G. G-protein-coupled receptors: an update. *Acta Physiol (Oxf)* 190: 3–7, 2007.

26. Fredholm BB, IJzerman AP, Jacobson KA, Linden J, Müller CE. International Union of Basic and Clinical Pharmacology. LXXXI. Nomenclature and classification of adenosine receptors–an update. *Pharmacol Rev* 63: 1–34, 2011.

27. Germaine M, Collins K, Shortall M. The effect of caffeine ingestion and carbohydrate mouth rinse on high-intensity running performance. *Sports* 7: E63, 2019.

28. Glade MJ. Caffeine-Not just a stimulant. *Nutrition* 26: 932–938, 2010.

29. Glaister M, Gissane C. Caffeine and physiological responses to submaximal exercise: A meta-analysis. *Int J Sports Physiol Perform* 13: 402–411, 2018.

30. Graham TE. Caffeine and exercise: metabolism, endurance and performance. *Sport Med* 31: 785–807, 2001.

31. Graham TE, Battram DS, Dela F, El-Sohemy A, Thong FSL. Does caffeine alter muscle carbohydrate and fat metabolism during exercise? *Appl Physiol Nutr Metab* 33: 1311–1318, 2008.

32. Grandner MA, Knutson KL, Troxel W, Hale L, Jean-Louis G, Miller KE. Implications of sleep and energy drink use for health disparities. *Nutr Rev* 72(Suppl 1): 14–22, 2014.

33. Grgic J. Caffeine ingestion enhances Wingate performance: a meta-analysis. *Eur J Sport Sci* 18: 219–225, 2018.

34. Grgic J, Mikulic P, Schoenfeld BJ, Bishop DJ, Pedisic Z. The influence of caffeine supplementation on resistance exercise: a review. *Sport Med* 49: 17–30, 2019.

35. Grgic J, Trexler ET, Lazinica B, Pedisic Z. Effects of caffeine intake on muscle strength and power: a systematic review and meta-analysis. *J Int Soc Sports Nutr* 15: 2018.

36. Gu L, Gonzalez FJ, Kalow W, Tang BK. Biotransformation of caffeine, paraxanthine, theobromine and theophylline by cDNA-expressed human CYP1A2 and CYP2E1. *Pharmacogenetics* 2: 73–77, 1992.

37. Guest N, Corey P, Vescovi J, El-Sohemy A. Caffeine, CYP1A2 genotype, and endurance performance in athletes. *Med Sci Sport Exerc* 50: 1570–1578, 2018.

38. Heaton K, Griffin R. The effects of caffeine use on driving safety among truck drivers who are habitual caffeine users. *Workplace Health Saf* 63: 333–341, 2015.

39. Higgins JP, Babu K, Deuster PA, Shearer J. Energy drinks: a contemporary issues paper. *Curr Sports Med Rep* 17: 65–72, 2018.

40. Higgins JP, Tuttle TD, Higgins CL. Energy beverages: content and safety. *Mayo Clin Proc* 85: 1033–1041, 2010.

41. Hurst P, Schipof-Godart L, Hettinga F, Roelands B, Beedie C. Improved 1000-m running performance and pacing strategy with caffeine and placebo: a balanced placebo design study. *Int J Sports Physiol Perform* 15: 483–488, 2019.

42. Jenkins NT, Trilk JL, Singhal A, O'Connor PJ, Cureton KJ. Ergogenic effects of low doses of caffeine on cycling performance. *Int J Sport Nutr Exerc Metab* 18: 328–342, 2008.

43. Juliano LM, Griffiths RR. A critical review of caffeine withdrawal: empirical validation of symptoms and signs, incidence, severity, and associated features. *Psychopharmacology (Berl)* 176: 1–29, 2004.

44. Kalow W, Tang B-K. Caffeine as a metabolic probe: exploration of the enzyme-inducing effect of cigarette smoking. *Clin Pharmacol Ther* 49: 44–48, 1991.

45. Kasper AM, Cocking S, Cockayne M, Barnard M, Tench J, Parker L, et al. Carbohydrate mouth rinse and caffeine improves high-intensity interval running capacity when carbohydrate restricted. *Eur J Sport Sci* 16: 560–568, 2016.

46. Keisler BD, Armsey TD. Caffeine as an ergogenic aid. *Curr Sports Med Rep* 5: 215–219, 2006.

47. Kim J, Park J, Lim K. Nutrition supplements to stimulate lipolysis: a review in relation to endurance exercise capacity. *J Nutr Sci Vitaminol (Tokyo)* 62: 141–161, 2016.

48. Kizzi J, Sum A, Houston FE, Hayes LD. Influence of a caffeine mouth rinse on sprint cycling following glycogen depletion. *Eur J Sport Sci* 16: 1087–1094, 2016.

49. Kuipers H. Letter to the editor. *Int J Sports Med* 28: 178, 2007.

50. Landi MT, Sinha R, Lang NP, Kadlubar FF. Human cytochrome P4501A2. *IARC Sci Publ*: 173–195, 1999.

51. Lane JD, Steege JF, Rupp SL, Kuhn CM. Menstrual cycle effects on caffeine elimination in the human female. *Eur J Clin Pharmacol* 43: 543–546, 1992.

52. Lazarus M, Chen JF, Huang ZL, Urade Y, Fredholm BB. Adenosine and sleep. *Handb Exp Pharmacol* 253: 359–381, 2019.

53. Lelo A, Miners JO, Robson RA, Birkett DJ. Quantitative assessment of caffeine partial clearances in man. *Br J Clin Pharmacol* 22: 183–186, 1986.

54. Liszt KI, Ley JP, Lieder B, Behrens M, Stöger V, Reiner A, et al. Caffeine induces gastric acid secretion via bitter taste signaling in gastric parietal cells. *Proc Natl Acad Sci* 114: E6260–E6269, 2017.

55. Lüttgau HC, Oetliker H. The action of caffeine on the activation of the contractile mechanism in striated muscle fibres. *J Physiol* 194: 51–74, 1968.

56. Lynge J, Hellsten Y. Distribution of adenosine A_1, A_{2A} and A_{2B} receptors in human skeletal muscle. *Acta Physiol Scand* 169: 283–290, 2000.

57. Russell M, Reynolds NA, Crewther BT, Cook CJ, Kilduff LP. The physiological and performance effects of caffeine gum consumed during a simulated half-time by professional academy rugby union players. *J Strength Cond Res* 34:145–151, 2020.

58. Madden R, Shearer J, Legg D, Parnell J. Evaluation of dietary supplement use in wheelchair rugby athletes. *Nutrients* 10: E1958, 2018.

59. Madden RF, Erdman KA, Shearer J, Spriet LL, Ferber R, Kolstad AT, et al. Effects of caffeine on exertion, skill performance and physicality in ice hockey. *Int J Sports Physiol Perform* 14: 1422–1429, 2019.

60. Madden RF, Shearer J, Parnell JA. Evaluation of dietary intakes and supplement use in Paralympic athletes. *Nutrients* 9: E1266, 2017.

61. Martyn D, Lau A, Richardson P, Roberts A. Temporal patterns of caffeine intake in the United States. *Food Chem Toxicol* 111: 71–83, 2018.

62. Maughan RJ, Burke LM, Dvorak J, Larson-Meyer DE, Peeling P, Phillips SM, et al. IOC consensus statement: dietary supplements and the high-performance athlete. *Int J Sport Nutr Exerc Metab* 28: 104–125, 2018.

63. Mclean CP, Zandberg L, Roache JD, Fitzgerald H, Pruiksma KE, Taylor DJ, et al, STRONG STAR Consortium. Caffeine use in military personnel with PTSD: prevalence and impact on sleep. *Behav Sleep Med* 17: 202–212, 2019.

64. McLellan TM, Caldwell JA, Lieberman HR. A review of caffeine's effects on cognitive, physical and occupational performance. *Neurosci. Biobehav. Rev* 71: 294–312, 2016.

65. Meeusen R, Roelands B, Spriet LL. Caffeine, exercise and the brain. *Nestle Nutr Inst Workshop Ser* 76:1–12, 2013.

66. Mielgo-Ayuso J, Marques-Jiménez D, Refoyo I, Del Coso J, León-Guereño P, Calleja-González J. Effect of caffeine supplementation on sports performance based on differences between sexes: a systematic review. *Nutrients* 11: E2313, 2019.

67. Mohr T, Van Soeren M, Graham TE, Kjaer M. Caffeine ingestion and metabolic responses of tetraplegic humans during electrical cycling. *J Appl Physiol* 85: 979–985, 1998.

68. Parnell JA, Lafave H, Wagner–Jones K, Madden RF, Erdman KA. Development of a questionnaire to assess dietary restrictions runners use to mitigate gastrointestinal symptoms. *J Int Soc Sports Nutr* 16: 11, 2019.

69. Peleli M, Fredholm BB, Sobrevia L, Carlström M. Pharmacological targeting of adenosine receptor signaling. *Mol Aspects Med* 55: 4–8, 2017.

70. Perera V, Gross AS, McLachlan AJ. Measurement of CYP1A2 activity: a focus on caffeine as a probe. *Curr Drug Metab* 13: 667–678, 2012.

71. Pickering C, Grgic J. Caffeine and exercise: what next? *Sport Med* 49: 1007–1030, 2019.

72. Pickering C, Kiely J. Are the current guidelines on caffeine use in sport optimal for everyone? Interindividual variation in caffeine ergogenicity, and a move towards personalised sports nutrition. *Sport Med* 48: 7–16, 2018.

73. Pickering C, Kiely J. What should we do about habitual caffeine use in athletes? *Sport Med* 49: 833–842, 2019.

74. Rasmussen BB, Brix TH, Kyvik KO, Brøsen K. The interindividual differences in the 3-demthylation of caffeine alias CYP1A2 is determined by both genetic and environmental factors. *Pharmacogenetics* 12: 473–478, 2002.

75. Reid JL, McCrory C, White CM, Martineau C, Vanderkooy P, Fenton N, et al. Consumption of caffeinated energy drinks among youth and young adults in Canada. *Prev Med Reports* 5: 65–70, 2017.

76. Revelle W, Condon DM, Wilt J. Caffeine. In: *Encyclopedia of Human Behavior* (2nd Edition). Cambridge: Elsevier Science & Technology, 2012, p. 423–429.

77. Ribeiro-Alves MA, Trugo LC, Donangelo CM. Use of oral contraceptives blunts the calciuric effect of caffeine in young adult women. *J Nutr* 133: 393–398, 2003.

78. Rivers WH, Webber HN. The action of caffeine on the capacity for muscular work. *J Physiol* 36: 33–47, 1907.

79. Rowe DJ, Watson ID, Williams J, Berry DJ. The clinical use and measurement of theophylline. *Ann Clin Biochem* 25: 4–26, 1988.

80. Sadek P, Pan X, Shepherd P, Malandain E, Carney J, Coleman H. A randomized, two-way crossover study to evaluate the pharmacokinetics of caffeine delivered using caffeinated chewing gum versus a marketed caffeinated beverage in healthy adult volunteers. *J Caffeine Res* 7: 125–132, 2017.

81. Shabir A, Hooton A, Tallis J, Higgins FM. The influence of caffeine expectancies on sport, exercise, and cognitive performance. *Nutrients* 10(10):1528, 2018.

82. Shearer J, Graham TE. Performance effects and metabolic consequences of caffeine and caffeinated energy drink consumption on glucose disposal. *Nutr Rev* 72: 121–136, 2014.

83. Southward K, Rutherfurd-Markwick K, Badenhorst C, Ali A. The role of genetics in moderating the inter-individual differences in the ergogenicity of caffeine. *Nutrients* 10: E1352, 2018.

84. Southward K, Rutherfurd-Markwick KJ, Ali A. The effect of acute caffeine ingestion on endurance performance: a systematic review and meta–analysis. *Sport Med* 48: 1913–1928, 2018.

85. Spriet LL. Exercise and sport performance with low doses of caffeine. *Sport Med* 44 Suppl 2: S175–S184, 2014.

86. Stephens MB, Attipoe S, Jones D, Ledford CJ, Deuster PA. Energy drink and energy shot use in the military. *Nutr Rev* 72(Suppl 1): 72–77, 2014.

87. Talanian JL, Spriet LL. Low and moderate doses of caffeine late in exercise improve performance in trained cyclists. *Appl Physiol Nutr Metab* 41: 850–855, 2016.

88. Tallis J, Duncan MJ, James RS. What can isolated skeletal muscle experiments tell us about the effects of caffeine on exercise performance? *Br J Pharmacol* 172: 3703–3713, 2015.

89. Tallis J, Duncan MJ, Wright SL, Eyre ELJ, Bryant E, Langdon D, et al. Assessment of the ergogenic effect of caffeine supplementation on mood, anticipation timing, and muscular strength in older adults. *Physiol Rep* 1, e00072, 2013.

90. Tang-Liu DD, Williams RL, Riegelman S. Disposition of caffeine and its metabolites in man. *J Pharmacol Exp Ther* 224: 180–185, 1983.

91. Temple JL, Bernard C, Lipshultz SE, Czachor JD, Westphal JA, Mestre MA. The safety of ingested caffeine: a comprehensive review. *Front Psychiatry* 8: 80, 2017.

92. Temple JL, Ziegler AM. Gender differences in subjective and physiological responses to caffeine and the role of steroid hormones. *J Caffeine Res* 1: 41–48, 2011.

93. Thorn CF, Aklillu E, McDonagh EM, Klein TE, Altman RB. PharmGKB summary: caffeine pathway. *Pharmacogenet. Genomics* 22: 389–395, 2012.

94. Tunnicliffe JM, Erdman KA, Reimer RA, Lun V, Shearer J. Consumption of dietary caffeine and coffee in physically active populations: physiological interactions. *Appl Physiol Nutr Metab* 33: 1301–1310, 2008.

95. Van Soeren MH, Sathasivam P, Spriet LL, Graham TE. Caffeine metabolism and epinephrine responses during exercise in users and nonusers. *J Appl Physiol (1985)* 75: 805–812, 1993.

96. Van Thuyne W, Delbeke F. Distribution of caffeine levels in urine in different sports in relation to doping control before and after the removal of caffeine from the WADA doping list. *Int J Sports Med* 27: 745–750, 2006.

97. Vitale K, Getzin A. Nutrition and supplement update for the endurance athlete: review and recommendations. *Nutrients* 11: E1289, 2019.

98. Wilson PB. 'I think I'm gonna hurl': a narrative review of the causes of nausea and vomiting in sport. *Sports (Basel)* 7: E162, 2019.

99. Yamakawa GR, Lengkeek C, Salberg S, Spanswick SC, Mychasiuk R. Behavioral and pathophysiological outcomes associated with caffeine consumption and repetitive mild traumatic brain injury (RmTBI) in adolescent rats. *PLOS ONE* 12: e0187218, 2017.

100. Zemková E, Kyselovičová O, Jeleň M, Kováčiková Z, Ollé G, Štefániková G, et al. Upper and lower body muscle power increases after 3-month resistance training in overweight and obese men. *Am J Mens Health* 11: 1728–1738, 2017.

101. Health Canada is advising Canadians about safe levels of caffeine consumption. (2017) https://healthycanadians.gc.ca/recall-alert-rappel-avis/hc-sc/2017/63362a-eng.php [24 Aug. 2019].

102. The Human Protein Atlas. ADORA2A protein expression summary - The Human Protein Atlas [Online]. [date unknown]. https://www.proteinatlas.org/ENSG00000128271-ADORA2A [26 Sep. 2019].

25

NUTRIGENOMICS FOR SPORT AND EXERCISE PERFORMANCE

Nanci S. Guest, Marc Sicova, and Ahmed El-Sohemy

Introduction

Nutrition can greatly affect sport and exercise performance. However, each individual can respond differently to the same dietary factors. This holds true across a variety of ages, ethnicities, training experience, and whether the goal is optimizing physical activity for health and fitness or for high-performance sport. The importance of a personalized sports nutrition plan was highlighted in the most recent "Nutrition and Athletic Performance" Joint Position Statement by the American College of Sports Medicine, the Academy of Nutrition and Dietetics, and the Dietitians of Canada, which states that "Nutrition plans need to be personalized to the individual athlete… and take into account specificity and uniqueness of responses to various strategies" (144). These strategies encompass overall dietary patterns, appropriate macronutrient ratios, micronutrient requirements, eating behaviours (e.g., nutrient timing), and the prudent use of supplements and ergogenic aids.

The paradigm shifts away from a universal, generic approach to dietary planning and toward personalization for the individual is moving nutrigenomics research from basic science into practice (37, 72). While it has long been recognized that genetics play an influential role in determining how an athlete responds to foods and nutrients, the surge in research into gene–diet interactions over the past decade has provided a scientific basis for this hypothesis through expanded research and the accretion of published studies (72). It is now widely recognized that genetic variants affect the way we absorb, metabolize, utilize, and excrete nutrients, and gene–diet interactions can affect metabolic pathways that are relevant to both health and performance (74). Personal genetic testing can provide information that will guide recommendations for dietary choices that are more effective at the individual level than current dietary advice, which has been set by government agencies and other health and sport organizations. Disclosure of genetic information has also been shown to enhance motivation and behaviour change and strengthen adherence to the dietary recommendations provided (24, 50, 80, 98, 109). Athletes tend to exhibit higher levels of motivation in general (36); however, nutrition professionals still encounter significant barriers to behaviour change when counselling athletes on improving their performance nutrition practices (31, 142). A recent systematic review found that when genetic information included actionable advice, individuals were more likely to change nutrition-related behaviours, including their dietary choices and intakes (82).

The demand for genetic testing for personalized sport is growing, and there is an increased need for dietitian-nutritionists, fitness professionals, coaches, and other sports medicine practitioners to understand the current evidence in this developing field (2, 3, 30, 88). Personalized nutrition, based on an individual's genotype, is not a novel concept, and there are several examples of rare (e.g., phenylketonuria) and common (e.g., lactose intolerance) genetic variants that require specific dietary strategies for their management (66). Genetic testing is well-established in the clinical setting; however, there are expanding opportunities to improve health, wellness, and performance in athletes and active individuals through nutrition-focused genetic testing.

Genes Associated with Sport Nutrition

The objective of this review is to outline the scientific evidence on specific nutrients and food bioactives whereby genetic variants appear to modify individual responses related to athlete health and athletic performance.

Caffeine

Caffeine has become ubiquitous in the sporting world and has dominated the ergogenic aids and sport supplements research domain over the past several decades (43, 58, 81). Along with increased coffee consumption, athletes have also increased their use of other caffeine-containing products, such as energy drinks (11, 130), "pre-workout supplements," chewing gum, energy gels and chews, aerosols, and many other novel caffeinated food products to boost performance (148). The form of caffeine used by most high-performance athletes and in most caffeine–exercise studies is anhydrous caffeine (capsule) (64, 68, 69, 95, 106, 113, 141), which allow more accurate standardizing of doses.

Numerous studies have investigated the effect of supplemental caffeine on exercise performance, but there is considerable interindividual variability in the magnitude of these effects (58, 69, 81) or in the lack of an effect (85, 127) when compared to placebo. These interindividual differences, along with other "health" responses to caffeine, appear to be partly due to genetic variation (153). Additional information on the biochemistry of caffeine and its influence on exercise performance can be found in Chapter 24.

Caffeine and Anxiety

In elite athletes, 50% face mental health issues some time during their career (6). Given that anxiety may be normalized in elite sports even at clinical levels, factors that contribute to anxiety should be mitigated whenever possible. Anxiety may be caused by stress-related disorders (i.e., burnout), poor quality sleep patterns, and possibly in response to caffeine (104). Caffeine is widely consumed across most sports both socially in the diet and as a performance-enhancing supplement (11, 58).

Caffeine blocks adenosine receptors, resulting in its stimulating effects (153). A common variation in the *ADORA2A* (adenosine A_{2A} receptor) gene contributes to the differences in subjective feelings of anxiety after caffeine ingestion (8, 28), especially in those who are habitually low caffeine consumers (128). This may be particularly relevant to athletes who possess the TT variant of rs5751876 in the *ADORA2A* gene. These individuals are likely to be more sensitive to the stimulating effects of caffeine and experience greater increases in feelings of anxiety after caffeine intake than do individuals with either the CT or CC variant (8, 28, 128).

Sport psychologists commonly work with athletes to help them overcome anxiety about performance during competitions. Anxiety before or during athletic competitions can interfere not only in performance but also increase injury risk (25). Athletes who are more prone to performance anxiety may exacerbate their risk for feelings of anxiety depending on their caffeine use and which variant of the *ADORA2A* gene they possess. Monitoring the actions of caffeine in those individuals who are susceptible may alleviate some of the related feeling of anxiety with caffeine use.

Caffeine and Performance: Interindividual Responses

Most studies on caffeine and performance do not explore the basis for the interindividual variation in response, which has been well-documented in several studies (44, 69, 86, 127, 149). For example,

Jenkins et al. (86) examined the effects of caffeine on exercise performance in 13 cyclists, and the interindividual range for performance change with caffeine at 1, 2, or 3 mg/kg compared with placebo was −7.9–17.8%. Similarly, Paton et al. (115) found that caffeinated (~3–4 mg/kg) chewing gum improved overall performance in a group of 20 male and female cyclists, but only 13 (65%) of the cyclists were considered "positive responders," while 5 (25%) experienced "negative" responses, and the remaining 2 (10%) experienced no observable effect on cycling performance.

Due to infrequent reporting of individual data, it is difficult to determine the extent to which variation in responses to caffeine or other ergogenic aids may be occurring. In the field of nutrigenomics, caffeine is the most widely researched compound, with several randomized controlled trials investigating the modifying effects of genetic variation on exercise performance (73, 114, 123, 151). These interindividual differences appear to be partly due to variations in genes such as *CYP1A2*, which is associated with caffeine metabolism and response (153). Over 95% of caffeine is metabolized by the CYP1A2 enzyme, which is encoded by the *CYP1A2* gene (15). The -163A>C (rs762551) single nucleotide polymorphism (SNP) has been shown to alter CYP1A2 enzyme inducibility and activity (41, 62) and has been used to identify and categorize individuals as "fast" or "slow" or sometimes "ultra-slow" (73) metabolizers of caffeine. The largest caffeine and exercise study to date (73) examined the effects of caffeine and *CYP1A2* genotype on 10 km cycling time in competitive male athletes (both endurance and power sports) after ingestion of caffeine at 0 mg, 2 mg (low dose), or 4 mg (moderate dose) per kg body mass. There was a 3% improvement in time-trial cycling time in the moderate dose in all subjects, which is consistent with previous studies using similar doses (40, 58). However, there was a significant caffeine–gene interaction where improvements in performance were seen at both caffeine doses, but only in those with the AA genotype who are "fast metabolizers" of caffeine. In that group, the 6.8% improvement in cycling time was observed at 4 mg/kg, which is greater than the 2–4% mean improvement seen in several other cycling time-trial studies using similar doses (20, 40, 58, 70, 86, 131, 138). Among those with the CC genotype, "slow metabolizers," 4 mg/kg caffeine impaired performance by 13.7%, and in those with the AC (heterozygous) genotype there was no effect of either dose (73). The findings are consistent with a previous study (151), which observed a caffeine–gene interaction and improved time-trial cycling performance with caffeine only in those with the AA genotype.

The effects of genotype on performance are most prominent during training or competition of longer duration or an accumulation of fatigue, i.e., muscular endurance, where caffeine appears to provide its greatest benefits and where the adverse effects to slow metabolizers are more likely to manifest (42, 134). In a study of basketball performance in elite players, caffeine improved repeated jumps (muscular endurance), but only in those with the AA genotype (122). Similarly, in a cross-over design of 30 resistance-trained men, caffeine ingestion resulted in a higher number of repetitions per sets and for total repetitions in three resistance exercises combined, which resulted in a greater volume of work compared to placebo conditions, but only in those with the *CYP1A2* AA genotype (123). There appears to be growing support for the role of *CYP1A2* in modifying the effects of caffeine ingestion on aerobic or muscular endurance-type exercise. From a practical perspective, this helps to determine which athletes may be impaired (73) or are most likely to benefit from caffeine and should experiment with its use. Caffeine is one of the few ergogenic aids/supplements that is considered both pharmacological, as anhydrous caffeine, and nutritional, as coffee, tea, and botanical, whose actions may be modified through genetic variation. This research provides a model for the study of other ergogenic aids.

Iron

Iron is an essential mineral required for the production of red blood cells (RBCs) (1) and supports the function of several endogenous proteins and enzymes (47). Due to iron's role in the production of RBCs, low iron status may result in impaired athletic performance (47, 101). The prevalence of low iron storage and anaemia is greater in elite athletes compared to the general population (47, 93, 101, 120). Iron requirements rise due to an increase in erythropoiesis as a result of high training intensity, and volume. The prevalence of iron deficiency is greater in females compared to males, which has previously been attributed to menstruation (93, 137). However, it has been proposed that the dysregulation of female sex hormones, rather than menstruation, may be the reason this is observed (124, 136). In sport, low energy intakes are common, which may result in iron deficiency (103, 108). Due to these risk factors, elite athletes are advised to regularly monitor their iron levels for optimal health and performance. Variation in the *TMPRSS6*, *TF*, and *TFR2* genes have been shown to influence one's susceptibility to low iron status (101).

TMPRSS6, TF, and TFR2 Genes

Three SNPs, *TMPRSS6* (rs4820268), *TF* (rs3811647), and *TFR2* (rs7385804), have been associated with low iron status and may modify an individual's risk for low iron status (101). The three SNPs are known to regulate the expression of the protein hepcidin (67, 124, 136). Hepcidin inhibits iron transport in the plasma by binding to ferroprotein, a transmembrane protein that transports iron from the inside to the outside of the cell (136). In addition, the oxygen carrying capacity of the two iron containing proteins, haemoglobin and myoglobin, is reduced due to low iron anaemia, impairing performance (27, 60). Low iron status can be predicted by certain combinations of genotypes within SNPs of the *TMPRSS6*, *TF*, and *TRF2* genes. Those with the GG genotype of *TMPRSS6* (rs4820268) possess an elevated risk for low transferrin saturation and haemoglobin, compared to A-allele carriers who possess a typical risk (46, 101). Those with the AA genotype of *TF* (rs3811647) are more likely to possess low ferritin but high transferrin saturations compared to G-allele carriers (101). Those with the CC genotype of *TFR2* (rs7385804) are more likely to experience decreased haematocrit, mean corpuscular volume, and RBC count compared to A-allele carriers. Genotyping of these three SNPs can be carried out and inputted into an algorithm to help predict individual risk for low iron status (17, 118). If an athlete is at risk for low iron, modifications can be made through diet or supplementation to offset their risk. Despite being at an increased risk for low iron status, athletes should monitor their supplemental iron intake and serum ferritin to ensure they are not consuming excessive amounts of iron. Indeed, variation in the *HFE* gene has been shown to influences one's susceptibility to iron overload (hemochromatosis) (16, 116).

HFE Gene

Many athletes choose to take iron supplements in order to prevent or treat low iron; however, they may be at risk of excessive intake (116). This may also negatively affect performance due to the tissue-damaging effects of excess iron (16) through the increased production of free radicals (51). Iron readily reacts with reactive oxygen species (ROS) such as hydrogen peroxide to produce free radicals (17, 51). This can arise when an individual possesses elevated iron levels, which occurs with conditions such as haemochromatosis. The gene associated with haemochromatosis is *HFE*, and there are two SNPs in this gene (rs1800562 and rs1799945) that can be used to predict the risk of haemochromatosis (103, 108). Those with the AA (rs1800562) and GG (rs1799945) genotypes of *HFE* possess the greatest risk for haemochromatosis (7, 79, 118). Those with the GA (rs1800562) and GC (rs1799945) genotypes are at a medium risk, and those with the GG (rs1800562) and CC (rs1799945) genotypes are at a low risk for haemochromatosis. Other combinations confer varying risks. Since athletes may be genetically at risk to possess higher iron levels, they possess a genetic advantage to excel in certain sports because of a greater oxygen–carrying capacity, and it has been observed that elite athletes possess the risk variant more so than the general population (74, 79). This benefit could also be a detriment if excessive iron levels persist and cause tissue damage (7, 79, 118). Athletes that possess an elevated risk of haemochromatosis should not consume iron supplements and ensure that they do not exceed the recommended daily intake to avoid iron overload (99). Supplements might not be avoided in those who do not have an elevated risk of haemochromatosis, although iron levels should be monitored to avoid consuming excessive amounts.

Lactate Production and Transport

Lactate is produced in the cell at the end of anaerobic glycolysis, when oxygen is not present (63). Pyruvate, the reagent present at the beginning of glycolysis, is converted into lactate by the enzyme lactate dehydrogenase (LDH) (63, 105). Muscle fatigue occurs due to the increased production and slow rate of removal of lactate and hydrogen ions (56). Lactate removal is regulated by monocarboxylate transporters (MCTs), which are lactate transporters found at the mitochondrial membrane (18). The MCT1 transporter is found in the muscle and modifies mitochondrial pH when altered (18, 34, 57, 119). During high-intensity exercise, mitochondrial pH decreases due to increased lactate and H^+ ion buildup (61). This results in decreased mitochondrial biogenesis, hindering performance (77, 152). Blood lactate concentration and the removal of lactate are associated with the MCT1 transporter (34, 71). To keep exercising at a specific intensity, lactate is transported across the plasma membrane into the mitochondria mainly through muscular contraction (4, 13, 63). This is important, as athletes must recover during interval training or in intermittent sports such as hockey and basketball (34, 100). Additionally, athletes that compete in multiple events over many days, such as the Tour de France and medal rounds of track and field must efficiently recover in a short duration (29). If the activity of MCT1 were to increase, lactate transport rates would rise, allowing athletes to recover within or between competition quickly. Variation in the *SLC16A1* gene has been shown to influence MCT1 transporter content and activity (12, 75).

SLC16A1 Gene

The *SLC16A1* gene encodes the MCT1 transporter, and a SNP (rs1049434) in this gene may modify lactate clearance (107). Individuals with the AA genotype of *SLC16A1* (rs1049434) possess an increased ability to clear lactate during high-intensity efforts compared to individuals with the TT genotype (32). The opposite was observed in a more recent study where those with the TT genotype possessed an increased ability to clear lactate, which the authors suggest is due to measurements in venous versus capillary (more arterialized) blood (33). That is, the less capillary lactate accumulation found in AA males would reflect an elevated lactate transport from arterial blood into the muscle fibres for its oxidation, indicating decreased MCT1 lactate transport in T-allele carriers (33, 34). This has been confirmed in wrestlers with the AA genotype, who experienced lower blood lactate levels after repeated sprints and a 30-second Wingate test (89). This is also consistent with additional research that individuals with the AA genotype are able to clear blood lactate at a faster rate compared to T-allele carriers (32, 33, 89, 102). The variants of *SLC16A1* seem to vary in the athletic population. The A-allele is more common in elite endurance rowers compared to the general population (54). Soccer players at the forward position possess the A-allele more than the general population (102). Anaerobic-based athletes possess the T-allele more than the general population, as well as endurance athletes (132). Anaerobic-based athletes produce more lactate, as their sport relies on anaerobic rather than aerobic glycolysis. Increased lactate is positively associated with anabolic hormones and muscle hypertrophy (19). Exercising individuals who consistently produce lactate have greater lean body mass and increased anaerobic performance due to an increased production of anabolic hormones (19, 132). Since individuals with the AA genotype are better able to clear lactate, those with the T-allele might respond best to buffering agents (32, 33, 89, 102). The two most prominent buffering supplements used in athletics are β-alanine and sodium bicarbonate (49, 92, 135). Additional information on these buffering supplements can be found in Chapter 22. The goal of buffering agents is to attenuate exercise-induced acidosis, thus improving high-intensity anaerobic performance and sprint efforts (19, 92, 132). The reason there are inconsistent effects of buffering supplements could be due to variability in *SLC16A1* (19, 132). Future trials must be designed where individuals are stratified based upon their *SLC16A1* genotype to determine the effects of different buffering agents across individuals.

Vitamin B$_{12}$

Individuals who are deficient in vitamin B$_{12}$ may experience megaloblastic anaemia and increased homocysteine levels (10, 78). Megaloblastic anaemia results in enlarged RBCs, thereby decreasing the oxygen-carrying capacity of the two proteins myoglobin and haemoglobin in the blood. Variation in the *FUT2* gene has been shown to influence one's susceptibility to vitamin B$_{12}$ deficiency (78, 90).

FUT2 Gene

Vitamin B$_{12}$ is absorbed and transported between cells by the fucosyltransferase 2 (FUT2) enzyme, which is encoded by the *FUT2* gene (78, 90). Individuals who possess the risk variant of *FUT2* may be at risk for B$_{12}$ deficiency if there is low B$_{12}$ in their diet. This is due to a SNP in *FUT2* (rs601338), which can alter vitamin B$_{12}$ absorption (10). The deficiency is observed more in vegetarian and vegan compared to omnivore athletes (10, 78). Individuals possess an elevated risk for B$_{12}$ deficiency if their diet is low in B$_{12}$, especially if they are a G-allele carrier, compared to those with the AA genotype of *FUT2* (rs601338) (78). Those with the AA genotype possess elevated B$_{12}$ levels in comparison to G-allele carriers. Highly bioavailable sources of vitamin B$_{12}$ such as meat and fish products can be consumed to ensure adequate vitamin B$_{12}$ levels. Vegan and vegetarian athletes may want to supplement with vitamin B$_{12}$ to ensure adequate levels.

Vitamin A

Vitamin A is a fat-soluble vitamin/antioxidant necessary to optimize immunity and vision (14, 22, 35). The bioavailable forms of vitamin A exist as retinal and retinoic acid (55, 56). Low vitamin A intake is associated with immune dysfunction (35). As an antioxidant, vitamin A reduces the risk of ocular diseases and may improve vision (22). The majority of sports require optimal vision and hand–eye coordination to excel (59). In sports such as ice hockey and baseball, the objects of interest, the puck and ball, respectively, rapidly move during play (59, 112). Athletes may be at a greater risk for a sport-related injury if they possess slow visuomotor reaction time (150).

Low vitamin A intake may result in an individual being more susceptible to infection due to immune dysfunction (22, 35). Low energy intake, in addition to physical/psychological stress, poor food choices, and jet lag, as well as exposure to foreign food, water, and pathogens, is common amongst athletes and has the potential to increase the likelihood of an infection (108, 146). Upper respiratory tract infections are more common in athletes following high-intensity and high-volume training programmes compared to sedentary individuals, as well as those who engage in moderate-intensity exercise programmes (146). Vitamin A is formed by the β-carotene mono-oxygenase 1 (BCMO1) enzyme expressed in enterocytes of the intestinal mucosa. Here, it converts dietary carotenoids, such as β-carotene, into vitamin A (96). However, β-carotene must then be converted to retinal or retinoic acid for vitamin A to exert its beneficial biological effects. Variation in the *BCMO1* gene has been shown to influence the conversion of carotenoids into the bioavailable form of vitamin A (55).

BCMO1 Gene

The *BCMO1* gene encodes the BCMO1 enzyme, which converts carotenoids into vitamin A's biologically active form (55). A SNP in *BCMO1* (rs11645428) can modify the conversion of carotenoids into vitamin A's biologically active form, increasing one's risk for low vitamin A levels. Those who possess the GG genotype of *BCMO1* (rs11645428) have a greater risk for vitamin A deficiency due to the poor conversion of carotenoids to the biologically active form of vitamin A (97). Those with the GG genotype may want to consume pre-formed vitamin A (found in animal products) in their diet to bypass the inefficient conversion of carotenoids into vitamin A (55, 96, 97). Alternatively, those who prefer to consume more of the plant-sourced vitamin A precursor, β-carotene, can increase their consumption of spinach and other vegetables and fruits that are orange-red in colour. This will ensure that vision and immune health are optimal for an athlete to perform in game and to ensure long-term viability without infection.

Vitamin C and Collagen

Vitamin C is a water-soluble vitamin that functions as an antioxidant (110). Exercise-induced muscle damage that occurs due to the production of free radicals may be decreased in the presence of vitamin C (45, 121). Exercising muscle produces more ROS than the non-exercising muscle due to increased oxygen uptake during exercise (45, 65, 125, 143). Exercise-induced free radical production at lower levels is viewed as a positive training stimulus (45). Excessive vitamin C intake may impair this process, preventing beneficial training adaptations (126). These training adaptations include increased muscle oxidative capacity and mitochondrial biogenesis (45, 65, 117, 145). Vitamin C intake of 250 mg through dietary sources, as opposed to supplements, is likely sufficient without blocking these physiological training adaptions from occurring (117). In addition to vitamin C's function as an antioxidant, it is necessary for the production of collagen, which is required for the formation of tendons, bones, and skin (21, 133). Vitamin C and collagen may assist with muscle repair and growth (117, 126, 145). Collagen synthesis is improved in athletes as a result of gelatin and vitamin C supplementation (133). This may assist athletes with injury prevention and increase the rate of musculoskeletal, ligament, or tendon tissue repair (21). However, some individuals may be at risk for vitamin C deficiency as a result of the *GSTT1* (Ins or Del) gene (23).

GSTT1 Gene

The *GSTT1* gene encodes a protein in the glutathione S-transferase enzyme, which mitigates oxidative stress through vitamin C status (23). Circulating levels of vitamin C can be modified due to a SNP in the *GSTT1* (Ins or Del) gene. Those with the Del/Del genotype of *GSTT1* possess an elevated risk for vitamin C deficiency compared to those with the Ins allele (83). Vitamin C is measured through ascorbic acid, and deficiencies are likely when intake is low. Vitamin C deficiency is characterized by the damage of healthy tissues, reduced connective tissue repair, and early exercise fatigue (23, 83). Athletes who possess the Ins allele of *GSTT1* are recommended to not consume vitamin C supplements, as it may negatively interfere with positive training adaptions that occur with low-level exercise-induced muscle damage (45, 65). Athletes can consume 250 mg daily without interfering with training adaptations (126). Those with the Del/Del genotype should ensure they consume adequate vitamin C and may also supplement to ensure optimal collagen production to repair muscles and tendons (133).

Vitamin D and Bone Health

Vitamin D is essential to calcium metabolism, increasing calcium absorption for optimal bone health, which is relevant to all athletes, but particularly those participating in sports with a high risk of stress fracture such as running (9, 76, 129, 139, 147). Two genes that have been shown to affect vitamin D status are the *GC* gene and the *CYP2R1* gene (139, 147).

GC and CYP2R1 Genes

Vitamin D 25-hydroxylase is the key enzyme that activates vitamin D from its pre-formed type, which is obtained through sun exposure and the diet (9, 76). This enzyme is encoded by the *CYP2R1* gene, and a variant of this gene has been associated with an increased risk of low circulating levels of vitamin D (139, 147). The *GC* gene encodes the vitamin D-binding protein, which binds vitamin D and transports it to tissues. A variant in this gene has also been associated with an increased risk of low circulating levels of vitamin D. In one study, individuals with the GG or GA genotype of *CYP2R1* were nearly four times more likely to have insufficient vitamin D levels compared to those with the AA genotype after vitamin D supplementation (139). Those with the GG genotype of the *GC* gene were significantly more likely to have low vitamin D levels compared to those with the TT genotype. These results were consistent with findings from previous research, including the Study of Underlying Genetic Determinants of Vitamin D and Highly Related Traits (SUNLIGHT), which found significance on a genome-wide basis in 15 cohorts with over 30,000 participants for three genetic variants, including *CYP2R1* (rs10741657) and *GC* (rs2282679), and vitamin D status (139, 147). Those with the risk variants may not efficiently absorb calcium, increasing their risk for stress and other bone fractures (53). Athletes who engage in weight-bearing repetitive-load sports, such as long-distance running, must monitor their vitamin D and calcium intake to decrease their risk of stress and other bone fractures (48, 91, 111).

Muscle Damage

Delayed-onset muscle soreness (DOMS) is commonly experienced in the days following unaccustomed or strenuous training, and it is characterized by tender, stiff muscles, which can also cause a temporary reduction in strength and range of motion (94). DOMS is a result of exercise-induced muscle damage, which at low levels, is a positive stimulus for muscle growth and increased strength (87). However, excessive damage or inadequate recovery may cause persistent and unnecessary soreness, which can impede strength gains or improvements in aerobic capacity and increase the risk of developing overuse injuries (84). DOMS is caused by oxidative stress, inflammation, and muscle protein degradation (26). There is considerable variability in an individual's response to muscle-damaging exercise due to factors such as age, training and sport history, and genetics (39). Research shows that variation in the *ACTN3* gene influences one's susceptibility to muscle damage after prolonged, strenuous, or unaccustomed exercise (38). The type of activity inducing the greatest muscle damage is most often high-intensity resistance or strength and power-type training.

ACTN3 Gene

The *ACTN3* (rs1815739) gene encodes the alpha-actin 3 protein, which plays a key role in the contraction of fast-twitch or power-type muscle fibres during short bursts of intense activities, such as sprinting or lifting heavy objects (154). Genetic variation in *ACTN3* affects the expression of the resulting protein in fast-twitch fibres, and individuals who carry at least one copy of the T variant produce a lower-functioning ACTN3 protein that has been linked to increased risk of muscle damage (52). For example, a recent study showed that experienced endurance athletes with the T variant had higher levels of markers of muscle damage after a competitive marathon (38) compared to individuals with the CC variant. A similar trend was observed in a study where healthy young men performed knee extension exercises, working the quadriceps, in a laboratory setting (39).

Athletes who are T-allele carriers for the *ACTN3* (rs1815739) gene have an increased susceptibility to muscle damage after strenuous or unaccustomed exercise. They may also be at greater risk of developing overuse injuries if not adequately recovered from the previous training sessions (5). Athletes who frequently experience more severe cases of DOMS should prioritize rest and recovery and also ensure an adequate total protein intake, as well as frequency of intake throughout the day for muscle repair (84). The consumption of plenty of antioxidant-rich plant foods such as fruits, vegetables, nuts, and seeds may help reduce inflammation (140) and mitigate the negative effects of oxidative stress caused by muscle damage (155).

Summary

This chapter provided an overview of the current science linking genetic variation to nutritional or supplemental needs with a focus on fitness and athletic performance. The ultimate goal of personalized sport nutrition is to design tailored dietary recommendations that may directly (performance) and indirectly (health) influence athletic performance.

Personalized nutrition pursuits should aim to aid in the development of more comprehensive and dynamic nutritional and supplement recommendations based on shifting and interacting parameters in an athlete's internal and external (sport) environment. Only a few gene–diet interaction studies have directly measured performance outcomes in competitive athletes (73, 123, 151), so this should be a focus of future research. Currently, the majority of studies associating nutrition to performance outcomes have not been intervention trials, but this is consistent with the field of nutrition as a whole. Nevertheless, it has been well-established in the literature that serum levels and/or dietary intakes of several nutrients and food bioactives can affect overall health, and in turn result in modest to sizable modifying effects in athletic performance. Personalized nutrition strategies for athletes will continue to develop as research identifies new genetic markers that enable these valuable targeted interventions.

Genetic testing for personalized sport nutrition is an effective tool that can be implemented into the practice of sport clinicians, nutritionists, and coaches to guide nutritional counselling and meal planning with the aim of optimizing athletic performance. A summary of the genetic markers reviewed in this chapter can be seen in Table 25.1.

Table 25.1 Summary of genetic variants that modify the effect of dietary factors or biological molecules on performance-related outcomes.

Gene (rs number)	Function	Dietary factor or biological molecule	Dietary sources or supplements	Performance-related outcome(s)
ADORA2A (rs5751876)	Regulates myocardial oxygen demand; increases coronary circulation via vasodilation	Caffeine	Coffee, tea, soda, energy drinks, caffeine supplements	Vigilance when fatigued, sleep quality, anxiety (8, 28, 128)
CYP1A2 (rs762551)	Encodes CYP1A2 liver enzyme: metabolizes caffeine; identifies individuals as fast or slow metabolizers	Caffeine	Coffee, tea, soda, energy drinks, caffeine supplements	Cardiovascular health, endurance performance (73, 114, 115, 123, 153)
TMPRSS6 (rs4820268), *TFR2* (rs7385804), *TF* (rs3811647)	Modifies iron absorption through regulating the protein hepcidin	Iron	Beef, chicken, fish, organ meats (haem iron); almonds, parsley, spinach (non-haem iron)	Iron-deficiency anaemia risk (16, 46, 118, 124, 136)
HFE (rs1800562 and rs1799945)	Regulates intestinal iron uptake	Iron	Beef, chicken, fish, organ meats (haem iron); almonds, parsley, spinach (non-haem iron)	Hereditary haemochromatosis (7, 17)
SLC16A1 (rs1049434)	Regulates lactate clearance from the muscle	Lactate	Beta alanine and sodium bicarbonate	Lactate clearance (33, 34, 107)

(Continued)

Table 25.1 (Continued)

Gene (rs number)	Function	Dietary factor or biological molecule	Dietary sources or supplements	Performance-related outcome(s)
FUT2 (rs602662)	Transport and absorption of vitamin B_{12}	Vitamin B_{12}	Clams, oysters, herring, nutritional yeast, beef, salmon	Megaloblastic anaemia and hyperhomocysteinemia (78)
BCMO1 (rs11645428)	Converts carotenoids to vitamin A	Vitamin A	Bluefin tuna, hard goat cheese, eggs, mackerel, carrots, sweet potato	Visuomotor skills and immunity (55, 96, 97)
GSTT1 (Ins/ Del)	Modifies glutathione S-transferase enzymes resulting in altered vitamin C utilization	Vitamin C and collagen	Red peppers, strawberries, pineapple, oranges, broccoli	Circulating ascorbic acid levels mitigate exercise-induced ROS production (23, 83)
GC (rs2282679)	Encodes vitamin D-binding protein, which transports vitamin D throughout the body; calcium absorption requires vitamin D	Calcium and vitamin D	Calcium: Yogurt, milk, cheese, firm tofu, canned salmon (with bones), edamame Vitamin D: Salmon, white fish, rainbow trout, halibut, milk	Bone/stress fracture risk (139, 147)
CYP2R1 (rs10741657)	Encodes vitamin D 25-hydroxylase which is the key enzyme that activates vitamin D from its pre-formed type.	Calcium and vitamin D	Calcium: Yogurt, milk, cheese, firm tofu, canned salmon (with bones), edamame Vitamin D: Salmon, white fish, rainbow trout, halibut, milk	Bone/stress fracture risk (139, 147)
ACTN3 (rs1815739)	Encodes the alpha-actin 3 protein, which is involved in the contraction of fast-twitch muscle fibres	Antioxidants/ protein	Bluefin tuna, hard goat cheese, eggs, mackerel, carrots, sweet potato, red peppers, strawberries, pineapple, oranges, broccoli	Modifies the susceptibility to muscle damage after strenuous or unaccustomed exercise (38, 39, 154)

References

1. Abbaspour N, Hurrell R, Kelishadi R. Review on iron and its importance for human health. *J Res Med Sci* 19: 164–174, 2014.
2. Abrahams M, Frewer LJ, Bryant E, Stewart-Knox B. Personalised nutrition technologies and innovations: a cross-national survey of registered dietitians. *Public Health Genomics* 22: 119–131, 2019.
3. Abrahams Mea. Factors determining the integration of nutritional genomics into clinical practice by registered dietitians. *Trends Food Sci Technol* 59: 139–147 2017.
4. Adeva-Andany M, Lopez-Ojen M, Funcasta-Calderon R, Ameneiros-Rodriguez E, Donapetry-Garcia C, Vila-Altesor M et al. Comprehensive review on lactate metabolism in human health. *Mitochondrion* 17: 76–100, 2014.
5. Aicale R, Tarantino D, Maffulli N. Overuse injuries in sport: a comprehensive overview. *J Orthop Surg Res* 13: 309, 2018.
6. Akesdotter C, Kentta G, Eloranta S, Franck J. The prevalence of mental health problems in elite athletes. *J Sci Med Sport* 23(4):329–335, 2019.
7. Allen KJ, Gurrin LC, Constantine CC, Osborne NJ, Delatycki MB, Nicoll AJ et al. Iron-overload-related disease in HFE hereditary hemochromatosis. *N Engl J Med* 358: 221–230, 2008.

8. Alsene K, Deckert J, Sand P, de Wit H. Association between A2a receptor gene polymorphisms and caffeine-induced anxiety. *Neuropsychopharmacology* 28: 1694–1702, 2003.

9. Angeline ME, Gee AO, Shindle M, Warren RF, Rodeo SA. The effects of vitamin D deficiency in athletes. *Am J Sports Med* 41: 461–464, 2013.

10. Aslinia F, Mazza JJ, Yale SH. Megaloblastic anemia and other causes of macrocytosis. *Clin Med Res* 4: 236–241, 2006.

11. Bailey RL, Saldanha LG, Dwyer JT. Estimating caffeine intake from energy drinks and dietary supplements in the United States. *Nutr Rev* 72(Suppl 1): 9–13, 2014.

12. Baker SK, McCullagh KJ, Bonen A. Training intensity-dependent and tissue-specific increases in lactate uptake and MCT-1 in heart and muscle. *J Appl Physiol (1985)* 84: 987–994, 1998.

13. Baldari C, Videira M, Madeira F, Sergio J, Guidetti L. Lactate removal during active recovery related to the individual anaerobic and ventilatory thresholds in soccer players. *Eur J Appl Physiol* 93: 224–230, 2004.

14. Beckerman S, Hitzeman SA. Sports vision testing of selected athletic participants in the 1997 and 1998 AAU junior Olympic games. *Optometry* 74: 502–516, 2003.

15. Begas E, Kouvaras E, Tsakalof A, Papakosta S, Asprodini EK. In vivo evaluation of CYP1A2, CYP2A6, NAT-2 and xanthine oxidase activities in a Greek population sample by the RP-HPLC monitoring of caffeine metabolic ratios. *Biomed Chromatogr* 21: 190–200, 2007.

16. Benyamin B, Ferreira MA, Willemsen G, Gordon S, Middelberg RP, McEvoy BP, et al. Common variants in TMPRSS6 are associated with iron status and erythrocyte volume. *Nat Genet* 41: 1173–1175, 2009.

17. Benyamin B, McRae AF, Zhu G, Gordon S, Henders AK, Palotie A, et al. Variants in TF and HFE explain approximately 40% of genetic variation in serum-transferrin levels. *Am J Hum Genet* 84: 60–65, 2009.

18. Bonen A. The expression of lactate transporters (MCT1 and MCT4) in heart and muscle. *Eur J Appl Physiol* 86: 6–11, 2001.

19. Bonen A, McCullagh KJ, Putman CT, Hultman E, Jones NL, Heigenhauser GJ. Short-term training increases human muscle MCT1 and femoral venous lactate in relation to muscle lactate. *Am J Physiol* 274: E102–107, 1998.

20. Bortolotti H, Altimari LR, Vitor-Costa M, Cyrino ES. Performance during a 20-km cycling time-trial after caffeine ingestion. *J Int Soc Sports Nutr* 11: 45, 2014.

21. Boyera N, Galey I, Bernard BA. Effect of vitamin C and its derivatives on collagen synthesis and cross-linking by normal human fibroblasts. *Int J Cosmet Sci* 20: 151–158, 1998.

22. Braakhuis A, Raman R, Vaghefi E. The association between dietary intake of antioxidants and ocular disease. *Diseases* 5(1):3, 2017.

23. Cahill LE, Fontaine-Bisson B, El-Sohemy A. Functional genetic variants of glutathione S-transferase protect against serum ascorbic acid deficiency. *Am J Clin Nutr* 90: 1411–1417, 2009.

24. Celis-Morales C, Marsaux CF, Livingstone KM, Navas-Carretero S, San-Cristobal R, Fallaize R, et al. Can genetic-based advice help you lose weight? Findings from the Food4Me European randomized controlled trial. *Am J Clin Nutr* 105: 1204–1213, 2017.

25. Chang C, Putukian M, Aerni G, Diamond A, Hong G, Ingram Y, et al. Mental health issues and psychological factors in athletes: detection, management, effect on performance and prevention: American Medical Society for Sports Medicine Position Statement-Executive summary. *Br J Sports Med* 54(4):216–220, 2019.

26. Cheung K, Hume P, Maxwell L. Delayed onset muscle soreness: treatment strategies and performance factors. *Sports Med* 33: 145–164, 2003.

27. Chicharro JL, Hoyos J, Gomez-Gallego F, Villa JG, Bandres F, Celaya P, et al. Mutations in the hereditary haemochromatosis gene HFE in professional endurance athletes. *Br J Sports Med* 38: 418–421, 2004.

28. Childs E, Hohoff C, Deckert J, Xu K, Badner J, de Wit H. Association between ADORA2A and DRD2 polymorphisms and caffeine-induced anxiety. *Neuropsychopharmacology* 33: 2791–2800, 2008.

29. Chycki J, Golas A, Halz M, et al. Chronic ingestion of sodium and potassium bicarbonate, with potassium, magnesium and calcium citrate improves anaerobic performance in elite soccer players. *Nutrients* 10: 2018.

30. Collins J, Adamski MM, Twohig C, Murgia C. Opportunities for training for nutritional professionals in nutritional genomics: What is out there? *Nutr Diet* 75: 206–218, 2018.

31. Costello N, McKenna J, Sutton L, Deighton K, Jones B. Using contemporary behavior change science to design and implement an effective nutritional intervention within professional rugby league. *Int J Sport Nutr Exerc Metab* 28: 553–557, 2018.

32. Cupeiro R, Benito PJ, Maffulli N, Calderon FJ, Gonzalez-Lamuno D. MCT1 genetic polymorphism influence in high intensity circuit training: a pilot study. *J Sci Med Sport* 13: 526–530, 2010.

33. Cupeiro R, Gonzalez-Lamuno D, Amigo T, Peinado AB, Ruiz JR, Ortega FB, et al. Influence of the MCT1-T1470A polymorphism (rs1049434) on blood lactate accumulation during different circuit weight trainings in men and women. *J Sci Med Sport* 15: 541–547, 2012.

34. Cupeiro R, Perez-Prieto R, Amigo T, Gortazar P, Redondo C, Gonzalez-Lamuno D. Role of the monocarboxylate transporter MCT1 in the uptake of lactate during active recovery. *Eur J Appl Physiol* 116: 1005–1010, 2016.

35. Czarnewski P, Das S, Parigi SM, Villablanca EJ. Retinoic acid and its role in modulating intestinal innate immunity. *Nutrients* 9(1):68, 2017.

36. De Francisco C, Arce C, Sanchez-Romero EI, Vilchez MP. The mediating role of sport self-motivation between basic psychological needs satisfaction and athlete engagement. *Psicothema* 30: 421–426, 2018.

37. de Toro-Martin J, Arsenault BJ, Despres JP, Vohl MC. Precision nutrition: a review of personalized nutritional approaches for the prevention and management of metabolic syndrome. *Nutrients* 9(8):913, 2017.

38. Del Coso J, Moreno V, Gutierrez-Hellin J, Baltazar-Martins G, Ruiz-Moreno C, Aguilar-Navarro M, et al. ACTN3 R577X genotype and exercise phenotypes in recreational marathon runners. *Genes (Basel)* 10(6):413, 2019.

39. Del Coso J, Valero M, Salinero JJ, Lara B, Diaz G, Gallo-Salazar C, et al. ACTN3 genotype influences exercise-induced muscle damage during a marathon competition. *Eur J Appl Physiol* 117: 409–416, 2017.

40. Desbrow B, Biddulph C, Devlin B, Grant GD, Anoopkumar-Dukie S, Leveritt MD. The effects of different doses of caffeine on endurance cycling time trial performance. *J Sports Sci* 30: 115–120, 2012.

41. Djordjevic N, Ghotbi R, Bertilsson L, Jankovic S, Aklillu E. Induction of CYP1A2 by heavy coffee consumption in Serbs and Swedes. *Eur J Clin Pharmacol* 64: 381–385, 2008.

42. Doherty M and Smith PM. Effects of caffeine ingestion on exercise testing: a meta-analysis. *Int J Sport Nutr Exerc Metab* 14: 626–646, 2004.

43. Doherty M and Smith PM. Effects of caffeine ingestion on rating of perceived exertion during and after exercise: a meta-analysis. *Scand J Med Sci Sports* 15: 69–78, 2005.

44. Doherty M, Smith PM, Davison RC, Hughes MG. Caffeine is ergogenic after supplementation of oral creatine monohydrate. *Med Sci Sports Exerc* 34: 1785–1792, 2002.

45. Draeger CL, Naves A, Marques N, Baptistella AB, Carnauba RA, Paschoal V, et al. Controversies of antioxidant vitamins supplementation in exercise: ergogenic or ergolytic effects in humans? *J Int Soc Sports Nutr* 11: 4, 2014.

46. Du X, She E, Gelbart T, Truksa J, Lee P, Xia Y, et al. The serine protease TMPRSS6 is required to sense iron deficiency. *Science* 320: 1088–1092, 2008.

47. Dubnov G, Foldes AJ, Mann G, Magazanik A, Siderer M, Constantini N. High prevalence of iron deficiency and anemia in female military recruits. *Mil Med* 171: 866–869, 2006.

48. Duckham RL, Peirce N, Meyer C, Summers GD, Cameron N, Brooke-Wavell K. Risk factors for stress fracture in female endurance athletes: a cross-sectional study. *BMJ Open* 2: 2012.

49. Edge J, Bishop D, Goodman C. Effects of chronic NaHCO3 ingestion during interval training on changes to muscle buffer capacity, metabolism, and short-term endurance performance. *J Appl Physiol (1985)* 101: 918–925, 2006.

50. El-Sohemy A. Only DNA-based dietary advice improved adherence to the Mediterranean diet score. *Am J Clin Nutr* 105: 770, 2017.

51. Emerit J, Beaumont C, Trivin F. Iron metabolism, free radicals, and oxidative injury. *Biomed Pharmacother* 55: 333–339, 2001.

52. Eynon N, Hanson ED, Lucia A, Houweling PJ, Garton F, North KN, et al. Genes for elite power and sprint performance: ACTN3 leads the way. *Sports medicine* 43: 803–817, 2013.

53. Fang Y, van Meurs JB, Arp P, van Leeuwen JP, Hofman A, Pols HA, et al. Vitamin D binding protein genotype and osteoporosis. *Calcif Tissue Int* 85: 85–93, 2009.

54. Fedotovskaya ON, Mustafina LJ, Popov DV, Vinogradova OL, Ahmetov, II. A common polymorphism of the MCT1 gene and athletic performance. *Int J Sports Physiol Perform* 9: 173–180, 2014.

55. Ferrucci L, Perry JR, Matteini A, Perola M, Tanaka T, Silander K, et al. Common variation in the beta-carotene 15,15'-monooxygenase 1 gene affects circulating levels of carotenoids: a genome-wide association study. *Am J Hum Genet* 84: 123–133, 2009.

56. Finsterer J. Biomarkers of peripheral muscle fatigue during exercise. *BMC Musculoskelet Disord* 13: 218, 2012.

57. Fishbein WN, Merezhinskaya N, Foellmer JW. Relative distribution of three major lactate transporters in frozen human tissues and their localization in unfixed skeletal muscle. *Muscle Nerve* 26: 101–112, 2002.

58. Ganio MS, Klau JF, Casa DJ, Armstrong LE, Maresh CM. Effect of caffeine on sport-specific endurance performance: a systematic review. *J Strength Cond Res* 23: 315–324, 2009.

59. Gao Y, Chen L, Yang SN, Wang H, Yao J, Dai Q, et al. Contributions of visuo-oculomotor abilities to interceptive skills in sports. *Optom Vis Sci* 92: 679–689, 2015.

60. Garvican L, Martin D, Quod M, Stephens B, Sassi A, Gore C. Time course of the hemoglobin mass response to natural altitude training in elite endurance cyclists. *Scand J Med Sci Sports* 22: 95–103, 2012

61. Genders AJ, Martin SD, McGee SL, Bishop DJ. A physiological drop in pH decreases mitochondrial respiration, and HDAC and Akt signaling, in L6 myocytes. *American Journal of Physiology-Cell Physiology* 316: C404–C414, 2019.

62. Ghotbi R, Christensen M, Roh HK, Ingelman-Sundberg M, Aklillu E, Bertilsson L. Comparisons of CYP1A2 genetic polymorphisms, enzyme activity and the genotype-phenotype relationship in Swedes and Koreans. *Eur J Clin Pharmacol* 63: 537–546, 2007.

63. Gladden LB. Lactate metabolism: a new paradigm for the third millennium. *J Physiol* 558: 5–30, 2004.

64. Goldstein ER, Ziegenfuss T, Kalman D, Kreider R, Campbell B, Wilborn C, et al. International society of sports nutrition position stand: caffeine and performance. *J Int Soc Sports Nutr* 7: 5, 2010.

65. Gomez-Cabrera MC, Domenech E, Romagnoli M, Arduini A, Borras C, Pallardo FV, et al. Oral administration of vitamin C decreases muscle mitochondrial biogenesis and hampers training-induced adaptations in endurance performance. *Am J Clin Nutr* 87: 142–149, 2008.

66. Gorman U, Mathers JC, Grimaldi KA, Ahlgren J, Nordstrom K. Do we know enough? A scientific and ethical analysis of the basis for genetic-based personalized nutrition. *Genes Nutr* 8: 373–381, 2013.

67. Govus AD, Garvican-Lewis LA, Abbiss CR, Peeling P, Gore CJ. Pre-altitude serum ferritin levels and daily oral iron supplement dose mediate iron parameter and hemoglobin mass responses to altitude exposure. *PLOS ONE* 10: e0135120, 2015.

68. Graham TE, Spriet LL. Metabolic, catecholamine, and exercise performance responses to various doses of caffeine. *J Appl Physiol (1985)* 78: 867–874, 1995.

69. Graham TE, Spriet LL. Performance and metabolic responses to a high caffeine dose during prolonged exercise. *J Appl Physiol (1985)* 71: 2292–2298, 1991.

70. Graham-Paulson T, Perret C, Goosey-Tolfrey V. Improvements in cycling but not handcycling 10 km time trial performance in habitual caffeine users. *Nutrients* 8(7):393, 2016.

71. Green H, Halestrap A, Mockett C, O'Toole D, Grant S, Ouyang J. Increases in muscle MCT are associated with reductions in muscle lactate after a single exercise session in humans. *Am J Physiol Endocrinol Metab* 282: E154–160, 2002.

72. Grimaldi KA, van Ommen B, Ordovas JM, Parnell LD, Mathers JC, Bendik I, et al. Proposed guidelines to evaluate scientific validity and evidence for genotype-based dietary advice. *Genes Nutr* 12: 35, 2017.

73. Guest N, Corey P, Vescovi J, El-Sohemy A. Caffeine, CYP1A2 genotype, and endurance performance in athletes. *Med Sci Sports Exerc* 50: 1570–1578, 2018.

74. Guest NS, Horne J, Vanderhout SM, El-Sohemy A. Sport nutrigenomics: personalized nutrition for athletic performance. *Front Nutr* 6: 8, 2019.

75. Halestrap AP, Price NT. The proton-linked monocarboxylate transporter (MCT) family: structure, function and regulation. *Biochem J* 343(Pt 2): 281–299, 1999.

76. Halliday TM, Peterson NJ, Thomas JJ, Kleppinger K, Hollis BW, Larson-Meyer DE. Vitamin D status relative to diet, lifestyle, injury, and illness in college athletes. *Med Sci Sports Exerc* 43: 335–343, 2011.

77. Hashimoto T, Hussien R, Oommen S, Gohil K, Brooks GA. Lactate sensitive transcription factor network in L6 cells: activation of MCT1 and mitochondrial biogenesis. *The FASEB Journal* 21: 2602–2612, 2007.

78. Hazra A, Kraft P, Selhub J, Giovannucci EL, Thomas G, Hoover RN, et al. Common variants of FUT2 are associated with plasma vitamin B12 levels. *Nat Genet* 40: 1160–1162, 2008.

79. Hermine O, Dine G, Genty V, Marquet LA, Fumagalli G, Tafflet M, et al. Eighty percent of French sport winners in Olympic, World and Europeans competitions have mutations in the hemochromatosis HFE gene. *Biochimie* 119: 1–5, 2015.

80. Hietaranta-Luoma HL, Tahvonen R, Iso-Touru T, Puolijoki H, Hopia A. An intervention study of individual, apoE genotype-based dietary and physical-activity advice: impact on health behavior. *J Nutrigenet Nutrigenomics* 7: 161–174, 2014.

81. Higgins S, Straight CR, Lewis RD. The effects of preexercise caffeinated coffee ingestion on endurance performance: an evidence-based review. *Int J Sport Nutr Exerc Metab* 26: 221–239, 2016.

82. Horne J, Madill J, O'Connor C, Shelley J, Gilliland J. A systematic review of genetic testing and lifestyle behaviour change: are we using high-quality genetic interventions and considering behaviour change theory? *Lifestyle Genom* 2018.

83. Horska A, Mislanova C, Bonassi S, Ceppi M, Volkovova K, Dusinska M. Vitamin C levels in blood are influenced by polymorphisms in glutathione S-transferases. *Eur J Nutr* 50: 437–446, 2011.

84. Howatson G, Van Someren KA. The prevention and treatment of exercise-induced muscle damage. *Sport Med* 38: 483–503, 2008.

85. Hunter AM, St Clair Gibson A, Collins M, Lambert M, Noakes TD. Caffeine ingestion does not alter performance during a 100-km cycling time-trial performance. *Int J Sport Nutr Exerc Metab* 12: 438–452, 2002.

86. Jenkins NT, Trilk JL, Singhal A, O'Connor PJ, Cureton KJ. Ergogenic effects of low doses of caffeine on cycling performance. *Int J Sport Nutr Exerc Metab* 18: 328–342, 2008.

87. Kanda K, Sugama K, Hayashida H, Sakuma J, Kawakami Y, Miura S, et al. Eccentric exercise-induced delayed-onset muscle soreness and changes in markers of muscle damage and inflammation. *Exerc Immunol Rev* 19:72–85, 2013.

88. Kicklighter JR, Dorner B, Hunter AM, Kyle M, Pflugh Prescott M, Roberts S, et al. Visioning report 2017: a preferred path forward for the nutrition and dietetics profession. *J Acad Nutr Diet* 117: 110–127, 2017.

89. Kikuchi N, Fuku N, Matsumoto R, Matsumoto S, Murakami H, Miyachi M, et al. The association between MCT1 T1470A polymorphism and power-oriented athletic performance. *Int J Sports Med* 38: 76–80, 2017.

90. King AJ, O'Hara JP, Arjomandkhah NC, Rowe J, Morrison DJ, Preston T, et al. Liver and muscle glycogen oxidation and performance with dose variation of glucose-fructose ingestion during prolonged (3 h) exercise. *Eur J Appl Physiol* 119: 1157–1169, 2019.

91. Kraus E, Tenforde AS, Nattiv A, Sainani KL, Kussman A, Deakins-Roche M, et al. Bone stress injuries in male distance runners: higher modified Female Athlete Triad Cumulative Risk Assessment scores predict increased rates of injury. *Br J Sports Med* 53: 237–242, 2019.

92. Lancha Junior AH, Painelli Vde S, Saunders B, Artioli GG. Nutritional strategies to modulate intracellular and extracellular buffering capacity during high-intensity exercise. *Sports Med* 45(Suppl 1): S71–81, 2015.

93. Latunde-Dada GO. Iron metabolism in athletes–achieving a gold standard. *Eur J Haematol* 90: 10–15, 2013.

94. Lewis PB, Ruby D, Bush-Joseph CA. Muscle soreness and delayed-onset muscle soreness. *Clin Sport Med* 31: 255–262, 2012.

95. Lieberman HR, Tharion WJ, Shukitt-Hale B, Speckman KL, Tulley R. Effects of caffeine, sleep loss, and stress on cognitive performance and mood during U.S. Navy SEAL training. Sea-Air-Land. *Psychopharmacology (Berl)* 164: 250–261, 2002.

96. Lietz G, Lange J, and Rimbach G. Molecular and dietary regulation of beta, beta-carotene 15,15'-monooxygenase 1 (BCMO1). *Arch Biochem Biophys* 502: 8–16, 2010.

97. Lietz G, Oxley A, Leung W, Hesketh J. Single nucleotide polymorphisms upstream from the beta-carotene 15,15'-monooxygenase gene influence provitamin a conversion efficiency in female volunteers. *J Nutr* 142: 161s–165s, 2012.

98. Livingstone KM, Celis-Morales C, Navas-Carretero S, San-Cristobal R, Macready AL, Fallaize R, et al. Effect of an Internet-based, personalized nutrition randomized trial on dietary changes associated with the Mediterranean diet: the Food4Me Study. *Am J Clin Nutr* 104: 288–297, 2016.

99. Lum JJ, Bui T, Gruber M, Gordan JD, DeBerardinis RJ, Covello KL, et al. The transcription factor HIF-1alpha plays a critical role in the growth factor-dependent regulation of both aerobic and anaerobic glycolysis. *Genes Dev* 21: 1037–1049, 2007.

100. Macutkiewicz D, Sunderland C. The use of GPS to evaluate activity profiles of elite women hockey players during match-play. *J Sports Sci* 29: 967–973, 2011.

101. Martinsson A, Andersson C, Andell P, Koul S, Engstrom G, Smith JG. Anemia in the general population: prevalence, clinical correlates and prognostic impact. *Eur J Epidemiol* 29: 489–498, 2014.

102. Massidda M, Mendez-Villanueva A, Gineviciene V, Proia P, Drozdovska SB, Dosenko V, et al. Association of monocarboxylate transporter-1 (MCT1) A1470T polymorphism (rs1049434) with forward football player status. *Int J Sports Med* 39: 1028–1034, 2018.

103. Mattei J, Qi Q, Hu FB, Sacks FM, Qi L. TCF7L2 genetic variants modulate the effect of dietary fat intake on changes in body composition during a weight-loss intervention. *Am J Clin Nutr* 96: 1129–1136, 2012.

104. Maughan RJ, Burke LM, Dvorak J, Larson-Meyer DE, Peeling P, Phillips SM, et al. IOC consensus statement: dietary supplements and the high-performance athlete. *Int J Sport Nutr Exerc Metab* 28: 104–125, 2018.

105. Maughan RJ, Depiesse F, Geyer H. The use of dietary supplements by athletes. *J Sports Sci* 25(Suppl 1): S103–113, 2007.

106. McNaughton LR, Lovell RJ, Siegler J, Midgley AW, Moore L, Bentley DJ. The effects of caffeine ingestion on time trial cycling performance. *Int J Sports Physiol Perform* 3: 157–163, 2008.

107. Merezhinskaya N, Fishbein WN, Davis JI, Foellmer JW. Mutations in MCT1 cDNA in patients with symptomatic deficiency in lactate transport. *Muscle Nerve* 23: 90–97, 2000.

108. Mountjoy M, Sundgot-Borgen J, Burke L, Carter S, Constantini N, Lebrun C, et al. The IOC consensus statement: beyond the Female Athlete Triad–Relative Energy Deficiency in Sport (RED-S). *Br J Sports Med* 48: 491–497, 2014.

109. Nielsen DE, El-Sohemy A. Disclosure of genetic information and change in dietary intake: a randomized controlled trial. *PLOS ONE* 9: e112665, 2014.

110. Nikolaidis MG, Kerksick CM, Lamprecht M, McAnulty SR. Does vitamin C and E supplementation impair the favorable adaptations of regular exercise? *Oxid Med Cell Longev* 2012: 707941, 2012.

111. Nose-Ogura S, Yoshino O, Dohi M, Kigawa M, Harada M, Hiraike O, et al. Risk factors of stress fractures due to the female athlete triad: differences in teens and twenties. *Scand J Med Sci Sports* 29: 1501–1510, 2019.

112. Palidis DJ, Wyder-Hodge PA, Fooken J, Spering M. Distinct eye movement patterns enhance dynamic visual acuity. *PLOS ONE* 12: e0172061, 2017.
113. Pasman WJ, van Baak MA, Jeukendrup AE, de Haan A. The effect of different dosages of caffeine on endurance performance time. *Int J Sports Med* 16: 225–230, 1995.
114. Pataky MW, Womack CJ, Saunders MJ, Goffe JL, D'Lugos AC, El-Sohemy A, et al. Caffeine and 3-km cycling performance: effects of mouth rinsing, genotype, and time of day. *Scand J Med Sci Sports* 26: 613–619, 2016.
115. Paton C, Costa V, Guglielmo L. Effects of caffeine chewing gum on race performance and physiology in male and female cyclists. *J Sports Sci* 33: 1076–1083, 2015.
116. Pedlar CR, Brugnara C, Bruinvels G, Burden R. Iron balance and iron supplementation for the female athlete: a practical approach. *Eur J Sport Sci* 18: 295–305, 2018.
117. Peternelj TT, Coombes JS. Antioxidant supplementation during exercise training: beneficial or detrimental? *Sports Med* 41: 1043–1069, 2011.
118. Pichler I, Minelli C, Sanna S, Tanaka T, Schwienbacher C, Naitza S, et al. Identification of a common variant in the TFR2 gene implicated in the physiological regulation of serum iron levels. *Hum Mol Genet* 20: 1232–1240, 2011.
119. Pilegaard H, Terzis G, Halestrap A, Juel C. Distribution of the lactate/H+ transporter isoforms MCT1 and MCT4 in human skeletal muscle. *Am J Physiol* 276: E843–848, 1999.
120. Piperno A, Galimberti S, Mariani R, Pelucchi S, Ravasi G, Lombardi C, et al. Modulation of hepcidin production during hypoxia-induced erythropoiesis in humans in vivo: data from the HIGHCARE project. *Blood* 117: 2953–2959, 2011.
121. Powers SK, Radak Z, Ji LL. Exercise-induced oxidative stress: past, present and future. *J Physiol* 594: 5081–5092, 2016.
122. Puente C, Abian-Vicen J, Del Coso J, Lara B, Salinero JJ. The CYP1A2 -163C>A polymorphism does not alter the effects of caffeine on basketball performance. *PLOS ONE* 13: e0195943, 2018.
123. Rahimi R. The effect of CYP1A2 genotype on the ergogenic properties of caffeine during resistance exercise: a randomized, double-blind, placebo-controlled, crossover study. *Ir J Med Sci* 188: 337–345, 2019.
124. Ravasi G, Pelucchi S, Buoli Comani G, Greni F, Mariani R, Pelloni I, et al. Hepcidin regulation in a mouse model of acute hypoxia. *Eur J Haematol* 100: 636–643, 2018.
125. Reid MB. Reactive oxygen species as agents of fatigue. *Med Sci Sports Exerc* 48: 2239–2246, 2016.
126. Roberts LA, Beattie K, Close GL, Morton JP. Vitamin C consumption does not impair training-induced improvements in exercise performance. *Int J Sports Physiol Perform* 6: 58–69, 2011.
127. Roelands B, Buyse L, Pauwels F, Delbeke F, Deventer K, Meeusen R. No effect of caffeine on exercise performance in high ambient temperature. *Eur J Appl Physiol* 111: 3089–3095, 2011.
128. Rogers PJ, Hohoff C, Heatherley SV, Mullings EL, Maxfield PJ, Evershed RP, et al. Association of the anxiogenic and alerting effects of caffeine with ADORA2A and ADORA1 polymorphisms and habitual level of caffeine consumption. *Neuropsychopharmacology* 35: 1973–1983, 2010.
129. Ruohola JP, Laaksi I, Ylikomi T, Haataja R, Mattila VM, Sahi T, et al. Association between serum 25(OH) D concentrations and bone stress fractures in Finnish young men. *J Bone Miner Res* 21: 1483–1488, 2006.
130. Rybak ME, Sternberg MR, Pao CI, Ahluwalia N, Pfeiffer CM. Urine excretion of caffeine and select caffeine metabolites is common in the U.S. population and associated with caffeine intake. *J Nutr* 145: 766–774, 2015.
131. Saunders B, de Oliveira LF, da Silva RP, de Salles Painelli V, Goncalves LS, Yamaguchi G, et al. Placebo in sports nutrition: a proof-of-principle study involving caffeine supplementation. *Scand J Med Sci Sports* 27: 1240–1247, 2017.
132. Sawczuk M, Banting LK, Cieszczyk P, Maciejewska-Karlowska A, Zarebska A, Leonska-Duniec A, et al. MCT1 A1470T: a novel polymorphism for sprint performance? *J Sci Med Sport* 18: 114–118, 2015.
133. Shaw G, Lee-Barthel A, Ross ML, Wang B, Baar K. Vitamin C-enriched gelatin supplementation before intermittent activity augments collagen synthesis. *Am J Clin Nutr* 105: 136–143, 2017.
134. Shen JG, Brooks MB, Cincotta J, Manjourides JD. Establishing a relationship between the effect of caffeine and duration of endurance athletic time trial events: A systematic review and meta-analysis. *J Sci Med Sport* 22: 232–238, 2019.
135. Siegler JC, Gleadall-Siddall DO. Sodium bicarbonate ingestion and repeated swim sprint performance. *J Strength Cond Res* 24: 3105–3111, 2010.
136. Sim M, Dawson B, Landers G, Trinder D, Peeling P. Iron regulation in athletes: exploring the menstrual cycle and effects of different exercise modalities on hepcidin production. *Int J Sport Nutr Exerc Metab* 24: 177–187, 2014.
137. Sim M, Garvican-Lewis LA, Cox GR, Govus A, McKay AKA, Stellingwerff T, et al. Iron considerations for the athlete: a narrative review. *Eur J Appl Physiol* 119: 1463–1478, 2019.

138. Skinner TL, Jenkins DG, Taaffe DR, Leveritt MD, Coombes JS. Coinciding exercise with peak serum caffeine does not improve cycling performance. *J Sci Med Sport* 16: 54–59, 2013.

139. Slater NA, Rager ML, Havrda DE, Harralson AF. Genetic variation in CYP2R1 and GC genes associated with vitamin D deficiency status. *J Pharm Pract* 30: 31–36, 2017.

140. Sousa M, Teixeira VH, Soares J. Dietary strategies to recover from exercise-induced muscle damage. *Int J Food Sci Nutr* 65: 151–163, 2014.

141. Spriet LL, MacLean DA, Dyck DJ, Hultman E, Cederblad G, Graham TE. Caffeine ingestion and muscle metabolism during prolonged exercise in humans. *Am J Physiol* 262: E891–898, 1992.

142. Spronk I, Heaney SE, Prvan T, O'Connor HT. Relationship between general nutrition knowledge and dietary quality in elite athletes. *Int J Sport Nutr Exerc Metab* 25: 243–251, 2015.

143. Taghiyar M, Darvishi L, Askari G, Feizi A, Hariri M, Mashhadi NS, et al. The effect of vitamin C and e supplementation on muscle damage and oxidative stress in female athletes: a clinical trial. *Int J Prev Med* 4: S16–23, 2013.

144. Thomas DT, Erdman KA, Burke LM. American college of sports medicine joint position statement. nutrition and athletic performance. *Med Sci Sports Exerc* 48: 543–568, 2016.

145. Vidal K, Robinson N, Ives SJ. Exercise performance and physiological responses: the potential role of redox imbalance. *Physiol Rep* 5(7):e13225, 2017.

146. Walsh NP, Gleeson M, Shephard RJ, Gleeson M, Woods JA, Bishop NC, et al. Position statement. Part one: Immune function and exercise. *Exerc Immunol Rev* 17: 6–63, 2011.

147. Wang TJ, Zhang F, Richards JB, Kestenbaum B, van Meurs JB, Berry D, et al. Common genetic determinants of vitamin D insufficiency: a genome-wide association study. *Lancet* 376: 180–188, 2010.

148. Wickham KA, Spriet LL. Administration of caffeine in alternate forms. *Sports Med* 48: 79–91, 2018.

149. Wiles JD, Coleman D, Tegerdine M, Swaine IL. The effects of caffeine ingestion on performance time, speed and power during a laboratory-based 1 km cycling time-trial. *J Sports Sci* 24: 1165–1171, 2006.

150. Wilkerson GB, Simpson KA, Clark RA. Assessment and training of visuomotor reaction time for football injury prevention. *J Sport Rehabil* 26: 26–34, 2017.

151. Womack CJ, Saunders MJ, Bechtel MK, Bolton DJ, Martin M, Luden ND, et al. The influence of a CYP1A2 polymorphism on the ergogenic effects of caffeine. *J Int Soc Sports Nutr* 9: 7, 2012.

152. Wu H, Kanatous SB, Thurmond FA, Gallardo T, Isotani E, Bassel-Duby R, et al. Regulation of mitochondrial biogenesis in skeletal muscle by CaMK. *Science* 296: 349–352, 2002.

153. Yang A, Palmer AA, de Wit H. Genetics of caffeine consumption and responses to caffeine. *Psychopharmacology (Berl)* 211: 245–257, 2010.

154. Yang N, MacArthur DG, Gulbin JP, Hahn AG, Beggs AH, Easteal S, et al. ACTN3 genotype is associated with human elite athletic performance. *Am J Hum Genet* 73: 627–631, 2003.

155. Yavari A, Javadi M, Mirmiran P, Bahadoran Z. Exercise-induced oxidative stress and dietary antioxidants. *Asian J Sport Med* 6(1):e24898, 2015.

SECTION IV

Exercise Biochemistry Relative to Health Through the Lifespan

Peter M. Tiidus

The last number of years have seen a tremendous increase in understanding and appreciation for the influence of exercise and physical activity on chronic and lifestyle-related diseases, ageing, and obesity. The positive effects of exercise have been firmly established for both the reduction in incidences and progression of chronic diseases such as cancers, cardiovascular conditions, type 2 diabetes, and osteoporosis. In addition, exercise has been demonstrated to improve the quality of health and life for individuals living with or being actively treated for these conditions.

The incidence and progression of childhood obesity, as well as the quality of life and functional capacity of those with childhood-onset type 1 diabetes, are also positively influenced by exercise and physical activity. Exercise has also been shown to have important positive influence on processes of ageing, longevity, and functional capacity of older adults. Physical activity plays a vital role in delaying ageing-related morbidity and is a likely factor in prolonging life. Exercise has a critically positive influence on mitochondrial function, vitality, and density in muscles, as well as other tissues, which contributes to many of these benefits, as well as being an important factor in influencing the progression of a number of other disease conditions.

This section deals specifically with important new understanding of how exercise influences the biochemistry of a number of chronic disease conditions, as well as ageing and some related c-morbidities such as osteoporosis as well as the propensity for obesity in children. This relatively new appreciation for the importance influence of regular exercise on disease incidence, severity, and progression and our growing understanding of the biochemical and cellular mechanisms involved in physiological adaptations to various forms of resistance, endurance, power, and movement-based exercise help to inform new therapeutic interventions and prophylactics for these diseases via exercise and lifestyle modifications. In addition, this research contributes significantly to understanding the basic science of such diseases and conditions, which can also inform investigations into other forms of treatments as well as pharmacological interventions. Understanding the biochemistry of exercise effects will also inform the efficacy of these treatments and how they contribute to improvements in individuals' quality of life in general as well as during active treatment.

The new and cutting-edge research outlined in the chapters in this section form a sound basis for understanding the complex and important biological effects of physical activity as preventive medicine as well as treatment for various diseases and other health-related issues, as well as enhanced-ageing related functionality and will prove to be a vital basis in moving forward with further research.

26

MITOCHONDRIAL DYSFUNCTION IN CHRONIC DISEASE

Christopher Newell, Heather Leduc-Pessah, Aneal Khan, and Jane Shearer

Introduction

Present in almost all eukaryotic cells, the mitochondrion is the organelle responsible for aerobic energy production via cellular respiration. Proper mitochondrial function is vital for metabolic homeostasis of the human body, whereas dysfunctional mitochondria, characterized by loss in the efficiency of the electron transport system and therefore a reduction in energy synthesis, has been linked to the ageing process (12) and a multitude of chronic disease states. These include neurodegenerative diseases (62), cardiovascular diseases (113), diabetes (112), cancers (109), musculoskeletal diseases (96), and gastrointestinal disorders (40), among others. Exercise is a well-known intervention proven to maintain mitochondrial function and density. This chapter highlights our current understanding of how mitochondria are affected by both exercise and chronic disease. There are also primary mitochondrial diseases that are a group of rare diseases which can be caused by mutations to either mitochondrial or nuclear DNA (mtDNA or nDNA) (106); however, these are beyond the scope of this chapter.

Mitochondrial Physiology

Anatomy of Mitochondria

The "bean-shaped" mitochondrion consist of outer and inner membranes made of proteins and phospholipid bilayers. The inner mitochondrial membrane (IMM) is folded into cristae which increase surface area, enabling increased capacity for energy production. The outer mitochondrial membrane (OMM) regulates the bidirectional movement of proteins, cellular signalling molecules, and metabolic intermediates. Between the IMM and OMM is the intermembrane space, whereas the innermost compartment surrounded by the IMM is called the matrix.

Inner Mitochondrial Membrane

Acting as a tight barrier to all ions and molecules from the matrix and intermembrane space, the IMM utilizes a proton gradient to drive ATP synthesis. Embedded in the IMM are a series of large enzyme complexes, which generate this proton gradient, collectively termed the electron transport system (ETS) (Figure 26.1). Once liberated from metabolic substrates, electrons are shuttled through the

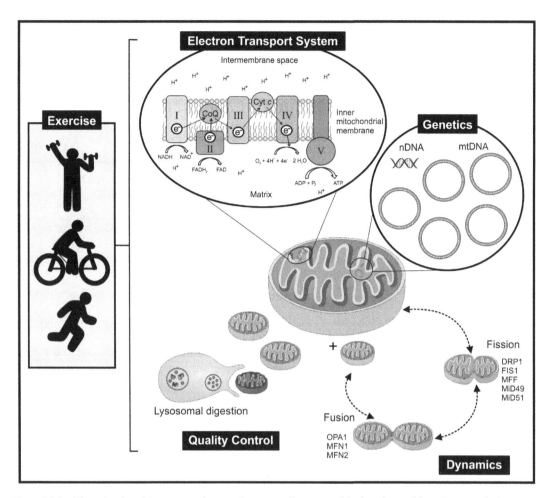

Figure 26.1 The mitochondria are a vastly complex organelle responsible for a host of functions regulating metabolic homeostasis

ETS via NADH dehydrogenase (Complex I) or succinate dehydrogenase (SDH; Complex II). Electrons are then carried by the mobile electron carrier ubiquinone (coenzyme Q or CoQ) to cytochrome *c* reductase (Complex III) before being transferred to cytochrome *c*, with cytochrome *c* oxidase (COX; Complex IV) eventually receiving the electrons. Complex IV enables O_2 to accumulate four electrons, which generates one molecule of H_2O. The drop in free energy that occurs drives proton pumping at Complexes I, III, and IV from the matrix into the mitochondrial intermembrane space. Complex II only transfers electrons to coenzyme Q and does not help generate the proton gradient. The proton redistribution established by mitochondrial respiration maintains and modulates the IMM proton gradient, which drives the formation of ATP via mitochondrial ATP synthase (Complex V). Interestingly, the organization of mitochondrial cristae is tightly linked to the location of ETS enzyme complexes embedded in the IMM (64).

Apart from ATP generation, the IMM is responsible for several other functions, including movement of ATP across the IMM via ADP/ATP translocase proteins (66), migration of proteins into the matrix through a translocase of the inner membrane (TIM) protein complexes (34), and transport of fatty acids into the mitochondrial matrix via carnitine acyltransferase (CAT) enzymes (9). In functional mitochondria, ATP synthase is arranged in a dimer at the hairpin of a cristae, while the cristae lumen is lined by ETS enzymes in supercomplexes (64). However, the cristae flatten with age, resulting in impaired ETS supercomplex activity, decreased ATP synthase activity, and culminate in IMM rupture and apoptosis (64). Contrarily, exercise has been shown to alter the fine structure of mitochondria resulting in increased mass and improved function (143).

Outer Mitochondrial Membrane

Separating the intermembrane space from the cytosol, the OMM is responsible for the exchange of information between the mitochondria and the cell. Embedded in the OMM are large numbers of voltage-dependent anion channel (VDAC) proteins, which regulate metabolic and energetic flux across the OMM (15). VDAC proteins maintain metabolic homeostasis by shuttling ATP, ADP, metabolites, and various enzymes, including creatine kinase and hexokinase, across the OMM (15). Larger proteins migrating from the cytosol into the mitochondria must enter through a translocase of the outer membrane (TOM) protein complex (57). In dysfunctional mitochondria, VDAC proteins play an important role in apoptosis through OMM permeabilization and release of cytochrome c (41). Specific to regulation of calcium signalling, the OMM is known to share structures with the endoplasmic reticulum (ER). The mitochondria-associated membranes (MAMs) are connections between the mitochondria and ER, which act as a signalling and metabolic interface (14, 26). In functional mitochondria, the MAMs maintain calcium homeostasis, lipid synthesis, and mitochondrial biogenesis (136). However, various stress response signals released by either the ER or dysfunctional mitochondria can initiate OMM permeabilization and apoptosis (136).

Mitochondrial Intermembrane Space

The intermembrane space is separated from the cytosol by the OMM, a permeable membrane to small molecules. The composition of ions is therefore the same between the cytosol and intermembrane space; however, larger proteins require transport across the OMM. The most studied component of the intermembrane space is the single electron carrier cytochrome c. Responsible for shuttling an electron between ETS Complexes III and IV, cytochrome c plays an integral role in maintaining oxidative capacity and has been identified as a reactive oxygen species (ROS) scavenger in functional mitochondria (52). Contrarily, the release of cytochrome c into the cytosol caused by dysfunctional mitochondria and permeabilization of the mitochondria is one of the most well-studied components of the apoptotic cascade (52).

Mitochondrial Matrix

As the innermost aspect of the mitochondria, the matrix contains the mitochondria's DNA, ribosomes, and many enzymes responsible for oxidative metabolism. Carbohydrates and amino acids enter the mitochondrial matrix, where the tricarboxylic acid (TCA) cycle occurs. The carbon-based derivatives of carbohydrates and amino acids are oxidized in the TCA cycle to generate the reducing equivalents nicotinamide adenine dinucleotide (NADH) and flavin adenine dinucleotide (FADH$_2$), biochemical redox cofactors capable of shuttling electrons to the ETS. Fats are also oxidized in the matrix, in a process termed β-oxidation. As a by-product of ATP production via ETS chemistry, mitochondria are responsible for generating ROS and reactive nitrogen species (92). Typically associated with mitochondrial dysfunction (73, 100), disease pathogenesis (102), and ageing (48), mitochondrial ROS are also a part of normal cellular signalling and the regulation of cellular communication machinery

(129). ROS are produced within the mitochondrial matrix when single electrons leak across the ETS to generate superoxide anions (O_2^-) (32). These superoxide anions are then either sequestered by anti-oxidant enzymes or cause damage to surrounding tissues, which may enable production of further reactive species.

Mitochondrial Genetics

Mitochondrial DNA

Adding to their complexity, mitochondria are under dual genetic control from both nDNA and mtDNA (Figure 26.1). nDNA encodes most of the eukaryotic genome and is contained in the cellular nucleus. Most proteins which comprise the mitochondria are encoded by nDNA and imported into the mitochondrion, with the remaining components being mtDNA derived (87). Fully identified in 1981, human mtDNA consists of a circular, double-stranded series of 16,596 DNA base pairs (3). Furthermore, mtDNA differs from nDNA by lacking non-coding introns (126), lacking histones for DNA packaging (1), is exclusively maternally inherited (148), and relies on a single enzyme for replication (DNA polymerase subunit gamma; POLG) (124). Although mtDNA lacks histones, mitochondrial transcription factor A (TFAM) is responsible for a protein–DNA complex which coats and packages mtDNA (94). mtDNA is structured as an outer ring of guanine-rich base pairs called the heavy (H) strand, which surrounds an inner ring of cytosine-rich base pairs called the light (L) strand. Lacking introns, mtDNA contains only a small section of non-coding base pairs. This region on the H-strand, named the D-loop, is 1.2 kb in length and contains one of the proposed replication origins for mtDNA replication (O_H), with the other replication origin being located on the L-strand (O_L) (133). Although the exact mechanism for mtDNA replication remains up for debate, the conventional theory follows a traditional leading-lagging strand mechanism. In this case, replication leads at the O_H origin, with the O_L lagging strand synthesis commencing shortly thereafter (144). The lagging strand is created in short Okazaki-like fragments, which are ultimately converted to DNA (144). This intricate replication complex includes the Twinkle helicase—which separates the two mtDNA strands, the mitochondrial single-stranded DNA binding protein—which stabilizes the unwound mtDNA, and the mtDNA replicating enzyme polymerase POLG (147).

mtDNA encodes for a total of 37 genes and several mitochondrially derived peptides, including the cytoprotective agent humanin (69) and the metabolic homeostasis regulator MOTS-c (70). Initially transcribed in the mitochondria, MOTS-c is then translated in the cytosol and regulates nuclear gene expression in response to metabolic stressors. These data indicate that nuclear and mitochondrial genomes regulate one another and this route of communication is genetically integrated (61). The 37 genes result in 13 proteins of the ETS, 2 ribosomal RNAs, and 22 transfer RNAs (8). The 13 ETS proteins correspond to Complexes I, III, IV, and V with the remaining ~70 proteins, including the entirety of Complex II, being encoded by nDNA and imported into the mitochondria for assembly. Transcription of mtDNA is controlled by a series of three promoters, heat shock proteins 1 and 2 (HSP1 and HSP2) which are found on the H-strand, and LSP which is found on the L-strand (7). LSP is responsible for transcribing the entire L-strand, and HSP2 transcribes nearly all the H-strand; HSP1 only transcribes for the two ribosomal RNA molecules. Although currently being debated, TFAM has been studied as another key contributor to mtDNA transcription. As the main factor responsible for packaging mtDNA into nucleoprotein complexes, TFAM also binds to mtDNA upstream of the three mtDNA promoters causing a bend in mtDNA, which may be vital for proper positioning of mtDNA transcription machinery (65, 120). Finally, the translation of mtDNA is the least understood maintenance process. Known to involve the importation of nDNA encoded factors (133), several elongation factors (72), a termination factor (142), and other molecular pieces, the mechanism is still poorly understood.

Mitochondrial Dynamics

Mitochondrial Fission and Fusion

Originally thought of as merely bean-shaped organelles, recent research has determined that mitochondria are actually highly dynamic (90, 95), continuously joining through the process of fusion and dividing through the process of fission (5) (Figure 26.1). The machinery responsible for fission and fusion processes dictate mitochondrial size and shape, and is tightly regulated alongside cellular signalling and stress response pathways (51). During steady state, there is a delicate balance between fission and fusion to maintain ATP production and optimal membrane potential of the mitochondrial population (27). However, unbalanced fission leads to mitochondrial fragmentation, and unbalanced fusion leads to mitochondrial elongation (18). Excessive fission has been linked to decreased ATP production, an increase in mitochondrial degradation (mitophagy), and a decrease in membrane potential (138)—collectively representing a "bad" mitochondrial phenotype. Conversely, excessive fusion has been shown to increase ATP production and inhibit mitophagy (134)—collectively representing a "good" mitochondrial phenotype. The impact of the imbalance in fission and fusion on chronic disease will be discussed in subsequent sections of this chapter.

Initially discovered in yeast, human homologues to the main components of both mitochondrial fission and fusion machinery have been identified along with their underlying mechanisms of action. In eukaryotes, mitochondrial fission is regulated by the proteins dynamin-related protein (DRP1), mitochondrial fission 1 protein (FIS1), mitochondrial fission factor (MFF), and mitochondrial dynamics proteins of 49 (MiD49) and 51 kDa (MiD51). Mitochondrial fusion is primarily regulated by the proteins mitofusin 1 (MFN1), mitofusin 2 (MFN2), and optic atrophy 1 (OPA1) (51). Fission involves the recruitment of the GTPase enzyme DRP1 from the cytosol to the OMM by MFF, FIS1, MiD49, and MiD51 (82). This recruitment stimulates DRP1 to form a helical assembly along the surface of the mitochondria and begins with constriction and culminates with the ultimate division of the mitochondria into two smaller, functional mitochondria (39). Research has also identified that the ER may have direct involvement in initiating fission by extending tubules which constrict the mitochondria prior to the recruitment of DRP1 (38). These ER tubules are extensions of the ER which wrap around neighbouring mitochondria and initiate a fission event.

In contrast to the work in yeast, DRP1 recruitment in mammals is achieved by MFF, MiD49, and MiD51, while FIS1 apparently plays only a minor role in the fission process (75). Fusion similarly requires the use of GTP hydrolyzing enzymes; however, this is a two-step process requiring cooperating enzymes on both the IMM and OMM. MFN1 and MFN2 reside on the OMM and are responsible for mediating OMM fusion (20). Existing in two isoforms (long and short), OPA1 is responsible for fusion of the IMM (122).

Exercise is a metabolically demanding process in which excessive stress is imparted on our cells to generate adequate energy to contract our skeletal musculature. Therefore, it is not surprising that exercise affects the mitochondrial fission and fusion processes. Early transmission electron microscopy showed that exercise altered mitochondrial morphology and caused increased mitochondrial mass and connectivity (60). Following discovery of the proteins responsible for mitochondrial fission and fusion, research identified that exercise increases both gene and protein expression of several fission and fusion mediators after as little as one exercise bout (17, 104, 132). Although there have been many studies investigating the impact of exercise on mitochondrial fission and fusion, the current consensus shows that long-term exercise training increases the expression of fusion proteins (132).

Mitochondrial Transport

Cells are constantly fine-tuning their energy requirements, namely during bouts of exercise. To generate enough ATP for each cell, mitochondria must be appropriately distributed throughout the cell.

Cytoskeleton components form a series of microtubule filaments using α- and β-tubulin subunits which act as a platform for mitochondrial transport (82). Heavily characterized in neuronal cultures (140), actin and intermediate filaments aid in the cytoskeletal distribution of mitochondria. Movement of the mitochondria is achieved through the attachment of motor proteins to the microtubule filaments (63). Kinesin motor proteins move the mitochondria in the anterograde (+) direction, while dynein motor proteins move mitochondria in the retrograde (-) direction (107). The connection between mitochondria and the aforementioned motor proteins is accomplished through the mitochondrial motor/adaptor complex (119). At this junction, kinesin/dynein motor proteins attach to the adaptor protein Milton, which then attaches to mitochondrial Rho GTPases 1 and 2 (MIRO1/2) on the OMM (119).

Mitochondrial Biogenesis

Representing the relationship between bioenergetic requirements and capacity, mitochondrial biogenesis is the process by which cells increase their number of mitochondria. An increase in mitochondrial self-replication is typically seen in response to elevated energy expenditure of the cell, requiring greater ATP output relative to baseline (118). Classically researchers have studied endurance exercise training as a means of inducing mitochondrial biogenesis. Although the mitochondria possesses its own genome (mtDNA), the vast majority of mitochondrial proteins are nuclear encoded and must therefore be targeted to and imported into the mitochondria (29, 83). All proteins migrating from the cytosol to the compartments of the mitochondria must enter through a TOM protein complex (57). Depending on their fate, migrating proteins may then further enter the matrix through a TIM protein complex or be integrated into a preceding mitochondrial compartment (34).

As the primary coactivator responsible for regulation of mitochondrial biogenesis, peroxisome proliferator-activated receptor-γ coactivator 1-α (PGC-1α) acts by regulating mitochondrial protein translation in response to energy balance fluctuations (23). PGC-1α is responsible for co-activating nuclear respiratory factor 2 (NRF2). Alongside NRF2, PGC-1α can then activate nuclear respiratory factor 1 (NRF1), which activates TFAM, a key activator of mitochondrial transcription within the nucleus (105) and regulator of mtDNA replication (35). Collectively, NRF1, NRF2, and TFAM ultimately enable regulation of nuclear encoded mitochondrial proteins in response to mitochondrial biogenesis, while also promoting mtDNA up-regulation to match increases in mitochondrial mass (53).

Responsible for regulating mitochondrial biogenesis, numerous studies have demonstrated a link between PGC-1α and exercise. Now accepted as dogma, both endurance and resistance exercise training have been shown to increase PGC-1α expression (50, 143). Furthermore, research investigating the impact of short exercise programmes have demonstrated that even single bouts of exercise increase PGC-1α expression in skeletal muscle, with markers of mitochondrial biogenesis being detected after three exercise bouts (104). This research also indicates that PGC-1α expression returns to baseline levels after each exercise bout, which suggests that PGC-1α senses the functional demands of exercise and responds accordingly by adjusting metabolic homeostasis. Interestingly, the influence of single exercise bouts on PGC-1α also results in an increased interaction of PGC-1α with TFAM and NRF1. This identifies that exercise both up-regulates the expression of PGC-1α and induces the translocation of PGC-1α to nuclear and mitochondrial transcription factors in order to stimulate biogenesis (116).

Mitochondrial Quality Control

Mitophagy

Mitochondrial maintenance also requires strict quality control. This process is facilitated by the marked localization of mitochondria to autophagosomes, followed by their lysosomal-dependent degradation (146) (Figure 26.1). This form of autophagy is activated in response to mitochondrial damage or excessive cellular stress. Specifically, mitophagy enables the high number of mitochondria present within each cell to be regulated in a selective process which marks specified mitochondria for breakdown (149). Potentially providing a quality control mechanism for recycling damaged mitochondria and mtDNA, the clinical efficiency of this process is still unknown, since several primary mitochondrial diseases are a result of accumulated mitochondrial dysfunction or mtDNA damage (138).

Several mitophagy pathways have been identified in mammals, with the PTEN-induced putative kinase 1 (PINK1)/Parkin pathway being the best characterized (22). In properly functioning mitochondria PINK1 is recruited to the OMM and imported into the mitochondria through a TOM protein complex. PINK1 is then cleaved and further translocated through a TIM protein complex and into the matrix where proteases can degrade PINK1 and maintain homeostasis (95). However, dysfunctional mitochondria are associated with depolarization across the IMM, which results in the inability of PINK1 to be successfully cleaved and imported through the TIM protein complex. PINK1 then accumulates on the OMM, and Parkin is recruited to the OMM in a PINK1-dependent manner (95). Parkin, a E3 ubiquitin ligase, is then able to ubiquitinate the OMM and facilitate lysosomal degradation of mitochondria by localizing microtubule-associated protein 1A/1B-light chain 3 to the outer mitochondrial membrane (111). Another commonly studied mitophagy pathway involves the BCL2/adenovirus E1B 19 kd-interacting protein 3 (BNIP3) receptor (91, 93). BNIP3 is an OMM localized mitophagy receptor which migrates to the OMM under conditions of cell stress (42). Following movement to the OMM, BNIP3 initiates binding with microtubule-associated protein 1A/1B-light chain 3, which is a potent recruitment molecule for autophagosomes, ultimately resulting in lysosomal mitophagy (127).

Critical to maintain skeletal muscle function, a functional mitochondrial population requires the removal of dysfunctional mitochondria via mitophagy. Only recently explored, research has identified that endurance exercise training is responsible for inducing mitophagy through increases in BNIP3 (74). Upstream from BNIP3 localization, these skeletal muscle mitophagy events seem to be linked to activation of 5' adenosine monophosphate–activated protein kinase (AMPK) and unc-51 like autophagy activating kinase 1 (ULK1) (68). In response to acute bouts of exercise, AMPK is responsible for the phosphorylation of ULK1, which culminates in mitophagy events. Further research has demonstrated that the AMPK-ULK1 mitophagy cascade occurs independently of PINK1 stabilization (30), although Parkin may be involved in exercise-induced mitophagy (19).

Mitochondrial Dysfunction: Potential Role in Ageing and Chronic Disease

Mitochondria and Ageing

The free-radical theory of ageing implies that humans age due to a build-up of free radical damage. Initially postulated in the 1950s (46), this theory was further developed in the early 1970s to highlight mitochondrial derived ROS as a primary contributor (47). Since this time, several studies have provided evidence of mitochondrial involvement in the ageing process.

As previously described, H_2O_2 and other peroxides are major contributors to ROS oxidative damage, which are sequestered by protective mitochondrial enzymes. However, the efficiency of these protective enzymes is not perfect, resulting in the gradual accumulation of ROS within cells. Over time, an accumulation of ROS can cause impairments in cellular function by creating a positive feedback loop of further ETS machinery damage, resulting in greater ROS generation (21)—this process is exacerbated with age. Of note, ROS damage appears to be more pronounced in tissues with a greater reliance on oxidative metabolism for ATP generation, such as the brain (117). Several neurological disease states have been shown to involve an accumulation of ROS as a hallmark phenotype (135). Ultimately resulting in widespread apoptosis, the clinical involvement of mitochondria in ageing showcases their importance in disease pathophysiology.

Relevant to ageing, exercise and physical activity induce oxidative stress in various tissues. It is now recognized that this stress is essential to mediating adaptive responses of tissues to exercise and is protective in mitigating ageing-induced declines in mitochondrial function. Essentially, exercise exposure improves resistance to cellular stress by increasing functional reserves and promoting mitochondrial health through biogenesis, enhancing mitochondrial turnover and the removal of damaged mitochondria (97).

Mitochondrial-Mediated Apoptosis

Apoptosis, or programmed cell death, is the process of cell turnover in a controlled manner. In mitochondrial-mediated necrotic cell death, the mitochondrial permeability transition pore (MPTP) initiates mitochondrial membrane permeabilization (67). The prolonged release of calcium, ROS, and other stimuli lead to MPTP opening and eventual mitochondrial membrane permeabilization, which results in cell rupture from a lack of cell membrane integrity (67). Differing from necrosis, apoptosis involves characteristic morphologic changes which culminate in the formation of apoptotic bodies – budding cellular fragments consisting of cytoplasm with tightly packed organelles which may contain a nuclear fragment (36). These apoptotic bodies are then targeted for breakdown by phagocytotic cells in the absence of further damaging responses to the neighbouring cellular populations (139). Characterized into intrinsic or extrinsic pathways, intrinsic refers to apoptosis activation by intracellular signals and protein release from the mitochondrial intermembrane space, while extrinsic refers to the role of extracellular ligands inducing apoptosis (36). Acting in response to mtDNA damage, metabolic stress accumulation, nDNA damage, and other cellular cues, the intrinsic apoptotic pathway can be initiated by permeabilization of the OMM. Associated with dissipation of mitochondrial membrane potential, pores in the OMM enable pro-apoptotic mediators to leak out (43). These pores are created by oligomerization of voltage-dependent anion channel 1 (VDAC1), the most abundant mitochondrial OMM protein (15). VDAC1 helps to regulate apoptosis through interaction with the pro-apoptotic Bcl-2 family of proteins and the anti-apoptotic hexokinase enzyme (15).

Hexokinase is an enzyme responsible for glycolysis initiation. As an anti-apoptotic mediator, VDAC1 enables hexokinase to bind to the OMM and access ATP for the generation of a concentration gradient that drives glycolysis (15). This mechanism is up-regulated in many malignant cancer cell lines, thus enabling sustained cell growth—the basis of the Warburg effect. Under conditions facilitating apoptosis, VDAC1 is hypothesized to interact with the monomeric cytosolic protein BAX and the OMM localized protein BAK (141). The BH3:groove model suggests that upstream regulation by BH3 and Bcl-2 proteins initiates a signalling cascade, which enables BAX to migrate to the OMM (141). Following migration of BAX to the OMM, BAX or BAK are able to self- or hetero-oligomerize, which results in mitochondrial permeabilization through formation of large oligomeric pore complexes (28). Interestingly, it is also proposed that the same protein grooves responsible for BAX and BAK apoptotic signalling may also be the site of pro-survival proteins which inhibit the oligomerization process from occurring (28). The formation of these mitochondrial pores enables cytochrome *c* to be released into the cytosol as a pro-apoptotic signalling molecule. Once released, cytochrome *c* cleaves and activates caspase 9, which perpetuates the apoptosis cascade and results in cell death (55).

The extrinsic apoptotic pathway is hypothesized to commence in response to activated macrophage release of the cytokine tumour necrosis factor-alpha (TNF-alpha) and the binding of the transmembrane protein First apoptosis signal (Fas) receptor to the Fas ligand (FasL) (36). Although this pathway is initiated outside the mitochondria, there are links to the intrinsic pathway. Specifically, binding of Fas and FasL results in release of caspases 8 and 10, which initiates extrinsic independent apoptosis in certain cells, termed type I cells (103). However, type II cells, including human hepatocytes, utilize mitochondrial-dependent apoptosis following Fas/FasL binding (103). While aspects of the connection between the intrinsic and extrinsic apoptotic pathways remains to be studied, there is no doubt that certain cell types require unique pathway variations.

Pathology of Dysfunctional Mitochondria

Tissues with high metabolic demands are abundant with mitochondria, such as cardiac muscle, skeletal muscle, the brain, and liver (37). In general, properly functioning mitochondrial oxidative machinery results in adequate metabolic function, and mitochondrial dysfunction can result in disease pathology (14, 88, 106). Furthermore, due to the widespread involvement of mitochondria in every major organ system, the accumulation of damaged or dysfunctional mitochondria can lead to varied disease phenotypes. The high susceptibility for mtDNA to accumulate mutations and damage results in significant clinical implications for organ systems affected.

Cell division, oxidative stress (mitochondrial ROS accumulations), metabolism (energy synthesis), and various disease states are all affected by unbalanced mitochondrial dynamics (51). In circumstances of mitochondrial dysfunction, functional and dysfunctional mitochondria may fuse in order to dilute the effect of the dysfunctional mitochondrial population on ETS machinery and therefore generate a sufficient quantity of ATP (5). Imbalances in the fission/fusion machinery of dysfunctional mitochondria can also result in excessive proliferation and resistance to apoptosis (5). Changing from a fission to fusion morphology prevents appropriate cell signalling and cell-mediated apoptosis machinery from identifying mutated mitochondria, therefore enabling the spread of the mutation (27).

Contributing to the body of literature examining mitochondrial dysfunction in disease, examination of aberrant mitochondrial dynamics has enabled further characterization of disease phenotypes. Although the link between human disease and mitochondrial dynamics is in its infancy, several diseases, including neuropathic, neurodegenerative, cardiovascular, musculoskeletal, gastrointestinal, endocrine, and cancers, have been implicated (5) (Figure 26.2, Table 26.1). As a front-line intervention for the prevention and treatment of many chronic diseases, the following paragraphs will also showcase evidence supporting exercise as a therapeutic modality in diseases which mitochondrial dysfunction is implicated.

Neurodegenerative Disease

Parkinson disease (PD) (24), Huntington disease (HD) (121), and Alzheimer disease (AD) (76) have all been linked to varying degrees of mitochondrial dysfunction, including excessive fission, impaired energy synthesis, and increased apoptotic signalling. PD is one of the most strongly associated neurodegenerative diseases with a mitochondrial fission abnormality. In the clinical setting patients often present with a parkinsonian syndrome, which includes bradykinesia, a resting tremor, rigidity, and gait disturbances (78). HD follows an autosomal dominant inheritance pattern and is caused by >40 CAG repeats in the Huntington gene (16). Patients with HD commonly present with chorea, altered mood, and altered cognition due to the neurodegeneration of the basal ganglia. Like PD, the neurodegeneration in HD is thought to be linked to neuronal apoptosis by abnormal calcium homeostasis, increased ROS production, and persistent mitochondrial fission morphology (56). Lastly, AD is a neurodegenerative disease involving destruction of cholinergic neurons (101). Mainly affecting cortical structures, AD is the most common cause of dementia. Analysis of tissues from AD patients has identified hypometabolism, decreased mitochondrial enzyme activities, and impaired mitochondrial transport in affected brain regions, implicating mitochondrial dysfunction in the pathogenesis of AD (101).

Physical exercise has long been associated with protection against acquired neurodegenerative disease (150). Those with high cardiovascular fitness have lower dementia risk and attenuated cognitive impairments compared to their sedentary counterparts. The mechanism(s) underlying this protection are diverse and include exercise-mediated blood-borne molecules such as BDNF (128), enhanced brain blood flow, and cerebrovascular reserve (25), as well as signalling and cellular adaptations (10). One such cellular adaptation involves the modulation of mitochondrial networks, function, and resilience wherein exercise-adapted mitochondria have a greater ability to counter insults such as oxidative stress (77). Beyond prevention, exercise is also an effective non-pharmacological strategy in the management of patients with neurodegenerative disorders.

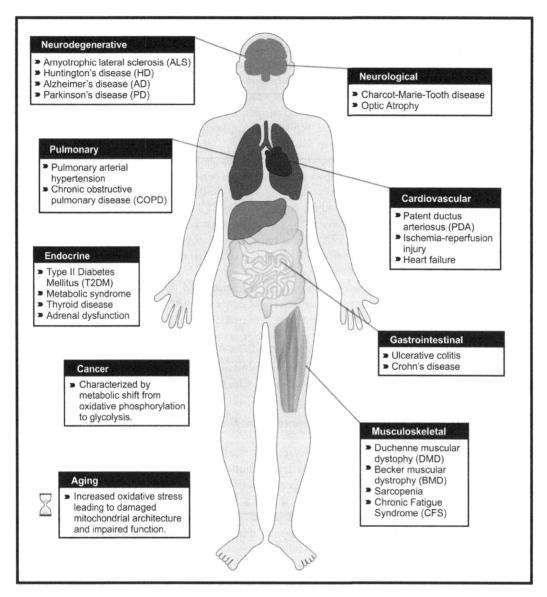

Figure 26.2 Mitochondrial dysfunction is implicated in a multitude of chronic diseases

Cardiovascular System

As an organ with high metabolism, the heart is known to contain large amounts of mitochondria. A down-regulation of genes involved with maintaining ETS machinery, as well as a decreased surface area of cristae, have been identified in heart failure patients and may contribute to decreased ATP production (113). Both pathologic and exercise-induced animal models of cardiac hypertrophy have confirmed a marked increase in mitochondrial biogenesis proportional to the change in heart size. In humans, patients with severe heart failure (NYHA Class IV) have decreased mitochondrial density (130), while patients with less severe heart failure (NYHA Class II) have minimal changes to mitochondrial density (citrate synthase) and minimal changes to mitochondrial activity (oxidative metabolism measurements) (31). Clinical research has also indicated that improvements in proxy measures of mitochondrial

Table 26.1 Mitochondrial abnormalities associated with chronic diseases

Ageing	Free-radical theory	Chen et al., 2003b
	↑ ROS production	
	↓ oxidative capacity	
Alzheimer disease	Generalized mitochondrial dysfunction	Manczak et al., 2012
(AD)	↓ oxidative capacity	Onyango et al., 2016
	Impaired mitochondrial transport	
Amyotrophic lateral	↑ mitochondrial fission	Smith et al., 2017
sclerosis (ALS)	↓ oxidative capacity	
	Impaired mitochondrial transport	
	Neuronal excitotoxicity	
Cancer	Metabolic shift from oxidative metabolism to glycolysis	Archer, 2013
	↑ mitochondrial fission	Rehman et al., 2012
	Inhibition of apoptosis	Porporato et al., 2018
Charcot–Marie–Tooth	↓ mitochondrial fusion	Archer, 2013
disease type 2A	Autosomal dominant missense mutation to *MFN2*	
Chronic fatigue	Generalized mitochondrial dysfunction	Myhill et al., 2009
syndrome (CFS)		
Chronic obstructive	↓ oxidative capacity	Meyer et al., 2013
pulmonary disease	↑ ROS production	
(COPD)	↓ mitochondrial biogenesis	
Heart failure	↓ oxidative capacity	Rosca et al., 2013
	↓ mitochondrial density	Toth et al., 2012
	↓ cristae surface area	Drexler et al., 1992
Huntington disease	↑ oxidative damage and ↑ mitochondrial fission	Song et al., 2011
(HD)	↑ ROS production and abnormal calcium homeostasis	Jodeiri et al., 2017
	cause neurodegeneration	
	Autosomal dominant CAG repeats in Huntington gene	
Inflammatory bowel	↑ ROS production	Guo et al., 2015
disease (IBD)	↑ mitochondrial fission	Novak et al., 2015
	↓ oxidative capacity	
	↓ cristae surface area	
Metabolic syndrome	↑ ROS production	Mitchell et al., 2012
	↓ oxidative capacity	
Muscular dystrophy	↑ mitochondrial-dependent apoptosis	Millay et al., 2008
	X-linked mutations in dystrophin	Kelly-Worden et al., 2014
Optic atrophy	↑ mitochondrial fission	Lenears et al., 2012
	Autosomal dominant mutation to *OPA1*	
Parkinson disease	↑ mitochondrial fission	Dagda et al., 2009
(PD)	Complex I deficiency	Bose et al., 2016
	Dopaminergic neurodegeneration	
	Autosomal recessive mutations in Parkin	
Patent ductus	↓ mitochondrial fission	Stoller et al., 2012
arteriosus (PDA)		Archer et al., 2004
Pulmonary arterial	↑ mitochondrial fission	Ryan et al., 2015
hypertension	Up-regulation of *DRP1* and down-regulation of *MFN2*	
Sarcopenia	↑ mitochondrial-dependent apoptosis	Alway et al., 2017
Thyroid disease and	Generalized mitochondrial dysfunction	Duarte et al., 2012
adrenal dysfunction	Loss of *MFN2* impairs steroid biosynthesis	Harper and Seifert, 2008
Type 2 diabetes	↑ mitochondrial fission	Rovira-Llopis et al.,
(T2DM)	↑ ROS production	2017
	Down-regulation of *MFN2* promotes fission morphology	Archer, 2013
	Metformin inhibits *DRP1*-mediated mitochondrial fission	Li et al., 2016

metabolism, namely peak oxygen consumption, lower the risk of cardiovascular mortality and all-cause mortality following a 3-month aerobic exercise programme (125). These data provide strong evidence that exercise training undoubtedly confers benefits to cardiovascular mitochondrial function, albeit, the duration and type of exercise training to confer said benefits require further investigation. Conversely, mitochondria have been found to contribute to physiological processes of the heart, such as closure of the patent ductus arteriosus (PDA) at birth, a cardiac shunt present in foetal circulation, has been linked to appropriate mitochondrial function. Acting as an oxygen sensor, smooth muscle cells may undergo a redox reaction to associated ROS signalling soon after birth in order to trigger alterations in vascular tone culminating in closure of the PDA (123). Through inhibition of mitochondrial fission this cascade can be inhibited in an ex vivo model, thus involving mitochondrial dynamics in pathologic cases involving PDA patency (6).

Respiratory System

Pulmonary arterial hypertension (PAH) is an idiopathic condition caused by vascular obstruction to the small pulmonary vessels. The clinical presentation of PAH is variable, although common symptoms include dyspnoea, lethargy, and fatigue. Biochemical and metabolic analyses of the smooth muscle cells in the arteries of PAH have demonstrated abnormal mitochondrial dynamics and oxygen sensing. Specifically, up-regulation of fission mediators, namely *DRP1*, and down-regulation of fusion mediators, namely *MFN2*, have resulted in a predominantly fission mitochondrial morphology (115). Given that, like heart failure, PAH is characterized by dyspnoea, fatigue, and exercise intolerance, clinical research has also investigated the role of exercise training to augment these clinical features. Notably, clinical data suggest that exercise training may improve survival and quality of life in patients with PAH when combined with standard medical therapy (44). Interestingly, analysis of the vastus lateralis and tibialis anterior muscles of patients with chronic obstructive pulmonary disease (COPD) has identified links to impairments in mitochondrial respiration, increased ROS production, and decreased mitochondrial biogenesis (79). As a common complication of COPD and prognostic factor, skeletal muscle dysfunction contributes to many of the symptoms such as dyspnoea, exercise intolerance, and fatigue. Furthermore, identification of mitochondrial dysfunction in skeletal muscle of COPD patients may provide a therapeutic target to delay progression (79). Although a paucity of research currently exists, possibly due to difficulties in compliance of exercise training programmes for patients with COPD, the efficacy of exercise training on localized muscle groups of COPD patients has been demonstrated (13). Interestingly, these data suggest that high-intensity exercise training of targeted muscle groups, as opposed to whole-body training, may restore skeletal muscle function in patients with COPD (13). Although this concept requires further investigation, these results also demonstrate the importance of personalized or disease-specific exercise training modules to accomplish the desired improvements in skeletal muscle function.

Musculoskeletal System

Myopathy is a hallmark of many primary mitochondrial diseases, although these are outside the scope of this current chapter. Apart from primary mitochondrial disease, mitochondrial dysfunction has been characterized in muscular dystrophy (59). Although many forms of muscular dystrophy exist, Duchenne (DMD) and Becker (BMD) muscular dystrophies are the most commonly studied and most severe forms. Caused by X-linked mutations to the dystrophin gene, DMD and BMD clinically present with progressive muscle weakness and fatigue. The dystrophin protein is a vital component in myofibril contractility and membrane stability. Dysfunctional dystrophin ultimately leads to porosity of the myofibril membranes, which permits calcium dysregulation and culminates in calcium overload of the mitochondria. Although not fully elucidated, existing animal research has implicated mitochondrial-dependent necrosis as a disease mechanism for muscular dystrophy (81). This cascade results in mitochondrial dysfunction and may ultimately trigger cellular apoptosis in a mitochondrially mediated fashion (59). Apart from muscular dystrophy, mitochondrial dysfunction is also linked to both sarcopenia and chronic fatigue syndrome (CFS). Sarcopenia is characterized by increased levels of apoptosis and reduced capacity for muscle regeneration, which leads to significant muscle wasting (2). As a working hypothesis to explain the development of sarcopenia, impairments in the clearance of damaged mitochondrial populations in neurons and myocytes leads to porosity of mitochondrial membranes, namely via opening of the MPTP (2). The release of mitochondrial contents into the cytosol triggers apoptosis and contributes to the loss of muscle tissue. CFS, on the other hand, is a multisystem disease which commonly presents with decreased stamina and increased levels of fatigue (86). Like sarcopenia the pathophysiology of CFS has yet to be determined; however, the existing metabolic hypothesis implicates dysfunctional mitochondria as the primary factor leading to widespread metabolic dysfunction (86). Therefore, existing research indicates that mitochondrial dysfunction may lead to various diseases affecting the musculoskeletal system. Unsurprisingly, exercise training has been shown to augment functional deficits in skeletal muscle function of various myopathies, including primary mitochondrial disease (89, 108) and sarcopenia (145). Mechanistically, exercise training improves the ability of skeletal muscle to utilize and extract oxygen through increased mitochondrial biogenesis and enhanced bioenergetic efficiency in healthy mitochondrial populations (108). Exercise is also clinically recommended in both DMD and BMD, although further research is warranted to definitively conclude the beneficial effects on clinical parameters (4).

Gastrointestinal System

As another hallmark symptom, gastrointestinal (GI) dysfunction has been commonly associated with primary mitochondrial disease. Inflammatory bowel disease (IBD) is divided into two chronic inflammatory diseases, ulcerative colitis and Crohn disease, which are characterized by diarrhoea, bloody stools, and abdominal pain (98). Interestingly, animal studies investigating mitochondrial ROS production have confirmed that oxidative stress contributes to inflammation of enterocytes and that lowering ROS production reduces the severity of drug-induced colitis (45). Clinically, mitochondria isolated from IBD enterocytes are fragmented (fission) with diminished cristae surface area, impaired energy synthesis, and increased ROS production (98). Collectively, these metabolic abnormalities identify mitochondrial dysfunction as a contributor to IBD pathogenesis.

Endocrine System

Type 2 diabetes mellitus (T2DM) is a progressive metabolic disease characterized by chronic hyperglycaemia, culminating in impaired insulin resistance and impaired insulin secretion. A chronic state of hyperglycaemia results in excessive ROS production via glucose oxidation, which leads to mitochondrial dysfunction. Impairments in mitochondrial function can then act in a cyclical manner and generate further ROS, resulting in accelerated mitochondrial dysfunction and insulin resistance (114). Mitochondrial dynamics are also altered through down-regulation of *MFN2*, promoting a fission morphology and leading to insulin intolerance (5). The importance of mitochondrial dynamics in T2DM is evidenced through the actions of metformin, a common first-line oral therapy for T2DM, which acts in part by inhibiting *DRP1*-mediated mitochondrial fission (71). On the other hand, type 1 diabetes (T1D) is an autoimmune condition resulting in destruction of the pancreatic beta cells and a loss of host insulin production. Notably, recent research has begun to characterize the role of skeletal muscle dysfunction in patients with T1D. Previously hypothesized to occur after the clinical onset of various complications of T1D, clinical and basic science studies have indicated that the function, structure, and mitochondrial metabolism of skeletal muscle are impaired in T1D prior to clinical symptoms (85). In a similar fashion, mitochondrial dysfunction is strongly associated with metabolic syndrome. Increased ROS production, decreased basal energy synthesis, and impaired mitochondrial dynamics have each been identified in the various facets of metabolic syndrome—high triglycerides, hypertension, visceral obesity, insulin resistance, and low high-density lipoprotein (HDL) cholesterol (84). Known to impart beneficial metabolic effects on mitochondrial populations found in skeletal musculature, exercise therapy has been studied as a potential therapeutic target for both diabetes and metabolic syndrome. Collectively, studies investigating exercise therapy in diabetes and metabolic syndrome have been shown to increase mitochondrial biogenesis, increase mitochondrial respiration, decrease ROS production, and increase mtDNA (11, 58). Furthermore, research also indicates that mitochondrial populations from adipose tissue also undergo metabolic adaptations in response to exercise training (131).

Another group of chronic diseases linked to mitochondrial dysfunction are those involving the adrenal and thyroid glands. Interestingly, all steroid hormones are produced in the mitochondria; therefore, dysfunctional mitochondria are likely to impair function of the adrenal cortex, a steroid hormone–secreting tissue. Furthermore, mitochondrial dynamics may act as the driving factor in steroidogenesis, since loss of *MFN2* is enough to impair steroid biosynthesis (33). Furthermore, a bidirectional relationship between mitochondrial energy synthesis and the production of thyroid hormones has been identified, although further exploration in human tissues is warranted (49).

Cancer

One of the hallmarks of cancer cells are their resistance to apoptosis and propensity for uncontrollable growth. Characterized by a metabolic shift from OXHPOS to glycolysis (Warburg effect), these alterations are facilitated in a mitochondrially dependent manner through the inhibition of pyruvate dehydrogenase, which inhibits oxidative metabolism (5). Undergoing distinct stages (initiation, growth, survival, and metastasis), tumorigenesis is known to require mitochondrial support at each stage. The initiation stage has been linked to excessive ROS production resulting in further genomic instability, whereas specific mutations to mitochondrial enzymes cause production of mitochondrial-derived signalling molecules termed oncometabolites (137). These oncometabolites, such as (R)-2-hydroxyglutarate, target TCA cycle enzymes by acting as competitive inhibitors and ultimately result in gene silencing (99). Tumour growth and survival also require aberrant mitochondrial function in order to serve the metabolic requirement of the tumour. The inhibition of apoptosis, alterations in mitochondrial biogenesis and dynamics, and mitochondrial signalling all contribute to tumour growth and survival (137). Human lung cancer models have identified that the mitochondrial population of tumours exhibits a fission morphology, which enables proliferation and confers resistance to targeted cytotoxic therapies (110). To exploit the role of mitochondria and the survival stage of tumorigenesis, current therapeutics are exploring stimulation of the pro-apoptotic cascade (109). However, existing therapeutic modalities, namely chemotherapy, also contribute to aberrant mitochondrial function through unintended damage to surrounding skeletal muscle. Commonly resulting in various degrees of fatigue, the skeletal muscle damage caused by chemotherapy has become a target for exercise therapy to maintain baseline skeletal muscle function. Research studies have shown that exercise training during chemotherapy for breast cancer has preserved skeletal muscle fibre architecture and mitochondrial content compared to control patients (80). Finally, mtDNA are known to confer metastatic potential. Research has indicated that mtDNA transplanted from malignant cells to non-malignant cells cause transference of malignant potential (54). This phenomenon demonstrates that mtDNA directly influences metastatic potential of tumour progression and that specific mtDNA mutations in tumours may act as targets for anti-cancer therapy.

Conclusion

Mitochondria are vital cellular organelles which have demonstrated pathological involvement in ageing and a multitude of chronic disease states. Prolonged mitochondrial dysfunction in which ATP generation is compromised connects aberrant mitochondrial function to the development of a diseased state. The involvement of mitochondria in all human organ systems and the variability of phenotypes require further investigation into the mechanisms of disease in order to exploit tangible mitochondrial therapeutic targets in the future. However, in order to effectively treat diseases involving mitochondrial dysfunction, we must cater therapies to the complex and dynamic nature of the mitochondrion. Although certain diseases, such as *OPA1*-dependent optic atrophy, appear to involve a single mitochondrial gene mutation, most diseases involving mitochondrial dysfunction are caused by multiple mitochondrial deficiencies. As a front-line intervention for the prevention and treatment of many chronic diseases, exercise is undoubtedly linked to proper mitochondrial function. Therefore, a comprehensive understanding of mitochondrial function will be required to provide the most successful clinical trials. Future studies investigating cancer therapies, for example, will require combinations which aim to target specified tumorigenesis stages through coordinated alterations to mitochondrial dynamics, signalling, biogenesis, metabolic regulation, exercise therapy, and others. This combination approach will be important to advance treatments for disease processes involving mitochondrial dysfunction.

References

1. Alexeyev M, Shokolenko I, Wilson G, LeDoux S. The maintenance of mitochondrial DNA integrity–critical analysis and update. *Cold Spring Harb Perspect Biol* 5: a012641, 2013.
2. Alway SE, Mohamed JS, Myers MJ. Mitochondria initiate and regulate sarcopenia. *Exerc Sport Sci Rev* 45: 58–69, 2017.
3. Anderson S, Bankier AT, Barrell BG, de Bruijn MHL, Coulson AR, Drouin J, et al. Sequence and organization of the human mitochondrial genome. *Nature* 290: 457–465, 1981.
4. Andrews JG, Wahl RA. Duchenne and Becker muscular dystrophy in adolescents: Current perspectives. *Adolesc Health Med Ther* 9: 53–63, 2018.
5. Archer SL. Mitochondrial dynamics–mitochondrial fission and fusion in human diseases. *N Engl J Med* 369: 2236–2251, 2013.
6. Archer SL, Wu X-C, Thébaud B, Moudgil R, Hashimoto K, Michelakis ED. O2 sensing in the human ductus arteriosus: Redox-sensitive K+ channels are regulated by mitochondria-derived hydrogen peroxide. *Biol Chem* 385: 205–216, 2004.
7. Asin-Cayuela J, Gustafsson CM. Mitochondrial transcription and its regulation in mammalian cells. *Trends Biochem Sci* 32: 111–117, 2007.
8. Ballard JW, Whitlock MC. The incomplete natural history of mitochondria. *Mol Ecol* 13: 729–744, 2004.
9. Bartlett K, Eaton S. Mitochondrial beta-oxidation. *Eur J Biochem* 271: 462–469, 2004.
10. Bernardo TC, Marques-Aleixo I, Beleza J, Oliveira PJ, Ascensão A, Magalhães J. Physical exercise and brain mitochondrial fitness: The possible role against alzheimer's disease. *Brain Pathol* 26: 648–663, 2016.
11. Bhatti JS, Bhatti GK, Reddy PH. Mitochondrial dysfunction and oxidative stress in metabolic disorders — A step towards mitochondria based therapeutic strategies. *Biochim. Biophys. Acta - Mol Basis Dis* 1663: 1066–1077, 2017.
12. Bratic I, Trifunovic A. Mitochondrial energy metabolism and ageing. *Biochim Biophys Acta - Bioenerg* 1797: 961–967, 2010.
13. Brønstad E, Rognmo O, Tjonna AE, Dedichen HH, Kirkeby-Garstad I, Håberg AK, et al. High-intensity knee extensor training restores skeletal muscle function in COPD patients. *Eur Respir J* 40: 1130–1136, 2012.
14. Camara AKS, Lesnefsky EJ, Stowe DF. Potential therapeutic benefits of strategies directed to mitochondria. *Antioxid Redox Signal* 13: 279–347, 2010.
15. Camara AKS, Zhou Y, Wen P-C, Tajkhorshid E, Kwok W-M. Mitochondrial VDAC1: A key gatekeeper as potential therapeutic target. *Front Physiol* 8: 460, 2017.
16. Carmo C, Naia L, Lopes C, Rego AC. Mitochondrial dysfunction in huntington's disease. In: *Advances in experimental medicine and biology*. 2018, p. 59–83.
17. Cartoni R, Léger B, Hock MB, Praz M, Crettenand A, Pich S, et al. Mitofusins 1/2 and ERRalpha expression are increased in human skeletal muscle after physical exercise. *J Physiol* 567: 349–358, 2005.
18. Chan DC. Mitochondrial fusion and fission in mammals. *Annu Rev Cell Dev Biol* 22: 79–99, 2006.
19. Chen CCW, Erlich AT, Crilly MJ, Hood DA. Parkin is required for exercise-induced mitophagy in muscle: Impact of aging. *Am J Physiol Metab* 315: E404–E415, 2018.
20. Chen H, Detmer SA, Ewald AJ, Griffin EE, Fraser SE, Chan DC. Mitofusins Mfn1 and Mfn2 coordinately regulate mitochondrial fusion and are essential for embryonic development. *J Cell Biol* 160: 189–200, 2003.
21. Chen Q, Vazquez EJ, Moghaddas S, Hoppel CL, Lesnefsky EJ. Production of reactive oxygen species by mitochondria: Central role of complex III. *J Biol Chem* 278: 36027–36031, 2003.

22. Chen Y, Dorn GW. PINK1-phosphorylated mitofusin 2 is a Parkin receptor for culling damaged mitochondria. *Science* 340: 471–475, 2013.

23. Dabrowska A, Venero JL, Iwasawa R, Hankir M-K, Rahman S, Boobis A, et al. PGC-1α controls mitochondrial biogenesis and dynamics in lead-induced neurotoxicity. *Aging (Albany NY)* 7: 629–647, 2015.

24. Dagda RK, Cherra SJ, Kulich SM, Tandon A, Park D, Chu CT. Loss of PINK1 function promotes mitophagy through effects on oxidative stress and mitochondrial fission. *J Biol Chem* 284: 13843–13855, 2009.

25. Davenport MH, Hogan DB, Eskes GA, Longman RS, Poulin MJ. Cerebrovascular reserve: The link between fitness and cognitive function? *Exerc Sport Sci Rev* 40: 153–158, 2012.

26. de Brito OM, Scorrano L. An intimate liaison: Spatial organization of the endoplasmic reticulum–mitochondria relationship. *EMBO J* 29: 2715–2723, 2010.

27. Detmer SA, Chan DC. Functions and dysfunctions of mitochondrial dynamics. *Nat Rev Mol Cell Biol* 8: 870–879, 2007.

28. Dewson G, Kluck RM. Mechanisms by which bak and bax permeabilise mitochondria during apoptosis. *J Cell Sci* 122: 2801–2808, 2009.

29. Dominy JE, Puigserver P. Mitochondrial biogenesis through activation of nuclear signaling proteins. *Cold Spring Harb Perspect Biol* 5, 2013.

30. Drake JC, Laker RC, Wilson RJ, Zhang M, Yan Z. Exercise-induced mitophagy in skeletal muscle occurs in the absence of stabilization of Pink1 on mitochondria. *Cell Cycle* 18: 1–6, 2019.

31. Drexler H, Riede U, Münzel T, König H, Funke E, Just H. Alterations of skeletal muscle in chronic heart failure. *Circulation* 85: 1751–1759, 1992.

32. Drose S, Brandt U. Molecular mechanisms of superoxide production by the mitochondrial respiratory chain. *Adv Exp Med Biol* 748: 145–169, 2012.

33. Duarte A, Poderoso C, Cooke M, Soria G, Cornejo Maciel F, Gottifredi V, et al. Mitochondrial fusion is essential for steroid biosynthesis. *PLOS ONE* 7: e45829, 2012.

34. Dudek J, Rehling P, van der Laan M. Mitochondrial protein import: Common principles and physiological networks. *Biochim Biophys Acta - Mol Cell Res* 1833: 274–285, 2013.

35. Ekstrand MI, Falkenberg M, Rantanen A, Park CB, Gaspari M, Hultenby K, et al. Mitochondrial transcription factor A regulates mtDNA copy number in mammals. *Hum Mol Genet* 13: 935–944, 2004.

36. Elmore S. Apoptosis: A review of programmed cell death. *Toxicol Pathol* 35: 495–516, 2007.

37. Forner F, Foster LJ, Campanaro S, Valle G, Mann M. Quantitative proteomic comparison of rat mitochondria from muscle, heart, and liver. *Mol Cell Proteomics* 5: 608–619, 2006.

38. Friedman JR, Lackner LL, West M, DiBenedetto JR, Nunnari J, Voeltz GK. ER tubules mark sites of mitochondrial division. *Science* 334: 358–362, 2011.

39. Friedman JR, Nunnari J. Mitochondrial form and function. *Nature* 505: 335–343, 2014.

40. Frye RE, Rossignol DA. Mitochondrial dysfunction can connect the diverse medical symptoms associated with autism spectrum disorders. *Pediatr Res* 69: 41R–47R, 2011.

41. Gellerich FN, Trumbeckaite S, Opalka JR, Seppet E, Rasmussen HN, Neuhoff C, et al. Function of the mitochondrial outer membrane as a diffusion barrier in health and diseases. *Biochem Soc Trans* 28: 164–169, 2000.

42. Glick D, Zhang W, Beaton M, Marsboom G, Gruber M, Simon MC, et al. BNip3 regulates mitochondrial function and lipid metabolism in the liver. *Mol Cell Biol* 32: 2570–2584, 2012.

43. Gonzalez D, Bejarano I, Barriga C, Rodriguez AB, Pariente JA. Oxidative stress-induced caspases are regulated in human myeloid HL-60 cells by calcium signal. *Curr Signal Transduct Ther* 5: 181–186, 2010.

44. Grünig E, Ehlken N, Ghofrani A, Staehler G, Meyer FJ, Juenger J, et al. Effect of exercise and respiratory training on clinical progression and survival in patients with severe chronic pulmonary hypertension. *Respiration* 81: 394–401, 2011.

45. Guo W, Liu W, Jin B, Geng J, Li J, Ding H, et al. Asiatic acid ameliorates dextran sulfate sodium-induced murine experimental colitis via suppressing mitochondria-mediated NLRP3 inflammasome activation. *Int Immunopharmacol* 24: 232–238, 2015.

46. Harman D. Aging: A theory based on free radical and radiation chemistry. *J Gerontol* 11: 298–300, 1956.

47. Harman D. The biologic clock: The mitochondria? *J Am Geriatr Soc* 20: 145–147, 1972.

48. Harman D. Free radical theory of aging. *Triangle* 12: 153–158, 1973.

49. Harper M-E, Seifert EL. Thyroid hormone effects on mitochondrial energetics. *Thyroid* 18: 145–156, 2008.

50. Hood DA. Mechanisms of exercise-induced mitochondrial biogenesis in skeletal muscle. *Appl Physiol Nutr Metab* 34: 465–472, 2009.

51. Hoppins S. The regulation of mitochondrial dynamics. *Curr Opin Cell Biol* 29C: 46–52, 2014.

52. Hüttemann M, Pecina P, Rainbolt M, Sanderson TH, Kagan VE, Samavati L, et al. The multiple functions of cytochrome c and their regulation in life and death decisions of the mammalian cell: From respiration to apoptosis. *Mitochondrion* 11: 369–381, 2011.

53. Ikeda M, Ide T, Fujino T, Arai S, Saku K, Kakino T, et al. Overexpression of TFAM or twinkle increases mtDNA copy number and facilitates cardioprotection associated with limited mitochondrial oxidative stress. *PLoS One* 10: e0119687, 2015.

54. Ishikawa K, Takenaga K, Akimoto M, Koshikawa N, Yamaguchi A, Imanishi H, et al. ROS-Generating mitochondrial DNA mutations can regulate tumor cell metastasis. *Science* 320: 661–664, 2008.

55. Jiang X, Wang X. Cytochrome c promotes caspase-9 activation by inducing nucleotide binding to apaf-1. *J Biol Chem* 275: 31199–31203, 2000.

56. Jodeiri Farshbaf M, Ghaedi K. Huntington's disease and mitochondria. *Neurotox Res* 32: 518–529, 2017.

57. Jornayvaz FR, Shulman GI. Regulation of mitochondrial biogenesis. *Essays Biochem* 47: 69–84, 2010.

58. Joseph AM, Hood DA. Relationships between exercise, mitochondrial biogenesis and type 2 diabetes. In: *Diabetes and Physical Activity* Goedecke JH, Ojuka EO. Eds., S. Karger AG, Basel, 2014, p. 48–61.

59. Kelly-Worden M, Thomas E. Mitochondrial dysfunction in Duchenne muscular dystrophy. *Open J Endocr Metab Dis* 4: 211–218, 2014.

60. Kiessling K-H, Piehl K, Lundquist C-G. *Effect of Physical Training on Ultrastructural Features in Human Skeletal Muscle.* Boston, MA: Springer, 1971, p. 97–101.

61. Kim KH, Son JM, Benayoun BA, Lee C. The mitochondrial-encoded peptide MOTS-c translocates to the nucleus to regulate nuclear gene expression in response to metabolic stress. *Cell Metab* 28: 516, 2018.

62. Koopman WJ, Distelmaier F, Smeitink JA, Willems PH. OXPHOS mutations and neurodegeneration. *EMBO J* 32: 9–29, 2013.

63. Kramer T, Enquist LW, Ashrafi G, Schlehe J, Wong YL, Selkoe D, et al. Alphaherpesvirus infection disrupts mitochondrial transport in neurons. *Cell Host Microbe* 11: 504–514, 2012.

64. Kühlbrandt W. Structure and function of mitochondrial membrane protein complexes. *BMC Biol* 13: 89, 2015.

65. Kukat C, Larsson N-G. mtDNA makes a U-turn for the mitochondrial nucleoid. *Trends Cell Biol* 23: 457–463, 2013.

66. Kunji ERS, Aleksandrova A, King MS, Majd H, Ashton VL, Cerson E, et al. The transport mechanism of the mitochondrial ADP/ATP carrier. *Biochim Biophys Acta - Mol Cell Res* 1863: 2379–2393, 2016.

67. Kwong JQ, Molkentin JD. Physiological and pathological roles of the mitochondrial permeability transition pore in the heart. *Cell Metab* 21: 206, 2015.

68. Laker RC, Drake JC, Wilson RJ, Lira VA, Lewellen BM, Ryall KA, et al. Ampk phosphorylation of Ulk1 is required for targeting of mitochondria to lysosomes in exercise-induced mitophagy. *Nat Commun* 8: 548, 2017.

69. Lee C, Yen K, Cohen P. Humanin: A harbinger of mitochondrial-derived peptides? *Trends Endocrinol Metab* 24: 222–228, 2013.

70. Lee C, Zeng J, Drew BG, Sallam T, Martin-Montalvo A, Wan J, et al. The mitochondrial-derived peptide MOTS-c promotes metabolic homeostasis and reduces obesity and insulin resistance. *Cell Metab* 21: 443–454, 2015.

71. Li A, Zhang S, Li J, Liu K, Huang F, Liu B. Metformin and resveratrol inhibit Drp1-mediated mitochondrial fission and prevent ER stress-associated NLRP3 inflammasome activation in the adipose tissue of diabetic mice. *Mol Cell Endocrinol* 434: 36–47, 2016.

72. Liao HX, Spremulli LL. Initiation of protein synthesis in animal mitochondria. Purification and characterization of translational initiation factor 2. *J Biol Chem* 266: 20714–20719, 1991.

73. Lin MT, Beal MF. Mitochondrial dysfunction and oxidative stress in neurodegenerative diseases. *Nature* 443: 787–795, 2006.

74. Lira VA, Okutsu M, Zhang M, Greene NP, Laker RC, Breen DS, et al. Autophagy is required for exercise training-induced skeletal muscle adaptation and improvement of physical performance. *FASEB J* 27: 4184–4193, 2013.

75. Losón OC, Song Z, Chen H, Chan DC. Fis1, Mff, MiD49, and MiD51 mediate Drp1 recruitment in mitochondrial fission. *Mol Biol Cell* 24: 659–667, 2013.

76. Manczak M, Reddy PH. Abnormal interaction between the mitochondrial fission protein Drp1 and hyperphosphorylated tau in Alzheimer's disease neurons: Implications for mitochondrial dysfunction and neuronal damage. *Hum Mol Genet* 21: 2538–2547, 2012.

77. Marques-Aleixo I, Santos-Alves E, Mariani D, Rizo-Roca D, Padrão AI, Rocha-Rodrigues S, et al. Physical exercise prior and during treatment reduces sub-chronic doxorubicin-induced mitochondrial toxicity and oxidative stress. *Mitochondrion* 20:22–33, 2015.

78. Massano J, Bhatia KP. Clinical approach to parkinson's disease: Features, diagnosis, and principles of management. *Cold Spring Harb Perspect Med* 2: a008870, 2012.

79. Meyer A, Zoll J, Charles AL, Charloux A, de Blay F, Diemunsch P, et al. Skeletal muscle mitochondrial dysfunction during chronic obstructive pulmonary disease: Central actor and therapeutic target. *Exp Physiol* 98: 1063–1078, 2013.

80. Mijwel S, Cardinale DA, Norrbom J, Chapman M, Ivarsson N, Wengström Y, et al. Exercise training during chemotherapy preserves skeletal muscle fiber area, capillarization, and mitochondrial content in patients with breast cancer. *FASEB J* 32: 5495–5505, 2018.

81. Millay DP, Sargent MA, Osinska H, Baines CP, Barton ER, Vuagniaux G, et al. Genetic and pharmacologic inhibition of mitochondrial-dependent necrosis attenuates muscular dystrophy. *Nat Med* 14: 442–447, 2008.

82. Mishra P, Chan DC. Mitochondrial dynamics and inheritance during cell division, development and disease. *Nat Rev Mol Cell Biol* 15: 634–646, 2014.

83. Mishra P, Chan DC. Metabolic regulation of mitochondrial dynamics. *J Cell Biol* 212: 379–387, 2016.

84. Mitchell T, Darley-Usmar V. Metabolic syndrome and mitochondrial dysfunction: Insights from preclinical studies with a mitochondrially targeted antioxidant. *Free Radic Biol Med* 52: 838–840, 2012.

85. Monaco CMF, Gingrich MA, Hawke TJ. Considering Type 1 Diabetes as a Form of Accelerated Muscle Aging. *Exerc Sport Sci Rev* 47: 98–107, 2019.

86. Myhill S, Booth NE, McLaren-Howard J. Chronic fatigue syndrome and mitochondrial dysfunction. *Int J Clin Exp Med* 2: 1–16, 2009.

87. Newell C, Hume S, Greenway SC, Podemski L, Shearer J, Khan A. Plasma-derived cell-free mitochondrial DNA: A novel non-invasive methodology to identify mitochondrial DNA haplogroups in humans. *Mol. Genet. Metab.* 125-332–337, 2018

88. Newell C, Khan A, Sinasac D, Shoffner J, Friederich MW, Van Hove JLK, et al. Hybrid gel electrophoresis using skin fibroblasts to aid in diagnosing mitochondrial disease. *Neurol Genet* 5: e336, 2019.

89. Newell C, Ramage B, Robu I, Shearer J, Khan A. Side alternating vibration training in patients with mitochondrial disease: A pilot study. *Arch Physiother* 7: 10, 2017.

90. Newell C, Sabouny R, Hittel DS, Shutt TE, Khan A, Klein MS, et al. Mesenchymal stem cells shift mitochondrial dynamics and enhance oxidative phosphorylation in recipient cells. *Front Physiol* 9: 1572, 2018.

91. Newell C, Shutt TE, Ahn Y, Hittel DS, Khan A, Rho JM, et al. Tissue specific impacts of a ketogenic diet on mitochondrial dynamics in the BTBR(T+tf/j) mouse. *Front Physiol* 7: 654, 2016.

92. Newsholme P, Gaudel C, Krause M. Mitochondria and diabetes. An intriguing pathogenetic role. *Adv Exp Med Biol* 942: 235–247, 2012.

93. Ney PA. Mitochondrial autophagy: Origins, significance, and role of BNIP3 and NIX. *Biochim Biophys Acta* 1853: 2775–2783, 2015.

94. Ngo HB, Lovely GA, Phillips R, Chan DC. Distinct structural features of TFAM drive mitochondrial DNA packaging versus transcriptional activation. *Nat Commun* 5: 3077, 2014.

95. Ni H-M, Williams JA, Ding W-X. Mitochondrial dynamics and mitochondrial quality control. *Redox Biol* 4: 6–13, 2015.

96. Nicolson GL. Mitochondrial dysfunction and chronic disease: Treatment with natural supplements. *Integr Med (Encinitas)* 13: 35–43, 2014.

97. Nilsson MI, Tarnopolsky MA. Mitochondria and aging—the role of exercise as a countermeasure. *Biology (Basel)* 2019.

98. Novak EA, Mollen KP. Mitochondrial dysfunction in inflammatory bowel disease. *Front cell Dev Biol* 3: 62, 2015.

99. Nowicki S, Gottlieb E. Oncometabolites: Tailoring our genes. *FEBS J* 282: 2796–2805, 2015.

100. Nyamandi VZ, Johnsen VL, Hughey CC, Hittel DS, Khan A, Newell C, et al. Enhanced stem cell engraftment and modulation of hepatic reactive oxygen species production in diet-induced obesity. *Obes. (Silver Spring)* 22:721–729, 2013.

101. Onyango IG, Dennis J, Khan SM. Mitochondrial dysfunction in alzheimer's disease and the rationale for bioenergetics based therapies. *Aging Dis* 7: 201–214, 2016.

102. Osborne NN, Alvarez CN, Del Olmo Aguado S. Targeting mitochondrial dysfunction as in aging and glaucoma. *Drug Discov Today* 19:613–1622, 2014)

103. Ozören N, El-Deiry WS. Defining characteristics of Types I and II apoptotic cells in response to TRAIL. *Neoplasia* 4: 551–557, 2002.

104. Perry CGR, Lally J, Holloway GP, Heigenhauser GJF, Bonen A, Spriet LL. Repeated transient mRNA bursts precede increases in transcriptional and mitochondrial proteins during training in human skeletal muscle. *J Physiol* 588: 4795–4810, 2010.

105. Picca A, Lezza AMS. Regulation of mitochondrial biogenesis through TFAM–mitochondrial DNA interactions: Useful insights from aging and calorie restriction studies. *Mitochondrion* 25: 67–75, 2015.

106. Pieczenik SR, Neustadt J. Mitochondrial dysfunction and molecular pathways of disease. *Exp Mol Pathol* 83: 84–92, 2007.

107. Pilling AD, Horiuchi D, Lively CM, Saxton WM. Kinesin-1 and dynein are the primary motors for fast transport of mitochondria in drosophila motor axons. *Mol Biol Cell* 17: 2057–2068, 2006.

108. Porcelli S, Grassi B, Poole DC, Marzorati M. Exercise intolerance in patients with mitochondrial myopathies: Perfusive and diffusive limitations in the O2 pathway. *Curr Opin Physiol* 10: 202–209, 2019.

109. Porporato PE, Filigheddu N, Pedro JMB-S, Kroemer G, Galluzzi L. Mitochondrial metabolism and cancer. *Cell Res* 28: 265–280, 2018.

110. Rehman J, Zhang HJ, Toth PT, Zhang Y, Marsboom G, Hong Z, et al. Inhibition of mitochondrial fission prevents cell cycle progression in lung cancer. *FASEB J* 26: 2175–2186, 2012.

111. Riley BE, Lougheed JC, Callaway K, Velasquez M, Brecht E, Nguyen L, et al. Structure and function of Parkin E3 ubiquitin ligase reveals aspects of RING and HECT ligases. *Nat Commun* 4: 1982, 2013.

112. Ritov VB, Menshikova E V, He J, Ferrell RE, Goodpaster BH, Kelley DE. Deficiency of subsarcolemmal mitochondria in obesity and type 2 diabetes. *Diabetes* 54: 8–14, 2005.

113. Rosca MG, Hoppel CL. Mitochondrial dysfunction in heart failure. *Heart Fail Rev* 18: 607–622, 2013.

114. Rovira-Llopis S, Bañuls C, Diaz-Morales N, Hernandez-Mijares A, Rocha M, Victor VM. Mitochondrial dynamics in type 2 diabetes: Pathophysiological implications. *Redox Biol* 11: 637–645, 2017.

115. Ryan J, Dasgupta A, Huston J, Chen K-H, Archer SL. Mitochondrial dynamics in pulmonary arterial hypertension. *J Mol Med* 93: 229–242, 2015.

116. Safdar A, Little JP, Stokl AJ, Hettinga BP, Akhtar M, Tarnopolsky MA. Exercise increases mitochondrial PGC-1α content and promotes nuclear-mitochondrial cross-talk to coordinate mitochondrial biogenesis. *J Biol Chem* 286: 10605–10617, 2011.

117. Salim S. Oxidative stress and the central nervous system. *J Pharmacol Exp Ther* 360: 201–205, 2017.

118. Sanchis-Gomar F, García-Giménez JL, Gómez-Cabrera MC, Pallardó F V. Mitochondrial biogenesis in health and disease. Molecular and therapeutic approaches. *Curr Pharm Des* 20: 5619–5633, 2014.

119. Schwarz TL. Mitochondrial trafficking in neurons. *Cold Spring Harb Perspect Biol* 5, 2013.

120. Shokolenko IN, Alexeyev MF. Mitochondrial transcription in mammalian cells. *Front Biosci (Landmark Ed)* 22: 835–853, 2017.

121. Song W, Chen J, Petrilli A, Liot G, Klinglmayr E, Zhou Y, et al, Bossy B, Perkins G, Bossy-Wetzel E. Mutant huntingtin binds the mitochondrial fission GTPase dynamin-related protein-1 and increases its enzymatic activity. *Nat Med* 17: 377–382, 2011.

122. Song Z, Chen H, Fiket M, Alexander C, Chan DC. OPA1 processing controls mitochondrial fusion and is regulated by mRNA splicing, membrane potential, and Yme1L. *J Cell Biol* 178, 2007.

123. Stoller JZ, Demauro SB, Dagle JM, Reese J. Current perspectives on pathobiology of the ductus arteriosus. *J Clin Exp Cardiolog* 8, 2012.

124. Stumpf JD, Saneto RP, Copeland WC. Clinical and molecular features of POLG-related mitochondrial disease. *Cold Spring Harb Perspect Biol* 5: a011395, 2013.

125. Swank AM, Horton J, Fleg JL, Fonarow GC, Keteyian S, Goldberg L, et al. Modest increase in peak VO2 is related to better clinical outcomes in chronic heart failure patients: Results from heart failure and a controlled trial to investigate outcomes of exercise training. *Circ Hear Fail* 5: 579–585, 2012.

126. Taanman J-W. The mitochondrial genome: Structure, transcription, translation and replication. *Biochim Biophys Acta - Bioenerg* 1410: 103–123, 1999.

127. Tanida I, Ueno T, Kominami E. LC3 and autophagy. In: *Methods in Molecular Biology (Clifton, N.J.)*. 2008, p. 77–88.

128. Tari AR, Norevik CS, Scrimgeour NR, Kobro-Flatmoen A, Storm-Mathisen J, Bergersen LH, et al. Are the neuroprotective effects of exercise training systemically mediated? *Prog Cardiovasc Dis* 2019.

129. Thannickal VJ, Fanburg BL. Reactive oxygen species in cell signaling. *Am J Physiol Lung Cell Mol Physiol* 279: L1005–L1028, 2000.

130. Toth MJ, Miller MS, Ward KA, Ades PA. Skeletal muscle mitochondrial density, gene expression, and enzyme activities in human heart failure: Minimal effects of the disease and resistance training. *J Appl Physiol* 112: 1864–1874, 2012.

131. Trevellin E, Scorzeto M, Olivieri M, Granzotto M, Valerio A, Tedesco L, et al. Exercise training induces mitochondrial biogenesis and glucose uptake in subcutaneous adipose tissue through eNOS-dependent mechanisms. *Diabetes* 63: 2800–2811, 2014.

132. Trewin A, Berry B, Wojtovich A. Exercise and mitochondrial dynamics: Keeping in shape with ROS and AMPK. *Antioxidants* 7: 7, 2018.

133. Tuppen HAL, Blakely EL, Turnbull DM, Taylor RW. Mitochondrial DNA mutations and human disease. *Biochim Biophys Acta - Bioenerg* 1797: 113–128, 2010.

134. Twig G, Shirihai OS. The interplay between mitochondrial dynamics and mitophagy. *Antioxid Redox Signal* 14: 1939–1951, 2011.

135. Valenti D, de Bari L, De Filippis B, Henrion-Caude A, Vacca RA. Mitochondrial dysfunction as a central actor in intellectual disability-related diseases: An overview of Down syndrome, autism, Fragile X and Rett syndrome. *Neurosci Biobehav Rev* 46: 202–217, 2014.

136. van Vliet AR, Agostinis P. Mitochondria-associated membranes and ER stress. In: *Current Topics in Microbiology and Immunology*. 2017, p. 73–102.

137. Vyas S, Zaganjor E, Haigis MC. Mitochondria and cancer. *Cell* 166: 555–566, 2016.

138. Wai T, Langer T. Mitochondrial dynamics and metabolic regulation. *Trends Endocrinol Metab* 27: 105–117, 2016.

139. Wang C, Youle RJ. The role of mitochondria in apoptosis*. *Annu Rev Genet* 43: 95–118, 2009.

140. Wang X, Schwarz TL. The mechanism of Ca2+ -dependent regulation of kinesin-mediated mitochondrial motility. *Cell* 136: 163–174, 2009.

141. Westphal D, Dewson G, Czabotar PE, Kluck RM. Molecular biology of Bax and Bak activation and action. *Biochim Biophys Acta - Mol Cell Res* 1813: 521–531, 2011.

142. Xin H, Woriax V, Burkhart W, Spremulli LL. Cloning and expression of mitochondrial translational elongation factor Ts from bovine and human liver. *J Biol Chem* 270: 17243–17249, 1995.

143. Yan Z, Lira VA, Greene NP. Exercise training-induced regulation of mitochondrial quality. *Exerc Sport Sci Rev* 40: 159–164, 2012.

144. Yasukawa T, Reyes A, Cluett TJ, Yang M-Y, Bowmaker M, Jacobs HT, et al. Replication of vertebrate mitochondrial DNA entails transient ribonucleotide incorporation throughout the lagging strand. *EMBO J* 25: 5358–5371, 2006.

145. Yoo SZ, No MH, Heo JW, Park DH, Kang JH, Kim SH, et al. Role of exercise in age-related sarcopenia. *J Exerc Rehabil* 14 Korean Society of Exercise Rehabilitation: 551–558, 2018.

146. Youle RJ, Narendra DP. Mechanisms of mitophagy. *Nat Rev Mol Cell Biol* 12: 9–14, 2011.

147. Young MJ, Humble MM, DeBalsi KL, Sun KY, Copeland WC. *POLG2* disease variants: analyses reveal a dominant negative heterodimer, altered mitochondrial localization and impaired respiratory capacity. *Hum Mol Genet* 24: 5184–5197, 2015.

148. Yu Z, O'Farrell PH, Yakubovich N, DeLuca SZ. The mitochondrial DNA polymerase promotes elimination of paternal mitochondrial genomes. *Curr Biol* 27: 1033–1039, 2017.

149. Zhang J. Autophagy and mitophagy in cellular damage control. *Redox Biol* 1: 19–23, 2013.

150. Zheng G, Xia R, Zhou W, Tao J, Chen L. Aerobic exercise ameliorates cognitive function in older adults with mild cognitive impairment: A systematic review and meta-analysis of randomised controlled trials. *Br J Sports Med* 50: 144301450, 2016.

27

EXERCISE TRAINING, MITOCHONDRIAL ADAPTATIONS, AND AGING

Nashwa Cheema, Matthew Triolo, and David A. Hood

Introduction

Mitochondria are the organelles that provide the energy for cell survival. They are remarkably complex metabolic machines that contain the enzymes of the electron transport chain and Krebs cycle for the oxidation of pyruvic acid, as well as β-oxidation enzymes for the breakdown of fatty acids from triglycerides. There are approximately 1,200 proteins within the matrix, inner and outer membranes, and intermembrane space compartments devoted to these metabolic tasks. While most of these are nuclear gene products which have to be imported into the organelle, a small number of mitochondrial proteins are transcribed from mitochondrial DNA (mtDNA). The oxidation of substrates by these proteins produces an electrochemical gradient across the inner membrane, which is used to drive the synthesis of adenosine triphosphate (ATP).

Because mitochondria are involved in energy production, it is perhaps not surprising that the mitochondrial content of cells is proportional to the energy demand of the tissue. For example, heart cells contain about 30% mitochondria by volume, the highest content of all organs within the body, as it continuously requires an elevated level of energy provision. Mitochondrial content in skeletal muscle is relatively low by comparison, as muscles are largely inactive until recruited for exercise purposes. Type I fibres generally have 5–7% mitochondria by volume, while the cell volume of mitochondria in type IIx fibres is only about 2–4% (74). However, this relatively low content compared to other tissues offers plenty of room for expansion, if the energy demands are elevated and consistent. Indeed, mitochondria exhibit considerable "plasticity" in skeletal muscle, a term coined to indicate the degree of organelle adaptability to exercise training. Mitochondria residing underneath the sarcolemma, termed "subsarcolemmal" (SS) mitochondria, adapt most readily to exercise, while those which provide energy for the myofibrils, termed intermyofibrillar, or IMF mitochondria, adapt less robustly. The increase in SS mitochondria as a result of training, for example, is about twice the response of IMF mitochondria.

The adaptive response of muscle mitochondria to exercise training has been established and characterized for over 50 years (71). Exercise training performed at an appropriately prescribed intensity, duration, and frequency per week, in combination with high-intensity intervals, can produce 50–100% increases in the level of oxidative enzymes per gram of muscle. Modest changes in mitochondrial composition favouring more densely packed electron transport chain proteins can also be observed occasionally, depending on the chronic nature of the training. It should be noted that the degree of adaptation depends also on the extent of motor unit recruitment. For example, type IIa and IIx fibres that are not recruited during low-intensity exercise will not adapt to the exercise programme. These fibres require more intense exercise for adaptations to become apparent, and this occurs in programmes of exercise training such as high-intensity interval training (HIIT). Any increase in mitochondrial content will have an impact on metabolism, leading to more favourable lipid oxidation, accompanied by reduced glycolytic flux and glycogen utilization. These physiological adaptations, along with reduced lactic acid production, contribute to the overall enhancement of endurance performance observed as a result of training. Of course, the cessation of training brings about the reverse: a decline in mitochondria and reduced endurance upon detraining.

While we have a considerable understanding of the degree of mitochondrial adaptations to exercise, it is vital to also comprehend the mechanisms of how these adaptations are induced. This would certainly facilitate potential pharmaceutical or nutritional interventions that could be added to exercise to increase mitochondrial biogenesis even further. This is also important for the ageing population, since mitochondrial content in muscle is reduced with age, a consequence of both inactivity and as age-specific reductions in the signalling pathways that trigger organelle biogenesis (73). Thus, this chapter will focus on the mechanisms of biogenesis and mitochondrial turnover that are activated by exercise and that appear to be deficient in ageing muscle.

Mitochondrial Biogenesis

Mitochondrial biogenesis refers to the expansion of the mitochondrial network within muscle. The processes that govern mitochondrial biogenesis are continuously ongoing in order to maintain organelle content and function (72, 88). In response to various stimuli, such as endurance exercise, mitochondrial biogenesis is enhanced, ultimately enhancing the metabolic health/capacity of the muscle. Understanding the processes that govern mitochondrial biogenesis in healthy skeletal muscle is important in developing interventions to prevent the progression of sarcopenia and metabolic disease.

Regulation of Biogenesis in the Nuclear Genome

Of the approximately 1200 proteins found within the mitochondria, only 1% (13 proteins) are encoded by the mitochondrial genome (161). The other proteins found within the organelle are transcribed from nuclear genes encoding mitochondrial proteins (NUGEMPs). Thus, mitochondria are created through an intricate process that requires the coordination of both the nuclear and mitochondrial genomes. The pre-millennial discovery of a cold-inducible protein, peroxisome proliferator-activated receptorPPAR) gamma coactivator 1α (PGC-1 α) (133), coupled with studies utilizing its overexpression (101, 111) and knockdown (48, 62, 63, 98, 190) have cumulatively shown that PGC-1 α is critical in determining the oxidative phenotype of muscle via its regulation of mitochondrial biogenesis. Interestingly, overexpression of PGC-1 α protects against denervation-induced skeletal muscle atrophy, signifying the importance of this co-activator in the maintenance of muscle mass (147, 167).

PGC-1 α is a transcriptional co-activator which serves to activate nuclear transcription factors such as nuclear respiratory factors 1 and 2 (NRF-1/2), PPARγ, and oestrogen-related receptors (ERR) to promote NUGEMP expression (131, 149, 150, 172). These proteins are imported into the mitochondria and incorporated into the organelle. One NUGEMP that is critical to the coordination of the nuclear and mitochondrial genomes is transcription factor A of the mitochondria (Tfam) (176), discussed later. In addition, PGC-1 α co-activates its own gene expression by positive feedback, thus acting to increase its protein content as well (5, 64). Activation of PGC-1 α and ultimately mitochondrial biogenesis, occurs in response to a variety of stimuli, many of which are induced with endurance-style exercise (72, 73).

Regulation of Biogenesis in the Mitochondrial Genome

Each mitochondrion possesses numerous copies of its own circular DNA (mtDNA), which is approximately 16.5 kb in size and contains 37 genes (6). The nuclear-encoded mitochondrial RNA polymerase

(POLRMT), mitochondrial transcription factors B1 and B2 (TFB1/2M), and Tfam mediate mtDNA transcription and replication (7, 46). Nuclear transcription of Tfam, TFB1M, and TFB2M are activated by NRF-1 and NRF-2 and co-activated by PGC-1 α. This represents an integral connection between the two genomes in the process of organelle synthesis (55, 176).

Tfam has been studied extensively in the context of muscle biology. Functionally, Tfam has high-mobility group (HGM)-box domains, which have the ability to induce a U-turn-like conformation of mtDNA allowing for the recruitment of TFB2M and POLRMT to the H and L promoters of mtDNA, ultimately promoting gene transcription (115, 140). In fact, various studies have reported that Tfam transcript levels, protein, and mitochondrial localization are enhanced when mitochondrial biogenesis is stimulated in skeletal muscle (32, 56, 94, 127, 166). Tfam also protects mtDNA from ROS-induced damage by packaging it into nucleoid-like structures (17, 116).

Regulation of Mitochondrial Biogenesis by p53

Commonly investigated for its role as a tumour suppressor, the transcription factor p53 is also identified as a regulator of mitochondrial biogenesis (10, 16, 45, 70, 107, 144). Specifically, an important feature of p53 is that it can localize within the cytoplasm, nucleus, and mitochondria to facilitate nuclear and mitochondrial gene expression (45, 70, 100, 145), likely promoting the coordinated expression of nuclear and mitochondrial genomes.

Within the nuclear genome, p53 supports mitochondrial biogenesis by up-regulating the expression of genes indicative of oxidative phenotypes such as PGC-1 α (15, 78), Tfam (15, 124, 143), and NRF-1 (143), as well as the ETC assembly protein synthesis of cytochrome C oxidase 2 (SOC2) (107). Within the mitochondrial genome, p53 induces the transcription of 16S rRNA (45) and cytochrome C oxidase subunit I (145), likely through interactions with Tfam (189). In addition to this transcriptional role, mitochondrial p53 interacts and stabilizes mtDNA (123). In fact, knockout of p53 in mice reduces basal mitochondrial content and leads to disrupted mitochondrial morphology with diminished function (15, 142, 146).

In response to acute endurance-style exercise, p53 undergoes post-translational modifications, including phosphorylation on serine15 (humans) or serine 18 (mice). This phosphorylation site is a target of both p38-MAPK (16, 155) and AMPK (16, 82). These are two kinases that are activated with endurance exercise and will be discussed in depth later in this chapter. In fact, with acute endurance exercise, p53 phosphorylation is enhanced (11, 12, 15, 142) and it becomes localized within the nucleus (59) and mitochondria (145). Importantly, although p53's absence alters basal mitochondrial health, it does not limit exercise-induced adaptations (15, 142), suggesting that there are overlapping mechanisms to promote mitochondrial biogenesis.

Mitochondrial Biogenesis and the Role of Exercise

A plethora of activators for mitochondrial biogenesis exist. This section will highlight those that relate to skeletal muscle physiology and exercise-induced mitochondrial biogenesis. It is well known that endurance-style exercise activates multiple intracellular signal transduction pathways which modulate the regulation of mitochondrial biogenesis, ultimately leading to the elevations in mitochondrial content that we observe with training regimens (72, 73). These pathways are summarized in Figure 27.1.

Perturbations in Cellular Energy Status

A potent inducer of mitochondrial biogenesis in skeletal muscle is a perturbation in cellular energy status. In particular, reductions in both intracellular ATP:AMP and NADH:NAD$^+$ are capable of promoting organelle synthesis through the activation of PGC-1 α (72, 88). In a "basal" state, PGC-1α remains dephosphorylated and acetylated, which ultimately holds it within the cytoplasm.

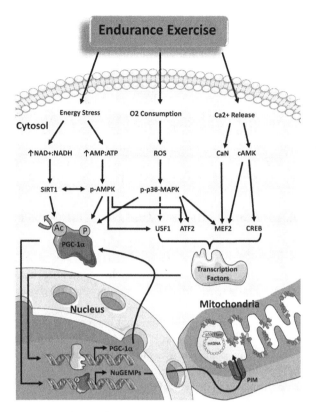

Figure 27.1 Exercise-mediated mitochondrial biogenesis. Endurance exercise leads to the activation of intracellular signalling cascades that converge to induce biogenesis through the transcription and activation of PGC-1α. PGC-1α promotes the expression of NUGEMPs. Perturbations in cellular energy status, as measured by increased NAD:NADH and AMP:ATP, activate SIRT1 and AMPK, respectively. SIRT1 deacetylates, whereas AMPK phosphorylates PGC-1a, leading to its activation and nuclear localization. Second, oxygen consumption is enhanced in working muscle leading to elevations in absolute ROS production. ROS activate p38-MAPK, which phosphorylates and stabilizes PGC-1α. p38 also activates transcription factors such as USF1, ATF2, and MEF2, which drive the transcription of PGC-1α. Third, Ca²⁺ is released from the sarcoplasmic reticulum during contraction, which acts as a secondary messenger activating the phosphatase calcineurin and Ca-calmodulin kinase, ultimately activating transcription factors such as MEF2 and CREB that promote PGC-1α transcription. Proteins will be translated within the cytosol and imported into the mitochondria by the protein import machinery (PIM), where it will drive mtDNA expression or be incorporated into the organelle, ultimately leading to the expansion of the mitochondrial network within the muscle

When cellular energy status is compromised, signified by elevations in intracellular AMP, AMP-activated protein kinase (AMPK) undergoes phosphorylation and activation (31, 58). Early reports confirmed that AMPK activation by pharmacological means enhanced skeletal muscle mitochondrial content in rats (14, 180) and mice (114), suggesting that AMPK triggers mitochondrial biogenesis. It was later confirmed that AMPK acts through the activating phosphorylation of PGC-1α on T-177 and S-538 (79). Others have also shown that AMPK activation is capable of enhancing PGC-1 α transcription (78, 79, 164), protein content (76), and activity (79). Importantly, studies that investigate loss of function or knockout of AMPK (118) have shown a failure to induce mitochondrial biogenesis in response to energy stress (195) and lower mitochondrial content. Similar deficits in mitochondrial content were found when the upstream kinase LKB1 was knocked out in skeletal muscle (80, 163). A number of studies that have used or modelled endurance exercise have shown that AMPK is activated (34, 42, 69, 76, 164, 192). There are reports that the magnitude of response is exercise intensity, duration, and modality dependent (69, 89). Importantly, inhibition of AMPK activity with compound C (CC) prevented stimulation-induced PGC-1α transcription in muscle cells (192). Similarly, AMPK knockout in muscle produces mice that are exercise-intolerant, likely due to reduced mitochondrial content (118). All these data suggest that AMPK stimulates mitochondrial biogenesis and this is likely mediated through the activation of PGC-1α.

In order for PGC-1α to enter and remain in the nucleus, it must also undergo de-acetylation via by silent mating type information regulation 2 homolog 1 (SIRT1). SIRT1 functions as a deacetylase that is sensitive to cellular energy status through elevations in NAD^+. When SIRT1 is active it deacetylates PGC-1α, promoting its nuclear localization and subsequent co-activation of NUGEMPs (26, 54, 60). Indeed, gain of function in SIRT1 promotes a slow-fibre type shift as the induction of markers of mitochondrial biogenesis (36, 175). Similarly, NAD+ precursors (28, 86, 169) which activate SIRT1 are capable of enhancing muscle mitochondrial content. In contrast, SIRT1 knockdown in muscle cells (54) and knockout in mice at both the whole-body (110) and muscle-specific (36) level reduce mitochondrial content and endurance capacity (36). Interestingly, AMPK and SIRT1 are interconnected, as AMPK activation is able to increase cellular NAD^+ levels thereby activating SIRT1, and vice versa (26, 27, 29, 135, 175). Cumulatively, these data signify the importance of SIRT1 in mediating organelle synthesis, likely through PGC1- α deacetylation. Concurrent with exercise-induced alterations in AMPK signalling, there are metabolic changes within the working muscle, in which NADH is oxidized to NAD+ to support the production of ATP by the ETC to fuel contraction. This NAD+, which increases with acute exercise (29) along with active AMPK, is capable of activating SIRT1, which can lead to PGC-1α acetylation, nuclear localization, and transcriptional activity (54). Thus, researchers have found changes in SIRT protein that acute exercise enhances SIRT1 activity and nuclear PGC-1α (61, 171).

Intracellular Calcium

Since calcium (Ca2+) is constantly in flux within skeletal muscle during contraction and relaxation cycles, researchers have tried to uncover if it plays a role in promoting an oxidative phenotype within muscle. In this context, parvalbumin binds and chaperones cytoplasmic Ca2+, thus reducing the free Ca2+ concentration in the cytoplasm within muscle. Parvalbumin knockout mice which have elevated free Ca2+ displayed higher mitochondrial content (40). The opposite was observed in parvalbumin-overexpressing mice (41). In addition, enhancement of cytosolic Ca2+ levels via pharmacological means increased mitochondria-related transcription and protein content in muscle cells (43, 50, 120). Ca2+/calmodulin dependent protein kinase (CaMK) was uncovered to be responsible for these changes via the up-regulation of PGC-1α transcriptional activity and ultimately protein content (49, 119, 138, 185, 192), and is enhanced with endurance training (137). Proposed mechanisms include CaMK's activation of cAMP response element-binding protein (CREB) and calcineurin A (CnA)'s activation of MEF2 and binding to the PGC-1α promoter (64). There is evidence that CaMK also promotes p38-MAPK activation to potentially induce mitochondrial biogenesis, as discussed later (182). In terms of exercise, when muscle cells are electrically stimulated in culture to mimic muscle contraction, there are increases in mitochondrial biogenesis, an adaptation which is prevented when the cells are co-treated with intracellular Ca2+ chelators (43, 192). This important evidence suggests that Ca2+ signalling contributes, at least in part, to mitochondrial biogenesis with exercise.

Reactive Oxygen Species

A by-product of mitochondrial respiration is the production of reactive oxygen species (ROS). Although harmful when in excess, transient elevations in ROS may be beneficial in promoting the synthesis of mitochondria through the induction of PGC-1 α expression (20, 187). For example, when skeletal muscle cells are treated with exogenous H_2O_2, PGC-1 α promoter activity and mRNA expression are enhanced (77), which may bring about elevations in mitochondrial biogenesis. One mechanism for this ROS-induced increase in organelle synthesis is via the activation of AMPK (77), which, as discussed earlier, can induce biogenesis. Uniquely, ROS can also promote biogenesis through the activation of p38-MAPK, which directly phosphorylates and stabilizes PGC-1 α (9, 47, 132). Alternatively, p38 also transcriptionally regulates PGC-1 through phosphorylation and activation of transcription factors such as MEF2 (193) and ATF2 (30), both of which regulate PGC-1α expression, as discussed later. Correspondingly, transgenic mice with overexpression of constitutively active p38-MAPK display enhanced PGC-1α expression and mitochondrial biogenesis, and mice that have inhibition of p38-MAPK show no change in PGC-1α promoter activity in response to biogenesis-inducing stimuli (2). In terms of exercise, voluntary wheel running in mice induces the activation of the p38MAPK pathway to stimulate PGC-1α expression (2). This is likely the result of ROS production during exercise (66, 130). In fact, antioxidant treatment in contracting muscle cells prevented activation of p38-MAPK and the regular contraction-induced increases in PGC-1α promoter activity (192). Similar results were also found when p38-MAPK was directly inhibited (192). Indeed, p38 is activated in response to contractile activity (34, 76, 192), muscle stretch (19), endurance exercise in humans (42, 125), and following marathon running in humans (18). Interestingly, it seems to be the p38 γisoform that is important in contraction-induced signalling, as its knockout prevents training-induced adaptations (128). Cumulatively, these data support the notion that p38-MAPK is important in the induction of mitochondrial biogenesis, particularly with exercise.

Exercise and the Regulation of PGC1- α *Expression*

As noted earlier, activation of PGC-1α is an important component of the signalling response to exercise. Exercise rapidly activates PGC-1α and promotes its nuclear localization via pathways highlighted earlier, ultimately leading to the transcription of NUGEMPs (183). This is supported by data that show that nuclear PGC-1 α is elevated in muscle taken immediately post-exercise (183) or in cells collected immediately post-stimulation (192). Additionally, PGC-1 α promoter activity is also enhanced post-contraction (34), which explains why transcript levels are elevated following muscle activity (34, 127, 164, 192). Accordingly, researchers have sought to determine how PGC-1α itself is regulated at the transcriptional level.

As with all genetic regulation, the PGC-1 α promoter has a variety of transcription factors that regulate its expression. Of these, cAMP responsive element binding protein (CREB), activating transcription factor 2 (ATF-2), myocyte enhancing factor 2 (MEF2), and upstream stimulatory factor 1 (USF1) have been investigated in the context of muscle and exercise. The activity of CREB is enhanced through Ca^{2+}–CaMK signalling, which allows it to bind to the CRE site in the PGC-1α promoter inducing transcription (64). In fact, the importance of CREB in contraction-induced PGC-1 α expression is shown in a study whereby mutations in the CRE region of the PGC-1α promoter reduce its transcription (3). ATF-2 is another cAMP-dependent transcription factor that binds to CRE in the PGC-1α promoter (2), and in response to wheel-running exercise, there is enhanced activation of ATF-2, likely promoting PGC-1 α expression (2). MEF is also involved, since site-directed mutagenesis of the MEF2 element within the PGC-1 α promoter prevented contractility-induced PGC-1α promoter activity (3). Finally, USF-1 binding to the PGC-1α promoter is enhanced both in response to treatment of muscle cells with H_2O_2 (77) and with AMPK activation (77, 78), both of which are enhanced with exercise, and this may further contribute to exercise induced-mitochondrial biogenesis. Thus, not only does exercise activate PGC-1α activation and ultimately NUGEMP expression, but it also increases PGC-1 α transcription, which will ultimately sustain elevated organelle synthesis.

Although these studies clearly show that PGC-1 α contributes to exercise-induced mitochondrial biogenesis, there are multiple reports that knockdown or silencing of PGC-1 α in vivo and in vitro does not abolish the ability of muscle to adapt to endurance exercise (1, 97, 139, 166). Thus, it seems that muscle activity stimulates independent pathways towards mitochondrial biogenesis, which have yet to be uncovered, but that can be activated when PGC-1 α is absent.

Mitochondrial Import and the Effects of Exercise

Since synthesizing mitochondria is a coordinated effort between nuclear and mitochondrial gene products, an extravagant mechanism has evolved for the over 1,200 nuclear-encoded proteins that must enter the mitochondria. This is termed the protein import machinery (PIM) pathway (179). This PIM consists of the translocase of the outer membrane (TOM) complex and the translocase of the inner membrane (TIM) complex (179). Nuclear gene products destined for the mitochondria contain a mitochondrial-targeting sequence, which signals the pre-protein to the correct location within the mitochondria. These pre-proteins can be localized to various areas of the mitochondria depending on their targeting sequence. In general, matrix-bound proteins enter through the TOM complex and they are shuttled through the TIM complex via the chaperone mtHsp70. The newly imported proteins are then processed by mitochondrial processing peptidase (MPP), and they are refolded into a mature form with the aid of mitochondrial chaperones (121, 178, 179). This import machinery is critically important, as many disorders are associated with its dysfunction (106). Endurance training has been shown to increase the expression of PIM components and enhance the kinetics of protein import into the mito-chondria (56, 84, 162). For example, Tfam import is accelerated by chronic exercise (56), and this serves to help coordinate the expression of mtDNA with that of nuclear gene expression.

Mitophagy

Mitochondrial biogenesis is important to the enhancement of oxidative capacity in muscle through ele-vating mitochondrial content. However, in order to maintain organelle health within the muscle, those that are damaged or dysfunctional must be removed (72, 165). In fact, when mitochondrial breakdown is inhibited in skeletal muscle, there is impaired muscle health.

The selective degradation of mitochondria utilizing the autophagy–lysosome system is termed mitophagy. Preceding the breakdown of these organelles, damaged mitochondrial segments are removed from the network of mitochondria through fission (122, 170). Following fission, a multistep process ensues. Briefly, this includes organelle targeting, engulfment in a double membrane autophagosome, and finally transport to and degradation within the lysosome (165).

Molecular Pathways Regulating Mitophagy

Targeting of mitochondria for breakdown occurs via several possible pathways, although only two have been investigated in muscle. The first, and simpler, method, is mediated by BCL2/adenovirus E1B 19kDA protein interacting 3 (BNIP3) (65, 134, 191, 194), a mitophagy receptor. This protein, when recruited to the outer mitochondrial membrane (OMM), interacts with autophagosome embedded proteins such as LC3 and GABARAP. Alternatively, a more intricate process begins with the OMM localization of PTEN-induced putative kinase (PINK1) (81, 92, 108, 113), a kinase that is normally imported into healthy mitochondria and degraded (81, 126). This active form of PINK1 recruits and phosphorylates the E3-ubiquitin ligase Parkin (92, 108, 113, 156), which poly-ubiquitinates OMM proteins (148). These poly-ubiquitin chains bind to adapter proteins such as SQSTM1 (also referred to as p62) (53) or optineurin (181), which act as a tethering point between the mitochondrion and the autophagosome through binding with the embedded LC3-II or GABARAP. Both processes ultimately lead to organelle degradation.

The Effect of Exercise on Mitophagy in Muscle

Various studies have examined the effects of acute exercise and endurance training on mitophagic signalling. For example, acute endurance exercise in humans at about 60% VO_2Max for 60 minutes increases muscle BNIP3 protein (21). This same study also reported that 8 weeks of cycle training increased whole muscle levels of BNIP3 protein (21). Other forms of training such as 4–5 weeks of voluntary wheel running (22, 186) or 9 days of chronic contractile activity (CCA) (33) led to elevations muscle BNIP3 protein. There is also evidence of increased BNIP3 in the mitochondrial fraction of mice following acute exercise (105).

Considerable work has been done investigating PINK1-Parkin–mediated mitophagic targeting with exercise. In wild-type mice, acute exercise results in elevated whole-muscle Parkin (188) and enhanced localization of Parkin and ubiquitin to mitochondria (38, 154, 168). In response to endurance training in rodents, there is elevated resting Parkin protein in the whole-muscle samples (22, 38) and in isolated mitochondria (38). Human subjects showed a similar response to training as well (21). Importantly, Parkin knockout mice have a blunted exercise-induced elevation in mitophagy and an attenuation of endurance training adaptations (38), signifying the importance of this system in exercise-induced mitochondrial adaptations.

In animal models of exercise, various techniques to measure mitophagy flux have been developed. Cumulatively, studies have shown that acute endurance exercise or muscle activity enhances mitophagy flux (38, 39, 87, 95, 168). This likely represents a signal to remove old/dysfunctional mitochondria with the aim of enhancing the health of the mitochondrial pool within the active muscle. In addition, in resting muscle following the cessation of endurance training in the form of 8-week swim training (85) or a period of CC (33, 87), there is reduced mitophagy flux vs. untrained counterparts. This adaptation occurs because training enhances the health of the organelle, thus eliminating the need to remove organelles. When acute exercise is performed following a training regimen in rodents and humans, the exercise-induced increase in mitophagy flux is ameliorated (38, 102) because the requirement to clear organelles in response to a stress, such as exercise, is diminished.

Impact of Ageing on Muscle and Mitochondria

Sarcopenia is defined as the age-related decline in skeletal muscle mass, function, and quality. The following section will discuss age-dependent alterations in muscle, specifically mitochondria, and the impact of exercise as a potential rejuvenator of aged muscle. An illustration of morphological changes to aged muscle is summarized in Figure 27.2.

Muscle Atrophy and Dysfunction

After the age of 50, a person loses 0.5–1% of muscle mass per year, resulting in a 40% decrease by 80 years old, and a 2- to 3-fold increase in functional disability (13). The elderly population (>65 years) with the least muscle strength are also at a higher risk of mortality, suggesting that strength is a strong predictor of healthy ageing (141). The age-related decline of strength can be attributed to multiple factors. Aged tissue is morphologically very different from young muscle. Alterations in muscle architecture such as increased fat infiltration and connective tissue reduce the overall quality of muscle (160). Single fibres have been isolated from muscle biopsies of young and old men, and the maximal force was reduced in aged myofibres (51). Contractile function is further exacerbated by muscle atrophy. In humans, the decline in muscle mass is due to a decrease in fibre number and an increase in fibre atrophy (99). Rodent studies indicate that the most significant declines in muscle mass are observed in the quadriceps muscles, with a concomitant decline in fibre number (24).

Quadriceps muscles are one of the largest muscle groups in the body involved in mild to vigorous activities. Muscle fibre type composition varies across the muscle groups, rendering some muscles more susceptible to sarcopenia. Fibres can be generally categorized as type I and type II fibres. Type I have reduced ATPase levels, slower contraction times, lower peak force, and increased resistance to fatigue compared to type II fibres. Due to these characteristics type I fibres are also known as "slow twitch," whereas type II are known as "fast twitch" fibres. Muscle atrophy is evident mainly in muscles composed of type II fibres such as the quadriceps muscles. Furthermore, the number of type II muscle

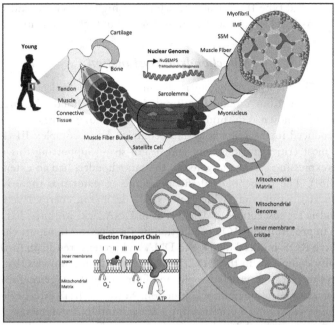

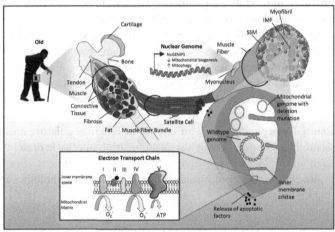

Figure 27.2 Skeletal muscle deterioration with ageing. Muscle undergoes a vast number of changes as an individual becomes older. Muscle is composed of fascicles, which are bundles of muscle fibres. In older people, there are fewer fibres in a fibre bundle, and fibres have a smaller cross-sectional area in comparison to young fibres. Aged fibres are also prone to regions of atrophy that differ along fibre length, which is evident in a longitudinal view of the muscle. Muscle is also composed of connective tissue, fat, and other cell types. Satellite cells are the resident pool of muscle stem cells required for regeneration. There is an age-dependent decline in satellite cell number and function, which exacerbates muscle atrophy. Satellite cells are naturally in a quiescent state but when activated, they fuse with existing myofibres to repair damage. The nuclei of satellite cells become an extension of the multinucleated fibre. A decline in myonuclear number is seen with age, partly due to smaller satellite cell numbers and increasing cell death from stress signals within the fibre. The muscle fibre is composed of myofilaments and mitochondria. Mitochondria that lie underneath the sarcolemma are termed subsarcolemmal (SS), whereas the mitochondrial pool between myofilaments are intermyofibrillar mitochondria (IMF). In young fibres, IMF mitochondria are fused, whereas in aged fibres they are more fragmented. Aged mitochondria also exhibit a loss of internal structure of their cristae, increasing ROS levels, and damage to mtDNA and are more susceptible to apoptosis. The electron transport chain is less efficient in producing ATP. Regulation of mitochondrial biogenesis by the nucleus is also reduced, and with increasing mitophagy the consequence is that aged muscle has reduced mitochondrial content

fibres declines with age, and type II–enriched muscles have higher levels of oxidative stress as well as increased susceptibility to apoptosis (35) and an abundance of mitochondrial abnormalities (24).

Mitochondrial Dysfunction

One of the most popular theories of ageing is the mitochondrial free radical theory. The theory postulates that ageing results from a gradual accumulation of mitochondrial damage from ROS. The free radical theory became known as the mitochondrial theory following the discovery that the majority of the ROS were produced in the mitochondria at complex I and complex III (112). Mitochondrial ROS production is most critical to longevity and health span. Supporting this theory, research on transgenic mice overexpressing catalase targeted to the mitochondria had an extension in median and maximal life span (151). The mitochondrial theory of ageing states that there is an age-dependent increase in mitochondrial dysfunction, which results in a decline in energy levels and an increase in cell death. Mitochondria are susceptible to damage, as mtDNA lacks histones, has an inefficient DNA repair system, and is in proximity to ROS production by the electron transport chain. A vicious cycle of events occurs, where ROS-induced damage to DNA and proteins results in further enhanced ROS production from faulty complexes in the ETC. With normal ageing, muscles that exhibit mitochondrial dysfunction have the greatest muscle atrophy and fibre loss (24), suggesting that the organelle can contribute to the age-related decline in muscle function. Mitochondria's direct role on sarcopenia was tested in transgenic mice expressing a proofreading-deficient mtDNA polymerase. The mice had high levels of mtDNA mutations and exhibited premature ageing phenotypes such as shortened life span, accelerated osteoporosis, weight loss, sarcopenia, and increased apoptosis (93).

Mitochondria from aged muscle exhibit a loss of internal cristae structure and are generally reduced in size and number. Smaller fragmented mitochondria have been observed in aged rats (75) and humans (83). The morphology of mitochondria is controlled by several factors. Fusion of the outer mitochondrial membranes is regulated by OPA1 and MFN1/2, while fragmentation of mitochondria is controlled by FIS1 and Drp1. In aged tissue, there is a decline of mitochondrial fusion proteins (83) and an increase in fission proteins (75), resulting in the age-dependent increase of fragmented mitochondria. Importantly, mitochondrial morphology plays an important role in regulating muscle mass. When the fission machinery was inhibited in mice, there was an attenuation in muscle mass loss (136). Along with increased fragmentation and reduced expression of fusion proteins, most studies indicate that mitochondrial function is also reduced in aged muscle, suggesting that morphology can regulate not only organelle function but also muscle mass.

Mitochondrial Quality Control

The quality of mitochondria is maintained via two major pathways: the generation of healthy mitochondria (mitochondrial biogenesis) and the degradation of dysfunctional mitochondria (mitophagy). In healthy muscle, both mechanisms work in tandem to maintain a steady-state level of mitochondrial content. However, in aged muscle reduced synthesis and/or increased mitophagy occurs, which skews the balance to reduce the content of organelles.

A lower mitochondrial content in aged muscle is likely due to declining levels of PGC-1α, a coactivator for NUGEMPs) (35, 104), a reduced drive for transcriptional activity of PGC-1α, and an instability of PGC-1α mRNA (34). Transgenic mice completely lacking PGC-1α have severe depletion of mitochondrial content, function, and increase in susceptibility to apoptosis (1), whereas animals overexpressing PGC-1α have increased mitochondrial content (25) and are protected from atrophy due to muscle disuse (177). Not only does PGC-1α regulate biogenesis but it also maintains mitochondrial homeostasis through the degradation of dysfunctional mitochondria via autophagy (167). In aged muscle, there is a greater localization of the autophagy and mitophagy markers LC3-II and PARKIN to the mitochondria, suggesting an increase in mitophagy (117). The application of colchicine, an autophagy inhibitor, can be used to evaluate autophagic flux in young and aged rodent models. Results indicated that autophagy flux was elevated with age (8, 90). To evaluate mitophagic flux, mitochondrial fraction is isolated from whole muscle from aged animals and the localization of mitophagy markers is assessed. Mitophagic flux was also elevated with age (33), suggesting that the mitophagy pathway may be a contributing factor to reduced mitochondrial content observed in ageing.

Mitochondrial DNA Mutations

Multiple copies of the mtDNA are present per organelle, giving rise to heteroplasmy, which is the mixture of wild-type and mutated genomes. As mutated mtDNA accumulate to high thresholds, phenotypical features of mitochondrial disease or ageing develop. The most frequently identified deletion mutation in mtDNA is the 4977 bp deletion that spans the major arc of the mitochondrial genome (103). The frequency of other, less common, deletion products also increases in aged muscle with a concomitant decline in mitochondrial activity (153). In tissue homogenates from aged muscle, the abundance of mtDNA deletions is very low (0.1-1.0%) (158). However, upon isolation of smaller fibre groups, the abundance of mtDNA deletions drastically increases (152). In single fibres from aged muscle, a unique mtDNA deletion clonally expands to an abundance level of >90% (67). Recent studies have employed techniques, such as digital polymerase chain reaction (PCR), where individual mtDNA deletion products undergo discrete PCR reactions to accurately measure mtDNA deletion frequency. In individual aged fibres, there is an age-dependent decline in mtDNA wild-type genomes, as well as an increase in mtDNA deletion frequency. The change in mitochondrial genomes is correlated with an increase in fibres with a deficient electron transport chain (68). Furthermore, muscle dysfunction was only present in homozygous mtDNA polymerase–deficient mice that had high levels of mtDNA deletions (174). Hence mitochondrial genomic integrity is essential in maintaining mitochondrial function and muscle health.

Mitochondrially Mediated Apoptosis

Mitochondria not only produce energy but also play an integral part in intracellular calcium regulation, the regulation of the membrane potential, steroid synthesis, hormone signalling, and apoptosis. Mitochondria have an important role in the intrinsic pathway of apoptosis, as the intermembrane space houses many proteins that are integral in initiating apoptosis. Once a cell death stimulus is received, apoptotic factors in the cytosol translocate to the mitochondria and permeabilize the outer mitochondrial membrane. Cytochrome c is released into the cytosol which cleaves procaspase 9, thus activating its caspase activity. A subsequent caspase cascade is initiated, which results in DNA fragmentation, the formation of apoptotic bodies, and ultimately cell death.

In aged muscle tissue, there is an increase in DNA stand breaks and proapoptotic factors such as cytosolic cytochrome c, procaspase-3, and APAF-1 (44). Myofibres undergoing cell death are abundant in mouse myopathy models, which are primarily characterized by progressive muscle weakness and wasting. Transgenic mice that express a deficient DNA polymerase exhibit extreme muscle wasting and significant amounts of apoptotic protein expression, suggesting a role of cell death in myofibre loss (93). These studies support the hypothesis that in normal ageing, cell death pathways may contribute to fibre loss and muscle atrophy.

Myofibres are multinucleated, and the loss of one nucleus causes decay of the cytoplasmic domain surrounding the nucleus, which results in localized fibre atrophy. Fibre atrophy can also occur via apoptosis of myonuclei. There is an age-dependant decline in the size of myonuclear domain (4), and aged myonuclei have high levels of DNA endonucleases (57), suggesting the loss of individual nuclei via apoptosis. Aged fibres that are mitochondrial dysfunctional are ~90% apoptotic and necrotic. The focal segment of a fibre that is apoptotic is also atrophic, suggesting that cell death pathways play a role in age-related fibre atrophy and loss (37). The loss of myonucleus may in part also be due to the lack of satellite cell activation. Satellite cells are the resident muscle stem cells that are activated when the muscle requires repair. They fuse with existing myofibres to provide additional nuclei. As a person ages the satellite number decreases, and this also contributes to fibre atrophy (173).

Exercise Benefits for Ageing

Exercise imparts a plethora of physiological and psychological benefits that have rejuvenating effects across the whole body. The following section will focus on the effects of exercise observed in aged muscle and the impact on mitochondria.

Impact on Muscle

Exercise is a powerful intervention in combatting age-associated diseases. Individuals that are sedentary have the highest mortality risk due to cardiovascular diseases and other age-related morbidities (159). Older individuals, (>65 years) that are moderately active have an attenuation of sarcopenic changes (96). Master athletes, participants of lifelong exercise, retain their lean muscle mass and specific muscle force with age (184). Endurance exercise training that stimulates an increase in heart rate and blood flow also has been shown to induce similar effects on muscle mass and function in aged individuals (157). Similarly, resistance exercise has proven to increase muscle mass, strength, and hypertrophy in old individuals. However, aged people over 80 years do not adapt as well as younger individuals, suggesting that there are intrinsic age-related effects which affect the adaptation response (129).

Impact on Mitochondria

Profound mitochondrial adaptations occur in the skeletal muscle of young and aged individuals following a regular exercise regimen. Exercise improves cardiovascular health and aerobic capacity in the elderly. This is correlated with a larger mitochondrial volume density (23). Furthermore, exercise reverses the aged transcriptome in physically active older subjects to the transcriptomic profile of a younger muscle. Most of the genes affected are involved in mitochondrial function and metabolism (109). Similarly, in rodent muscle, training reverses the ageing phenotypes typically observed. Skeletal muscle from trained rats have an increase in protein abundances of PGC-1α, increases in mtDNA, mitochondrial mass, complexes in the ETC, and mitochondrial transcriptional regulators such as Tfam (91). Experiments using chronic contractile activity (CCA) as a model of exercise in rodents have indicated that in aged muscle, CCA for 7 days can attenuate the decline in PGC-1α along with mitochondrial dysfunction. Chronic exercise restored mitochondrial activity and function in aged rodents (34). In mice, lifelong exercise induced mitochondrial biogenesis, prevented symptoms of muscle frailty, and improved the overall healthspan with no change in lifespan (52). Despite these rejuvenating effects on mitochondria and overall health, mitochondrial adaptations to exercise in aged muscle are not as robust to what is observed in young muscle (104), suggesting that some mitochondrial dysfunction is inherent to the ageing phenotype and not due to muscle disuse that accompanies the physical inactivity with age.

References

1. Adhihetty PJ, Uguccioni G, Leick L, Hidalgo J, Pilegaard H, Hood DA. The role of PGC-1alpha on mitochondrial function and apoptotic susceptibility in muscle. *Am J Physiol Cell Physiol* 297: C217–C225, 2009.
2. Akimoto T, Pohnert SC, Li P, Zhang M, Gumbs C, Rosenberg PB, et al. Exercise stimulates Pgc-1α transcription in skeletal muscle through activation of the p38 MAPK pathway. *J Biol Chem* 280: 19587–19593, 2005.
3. Akimoto T, Sorg BS, Yan Z. Real-time imaging of peroxisome proliferator-activated receptor-γ coactivator-1α promoter activity in skeletal muscles of living mice. *Am J Physiol Physiol* 287: C790–C796, 2004.
4. Alway SE, Siu PM. Nuclear apoptosis contributes to sarcopenia. *Exerc Sport Sci Rev* 36: 51–7, 2008.

5. Amat R, Planavila A, Chen SL, Iglesias R, Giralt M, Villarroya F. SIRT1 controls the transcription of the peroxisome proliferator-activated receptor-gamma Co-activator-1alpha (PGC-1alpha) gene in skeletal muscle through the PGC-1alpha autoregulatory loop and interaction with MyoD. *J Biol Chem* 284: 21872–80, 2009.

6. Anderson S, Bankier AT, Barrell BG, de Bruijn MH, Coulson AR, Drouin J, et al. Sequence and organization of the human mitochondrial genome. *Nature* 290: 457–465, 1981.

7. Arnold JJ, Smidansky ED, Moustafa IM, Cameron CE. Human mitochondrial RNA polymerase: structure-function, mechanism and inhibition. *Biochim Biophys Acta - Gene Regul Mech* 1819: 948–960, 2012.

8. Baehr LM, West DWD, Marcotte G, Marshall AG, De Sousa LG, Baar K, et al. Age-related deficits in skeletal muscle recovery following disuse are associated with neuromuscular junction instability and ER stress, not impaired protein synthesis. *Aging (Albany NY)* 8: 127–146, 2016.

9. Barger PM, Browning AC, Garner AN, Kelly DP. P38 mitogen-activated protein kinase activates peroxisome proliferator-activated receptor alpha: a potential role in the cardiac metabolic stress response. *J Biol Chem* 276: 44495–501, 2001.

10. Bartlett JD, Close GL, Drust B, Morton JP. The emerging role of p53 in exercise metabolism. *Sport Med* 44: 303–309, 2014.

11. Bartlett JD, Hwa Joo C, Jeong T-S, Louhelainen J, Cochran AJ, Gibala MJ, et al. Matched work high-intensity interval and continuous running induce similar increases in PGC-1 mRNA, AMPK, p38, and p53 phosphorylation in human skeletal muscle. *J Appl Physiol* 112: 1135–1143, 2012.

12. Bartlett JD, Louhelainen J, Iqbal Z, Cochran AJ, Gibala MJ, Gregson W, et al. Reduced carbohydrate availability enhances exercise-induced p53 signaling in human skeletal muscle: implications for mitochondrial biogenesis. *Am J Physiol Regul Integr Comp Physiol* 304: R450–R458, 2013.

13. Baumgartner RN, Koehler KM, Gallagher D, Romero L, Heymsfield SB, Ross RR, et al. Epidemiology of sarcopenia among the elderly in New Mexico. *Am J Epidemiol* 147: 755–763, 1998.

14. Bergeron R, Ren JM, Cadman KS, Moore IK, Perret P, Pypaert M, et al. Chronic activation of AMP kinase results in NRF-1 activation and mitochondrial biogenesis. *Am J Physiol - Endocrinol Metab* 281; E1340-E1346, 2001.

15. Beyfuss K, Erlich AT, Triolo M, Hood DA. The role of p53 in determining mitochondrial adaptations to endurance training in skeletal muscle. *Sci Rep* 8: 14710, 2018.

16. Beyfuss K, Hood DA. A systematic review of p53 regulation of oxidative stress in skeletal muscle. *Redox Rep* 23: 100–117, 2018.

17. Bogenhagen DF. Mitochondrial DNA nucleoid structure. *Biochim Biophys Acta - Gene Regul Mech* 1819: 914–920, 2012.

18. Boppart MD, Asp S, Wojtaszewski JFP, Fielding RA, Mohr T, Goodyear LJ. Marathon running transiently increases c-Jun NH2-terminal kinase and p38γ activities in human skeletal muscle. *J Physiol* 526: 663, 2000.

19. Boppart MD, Hirshman MF, Sakamoto K, Fielding RA, Goodyear LJ. Static stretch increases c-Jun NH$_2$-terminal kinase activity and p38 phosphorylation in rat skeletal muscle. *Am J Physiol Physiol* 280: C352–C358, 2001.

20. Bouchez C, Devin A. Mitochondrial biogenesis and mitochondrial Reactive Oxygen Species (ROS): a complex relationship regulated by the cAMP/PKA signaling pathway. *Cells* 8:287, 2019.

21. Brandt N, Gunnarsson TP, Bangsbo J, Pilegaard H. Exercise and exercise training-induced increase in autophagy markers in human skeletal muscle. *Physiol Rep* 6: e13651, 2018.

22. Brandt N, Nielsen L, Thiellesen Buch B, Gudiksen A, Ringholm S, Hellsten Y, et al. Impact of β-adrenergic signaling in PGC-1α-mediated adaptations in mouse skeletal muscle. *Am J Physiol Metab* 314: E1–E20, 2018.

23. Broskey NT, Greggio C, Boss A, Boutant M, Dwyer A, Schlueter L, et al. Skeletal muscle mitochondria in the elderly: effects of physical fitness and exercise training. *J Clin Endocrinol Metab* 99: 1852–1861, 2014.

24. Bua EA, McKiernan SH, Wanagat J, McKenzie D, Aiken JM. Mitochondrial abnormalities are more frequent in muscles undergoing sarcopenia. *J Appl Physiol* 92: 2617–2624, 2002.

25. Calvo JA, Daniels TG, Wang X, Paul A, Lin J, Spiegelman BM, et al. Muscle-specific expression of PPARgamma coactivator-1alpha improves exercise performance and increases peak oxygen uptake. *J Appl Physiol* 104: 1304–1312, 2008.

26. Cantó C, Auwerx J. PGC-1alpha, SIRT1 and AMPK, an energy sensing network that controls energy expenditure. *Curr Opin Lipidol* 20: 98–105, 2009.

27. Cantó C, Gerhart-Hines Z, Feige JN, Lagouge M, Noriega L, Milne JC, et al. AMPK regulates energy expenditure by modulating NAD+ metabolism and SIRT1 activity. *Nature* 458: 1056–60, 2009.

28. Cantó C, Houtkooper RH, Pirinen E, Youn DY, Oosterveer MH, Cen Y, et al. The NAD+ precursor nicotinamide riboside enhances oxidative metabolism and protects against high-fat diet-induced obesity. *Cell Metab* 15: 838–847, 2012.

29. Cantó C, Jiang LQ, Deshmukh AS, Mataki C, Coste A, Lagouge M, et al. Interdependence of AMPK and SIRT1 for metabolic adaptation to fasting and exercise in skeletal muscle. *Cell Metab* 11: 213–219, 2010.

30. Cao W, Daniel KW, Robidoux J, Puigserver P, Medvedev AV, Bai X, et al. P38 mitogen-activated protein kinase is the central regulator of cyclic AMP-dependent transcription of the brown fat uncoupling protein 1 gene. *Mol Cell Biol* 24: 3057–3067, 2004.

31. Carling D. The AMP-activated protein kinase cascade – a unifying system for energy control. *Trends Biochem Sci* 29: 18–24, 2004.

32. Carter HN, Hood DA. Contractile activity-induced mitochondrial biogenesis and mTORC1. *AJP Cell Physiol* 303: C540–C547, 2012.

33. Carter HN, Kim Y, Erlich AT, Zarrin-khat D, Hood DA. Autophagy and mitophagy flux in young and aged skeletal muscle following chronic contractile activity. *J Physiol* 596: 3567–3584, 2018.

34. Carter HN, Pauly M, Tryon LD, Hood DA. Effect of contractile activity on PGC-1 transcription in young and aged skeletal muscle. *J Appl Physiol* 124: 1605–1615, 2018.

35. Chabi B, Ljubicic V, Menzies KJ, Huang JH, Saleem A, Hood DA. Mitochondrial function and apoptotic susceptibility in aging skeletal muscle. *Aging Cell* 7: 2–12, 2008.

36. Chalkiadaki A, Igarashi M, Nasamu AS, Knezevic J, Guarente L. Muscle-specific SIRT1 gain-of-function increases slow-twitch fibers and ameliorates pathophysiology in a mouse model of duchenne muscular dystrophy. *PLOS Genet* 10: e1004490, 2014.

37. Cheema N, Herbst A, Mckenzie D, Aiken JM. Apoptosis and necrosis mediate skeletal muscle fiber loss in age-induced mitochondrial enzymatic abnormalities. *Aging Cell* 14: 1085–1093, 2015.

38. Chen CC, Erlich AT, Hood DA. Role of parkin and endurance training on mitochondrial turnover in skeletal muscle. *Skelet Muscle* 8: 1–14, 2018.

39. Chen CCW, Erlich AT, Crilly MJ, Hood DA. Parkin is required for exercise-induced mitophagy in muscle: impact of aging. *Am J Physiol Metab* 315: E404–E415, 2018.

40. Chen G, Carroll S, Racay P, Dick J, Pette D, Traub I, et al. Deficiency in parvalbumin increases fatigue resistance in fast-twitch muscle and upregulates mitochondria. *Am J Physiol Cell Physiol* 281: C114–122, 2001.

41. Chin ER, Grange RW, Viau F, Simard AR, Humphries C, Shelton J, et al. Alterations in slow-twitch muscle phenotype in transgenic mice overexpressing the Ca2+buffering protein parvalbumin. *J Physiol* 547: 649–663, 2003.

42. Combes A, Dekerle J, Webborn N, Watt P, Bougault V, Daussin FN. Exercise-induced metabolic fluctuations influence AMPK, p38-MAPK and CaMKII phosphorylation in human skeletal muscle. *Physiol Rep* 3:e12462, 2015.

43. Connor MK, Irrcher I, Hood DA. Contractile activity-induced transcriptional activation of cytochrome C involves Sp1 and is proportional to mitochondrial ATP synthesis in C2C12 muscle cells. *J Biol Chem* 276: 15898–15904, 2001.

44. Dirks AJ, Leeuwenburgh C. Aging and lifelong calorie restriction result in adaptations of skeletal muscle apoptosis repressor, apoptosis-inducing factor, X-linked inhibitor of apoptosis, caspase-3, and caspase-12. *Free Radic Biol Med* 36: 27–39, 2004.

45. Donahue RJ, Razmara M, Hoek JB, Knudsen TB. Direct influence of the p53 tumor suppressor on mitochondrial biogenesis and function. *FASEB J* 15: 635–644, 2001.

46. Falkenberg M, Larsson N-G, Gustafsson CM. DNA replication and transcription in mammalian mitochondria. *Annu Rev Biochem* 76: 679–699, 2007.

47. Fan M, Rhee J, St-Pierre J, Handschin C, Puigserver P, Lin J, et al. Suppression of mitochondrial respiration through recruitment of p160 myb binding protein to PGC-1α: modulation by p38 MAPK. *Genes Dev* 18: 278–289, 2004.

48. Finley LWS, Lee J, Souza A, Desquiret-Dumas V, Bullock K, Rowe GC, et al. Skeletal muscle transcriptional coactivator PGC-1α mediates mitochondrial, but not metabolic, changes during calorie restriction. *Proc Natl Acad Sci U S A* 109: 2931–6, 2012.

49. Freyssenet D, Di Carlo M, Hood DA. Calcium-dependent regulation of cytochrome c gene expression in skeletal muscle cells. Identification of a Protein Kinase C-Dependent Pathway. *J Biol Chem* 274: 9305–9311, 1999.

50. Freyssenet D, Irrcher I, Connor MK, Di Carlo M, Hood D a. Calcium-regulated changes in mitochondrial phenotype in skeletal muscle cells. *Am J Physiol Cell Physiol* 286: C1053–C1061, 2004.

51. Frontera WR, Hughes VA, Fielding RA, Fiatarone MA, Evans WJ, Roubenoff R. Aging of skeletal muscle: a 12-yr longitudinal study. *J Appl Physiol* 88: 1321–1326, 2000.

52. Garcia-Valles R, Gomez-Cabrera M, Rodriguez-Mañas L, Garcia-Garcia FJ, Diaz A, Noguera I, et al. Lifelong spontaneous exercise does not prolong lifespan but improves health span in mice. *Longev Heal* 2: 14, 2013.

53. Geisler S, Holmström KM, Skujat D, Fiesel FC, Rothfuss OC, Kahle PJ, et al. PINK1/parkin-mediated mitophagy is dependent on VDAC1 and p62/SQSTM1. *Nat Cell Biol* 12: 119–131, 2010.

54. Gerhart-Hines Z, Rodgers JT, Bare O, Lerin C, Kim S-H, Mostoslavsky R, et al. Metabolic control of muscle mitochondrial function and fatty acid oxidation through SIRT1/PGC-1alpha. *EMBO J* 26: 1913–1923, 2007.

55. Gleyzer N, Vercauteren K, Scarpulla RC. Control of mitochondrial transcription specificity factors (TFB1M and TFB2M) by nuclear respiratory factors (NRF-1 and NRF-2) and PGC-1 family coactivators. *Mol Cell Biol* 25: 1354–1366, 2005.

56. Gordon JW, Rungi AA, Inagaki H, Hood DA. Effects of contractile activity on mitochondrial transcription factor a expression in skeletal muscle. *J Appl Physiol* 90: 389–396, 2001.

57. Gouspillou G, Sgarioto N, Kapchinsky S, Purves-Smith F, Norris B, Pion CH, et al. Increased sensitivity to mitochondrial permeability transition and myonuclear translocation of endonuclease G in atrophied muscle of physically active older humans. *FASEB J* 28: 1621–1633, 2014.

58. Gowans GJ, Hawley SA, Ross FA, Hardie DG. AMP is a true physiological regulator of amp-activated protein kinase by both allosteric activation and enhancing net phosphorylation. *Cell Metab* 18: 556–566, 2013.

59. Granata C, Oliveira RSF, Little JP, Renner K, Bishop DJ. Sprint-interval but not continuous exercise increases PGC-1α protein content and p53 phosphorylation in nuclear fractions of human skeletal muscle. *Sci Rep* 7: 44227, 2017.

60. Gurd BJ. Deacetylation of PGC-1α by SIRT1: importance for skeletal muscle function and exercise-induced mitochondrial biogenesis. *Appl Physiol Nutr Metab* 36: 589–597, 2011.

61. Gurd BJ, Yoshida Y, McFarlan JT, Holloway GP, Moyes CD, Heigenhauser GJF, et al. Nuclear SIRT1 activity, but not protein content, regulates mitochondrial biogenesis in rat and human skeletal muscle. *Am J Physiol - Regul Integr Comp Physiol* 301: R67–R75, 2011.

62. Handschin C, Cheol SC, Chin S, Kim S, Kawamori D, Kurpad AJ, et al. Abnormal glucose homeostasis in skeletal muscle-specific PGC-1α knockout mice reveals skeletal muscle-pancreatic β cell crosstalk. *J Clin Invest* 117: 3463–3474, 2007.

63. Handschin C, Chin S, Li P, Liu F, Maratos-Flier E, LeBrasseur NK, et al. Skeletal muscle fiber-type switching, exercise intolerance, and myopathy in PGC-1α muscle-specific knock-out animals. *J Biol Chem* 282: 30014–30021, 2007.

64. Handschin C, Rhee J, Lin J, Tarr PT, Spiegelman BM. An autoregulatory loop controls peroxisome proliferator-activated receptor gamma coactivator 1alpha expression in muscle. *Proc Natl Acad Sci U S A* 100: 7111–6, 2003.

65. Hanna RA, Quinsay MN, Orogo AM, Giang K, Rikka S, Gustafsson ÅB. Microtubule-associated protein 1 light chain 3 (LC3) interacts with Bnip3 protein to selectively remove endoplasmic reticulum and mitochondria via autophagy. *J Biol Chem* 287: 19094–19104, 2012.

66. He F, Li J, Liu Z, Chuang CC, Yang W, Zuo L. Redox mechanism of reactive oxygen species in exercise. *Front Physiol* 7: 1–10, 2016.

67. Herbst A, Pak JW, McKenzie D, Bua E, Bassiouni M, Aiken JM. Accumulation of mitochondrial DNA deletion mutations in aged muscle fibers: evidence for a causal role in muscle fiber loss. *Journals Gerontol - Ser A Biol Sci Med Sci* 62: 235–245, 2007.

68. Herbst A, Widjaja K, Nguy B, Lushaj EB, Moore TM, Hevener AL, et al. Digital PCR quantitation of muscle mitochondrial DNA: age, fiber type, and mutation-induced changes. *Journals Gerontol - Ser A Biol Sci Med Sci* 72: 1327–1333, 2017.

69. Herzig S, Shaw RJ. AMPK: guardian of metabolism and mitochondrial homeostasis. *Nat Rev Mol Cell Biol* 19: 121–135, 2018.

70. Heyne K, Mannebach S, Wuertz E, Knaup KX, Mahyar-Roemer M, Roemer K. Identification of a putative p53 binding sequence within the human mitochondrial genome. *FEBS Lett* 578: 198–202, 2004.

71. Holloszy JO. Biochemical adaptations in muscle. *J Biol Chem* 242: 2278–2282, 1967.

72. Hood DA, Memme JM, Oliveira AN, Triolo M. Maintenance of skeletal muscle mitochondria in health, exercise, and aging. *Annu Rev Physiol* 81:19–41, 2019.

73. Hood DA, Tryon LD, Carter HN, Kim Y, Chen CCW. Unravelling the mechanisms regulating muscle mitochondrial biogenesis. *Biochem J* 473: 2295–2314, 2016.

74. Hoppeler H. Exercise-induced ultrastructural changes in skeletal muscle. *Int J Sports Med* 07: 187–204, 1986.

75. Iqbal S, Ostojic O, Singh K, Joseph A-M, Hood DA. Expression of mitochondrial fission and fusion regulatory proteins in skeletal muscle during chronic use and disuse. *Muscle Nerve* 48: 963–970, 2013.

76. Irrcher I, Adhihetty PJ, Sheehan T, Joseph A-M, Hood DA. PPARγ coactivator-1α expression during thyroid hormone- and contractile activity-induced mitochondrial adaptations. *Am J Physiol Physiol* 284: C1669–C1677, 2003.

77. Irrcher I, Ljubicic V, Hood DA. Interactions between ROS and AMP kinase activity in the regulation of PGC-1alpha transcription in skeletal muscle cells. *Am J Physiol Cell Physiol* 296: C116–23, 2009.
78. Irrcher I, Ljubicic V, Kirwan AF, Hood DA. AMP-activated protein kinase-regulated activation of the PGC-1αpromoter in skeletal muscle cells. *PLOS ONE* 3: e3614, 2008.
79. Jäger S, Handschin C, St-Pierre J, Spiegelman BM. AMP-activated protein kinase (AMPK) action in skeletal muscle via direct phosphorylation of PGC-1alpha. *Proc Natl Acad Sci U S A* 104: 12017–12022, 2007.
80. Jeppesen J, Maarbjerg SJ, Jordy AB, Fritzen AM, Pehmøller C, Sylow L, et al. LKB1 regulates lipid oxidation during exercise independently of AMPK. *Diabetes* 62: 1490–1499, 2013.
81. Jin SM, Lazarou M, Wang C, Kane LA, Narendra DP, Youle RJ. Mitochondrial membrane potential regulates PINK1 import and proteolytic destabilization by PARL. *J Cell Biol* 191: 933–942, 2010.
82. Jones RG, Plas DR, Kubek S, Buzzai M, Mu J, Xu Y, et al. AMP-activated protein kinase induces a p53-dependent metabolic checkpoint. *Mol Cell* 18: 283–293, 2005.
83. Joseph A-M, Adhihetty PJ, Buford TW, Wohlgemuth SE, Lees HA, Nguyen LM-D, et al. The impact of aging on mitochondrial function and biogenesis pathways in skeletal muscle of sedentary high- and low-functioning elderly individuals. *Aging Cell* 11: 801–9, 2012.
84. Joseph A, Hood DA. Mitochondrion plasticity of TOM complex assembly in skeletal muscle mitochondria in response to chronic contractile activity. *Mitochondrion* 12: 305–312, 2012.
85. Ju J, Jeon S, Park J, Lee J, Lee S, Cho K, et al. Autophagy plays a role in skeletal muscle mitochondrial biogenesis in an endurance exercise-trained condition. *J Physiol Sci* 66: 417–430, 2016.
86. Khan NA, Auranen M, Paetau I, Pirinen E, Euro L, Forsström S, et al. Effective treatment of mitochondrial myopathy by nicotinamide riboside, a vitamin B3. *EMBO Mol Med* 6: 721–731, 2014.
87. Kim Y, Triolo M, Erlich AT, Hood DA. Regulation of autophagic and mitophagic flux during chronic contractile activity-induced muscle adaptations. *Pflügers Arch - Eur J Physiol* 471: 431–440, 2019.
88. Kim Y, Triolo M, Hood DA. Impact of aging and exercise on mitochondrial quality control in skeletal muscle. *Oxid Med Cell Longev* 2017: 3165396, 2017.
89. Kjøbsted R, Hingst JR, Fentz J, Foretz M, Sanz MN, Pehmøller C, et al. AMPK in skeletal muscle function and metabolism. *FASEB J* 32: 1741–1777, 2018.
90. Klionsky DJ, Abdelmohsen K, Abe A, Abedin MJ, Abeliovich H, Al E. Guidelines for the use and interpretation of assays for monitoring autophagy. *Autophagy* 12: 1, 2016.
91. Koltai E, Hart N, Taylor AW, Goto S, Ngo JK, Davies KJA, et al. Age-associated declines in mitochondrial biogenesis and protein quality control factors are minimized by exercise training. *Am J Physiol Regul Integr Comp Physiol* 303: R127–34, 2012.
92. Kondapalli C, Kazlauskaite A, Zhang N, Woodroof HI, Campbell DG, Gourlay R, et al. PINK1 is activated by mitochondrial membrane potential depolarization and stimulates parkin E3 ligase activity by phosphorylating serine 65. *Open Biol* 2: 120080, 2012.
93. Kujoth CC, Hiona A, Pugh TD, Someya S, Panzer K, Wohlgemuth SE, et al. Medicine: mitochondrial DNA mutations, oxidative stress, and apoptosis in mammalian aging. *Science* 309: 481–484, 2005.
94. Lai RYJ, Ljubicic V, D'souza D, Hood DA. Effect of chronic contractile activity on mRNA stability in skeletal muscle. *Am J Physiol Cell Physiol* 299: C155–163, 2010.
95. Laker RC, Drake JC, Wilson RJ, Lira VA, Lewellen BM, Ryall KA, et al. Ampk phosphorylation of Ulk1 is required for targeting of mitochondria to lysosomes in exercise-induced mitophagy. *Nat Commun* 8: 548, 2017.
96. Lee JSW, Auyeung TW, Kwok T, Lau EMC, Leung PC, Woo J. Associated factors and health impact of sarcopenia in older Chinese men and women: a cross-sectional study. *Gerontology* 53: 404–410, 2008.
97. Leick L, Wojtaszewski JFP, Johansen SJ, Kiilerich K, Comes J, Hellsten Y, et al. PGC-1α is not mandatory for exercise-and training-induced adaptive gene responses in mouse skeletal muscle. *Am J Physiol Endocrinol Metab* 294: 463–474, 2008.
98. Leone TC, Lehman JJ, Finck BN, Schaeffer PJ, Wende AR, Boudina S, et al. PGC-1alpha deficiency causes multi-system energy metabolic derangements: muscle dysfunction, abnormal weight control and hepatic steatosis. *PLOS Biol* 3: e101, 2005.
99. Lexell J, Taylor CC, Sjöström M. What is the cause of the ageing atrophy?. Total number, size and proportion of different fiber types studied in whole vastus lateralis muscle from 15- to 83-year-old men. *J Neurol Sci* 84: 275–294, 1988.
100. Liang S-H, Clarke MF. Regulation of p53 localization. *Eur J Biochem* 268: 2779–2783, 2001.
101. Lin J, Wu H, Tarr PT, Zhang C-Y, Wu Z, Boss O, et al. Transcriptional co-activator PGC-1 alpha drives the formation of slow-twitch muscle fibres. *Nature* 418: 797–801, 2002.
102. Line Schwalm C, Deldicque L, Francaux M. Lack of activation of mitophagy during endurance exercise in human. *Sci Sport Exerc* 49: 1552–1561, 2017.

103. Linnane AW, Baumer A, Maxwell RJ, Preston H, Zhang CF, Marzuki S. Mitochondrial gene mutation: the ageing process and degenerative diseases. *Biochem Int* 22: 1067–1076, 1990.

104. Ljubicic V, Joseph A-M, Adhihetty PJ, Huang JH, Saleem A, Uguccioni G, et al. Molecular basis for an attenuated mitochondrial adaptive plasticity in aged skeletal muscle. *Aging (Albany NY)* 1: 818–830, 2009.

105. Lo Verso F, Carnio S, Vainshtein A, Sandri M. Autophagy is not required to sustain exercise and PRKAA1/ AMPK activity but is important to prevent mitochondrial damage during physical activity. *Autophagy* 10: 1883–1894, 2014.

106. MacKenzie JA, Payne RM. Mitochondrial protein import and human health and disease. *Biochim Biophys Acta - Mol Basis Dis*. 1772: 509–523, 2007.

107. Matoba S, Kang J-G, Patino WD, Wragg A, Boehm M, Gavrilova O, et al. P53 regulates mitochondrial metabolism. *Science* 312: 1650–1653, 2006.

108. Matsuda N, Sato S, Shiba K, Okatsu K, Saisho K, Gautier CA, et al. PINK1 stabilized by mitochondrial depolarization recruits Parkin to damaged mitochondria and activates latent parkin for mitophagy. *J Cell Biol* 189: 211–221, 2010.

109. Melov S, Tarnopolsky MA, Beckman K, Felkey K, Hubbard A. Resistance exercise reverses aging in human skeletal muscle. *PLOS ONE* 2: e465, 2007.

110. Menzies KJ, Singh K, Saleem A, Hood DA. Sirtuin 1-mediated effects of exercise and resveratrol on mitochondrial biogenesis. *J Biol Chem* 288: 6968–6979, 2013.

111. Mortensen OH, Frandsen L, Schjerling P, Nishimura E, Grunnet N. PGC-1α and PGC-1β have both similar and distinct effects on myofiber switching toward an oxidative phenotype. *Am J Physiol Metab* 291: E807–E816, 2006.

112. Muller FL, Liu Y, Van Remmen H. Complex III releases superoxide to both sides of the inner mitochondrial membrane. *J Biol Chem* 279: 49064–49073, 2004.

113. Narendra DP, Jin SM, Tanaka A, Suen D-F, Gautier CA, Shen J, et al. PINK1 is selectively stabilized on impaired mitochondria to activate parkin. *PLOS Biol* 8: e1000298, 2010.

114. Narkar VA, Downes M, Yu RT, Embler E, Wang YX, Banayo E, et al. AMPK and PPARδ agonists are exercise mimetics. *Cell* 134: 405–415, 2008.

115. Ngo HB, Kaiser JT, Chan DC. The mitochondrial transcription and packaging factor Tfam imposes a U-turn on mitochondrial DNA. *Nat Struct {&} Mol Biol* 18: 1290–1296, 2011.

116. Ngo HB, Lovely GA, Phillips R, Chan DC. Distinct structural features of TFAM drive mitochondrial DNA packaging versus transcriptional activation. *Nat Commun* 5: 3077, 2014.

117. O'Leary MF, Vainshtein A, Iqbal S, Ostojic O, Hood DA. Adaptive plasticity of autophagic proteins to denervation in aging skeletal muscle. *Am J Physiol Cell Physiol* 304: C422–30, 2013.

118. O'Neill HM, Maarbjerg SJ, Crane JD, Jeppesen J, Jørgensen SB, Schertzer JD, et al. AMP-activated protein kinase (AMPK) beta1beta2 muscle null mice reveal an essential role for AMPK in maintaining mitochondrial content and glucose uptake during exercise. *Proc Natl Acad Sci U S A* 108: 16092–16097, 2011.

119. Ojuka EO, Jones TE, Han D-H, Chen M, Holloszy JO. Raising Ca2+ in L6 myotubes mimics effects of exercise on mitochondrial biogenesis in muscle. *FASEB J* 17: 675–681, 2003.

120. Ojuka EO, Jones TE, Han D-H, Chen M, Wamhoff BR, Sturek M, et al. Intermittent increases in cytosolic Ca $^{2+}$ stimulate mitochondrial biogenesis in muscle cells. *Am J Physiol Metab* 283: E1040–E1045, 2002.

121. Opalińska M, Meisinger C. Metabolic control via the mitochondrial protein import machinery. *Curr Opin Cell Biol* 33: 42–48, 2015.

122. Pagliuso A, Cossart P, Stavru F. The ever-growing complexity of the mitochondrial fission machinery. *Cell Mol Life Sci* 75: 355–374, 2018.

123. Park J-H, Zhuang J, Li J, Hwang PM. P53 as guardian of the mitochondrial genome. *FEBS Lett* 590: 924–934, 2016.

124. Park J-Y, Wang P-Y, Matsumoto T, Sung HJ, Ma W, Choi JW, et al. P53 improves aerobic exercise capacity and augments skeletal muscle mitochondrial DNA content. *Circ Res* 105: 705–712, 2009.

125. Parker L, Trewin A, Levinger I, Shaw CS, Stepto NK. The effect of exercise-intensity on skeletal muscle stress kinase and insulin protein signaling. *PLoS One* 12, 2017.

126. Pickles S, Vigié P, Youle RJ. Mitophagy and quality control mechanisms in mitochondrial maintenance. *Curr Biol* 28: R170–R185, 2018.

127. Pilegaard H, Saltin B, Neufer PD. Exercise induces transient transcriptional activation of the PGC-1α gene in human skeletal muscle. *J Physiol* 546: 851–858, 2003.

128. Pogozelski AR, Geng T, Li P, Yin X, Lira VA, Zhang M, et al. P38 mitogen-activated protein kinase is a key regulator in skeletal muscle metabolic adaptation in mice. *PLOS One* 4: e7934, 2009.

129. Power GA, Minozzo FC, Spendiff S, Filion ME, Konokhova Y, Purves-Smith MF, et al. Reduction in single muscle fiber rate of force development with aging is not attenuated in world class older masters athletes. *Am J Physiol - Cell Physiol* 310: C318–C327, 2016.

130. Powers SK, Ji LL, Kavazis AN, Jackson MJ. Reactive oxygen species: impact on skeletal muscle. *Compr Physiol* 1: 941–969, 2011.

131. Puigserver P, Adelmant G, Wu Z, Fan M, Xu J, O'Malley B, et al. Activation of PPARgamma coactivator-1 through transcription factor docking. *Science* 286: 1368–71, 1999.

132. Puigserver P, Rhee J, Lin J, Wu Z, Yoon JC, Zhang C, et al. Cytokine stimulation of energy expenditure through p38 MAP kinase activation of PPARgamma coactivator-1. *Mol Cell* 8: 971–982, 2001.

133. Puigserver P, Wu Z, Park CW, Graves R, Wright M, Spiegelman BM. A cold-inducible coactivator of nuclear receptors linked to adaptive thermogenesis. *Cell* 92: 829–839, 1998.

134. Quinsay MN, Thomas RL, Lee Y, Gustafsson AB. Bnip3-mediated mitochondrial autophagy is independent of the mitochondrial permeability transition pore. *Autophagy* 6: 855–62, 2010.

135. Rafaeloff-Phail R, Ding L, Conner L, Yeh W-K, McClure D, Guo H, et al. Biochemical regulation of mammalian AMP-activated protein kinase activity by NAD and NADH. *J Biol Chem* 279: 52934–52939, 2004.

136. Romanello V, Guadagnin E, Gomes L, Roder I, Sandri C, Petersen Y, et al. Mitochondrial fission and remodelling contributes to muscle atrophy. *EMBO J* 29: 1774–85, 2010.

137. Rose AJ, Frosig C, Kiens B, Wojtaszewski JFP, Richter EA. Effect of endurance exercise training on Ca2+-calmodulin-dependent protein kinase II expression and signalling in skeletal muscle of humans. *J Physiol* 583: 785–795, 2007.

138. Rose AJ, Hargreaves M. Exercise increases Ca2+-calmodulin-dependent protein kinase II activity in human skeletal muscle. *J Physiol* 553: 303–309, 2003.

139. Rowe GC, El-Khoury R, Patten IS, Rustin P, Arany Z. PGC-1 a is dispensable for exercise-induced mitochondrial biogenesis in skeletal muscle. *PLOS ONE* 7: e41817, 2012.

140. Rubio-Cosials A, Sidow JF, Jiménez-Menéndez N, Fernández-Millán P, Montoya J, Jacobs HT, et al. Human mitochondrial transcription factor a induces a U-turn structure in the light strand promoter. *Nat Struct {&} Mol Biol* 18: 1281–1289, 2011.

141. Ruiz JR, Sui X, Lobelo F, Morrow JR, Jackson AW, Sjöström M, et al. Association between muscular strength and mortality in men: prospective cohort study. *BMJ* 337: 92–95, 2008.

142. Saleem A, Adhihetty PJ, Hood DA. Role of p53 in mitochondrial biogenesis and apoptosis in skeletal muscle. *Physiol Genomics* 3: 58–66, 2009.

143. Saleem A, Carter HN, Hood DA. P53 is necessary for the adaptive changes in the cellular milieu subsequent to an acute bout of endurance exercise. *Am J Physiol Cell Physiol* 306: C241–249, 2014.

144. Saleem A, Carter HN, Iqbal S, Hood DA. Role of p53 within the regulatory network controlling muscle mitochondrial biogenesis. *Exerc Sport Sci Rev* 39: 199–205, 2011.

145. Saleem A, Hood DA. Acute exercise induces tumour suppressor protein p53 translocation to the mitochondria and promotes a p53-Tfam-mitochondrial DNA complex in skeletal muscle. *J Physiol* 591: 3625–3636, 2013.

146. Saleem A, Iqbal S, Zhang Y, Hood DA. Effect of p53 on mitochondrial morphology, import and assembly in skeletal muscle. *Am J Physiol Cell Physiol* 308: C319–C329, 2015.

147. Sandri M, Lin J, Handschin C, Yang W, Arany ZP, Lecker SH, et al. PGC-1alpha protects skeletal muscle from atrophy by suppressing FoxO3 action and atrophy-specific gene transcription. *Proc Natl Acad Sci U S A* 103: 16260–16265, 2006.

148. Sarraf SA, Raman M, Guarani-Pereira V, Sowa ME, Huttlin EL, Gygi SP, et al. Landscape of the PARKIN-dependent ubiquitylome in response to mitochondrial depolarization. *Nature* 496: 372–376, 2013.

149. Schreiber SN, Emter R, Hock MB, Knutti D, Cardenas J, Podvinec M, et al. The estrogen-related receptor alpha (ERRalpha) functions in PPARgamma coactivator 1alpha (PGC-1alpha)-induced mitochondrial biogenesis. *Proc Natl Acad Sci U S A* 101: 6472–6477, 2004.

150. Schreiber SN, Knutti D, Brogli K, Uhlmann T, Kralli A. The transcriptional coactivator PGC-1 regulates the expression and activity of the orphan nuclear receptor estrogen-related receptor alpha (ERRalpha). *J Biol Chem* 278: 9013–9018, 2003.

151. Schriner SE, Linford NJ, Martin GM, Treuting P, Ogburn CE, Emond M, et al. Medicine extension of murine life span by overexpression of catalase targeted to mitochondria. *Science* 308: 1909–1911, 2005.

152. Schwarze SR, Lee CM, Chung SS, Roecker EB, Weindruch R, Aiken JM. High levels of mitochondrial DNA deletions in skeletal muscle of old rhesus monkeys. *Mech Ageing Dev* 83: 91–101, 1995.

153. Shah VO, Scariano J, Waters D, Qualls C, Morgan M, Pickett G, et al. Mitochondrial DNA deletion and sarcopenia. *Genet Med* 11: 147–152, 2009.

154. Shang H, Xia Z, Bai S, Zhang HE, Gu B, Wang R. Downhill running acutely elicits mitophagy in rat soleus muscle. *Med Sci Sports Exerc* 51: 1396–1403, 2019.

155. She Q-B, Bode AM, Ma W-Y, Chen N-Y, Dong Z. Resveratrol-induced activation of p53 and apoptosis is mediated by extracellular- signal-regulated protein kinases and p38 kinase. *Cancer Res* 61: 1604–1610, 2001.

156. Shiba-Fukushima K, Imai Y, Yoshida S, Ishihama Y, Kanao T, et al. PINK1-mediated phosphorylation of the parkin ubiquitin-like domain primes mitochondrial translocation of parkin and regulates mitophagy. *Sci Rep* 2: 1002, 2012.

157. Short KR, Vittone JL, Bigelow ML, Proctor DN, Rizza RA, Coenen-Schimke JM, et al. Impact of aerobic exercise training on age-related changes in insulin sensitivity and muscle oxidative capacity. *Diabetes* 52: 1888–1896, 2003.

158. Simonetti S, Chen X, DiMauro S, Schon EA. Accumulation of deletions in human mitochondrial DNA during normal aging: analysis by quantitative PCR. *BBA - Mol Basis Dis* 1180: 113–122, 1992.

159. Stamatakis E, Gale J, Bauman A, Ekelund U, Hamer M, Ding D. Sitting time, physical activity, and risk of mortality in adults. *J Am Coll Cardiol* 73: 2062–2072, 2019.

160. Taaffe DR, Henwood TR, Nalls MA, Walker DG, Lang TF, Harris TB. Alterations in muscle attenuation following detraining and retraining in resistance-trained older adults. *Gerontology* 55: 217–223, 2009.

161. Taanman J-W. The mitochondrial genome: structure, transcription, translation and replication. *Biochim Biophys Acta - Bioenerg* 1410: 103–123, 1999.

162. Takahashi M, Chesley A, Freyssenet D, Hood DA. Contractile activity-induced adaptations in the mitochondrial protein import system. *Am J Physiol* 274: C1380–1387, 1998.

163. Tanner CB, Madsen SR, Hallowell DM, Goring DMJ, Moore TM, Hardman SE, et al. Mitochondrial and performance adaptations to exercise training in mice lacking skeletal muscle LKB1. *Am J Physiol - Endocrinol Metab* 305, 2013.

164. Terada S, Goto M, Kato M, Kawanaka K, Shimokawa T, Tabata I. Effects of low-intensity prolonged exercise on PGC-1 mRNA expression in rat epitrochlearis muscle. *Biochem Biophys Res Commun* 296: 350–354, 2002.

165. Triolo M, Hood DA. Mitochondrial breakdown in skeletal muscle and the emerging role of the lysosomes. *Arch Biochem Biophys* 661:66-73, 2019.

166. Uguccioni G, Hood DA. The importance of PGC-1α in contractile activity-induced mitochondrial adaptations. *Am J Physiol Endocrinol Metab* 300: E361–E371, 2011.

167. Vainshtein A, Desjardins EM, Armani A, Sandri M, Hood DA. PGC-1α modulates denervation-induced mitophagy in skeletal muscle. *Skelet Muscle* 5: 9, 2015.

168. Vainshtein A, Tryon LD, Pauly M, Hood DA. Role of PGC-1α during acute exercise-induced autophagy and mitophagy in skeletal muscle. *Am J Physiol Cell Physiol* 308: C710–719, 2015.

169. Van De Weijer T, Phielix E, Bilet L, Williams EG, Ropelle ER, Bierwagen A, et al. Evidence for a direct effect of the NAD+ precursor acipimox on muscle mitochondrial function in humans. *Diabetes* 64: 1193–1201, 2015.

170. van der Bliek AM, Shen Q, Kawajiri S. Mechanisms of mitochondrial fission and fusion. *Cold Spring Harb Perspect Biol* 5: a011072, 2013.

171. Vargas-Ortiz K, Pérez-Vázquez V, Macías-Cervantes MH. Exercise and sirtuins: a way to mitochondrial health in skeletal muscle. *Int J Mol Sci* 20: 2717, 2019.

172. Vega RB, Huss JM, Kelly DP. The coactivator PGC-1 cooperates with peroxisome proliferator-activated receptor alpha in transcriptional control of nuclear genes encoding mitochondrial fatty acid oxidation enzymes. *Mol Cell Biol* 20: 1868–1876, 2000.

173. Verdijk LB, Snijders T, Drost M, Delhaas T, Kadi F, Van Loon LJC. Satellite cells in human skeletal muscle; from birth to old age. *Age (Omaha)* 36: 545–557, 2014.

174. Vermulst M, Wanagat J, Kujoth GC, Bielas JH, Rabinovitch PS, Prolla TA, et al. DNA deletions and clonal mutations drive premature aging in mitochondrial mutator mice. *Nat Genet* 40: 392–394, 2008.

175. Vil L, Roca C, Elias I, Casellas A, Lage R, Franckhauser S, et al. AAV-mediated sirt1 overexpression in skeletal muscle activates oxidative capacity but does not prevent insulin resistance. *Mol Ther - Methods Clin Dev* 3: 16072, 2016.

176. Virbasius J V, Scarpulla RC. Activation of the human mitochondrial transcription factor a gene by nuclear respiratory factors: a potential regulatory link between nuclear and mitochondrial gene expression in organelle biogenesis. *Proc Natl Acad Sci U S A* 91: 1309–1313, 1994.

177. Wang J, Wang F, Zhang P, Liu H, He J, Zhang C, et al. PGC-1α over-expression suppresses the skeletal muscle atrophy and myofiber-type composition during hindlimb unloading. *Biosci Biotechnol Biochem* 81: 500–513, 2017.

178. Wenz LS, Opaliński Ł, Wiedemann N, Becker T. Cooperation of protein machineries in mitochondrial protein sorting. *Biochim Biophys Acta - Mol Cell Res* 1853: 1119–1129, 2015.

179. Wiedemann N, Pfanner N. Mitochondrial machineries for protein import and assembly. *Annu Rev Biochem* 86: 685–714, 2017.

180. Winder WW, Holmes BF, Rubink DS, Jensen EB, Chen M, Holloszy JO. Activation of AMP-activated protein kinase increases mitochondrial enzymes in skeletal muscle. *J Appl Physiol* 88: 2219–2226, 2000.

181. Wong YC, Holzbaur ELF. Optineurin is an autophagy receptor for damaged mitochondria in parkin-mediated mitophagy that is disrupted by an ALS-linked mutation. *Proc Natl Acad Sci U S A* 111: E4439–4448, 2014.

182. Wright DC, Geiger PC, Han DH, Jones TE, Holloszy JO. Calcium induces increases in peroxisome proliferator-activated receptor gamma coactivator-1alpha and mitochondrial biogenesis by a pathway leading to p38 mitogen-activated protein kinase activation. *J Biol Chem* 282: 18793–18799, 2007.

183. Wright DC, Han D, Garcia-Roves PM, Geiger PC, Jones TE, Holloszy JO. Exercise-induced mitochondrial biogenesis begins before the increase in muscle PGC-1 alpha expression. *J Biol Chem* 282: 194–199, 2007.

184. Wroblewski AP, Amati F, Smiley MA, Goodpaster B, Wright V. Chronic exercise preserves lean muscle mass in masters athletes. *Phys Sportsmed* 39: 62, 2011.

185. Wu H, Kanatous SB, Thurmond FA, Gallardo T, Isotani E, Bassel-Duby R, et al. Regulation of mitochondrial biogenesis in skeletal muscle by CaMK. *Science* 296: 349–352, 2002.

186. Yan Z, Lira VA, Greene NP. Exercise training-induced regulation of mitochondrial quality. *Exerc Sport Sci Rev* 40:159–164, 2012.

187. Yoboue ED, Devin A. Reactive oxygen species-mediated control of mitochondrial biogenesis. *Int J Cell Biol* 2012: 1–8, 2012.

188. Yoo S-Z, No M-H, Heo J-W, Park D-H, Kang J-H, Kim J-H, et al. Effects of acute exercise on mitochondrial function, dynamics, and mitophagy in rat cardiac and skeletal muscles. *Int Neurourol J* 23: S22–31, 2019.

189. Yoshida Y, Izumi H, Torigoe T, Ishiguchi H, Itoh H, Kang D, et al. P53 physically interacts with mitochondrial transcription factor a and differentially regulates binding to damaged DNA. *Cancer Res* 63: 3729–3734, 2003.

190. Zechner C, Lai L, Zechner JF, Geng T, Yan Z, Rumsey JW, et al. Total skeletal muscle PGC-1 deficiency uncouples mitochondrial derangements from fiber type determination and insulin sensitivity. *Cell Metab* 12: 633–42, 2010.

191. Zhang H, Bosch-Marce M, Shimoda LA, Tan YS, Baek JH, Wesley JB, et al. Mitochondrial autophagy is an HIF-1-dependent adaptive metabolic response to hypoxia. *J Biol Chem* 283: 10892–903, 2008.

192. Zhang Y, Uguccioni G, Ljubicic V, Irrcher I, Iqbal S, Singh K, et al. Multiple signaling pathways regulate contractile activity-mediated PGC-1 gene expression and activity in skeletal muscle cells. *Physiol Rep* 2: e12008–e12008, 2014.

193. Zhao M, New L, Kravchenko VV, Kato Y, Gram H, di Padova F, et al. Regulation of the MEF2 family of transcription factors by p38. *Mol Cell Biol* 19: 21–30, 1999.

194. Zhu Y, Massen S, Terenzio M, Lang V, Chen-Lindner S, Eils R, et al. Modulation of serines 17 and 24 in the LC3-interacting region of Bnip3 determines pro-survival mitophagy versus apoptosis. *J Biol Chem* 288: 1099–113, 2013.

195. Zong H, Ren JM, Young LH, Pypaert M, Mu J, Birnbaum MJ, et al. AMP kinase is required for mitochondrial biogenesis in skeletal muscle in response to chronic energy deprivation. *Proc Natl Acad Sci U S A* 99: 15983–15987, 2002.

28
BIOCHEMISTRY OF EXERCISE EFFECTS IN TYPE 2 DIABETES

Barry Braun, Karyn L. Hamilton, Dan S. Lark,
and Alissa Newman

Overall Benefits of Exercise

Numerous epidemiological and experimental studies, in both animals and humans across sexes and in a variety of ethnicities, races, and geographic locations, strongly indicate a positive and roughly dose-response relationship between physical activity and prevention/management of type 2 diabetes (6, 98, 122). Physical activity contributes to the prevention, management, and (potentially) reversal of type 2 diabetes (T2D), at least in part by directly increasing the transport of glucose from blood to tissues and by opposing the insulin resistance that underlies the pathophysiology of the majority of individuals with T2D. In individuals with T2D, insulin produced by pancreatic beta cells binds to receptors (e.g., SkM, adipose, liver) but the cellular responses are attenuated. Most of the post-receptor binding attention has been focused on the migration of GLUT-4 transporters from the intracellular vesicle to the plasma membrane where they facilitate glucose transport from the blood to the intracellular environment, but hepatic glucose production, triacylglycerol synthesis/lipolysis, and protein turnover are altered as well. In pre-diabetes and in the early progression of T2D, beta cells secrete more insulin, and this compensatory hyperinsulinemia constrains dramatic elevations in fasting and post-meal glycemia. In many individuals, however, the beta cells fail to maintain the prodigious insulin supply to meet the excessive demand incurred by insulin resistance, resulting in a transition to glucose intolerance, elevated fasting glucose, and eventually, overt T2D.

In response to the immense repository of data available, the American Diabetes Association (ADA) creates recommendations for physical activity among people with pre-diabetes and diabetes and updates them regularly. Currently (34), the American Diabetes Association makes the following exercise/physical activity recommendations:

- Daily exercise, or at least not allowing more than 2 days to elapse between exercise sessions, is recommended to enhance insulin action; adults should perform both aerobic and resistance training for optimal glycaemic and health outcomes; structured interventions should include at least 150 minutes of physical activity (34).
- Reduced sedentary time and prolonged sitting should be interrupted with bouts of light activity every 30 min for blood glucose benefits; these are in addition to, and not a replacement for, increased structured exercise and incidental movement (34).

The benefits of physical activity and minimizing sedentary behaviour are manifested both acutely, i.e., during and for up to 48–72 hours post-exercise, and in response to habitual activity that occurs over the

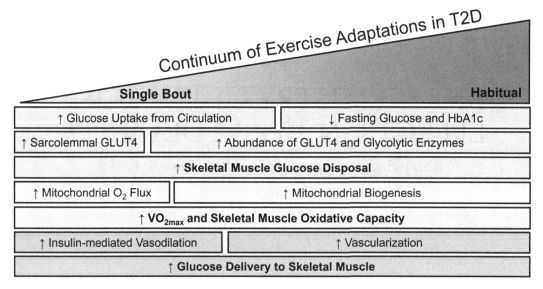

Figure 28.1   Continuum of exercise adaptations in type 2 diabetes

course of weeks, months, and years. The distinction between acute and habitual exercise is important because the management of diabetes occurs in both the short term (blood glucose in the daytime fasted, fed, and overnight conditions) and long term (blood glucose control over months and years). In the short term, there is potential for medical issues resulting from both hyperglycaemia (ketoacidosis) and hypoglycaemia (cognitive and motor impairment, coma, even death). In the long term, the risk for complications like amputation, blindness, and kidney, liver, and/or cardiovascular disease is strongly influenced by "average" glycemia as reflected in HbA1c (although there is increasing attention to the role of glycaemic variability independent of average glycemia). Therefore, to fully understand the biochemistry of exercise for T2D, it is necessary to consider both the acute and habitual contexts (Figure 28.1). In the sections that follow, we summarize key animal and human subjects research literature focused on the biochemistry of both acute and habitual exercise. It is important to note that humans have ~10 times more muscle glycogen than mice (109, 142) and therefore, rodent exercise studies should be interpreted in light of this consideration. We conclude with some clinical considerations including exercise timing and interaction with T2DM pharmacology.

Acute Exercise

A single bout of exercise elicits robust benefits for whole-body glucose homeostasis. Skeletal muscle (SkM) is the primary site of glucose disposal during exercise and in response to insulin (39), and thus is the primary actor in the glucose-lowering effects of exercise. During exercise, SkM glycogen is consumed to support contraction, requiring increased uptake of glucose from the circulation. This process involves three coordinated steps: delivery, transport, and phosphorylation. All three steps are augmented by insulin; in T2D, insulin resistance (IR) is observed in the cells and pathways involved in regulation of these steps (40). Importantly, however, exercise enhances SkM glucose uptake by circumventing IR *during* exercise and attenuating IR *after* exercise.

Skeletal Muscle Glucose Disposal During Exercise

Skeletal muscle contraction results in adenosine triphosphate (ATP) hydrolysis to support myosin–actin cross-bridge cycling and a variety of other concurrent processes (i.e., calcium handling, phosphorylation events, etc.). Glucose is a major source of fuel utilized by anaerobic (i.e., lactate) or aerobic (i.e., oxidative phosphorylation) pathways to replenish ATP. Glucose can either be liberated from intracellular glycogen stores or extracted from the blood. Glycogen is the preferred source of glucose during exercise at intensities above 70% of maximal oxygen uptake (VO2max) (185, 212); however, depletion of intramuscular glycogen increases the need for circulating glucose. Consistent with this principle, glucose uptake from the circulation during exercise increases as a function of both the duration and intensity of physical activity (217).

In order for glucose to reach a SkM fibre, it must first travel through the vasculature, traverse the endothelium, and reach the interstitial space between the vasculature and SkM. Glucose delivery to the SkM tissue is a function of limb blood flow (10); insulin serves as a potent vasodilator in SkM and stimulates the release of nitric oxide from the vascular endothelium, which results in relaxation of capillaries. This increase in local blood flow through capillaries enhances glucose delivery to the tissue. Unfortunately, IR and T2D impair insulin-stimulated vasodilation (152).

The mechanisms linking T2D to vascular dysfunction have been described in detail elsewhere (225). Briefly, reduced expression of endothelial nitric oxide synthase (eNOS) (177) is implicated, which may explain reduced insulin-stimulated vasodilation. Studies in diet-induced obese rodents demonstrate that glucose delivery is the rate-limiting step for insulin-stimulated glucose uptake (71). Like insulin, exercise increases local blood flow and enhances glucose delivery both during (4, 72) and after exercise (9), and pre-clinical studies provide evidence that exercise can restore or reverse the microvascular dysfunction imposed by diabetes (143, 157).

Once glucose reaches the interstitial space, it must be transported across the sarcolemma into the cell. Insulin-stimulated glucose transport, even at supraphysiological doses of insulin, has been shown to be impaired with T2D (219, 229). Exercise increases SkM glucose transport (91, 126, 169, 218), and this exercise-induced increase in glucose transport is not impaired in subjects with T2D (149). How exercise increases glucose transport is incompletely defined, although recent work has made great strides towards unravelling this complex process.

Glucose transporter 4 (GLUT4) is the primary glucose transporter in SkM. Translocation of GLUT4 from intracellular vesicles to the sarcolemma facilitates glucose transport in response to insulin or contraction (180, 181). Under resting conditions, GLUT4 is embedded in intracellular vesicles that are proximal to the sarcolemma (170). Exocytosis of GLUT4-containing vesicles results in GLUT4 becoming embedded in the sarcolemma, while endocytosis of GLUT4 decreases its presence at the sarcolemma. For a contemporary review of GLUT4 trafficking, see (120). It is the balance between these two processes that determines GLUT4 abundance, and thus, glucose transport (190). Insulin increases sarcolemmal GLUT4 abundance (111) largely via exocytosis (227), whereas exercise preserves GLUT4 abundance by reducing endocytosis (178). While SkM GLUT4 levels are typically maintained (230), T2D causes a decrease in GLUT4 translocation to the sarcolemma (186, 230). Increased GLUT4 activity, as opposed to abundance, has also been proposed as a mechanism contributing to enhanced glucose transport, but its role is less defined (95, 201).

Contraction-mediated GLUT4 translocation can be stimulated by both metabolic and mechanical alterations in SkM. For example, the increase in metabolic demand caused by exercise, specifically an increase in the ratio of adenosine monophosphate (AMP) to adenosine triphosphate (ATP), results in the activation of AMP-activated protein kinase (AMPK). AMPK is a heterotrimer with a catalytic alpha subunit and regulatory beta and gamma subunits. For a comprehensive discussion on the role of AMPK on metabolism, readers are directed to the following review: (86). The role of AMPK in contraction-mediated glucose uptake was first described in 1998 using the AMPK agonist 5-aminoimidazole-4-carboxamide ribonucleoside (AICAR) (80). Further, this study revealed that AMPK, via AICAR, promotes glucose uptake independent of insulin. This study was the catalyst for a vigorous pursuit to better understand how metabolic state stimulates glucose uptake in the absence of insulin.

While AMPK has emerged as an important regulator of exercise-stimulated glucose uptake, calcium released from the sarcoplasmic reticulum in response to an action potential activates calcium calmodulin kinase 2 (CAMK-II), another important potential regulator of exercise-mediated glucose uptake. In this paradigm, calcium binds to calmodulin, which in turn activates CAMK-II. Mouse studies have demonstrated that CAMK-II is responsible for the regulation of contraction-stimulated glucose uptake, but not in response to insulin (224). Surprisingly, CAMK-II promotes glucose uptake independent of both AMPK and Akt (223).

Phosphorylation is the first chemical modification that occurs to glucose once inside the cell. Glucose phosphorylation occurs via the enzyme hexokinase, and the conversion of glucose to glucose-6-phosphate by hexokinase effectively traps glucose within the cell (174). Glucose phosphorylation during an insulin clamp is decreased in humans with (66) suggesting a functional barrier to glucose phosphorylation in vivo. Exercise acutely increases the activity of hexokinase-2, which increases the capacity for glucose phosphorylation (124). Through modulating hexokinase-2 gene expression in mice, glucose phosphorylation was shown to be the rate-limiting step for both insulin- and exercise-stimulated SkM glucose uptake in mice fed a normal chow diet (54, 55, 73). In diet-induced obese mice, glucose phosphorylation is only a rate-limiting step for exercise-induced glucose uptake (53), suggesting that transport and/or delivery are the primary barriers to insulin-stimulated glucose uptake in human T2D.

Skeletal Muscle Glucose Metabolism After Exercise

In addition to increased glucose disposal during exercise, there is a residual improvement in insulin sensitivity following exercise. The insulin-sensitizing impact of each individual exercise bout lasts for somewhere between 24 and 72 hours, depending on the "usual suspects" of intensity, duration, and total energy expenditure (18, 62, 108, 116, 117). Intense, long-duration, glycogen-depleting exercise can exert potent effects on whole-body insulin sensitivity for up to 3 days post exercise, whereas the residual effects of a bout of exercise that only just meets the physical activity recommendations (e.g., 30 min of walking) will dissipate in far less time. In this manner, exercise can be viewed similarly to medication (i.e., taken at sufficient doses) and its metabolic benefits will wane over time, requiring recurrent subsequent doses to maintain the positive effects. The intensity, duration, frequency, and mode can be tailored to optimize the beneficial impact of exercise in order to prevent or delay the transition from pre-diabetes to T2D.

As with medication (discussed later in the chapter), the nutritional environment in which the exercise dose is administered can greatly modulate the insulin-sensitizing effect that follows a bout of exercise. Irrespective of appreciable weight loss or gain, it is apparent that changes in energy balance and/or carbohydrate availability modulate the metabolic response to exercise. Energy and/or carbohydrate deficit will prolong the insulin sensitivity enhancement, where energy intake (and restored energy balance) may blunt the effect. Even minor deficits or surpluses can have a profound effect on the duration and magnitude of the metabolic responses to exercise (203). Carbohydrate deficit/balance may be of more importance than energy status per se; several studies have evaluated the effect of restoring energy balance but restricting carbohydrate (50, 93, 162, 194) and found that the duration and magnitude of enhanced insulin sensitivity are maintained.

What Is the Relationship Between Acute and Habitual Exercise?

The effects of an acute bout of exercise can last for hours to days after the exercise session. Therefore, it is possible that some of the benefits attributed to habitual exercise or exercise training may actually be residual effects of individual exercise sessions (132). Additionally, exercise training increases the capacity for exercise, which in turn, may allow for longer or more intense exercise bouts, eliciting a greater acute effect (206).

Many researchers have used an exercise model that consists of 2–7 consecutive days of activity to test for effects of "exercise" (19, 25, 107, 155). Is this acute exercise or habitual activity? It seems likely that there are adaptations to multiple bouts of exercise at the cellular or subcellular level that exceed those attributable to a single exercise bout. But some of the hallmark effects of weeks/months/years of activity, such as reduced visceral fat, increased cardiorespiratory fitness, angiogenesis resulting in higher capillary density, and changes in SkM fibre subtype or total area, are unlikely to be evident after a few bouts of activity. Therefore, we are generally considering short-term training of a week or less to be more similar to acute exercise than habitual activity. We will point out instances where this is likely not the case.

For the purposes of this review, we define habitual exercise as regular physical activity that meets or exceeds the recommendations of 150 minutes/week of moderate activity or a rough equivalent based on less time/more intensity. Given that the effects of an individual bout of exercise can last for no more than 72 hours and many training adaptations are measurable after 8 weeks or so, there is a logical rationale to define habitual exercise as taking place for 3 or more days per week for at least 8 weeks.

Habitual Exercise

An important piece of context that complicates how we define adaptations to habitual activity is the role of weight loss. In the Diabetes Prevention Program (DPP), greater weight loss was associated with greater decreases in risk of developing T2D (122). However, regular physical activity can elicit beneficial effects, even in the absence of weight loss (21, 58). The composition of the weight lost is a critical variable, as fat loss is clearly more relevant than gross change in body weight, and loss of visceral and/or ectopic fat is particularly relevant to metabolic benefits (13, 118). At a simplistic level, the adaptations to physical activity appear to be accentuated when activity results in fat loss but teasing apart the biochemistry of physical activity per se versus weight/fat loss is beyond the scope of this review.

Glucoregulatory Benefits of Habitual Physical Activity

In children and adults, habitual physical activity is linked to a wide variety of physiological benefits, including improved cardiovascular function (85, 184), improved mental health (163, 182), and improved glucose tolerance (82, 183). Here we focus on the glucoregulatory benefits of exercise training, particularly in SkM.

Habitual activity increases the delivery of both nutrients and oxygen to SkM and the capacity of SkM mitochondria to use oxygen to support metabolism (89). Furthermore, exercise training increases SkM glucose disposal through myriad processes, including changes in post-receptor insulin signalling pathways. For example, exercise training in participants with T2D improved the insulin-stimulated phosphorylation of Akt and AS160 in response to insulin (78). However, some of these studies (52) also noted that blood flow increased. Since insulin is a vasodilator (31, 104), this observation led to increased interest in changes in limb blood flow in response to habitual exercise. Indeed, more recent work demonstrated that exercise training augments insulin-stimulated blood flow and, thus, likely contributes to improved insulin-stimulated glucose disposal (228). Habitual exercise also improves the regulation of SkM blood flow (33, 77, 81, 103, 179). Mechanistically, this can occur via improved insulin-stimulated vasodilation (38) and/or increased SkM capillarization (175).

While an acute bout of exercise can enhance insulin sensitivity in the short term, there is also an effect of habitual exercise on insulin sensitivity that is greater than the sum of accumulated bouts of exercise. After 7 days of inactivity, the improvements in insulin sensitivity resulting from training dissipate (27), but maximal insulin-stimulated glucose disposal is preserved for at least 10 days (116).

One benefit of enhanced peripheral and hepatic insulin sensitivity is the lower demand for insulin that results from a greater capacity for glucose disappearance (or more constrained hepatic production per unit circulating insulin). Lower demand means less need for beta cells to make insulin, which may preserve beta cell function over time and delay or prevent requirements for patients to use insulin to manage T2D. Note that recent evidence suggests that insulin supply and demand can be affected by short-term (e.g., 7 days or less) exercise and by physical inactivity via increased hepatic insulin extraction with exercise and decreased extraction with inactivity (216). This may be a way to match insulin demand and supply without up- or down-regulating the beta cell insulin synthesizing machinery (14, 216).

Oxidative Metabolic Adaptations to Habitual Physical Activity

Habitual exercise also has clear benefits for oxidative metabolism in those with T2D. Exercise itself increases metabolic rate, which consumes SkM glycogen. This glycogen is replaced through the extraction of glucose from the blood. Furthermore, habitual exercise causes remodelling of SkM to increase energetic efficiency (20) and increased enzymatic activity between bouts of exercise (51).

Whole-body metabolic adaptations to habitual exercise include (1) increased reliance on fatty acids (92, 119, 208); (2) improved pulmonary function (87); and (3) in some cases, increased maximal oxygen consumption (67). The increased reliance on fatty acids, particularly following endurance exercise training, is conferred by increased mitochondrial content (90) and greater abundance of enzymes involved in beta oxidation (69). Accompanying this increased utilization of fatty acids is an increased in intramuscular triglycerides (195). There is also an increase in intramuscular fatty acids with obesity and T2D, a phenomenon termed the "Athlete's Paradox" (213). While both scenarios involved elevated intramuscular lipids, recent work has revealed important distinctions. In highly trained athletes, lipids (mainly triglycerides) are sequestered in inert lipid droplets (135) and intramuscular triglyceride synthesis is linked to greater insulin sensitivity (12). Although triglyceride synthesis rates in SkM were positively correlated with insulin sensitivity, they were negatively correlated with the abundance of ceramide, a lipid intermediate implicated in the development of insulin resistance (1). By contrast, accumulation of saturated triglycerides in SkM is associated with insulin resistance (191). In diet-induced obesity, incompletely oxidized fatty acids accumulate within the cytoplasm and mitochondria of SkM and contribute to insulin resistance (125). There are two lines of evidence regarding how lipid intermediates contribute to IR. First, intermediates like ceramide and diacylglycerol can disrupt insulin signalling through activation of PKC-theta (70, 114, 226). A second line of work has demonstrated that lipid intermediates are evidence of excessive beta oxidation by mitochondria and lead to an increased generation of reactive oxygen species (ROS) like hydrogen peroxide that contribute to insulin resistance (5). Furthermore, incomplete fat oxidation can explain severe insulin resistance in poorly controlled T2D (60).

Individuals with T2D tend to have smaller, damaged, and dysfunctional mitochondria (65), and restoration of mitochondrial function via habitual exercise is associated with improvements in SkM insulin sensitivity (141, 153), although it is not clear if the mitochondrial dysfunction precedes the development of T2D or if T2D leads to the mitochondrial impairment. An ongoing debate in the study of fat metabolism and T2D is whether or not impairments in mitochondrial oxidative capacity contribute to the IR observed in T2D. On one hand, T2D can impair mitochondrial respiratory capacity (110, 168). However, an abundance of work in both animals and humans illustrates a more complex role for mitochondria. For example, there are a number of studies demonstrating that short-term consumption of a hypercaloric diet rich in fatty acids elicits IR without an impairment in mitochondrial energetics (74, 209). Research in humans (188, 207) has demonstrated that consumption of a hypercaloric diet rich in fatty acids causes IR without an impairment in mitochondrial energetics. Recent work has suggested that observed reductions in mitochondrial respiratory capacity seen in some high-fat diet studies could be in fact due to a reduced sensitivity of mitochondria to ADP, the molecule that drives oxidative phosphorylation (156). Furthermore, transgenic mouse studies in which fatty acid transport is blocked surprisingly show improvements in glucose tolerance and insulin sensitivity (61, 115). Finally, there is evidence from human studies that impaired mitochondrial respiratory capacity is not always present in T2D (48, 160). In light of these studies, it is likely that impaired mitochondrial respiration contributes to T2D pathology in certain cases, but is not a ubiquitous mechanism for T2D pathogenesis.

Impact of Exercise Mode/Intensity/Duration/Volume

Low to moderate intensity aerobic exercise has been established as an effective strategy to improve the metabolic health of people with T2D (75). Higher intensity or longer duration exercise, resulting in greater total energy expenditure (8, 25, 29, 33, 77), accentuates the magnitude of the insulin-sensitizing effect.

There is mixed evidence regarding the independent (i.e., holding energy expenditure constant) effects of exercise intensity on metabolic health. Some research suggests that the total volume of exercise (i.e., total kcal expenditure regardless of components) is the most important driver of adaptations and that duration may even play a more specific role than intensity (94, 103). However, there is also evidence that long-duration, low-intensity activity (such as walking) is an insufficient stimulus for increasing cardiorespiratory fitness, which is closely related to insulin sensitivity/glucose tolerance (200).

Much prior research has not uncovered mechanisms to support a strong independent effect of exercise intensity (e.g., via greater depletion of SkM glycogen or increased up-regulation of intracellular mediators like AMPK-activated protein kinase or PGC-1 alpha, etc.) or duration (longer exposure to factors like ROS signalling or endocrine factors that stimulate mitochondrial biogenesis). However, a growing body of studies using high-intensity interval exercise (HIIE, also called high-intensity training [HIT] or sprint-interval training [SIT]) indicate that repeated applications of very high-intensity activity, even as little as a few minutes per day (2, 62, 63, 139), can have potent beneficial effects on metabolic health (100). Experimentally, early studies utilized repeated Wingate tests (30-sec exercise bouts at maximum intensity; 5–6 bouts per session) with ~4-minute periods of light recovery exercise in between bouts. Indeed, this mode of exercise is effective at improving glucose tolerance in those with T2D (7, 63, 140). However, although the "time active" in this paradigm is much less than conventional continuous exercise programmes, the overall time spent exercising is still ~30 minutes. More recent work using SIT (62) or HIIT (112, 220) has focused on reducing the overall time spent active. In sedentary, but otherwise healthy men, 12 weeks of SIT (3 × 20-second bouts of maximal sprinting interspersed with 2 minutes of light cycling three times per week; ~7 minutes spent active per session) improved glucose tolerance to a similar degree to 45 minutes of moderate intensity cycling (~70% maximum heart rate) (64). How much of the effects are attributable to the frequent "on-off" cycles between high- and low-intensity activity and the mechanistic underpinnings for these benefits is an area of great research interest

In addition to aerobic exercise, individuals with T2D are encouraged to participate in regular resistance training. The combination of aerobic and resistance training has been shown to be more beneficial than either one alone. An in-depth discussion of this area is beyond the scope of this chapter and we refer the reader to several reviews (102, 148, 197).

Physical Activity versus Breaking Up Sedentary Behaviour?

The past 10–15 years have brought increasing attention to sedentary behaviour and physical inactivity (42, 202, 221). In this context, inactivity is not just a lack of the positive effects of being physically active; strong research has shown that prolonged sitting results in negative health consequences, including heightened risk for T2D, obesity, and cardiovascular diseases, with distinct mechanistic underpinnings (11, 166).

Akin to exercise studies, the nutritional context plays a very important role in modulating the metabolic response to prolonged inactivity. Studies of bed rest or prolonged sitting designed to mimic sedentary behaviour are almost invariably confounded by positive energy balance unless strict care is taken to lower energy intake to match the low expenditure. The danger to clear interpretation of results is that "positive energy balance due to overfeeding is a confounding variable that exaggerates the deleterious effects of physical inactivity" (17). However, there are studies that have examined inactivity in the context of energy balance and show that inactivity (i.e., prolonged sitting) is detrimental to metabolic health. For example, Stephens et al. (204) found that a day of sitting combined with energy surplus reduced insulin action by 39% relative to an active control condition (standing, walking, and very little sitting but without structured exercise); this effect was blunted, but not prevented entirely, by matching energy intake to expenditure. Over the course of 10 days, Winn et al. (222) found that individuals who were relatively inactive (~4,000 steps per day) and in positive energy balance exhibited increased body weight, body fat, and impaired insulin sensitivity. However, individuals who were relatively inactive but in energy balance and/or a slight deficit did not experience these impairments. On the extreme end of inactivity, bed rest, even in the context of energy balance, impairs insulin sensitivity (15, 16).

There are a number of benefits associated with increasing movement and decreasing sedentary behaviour, outside of structured exercise. The interruption of prolonged sitting with light intensity movement may be sufficient to induce some favourable metabolic changes in people who are inactive with or without T2D (11). Short bouts of activity (41, 42) and/or "sitting less" (i.e., 4.7 hours of sitting replaced with 2.5 hours of standing and 2.2 hours of light-intensity walking) can improve glucose control and insulin sensitivity (43).

Some of these favourable adaptations to increasing movement may be mediated by changes in the expression of SkM genes involved in cellular development, growth and proliferation, and lipid and carbohydrate metabolism (131). Additionally, breaking up prolonged sitting favourably alters adipose gene expression associated with macronutrient metabolism and ATP synthesis, immune function, signal transduction, and cell cycle regulation (68).

Clinical Considerations

While it is clear that exercise contributes to improved glucose homeostasis in T2D, it is important to understand factors that can modify adaptations to exercise, and therefore exercise-induced improvements in glucose homeostasis. As with the nutrition/energy balance examples offered in a prior section, the pharmacologic and circadian contexts in which exercise takes place can modulate the resulting beneficial adaptations. Here we review some of the salient research that defines current understanding of circadian clocks and pharmacology as modulators of metabolic adaptations to habitual exercise.

Exercise and Molecular Clocks: Timing of Habitual Exercise Matters

Cells have internal molecular or circadian clocks that play an important role in driving metabolism. Circadian rhythms are the product of a transcription–translation feedback loop. The positive limb of the loop is regulated by the brain and SkM arnt-like protein 1 (Bmal1) and circadian locomotor output cycles kaput (Clock), while the negative limb of the loop is under the control of period (period 1 and 2 (Per 1/2)) and cryptochrome (Cry1/2) (127, 199). Orchestrated regulation via this feedback loop, reviewed in detail elsewhere (57, 59), results in a 24-hour rhythm that can also influence physiology and behaviour.

It is now well-established that disruption of circadian clocks results in tissue-specific metabolic changes that have the potential to contribute to chronic disease. The relationship between circadian clock disruption and chronic diseases comes in part from observations in both children and adults that insufficient periods of sleep are associated with increased risk for obesity [reviewed in (26)], diabetes (215), and cardiovascular disease (113). Additional evidence that circadian misalignment can contribute to metabolic diseases comes from controlled trials inducing misalignment between fasting/feeding cycles and sleep/wake cycles (193). Preclinical trials using loss-of-function models establish that, indeed, disruption of cellular regulators of the circadian rhythm results in tissue and system glucose dyshomeostasis (44, 76, 196). For example, use of a murine model of SkM-specific Bmal1 deletion helped to establish that the SkM molecular clock is important not only for maintaining glucose tolerance (76) but also for regulating total sleep amount (45). These and many other preclinical and clinical studies provide compelling evidence that disruption of circadian rhythms, such as occurs chronically with shift work and acutely with "jet lag," can impose increased risk for obesity and glucose dyshomeostasis.

Evidence suggests that physical activity can change the activity of peripheral circadian clocks, underscoring the interconnectedness of peripheral circadian clocks and metabolic regulation. There is some suggestion that circadian misalignment can alter the response to exercise (57). One potential mechanism for an interference with exercise adaptation is via stability of Cry1 and PER2, which can reportedly be altered by energy sensing via AMPK activation (128). Additionally, Cry1/2 can interact with the lipid-sensing peroxisome proliferator-activated receptor-δ (PPARδ), resulting in decreased PPARδ activation and exercise capacity (105). However, there is also evidence that exercise may be able to protect against disruption of circadian rhythm by entraining molecular clocks. Specifically, in a pre-clinical study, voluntary exercise increased Bmal1 and Clock abundance, with a reduction in body weight gain on a high-fat diet that was dependent on the time of day in which exercise occurred (36).

The circadian rhythm of glucose tolerance is indeed an important consideration for the timing of exercise to achieve the most beneficial glucose homeostatic adaptations in humans. Both historic and recent data describe a diurnal variation in glucose tolerance in the absence of T2D, with a peak in the morning and the greatest impairment later in the day (99, 187). This rhythm of glucose control can be explained in large part by variations in the insulin secretory response, which is greater in the morning than in the evening, and alterations in hepatic insulin extraction, which seems to be lower in the morning than it is later in the day (158, 187). One hypothesis is that T2D is associated with a "flipped" circadian rhythm of insulin sensitivity, that is best during evening hours with gradual worsening overnight resulting in abnormally elevated morning glucose (83). Therefore, as discussed in a review by Heden and Kanaley (83), timing exercise to occur later in the day in people with T2D should logically bring the most benefit both for glucose control after the evening meal, as well as for overnight insulin sensitivity and morning glycemia. Indeed, most studies show that timing exercise to occur after meals in people with T2D is more beneficial than exercise before meals for post-prandial glucose control (35, 79, 84, 129, 130, 171, 172, 176). Additional support for this notion comes from evidence that exercise after a midday meal results in little improvement in glycaemic control (79), while evening exercise beneficially affects glucose homeostasis overnight (35, 84). A recent clinical trial investigated the influence of time of day on metabolic adaptations to high-intensity interval exercise in people with T2D. Savikj and colleagues reported that afternoon exercise training resulted in significantly greater improvements in blood glucose regulation compared to morning exercise which, in fact, acutely increased blood glucose (192). Collectively, these human studies suggest that time of day is emerging as a critical contextual consideration for maximizing beneficial metabolic adaptations to exercise (189), though current understanding about the circadian biology of IR is in its infancy.

Exercise and Diabetes Pharmacology: A Complicated Interaction

Currently nine groups of drugs comprise the non-insulin pharmacological arsenal to manage T2D: metformin, thiazolidinediones, sulfonylureas, glinides, α-glucosidase inhibitors, dipeptidyl peptidase-4 inhibitors, sodium–glucose cotransporter 2 inhibitors, glucagon-like peptide-1 receptor agonists, and insulin. When diagnosed with T2D, the clinical advice provided is typically to increase habitual physical activity and begin a prescription of a glucose-lowering drug. The pharmacotherapeutics with beneficial cardiovascular and renal outcomes, in addition to improved glucose control (metformin, sodium–glucose cotransporter 2 inhibitors, glucagon-like peptide-1 receptor agonists), tend to be most frequently prescribed. However, the body of literature aimed at identifying interactions between exercise and the pharmacology prescribed for T2D is surprisingly sparse.

The biguanide drug metformin is the most frequently prescribed pharmaceutical treatment for T2D (97), with many years of established safety and efficacy and availability at a low cost. The enigmatic mechanism(s) by which metformin so effectively lowers blood glucose have been debated and somewhat elusive despite over 50 years of research. The legacy has predominantly been that metformin improves glucose homeostasis by inhibiting hepatic glucose production via AMPK activation (56) and perhaps by inhibiting hepatocellular respiration through mitochondrial complex I inhibition (46, 164). However, there are challenges to assessing hepatic AMPK regulation in laboratory animal models, and not all evidence points toward metformin being a potent AMPK activator (49) or toward mitochondria being the primary target (167). Interestingly, relatively recent studies have dissociated the glucose-lowering effect of metformin from plasma concentrations, providing compelling evidence that it is predominantly mediated in the lower bowel (28). The intestinal hypotheses about metformin's mechanism of action can be explained by via increased intestinal release of glucagon-like peptide-1 (144, 159), stimulating insulin and inhibiting glucagon release. Additionally, mounting evidence establishes the possibility of improved glucose homeostasis resulting from microbiota-mediated effects of metformin (173). Recently, an elegant study showed that the AMP-inhibited enzyme fructose-1,6-bisphosphatase-1, a rate-controlling enzyme in gluconeogenesis, represents a significant contributor to glucose lowering by metformin (96). Despite the still incompletely understood mechanism of action, metformin remains a major player in the clinical treatment of T2D. However, the interplay between metformin and the other prong of the clinical approach to T2D management, habitual physical activity, seems to be quite complex.

Because metformin decreases blood glucose primarily by restraining hepatic gluneogenesis (164), while exercise results in metabolic adaptations that also include improvements in insulin sensitivity in both SkM and adipose tissue, it is logical to posit that combining metformin treatment with exercise training could result in additive improvements in glucose homeostasis. However, both pre-clinical and clinical studies establish that this is not the case. For example, in a pre-clinical model of T2D and non-alcoholic fatty liver disease, exercise training led to greater improvements in glycaemic control, liver diacylglycerol content, and hepatic mitochondrial function, as well as greater attenuation of hepatic fatty acids than metformin (137). Adding metformin to exercise training offered essentially no benefit and in fact, resulted in an attenuation of exercise-induced increases in mitochondrial function (137). Clinical findings parallel these preclinical outcomes quite closely. In people with pre-diabetes, exercise training resulted in the expected improvements in whole-body insulin sensitivity; however, adding metformin blunted this beneficial exercise adaptation (146). In studies assessing cardiovascular disease (CVD) risk in people with impaired glucose tolerance, only exercise training or metformin alone improved blood pressure and the inflammatory marker C-reactive protein. Co-treatment with exercise and metformin did not provide greater improvements in circulating lipids (137, 147) or metabolic syndrome (147) compared to either monotreatment. In fact, combining the two treatments attenuated the beneficial effects on CVD risk and metabolic syndrome severity (147). Consistent with these findings, metformin diminished the improvement in insulin sensitivity and cardiorespiratory fitness after exercise training in older people at risk for T2D, with concomitant inhibition of beneficial exercise adaptations in SkM mitochondrial respiration (123).

The collective evidence (summarized in Table 28.1) suggests that while metformin is an effective drug for treating T2DM, it can also blunt exercise-induced improvements in SkM mitochondrial function,

Table 28.1 Summary of published interactions between exercise and metformin treatment in people at risk for type 2 diabetes and in people with impaired glucose tolerance

	Exercise	*Metformin*	*Exercise+Metformin*
Whole Body Insulin Sensitivity	↑↑	↑↑	--
Hepatic Insulin Sensitivity	↑↑	↑	--
AMPK Activation	↑↑	↑	↑
Muscle Mitochondrial Function	↑↑		--
Cardiovascular Disease Risk	↓↓	↓	--
Whole Body VO2max	↑↑	-- or ↓	↑

glucose homeostasis, CVD risk, and cardiorespiratory capacity (22–24, 32, 123, 137, 145, 198). Without question, this underscores the importance of carefully considering the pharmacotherapeutic approach used for treating people with T2D who are likely to also adhere to an exercise prescription. While the mounting evidence points toward some interactions between metformin and exercise that are antagonistic for promoting beneficial outcomes, including improved glucose homeostasis, decreased metabolic syndrome, and even SkM mitochondrial adaptations to exercise, the molecular underpinnings of this drug–exercise interaction are incompletely understood. Furthermore, it is not known if initiating metformin treatment in people who are already engaging is habitual exercise elicits similar interactions as initiating the pharmacotherapy prior to beginning an exercise prescription. Whether there is a specific phenotype or genotype that is more likely to be associated with an antagonistic interaction between metformin and exercise is also completely unknown. Finally, the effect of both dose and timing of exercise and metformin on their interaction are still underexplored. However, this growing body of literature certainly underscores the need for investigating alternative T2D pharmacotherapies and their interaction with exercise.

A newer class of diabetes oral pharmaceutics, the sodium-glucose cotransporter-2 inhibitors (SGLT2i), are emerging as candidates for not only improving glucose homeostasis (37, 133) but also for promoting cardiovascular and cardiorenal benefits (101, 121, 136, 151). The interest in SGLT2i efficacy has risen sharply as evidenced by only 1 PubMed manuscript in 2006 and 551 in 2018. However, little research has been carried out to date on the interaction of SGLT2i treatment with habitual exercise. In a pre-clinical model of T2D, both endurance exercise training and treatment with the SGLT2i canagliflozin independently improved indices of glycaemic control (138). The combination of SGLT2i treatment and exercise further improved glucose tolerance and insulin responses during an oral glucose challenge. Only the treatment combination decreased body weight (on a high-fat diet). Surprisingly, exercise-trained animals treated with SGLT2i had greater submaximal exercise capacity compared to exercise training alone (138). The metabolic adaptations with SGLT2i treatment in this study deserve further interrogation, as increased ketone production and a greater reliance on fat as a source of energy during both normal activity and during exercise may be important for this potential additive effect of habitual exercise and SGLT2i treatment. Whether or not the findings of this pre-clinical study (138) will translate to a clinical T2D setting remains unknown. However, a recent study with sedentary overweight and obese human participants investigated the effects of 12 weeks of supervised endurance exercise training, with daily doses of the SGLT2i dapagliflozin or placebo (161). While exercise resulted in all of the expected favourable adaptations including in body mass and composition, cardiorespiratory fitness, insulin sensitivity, and SkM citrate synthase activity, SGLT2i did not. In fact, after endurance exercise training, fasting blood glucose was greater with SGLT2i compared to placebo, and the exercise-induced improvements in insulin sensitivity were abrogated with SGLT2i (161). Whether or not this unfavourable interaction of exercise and SGLT2i pharmacotherapy would persist in a clinical population with T2D is not known. Embarking on a study to address this important question is complicated by the fact that most people with T2D are first prescribed metformin, so recruiting a "pharmacotherapy-naïve" clinical population will be difficult.

Glucagon-like peptide-1 (GLP-1), already mentioned earlier, is an incretin hormone released from intestinal cells that stimulates insulin and inhibits glucagon release, thereby playing an important role in glucose homeostasis (3). Whether or not GLP-1 secretion is decreased in T2D, and if this is a cause or consequence, seems debated (214). However, GLP-1 receptor agonists have emerged as a promising treatment for T2D with, as mentioned previously, additional evidence of beneficial cardiovascular effects in addition to improved glucose homeostasis (30). Interestingly, there is some evidence to suggest that exercise can increase GLP-1 in healthy, overweight, and obese persons (88, 150, 210, 211), though less is known about the effects of exercise on GLP-1 in T2D (47, 134). In people with T2D who engaged in supervised endurance and resistance exercise, treatment with the GLP-1 receptor agonist liraglutide reportedly resulted in greater improvements in HbA1c, body weight and composition, fasting blood glucose, and blood pressure compared to the exercise regimen alone (154).

However, some of the beneficial cardiovascular adaptations to exercise training, in particular left ventricular (LV) diastolic function, can be attenuated during co-treatment with liraglutide LV diastolic function (106). These divergent outcomes, suggesting both benefits and detriments to adding GLP-1 receptor agonist treatment to an exercise prescription in T2D, underscore the need to carry out pre-clinical work to identify mechanisms of this apparent drug–exercise interaction, as well as more clinical investigations into the populations who may be best suited for monotherapy versus co-treatment.

Endogenous GLP-1 is important for glucose homeostatic maintenance but has a very short physiological half-life because it is rapidly degraded by dipeptidyl peptidase-4 (DPP-4). Therefore, DPP-4 inhibitors were developed to enhance insulin secretion by preventing GLP-1 degradation. To investigate the drug–exercise interaction, treatment with a DPP-4 inhibitor, treadmill exercise training, or a combination of both exercise and the DPP-4 inhibitor were compared in a murine model of diabetes. The combination treatment was effective against high-fat diet-induced hepatic lipid accumulation and decreased fasting insulin compared to untreated controls. Both exercise and the combined treatment improved the response to a glucose challenge (205). However little is known about interactions between DPP-4 inhibitor treatment with exercise in humans with T2D. In patients with T2D inadequately controlled by diet and exercise, the DPP-4 inhibitor evogliptin significantly decreased HbA1c compared to placebo, without increased incidence of hypoglycaemia (165). However, exercise was not part of the controlled intervention, and no exercise adaptations were evaluated.

Drug combination therapies hold promise for maximizing pharmacological management of T2D while minimizing potential untoward effects. Combinations of pharmacotherapies also hold potential for capitalizing on drugs that may potentiate the beneficial adaptations to exercise, while minimizing any antagonism between exercise and pharmacology. At present, this is essentially uncharted research territory.

Summary and Suggestions for Future Research

The broad strokes of the "biochemistry of exercise for T2D" are reasonably clear. Acutely, exercise enhances up-regulated contraction-mediated glucose uptake via mechanisms linked to AMPK and CAMKII. After exercise, glucose uptake via those pathways dissipates over the course of several hours but glucose uptake remains elevated over "no prior exercise" conditions by an increase to insulin-mediated glucose uptake via mechanisms that are well characterized. The persistence of these post-exercise effects is modulated by the intensity/duration of the exercise and the post-exercise nutritional environment, particularly energy balance and carbohydrate intake. Habitual exercise benefits glycemia in a host of ways, attenuating the mitochondrial dysfunction that may be a cause or an effect of IR (or likely, both), directing fatty acids to oxidation rather than other metabolic fates and increasing capillary density to allow better perfusion of skeletal muscle, among other adaptations to training. Sedentary behaviour strongly contributes to insulin resistance, and interrupting sedentary behaviour with short bouts of activity appears to have efficacy that is roughly similar to exercise in opposing IR. The magnitude of the effects of interrupting sitting are out of proportion to the actual energy expenditure, suggesting that, possibly akin to HIIT, there is a value to the frequent "on-off" cycles to mobilize cellular glucose uptake. Understanding how both interrupting sitting and HIIT can so efficiently drive greater insulin sensitivity and glycaemic control is a promising area for future research.

The nutritional, circadian, and pharmacologic contexts in which exercise takes place have been understudied and are ripe for both basic and translational research. There is no doubt that all three are important modulators of exercise effects with the potential to accentuate (energy deficit, carbohydrate restriction, timing of exercise to circadian clocks, ensuring optimal sleep along with physical activity, hints that GLP1 agonists may potentiate) or blunt (energy excess, high carbohydrate intake, mistiming exercise with circadian clocks, inadequate sleep quantity or quality, addition of metformin or SGLT2 inhibitors) the beneficial effects of acute exercise and habitual physical activity. Although it is difficult to do studies, particularly in humans, that complicate an "exercise or no-exercise" design by either introducing these elements or trying to control for them as confounding variables, they are necessary to provide the nuanced understanding necessary to best apply exercise as a therapeutic modality for type 2 diabetes.

References

1. Aburasayn H, Al Batran R, Ussher JR. Targeting ceramide metabolism in obesity. *Am J Physiol Endocrinol Metab* 311: E423–435, 2016.
2. Adams OP. The impact of brief high-intensity exercise on blood glucose levels. *Diabetes Metab Syndr Obes* 6: 113–122, 2013.
3. Andersen A, Lund A, Knop FK, Vilsboll T. Glucagon-like peptide 1 in health and disease. *Nat Rev Endocrinol* 14: 390–403, 2018.
4. Andersen P, Saltin B. Maximal perfusion of skeletal muscle in man. *J Physiol* 366: 233–249, 1985.
5. Anderson EJ, Lustig ME, Boyle KE, Woodlief TL, Kane DA, Lin CT, et al. Mitochondrial H2O2 emission and cellular redox state link excess fat intake to insulin resistance in both rodents and humans. *J Clin Invest* 119: 573–581, 2009.
6. Aune D, Norat T, Leitzmann M, Tonstad S, Vatten LJ. Physical activity and the risk of type 2 diabetes: A systematic review and dose–response meta-analysis. *Eur J Epidemol* 30: 529–542, 2015.
7. Babraj JA, Vollaard NBJ, Keast C, Guppy FM, Cottrell G, Timmons JA. Extremely short duration high intensity interval training substantially improves insulin action in young healthy males. *BMC Endocrine Disorders* 9: 3, 2009.
8. Bajpeyi S, Tanner CJ, Slentz CA, Duscha BD, McCartney JS, Hickner RC, et al. Effect of exercise intensity and volume on persistence of insulin sensitivity during training cessation. *J Appl Physiol (1985)* 106: 1079–1085, 2009.
9. Bangsbo J, Hellsten Y. Muscle blood flow and oxygen uptake in recovery from exercise. *Acta Physiol Scand* 162: 305–312, 1998.
10. Baron AD, Steinberg H, Brechtel G, Johnson A. Skeletal muscle blood flow independently modulates insulin-mediated glucose uptake. *Am J Physiol Endocrinol Metab* 266: E248–E253, 1994.
11. Benatti F, Ried-Larsen, M. The effects of breaking up prolonged sedentary time: a review of experimental studies. *Med Sci Sport Exer* 47: 2053–2061, 2015.
12. Bergman BC, Perreault L, Strauss A, Bacon S, Kerege A, Harrison K, et al. Intramuscular triglyceride synthesis: importance in muscle lipid partitioning in humans. *Am J Physiol Endocrinol Metab* 314: E152–E164, 2018.
13. Bergman RN, Kim SP, Catalano KJ, Hsu IR, Chiu JD, Kabir M, et al. Why visceral fat is bad: mechanisms of the metabolic syndrome. *Obesity* 14: 16S–19S, 2006.
14. Bergman RN, Piccinini F, Kabir M, Kolka CM, Ader M. Hypothesis: role of reduced hepatic insulin clearance in the pathogenesis of type 2 diabetes. *Diabetes* 68: 1709–1716, 2019.
15. Bergouignan A, Schoeller DA, Normand S, Gauquelin-Koch G, Laville M, Shriver T, et al. Effect of physical inactivity on the oxidation of saturated and monounsaturated dietary Fatty acids: results of a randomized trial. *PLOS Clin Trials* 1: e27 (1–10) 2006.
16. Bergouignan A, Trudel G, Simon C, Chopard A, Schoeller DA, Momken I, et al. Physical inactivity differentially alters dietary oleate and palmitate trafficking. *Diabetes* 58: 367–376, 2009.
17. Biolo G, Agostini F, Simunic B, Sturma M, Torelli L, Preiser JC, et al. Positive energy balance is associated with accelerated muscle atrophy and increased erythrocyte glutathione turnover during 5 wk of bed rest. *Am J Clin Nutr* 88: 950–958, 2008.
18. Bird SR, Hawley JA. Exercise and type 2 diabetes: new prescription for an old problem. *Maturitas* 72: 311–316, 2012.
19. Black SE, Mitchell E, Freedson PS, Chipkin SR, Braun B. Improved insulin action following short-term exercise training: role of energy and carbohydrate balance. *J Appl Physiol* 99: 2285–2293, 2005.
20. Booth FW, Thomason DB. Molecular and cellular adaptation of muscle in response to exercise: perspectives of various models. *Physiol Rev* 71: 541–585, 1991.
21. Boulé NG, Haddad E, Kenny GP, Wells GA, Sigal RJ. Effects of exercise on glycemic control and body mass in type 2 diabetes mellitus: a meta-analysis of controlled clinical trials. *JAMA* 286: 1218–1227, 2001.
22. Boule NG, Kenny GP, Larose J, Khandwala F, Kuzik N, Sigal RJ. Does metformin modify the effect on glycaemic control of aerobic exercise, resistance exercise or both? *Diabetologia* 56: 2378–2382, 2013.
23. Boule NG, Robert C, Bell GJ, Johnson ST, Bell RC, Lewanczuk RZ, et al. Metformin and exercise in type 2 diabetes: examining treatment modality interactions. *Diabetes Care* 34: 1469–1474, 2011.

24. Braun B, Eze P, Stephens BR, Hagobian TA, Sharoff CG, Chipkin SR, et al. Impact of metformin on peak aerobic capacity. *Appl Physiol Nutr Metab* 33: 61–67, 2008.

25. Braun B, Zimmermann MB, Kretchmer N. Effects of exercise intensity on insulin sensitivity in women with non-insulin-dependent diabetes mellitus. *J Appl Physiol* 78: 300–306, 1995.

26. Broussard JL, Van Cauter E. Disturbances of sleep and circadian rhythms: novel risk factors for obesity. *Curr Opin Endocrinol Diabetes Obes* 23: 353–359, 2016.

27. Burstein R, Polychronakos C, Toews CJ, MacDougall JD, Guyda HJ, Posner BI. Acute reversal of the enhanced insulin action in trained athletes: association with insulin receptor changes. *Diabetes* 34: 756–760, 1985.

28. Buse JB, DeFronzo RA, Rosenstock J, Kim T, Burns C, Skare S, et al. The primary glucose-lowering effect of metformin resides in the gut, not the circulation: results from short-term pharmacokinetic and 12-week dose-ranging studies. *Diabetes Care* 39: 198–205, 2016.

29. Cartee GD, Holloszy JO. Exercise increases susceptibility of muscle glucose transport to activation by various stimuli. *Am J Physiol Endocrinol Metab* 258: E390–E393, 1990.

30. Chatterjee S, Ghosal S, Chatterjee S. Glucagon-like peptide-1 receptor agonists favorably address all components of metabolic syndrome. *World J Diabetes* 7: 441–448, 2016.

31. Chen YL, Messina EJ. Dilation of isolated skeletal muscle arterioles by insulin is endothelium dependent and nitric oxide mediated. *Am J Physiol* 270: H2120–2124, 1996.

32. Clarson CL, Mahmud FH, Baker JE, Clark HE, McKay WM, Schauteet VD, et al. Metformin in combination with structured lifestyle intervention improved body mass index in obese adolescents, but did not improve insulin resistance. *Endocrine* 36: 141–146, 2009.

33. Colberg SR, Sigal RJ, Fernhall B, Regensteiner JG, Blissmer BJ, Rubin RR, et al, American College of Sports M, American Diabetes A. exercise and type 2 diabetes: the American College of Sports Medicine and the American Diabetes Association: Joint position statement executive summary. *Diabetes Care* 33: 2692–2696, 2010.

34. Colberg SR, Sigal RJ, Yardley JE, Riddell MC, Dunstan DW, Dempsey PC, et al. Physical activity/exercise and diabetes: a position statement of the American Diabetes Association. *Diabetes Care* 39: 2065–2079, 2016.

35. Colberg SR, Zarrabi L, Bennington L, Nakave A, Thomas Somma C, Swain DP, et al. Postprandial walking is better for lowering the glycemic effect of dinner than pre-dinner exercise in type 2 diabetic individuals. *J Am Med Dir Assoc* 10: 394–397, 2009.

36. Dalbram E, Basse AL, Zierath JR, Treebak JT. Voluntary wheel running in the late dark phase ameliorates diet-induced obesity in mice without altering insulin action. *J Appl Physiol (1985)* 126: 993–1005, 2019.

37. Davies MJ, D'Alessio DA, Fradkin J, Kernan WN, Mathieu C, Mingrone G, et al. Management of hyperglycemia in type 2 diabetes, 2018. a consensus report by the american diabetes association (ADA) and the European association for the study of diabetes (EASD). *Diabetes Care* 41: 2669–2701, 2018.

38. De Filippis E, Cusi K, Ocampo G, Berria R, Buck S, Consoli A, et al. Exercise-induced improvement in vasodilatory function accompanies increased insulin sensitivity in obesity and type 2 diabetes mellitus. *J Clin Endocrinol Metab* 91: 4903–4910, 2006.

39. DeFronzo RA, Ferrannini E, Sato Y, Felig P, Wahren J. Synergistic interaction between exercise and insulin on peripheral glucose uptake. *J Clin Invest* 68: 1468–1474, 1981.

40. DeFronzo RA, Tripathy D. Skeletal muscle insulin resistance is the primary defect in type 2 diabetes. *Diabetes Care* 32(Suppl 2): S157–163, 2009.

41. Dempsey PC, Larsen RN, Sethi P, Sacre JW, Straznicky NE, Cohen ND, et al. Benefits for type 2 diabetes of interrupting prolonged sitting with brief bouts of light walking or simple resistance activities. *Diabetes Care* 39: 964–972, 2016.

42. Dunstan DW, Howard B, Healy GN, Owen N. Too much sitting – A health hazard. *Diabetes Rs Clin Pract* 97: 368–376, 2012.

43. Duvivier BMFM, Schaper NC, Koster A, van Kan L, Peters HPF, Adam JJ, et al. Benefits of substituting sitting with standing and walking in free-living conditions for cardiometabolic risk markers, cognition and mood in overweight adults. *Front Physiol* 8: 353–353, 2017.

44. Dyar KA, Ciciliot S, Wright LE, Bienso RS, Tagliazucchi GM, Patel VR, et al. Muscle insulin sensitivity and glucose metabolism are controlled by the intrinsic muscle clock. *Mol Metab* 3: 29–41, 2014.

45. Ehlen JC, Brager AJ, Baggs J, Pinckney L, Gray CL, DeBruyne JP, et al. Bmal1 function in skeletal muscle regulates sleep. *Elife* 6: 2017.

46. El-Mir MY, Nogueira V, Fontaine E, Averet N, Rigoulet M, Leverve X. Dimethylbiguanide inhibits cell respiration via an indirect effect targeted on the respiratory chain complex I. *J Biol Chem* 275: 223–228, 2000.

47. Eshghi SR, Bell GJ, Boule NG. Effects of aerobic exercise with or without metformin on plasma incretins in type 2 diabetes. *Can J Diabetes* 37: 375–380, 2013.

48. Fisher-Wellman KH, Weber TM, Cathey BL, Brophy PM, Gilliam LAA, Kane CL, et al. Mitochondrial respiratory capacity and content are normal in young insulin-resistant obese humans. *Diabetes* 63: 132–141, 2014.

49. Foretz M, Hebrard S, Leclerc J, Zarrinpashneh E, Soty M, Mithieux G, et al. Metformin inhibits hepatic gluconeogenesis in mice independently of the LKB1/AMPK pathway via a decrease in hepatic energy state. *J Clin Invest* 120: 2355–2369, 2010.

50. Fox AK, Kaufman AE, Horowitz JF. Adding fat calories to meals after exercise does not alter glucose tolerance. *J Appl Physiol* 97: 11–16, 2004.

51. Frøsig C, Jørgensen SB, Hardie DG, Richter EA, Wojtaszewski JFP. 5′-AMP-activated protein kinase activity and protein expression are regulated by endurance training in human skeletal muscle. *Am J Physiol Endocrinol Metab* 286: E411–E417, 2004.

52. Frosig C, Rose AJ, Treebak JT, Kiens B, Richter EA, Wojtaszewski JF. Effects of endurance exercise training on insulin signaling in human skeletal muscle: Interactions at the level of phosphatidylinositol 3-kinase, Akt, and AS160. *Diabetes* 56: 2093–2102, 2007.

53. Fueger PT, Bracy DP, Malabanan CM, Pencek RR, Granner DK, Wasserman DH. Hexokinase II overexpression improves exercise-stimulated but not insulin-stimulated muscle glucose uptake in high-fat-fed C57BL/6J mice. *Diabetes* 53: 306–314, 2004.

54. Fueger PT, Heikkinen S, Bracy DP, Malabanan CM, Pencek RR, Laakso M, et al. Hexokinase II partial knockout impairs exercise-stimulated glucose uptake in oxidative muscles of mice. *Am J Physiol Endocrinol Metab* 285: E958–963, 2003.

55. Fueger PT, Hess HS, Posey KA, Bracy DP, Pencek RR, Charron MJ, et al. Control of exercise-stimulated muscle glucose uptake by GLUT4 is dependent on glucose phosphorylation capacity in the conscious mouse. *J Biol Chem* 279: 50956–50961, 2004.

56. Fullerton MD, Galic S, Marcinko K, Sikkema S, Pulinilkunnil T, Chen ZP, et al Single phosphorylation sites in Acc1 and Acc2 regulate lipid homeostasis and the insulin-sensitizing effects of metformin. *Nat Med* 19: 1649–1654, 2013.

57. Gabriel BM, Zierath JR. Circadian rhythms and exercise - re-setting the clock in metabolic disease. *Nat Rev Endocrinol* 15: 197–206, 2019.

58. Gaesser GA, Angadi SS, Sawyer BJ. Exercise and diet, independent of weight loss, improve cardiometabolic risk profile in overweight and obese individuals. *Phys Sportsmed* 39: 87–97, 2011.

59. Gallego M, Virshup DM. Post-translational modifications regulate the ticking of the circadian clock. *Nat Rev Mol Cell Biol* 8: 139–148, 2007.

60. Gavin TP, Ernst JM, Kwak HB, Caudill SE, Reed MA, Garner RT, et al. High incomplete skeletal muscle fatty acid oxidation explains low muscle insulin sensitivity in poorly controlled T2D. *J Clin Endocrinol Metab* 103: 882–889, 2018.

61. Ghosh S, Wicks SE, Vandanmagsar B, Mendoza TM, Bayless DS, Salbaum JM, et al. Extensive metabolic remodeling after limiting mitochondrial lipid burden is consistent with an improved metabolic health profile. *J Biol Chem* 294: 12313–12327, 2019.

62. Gibala MJ, Little JP, Macdonald MJ, Hawley JA. Physiological adaptations to low-volume, high-intensity interval training in health and disease. *J Physiol* 590: 1077–1084, 2012.

63. Gillen JB, Little JP, Punthakee Z, Tarnopolsky MA, Riddell MC, Gibala MJ. Acute high-intensity interval exercise reduces the postprandial glucose response and prevalence of hyperglycaemia in patients with type 2 diabetes. *Diabetes, Obes Metab* 14: 575–577, 2012.

64. Gillen JB, Martin BJ, MacInnis MJ, Skelly LE, Tarnopolsky MA, Gibala MJ. Twelve weeks of sprint interval training improves indices of cardiometabolic health similar to traditional endurance training despite a five-fold lower exercise volume and time commitment. *PLOS ONE* 11: e0154075, 2016.

65. Gonzalez-Franquesa A, Patti M-E. Insulin Resistance and Mitochondrial Dysfunction. In: *Mitochondrial Dynamics in Cardiovascular Medicine*, edited by Santulli G. Cham: Springer International Publishing, 2017, p. 465–520.

66. Goodpaster BH, Bertoldo A, Ng JM, Azuma K, Pencek RR, Kelley C, et al. Interactions among glucose delivery, transport, and phosphorylation that underlie skeletal muscle insulin resistance in obesity and type 2 Diabetes: studies with dynamic PET imaging. *Diabetes* 63: 1058–1068, 2014.

67. Gormley S, Swain P, High R, Spina R, Dowling E, Kotipalli U, Gandrakota R. Effect of intensity of aerobic training on VO2max. *Med Sci Sport Exer* 40: 1336–1343, 2008.

68. Grace MS, Formosa MF, Bozaoglu K, Bergouignan A, Brozynska M, Carey AL, et al. Acute effects of active breaks during prolonged sitting on subcutaneous adipose tissue gene expression: an ancillary analysis of a randomised controlled trial. *Sci Rep* 9: 3847–3847, 2019.

69. Granata C, Jamnick NA, Bishop DJ. Training-induced changes in mitochondrial content and respiratory function in human skeletal muscle. *Sports Med* 48: 1809–1828, 2018.

70. Griffin ME, Marcucci MJ, Cline GW, Bell K, Barucci N, Lee D, et al. Free fatty acid-induced insulin resistance is associated with activation of protein kinase C theta and alterations in the insulin signaling cascade. *Diabetes* 48: 1270–1274, 1999.

71. Halseth AE, Bracy DP, Wasserman DH. Limitations to basal and insulin-stimulated skeletal muscle glucose uptake in the high-fat-fed rat. *Am J Physiol Endocrinol Metab* 279: E1064–1071, 2000.

72. Halseth AE, Bracy DP, Wasserman DH. Limitations to exercise- and maximal insulin-stimulated muscle glucose uptake. *J Appl Physiol (1985)* 85: 2305–2313, 1998.

73. Halseth AE, Bracy DP, Wasserman DH. Overexpression of hexokinase II increases insulin and exercise-stimulated muscle glucose uptake in vivo. *Am J Physiol* 276: E70–77, 1999.

74. Hancock CR, Han D-H, Chen M, Terada S, Yasuda T, Wright DC, et al. High-fat diets cause insulin resistance despite an increase in muscle mitochondria. *Proc Natl Acad Sci U S A* 105: 7815–7820, 2008.

75. Hansen D, Dendale P, Jonkers RAM, Beelen M, Manders RJF, Corluy L, et al. Continuous low- to moderate-intensity exercise training is as effective as moderate- to high-intensity exercise training at lowering blood HbA(1c) in obese type 2 diabetes patients. *Diabetologia* 52: 1789–1797, 2009.

76. Harfmann BD, Schroder EA, Kachman MT, Hodge BA, Zhang X, Esser KA. Muscle-specific loss of Bmal1 leads to disrupted tissue glucose metabolism and systemic glucose homeostasis. *Skelet Muscle* 6: 12, 2016.

77. Hawley JA, Gibala MJ. What's new since Hippocrates? Preventing type 2 diabetes by physical exercise and diet. *Diabetologia* 55: 535–539, 2012.

78. Hawley JA, Lessard SJ. Exercise training-induced improvements in insulin action. *Acta Physiol (Oxf)* 192: 127–135, 2008.

79. Haxhi J, Leto G, di Palumbo AS, Sbriccoli P, Guidetti L, Fantini C, et al. Exercise at lunchtime: effect on glycemic control and oxidative stress in middle-aged men with type 2 diabetes. *Eur J Appl Physiol* 116: 573–582, 2016.

80. Hayashi T, Hirshman MF, Kurth EJ, Winder WW, Goodyear LJ. Evidence for 5' AMP-activated protein kinase mediation of the effect of muscle contraction on glucose transport. *Diabetes* 47: 1369–1373, 1998.

81. Hayes C, Kriska A. Role of physical activity in diabetes management and prevention. *J Am Diet Assoc* 108: S19–S23, 2008.

82. Heath GW, Gavin JR, Hinderliter JM, Hagberg JM, Bloomfield SA, Holloszy JO. Effects of exercise and lack of exercise on glucose tolerance and insulin sensitivity. *J Appl Physiol* 55: 512–517, 1983.

83. Heden TD, Kanaley JA. Syncing exercise with meals and circadian clocks. *Exerc Sport Sci Rev* 47: 22–28, 2019.

84. Heden TD, Winn NC, Mari A, Booth FW, Rector RS, Thyfault JP, et al. Postdinner resistance exercise improves postprandial risk factors more effectively than predinner resistance exercise in patients with type 2 diabetes. *J Appl Physiol (1985)* 118: 624–634, 2015.

85. Hellsten Y, Nyberg M. Cardiovascular adaptations to exercise training. *Compr Physiol* 6: 1–32, 2015.

86. Herzig S, Shaw RJ. AMPK: Guardian of metabolism and mitochondrial homeostasis. *Nat Rev Mol Cell Biol* 19: 121–135, 2018.

87. Hickam JB, Cargill WH. EFFECT of exercise on cardiac output and pulmonary arterial pressure in normal persons and in patients with cardiovascular disease and pulmonary emphysema. *J Clin Invest* 27: 10–23, 1948.

88. Holliday A, Blannin A. Appetite, food intake and gut hormone responses to intense aerobic exercise of different duration. *J Endocrinol* 235: 193–205, 2017.

89. Holloszy JO. Biochemical adaptations in muscle: effects of exercise on mitochondrial oxygen uptake and respiratory enzyme activity in skeletal muscle. *J Biol Chem* 242: 2278–2282, 1967.

90. Holloszy JO, Booth FW. Biochemical adaptations to endurance exercise in muscle. *Annu Rev Physiol* 38: 273–291, 1976.

91. Holloszy JO, Constable SH, Young DA. Activation of glucose transport in muscle by exercise. *Diabetes Metab Rev* 1: 409–423, 1986.

92. Holloszy JO, Coyle EF. Adaptations of skeletal muscle to endurance exercise and their metabolic consequences. *J Appl Physiol* 56: 831–838, 1984.

93. Host HH, Hansen PA, Nolte LA, Chen MM, Holloszy JO. Glycogen supercompensation masks the effect of a training induced increase in GLUT-4 on muscle glucose transport. *J Appl Physiol* 85: 133–138, 1998.

94. Houmard JA, Tanner CJ, Slentz CA, Duscha BD, McCartney JS, Kraus WE. Effect of the volume and intensity of exercise training on insulin sensitivity. *J Appl Physiol* 96: 101–106, 2004.

95. Huang C, Somwar R, Patel N, Niu W, Torok D, Klip A. Sustained exposure of L6 myotubes to high glucose and insulin decreases insulin-stimulated GLUT4 translocation but upregulates GLUT4 activity. *Diabetes* 51: 2090–2098, 2002.

96. Hunter RW, Hughey CC, Lantier L, Sundelin EI, Peggie M, Zeqiraj E, et al. Metformin reduces liver glucose production by inhibition of fructose-1-6-bisphosphatase. *Nat Med* 24: 1395–1406, 2018.

97. Inzucchi SE, Bergenstal RM, Buse JB, Diamant M, Ferrannini E, Nauck M, et al, American diabetes a, European association for the study of D. management of hyperglycemia in type 2 diabetes: a patient-centered approach: Position statement of the American diabetes association (ADA) and the European association for the study of diabetes (EASD). *Diabetes Care* 35: 1364–1379, 2012.

98. Jadhav RA, Hazari A, Monterio A, Kumar S, Maiya AG. Effect of physical activity intervention in prediabetes: a systematic review with meta-analysis. *J Phys Act Health* 14: 745–755, 2017.

99. Jarrett RJ, Baker IA, Keen H, Oakley NW. Diurnal variation in oral glucose tolerance: blood sugar and plasma insulin levels morning, afternoon, and evening. *Br Med J* 1: 199–201, 1972.

100. Jelleyman C, Yates T, O'Donovan G, Gray LJ, King JA, Khunti K, et al. The effects of high-intensity interval training on glucose regulation and insulin resistance: a meta-analysis. *Obesity Reviews* 16: 942–961, 2015.

101. Jensen J, Omar M, Kistorp C, Poulsen MK, Tuxen C, Gustafsson I, et al. Empagliflozin in heart failure patients with reduced ejection fraction: a randomized clinical trial (Empire HF). *Trials* 20: 374, 2019.

102. Johannsen NM, Swift DL, Lavie CJ, Earnest CP, Blair SN, Church TS. Combined aerobic and resistance training effects on glucose homeostasis, fitness, and other major health indices: a review of current guidelines. *Sport Med* 46: 1809–1818, 2016.

103. Johnson JL, Slentz CA, Houmard JA, Samsa GP, Duscha BD, Aiken LB, et al. Exercise training amount and intensity effects on metabolic syndrome (from studies of a targeted risk reduction intervention through defined exercise). *Am J Cardiol* 100: 1759–1766, 2007.

104. Johnstone MT, Creager SJ, Scales KM, Cusco JA, Lee BK, Creager MA. Impaired endothelium-dependent vasodilation in patients with insulin-dependent diabetes mellitus. *Circulation* 88: 2510–2516, 1993.

105. Jordan SD, Kriebs A, Vaughan M, Duglan D, Fan W, Henriksson E, et al. CRY1/2 selectively repress PPARdelta and limit exercise capacity. *Cell Metab* 26: 243–255 e246, 2017.

106. Jorgensen PG, Jensen MT, Mensberg P, Storgaard H, Nyby S, Jensen JS, et al. Effect of exercise combined with glucagon-like peptide-1 receptor agonist treatment on cardiac function: a randomized double-blind placebo-controlled clinical trial. *Diabetes Obes Metab* 19: 1040–1044, 2017.

107. Kang J, Robertson RJ, Hagberg JM, Kelley DE, Goss FL, Dasilva SG, et al. Effect of exercise intensity on glucose and insulin metabolism in obese individuals and obese NIDDM patients. *Diabetes Care* 19: 341–349, 1996.

108. Karstoft K, Winding K, Knudsen SH, Nielsen JS, Thomsen C, Pedersen BK, et al. The effects of free-living interval-walking training on glycemic control, body composition, and physical fitness in type 2 diabetic patients: a randomized, controlled trial. *Diabetes Care* 36: 228–236, 2013.

109. Kasuga M, Ogawa W, Ohara T. Tissue glycogen content and glucose intolerance. *J Clin Invest* 111: 1282–1284, 2003.

110. Kelley DE, He J, Menshikova EV, Ritov VB. Dysfunction of mitochondria in human skeletal muscle in type 2 diabetes. *Diabetes* 51: 2944–2950, 2002.

111. Kern M, Wells JA, Stephens JM, Elton CW, Friedman JE, Tapscott EB, et al. Insulin responsiveness in skeletal muscle is determined by glucose transporter (Glut4) protein level. *Biochem J* 270: 397–400, 1990.

112. Kessler HS, Sisson SB, Short KR. The potential for high-intensity interval training to reduce cardiometabolic disease risk. *Sport Med* 42: 489–509, 2012.

113. Khan MS, Aouad R. The effects of insomnia and sleep loss on cardiovascular disease. *Sleep Med Clin* 12: 167–177, 2017.

114. Kim JK, Fillmore JJ, Sunshine MJ, Albrecht B, Higashimori T, Kim DW, et al. PKC-theta knockout mice are protected from fat-induced insulin resistance. *J Clin Invest* 114: 823–827, 2004.

115. Kim T, He L, Johnson MS, Li Y, Zeng L, Ding Y, et al. Carnitine palmitoyltransferase 1b deficiency protects mice from diet-induced insulin resistance. *J Diabetes Metab* 5: 361, 2014.

116. King DS, Dalsky GP, Clutter WE, Young DA, Staten MA, Cryer PE, et al. Effects of exercise and lack of exercise on insulin sensitivity and responsiveness. *J Appl Physiol* 64: 1942–1946, 1988.

117. King DS, Dalsky GP, Clutter WE, Young DA, Staten MA, Cryer PE, et al. Effects of lack of exercise on insulin secretion and action in trained subjects. *Am J Physiol Endocrinol Metab* 254: E537–E542, 1988.

118. Klein S. Is visceral fat responsible for the metabolic abnormalities associated with obesity?: implications of omentectomy. *Diabetes Xare* 33: 1693–1694, 2010.

119. Klein S, Coyle EF, Wolfe RR. Fat metabolism during low-intensity exercise in endurance-trained and untrained men. *Am J Physiol Endocrinol Metab* 267: E934–E940, 1994.

120. Klip A, McGraw TE, James DE. Thirty sweet years of GLUT4. *J Biol Chem* 294: 11369–11381, 2019.

121. Kluger AY, Tecson KM, Barbin CM, Lee AY, Lerma EV, Rosol ZP, et al. Cardiorenal outcomes in the CANVAS, DECLARE-TIMI 58, and EMPA-REG OUTCOME Trials: a systematic review. *Rev Cardiovasc Med* 19: 41–49, 2018.

122. Knowler WC, Barrett-Connor E, Fowler SE, Hamman RF, Lachin JM, Walker EA, et al, Diabetes prevention program research G. Reduction in the incidence of type 2 diabetes with lifestyle intervention or metformin. *N Engl J Med* 346: 393–403, 2002.

123. Konopka AR, Laurin JL, Schoenberg HM, Reid JJ, Castor WM, Wolff CA, et al. Metformin inhibits mitochondrial adaptations to aerobic exercise training in older adults. *Aging Cell* 18: e12880, 2019.

124. Koval JA, DeFronzo RA, O'Doherty RM, Printz R, Ardehali H, Granner DK, et al. Regulation of hexokinase II activity and expression in human muscle by moderate exercise. *Am J Physiol* 274: E304–308, 1998.

125. Koves TR, Ussher JR, Noland RC, Slentz D, Mosedale M, Ilkayeva O, et al. Mitochondrial overload and incomplete fatty acid oxidation contribute to skeletal muscle insulin resistance. *Cell Metab* 7: 45–56, 2008.

126. Kristiansen S, Hargreaves M, Richter EA. Exercise-induced increase in glucose transport, GLUT-4, and VAMP-2 in plasma membrane from human muscle. *Am J Physiol* 270: E197–201, 1996.

127. Kume K, Zylka MJ, Sriram S, Shearman LP, Weaver DR, Jin X, et al, Reppert SM. mCRY1 and mCRY2 are essential components of the negative limb of the circadian clock feedback loop. *Cell* 98: 193–205, 1999.

128. Lamia KA, Sachdeva UM, DiTacchio L, Williams EC, Alvarez JG, Egan DF, et al. AMPK regulates the circadian clock by cryptochrome phosphorylation and degradation. *Science* 326: 437–440, 2009.

129. Larsen JJ, Dela F, Kjaer M, Galbo H. The effect of moderate exercise on postprandial glucose homeostasis in NIDDM patients. *Diabetologia* 40: 447–453, 1997.

130. Larsen JJ, Dela F, Madsbad S, Galbo H. The effect of intense exercise on postprandial glucose homeostasis in type II diabetic patients. *Diabetologia* 42: 1282–1292, 1999.

131. Latouche C, Jowett JBM, Carey AL, Bertovic DA, Owen N, Dunstan DW, et al. Effects of breaking up prolonged sitting on skeletal muscle gene expression. *J Appl Physiol* 114: 453–460, 2013.

132. Laurie J. Goodyear P, Barbara B. Kahn M. Exercise, glucose transport, and insulin sensitivity. *Annu Rev Med* 49: 235–261, 1998.

133. Lee S. Update on SGLT2 Inhibitors-new data released at the American diabetes association. *Crit Pathw Cardiol* 16: 93–95, 2017.

134. Lee SS, Yoo JH, So YS. Effect of the low- versus high-intensity exercise training on endoplasmic reticulum stress and GLP-1 in adolescents with type 2 diabetes mellitus. *J Phys Ther Sci* 27: 3063–3068, 2015.

135. Li X, Li Z, Zhao M, Nie Y, Liu P, Zhu Y, et al. Skeletal muscle lipid droplets and the Athlete's paradox. *Cells* 8: 249, 2019.

136. Lim S. Effects of sodium-glucose cotransporter inhibitors on cardiorenal and metabolic systems: Latest perspectives from the outcome trials. *Diabetes Obes Metab* 21(Suppl 2): 5–8, 2019.

137. Linden MA, Fletcher JA, Morris EM, Meers GM, Kearney ML, Crissey JM, et al. Combining metformin and aerobic exercise training in the treatment of type 2 diabetes and NAFLD in OLETF rats. *Am J Physiol Endocrinol Metab* 306: E300–310, 2014.

138. Linden MA, Ross TT, Beebe DA, Gorgoglione MF, Hamilton KL, Miller BF, et al. The combination of exercise training and sodium-glucose cotransporter-2 inhibition improves glucose tolerance and exercise capacity in a rodent model of type 2 diabetes. *Metabolism* 97: 68–80, 2019.

139. Little JP, Francois ME. High-intensity interval training for improving postprandial hyperglycemia. *Res Q Exer Sport* 85: 451–456, 2014.

140. Little JP, Gillen JB, Percival ME, Safdar A, Tarnopolsky MA, Punthakee Z, et al. Low-volume high-intensity interval training reduces hyperglycemia and increases muscle mitochondrial capacity in patients with type 2 diabetes. *J Appl Physiol* 111: 1554–1560, 2011.

141. Lumini JA, Magalhães J, Oliveira PJ, Ascensão A. Beneficial effects of exercise on muscle mitochondrial function in diabetes mellitus. *Sport Med* 38: 735–750, 2008.

142. Lyon JB, Jr. Muscle and liver glycogen levels in lean and obese strains of mice. *Am J Physiol* 190: 434–438, 1957.

143. Machado MV, Martins RL, Borges J, Antunes BR, Estato V, Vieira AB, et al. Exercise training reverses structural microvascular rarefaction and improves endothelium-dependent microvascular reactivity in rats with diabetes. *Metab Syndr Relat Disord* 14: 298–304, 2016.

144. Maida A, Lamont BJ, Cao X, Drucker DJ. Metformin regulates the incretin receptor axis via a pathway dependent on peroxisome proliferator-activated receptor-alpha in mice. *Diabetologia* 54: 339–349, 2011.

145. Malin SK, Braun B. Effect of metformin on substrate utilization after exercise training in adults with impaired glucose tolerance. *Appl Physiol Nutr Metab* 38: 427–430, 2013.

146. Malin SK, Gerber R, Chipkin SR, Braun B. Independent and combined effects of exercise training and metformin on insulin sensitivity in individuals with prediabetes. *Diabetes Care* 35: 131–136, 2012.

147. Malin SK, Nightingale J, Choi SE, Chipkin SR, Braun B. Metformin modifies the exercise training effects on risk factors for cardiovascular disease in impaired glucose tolerant adults. *Obesity (Silver Spring)* 21: 93–100, 2013.

148. Mann S, Beedie C, Balducci S, Zanuso S, Allgrove J, Bertiato F, et al. Changes in insulin sensitivity in response to different modalities of exercise: a review of the evidence. *Diabetes/Metabolism Research and Reviews* 30: 257–268, 2014.

149. Martin IK, Katz A, Wahren J. Splanchnic and muscle metabolism during exercise in NIDDM patients. *Am J Physiol Endocrinol Metab* 269: E583–E590, 1995.

150. Martins C, Stensvold D, Finlayson G, Holst J, Wisloff U, Kulseng B, et al. Effect of moderate- and high-intensity acute exercise on appetite in obese individuals. *Med Sci Sports Exerc* 47: 40–48, 2015.

151. McMurray JJV, DeMets DL, Inzucchi SE, Kober L, Kosiborod MN, Langkilde AM, et al, Committees D-H, Investigators. The dapagliflozin and prevention of adverse-outcomes in heart failure (DAPA-HF) trial: Baseline characteristics. *Eur J Heart Fail 21:1402-1411*, 2019.

152. McVeigh GE, Gibson W, Hamilton PK. Cardiovascular risk in the young type 1 diabetes population with a low 10-year, but high lifetime risk of cardiovascular disease. *Diabetes, Obes Metab* 15: 198–203, 2013.

153. Meex RCR, Schrauwen-Hinderling VB, Moonen-Kornips E, Schaart G, Mensink M, Phielix E, et al. Restoration of muscle mitochondrial function and metabolic flexibility in type 2 diabetes by exercise training is paralleled by increased myocellular fat storage and improved insulin sensitivity. *Diabetes* 59: 572–579, 2010.

154. Mensberg P, Nyby S, Jorgensen PG, Storgaard H, Jensen MT, Sivertsen J, et al. Near-normalization of glycaemic control with glucagon-like peptide-1 receptor agonist treatment combined with exercise in patients with type 2 diabetes. *Diabetes Obes Metab* 19: 172–180, 2017.

155. Mikus CR, Oberlin DJ, Libla J, Boyle LJ, Thyfault JP. Glycaemic control is improved by 7 days of aerobic exercise training in patients with type 2 diabetes. *Diabetologia* 55: 1417–1423, 2012.

156. Miotto PM, LeBlanc PJ, Holloway GP. High-fat diet causes mitochondrial dysfunction as a result of impaired ADP sensitivity. *Diabetes* 67: 2199–2205, 2018.

157. Moien-Afshari F, Ghosh S, Elmi S, Rahman MM, Sallam N, Khazaei M, et al. Exercise restores endothelial function independently of weight loss or hyperglycaemic status in db/db mice. *Diabetologia* 51: 1327–1337, 2008.

158. Morris CJ, Yang JN, Garcia JI, Myers S, Bozzi I, Wang W, et al. Endogenous circadian system and circadian misalignment impact glucose tolerance via separate mechanisms in humans. *Proc Natl Acad Sci U S A* 112: E2225–2234, 2015.

159. Mulherin AJ, Oh AH, Kim H, Grieco A, Lauffer LM, Brubaker PL. Mechanisms underlying metformin-induced secretion of glucagon-like peptide-1 from the intestinal L cell. *Endocrinology* 152: 4610–4619, 2011.

160. Nair KS, Bigelow ML, Asmann YW, Chow LS, Coenen-Schimke JM, Klaus KA, et al. Asian Indians Have enhanced skeletal muscle mitochondrial capacity to produce ATP in association with severe insulin resistance. *Diabetes* 57: 1166–1175, 2008.

161. Newman AA, Grimm NC, Wilburn JR, Schoenberg HM, Trikha SRJ, Luckasen GJ, et al. Influence of sodium glucose cotransporter 2 inhibition on physiological adaptation to endurance exercise training. *J Clin Endocrinol Metab* 104: 1953–1966, 2019.

162. Newsom SA, Schenk S, Thomas KM, Harber MP, Knuth ND, Goldenberg N, et al. Energy deficit after exercise augments lipid mobilization but does not contribute to the exercise-induced increase in insulin sensitivity. *J Appl Physiol (1985)* 108: 554–560, 2010.

163. O'Keefe EL, O'Keefe JH, Lavie CJ. Exercise counteracts the cardiotoxicity of psychosocial stress. *Mayo Clin Proc* 94: 1852–1864, 2019.

164. Owen MR, Doran E, Halestrap AP. Evidence that metformin exerts its anti-diabetic effects through inhibition of complex 1 of the mitochondrial respiratory chain. *Biochem J* 348(Pt 3): 607–614, 2000.

165. Park J, Park SW, Yoon KH, Kim SR, Ahn KJ, Lee JH, et al. Efficacy and safety of evogliptin monotherapy in patients with type 2 diabetes and moderately elevated glycated haemoglobin levels after diet and exercise. *Diabetes Obes Metab* 19: 1681–1687, 2017.

166. Patel AV, Maliniak ML, Rees-Punia E, Matthews CE, Gapstur SM. Prolonged leisure time spent sitting in relation to cause-specific mortality in a large US cohort. *Am J Epidemiol* 187: 2151–2158, 2018.

167. Pecinova A, Brazdova A, Drahota Z, Houstek J, Mracek T. Mitochondrial targets of metformin-Are they physiologically relevant? *Biofactors* 2019.

168. Petersen KF, Befroy D, Dufour S, Dziura J, Ariyan C, Rothman DL, et al. Mitochondrial dysfunction in the elderly: possible role in insulin resistance. *Science* 300: 1140–1142, 2003.

169. Ploug T, Galbo H, Vinten J, Jorgensen M, Richter EA. Kinetics of glucose transport in rat muscle: effects of insulin and contractions. *Am J Physiol* 253: E12–20, 1987.

170. Ploug T, van Deurs B, Ai H, Cushman SW, Ralston E. Analysis of GLUT4 distribution in whole skeletal muscle fibers: identification of distinct storage compartments that are recruited by insulin and muscle contractions. *J Cell Biol* 142: 1429–1446, 1998.

171. Poirier P, Mawhinney S, Grondin L, Tremblay A, Broderick T, Cleroux J, et al. Prior meal enhances the plasma glucose lowering effect of exercise in type 2 diabetes. *Med Sci Sports Exerc* 33: 1259–1264, 2001.

172. Poirier P, Tremblay A, Catellier C, Tancrede G, Garneau C, Nadeau A. Impact of time interval from the last meal on glucose response to exercise in subjects with type 2 diabetes. *J Clin Endocrinol Metab* 85: 2860–2864, 2000.

173. Prattichizzo F, Giuliani A, Mensa E, Sabbatinelli J, De Nigris V, Rippo MR, et al. Pleiotropic effects of metformin: Shaping the microbiome to manage type 2 diabetes and postpone ageing. *Ageing Res Rev* 48: 87–98, 2018.

174. Price WH, Cori CF, Colowick SP. The effect of anterior pituitary extract and of insulin on the hexokinase reaction. *J Biol Chem* 160: 633, 1945.

175. Prior SJ, Goldberg AP, Ortmeyer HK, Chin ER, Chen D, Blumenthal JB, et al. Increased skeletal muscle capillarization independently enhances insulin sensitivity in older adults after exercise training and detraining. *Diabetes* 64: 3386–3395, 2015.

176. Reynolds AN, Mann JI, Williams S, Venn BJ. Advice to walk after meals is more effective for lowering postprandial glycaemia in type 2 diabetes mellitus than advice that does not specify timing: a randomised crossover study. *Diabetologia* 59: 2572–2578, 2016.

177. Reynolds LJ, Credeur DP, Manrique C, Padilla J, Fadel PJ, Thyfault JP. Obesity, type 2 diabetes, and impaired insulin-stimulated blood flow: role of skeletal muscle NO synthase and endothelin-1. *J Appl Physiol (1985)* 122: 38–47, 2017.

178. Richter EA, Hargreaves M. Exercise, GLUT4, and skeletal muscle glucose uptake. *Physiological Reviews* 93: 993–1017, 2013.

179. Roberts C, Little J, Thyfault J. Modification of insulin sensitivity and glycemic control by activity and exercise. *Med Sci Sport Exer* 45: 1868–1877, 2013.

180. Rodnick KJ, Henriksen EJ, James DE, Holloszy JO. Exercise training, glucose transporters, and glucose transport in rat skeletal muscles. *Am J Physiol* 262: C9–14, 1992.

181. Rodnick KJ, Slot JW, Studelska DR, Hanpeter DE, Robinson LJ, Geuze HJ, et al. Immunocytochemical and biochemical studies of GLUT4 in rat skeletal muscle. *J Biol Chem* 267: 6278–6285, 1992.

182. Rodriguez-Ayllon M, Cadenas-Sanchez C, Estevez-Lopez F, Munoz NE, Mora-Gonzalez J, Migueles JH, et al. Role of physical activity and sedentary behavior in the mental health of preschoolers, children and adolescents: a systematic review and meta-analysis. *Sports Med* 49: 1383–1410, 2019.

183. Rogers MA, Yamamoto C, King DS, Hagberg JM, Ehsani AA, Holloszy JO. Improvement in glucose tolerance after 1 Wk of exercise in patients with mild NIDDM. *Diabetes Care* 11: 613–618, 1988.

184. Romero SA, Minson CT, Halliwill JR. The cardiovascular system after exercise. *J Appl Physiol (1985)* 122: 925–932, 2017.

185. Romijn JA, Coyle EF, Sidossis LS, Gastaldelli A, Horowitz JF, Endert E, et al. Regulation of endogenous fat and carbohydrate metabolism in relation to exercise intensity and duration. *Am J Physiol Endocrinol Metab* 265: E380–E391, 1993.

186. Ryder JW, Yang J, Galuska D, Rincón J, Björnholm M, Krook A, et al. Use of a novel impermeable biotinylated photolabeling reagent to assess insulin- and hypoxia-stimulated cell surface GLUT4 content in skeletal muscle from type 2 diabetic patients. *Diabetes* 49: 647–654, 2000.

187. Saad A, Dalla Man C, Nandy DK, Levine JA, Bharucha AE, Rizza RA, et al. Diurnal pattern to insulin secretion and insulin action in healthy individuals. *Diabetes* 61: 2691–2700, 2012.

188. Samocha-Bonet D, Campbell LV, Mori TA, Croft KD, Greenfield JR, Turner N, et al. Overfeeding reduces insulin sensitivity and increases oxidative stress, without altering markers of mitochondrial content and function in humans. *PLoS One* 7: e36320, 2012.

189. Sato S, Basse AL, Schonke M, Chen S, Samad M, Altintas A, et al. Time of exercise specifies the impact on muscle metabolic pathways and systemic energy homeostasis. *Cell Metab* 30: 92–110, 2019.

190. Satoh S, Nishimura H, Clark AE, Kozka IJ, Vannucci SJ, Simpson IA, et al D. Use of bismannose photolabel to elucidate insulin-regulated GLUT4 subcellular trafficking kinetics in rat adipose cells. Evidence that exocytosis is a critical site of hormone action. *J Biol Chem* 268: 17820–17829, 1993.

191. Savage DB, Watson L, Carr K, Adams C, Brage S, Chatterjee KK, et al. Accumulation of saturated intramyocellular lipid is associated with insulin resistance. *J Lipid Res* 60: 1323–1332, 2019.

192. Savikj M, Gabriel BM, Alm PS, Smith J, Caidahl K, Bjornholm M, et al. Afternoon exercise is more efficacious than morning exercise at improving blood glucose levels in individuals with type 2 diabetes: a randomised crossover trial. *Diabetologia* 62: 233–237, 2019.

193. Scheer FA, Hilton MF, Mantzoros CS, Shea SA. Adverse metabolic and cardiovascular consequences of circadian misalignment. *Proc Natl Acad Sci U S A* 106: 4453–4458, 2009.

194. Schenk S, Cook JN, Kaufman AE, Horowitz JF. Postexercise insulin sensitivity is not impaired after an overnight lipid infusion. *Am J Physiol Endocrinol Metab* 288: E519–E525, 2005.

195. Schenk S, Horowitz JF. Acute exercise increases triglyceride synthesis in skeletal muscle and prevents fatty acid-induced insulin resistance. *J Clin Invest* 117: 1690–1698, 2007.
196. Schiaffino S, Blaauw B, Dyar KA. The functional significance of the skeletal muscle clock: Lessons from Bmal1 knockout models. *Skelet Muscle* 6: 33, 2016.
197. Schwingshackl L, Missbach B, Dias S, König J, Hoffmann G. Impact of different training modalities on glycaemic control and blood lipids in patients with type 2 diabetes: A systematic review and network meta-analysis. *Diabetologia* 57: 1789–1797, 2014.
198. Sharoff CG, Hagobian TA, Malin SK, Chipkin SR, Yu H, Hirshman MF, et al. Combining short-term metformin treatment and one bout of exercise does not increase insulin action in insulin-resistant individuals. *Am J Physiol Endocrinol Metab* 298: E815–823, 2010.
199. Shearman LP, Sriram S, Weaver DR, Maywood ES, Chaves I, Zheng B, et al. Interacting molecular loops in the mammalian circadian clock. *Science* 288: 1013–1019, 2000.
200. Solomon TPJ, Malin SK, Karstoft K, Knudsen SH, Haus JM, Laye MJ, et al. Association between cardio-respiratory fitness and the determinants of glycemic control across the entire glucose tolerance continuum. *Diabetes care* 38: 921–929, 2015.
201. Somwar R, Kim DY, Sweeney G, Huang C, Niu W, Lador C, et al. GLUT4 translocation precedes the stimulation of glucose uptake by insulin in muscle cells: Potential activation of GLUT4 via p38 mitogen-activated protein kinase. *Biochem J* 359: 639–649, 2001.
202. Staiano AE, Harrington DM, Barreira TV, Katzmarzyk PT. Sitting time and cardiometabolic risk in US adults: associations by sex, race, socioeconomic status and activity level. *Br J Sports Med* 48: 213–219, 2014.
203. Stephens BR, Braun B. Impact of nutrient intake timing on the metabolic response to exercise. *Nutrition Reviews* 66: 473–476, 2008.
204. Stephens BR, Granados K, Zderic TW, Hamilton MT, Braun B. Effects of 1 day of inactivity on insulin action in healthy men and women: interaction with energy intake. *Metabolism* 60: 941–949, 2011.
205. Tanimura Y, Aoi W, Mizushima K, Higashimura Y, Naito Y. Combined treatment of dipeptidyl peptidase-4 inhibitor and exercise training improves lipid profile in KK/Ta mice. *Exp Physiol* 104: 1051–1060, 2019.
206. Thompson P, Crouse S, Goodpaster B, Kelley D, Moyna N, Pescatello L. The acute versus the chronic response to exercise. *Med Sci Sport Exer* 33: S438–S445, 2001.
207. Toledo FGS, Johannsen DL, Covington JD, Bajpeyi S, Goodpaster B, Conley KE, et al. Impact of prolonged overfeeding on skeletal muscle mitochondria in healthy individuals. *Diabetologia* 61: 466–475, 2018.
208. Turcotte LP, Richter EA, Kiens B. Increased plasma FFA uptake and oxidation during prolonged exercise in trained vs. untrained humans. *Am J Physiol Endocrinol Metab* 262: E791–E799, 1992.
209. Turner N, Bruce CR, Beale SM, Hoehn KL, So T, Rolph MS, et al. Excess lipid availability increases mito-chondrial fatty acid oxidative capacity in muscle. *Evidence Against a Role for Reduced Fatty Acid Oxidation in Lipid-Induced Insulin Resistance in Rodents Diabetes* 56: 2085–2092, 2007.
210. Ueda SY, Yoshikawa T, Katsura Y, Usui T, Fujimoto S. Comparable effects of moderate intensity exercise on changes in anorectic gut hormone levels and energy intake to high intensity exercise. *J Endocrinol* 203: 357–364, 2009.
211. Ueda SY, Yoshikawa T, Katsura Y, Usui T, Nakao H, Fujimoto S. Changes in gut hormone levels and nega-tive energy balance during aerobic exercise in obese young males. *J Endocrinol* 201: 151–159, 2009.
212. van Loon LJ, Greenhaff PL, Constantin-Teodosiu D, Saris WH, Wagenmakers AJ. The effects of increasing exercise intensity on muscle fuel utilisation in humans. *J Physiol* 536: 295–304, 2001.
213. van Loon LJC, Goodpaster BH. Increased intramuscular lipid storage in the insulin-resistant and endurance-trained state. *Pflügers Archiv* 451: 606–616, 2006.
214. Vella A, Cobelli C. Defective glucagon-like peptide 1 secretion in prediabetes and type 2 diabetes is influenced by weight and sex. chicken, egg, or none of the above? *Diabetes* 64: 2324–2325, 2015.
215. Vetter C, Devore EE, Ramin CA, Speizer FE, Willett WC, Schernhammer ES. Mismatch of sleep and work timing and risk of type 2 diabetes. *Diabetes Care* 38: 1707–1713, 2015.
216. Viskochil R, Lyden K, Staudenmayer J, Keadle SK, Freedson PS, Braun B. Elevated insulin levels following 7 days of increased sedentary time are due to lower hepatic extraction and not higher insulin secretion. *Applied Physiology, Nutrition, and Metabolism* 44: 1020–1023, 2019.
217. Wahren J, Felig P, Ahlborg G, Jorfeldt L. Glucose metabolism during leg exercise in man. *J Clin Invest* 50: 2715–2725, 1971.
218. Wallberg-Henriksson H. Repeated exercise regulates glucose transport capacity in skeletal muscle. *Acta Physiol Scand* 127: 39–43, 1986.
219. Wallberg-Henriksson H, Holloszy JO. Activation of glucose transport in diabetic muscle: responses to con-traction and insulin. *Am J Physiol* 249: C233–237, 1985.
220. Weston KS, Wisløff U, Coombes JS. High-intensity interval training in patients with lifestyle-induced cardiometabolic disease: a systematic review and meta-analysis. *Br J Sport Med* 48: 1227–1234, 2014.

221. Wilmot EG, Edwardson CL, Achana FA, Davies MJ, Gorely T, Gray LJ, et al. Sedentary time in adults and the association with diabetes, cardiovascular disease and death: systematic review and meta-analysis. *Diabetologia* 55: 2895–2905, 2012.

222. Winn N, Pettit-Mee R, Walsh L, Restaino R, Ready S, Padilla J, et al. Metabolic implications of diet and energy intake during physical inactivity. *Med Sci Sport Exer* 51: 995–1005, 2019.

223. Witczak CA, Fujii N, Hirshman MF, Goodyear LJ. Ca2+/calmodulin-dependent protein kinase kinase-alpha regulates skeletal muscle glucose uptake independent of AMP-activated protein kinase and Akt activation. *Diabetes* 56: 1403–1409, 2007.

224. Witczak CA, Jessen N, Warro DM, Toyoda T, Fujii N, Anderson ME, et al. CaMKII regulates contraction- but not insulin-induced glucose uptake in mouse skeletal muscle. *Am J Physiol Endocrinol Metab* 298: E1150–1160, 2010.

225. Woodman RJ, Chew GT, Watts GF. Mechanisms, significance and treatment of vascular dysfunction in type 2 diabetes mellitus. *Drugs* 65: 31–74, 2005.

226. Yu C, Chen Y, Cline GW, Zhang D, Zong H, Wang Y, et al. Mechanism by which fatty acids inhibit insulin activation of insulin receptor substrate-1 (IRS-1)-associated phosphatidylinositol 3-kinase activity in muscle. *J Biol Chem* 277: 50230–50236, 2002.

227. Zeigerer A, McBrayer MK, McGraw TE. Insulin stimulation of GLUT4 exocytosis, but not its inhibition of endocytosis, is dependent on RabGAP AS160. *Mol Biol Cell* 15: 4406–4415, 2004.

228. Zheng C, Liu Z. Vascular function, insulin action, and exercise: an intricate interplay. *Trends Endocrinol Metab* 26: 297–304, 2015.

229. Ziel FH, Venkatesan N, Davidson MB. Glucose transport is rate limiting for skeletal muscle glucose metabolism in normal and STZ-induced diabetic rats. *Diabetes* 37: 885–890, 1988.

230. Zierath JR, Krook A, Wallberg-Henriksson H. Insulin action and insulin resistance in human skeletal muscle. *Diabetologia* 43: 821–835, 2000.

29

BIOCHEMISTRY OF EXERCISE TRAINING AND MITIGATION OF CARDIOVASCULAR DISEASE

Barry A. Franklin and John C. Quindry

In 1953, Morris et al. reported that physically active bus conductors and mail delivery postmen demonstrated a 50% lower event rate from coronary artery disease (CAD) compared with their sedentary counterparts, that is, bus drivers and clerical postal workers, respectively (108). Because epidemiologic data indicate that habitually sedentary individuals have an increased prevalence of 25 chronic diseases, the phrase "sedentary death syndrome" was promulgated to highlight the emerging entity of sedentary lifestyle–mediated unhealthy conditions, almost all of which are chronic diseases or risk factors for chronic diseases that ultimately result in increased mortality (17). Accordingly, physical inactivity increases the relative risk of CAD, stroke, hypertension, and osteoporosis by ~30–60% (18). Due to contemporary technologic advances which provide causative insights into the leading forms of morbidity and mortality, the U.S. Bureau of Labour Statistics now lists sedentary behaviour as the most common shared occupational health risk. Collectively, these data and related reports suggest that deaths attributable to physical inactivity may soon exceed those due to cigarette smoking (91). For these reasons, the global prevalence of physical inactivity is increasingly recognized as a pandemic, with far-reaching health, economic, environmental, and social consequences (8).

In an early meta-analysis of 43 studies of the relation between physical activity (PA) and coronary heart disease (CHD) incidence, the relative risk of CHD corresponding to physical inactivity ranged from 1.5 to 2.4, with a median value of 1.9 (118). Moreover, the relative risk of a sedentary lifestyle appeared to be similar in magnitude to that associated with other major CHD risk factors. Another systematic review and meta-analysis of 33 PA studies including 883,372 participants reported pooled risk reductions of 35% and 33% for cardiovascular disease (CVD) and all-cause mortality, respectively, among the most physically active cohorts (113).

Relative to longevity, regular exercisers and endurance athletes live, on average, 3–6 years longer than the general population (32, 76, 97). More recently, researchers estimated the influence of five low-risk lifestyle factors (never smoking, body mass index [BMI] of 18.5–24.9 kg/m^2, ≥30 minutes per day of moderate-to-vigorous PA, moderate alcohol intake, and a healthy diet score [upper 40%]) on premature mortality and life expectancy in the U.S. population. During the follow-up period, which extended 34 years for some participants, adherence to all five low-risk lifestyle-related factors prolonged the life expectancy at age 50 years by 14.0 and 12.2 years for female and male U.S. adults, respectively, as compared with those who adopted "zero" low-risk lifestyle factors. Interestingly, the most physically active cohorts of men and women demonstrated 7- to 8-year gains in life expectancy (95)!

Cardioprotective Benefits of Regular Physical Activity: Potential Underlying Mechanisms

According to two scientific statements from the American Heart Association, published data from epidemiologic and related experimental research satisfy the criteria required to infer a causal relation such that physical inactivity is now designated as a major CHD risk factor (94, 150). These and other relevant reports (10, 84, 85, 90, 132), when combined with experimental and clinical investigations providing biologic plausibility (68, 121), strongly support the recommendation that habitual occupational and/or leisure-time PA reduces the incidence of CHD.

Regular moderate-to-vigorous PA, structured exercise, or both can decrease the risk of initial recurrent cardiovascular events, presumably from multiple mechanisms, including anti-atherosclerotic, anti-ischemic, anti-arrhythmic, anti-thrombotic, and improved psychologic effects (Figure 29.1). Biochemical cardiac pre-conditioning against ischemic damage also has a significant cardioprotective role (121).

Anti-atherosclerotic Effects

Chronic aerobic exercise can result in modest-to-moderate reductions in body weight and fat stores. Endurance exercise can also promote decreases in blood pressure (particularly in hypertensives) (116) and in serum triglycerides (75) and increases in cardiorespiratory fitness (CRF) (10, 84, 85, 90, 132) and the "anti-atherogenic" high-density lipoprotein subfraction (75). Exercise also has favourable effects on glucose and insulin homeostasis (19, 80, 156) and inflammatory markers, including C-reactive protein (31, 45, 89).

Anti-ischemic Effects

Specific anti-ischemic effects of regular exercise include reducing the rate-pressure product and associated myocardial oxygen demands by lowering heart rate and systolic blood pressure at rest and at

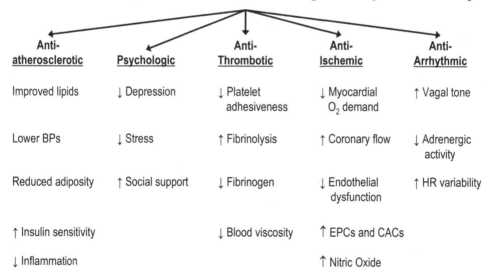

Figure 29.1 Multiple mechanisms by which moderate-to-vigorous exercise training may reduce the risk for non-fatal and fatal cardiovascular events. BP, blood pressure; CACs, cultured/circulating angiogenic cells; EPC, endothelial progenitor cells; HR, heart rate; O_2, oxygen; ↑, increased; and ↓, decreased

any given sub-maximal workload, as well as increasing the period of diastole, during which coronary perfusion predominates. Accordingly, vagal tone is enhanced at rest, while sympathetic drive (circulating catecholamine levels, particularly norepinephrine) is reduced during sub-maximal intensity exercise. Additional physiologic benefits include improved coronary blood flow and endothelial function (59), as well as the production of endothelial progenitor cells and increased delivery of the vasoactive compound, nitric oxide. The beneficial effects of exercise training on myocardial perfusion and/or indices of myocardial ischemia include less ST-segment depression during exercise testing, training, and ambulatory electrocardiographic monitoring. Furthermore, the benefits of exercise training in those with advanced CVD manifest as reduced anginal symptoms at all exercise workloads and a delay in the onset of angina during incremental exercise testing. Finally, and perhaps most remarkably, exercise training is associated with partial or complete resolution of reversible myocardial perfusion imaging defects in those with suspected or known CVD (136). Although conventional scientific and medical wisdom held that exercise per se had little or no influence on increasing coronary collateral circulation in humans (46), a non-randomized clinical trial in 40 patients challenged this tentative hypothesis (167). Moreover, in the randomized EXCITE trial investigators reported that both moderate- and high-intensity exercise performed for 10 hours per week resulted in an improvement of coronary collateral flow index after 4 weeks (104).

Antiarrhythmic Effects

Decreased vulnerability to threatening ventricular arrhythmias and increased resistance to ventricular fibrillation have also been postulated to reflect exercise-related adaptations in autonomic control, including reduced sympathetic drive and increased vagal tone. Exercise has also been suggested as a benign form of ischemic pre-conditioning that attenuates the effects of subsequent ischemia in experimental models of CVD (78). Ischemic pre-conditioning refers to the observation, primarily in animal models, that brief periods of myocardial ischemia before coronary occlusion can reduce subsequent infarct size and/or the potential for malignant ventricular arrhythmias.

In 1984, Billman et al. reported that a 6-week daily exercise regimen prevented exercise-triggered ventricular tachycardia following experimentally induced myocardial ischemia in a sub-group of dogs with a healed myocardial infarction identified to be at high risk of sudden cardiac death (SCD) (7). To clarify the potential mechanisms that may be responsible for the protection from arrhythmogenic death, Hull and associates replicated this classic experiment and reported significant increases in baroreflex sensitivity, heart rate variability, and repetitive extra systole threshold (66). In this study, daily exercise exerted a powerful anti-fibrillatory effect, as all animals survived. Other studies in persons with and without CAD have confirmed that endurance exercise training increases baroreflex sensitivity and heart rate variability, both of which are considered cardioprotective adaptations (67). Collectively, these studies (6) and other recent reports (121) suggest that aerobic exercise conditioning provides a non-pharmacological anti-arrhythmic intervention by enhancing cardiac electrical stability and preventing SCD. Collectively, these findings are remarkable given that an acute exercise bout increases the myocardial supply–demand mismatch in hearts with coronary perfusion deficits.

Antithrombotic Effects

Increasing scientific evidence suggests that aerobic exercise training improves blood rheology in individuals with and without CAD. Vigorous endurance exercise in young, middle-aged, and older individuals has been shown to improve haemostatic/fibrinolytic parameters, with decreases in plasma fibrinogen levels, platelet aggregability, and haematocrit standardized blood viscosity and increases in fibrinolysis (136). Low-load resistance exercise also favourably modifies thrombogenesis by reducing inflammatory processes and potentiating fibrinolytic features (28). In aggregate, these adaptations may serve to reduce the short-term and long-term likelihood for coronary events through the potential of acute thrombosis and the prevention of plaque expansion.

Psychologic Effects

Although behaviour modification, stress management, relaxation techniques, and drug treatment (e.g., sertraline) have been suggested as therapeutic interventions to reduce the psychologic stressors associated with CAD, well-designed studies now highlight the value of regular aerobic exercise in reducing chronic stress, anxiety, and depression (12).

Biochemical Cardiac Pre-conditioning

The physiological basis and rationale for exercise-induced biochemical cardiac pre-conditioning is discussed in several excellent reviews (22, 120, 125, 143) as well as a detailed section on this phenomenon later in the chapter. In essence, biochemical cardiac pre-conditioning occurs in response to each bout of exercise. Specifically, acute bouts of exercise impose a hermetic stress on the heart such that cellular biochemistry is favourably altered and an ischemic-resistant phenotype is conferred, at least temporarily (121).

Cardioprotective Benefits of Vigorous Versus Moderate-Intensity Physical Activity

Relative to the all-cause and cardiovascular mortality reduction associated with regular exercise, intensity and duration appear to be inversely related. The mortality reduction associated with a regular 5-minute run approximates a 15-minute walk and a 25-minute run is comparable to a 105-minute walk (157). Thus, for those seeking a time-saving alternative to moderate-intensity continuous training, vigorous exercise, specifically jogging, running, or walking up a treadmill grade or incline, may be preferred over level walking.

Why vigorous-intensity exercise provides greater cardiovascular benefits than moderate-intensity PA, even when the energy expenditure is equated (146), may be due to several factors. Vigorous exercise intensities are more effective than moderate intensities at increasing CRF (165), especially for individuals with higher baseline CRF (145, 147). This understanding has additional prognostic significance, since the level of CRF, expressed as millilitres of oxygen per kilogram body weight per minute (mL/kg/min) or as metabolic equivalents (METs; 1 MET = 3.5 mL/kg/min), is inversely related to the risk of cardiovascular morbidity and mortality (47). Other possible mechanisms associated with the added cardioprotective benefits of vigorous-intensity exercise training include decreased inflammation and endothelial dysfunction, as well as increased arterial compliance and parasympathetic tone, among many others (50). In addition, escalating reliance on carbohydrate use over fat metabolism evoked by increased adrenergic stimulation at higher exercise intensities may be the mechanism underlying improvements in insulin sensitivity after vigorous-intensity training in obese individuals with and without diabetes mellitus (70).

Cardiorespiratory Fitness and Physical Activity as Separate Heart Disease Risk Factors

Comparative Benefits

Numerous studies now suggest that CRF is one of the strongest prognostic markers in persons with and without chronic disease, including CAD (9, 11, 39, 47, 58, 72, 73, 112, 154). In fact, higher levels of CRF are associated with a reduced risk of developing hypertension, type 2 diabetes, atrial fibrillation, chronic kidney disease, and major adverse cardiovascular events, including heart failure, myocardial infarction, stroke, and coronary artery bypass grafting (86). Williams reported that increasing levels of PA and CRF had significantly different relationships to CVD (161). There was a 64% decline in the risk of heart disease from the least to the most fit, with a precipitous drop in risk when comparing the lowest (0) to the next lowest fitness category (i.e., 25th percentile), but only a 30% decline from the least to the most physically active. Thus, individuals with the highest levels of CRF demonstrated more than twice the reduction in risk. Collectively, these data suggest that being unfit warrants consideration as an independent risk factor and that a low level of CRF or aerobic capacity increases the risk of CVD to a greater extent than merely being physically inactive. Although the cut-points vary slightly depending on age and gender, an exercise capacity <5 METs generally indicates a higher mortality group, whereas an exercise capacity ≥10 METs identifies a group with an excellent long-term prognosis, regardless of the underlying extent of CAD (47).

These epidemiologic analyses and other relevant reports (10, 84, 85) empirically support a cause-and-effect relationship between increased levels of PA and CRF and reduced CVD mortality, rather than merely associations between these variables. For the primary and secondary prevention of CAD, each 1 MET increase in CRF confers a ~15% decrease in mortality up to about 10 METs (13, 81), which compares favourably with the survival benefit conferred by the independent use of low-dose aspirin, statins, β-blockers, and angiotensin-converting enzyme inhibitors after acute myocardial infarction. Moreover, Dutcher et al., using the well-described primary angioplasty in acute myocardial infarction (PAMI-2) database, reported that exercise capacity more accurately predicts 2- and 5-year mortality than does left ventricular ejection fraction in patients with ST-elevation myocardial infarction treated with percutaneous coronary intervention (42). Those who had an exercise capacity ≥4 METs had excellent long-term survival, regardless of their ejection fraction. In contrast, those with an exercise capacity <4 METs were at a substantially increased risk of mortality, which was exacerbated in the presence of left ventricular dysfunction (ejection fraction <40%). Accordingly, these data have important implications for the medical management and triaging of post–myocardial infarction patients who may benefit the most from an exercise-based cardiac rehabilitation programme.

Finally, individuals with low PA and/or CRF levels have higher annual health care costs (27, 111, 131), higher rates of incident heart failure (82), increased cardiovascular events at any given coronary artery calcium level (129), and are two to three times more likely to die prematurely than their risk factor–matched fitter counterparts (112, 159). Increased levels of PA and/or CRF before hospitalization for acute coronary syndromes (117) and elective or emergent surgical procedures also appear to confer more favourable short-term outcomes (69, 132). Complications after surgery, including bariatric surgery (99) and coronary artery bypass grafting (140), have also been linked to reduced pre-operative levels of PA or CRF (64). Collectively, these data and other recent reports suggest that the primary beneficiaries of regular exercise appear to be those comprising the bottom 20% of the CRF/PA continuum.

Mechanisms of Cardiac Ischemic Injury

Ischemic injury of the myocardium reflects the convergence of two fundamental tenets of cardiac physiology: (1) it is biologically necessary for the heart to beat continuously and (2) even a momentary oxygen supply–demand mismatch may be deleterious to the preservation of cardiac structure and function. The magnitude of the ischemic insult accrues in a time-dependent manner, and the injury process is evolutionary in nature (79). Upon a sufficiently reduced or occluded blood flow to a portion of the left ventricle, the earliest manifestation (1–5 minutes) of a supply–demand mismatch involves electrical abnormalities that are readily identifiable on an electrocardiogram (ECG). As the ischemic duration exceeds ~5 minutes, the heart exhibits a temporary loss in ventricular contractility called myocardial stunning. Individual symptomology of myocardial stunning is highly variable, but may include light-headedness and fainting. Importantly, the ventricular arrhythmias and myocardial stunning that occur during the early phases of an ischemic cardiac event are considered reversible with appropriate medical attention, including restoration of coronary blood flow (e.g., emergent coronary revascularization).

After ~20 minutes, however, unremitting cardiac ischemia is marked by myocardial infarction and tissue death (25).

From a cellular perspective, ischemic pathology reflects three distinct outcomes: (1) bioenergetic distress, (2) calcium dyshomeostasis, and (3) oxidative stress. Metabolic distress, characterized by cessation of oxidative phosphorylation, occurs rapidly upon the obstruction of adequate blood flow to the heart. While the heart exhibits a biological propensity for "metabolic flexibility," the anaerobic production of adenosine triphosphate (ATP) via glycolytic means is insufficient to meet the continued energy requirements of the critically ischemic heart (24). A direct consequence of the precipitous drop in cellular ATP levels is that ionic dysregulation rapidly ensues. Although ionic instability in excitable cardiac cells is faceted and includes catastrophic changes in the otherwise tight regulation of [K^+], [Na^+], and [H^+], it is the inability to re-sequester Ca^{2+} on a beat-by-beat basis that appears to initiate the immediate cellular decline (37). Concomitantly, ischemic myocytes exhibit a pathological oxidative stress, or an imbalance between the production of free radicals (and reactive oxygen/nitrogen species) and antioxidants, their molecular counterparts (41).

Ca^{2+} dyshomeostasis and oxidative stress are secondary to the bioenergetic distress caused by an ischemic episode, and these two mechanisms work synergistically to advance ischemic pathology through a series of enzymatic interactions (16). Perhaps most alarming, and while cardiac reperfusion is a necessary prerequisite to long-term survivability, it is the very process of reperfusion (via revascularization, anti-thrombolytic therapy, etc.) that produces that greatest injury via Ca^{2+} overload and oxidative stress. Accordingly, the collective pathology is described as *ischemia-reperfusion* injury. In reference to this response, viable countermeasures against ischemic heart disease must improve bioenergetic efficiency while simultaneously mitigating Ca^{2+} overload and oxidative stress within the heart muscle cells. To this end, the pre-clinical strategies for cardioprotection first appeared in the mid-1980s with the discovery of cardiac pre-conditioning.

Cardiac Pre-conditioning

To understand exercise-induced cardioprotection, one must first consider the broader topic of cardiac pre-conditioning against ischemic injury. Pre-conditioning refers to biochemical alterations within cardiac tissues that confer cellular protection against a host of subsequent physiologic challenges, including myocardial ischemia. For decades, both clinical and epidemiologic studies hinted at the concept of cardiac pre-conditioning, but the first direct evidence, in 1986, was provided by a classic investigation (110). In this study, anesthetized dogs were exposed to surgical ligation of the left anterior descending (LAD) coronary artery as an experimental surrogate to the spontaneous clots and plaque rupture that produce myocardial infarction in humans. However, there was an experimental twist that forever changed our collective understanding of cardiac biochemistry. This investigation exposed dogs in the experimental group to a few rounds of sub-lethal myocardial ischemia for only a few minutes at a time. The following day, the same experimental animals were anesthetized once again, but this time they received a long-duration surgical ligation of the same coronary artery in order to mimic an extended duration heart attack as occurs in humans. When the hearts from these dogs were compared in postmortem analyses to hearts from a control group that received the long-duration ischemic insult without the ischemic stimulus, it was discovered that the experimental group fared much better in terms of reduced infarct area (110). Thus, the hearts from experimental animals were *pre-conditioned* by the short-duration ischemia and subsequently experienced a smaller-magnitude heart attack despite the fact that the ischemic area and the ischemic duration were identical between the two groups. This finding was the first of what is now commonly described as the late-phase window of protection (lasting for days following the stimulus) due to an ischemic stimulus (15, 110).

Given that most of this research has been performed in rodent models of ischemic injury, Figure 29.2 presents the conceptual research approach for ischemic pre-conditioning. Based upon this general

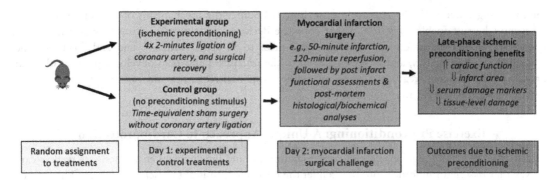

Figure 29.2 Study design for ischemic pre-conditioning research

model, many generations of research studies have followed the approach first used in this investigation (110). Animals are assigned to ischemic pre-conditioning or sham control groups, with the respective surgeries occurring on day 1 of the study. Day 2 involves a lengthy ischemic insult that replicates a clinical heart attack in humans. Animals are then euthanized under humane conditions either on day 2, or in other studies, days to weeks after the myocardial infarction. Tissues, including the heart, are then saved for subsequent histological, biochemical, and molecular biology analyses so that postmortem outcomes can be compared to clinically directed measures of cardiac function (echocardiography, etc.).

Perhaps the most important discovery of this research is the observation that the ischemic pre-conditioning and the surgical heart attack were separated by only 24 hours. Thus, the only plausible explanation for the marked infarct protection observed in the experimental group was that ischemic pre-conditioning must have promoted up-regulation of a biochemical mechanism, or mechanisms, that are cardioprotective. Stated differently, because of the short duration of these experiments (110), and in the many studies that have followed, there was not time to revascularize or remodel the heart. Accordingly, the protective outcomes must be due to biochemical changes that can occur in the minutes to hours following the pre-conditioning stimulus. Indeed, in the decades since that first observation of cardiac pre-conditioning (110), many mechanisms of cardioprotection against an ischemic insult have been identified (15, 57). Perhaps not surprisingly, these protective mechanisms at work in the pre-conditioned hearts act to counter the various aspects of cellular pathology previously described. With this collective knowledge, the overarching goal of pre-conditioning research has been to "reverse engineer" a pharmacologic counter-therapy for those at the highest risk for a myocardial infarction. Unfortunately, the mechanisms of cardiac pre-conditioning against ischemic injury do not appear to be "druggable" as first hoped (15). While beyond the scope of the current chapter, several reviews provide thought-provoking explanations regarding the challenges in translating pre-conditioning research into a pharmacologic countermeasure (23, 121, 125).

One of the key limiting factors to translating ischemic pre-conditioning into a therapeutic intervention is that chronic ischemia is not biologically intended as an extended cardioprotective stimulus (163). Stated differently, while non-lethal ischemia temporarily cardioprotects the myocardium, the cellular pathways are inflammatory in nature (15, 16). Accordingly, any therapeutic effect resulting from this approach would presumably mimic an unsustainable inflammatory stimulus and likely result in pathological remodelling of the heart, including the potential development of congestive heart failure. An additional barrier to clinical translation of ischemic pre-conditioning research is that the timing of spontaneous myocardial infarctions is difficult to predict. Thus, it is not possible to deliver a pre-conditioning agent in advance of the insult because these agents are not therapeutically sustainable. Hence, any cardioprotective antidote developed from pre-conditioning research must meet the following criteria: (1) the approach must directly counter the mechanisms of ischemic pathology; (2) it must be sustainable—a stimulus that could be delivered indefinitely without long-term consequence; (3) it must be pragmatic and deliverable prior to an acute cardiac event; and (4) it must be cost-effective. Fortunately, and in stark contrast to the unfruitful efforts to develop a pharmacological pre-conditioning agent, regular exercise meets these essential requisites and can uniquely be used to cardioprotect the heart against ischemic insults.

Exercise Pre-conditioning: A Unique Approach to Cardioprotection

The robust benefits of regular exercise confer anatomical and biochemical adaptations, as well as cardiovascular risk factor modifications that render the heart more resistant to ischemic injury. These three cardioprotective facets highlight disease prevention within the exercised heart, but should not overshadow the fact that rehabilitative exercise also prevents recurrent cardiac events and can slow, halt, and even reverse some aspects of pathology in those with CVD. While beyond the scope of this chapter, we have recently reviewed the topic of exercise-induced cardioprotection against ischemic heart disease within the context of both pharmacologic agents and exercise-based cardiac rehabilitation (121, 122). Nonetheless, research over the last 2 decades has shown that even a few bouts of exercise (one to three sessions) can pre-condition the heart against myocardial infarction. As a scientific observation, exercise-induced cardioprotection of the pre-conditioned heart is among the most reproducible physiologic responses and has significant clinical implications.

The phenomenon of exercise pre-conditioning has been well described over the last 30 years, primarily in animal models including rats, mice, and other mammalian species. Figure 29.3 presents the typical methodologic approach to research studies evaluating cardioprotective exercise pre-conditioning. While the overall study design is similar to ischemic pre-conditioning, between 1 and 3 days of exercise are used to induce a protective stimulus. Similar to ischemic pre-conditioning research, the exercise studies utilize surgical models of infarction in either isolated hearts or in vivo models of coronary artery ligation in anesthetized animals.

While the most salient observational and mechanistic findings from exercise pre-conditioning research are summarized herein, the reader is also directed to several relevant authoritative reviews (23, 120, 125, 143). Exercise pre-conditioning favourably influences numerous clinically directed outcome variables, including the ECG (61, 128), ventricular contractility (142, 144, 148), preservation of ventricular pump function (36, 119, 60), circulating markers of cardiac damage (92), and measures of infarct size (126, 127).

Table 29.1 summarizes the most important phenomena observed with exercise pre-conditioning in countering an ischemic insult. Extending upon prior comparisons and contrasts with ischemic pre-conditioning, exercise confers a biphasic cardioprotection, with an early-phase window of ischemic

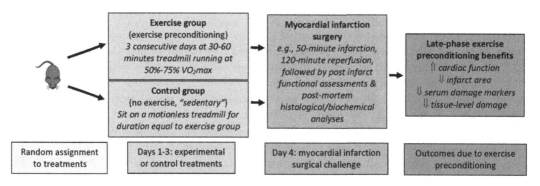

Figure 29.3 Study design for exercise pre-conditioning research

Table 29.1 The phenomenology of exercise pre-conditioning against ischemic insults in the heart
The key observations of exercise induced pre-conditioning include a biphasic time course for cardioprotection. Exercise pre-conditioning appears to be threshold-dependent, with various exercise modalities, intensities, and durations yielding equivalent levels of protection. Early findings suggest strength training protects the heart in a similar fashion to aerobic exercise. Exercise pre-conditioning occurs regardless of age or sex

Pre-conditioning Time Course

- An early-phase window of protection is observed 30 minutes to 180 minutes following exercise
- A robust-late phase window of protection is observed 24 hours following a bout of exercise and appears to be responsible for the phenomena associated with exercise pre-conditioning
- Pre-conditioning associated with late-phase pre-conditioning persists for up to 9 days following the cessation of exercise

Exercise Training Specifications

- One to three individual bouts of exercise cardioprotect against ischemic injury to the same extent as weeks to months of exercise training
- Various aerobic exercise modalities appear to confer identical levels of cardioprotection (e.g., treadmill running, swimming, etc.)
- Moderate- and vigorous-intensity exercise appear to confer identical levels of protection
- Exercise durations of 20–60 minutes, in addition to discontinuous aerobic exercise, protect the heart to a similar degree
- Preliminary findings suggest that strength/resistance-type exercise produce a cardioprotective phenotype similar to aerobic exercise approaches

Characteristic Aspects of Exercise Pre-conditioning

- Cardioprotection occurs independent of age
- Male and female hearts are equally protected

---

resistance occurring in the minutes after exercise and a more robust late-phase window of protection occurring ~24 hours after an exercise bout (119, 166), which is thought to provide the most resiliency to the exercised heart.

Among the most important descriptive aspects of exercise pre-conditioning is that the stimulus appears to be *threshold-dependent*. First, and perhaps foremost, one to three individual bouts of exercise are equally protective against an ischemic injury, as are weeks to months of regimented exercise training (36, 119). Moreover, a few days of moderate-intensity (55% VO_2max) or vigorous aerobic exercise (75% VO_2max) appear to be equally protective against an ischemic insult (92). In addition, both sexes exhibit a similar infarct-sparing phenotype when first exposed to an exercise pre-conditioning stimulus (22, 30). While some may be sceptical of the animal exercise methodologies used in these studies, it is important to recognize that the volume of self-selected running wheel distances (96) closely approximates those of forced exercise (e.g., rodent treadmills with electric shockers). Moreover, caged rodents given access to running wheels exhibit a cardioprotected phenotype comparable to those performing forced exercise (33).

In regard to our descriptive understanding of exercise pre-conditioning, there are several notable differences when compared with ischemic pre-conditioning. First, the exercise pre-conditioning phenotype persists for ~9 days after the cessation of exercise (93), whereas protection following an ischemic stimulus lasts just 3–4 days (15). Perhaps more importantly from a clinical perspective, aged hearts are readily protected against ischemic injury when first exposed to exercise (123), but aged hearts are unable to maintain protection when ischemia-reperfusion is the pre-conditioning stimulus (134).

Biochemical Mechanisms of Exercise Pre-conditioning

A series of important reductionist experiments have been conducted over the last 15 years to clarify why and how exercise is cardioprotective. The time course of late-phase cardioprotective responses indicates that the protective phenotype is biochemical in nature. Moreover, with our understanding of the pathological underpinnings of ischemic injury, the protective mechanisms due to exercise are likely to affect bioenergetics, calcium handling, and oxidative stress. Accordingly, there is evidence that adaptive responses to exercise pre-conditioning include fortification of the bioenergetic processes (20). Although it is clear that exercise bolsters mitochondrial sub-populations (sub-sarcolemmal mitochondria and intramyofibrillar mitochondria) in exercised hearts (74), the exact mechanism, or more likely mechanisms, are not fully understood. One possibility, however, is that cellular metabolism is improved by pre-emptive opening of ATP-sensitive potassium channels found at both the sarcolemma and within the mitochondria (22, 127, 128). Collectively, it appears that exercised hearts exhibit improved bioenergetic control in the face of an ischemic insult.

The fact that metabolic activity in exercised hearts is improved during an ischemic challenge suggests that calcium handling is also improved and oxidative stress is mitigated. Indeed, strong evidence indicates that exercise pre-conditioning preserves calcium control during ischemia (20), although the protection is attenuated when compared with the unstressed heart (141). Preservation of cellular calcium transients is at least modestly improved by the fact that the sarcoplasmic endoplasmic calcium ATPase-2A (SERCA2A) structure is partially preserved in exercise pre-conditioned hearts (53, 54). The observation that the SERCA2A is protected against ischemic modification in exercised hearts may also suggest an interface between Ca^{2+} mechanisms and prevention of oxidative stress. Indeed, investigators demonstrated a strong association between antioxidant capacity, oxidative stress prevention, and preservation of SERCA2A damage in exercised hearts exposed to an ischemic insult (53, 54). Although the specific antioxidants that are responsible for these anti-infarct responses remain elusive, it is clear that an isoform of the endogenous antioxidant superoxide dismutase-2 (SOD2), found in the mitochondria, is rapidly overexpressed and allosterically activated following exercise pre-conditioning (61, 166). Moreover, since antioxidants suppress free radicals and other radical species through a network of chemical reactions, it is unlikely that SOD2 is preventing oxidative stress on its own. In support, a series of well-designed experiments demonstrated that the glutathione system is essential in protecting the exercise pre-conditioned heart in cooperation with SOD2, and perhaps other endogenous antioxidants found in ventricular myocytes (55, 56). It is also possible that antioxidant protection may be provided to the exercised heart through up-regulation of non-traditional antioxidants such as heat shock proteins. Indeed, numerous studies have now demonstrated that a family of heat shock proteins are overexpressed in the hearts of exercised animals, although their essentiality to the exercise pre-conditioning response remains unproven (35, 62, 126).

Previous research suggests that the biochemical adaptations responsible for exercise pre-conditioning against ischemic reperfusion injury are a result of localized, endogenous cellular cardiac adaptations. However, there is recent scientific evidence that other tissues might signal cardioprotection through a circulating factor or factors. Accordingly, researchers reported that delta opioid receptors appeared to mediate receptor-based cardioprotection following an exercise pre-conditioning stimulus (38). Interestingly, a follow-up study suggested that the endogenous opiates responsible for this protection were generated in the heart and confer cardioprotection through either autocrine or paracrine effects (102). It is important to note that the chemical makeup of the endogenous opioids are enkephalins rather than the more commonly known endorphins, which are released following prolonged endurance exercise. This point validates the experimental approach to exercise pre-conditioning in that the duration of cardioprotective exercise is well below the threshold needed to evoke an increase in circulating endorphins. Nonetheless, it is biologically plausible that endorphins may also signal cardioprotection as part of a redundant pre-conditioning process, although this notion requires additional confirmation.

464

Finally, it has been hypothesized that exercised skeletal muscle may release a myokine, or other factor, that pre-conditions the exercised heart through a receptor-mediated process. If correct, this finding would reinforce considerable evidence that tissue-to-tissue crosstalk is essential to exercise adaptations and good health in physically active individuals (71, 115). To that end, investigators found that inter-leukin-6 (IL-6) mediates exercise pre-conditioning against multiple forms of ischemic injury, including ventricular abnormalities and tissue death (100).

In summary, exercise pre-conditions the heart against ischemic injury through the up-regulation of multiple endogenous factors that improve bioenergetics while simultaneously preventing calcium overload and oxidative stress. The cardioprotective effect appears to be highly potent because many cellular mediators of pre-conditioning work synergistically to counter ischemic damage. In addition, certain factors responsible for exercise pre-conditioning appear to offer redundant protection, indicating that if one or more factors are not present in the exercised heart, other up-regulated mediators will prevent ischemic damage. This understanding of exercise pre-conditioning contrasts with ischemic pre-conditioning, where the descriptive data regarding cardioprotection are less robust. In this regard, there is also evidence that the mechanisms of cardioprotection are at least partially different in exercised hearts as compared to ischemic pre-conditioning. Indeed, pre-conditioning due to an ischemic stimulus is dependent upon up-regulation of inflammatory mediators, including inducible nitric oxide synthase (iNOS) and cyclooxygenase-2 (COX2) (137-139); however, these compounds are not essential for exercise pre-conditioning and are not altered in the exercised heart (100, 124).

Clinical Verification of Exercise Pre-conditioning in Humans

As remarkable as the earlier referenced findings of exercise pre-conditioning are, these data are of limited value without confirmatory evidence that the same mechanisms are generalizable to humans. Fortunately, a series of recent clinical investigations of exercise pre-conditioning supports the key findings from relevant animal experiments. To this end, the reader is directed to a recent review that comprehensively summarizes current findings from human clinical studies (149), supporting the threshold effect of late-phase exercise pre-conditioning. Moreover, numerous lines of evidence now strongly substantiate that the mechanisms responsible for endogenous and exogenous exercise-induced cardioprotection observed in animal studies are also cardioprotective in humans (149).

High-Volume and High-Intensity Endurance Training and Potential Adverse Cardiovascular Maladaptations

There is a wealth of epidemiologic and observational studies demonstrating that regular moderate-to-vigorous intensity PA is a powerful intervention in the prevention and treatment of many common chronic diseases—obesity, diabetes, metabolic syndrome, atherosclerotic CVD, and some cancers (48, 86, 113). These data, coupled with the finding that regular exercise prevents cellular senescence in animals and humans, as suggested by differences in telomere length (29, 158), have led an increasing number of middle-aged and older adults to the conclusion that "more exercise is better." However, emerging evidence in cohorts of endurance athletes now suggest that potentially adverse cardiovascular manifestations may occur following high-volume and/or high-intensity long-term exercise training/competition, which may attenuate the health benefits of a physically active lifestyle. Accelerated coronary artery calcification (CAC), exercise-induced cardiac biomarker release, evidence of transient myocardial dysfunction using echocardiographic studies or cardiovascular magnetic resonance imaging, myocardial fibrosis, atrial fibrillation (AF), and even rare instances of SCD have been reported in endurance athletes (43). These reports should also be considered when recommending strenuous leisure time or exercise interventions. If the current mantra "exercise is medicine" is embraced, underdosing and overdosing are possible. Thus, exercise may have a typical dose-response curve with a plateau in benefit or even adverse effects in some individuals at more extreme levels.

Accelerated Coronary Artery Calcification

Several studies have reported a higher prevalence of elevated CAC among middle-aged and older endurance athletes versus age- and gender-matched controls. Möhlenkamp et al. (105) found a higher prevalence of elevated CAC scores (≥100 Agatston units) among 108 marathon runners ≥50 years of age compared with an age- and risk factor–matched control group from the general population, 36% versus 22%, respectively. Interestingly, 8% of the marathon runners with CAC 100 to <400 required coronary revascularization during a 2-year follow-up. The investigators concluded that advanced CAC scores, even in highly trained endurance athletes, seem to contribute to increased myocardial damage and adverse cardiovascular outcomes. Others have reported that individuals who participate in three times the recommended PA guidelines (88) and marathon runners (21, 135) are more likely to develop CAC and higher total coronary plaque volume than their sedentary or less active control counterparts.

Recent studies have provided important novel insights regarding the accelerated coronary artery atherosclerosis commonly reported in endurance athletes. Aengevaeren et al. (4) examined the dose-response relationship between lifelong PA volume and characteristics of coronary artery atherosclerosis in a cohort of 284 male amateur athletes. The most active athletes had a higher CAC prevalence, a lower prevalence of mixed plaques, and more often had only calcified plaques compared with the least active athletes. A similar investigation of 152 veteran masters endurance athletes revealed that the athletes more often had atherosclerotic plaques, which were predominantly calcified, and a higher prevalence of CAC >300, when compared with an age and risk factor–matched sedentary control group (101). These reports have important clinical relevance, as mixed plaques are associated with a greater likelihood of future cardiovascular events compared with calcified plaques (38% versus 6%) (65).

In aggregate, athletes with CAC are at higher risk for mortality and cardiovascular events compared to athletes without CAC. However, the risk for adverse cardiovascular outcomes is lower in active and/or aerobically fit persons compared to inactive and/or unfit persons with a comparable CAC score (34, 129). Indeed, Radford et al. (129) found that after adjusting for CAC level (scores of 0, 1–99, 100–399, and ≥400), for each additional 1 MET increase in CRF there was an 11% lower risk for subsequent cardiovascular events during an average follow-up of 8.4 years. Apparently, exercise-induced cardioprotective adaptations such as a lower prevalence of unstable mixed plaques, increased coronary artery size and dilating capacity, and higher levels of CRF may offset the negative implications of a higher CAC score (52).

Transient Cardiac Dysfunction and Increased Myocardial Fibrosis

In recent years, considerable attention has focused on the post-exercise rise in cardiac biomarkers, such as troponin, a marker of cardiomyocyte damage, and B-type natriuretic peptide (BNP), a marker of myocardial stress, as well as evidence of transient myocardial dysfunction using echocardiographic studies or cardiovascular magnetic resonance imaging (MRI) in both elite and recreational athletes. Douglas et al. (40) first reported abnormalities in left ventricular systolic and diastolic function after an ultra-endurance race that included a 2.4-, 112-, and 26.2-mile swim; bike ride; and run, respectively. Similarly, La Gerche et al. (87) observed striking increases in cardiac troponin and BNP in the immediate post-race setting and echocardiographic evidence of both left and right ventricular dysfunction in 27 athletes competing in a triathlon. Although evidence of myocardial injury/damage resolved after 7 days, the authors speculated that long-term intense endurance exercise may, at least in some athletes, generate scar tissue and create a substrate for threatening ventricular arrhythmias. While this tentative conclusion requires additional study to confirm, existing research appears to support the notion that prolonged endurance exercise may provoke pathological cardiac remodelling. To this end, Trivax et al. (151) reported that marathon running causes acute dilation of the right atrium and right ventricle, a transient reduction of the right ventricular ejection fraction, and elevations in cardiac troponin I and BNP. Whether these abnormal findings represent possible harbingers of long-term sequelae, including cardiac fibrosis, or are simply part of the normal physiological process of stress, repair, and recovery remains uncertain. Nevertheless, investigators recently reported that exercise-induced troponin I elevations above the 99th percentile independently predicted higher mortality and cardiovascular events in older long-distance walkers (3).

Emergent evidence that prolonged exercise may lead to deleterious cardiac remodelling is potentially alarming, but clinical relevance is ultimately dependent upon the rates of occurrence and the populations most at risk. Previous studies using MRI in endurance athletes reported that the prevalence of myocardial fibrosis varied substantially between study populations. One systematic review found evidence of myocardial fibrosis in only 30 of 509 scanned athletes (5.9%), the presence of which was strongly associated with the cumulative exercise dose (153). Other recent studies support the fact that myocardial fibrosis is a notably rare finding among endurance athletes (2, 14). On the other hand, Wilson and associates (164) used delayed gadolinium enhancement on cardiovascular MRI to describe diverse patterns of myocardial fibrosis in 6 of 12 highly trained veteran endurance athletes. The discordant prevalence rates of myocardial fibrosis are likely due to the differing age and training characteristics/ duration (years) of the study populations or to survival bias, highlighting the need for additional prospective studies to further clarify these associations.

Exercise and Atrial Fibrillation

Atrial Fibrillation (AF) is a cardiac arrhythmia during which the heart's two upper chambers (the atria) may contract very rapidly and irregularly. The incomplete contractions allow blood to pool and clots to form in the auricles of the upper chambers. Clinical risk is proportional to the size of the resultant clots, in that portions of the inherently unstable blood clot can break loose and leave the heart. Once a piece of the clot enters the bloodstream, it can travel to the brain, lung, or periphery and cause a stroke, pulmonary embolism, or other life-threatening vascular event, respectively.

Today, AF is the most commonly treated cardiac rhythm disorder in clinical practice, accounting for approximately one-third of U.S. hospital admissions for cardiac arrhythmias. Conventional risk factors for AF include increasing age, structural heart disease, hypertension, overweight/obesity, metabolic abnormalities (e.g., diabetes mellitus), excessive alcohol intake, and obstructive sleep apnoea. However, recent studies suggest that high-volume, high-intensity endurance exercise training can also increase the likelihood of developing AF independent of these more "traditional" contributing factors.

A landmark observational study of 5,446 older men and women (≥65 years) investigated associations of leisure-time physical activity and the incidence of AF (109). Overall, 20% of the study subjects developed AF during a 12-year follow-up. As compared with no regular exercise, AF incidence was lower with light- and moderate-intensity physical activity (HR, 0.72; 95% confidence interval [CI]: 0.58–0.89), particularly leisure-time activity and walking, but not with high-intensity exercise (HR, 0.87; 95% CI: 0.64–1.19), demonstrating that in older adults exercise intensity showed the familiar J-shaped relationship with the risk of AF (Figure 29.4). The investigators concluded that up to one-fourth of new cases of AF in older adults may be attributed to their sedentary lifestyle and that regular walking at a light-to-moderate intensity and distance may be helpful in preventing this common and potentially serious heart arrhythmia.

Numerous epidemiologic and observational studies have similarly reported a statistically significant association between chronic high-volume, high-intensity exercise training and a heightened risk of developing AF (43, 114). An investigation of 52,755 long-distance cross-country skiers found over a nearly 10-year follow-up that those who completed the highest number of races and those with the fastest finishing times had the highest risk for developing AF (HR, 1.29; 95% CI: 1.04–1.61 and HR,

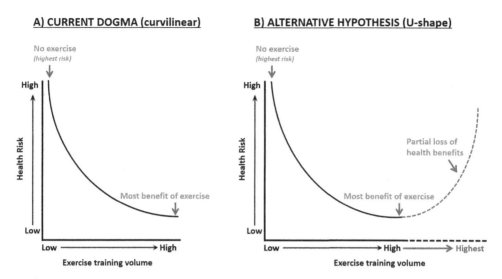

Figure 29.4 Conceptual overview of the dose-response association between exercise training volume and cardiovascular health outcomes in line with Panel A, the current dogma, and Panel B, and alternative hypothesis (reverse J-shaped or U-shaped curves)

1.20; 95% CI: 0.93–1.55), respectively (5). One systematic literature review and meta-analysis of six case-control studies found that the overall risk of AF was significantly higher in athletes ($n = 655$) than controls ($n = 895$), with a 5.29 odds ratio (95% CI: 3.57–7.85), P = 0.0001 (1). Similarly, others have reported that regular endurance exercise increases the probability of experiencing AF by 2-to-10 fold, even after adjusting for potential confounding variables and other contributing risk factors (107). In another prospective case-control study including 115 cases and 57 controls, investigators reported that the lifetime-accumulated hours of vigorous endurance training, specifically ≥2,000 hours, was the most powerful predictor of incident, exercise-related AF (26). Although the underlying mechanisms remain unclear, the repeated cardiovascular stresses of extreme endurance exercise over time likely impart some of the increased risk for AF (Figure 29.5) (43). Fortunately, much of the risk seems to resolve with

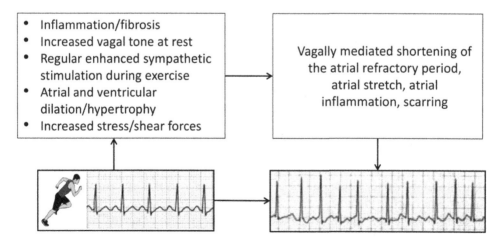

Figure 29.5 Potential mechanisms and associated sequelae for atrial fibrillation induced by regular strenuous endurance exercise and competitive athletic events

detraining and/or exercising at more moderate intensities, presumably because of the normalization of atrial structure and neural tone (114).

Collectively, these findings suggest that regular exercise both protects against and provokes AF, with light-to-moderate amounts of exercise decreasing disease incidence, but larger volumes or higher intensities of exercise increasing the risk of developing AF. Accordingly, it is generally recommended that previously sedentary, otherwise healthy young-to-middle-aged patients participate in a progressive moderate-to-vigorous PA programme, provided they remain asymptomatic. In contrast, light-to-moderate intensity PA is preferred for higher-risk, older patients to achieve a reasonable level of fitness when the goals are prevention of AF and the maintenance or improvement of cardiovascular health.

Sudden Cardiac Death

Although vigorous PA acutely increases the relative risk of acute myocardial infarction and/or SCD by ~2 to 107-fold compared with non-vigorous exercise or rest, the relative risk is greatest with unaccustomed strenuous exertion and decreases with increasing frequencies of vigorous weekly exercise (49, 103).

Atherosclerotic CAD is the most common autopsy finding in individuals aged >40 years who experience exertion-related cardiac arrest and SCD (155). In contrast, structural cardiovascular abnormalities, most notably, hypertrophic cardiomyopathy (HCM), are a commonly cited cause of SCD during vigorous-to-high intensity physical activity in younger individuals (98). However, recent studies of young exercise-related SCD victims have often revealed no structural abnormalities at autopsy, classifying these as either sudden arrhythmic death or SCD with a structurally normal heart (152). Despite the absence of absolute proof from randomized controlled clinical trials, the deleterious effect of extreme endurance exercise training on arrhythmogenic right ventricular cardiomyopathy is now well accepted (52). It is important to recognize that while this conclusion is scientifically tentative, it is not premature, as recent guidelines formulated by eminent experts in the field recommend avoiding strenuous endurance exercise in patients with compromised right heart function. Whether high-volume, high-intensity endurance exercise can accelerate disease development and severity in other genetic cardiac conditions is unknown; however, preliminary studies suggest potential deleterious effects in patients with long QT syndrome and inherited disorders of cardiac membrane structural proteins such as lamin A/C mutations (52).

Despite the potential cardioprotective and anti-ageing effects of regular, moderate-to-vigorous intensity exercise, numerous anecdotal reports of acute cardiac events occur in marathon runners and triathlon participants each year. In 2009, three runners died within 15 minutes of each other while competing in the Detroit Free Press Flagstar Marathon (160). These unexpected tragedies attract considerable media attention and have led to escalating concerns regarding the health risks of these highly competitive activities. Fuelling this concern, recent studies have reported that in response to more extreme vigorous- to high-intensity exercise, there can be a deleterious inflammatory milieu in the circulation (28). For instance, the normally cardioprotective release of the myokine IL-6, produced by exercised skeletal muscle, can promote counter-productive inflammatory responses when combined with elevated levels of tumour necrosis factor alpha (TNF-a) (100). Indeed, a post-exercise inflammatory milieu is linked to untoward cardiovascular profiles when further combined with the release of acute-phase reactant proteins from the liver, such as C-reactive protein (CRP) (28). Thus, a heightened inflammation response post-exercise can stimulate a cascade of signalling events that are potentially maladaptive, including an increase in monocyte tissue factor production, provocation of platelet hyperreactivity, increased fibrinogen biosynthesis, and enhanced microparticle formation and erythrocyte aggregability, triggering a prothrombotic state (28).

To clarify the risk of cardiac arrest associated with marathon and half-marathon races in the United States from January 1, 2000, to May 31, 2010, investigators reported on the incidences and outcomes of events among 10.9 million registered marathon runners (77). Of the 59 cases of cardiac arrest (mean ± SD age: 42 ± 13 years; 51 men), 42 (71%) were fatal. The final mile, <50% of the entire marathon distance, accounted for ~50% of the SCDs. In addition, the most frequent clinical and autopsy findings were HCM and atherosclerotic CAD, respectively. More recently, investigators reported on death and cardiac arrest in >9 million triathlon participants over a 30-year period (63). A total of 135 SCDs occurred, with an incidence of 1.74 per 100,000—exceeding the incidence reported for marathon racing (1 per 100,000). Interestingly, during ultra-endurance triathlon events, most SCDs and cardiac arrests occurred during the swim segment (*n* = 90; 67%); the others occurred during bicycling (*n* = 22; 16%), running (*n* = 15; 11%), and post-race recovery (*n* = 8; 6%). Among these SCD victims, 68 of the participants whose previous race experience was known, 26 (38%) were competing in their first triathlon. Among the autopsies conducted, 44% had clinically relevant cardiovascular abnormalities, most frequently atherosclerotic CAD or cardiomyopathy. Collectively, these studies suggest that cardiac arrest and SCD during marathon running and triathlon participation are infrequent, that inadequate training or race preparation may be linked to some inaugural fatalities, and that clinicians evaluating potential race participants should be aware of the risks of HCM and atherosclerotic CAD in this patient population, both of which can often be detected via appropriate medical screening.

Conclusions

In summary, higher levels of regular PA and CRF are associated with a reduced risk of developing hypertension, obesity, type 2 diabetes, atrial fibrillation, chronic kidney disease, heart failure, and major cardiovascular events, including myocardial infarction, coronary artery bypass graft surgery, stroke, and SCD (86). Relative to CVD, the inverse association of lower incidence of type 2 diabetes with PA or CRF has also been noted against the diabetogenic effects of cholesterol-lowering statins (133). These findings suggest that regular exercise appears to more than compensate for the purported modest increase in diabetes risk from statin use (51, 83, 162). Moreover, in a recent report of patients with known CVD, maintaining or increasing PA at or above the recommended guidelines resulted in lower all-cause and CVD mortality rates (106). In contrast, weight loss in this cohort was not associated with improved survival.

The beneficial cardiovascular outcomes resulting from regular PA, increased CRF, or both are generally attributed to multiple mechanisms, including anti-atherosclerotic, anti-ischemic, anti-arrhythmic, anti-thrombotic, and psychological effects. In addition, ischemic and biochemical cardiac preconditioning offers a unique and undervalued nonpharmacological approach to prevent and attenuate acute coronary syndromes (7, 23, 66, 120, 121, 125, 143). Accordingly, it appears that regular increases in heart rate and metabolism evoked by moderate-to-vigorous PA can reduce subsequent infarct size and/or the potential for malignant ventricular arrhythmias triggered by acute myocardial ischemia.

Although vigorous exercise is more protective than moderate-intensity PA (146, 157), it is also associated with increased cardiovascular events, especially in persons with known or occult CVD who were participating in unaccustomed strenuous physical exertion (103). However, fatal exercise-related acute cardiovascular events also occur each year in highly trained endurance athletes participating in marathons and triathlons (63, 77). Autopsies in these individuals invariably reveal underlying atherosclerotic CVD or structural cardiovascular abnormalities, most notably HCM, in the vast majority.

Despite the well-documented effects of regular moderate-to-vigorous PA and increased CRF, emerging evidence in cohorts of middle-aged and older endurance athletes now suggest that potentially adverse cardiovascular adaptations may occur following high-volume, high-intensity long-term training regimens and competition, especially increased CAC and incident AF (43, 52). Although the deleterious effect of vigorous- to high-intensity endurance training on arrhythmogenic right ventricular cardiomyopathy is now well accepted (52), whether extreme exercise regimens can accelerate disease development and severity in those with other genetic cardiac conditions is unknown. Nevertheless, preliminary studies suggest potentially unfavourable effects in patients with long QT syndrome and other inherited disorders of cardiac membrane structural proteins such as lamin A/C mutations (52).

In closing, perhaps William C. Roberts, MD, editor of the *American Journal of Cardiology*, summed it up best when he commented on the medicinal properties of exercise as "an agent with lipid-lowering, antihypertensive, positive inotropic, negative chronotropic, vasodilating, diuretic, anorexigenic, weight-reducing, cathartic, hypoglycaemic, tranquilizing, hypnotic and anti-depressive qualities" (130). Certainly, at the population level, more rigorous promotion of regular PA is needed to combat, at least in part, contemporary technologic advancements that have contributed to our increasingly hypokinetic lifestyle (44).

Acknowledgments

The authors acknowledge the facilities and staff of the Department of Preventive Cardiology/Cardiac Rehabilitation, William Beaumont Hospital, Royal Oak, Michigan and the School of Integrative Physiology and Athletic Training at University of Montana. Additional thanks are offered to affiliations with the International Heart Institute, Missoula, Montana, and to Brenda White for her assistance with the preparation of this manuscript, laboriously checking the accuracy and placement of our references.

References

1. Abdulla J, Nielsen JR. Is the risk of atrial fibrillation higher in athletes than in the general population? A systematic review and meta-analysis. *Europace* 11: 1156–1159, 2009
2. Abdullah SM, Barkley KW, Bhella PS, Hastings JL, Matulevicius S, Fujimoto N, et al. Lifelong physical activity regardless of dose is not associated with myocardial fibrosis. *Circ Cardiovasc Imaging* 9: 2016. doi: 10.1161/CIRCIMAGING.116.005511.
3. Aengevaeren VL, Hopman MTE, Thompson PD, Bakker EA, George KP, Thijssen DHJ, et al. Exercise-induced cardiac troponin i increase and incident mortality and cardiovascular events. *Circulation* 140: 804–814, 2019.
4. Aengevaeren VL, Mosterd A, Braber TL, Prakken NHJ, Doevendans PA, Grobbee DE, et al. Relationship between lifelong exercise volume and coronary atherosclerosis in athletes. *Circulation* 136: 138–148, 2017.
5. Andersen K, Farahmand B, Ahlbom A, Held C, Ljunghall S, Michaëlsson K, et al. Risk of arrhythmias in 52 755 long-distance cross-country skiers: a cohort study. *Eur Heart J* 34: 3624–3631, 2013.
6. Billman GE. Aerobic exercise conditioning: a nonpharmacological antiarrhythmic intervention. *J Appl Physiol (1985)* 92: 446–454, 2002.
7. Billman GE, Schwartz PJ, Stone HL. The effects of daily exercise on susceptibility to sudden cardiac death. *Circulation* 69: 1182–1189, 1984.
8. Blair SN. Physical inactivity: the biggest public health problem of the 21st century. *Br J Sports Med* 43: 1–2, 2009.
9. Blair SN, Kampert JB, Kohn HW III, Barlow CE, Macera CA, Paffenbarger RS Jr, et al. Influences of cardiorespiratory fitness and other precursors on cardiovascular disease and all-cause mortality in men and women. *JAMA* 276: 205–210, 1996.
10. Blair SN, Kohl HW III, Barlow CE, Paffenbarger RS Jr, Gibbons LW, Macera CA. Changes in physical fitness and all-cause mortality: a prospective study of healthy and unhealthy men. *JAMA* 273: 1093–1098, 1995.
11. Blair SN, Kohl HW III, Paffenbarger RS Jr, Clark DG, Cooper KH, Gibbons LW. Physical fitness and all-cause mortality: a prospective study of healthy men and women. *JAMA* 262: 2395–2401, 1989.
12. Blumenthal JA, Babyak MA, Moore KA, Craighead WE, Herman S, Khatri P, et al. Effects of exercise training on older adults with major depression. *Arch Intern Med* 159:2349–2356, 1999.
13. Boden WE, Franklin BA, Wenger NK. Physical activity and structured exercise for patients with stable ischemic heart disease. *JAMA* 309: 143–144, 2013..

14. Bohm P, Schneider G, Linneweber L, Rentzsch A, Krämer N, Abdul-Khalig H, et al. Right and left ventricular function and mass in male elite master athletes: a controlled contrast-enhanced cardiovascular magnetic resonance study. *Circulation* 133: 1927–1935, 2016.

15. Bolli R, Becker L, Gross G, Mentzer R Jr, Balshaw D, Lathrop DA; NHLBI Working Group on the Translation of Therapies for Protecting the Heart from Ischemia. Myocardial protection at a crossroads: the need for translation into clinical therapy. *Circ Res* 95: 125–134, 2004.

16. Bolli R, Marbán E. Molecular and cellular mechanisms of myocardial stunning. *Physiol Rev* 79: 609–634, 1999.

17. Booth FW, Gordon SE, Carlson CJ, Hamilton MT. Waging war on modern chronic diseases: primary prevention through exercise biology. *J Appl Physiol (1985)* 88: 774–87, 2000.

18. Booth FW, Lees SJ. Fundamental questions about genes, inactivity, and chronic disease. *Physiol Genomics* 28: 146–157, 2007.

19. Boulé NG, Haddad E, Kenny GP, Wells GA, Sigal RJ. Effects of exercise on glycemic control and body mass in type 2 diabetes mellitus: a meta-analysis of controlled clinical trials. *JAMA* 286: 1218–1227, 2001.

20. Bowles DK, Starnes JW. Exercise training improves metabolic response after ischemia in isolated working rat heart. *J Appl Physiol (1985)* 76: 1608–1614, 1994.

21. Breuckmann F, Möhlenkamp S, Nassenstein K, Lehmann N, Ladd S, Schmermund A, et al. Myocardial late gadolinium enhancement: prevalence, pattern, and prognostic relevance in marathon runners. *Radiology* 251: 50–57, 2009.

22. Brown DA, Chicco AJ, Jew KN, Johnson MS, Lynch JM, Watson PA, et al. Cardioprotection afforded by chronic exercise is mediated by the sarcolemmal, and not the mitochondrial, isoform of the KATP channel in the rat. *J Physiol* 569: 913–924, 2005.

23. Brown DA, Moore RL. Perspectives in innate and acquired cardioprotection: cardioprotection acquired through exercise. *J Appl Physiol (1985)* 103: 1894–1899, 2007.

24. Buja LM. Myocardial ischemia and reperfusion injury. *Cardiovasc Pathol* 14: 170–175, 2005.

25. Buja LM, Weerasinghe P. Unresolved issues in myocardial reperfusion injury. *Cardiovasc Pathol* 19: 29–35, 2010.

26. Calvo N, Ramos P, Montserrat S, Guasch E, Coll-Vinent B, Domenech M, et al. Emerging risk factors and the dose-response relationship between physical activity and lone atrial fibrillation: a prospective case-control study. *Europace* 18: 57–63, 2016.

27. Carlson SA, Fulton JE, Pratt M, Yang Z, Adams EK. Inadequate physical activity and health care expenditures in the United States. *Prog Cardiovasc Dis* 57: 315–323, 2015.

28. Chen YW, Apostolakis S, Lip GYH. Exercise-induced changes in inflammatory processes: Implications for thrombogenesis in cardiovascular disease. *Ann Med* 46: 439–455, 2014.

29. Cherkas LF, Hunkin JL, Kato BS, Richards JB, Gardner JP, Surdulescu GL, et al. The association between physical activity in leisure time and leukocyte telomere length. *Arch Intern Med* 168: 154–158, 2008.

30. Chicco AJ, Johnson MS, Armstrong CJ, Lynch JM, Gardner RT, Fasen GS, et al. Sex-specific and exercise-acquired cardioprotection is abolished by sarcolemmal KATP channel blockade in the rat heart. *Am J Physiol Heart Circ Physiol* 292: H2432–2437, 2007.

31. Church TS, Barlow CE, Earnest CP, Kampert JB, Priest EL, Blair SN. Associations between cardiorespiratory fitness and C-reactive protein in men. *Arterioscler Thromb Vasc Biol* 22: 1869–1876, 2002.

32. Clarke PM, Walter SJ, Hayen A, Mallon WJ, Heijmans J, Studdert DM. Survival of the fittest: retrospective cohort study of the longevity of Olympic medallists in the modern era. *Br J Sports Med* 49: 898–902, 2015.

33. Collins HL, Loka AM, Dicarlo SE. Daily exercise-induced cardioprotection is associated with changes in calcium regulatory proteins in hypertensive rats. *Am J Physiol Heart Circ Physiol* 288: H532–540, 2005.

34. DeFina LF, Radford NB, Barlow CE, Willis BL, Leonard D, Haskell WL, et al. Association of all-cause and cardiovascular mortality with high levels of physical activity and concurrent coronary artery calcification. *JAMA Cardiol* 4: 174–181, 2019.

35. Demirel HA, Hamilton KL, Shanely RA, Tümer N, Koroly MJ, Powers SK. Age and attenuation of exercise-induced myocardial HSP72 accumulation. *Am J Physiol Heart Circ Physiol* 285: H1609–1615, 2003.

36. Demirel HA, Powers SK, Zergeroglu MA, Shanely RA, Hamilton K, Coombes J, et al. Short-term exercise improves myocardial tolerance to in vivo ischemia-reperfusion in the rat. *J Appl Physiol (1985)* 91: 2205–2212, 2001.

37. Dhalla NS, Temsah RM, Netticadan T, Sandhu MS. Calcium overload in ischemia/reperfusion injury. In: *Heart Physiology and Pathophysiology, edited by* Sperelakis N, Kurachi Y, Terzic A, Cohen MV. San Diego, CA: Academic Press, 2001, pp. 949–965.

38. Dickson EW, Hogrefe CP, Ludwig PS, Ackermann LW, Stoll LL, Denning GM. Exercise enhances myocardial ischemic tolerance via an opioid receptor-dependent mechanism. *Am J Physiol Heart Circ Physiol* 294: H402–408, 2008.

39. Dorn J, Naughton J, Imamura D, Trevisan M. Results of a multicenter randomized clinical trial of exercise and long-term survival in myocardial infarction patients: the national exercise and heart disease project (NEHDP). *Circulation* 100: 1764–1769, 1999.

40. Douglas PS, O'Toole ML, Hiller WD, Hackney K, Reichek N. Cardiac fatigue after prolonged exercise. *Circulation* 76: 1206–1213, 1987.

41. Downey JM. Free radicals and their involvement during long-term myocardial ischemia and reperfusion. *Annu Rev Physiol* 52: 487–504, 1990.

42. Dutcher JR, Kahn J, Grines C, Franklin B. Comparison of left ventricular ejection fraction and exercise capacity as predictors of two- and five-year mortality following acute myocardial infarction. *Am J Cardiol* 99: 436–441, 2007.

43. Eijsvogels TMH, Thompson PD, Franklin BA. The "extreme exercise hypothesis": recent findings and cardiovascular health implications. *Curr Treat Options Cardiovasc Med* 20: 84, 2018.

44. Fletcher GF, Landolfo C, Niebauer J, Ozemek C, Arena R, Lavie CJ. Promoting physical activity and exercise: JACC Health Promotion Series. *J Am Coll Cardiol* 72: 1622–1639, 2018.

45. Ford ES. Does exercise reduce inflammation? Physical activity and C-reactive protein among U.S. adults. *Epidemiology* 13: 561–568, 2002.

46. Franklin BA. Exercise training and coronary collateral circulation. *Med Sci Sports Exerc* 23: 648–653, 1991.

47. Franklin BA. Survival of the fittest: evidence for high-risk and cardioprotective fitness levels. *Cur Sports Med Rep* 1: 257–259, 2002.

48. Franklin BA. Physical activity to combat chronic diseases and escalating health care costs: the unfilled prescription. *Curr Sports Med Reports* 7: 122–125, 2008.

49. Franklin BA. Preventing exercise-related cardiovascular events: is a medical examination more urgent for physical activity or inactivity? *Circulation* 129: 1081–1084, 2014.

50. Franklin BA, Kaminsky LA, Kokkinos P. Quantitating the dose of physical activity in secondary prevention: relation of exercise intensity to survival. *Mayo Clin Proc* 93: 1158–1163, 2018.

51. Franklin BA, Lavie CJ. Impact of statins on physical activity and fitness: ally or adversary? *Mayo Clin Proc* 90: 1314–1319, 2015.

52. Franklin BA, Thompson PD, Al-Zaiti SS, Albert CM, Hiveret M-F, Levine BD, et al; on behalf of the American Heart Association Physical Activity Committee of the Council on Lifestyle and Cardiometabolic Heath, Council on Cardiovascular and Stroke Nursing, Council on Clinical Cardiology and Stroke Council. Exercise-related acute cardiovascular events and potential deleterious adaptations following long-term exercise training: Placing the risks into perspective – an update. *Circulation* 141: 00–00, 2020 (In press).

53. French JP, Hamilton KL, Quindry JC, Lee Y, Upchurch PA, Powers SK. Exercise-induced protection against myocardial apoptosis and necrosis: MnSOD, calcium-handling proteins, and calpain. *FASEB J* 22: 2862–2871, 2008.

54. French JP, Quindry JC, Falk DJ, Staib JL, Lee Y, Wang KK, et al. Ischemia-reperfusion-induced calpain activation and SERCA2a degradation are attenuated by exercise training and calpain inhibition. *Am J Physiol Heart Circ Physiol* 290: H128–136, 2006.

55. Frasier CR, Moukdar F, Patel HD, Sloan RC, Stewart LM, Alleman RJ, et al. Redox-dependent increases in glutathione reductase and exercise preconditioning: role of NADPH oxidase and mitochondria. *Cardiovasc Res* 98: 47–55, 2013.

56. Frasier CR, Sloan RC, Bostian PA, Gonzon MD, Kurowicki J, Lopresto SJ, et al. Short-term exercise preserves myocardial glutathione and decreases arrhythmias after thiol oxidation and ischemia in isolated rat hearts. *J Appl Physiol (1985)* 111: 1751–1759, 2011.

57. Gross ER, Gross GJ. Pharmacologic therapeutics for cardiac reperfusion injury. *Expert Opin Emerg Drugs* 12: 367–388, 2007.

58. Gulati M, Pandey DK, Arnsdorf MF, Lauderdale DS, Thisted RA, Wicklund RH, et al. Exercise capacity and the risk of death in women: the St James Women Take Heart Project. *Circulation* 108: 1554–1559, 2003.

59. Hambrecht R, Wolf A, Gielen S, Linke A, Hofer J, Erbs S, et al. Effect of exercise on coronary endothelial function in patients with coronary artery disease. *N Engl J Med* 342: 454–460, 2000.

60. Hamilton KL, Powers SK, Sugiura T, Kim S, Lennon S, Tumer N, et al. Short-term exercise training can improve myocardial tolerance to I/R without elevation in heat shock proteins. *Am J Physiol Heart Circ Physiol* 281: H1346–1352, 2001.

61. Hamilton KL, Quindry JC, French JP, Staib J, Hughes J, Mehta JL, et al. MnSOD antisense treatment and exercise-induced protection against arrhythmias. *Free Radic Biol Med* 37: 1360–1368, 2004.

62. Hamilton KL, Staib JL, Phillips T, Hess A, Lennon SL, Powers SK. Exercise, antioxidants, and HSP72: protection against myocardial ischemia/reperfusion. *Free Radic Biol Med* 34: 800–809, 2003.

63. Harris KM, Creswell LL, Haas TS, Thomas T, Tung M, Isaacson E, et al. Death and cardiac arrest in U.S. triathlon participants, 1985 to 2016: a case series. *Ann Intern Med* 167: 529–535, 2017.

64. Hoogeboom TJ, Dronkers JJ, Hulzebos EH, van Meeteren NL. Merits of exercise therapy before and after major surgery. *Curr Opin Anaesthesiol* 27:161–166, 2014.

65. Hou ZH, Lu B, Gao Y, Jiang SL, Wang Y, Li W, et al. Prognostic value of coronary CT angioplasty and calcium score for major adverse cardiac events in outpatients. *JACC Cardiovasc Imaging* 5: 990–999, 2012.

66. Hull SS Jr, Vanoli E, Adamson PB, Verrier RL, Foreman RD, Schwartz PJ. Exercise training confers anticipatory protection from sudden death during acute myocardial ischemia. *Circulation* 89: 548–552, 1994.

67. Iellamo F, Legramante JM, Massaro M, Raimondi G, Galante A. Effects of a residential exercise training on baroreflex sensitivity and heart rate variability in patients with coronary artery disease: a randomized, controlled study. *Circulation* 102: 2588–2592, 2000.

68. Joyner MJ, Green DJ. Exercise protects the cardiovascular system: effects beyond traditional risk factors. *J Physiol* 587: 5551–5558, 2009.

69. Kaminsky LA, Arena R, Beckie TM, Brubaker PH, Church TS, Forman DE, et al; American Heart Association Advocacy Coordinating Committee, Council on Clinical Cardiology, and Council on Nutrition, Physical Activity and Metabolism. The importance of cardiorespiratory fitness in the United States: the need for a national registry. A policy statement from the American Heart Association. *Circulation* 127: 652–662, 2013.

70. Kang J, Robertson RJ, Hagberg JM, Kelley DE, Goss FL, DaSilva SG, et al. Effect of exercise intensity on glucose and insulin metabolism in obese individuals and obese NIDDM patients. *Diabetes Care* 19: 341–349, 1996.

71. Karstoft K, Pedersen BK. Skeletal muscle as a gene regulatory endocrine organ. *Curr Opin Clin Nutr Metab Care* 19: 270–275, 2016.

72. Kavanagh T, Mertens DJ, Hamm LF, Beyene J, Kennedy J, Corey P, et al. Prediction of long-term prognosis in 12 169 men referred for cardiac rehabilitation. *Circulation* 106: 666–671, 2002.

73. Kavanagh T, Mertens DJ, Hamm LF, Beyene J, Kennedy J, Corey P, et al. Peak oxygen intake and cardiac mortality in women referred for cardiac rehabilitation. *J Am Coll Cardiol* 42: 2139–2143, 2003.

74. Kavazis AN, McClung JM, Hood DA, Powers SK. Exercise induces a cardiac mitochondrial phenotype that resists apoptotic stimuli. *Am J Physiol Heart Circ Physiol* 294: H928–935, 2008.

75. Kelly GA, Kelley KS, Franklin B. Aerobic exercise and lipids and lipoproteins in patients with cardiovascular disease: a meta-analysis of randomized controlled trials. *J Cardiopulm Rehabil* 26: 131–139, 2006.

76. Kettunen JA, Kujala UM, Kaprio J, Bäckmand H, Peltonen M, Eriksson JG, et al. All-cause and disease-specific mortality among male, former elite athletes: an average 50-year follow-up. *Br J Sports Med* 49: 893–897, 2015.

77. Kim JH, Malhotra R, Chiampas G, d'Hemecourt P, Troyanos C, Cianca J, et al; Race Associated Cardiac Arrest Event Registry RACER) Study. Cardiac arrest during long-distance running races. *N Engl J Med* 366: 130–140, 2012.

78. Kloner RA, Bolli R, Marban E, Reinlib L, Braunwald E. Medical and cellular implications of stunning, hibernation, and preconditioning: an NHLBI workshop. *Circulation* 97:1848–1867, 1998.

79. Kloner RA, Jennings RB. Consequences of brief ischemia: stunning, preconditioning, and their clinical implications (Part 1). *Circulation* 104: 2981–2989, 2001.

80. Knowler WC, Barrett-Connor E, Fowler SE, Hamman RF, Lachin JM, Walker EA, et al; Diabetes Prevention Program Research Group. Reduction in the incidence of type 2 diabetes with lifestyle intervention or metformin. *N Engl J Med* 346: 393–403, 2002.

81. Kodama S, Saito K, Tanaka S, Maki M, Yachi Y, Asumi M, et al. Cardiorespiratory fitness as a quantitative predictor of all-cause mortality and cardiovascular events in healthy men and women: a meta-analysis. *JAMA* 301: 2024–2035, 2009.

82. Kokkinos P, Faselis C, Franklin B, Lavie CJ, Sidossis L, Moor H, et al. Cardiorespiratory fitness, body mass index and heart failure incidence. *Eur J Heart Fail* 21: 436–444, 2019.

83. Kokkinos P, Faselis C, Narayan P, Myers J, Nylen E, Sui X, et al. Cardiorespiratory fitness and incidence of type 2 diabetes in United States veterans on statin therapy. *Am J Med* 130: 1192–1198, 2017.

84. Kokkinos P, Myers J. Exercise and physical activity: clinical outcomes and applications. *Circulation* 122:1637–1648, 2010.

85. Kokkinos P, Myers J, Faselis C, Panagiotakos DB, Doumas M, Pittaras A, et al. Exercise capacity and mortality in older men: a 20-year follow-up study. *Circulation* 122: 790–797, 2010.

86. Kokkinos P, Narayan P, Myers J, Franklin B. Cardiorespiratory fitness and the incidence of chronic disease. *J Clin Exer Physiol* 7: 37–45, 2018.

87. La Gerche A, Prior DL. Exercise—is it possible to have too much of a good thing? *Heart Lung Circ* 16: S102–104, 2007.

88. Laddu DR, Rana JS, Murillo R, Sorel ME, Quesenberry CP Jr, Allen NB, et al. 25-year physical activity trajectories and development of subclinical coronary artery disease as measured by coronary artery calcium: the coronary artery risk development in young adults (CARDIA) study. *Mayo Clin Proc* 92: 1660–1670, 2017.

89. LaMonte MJ, Durstine JL, Yanowitz FG, Lim T, DuBose KD, et al. Cardiorespiratory fitness and C-reactive protein among a tri-ethnic sample of women. *Circulation* 106: 403–406, 2002.

90. Lavie CJ, Arena R, Swift DL, Johannsen NM, Sui X, Lee DC, et al. Exercise and the cardiovascular system: clinical science and cardiovascular outcomes. *Cir Res* 117: 207–219, 2015.

91. Lee IM, Shiroma EJ, Lobelo F, Puska P, Blair SN, Katzmarzyk PT; Lancet Physical Activity Series Working Group. Effect of physical inactivity on major non-communicable diseases worldwide: an analysis of burden of disease and life expectancy. *Lancet* 380: 219–229, 2012.

92. Lennon SL, Quindry JC, French JP, Kim S, Mehta JL, Powers SK. Exercise and myocardial tolerance to ischaemia-reperfusion. *Acta Physiol Scand* 182: 161–169, 2004.

93. Lennon SL, Quindry J, Hamilton KL, French J, Staib J, Mehta JL, et al. Loss of exercise-induced cardioprotection after cessation of exercise. *J Appl Physiol (1985)* 96: 1299–1305, 2004.

94. Leon AS, Franklin BA, Costa F, Balady GJ, Berra KA, Stewart KJ, et al; American Heart Association; Council on Clinical Cardiology (Subcommittee on Exercise, Cardiac Rehabilitation, and Prevention); Council on Nutrition, Physical Activity, and Metabolism (Subcommittee on Physical Activity); American Association of Cardiovascular and Pulmonary Rehabilitation. Cardiac rehabilitation and secondary prevention of coronary heart disease: an American heart association scientific statement from the council on clinical cardiology (Subcommittee on exercise, cardiac rehabilitation, and prevention) and the council on nutrition, physical activity, and metabolism (subcommittee on physical activity), in collaboration with the American Association of cardiovascular and pulmonary rehabilitation. *Circulation* 111: 369–376, 2005.

95. Li Y, Pan A, Wang DD, Wang DD, Liu X, Dhana K, et al. Impact of healthy lifestyle factors on life expectancies in the US population. *Circulation* 138: 345–355, 2018.

96. Lightfoot JT, Leamy L, Pomp D, Turner MJ, Fodor AA, Knab A, et al. Strain screen and haplotype association mapping of wheel running in inbred mouse strains. *J Appl Physiol (1985)* 109: 623–634, 2010.

97. Marijon E, Tafflet M, Antero-Jacquemin J, El Helou N, Berthelot G, Celermajer DS, et al. Mortality of French participants in the tour de France (1947-2012). *Eur Heart J* 34: 3145–3150, 2013.

98. Maron BJ, Shirani J, Poliac LC, Mathenge R, Roberts WC, Mueller FO. Sudden death in young competitive athletes: clinical, demographic, and pathological profiles. *JAMA* 276: 99–204, 1996.

99. McCullough PA, Gallagher MJ, deJong AT, Sandberg KR, Trivax JE, Alexander D, et al. Cardiorespiratory fitness and short-term complications after bariatric surgery. *Chest* 130: 517–525, 2006.

100. McGinnis GR, Ballmann C, Peters B, Nanayakkara G, Roberts M, Amin R, et al. Interleukin-6 mediates exercise preconditioning against myocardial ischemia reperfusion injury. *Am J Physiol Heart Circ Physiol* 308: H1423–1433, 2015.

101. Merghani A, Maestrini V, Rosmini S, Cox AT, Dhutia H, Bastiaenan R, et al. Prevalence of subclinical coronary artery disease in masters endurance athletes with a low atherosclerotic risk profile. *Circulation* 136: 126–137, 2017.

102. Miller LE, McGinnis GR, Peters BA, Ballmann CG, Nanayakkara G, Amin R, et al. Involvement of the δ-opioid receptor in exercise-induced cardioprotection. *Exp Physiol* 100: 410–421, 2015.

103. Mittleman MA, Maclure M, Tofler GH, Sherwood JB, Goldberg RJ, Muller JE. Triggering of acute myocardial infarction by heavy physical exertion: protection against triggering by regular exertion. Determinants of myocardial infarction onset study investigators. *N Engl J Med* 329: 1677–1683, 1993.

104. Möbius-Winkler S, Uhlemann M. Adams V, Sandri M, Erbs S, Lenk K, et al. Coronary collateral growth induced by physical exercise: results of the impact of intensive exercise training on coronary collateral circulation in patients with stable coronary artery disease (EXCITE) trial. *Circulation* 133: 1438–1448, 2016.

105. Möhlenkamp S, Lehmann N, Breuckmann F, Bröcker-Preuss M, Nassenstein K, Halle M, et al.; Marathon Study Investigators; Heinz Nixdorf Recall Study Investigators. Running: the risk of coronary events: Prevalence and prognostic relevance of coronary atherosclerosis in marathon runners. *Eur Heart J* 29: 1903–1910, 2008.

106. Moholdt T, Lavie CJ, Nauman J. Sustained physical activity, not weight loss, associated with improved survival in coronary heart disease. *J Am Coll Cardiol* 71: 1094–1101, 2018.

107. Mont L, Elosua R, Brugada J. Endurance sport practice as a risk factor for atrial fibrillation and atrial flutter. *Europace* 11: 11–17, 2009.

108. Morris JN, Heady JA, Raffle PA, Roberts CG, Parks JW. Coronary heart-disease and physical activity of work. *Lancet* 262: 1111–1120, 1953.

109. Mozaffarian D, Furberg CD, Psaty BM, Siscovick D. Physical activity and incidence of atrial fibrillation in older adults: the Cardiovascular Health Study. *Circulation* 228: 800–807, 2008.

110. Murry CE, Jennings RB, Reimer KA. Preconditioning with ischemia: a delay of lethal cell injury in ischemic myocardium. *Circulation* 74: 1124–1136, 1986.

111. Myers J, Doom R, King R, Fonda H, Chan K, Kokkinos P, et al. Association between cardiorespiratory fitness and health care costs: the veterans exercise testing study. *Mayo Clin Proc* 93: 48–55, 2018.

112. Myers J, Prakash M, Froelicher V, Do D, Partington S, Atwood JE. Exercise capacity and mortality among men referred for exercise testing. *N Engl J Med* 346: 793–801, 2002.

113. Nocon M, Hiemann T. Müller-Riemenschneider F, Thalau F, Roll S, Willich SN. Association of physical activity with all-cause and cardiovascular mortality: a systematic review and meta-analysis. *Eur J Cardiovasc Prev Rehabil* 15: 239–246, 2008.

114. O'Keefe JH, Franklin B, Lavie CJ. Exercising for health and longevity vs peak performance: different regimens for different goals. *Mayo Clin Proc* 89: 1171–1175, 2014.

115. Pedersen BK. Edward F. Adolph distinguished lecture: muscle as an endocrine organ: IL-6 and other myokines. *J Appl Physiol (1985)* 107: 1006–1014, 2009.

116. Pescatello LS, Franklin BA, Fagard R, Farquhar WB, Kelley GA, Ray CA; American College of Sports Medicine. Exercise and hypertension. American college of sports medicine position stand. *Med Sci Sports Exerc* 36: 533–553, 2004.

117. Pitsavos C, Kavouras SA, Panagiotakos DB, Arapi S, Anastasiou CA, Zombolos S, et al.; GRECS Study Investigators. Physical activity status and acute coronary syndromes survival: the GREECS (greek study of acute coronary syndromes) study. *J Am Coll Cardiol* 51: 2034–2039, 2008.

118. Powell KE, Thompson PD, Caspersen CJ, Kendrick JS. Physical activity and the incidence of coronary heart disease. *Annu Rev Public Health* 8: 253–287, 1987.

119. Powers SK, Demirel HA, Vincent HK, Coombes JS, Naito H, Hamilton KL, et al. Exercise training improves myocardial tolerance to in vivo ischemia-reperfusion in the rat. *Am J Physiol* 275: R1468–1477, 1998.

120. Powers SK, Smuder AJ, Kavazis AN, Quindry JC. Mechanisms of exercise-induced cardioprotection. *Physiology (Bethesda)* 29: 27–38, 2014.

121. Quindry JC, Franklin BA. Cardioprotective exercise and pharmacologic interventions as complementary antidotes to cardiovascular disease. *Exerc Sport Sci Rev* 46:5–17, 2018.

122. Quindry JC, Franklin BA, Chapman M, Humphrey R, Mathis S. Benefits and risks of high-intensity interval training in patients with coronary artery disease. *Am J Cardiol* 123: 1370–1377, 2019.

123. Quindry J, French J, Hamilton K, Lee Y, Mehta JL, Powers S. Exercise training provides cardioprotection against ischemia-reperfusion induced apoptosis in young and old animals. *Exp Gerontol* 40: 416–425, 2005.

124. Quindry JC, French J, Hamilton KL, Lee Y, Selsby J, Powers S. Exercise does not increase cyclooxygenase-2 myocardial levels in young or senescent hearts. *J Physiol Sci* 60: 181–186, 2010.

125. Quindry JC, Hamilton KL. Exercise and cardiac preconditioning against ischemia reperfusion injury. *Curr Cardiol Rev* 9: 220–229, 2013.

126. Quindry JC, Hamilton KL, French JP, Lee Y, Murlasits Z, Tumer N, et al. Exercise-induced HSP-72 elevation and cardioprotection against infarct and apoptosis. *J Appl Physiol (1985)* 103: 1056–1062, 2007.

127. Quindry JC, Miller L, McGinnis G, Kliszczewicz B, Irwin JM, Landram M, et al. Ischemia reperfusion injury, KATP channels, and exercise-induced cardioprotection against apoptosis. *J Appl Physiol (1985)* 113: 498–506, 2012.

128. Quindry JC, Schreiber L, Hosick P, Wrieden J, Irwin JM, Hoyt E. Mitochondrial KATP channel inhibition blunts arrhythmia protection in ischemic exercised hearts. *Am J Physiol Heart Circ Physiol* 299: H175–183, 2010.

129. Radford NB, DeFina LF, Leonard D, Barlow CE, Willis BL, Gibbons LW, et al. Cardiorespiratory fitness, coronary artery calcium, and cardiovascular disease events in a cohort of generally healthy middle-age men: results from the cooper center longitudinal study. *Circulation* 137: 1888–1895, 2018.

130. Roberts WC. An agent with lipid-lowering, antihypertensive, positive inotropic, negative chronotropic, vasodilating, diuretic, anorexigenic, weight-reducing, cathartic, hypoglycemic, tranquilizing, hypnotic and antidepressive qualities. *Am J Cardiol* 53: 261–262, 1984.

131. Rosenberg D, Cook A, Gell N, Lozano P, Grothaus L, Arterburn D. Relationships between sitting time and health indicators, costs, and utilization in older adults. *Prev Med Rep* 2: 247–249, 2015.

132. Ross R, Blair SN, Arena R, Church TS, Després JP, Franklin BA, et al.; American Heart Association Physical Activity Committee of the Council on Lifestyle and Cardiometabolic Health; Council on Clinical Cardiology; Council on Epidemiology and Prevention; Council on Cardiovascular and Stroke Nursing; Council on Functional Genomics and Translational Biology; Stroke Council. Importance of assessing cardiorespiratory fitness in clinical practice: a case for fitness as a clinical vital sign: a scientific statement from the American heart association. *Circulation* 134: e653–e699, 2016.

133. Sattar N, Preiss D, Murray HM, Welsh P, Buckley BM, de Craen AJ, et al. Statins and risk of incident diabetes: a collaborative meta-analysis of randomized statin trials. *Lancet* 375: 735–742, 2010.

134. Schulman D, Latchman DS, Yellon DM. Effect of aging on the ability of preconditioning to protect rat hearts from ischemia-reperfusion injury. *Am J Physiol Heart Circ Physiol* 281: H1630–1636, 2001.

135. Schwartz RS, Kraus SM, Schwartz JG, Wickstrom KK, Peichel G, Garberich RF, et al. Increased coronary artery plaque volume among male marathon runners. *Mo Med* 111: 89–94, 2014.

136. Shephard RJ, Balady GJ. Exercise as cardiovascular therapy. *Circulation* 99: 963–972, 1999.

137. Shinmura K, Nagai M, Tamaki K, Tani M, Bolli R. COX-2-derived prostacyclin mediates opioid-induced late phase of preconditioning in isolated rat hearts. *Am J Physiol Heart Circ Physiol* 283: H2534–2543, 2002.

138. Shinmura K, Tang XL, Wang Y, Xuan YT, Liu SQ, Takano H, et al. Cyclooxygenase-2 mediates the cardioprotective effects of the late phase of ischemic preconditioning in conscious rabbits. *Proc Natl Acad Sci U S A* 97: 10197–10202, 2000.

139. Shinmura K, Xuan YT, Tang XL, Kodani E, Han H, Zhu Y, et al. Inducible nitric oxide synthase modulates cyclooxygenase-2 activity in the heart of conscious rabbits during the late phase of ischemic preconditioning. *Circ Res* 90:602–608, 2002.

140. Smith JL, Verrill TA, Boura JA, Sakwa MP, Shannon FL, et al. Effect of cardiorespiratory fitness on short-term morbidity and mortality after coronary artery bypass grafting. *Am J Cardiol* 112: 1104–1109, 2013.

141. Starnes JW, Barnes BD, Olsen ME. Exercise training decreases rat heart mitochondria free radical generation but does not prevent Ca^{2+}-induced dysfunction. *J Appl Physiol (1985)* 102: 1793–1798, 2007.

142. Starnes JW, Bowles DK. Role of exercise in the cause and prevention of cardiac dysfunction. *Exerc Sport Sci Rev* 23: 349–373, 1995.

143. Starnes JW, Taylor RP. Exercise-induced cardioprotection: endogenous mechanisms. *Med Sci Sports Exerc* 39: 1537–1543, 2007.

144. Starnes JW, Taylor RP, Park Y. Exercise improves postischemic function in aging hearts. *Am J Physiol Heart Circ Physiol* 285: H347–451, 2003.

145. Swain DP. Moderate or vigorous intensity exercise: which is better for improving aerobic fitness? *Prev Cardiol* 8: 55–58, 2005.

146. Swain DP, Franklin BA. Comparison of cardioprotective benefits of vigorous versus moderate intensity aerobic exercise. *Am J Cardiol* 97: 141–147, 2006.

147. Swain DP, Franklin BA. VO_2 reserve and the minimal intensity for improving cardiorespiratory fitness. *Med Sci Sports Exerc* 34: 152–157, 2002.

148. Taylor RP, Harris MB, Starnes JW. Acute exercise can improve cardioprotection without increasing heat shock protein content. *Am J Physiol* 276: H1098–1102, 1999.

149. Thijssen DHJ, Redington A, George KP, Hopman MTE, Jones H. Association of exercise preconditioning with immediate cardioprotection: a review. *JAMA Cardiol* 3: 169–176, 2018.

150. Thompson PD, Buchner D, Pina IL, Balady GJ, Williams MA, Marcus BH, et al.; American Heart Association Council on Clinical Cardiology Subcommittee on Exercise, Rehabilitation, and Prevention; American Heart Association Council on Nutrition, Physical Activity and Metabolism Subcommittee on Physical Activity. Exercise and physical activity in the prevention and treatment of atherosclerotic cardiovascular disease: a statement from the council on clinical cardiology (subcommittee on exercise, rehabilitation, and prevention) and the council on nutrition, physical activity, and metabolism (subcommittee on physical activity. *Circulation* 107: 3109–3116, 2003.

151. Trivax JE, Franklin BA, Goldstein JA, Chinnaiyan KM, Gallagher MJ, deJong AT, et al. Acute cardiac effects of marathon running. *J Appl Physiol (1985)* 108: 1148–1153, 2010.

152. Ullal AJ, Abdelfattah RS, Ashley EA, Froelicher VF. Hypertrophic cardiomyopathy as a cause of sudden cardiac death in the young: a meta-analysis. *Am J Med* 129: 486–496.e2, 2016.

153. van de Schoor FR, Aengevaeren VL, Hopman MT, Oxborough DL, George KP, Thompson PD. Myocardial fibrosis in athletes. *Mayo Clin Proc* 91; 1617–1631, 2016.

154. Vanhees L, Fagard R, Thijs L, Staessen J, Amery A. Prognostic significance of peak exercise capacity in patients with coronary artery disease. *J Am Coll Cardiol* 23: 358–363, 1994.

155. Waller BF, Roberts WC. Sudden death while running in conditioned runners aged 40 years or over. *Am J Cardiol* 45: 1292–1300, 1980.

156. Wei M, Gibbons LW, Mitchell TL, Kampert JB, Lee CD, Blair SN. The association between cardiorespiratory fitness and impaired fasting glucose and type 2 diabetes mellitus in men. *Ann Intern Med* 130: 89–96, 1999.

157. Wen CP, Wai JP, Tsai MK, Yang YC, Cheng TY, Lee MC, et al. Minimum amount of physical activity for reduced mortality and extended life expectancy: a prospective cohort study. *Lancet* 378: 1244–1253, 2011.

158. Werner C, Füster T, Widmann T, Pöss J, Roggia C, Hanhoun M, et al. Physical exercise prevents cellular senescence in circulating leukocytes and in the vessel wall. *Circulation* 120: 2438–2447, 2009.

159. Wickramasinghe CD, Ayers CR, Das S, de Lemos JA, Willis BL, Berry JD. Prediction of 30-year risk for cardiovascular mortality by fitness and risk factor levels: the cooper center longitudinal study. *Cir Cardiovasc Qual Outcomes* 7: 497–602, 2014.

160. Wilkins S. 32ndFree Press/Flagstar marathon, triumph and tragedy – record field but 3 deaths in annual race. *The Detroit Free Press*, 19 October 2009, pp. A1.

161. Williams PT. Physical fitness and activity as separate heart disease risk factors: a meta-analysis. *Med Sci Sports Exerc* 33: 754–761, 2001.

162. Williams PT, Franklin BA. Incident diabetes mellitus, hypertension, and cardiovascular disease risk in exercising hypercholesterolemic patients. *Am J Cardiol* 116: 1516–1520, 2015.

163. Wilson EM, Diwan A, Spinale FG, Mann DL. Duality of innate stress responses in cardiac injury, repair, and remodeling. *J Mol Cell Cardiol* 37: 801–811, 2004.

164. Wilson M, O'Hanlon R, Prasad S, Deighan A, Macmillan P, Oxborough D, et al. Dverse patterns of myocardial fibrosis in lifelong, veteran endurance athletes. *J Appl Physiol (1985)* 110: 1622–1626, 2011.

165. Wislöff U, Stöylen A, Loennechen JP, Bruvold M, Rognmo Ø, Haram PM, et al. Superior cardiovascular effect of aerobic interval training versus moderate continuous training in heart failure patients: a randomized study. *Circulation* 115: 3086–3094, 2007.

166. Yamashita N, Hoshida S, Otsu K, Asahi M, Kuzuya T, Hori M. Exercise provides direct biphasic cardioprotection via manganese superoxide dismutase activation. *J Exp Med* 189: 1699–1706, 1999.

167. Zbinden R, Zbinden S, Meier P, Hutter D, Billinger M, Wahl A, et al. Coronary collateral flow in response to endurance exercise training. *Eur J Cardiovasc Prev Rehabil* 14: 250–257, 2007.

30

BIOCHEMISTRY OF EXERCISE TRAINING AND TYPE 1 DIABETES

Sam N. Scott, Matt Cocks, Anton J. M. Wagenmakers,
Sam O. Shepherd, and Michael C. Riddell

Introduction

Type 1 diabetes (T1D), previously known as insulin-dependent diabetes mellitus or juvenile diabetes, is an autoimmune disease whereby the insulin-producing β-cells of the pancreas are destroyed (6, 50). This leads to little or no insulin production, making it a challenge to maintain euglycaemia (blood glucose concentration 4–8 mmol/L) through exogenous insulin administration (by either insulin pump or injection), regular blood glucose monitoring, and dietary control. As such, T1D increases the risk of acute and long-term complications because of the difficulties of regulating blood glucose concentrations. Acute complications include diabetic ketoacidosis (i.e., hyperglycaemia, hyperketonaemia, and metabolic acidosis) and hypoglycaemia, which can be potentially life threatening. Long-term complications caused through lifelong exposure to dysglycaemia (113) include neuropathy (nerve damage), nephropathy (kidney damage), retinopathy (damage to the eyes), heart disease, stroke, and foot ulcers, the latter of which may lead to foot amputation if prolonged infection and tissue necrosis exist.

The cause of T1D remains unknown, but there is a strong genetic component, thought to be controlled by a number of susceptibility genes (i.e., certain variants of the human leukocyte antigen [HLA] complex), that require exposure to one or more environmental triggers such as a virus, environmental toxins, or certain foods (7). T1D can be diagnosed at any age, although the incidence is highest during childhood and adolescence (144). When T1D develops in adulthood, individuals are frequently misdiagnosed initially as having type 2 diabetes (143). The incidence of T1D is increasing annually by 3–5%, presumably due to unidentified environmental factors such as the obesity epidemic or increases in human hygiene (32, 115), although mechanisms for this are speculative at present. There is also a trend towards earlier onset of the disease (136) and a greater preponderance in males than in females (143). The incidence of T1D is highly variable between geographical locations and ethnic populations (51, 109), with the lowest recorded incidence of 0.1/100,000 people diagnosed per year in the Zunyi region in China and the highest rates of >40/100,000 people per year in Finland (1, 97, 132). Although there are no available statistics for all worldwide cases of T1D, the International Diabetes Federation estimates that there are currently over 1 million youth worldwide living with T1D (89).

People with T1D are recommended to engage in regular exercise for the maintenance of overall health and to reduce the risk of macrovascular and microvascular complications (40, 129, 188). The current guidelines are to accumulate 150 minutes of moderate- to vigorous-intensity aerobic exercise per week, spread over at least 3 days, with no more than 2 consecutive days without activity (40). However, many people with T1D lead a sedentary lifestyle and fail to meet these guidelines (119, 170, 183), in part because of the considerable challenge of managing blood glucose concentration around exercise and fear of hypoglycaemia. An understanding of glucose targets for safe and effective exercise and the neurohormonal responses to different forms of exercise is important.

This chapter will outline the importance of maximizing time in the target blood glucose range to reduce the risk of acute and long-term complications. The chapter will then describe the hormonal and glycaemic responses to a single bout of exercise. The final section will provide an overview of what is known about the adaptations to exercise training in people with T1D.

The Importance of Glucose Homeostasis

In healthy individuals without T1D, tight neuroendocrine control mechanisms exist so that glucose uptake into peripheral tissues is precisely matched by the rate of endogenous (hepatic) glucose production to maintain plasma glucose concentration between 4 and 8 mmol/L (64). Glucose is the primary fuel source of the brain, so hypoglycaemia is deleterious to brain function (146). Conversely, prolonged and/or recurrent exposure to raised blood glucose levels leads to tissue damage throughout the body (25). Importantly for people with T1D, in addition to overexposure to hyperglycaemia in general, glucose variability and rate of change in blood glucose concentrations have independent and clinically important roles in the risk of developing complications (113). Oxidative stress is postulated to be the key mechanism by which hyperglycaemia causes vascular damage due to formation of advanced glycated end products (AGEs), which leads to the production of cytokines, which cause inflammation and tissue damage (25, 73). The pathological consequences of hyperglycaemia are classified as either macrovascular (coronary artery disease, peripheral artery disease, stroke) or microvascular complications (diabetic nephropathy, neuropathy, retinopathy). Increasing time in the target glycaemic range (4–10 mmol/L) is associated with reduced risk of these comorbidities in people with T1D (71).

Mild hypoglycaemia is defined as a blood glucose concentration of 3.0–3.9 mmol/L; serious or clinically important hypoglycaemia can be defined as a blood glucose concentration ≤2.9 mmol/L; while severe hypoglycaemia is defined as the patient requiring assistance from another for recovery (90). Interestingly, symptoms of hypoglycaemia (i.e., shakiness, hunger, confusion) can occur at blood glucose levels above 3.9 mmol/L, particularly in individuals recently diagnosed with T1D and who have been in a state of chronic hyperglycaemia (156). However, it is also important to note that in individuals with hypoglycaemia unawareness, symptoms are not triggered until blood glucose levels are very low, often after cognitive function is impaired (78). The symptoms of hypoglycaemia can range in seriousness from mild tremor, loss of coordination, and mental confusion to convulsions, unconsciousness, brain damage, and even death (15, 46). Reports estimate that people with T1D are exposed to, on average, 3.5–7.2 episodes of symptomatic hypoglycaemia per month (24, 70, 135), although studies using continuous glucose monitors show higher unnoticed (often nocturnal) incidents (93, 105). On average, around 12% of adults living with T1D experience at least one severe temporarily disabling episode of hypoglycaemia per year (79, 116, 190, 198).

Living with T1D can be described as being like walking a constant tightrope between hyperglycaemia and hypoglycaemia whereby the patient must balance numerous factors that influence their blood glucose concentration to reduce the risk of acute and long-term complications (Figure 30.1). Exercise can be particularly challenging for this population because of the increased risk of hypoglycaemia both during the exercise and up to 48 hours post exercise (21, 100, 111, 139). Within any given exercise bout, numerous factors can have an impact on glycaemia, including exercise type, duration, and intensity; level of circulating exogenous insulin during and after exercise; and pre-exercise blood glucose concentration (Figure 30.2)The following section will provide an overview of the neurohormonal responses to exercise in individuals with and without T1D.

Endocrine Responses During Exercise

When a healthy individual who does not have T1D performs a bout of exercise, several counterregulatory mechanisms are activated in a stepwise and hierarchical fashion so that glucose utilization by the muscles is matched by glucose provision by the liver and/or gut. These mechanisms

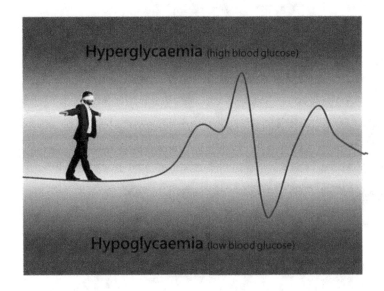

- Ambient temperature

- composition of last meal

- amount of circulating insulin

- location of insulin delivery

- Type, duration, intensity of exercise

- pre-exercise blood glucose concentration

- competition stress, time of day

- time of day

Figure 30.1 Living with type 1 diabetes (T1D) is like walking a constant tightrope between hyperglycaemia and hypoglycaemia

ensure that glucose uptake and production are precisely matched to prevent hypoglycaemia (43). Exercise is generally classified as "aerobic" or "anaerobic," depending on the predominant energy systems used, although many forms of exercise use a combination of the two systems. Aerobic exercise, defined here as prolonged (>30 minutes) activity performed at 50–80% of maximal aerobic capacity ($\dot{V}O_{2max}$), typically uses large muscle groups in a continuous manner (e.g., running, cycling, or swimming). High-intensity or anaerobic exercise (>80% $\dot{V}O_{2max}$) cannot be maintained for long, especially if the individual is untrained. However, activities performed at efforts >80% $\dot{V}O_{2max}$ may still be aerobic in nature but with additional energy supplied from anaerobic glycolysis. Few activities have little or no aerobic component, except for burst activities like maximal-intensity sprinting (69). In the following sections the focus will be on prolonged moderate- and high-intensity exercise with a highly aerobic component.

It is important to understand the normal counter-regulatory responses to exercise before one can compare this to the response in someone with T1D. Because an individual with T1D relies on exogenous insulin, these counterregulatory mechanisms are impaired and they are at greater risk of hyper- or hypoglycaemia. Figures 30.3 and 30.4 describe the hormonal responses to moderate- and high-intensity exercise in an individual without T1D and in someone with T1D. Following an exercise bout, the increased risk of hypoglycaemia is primarily due to increased insulin sensitivity, which can vary according to the duration and intensity of exercise that was performed. The increased insulin sensitivity and continued extraction of glucose from the circulation may be due to increased glycogen synthase activity to replenish glycogen stores (20, 30, 164). Enhanced glucose transporter 4 (GLUT4) translocation and muscle microvascular perfusion are also important (164, 185, 186). Special care may be required to prevent post-exercise hypoglycaemia following afternoon or evening exercise because there is a greater risk of nocturnal hypoglycaemia (74, 91, 121, 172).

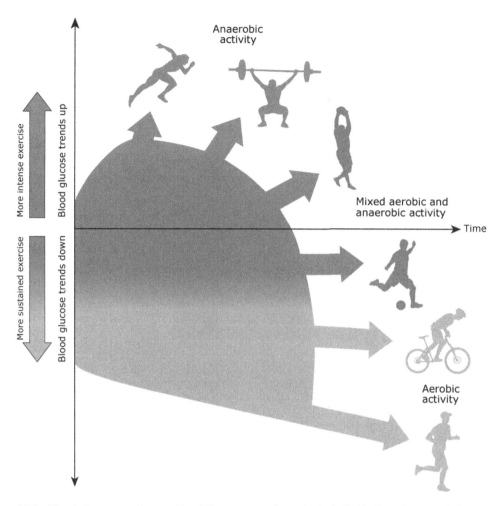

Figure 30.2 Blood glucose trends caused by different types of exercise in individuals with type 1 diabetes (T1D)

Additional Factors to Consider

In addition to the effect of type, duration, and intensity of exercise, there are many other interindividual and intraindividual factors for people with T1D to consider (Figure 30.1). The location of insulin delivery, amount of insulin in the circulation, blood glucose concentration before exercise, and composition of the last meal can all influence glycaemic response (2, 39, 77). The site and depth of insulin injection also affect the absorption characteristics (62, 87). Injecting insulin into a location used during exercise can increase the rate of absorption and cause more rapid decreases in blood glucose concentration (e.g., injecting the thigh before cycling). Higher ambient temperature increases skin temperature, which enhances subcutaneous blood flow and accelerates insulin absorption, increasing the risk of hypoglycaemia compared to cooler temperatures (2, 77, 85).

Antecedent hypoglycaemia and exercise, along with competition stress, also affect glycaemia due to differences in hormonal responses (10, 23, 67). Antecedent hypoglycaemia shifts the glycaemic threshold for counter-regulatory response to lower glucose values, leading to a vicious cycle of recurrent hypoglycaemia and further impairments of glucose counter-regulation (22, 45, 49). This is a condition referred to as hypoglycaemia-associated autonomic failure (HAAF) (44, 47), whereby there is an attenuated

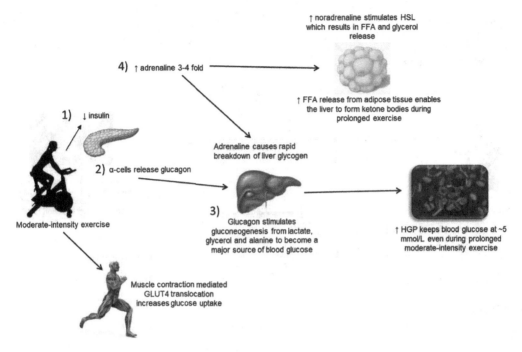

Figure 30.3a

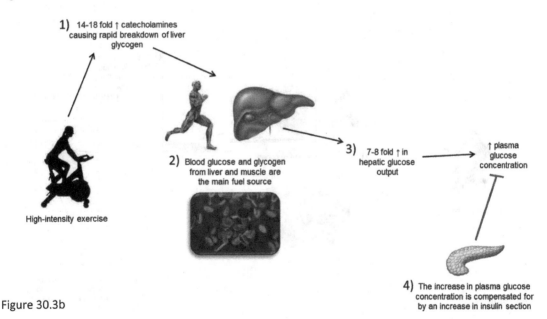

Figure 30.3b

Figure 30.3 (a) Glucoregulatory responses to moderate-intensity exercise (50–80% of $\dot{V}O_{2max}$) in a healthy individual without type 1 diabetes (T1D). (b) Glucoregulatory responses to high-intensity exercise (>80% of $\dot{V}O_{2max}$) in healthy individuals without diabetes

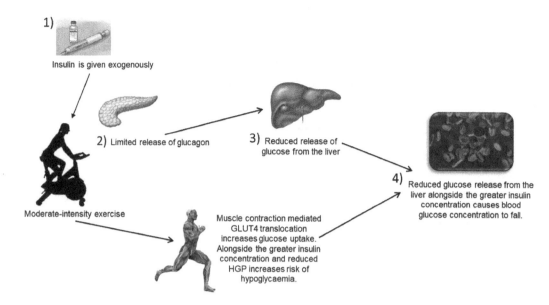

Figure 30.4a

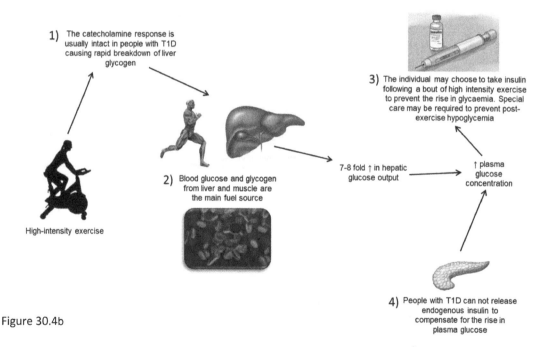

Figure 30.4b

Figure 30.4 (a) Glucoregulatory responses to moderate–intensity exercise (50–80% of $\dot{V}O_{2max}$) in individuals with T1D. (b) Glucoregulatory responses to high-intensity exercise in an individual with type 1 diabetes (T1D)

epinephrine response to hypoglycaemia as well as hypoglycaemia unawareness, leading to loss of warning and compromises in behavioural responses (e.g., carbohydrate ingestion) (45). Antecedent exercise (i.e., performing a prior bout of exercise the day before or a few hours before a subsequent bout of exercise) reduces counter-regulatory responses to subsequent hypoglycaemia in a similar manner to antecedent hypoglycaemia (65).

The time of day that exercise is performed can also alter the glycaemic responses to exercise, particularly if the individual is fasting (60). As briefly mentioned, during studies of afternoon resistance exercise in people with T1D, declines in blood glucose were observed (192, 193), whereas an almost identical resistance exercise protocol performed in the morning under fasting conditions resulted in either no change (175) or a mean increase (174) in blood glucose during the exercise session. Similar outcomes were found using a repeated measures design of fasting morning and afternoon resistance exercise, where the morning fasting exercise led to an increasing trend in blood glucose, while blood glucose levels declined with afternoon exercise following a standardized snack (60). There have also been similar findings with fasting aerobic exercise. For example, Ruegemer et al. (149) observed a decline in blood glucose level with 30 minutes of aerobic exercise in the afternoon, with the same participants having an increase in blood glucose level when the same exercise was performed fasted in the morning. Scott et al. (154) also observed that participants with T1D performing both moderate aerobic and high-intensity interval training (HIIT) in the fasted state did not have a decline in blood glucose during either exercise protocol. These findings contrast with the declines in blood glucose found during later day (fed state) aerobic exercise (28, 80, 121, 127, 191, 197) and interval-style exercise (81, 121, 127).

There are several possible explanations for this phenomenon observed with fasted exercise performed in the morning. The first is that lower circulating insulin levels during fasted exercise increase hepatic glycogenolysis and consequently help to maintain blood glucose concentration during exercise. In addition, when exercise is performed in the morning, individuals with T1D may experience the "dawn phenomenon" (153), an early morning rise in blood glucose possibly due to an increase in circulating growth hormone and/or cortisol (29, 48, 58). Previous T1D exercise studies suggest that higher growth hormone levels could limit the drop in blood glucose level during exercise (193, 194) by stimulating more lipolysis (76). While these theories remain unconfirmed, it can still be suggested that those struggling with hypoglycaemia during exercise and/or those trying to avoid additional carbohydrates to aid weight management may have greater success with early morning/fasted exercise than they would with exercise later in the day.

Using exercise diaries or smartphone-based applications to carefully monitor the effects of carbohydrate intake, insulin dosage, and type of exercise on glycaemia can help the individual with T1D to improve glycaemic control with practice. This information may be particularly useful for people with T1D who train or compete regularly, so they can devise a routine that works for them. More research using larger sample sizes is needed to investigate the reproducibility of blood glucose responses to different types of exercise under varying conditions. This will help health care professionals provide more accurate evidence-based advice to their patients with T1D and will also help researchers with the development of algorithms for use with the artificial pancreas.

The Importance of Regular Exercise in People with Type 1 Diabetes

People with T1D are recommended to engage in regular exercise for the maintenance of overall health and prevention of macrovascular and microvascular complications, which are a major cause of mortality and morbidity (36, 129, 188). Although there is no general consensus as to whether exercise improves glycaemic control, studies have demonstrated other health benefits of exercise for those with T1D, including improved cardiovascular disease risk profile (124), body composition, cardiorespiratory fitness (155), endothelial function (63), blood lipid profile (36, 37, 119), and reduced insulin dose requirements (63, 195). The following section provides an overview of the adaptations to regular exercise in people with T1D and is summarized in Figure 30.5. T1D is associated with increased risk of complications and impaired metabolic health in almost all organ systems; therefore, it is important to understand that the benefits will be on a whole-body level e.g., adaptations to the microvasculature will positively affect the kidneys and eyes and improve skeletal muscle health.

Macrovascular complications, such as cardiovascular disease and stroke, are the most common cause of mortality in people with T1D (107, 165). Microvascular dysfunction causes complications that include damage to eyes (diabetic retinopathy); kidney damage (diabetic nephropathy); and nerve damage (diabetic neuropathy), which leads to loss of sensation in the feet, increasing the risk of foot ulcers and lower limb amputations. The elevated risk of cardiovascular disease in people with T1D is likely linked to alterations in several predisposing factors, including the tendency for suboptimal glycaemic control, hypertension, elevated triacylglyceride, and low-density lipoprotein cholesterol levels, along with lower high-density lipoprotein cholesterol levels (165, 166). Regular exercise has beneficial effects on lipid levels (63, 106, 196), which are similar to the benefits observed in those without T1D and appear to be

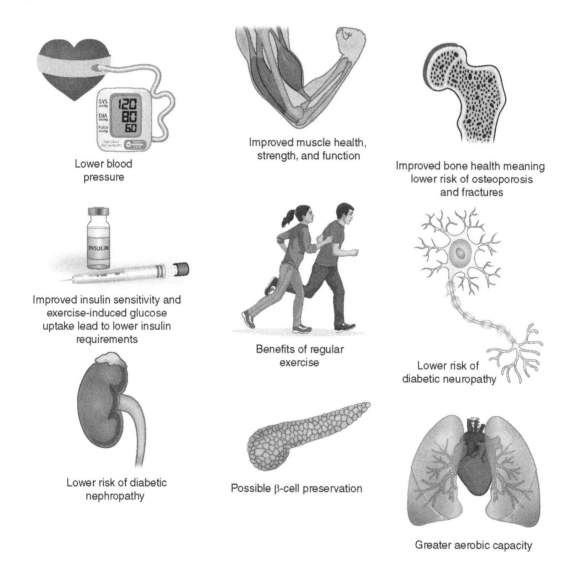

Figure 30.5 Summary of benefits of regular exercise in people with type 1 diabetes

independent of changes in glycaemic control (36). The Pittsburgh Insulin-Dependent Diabetes Mellitus Morbidity and Mortality study demonstrated that men with T1D that had participated in team sports while at school were three times less likely to report macrovascular disease than those who did not participate in sport (108). Further follow-up in this investigation showed that level of physical activity participation in adulthood predicted mortality 6 years later, as sedentary men were three times more likely to die than active men (129). Exercise training has been shown to improve endothelial function in people with T1D (19, 63, 157, 171), which is important, as endothelial dysfunction is related to the development of atherosclerosis (33).

Diabetic nephropathy (kidney disease) results from a greater incidence of hypertension in people with T1D than the general population and can lead to end-stage renal disease (151). In addition to hypertension and elevated glucose exposure, kidney disease progression is linked to increased inflammatory markers in T1D (8). One large cohort study by Wadén et al. (184) showed that greater leisure-time physical activity, particularly of a higher intensity, was associated with a lower risk of developing diabetic kidney disease. Similarly, cross-sectional data from Bjornstad et al. (17) has shown a strong association between exercise capacity and renal health in adolescents with T1D. Possible protective mechanisms include lowering of blood pressure, along with improved blood lipid profile, glycaemic control, and endothelial function. Improved insulin sensitivity may also be important due to the association between insulin resistance and microalbuminuria (59, 133).

Autonomic neuropathy (damage to nerves) is a complication of T1D that affects multiple organ systems and has widespread clinical manifestations. There are two major classes of diabetic neuropathies: sensorimotor and autonomic. Cardiovascular autonomic neuropathy is characterized by damage of the autonomic nerve fibres innervating the heart and blood vessels leading to abnormalities in heart rate control and vascular dynamics leading to exercise intolerance, orthostatic hypotension, decreased peripheral blood flow to skeletal muscle, and reduced heart rate response and cardiac output (86). Impaired cardiovascular autonomic neuropathy is associated with increased risk of mortality in people with T1D (5, 122, 199). The second form of neuropathy is diabetic polyneuropathy (peripheral neuropathy), which is typically characterized by significant deficits in tactile sensitivity, vibration sense, lower limb proprioception, and kinaesthesia due to damage to the peripheral nerves. Reduced or absent sensation in the feet can increase the risk of injury and wounds that may develop into serious infections requiring amputation. The Diabetes Control and Complications Trial (DCCT) demonstrated that intensive glycaemic control implemented early after diagnosis delayed polyneuropathy. Although exercise has been shown to be beneficial for diabetes control, its effects on diabetic peripheral neuropathy are not clear. Because poor glycaemic control leading to nerve damage is one of the main causes of diabetic neuropathy, it is possible that exercise would offer protection. Exercise may target diabetic peripheral neuropathy by altering the microvascular components of diabetes. From this we may infer that exercise has the potential to improve the impaired blood supply to the peripheral nerves; however, further research is needed in this area.

Similarly to the general population, insulin resistance is common in people with T1D and the incidence is rising, reflecting the rising rates of inactivity and obesity (52, 101, 125). This fact is important given that insulin resistance is an additional independent risk factor for microvascular and macrovascular complications in those with T1D (34, 72, 101, 133, 134, 169). Little information exists on the mechanisms of insulin resistance in people with T1D; therefore, much must be inferred from what is known in people without T1D. Lipid-induced insulin resistance in skeletal muscle due to intramuscular triglyceride (IMTG) accumulation has been hypothesized to be one mechanism responsible for the development of insulin resistance in T2D. A full description of lipid-induced insulin resistance is beyond the scope of this chapter; therefore, readers are referred to reviews by Tumova et al. (173) and Shaw et al. (159). Overall, the current evidence suggests that obesity and inactivity lead to accumulation of lipids within the skeletal muscle and reduced access of the lipid droplets to the mitochondria for oxidation, which suggests impaired metabolic flexibility. It is important to note that endurance-trained athletes have equal or even higher IMTG content than obese individuals or people with T2D, despite being insulin sensitive (75). This phenomenon has been termed the "athletes' paradox" (75). The elevated IMTG storage in endurance-trained individuals appears to represent an important metabolic adaptation to endurance training (3, 177), as the IMTG pool makes a significant contribution to total substrate oxidation during a bout of endurance exercise (178). With exercise training there will be increased IMTG turnover (greater lipolysis compared with lipid synthesis) resulting in reduced accumulation of lipid metabolites such as ceramides, LCFA-CoA, and DAG that can impair insulin signalling at IRS-1 and Akt/PKB (3, 159, 161), eventually leading to improved insulin sensitivity (160). Furthermore, mitochondrial dysfunction, which has been reported in people with T1D (126), is proposed to decrease the rate of β-oxidation, which leads to accumulation of lipid metabolites that disrupt insulin signalling (114).

People with T1D have higher IMTG content than weight- and activity-matched people without diabetes, and this is associated with impaired insulin sensitivity (54, 137). Studies using nuclear magnetic resonance spectrometry (137), computed tomography (54), and biochemical assays of the lipid concentration from muscle biopsies (56) have shown that skeletal muscle from people with T1D typically contains more IMTG compared to non-diabetic muscle. It is assumed that as IMTG deposition increases in people with T1D, the ensuing lipotoxicity enhances stress on the tissue (176). A chronic hyperglycaemic state may be a relevant mechanism for exaggerated IMTG accumulation in those with T1D, as Perseghin et al. (137) found that patients with better (HbA1c <7.5%) metabolic control possessed a higher insulin-stimulated glucose metabolic clearance rate in association with lower IMTG compared to those with poorer (>7.6%) metabolic control. These outcomes suggest that when good glucose control is achieved, these abnormalities may be partially reversed, and this is supported by Kacerovsky et al. (96), who found IMTG content did not differ between people with well-controlled T1D and a control group without T1D. Studies in people without T1D demonstrate that exercise training causes remodelling of IMTG-containing lipid droplets, which is associated with improved insulin sensitivity (160).

Physically inactive people with T1D may have lower skeletal muscle health (quantity and quality of skeletal muscle) compared to those without diabetes who are also inactive, due to increased metabolic stress, vascular impairments, and insulin resistance (41). These impairments, along with altered mitochondrial morphology and function in young people with T1D, may lead to a vicious cycle of insulin resistance, impaired glucose and lipid disposal, and reduced basal metabolic rate. All of these factors may affect blood glucose management (104, 126), as the muscle cannot respond optimally to stressors or combat elevated glycaemic and lipid loads frequently experienced in T1D. In addition, impaired insulin-stimulated vasodilation can reduce blood flow and therefore glucose delivery for extraction in skeletal muscle (13, 118). As exercise improves skeletal muscle health, it may contribute to delaying complications in those with T1D.

Increased whole-body inflammation and oxidative stress are also common in T1D (26). Excessive plasma glucose promotes reactive oxygen species production and the expression of inflammatory cytokines (41, 150). Oxidative stress likely contributes to diabetic myopathy through up-regulation of atrophy-related genes (4) and is a key driver of impaired vascular function (98), leading to microvascular and macrovascular complications (33). High oxidative stress can also affect the transcription of glucose transporters, contributing to the development of insulin resistance (18). Interleukin-6 (IL-6), an inflammatory cytokine, has been linked with numerous atrophic states and is elevated in children with T1D (68, 147, 148). Single bouts of exercise elicit anti-inflammatory effects, and exercise training may decrease basal IL-6 levels (61). The anti-inflammatory effects of exercise may also benefit β-cell mass due to increases in circulating growth hormone, insulin-like growth factor 1, glucagon-like peptide-1, and IL-1 receptor agonist. Emerging evidence suggests that regular physical activity/exercise training may preserve β-cell function in people recently diagnosed with T1D (35, 130). Preservation of pancreatic β-cells has important clinical benefits due to overall better glycaemic control alongside decreased insulin requirements, which would reduce the risk of hypoglycaemia and risk of diabetic complications (167).

Loss of bone mineral density, osteoporosis, and increased risk of fracture are common in inactive people with T1D, particularly in the presence of sub-optimal glucose control and neuropathy (92, 99, 158), and this increases the risk of osteoporosis and fractures (83). Exercise is beneficial for osteoporosis risk and bone health in people without T1D (12), suggesting the same would be true for people with T1D. Resistance exercise is known to have a positive impact on all of these factors, and therefore may play an especially important role in people with T1D (40). However, the impact of resistance training on long-term blood glucose control is still under some debate (55, 128, 140).

Does Type 1 Diabetes Affect Physical Performance?

It is currently unclear how T1D can affect exercise and sport performance, although it is clear that exceptional athletes live and compete with a diagnosis of T1D (see https://integrateddiabetes.com/athletes-with-type-1-diabetes and www.teamnovonordisk.com/teams/pro-team for a partial list). Nevertheless, even those that achieve elite athlete status can struggle with glucose control around exercise, which may affect their performance (141). The athlete with T1D will recognize the importance of individualizing their insulin regimen and diet according to their sporting event, training schedule, and personal experiences.

There are reports that people with T1D in general have lower age- and activity- matched $\dot{V}O_{2max}$ scores than those without T1D (11, 82, 88, 102, 138). Several cardiovascular, muscular, and metabolic impairments have been suggested to explain the potential decrement in aerobic and anaerobic performance. End diastolic volume and left ventricular ejection fraction fail to increase normally during exercise in young people with T1D (110), and there are differences in glycolytic metabolism that reflect an earlier onset of glycolysis in individuals with T1D (42), which could be a consequence of alterations in the bioenergetics and ultrastructure of skeletal muscle mitochondria that has been observed in skeletal muscle of people with T1D (126). However, Nugent et al. (131) found no differences in $\dot{V}O_{2peak}$ in adults with long-standing T1D compared to healthy controls, and observations in professional cyclists with T1D suggest no impairment in maximal exercise performance (57). Similarly, Veves et al. (180) observed that only inactive adults with neuropathic complications or a sedentary lifestyle demonstrated decreased $\dot{V}O_{2max}$, suggesting T1D per se does not directly affect exercise capacity in trained individuals. If impairments in physical capacity do exist in those with T1D, it is likely related to the patient's level of glycaemic control over the last several days, months, and years, which can have subtle effects on muscle (104, 126) and/or performance (66). Huttunen et al. (88) and Poortmans et al. (138) both reported that physical capacity was inversely related to the level of metabolic control as indicated by HbA1c.

Blood glucose concentration during a given bout of exercise may affect metabolism; however, the degree to which acute changes in blood glucose levels influence sports performance is unclear. Stettler and colleagues (168) compared the effects of euglycaemia (5.3 ± 0.6 mmol/L) and hyperglycaemia (12.4 ± 2.1 mmol/L) on exercise capacity in people with T1D and found that plasma glucose availability did not have an impact on peak power output, heart rate, lactate levels, or respiratory exchange ratio. Jenni et al. (94) investigated fuel metabolism during 120 min of aerobic exercise (55–60% $\dot{V}O_{2max}$) at euglycaemia (5.3 ± 0.6 mmol/L) or hyperglycaemia (11.0 ± 0.3 mmol/L) with identical insulin levels. Substrate oxidation during exercise in the participants with T1D was similar to that observed in healthy individuals without T1D (84) at euglycaemia whereby there was shift to lipid oxidation. In the hyperglycaemic condition (94) there was greater carbohydrate oxidation and no sparing of intramyocellular glycogen. The authors (94) were unable to pinpoint the mechanisms for these findings, as there were no differences in insulin, glucagon, or catecholamines between the euglycaemic and hyperglycaemic conditions in the participants with T1D. Exercising with higher blood glucose concentration increases reliance on muscle glycogen compared to euglycaemia (94), which may limit the capacity to switch from carbohydrate to lipid metabolism. Patients are also more prone to early dehydration and acidosis when exercising with high blood glucose (117). These factors may promote early fatigue, consequently decreasing endurance. Prolonged hypoinsulinaemia/hyperglycaemia would presumably lower muscle glycogen levels, reduce muscle strength, and lead to dehydration and electrolyte imbalance (95). As such, it is likely that euglycaemia promotes the best performance.

Conclusions

There is little doubt that regular exercise is beneficial for the maintenance of cardio-metabolic health in people with T1D and so should be encouraged. Research has demonstrated that exercise improves cardiorespiratory fitness and blood lipid profile, increases endothelial function, and reduces insulin requirements. However, managing glycaemia during and after exercise represents a considerable challenge for the individual with T1D and the health care provider. As discussed, in addition to the effect of type, duration, and intensity of the exercise performed, people with T1D must consider a host of other variables, including the location of insulin delivery, amount of insulin in the circulation, blood glucose concentration before exercise, and composition of the last meal. The individual with T1D needs an understanding of the glycaemic responses to exercise and strategies to increase the time spent in the euglycaemic range in order to exercise safely.

References

1. Variation and trends in incidence of childhood diabetes in Europe. EURODIAB ACE Study Group. *Lancet (London, England)* 355: 873–876, 2000.
2. Al-Qaissi A, Papageorgiou M, Javed Z, Heise T, Rigby AS, Garrett AT, et al. Environmental effects of ambient temperature and relative humidity on insulin pharmacodynamics in adults with type 1 diabetes mellitus. *Diabetes Obes Metab* 21: 569–574, 2019.
3. Amati F, Dubé JJ, Alvarez-Carnero E, Edreira MM, Chomentowski P, Coen PM, et al. Skeletal muscle triglycerides, diacylglycerols, and ceramides in insulin resistance: another paradox in endurance-trained athletes? *Diabetes* 60: 2588–2597, 2011.
4. Arthur PG, Grounds MD, Shavlakadze T. Oxidative stress as a therapeutic target during muscle wasting: considering the complex interactions. *Curr Opin Clin Nutr Metab Care* 11: 408–416, 2008.
5. Astrup AS, Tarnow L, Rossing P, Hansen BV, Hilsted J, Parving H-H. Cardiac autonomic neuropathy predicts cardiovascular morbidity and mortality in type 1 diabetic patients with diabetic nephropathy. *Diabetes Care* 29: 334–339, 2006.
6. Atkinson MA, Eisenbarth GS. Type 1 diabetes: new perspectives on disease pathogenesis and treatment. *Lancet* 358: 221–229, 2001.
7. Atkinson MA, Maclaren NK. The pathogenesis of insulin-dependent diabetes mellitus. *N Engl J Med* 331: 1428–1436, 1994.
8. Baker NL, Hunt KJ, Stevens DR, Jarai G, Rosen GD, Klein RL, et al. Association between inflammatory markers and progression to kidney dysfunction: examining different assessment windows in patients with type 1 diabetes. *Diabetes Care* 41: 128–135, 2018.
9. Bally L, Zueger T, Buehler T, Dokumaci AS, Speck C, Pasi N, et al. Metabolic and hormonal response to intermittent high-intensity and continuous moderate intensity exercise in individuals with type 1 diabetes: a randomised crossover study. *Diabetologia* 59: 776–784, 2016.
10. Bao S, Briscoe VJ, Tate DB, Davis SN. Effects of differing antecedent increases of plasma cortisol on counterregulatory responses during subsequent exercise in type 1 diabetes. *Diabetes* 58: 2100–2108, 2009.
11. Baraldi E, Monciotti C, Filippone M, Santuz P, Magagnin G, Zanconato S, et al. Gas exchange during exercise in diabetic children. *Pediatr Pulmonol* 13: 155–160, 1992.
12. Barlet JP, Coxam V, Davicco MJ. [Physical exercise and the skeleton]. *Arch Physiol Biochem* 103: 681–698, 1995.
13. Baron AD, Laakso M, Brechtel G, Edelman SV. Mechanism of insulin resistance in insulin-dependent diabetes mellitus: a major role for reduced skeletal muscle blood flow. *J Clin Endocrinol Metab* 73: 637–643, 1991.
14. Bartness TJ, Liu Y, Shrestha YB, Ryu V. Neural innervation of white adipose tissue and the control of lipolysis. *Front Neuroendocrinol* 35: 473–493, 2014.
15. Becker DJ, Ryan CM. Hypoglycemia: a complication of diabetes therapy in children. *Trends Endocrinol Metab* 11: 198–202, 2000.
16. Berger M, Berchtold P, Cüppers HJ, Drost H, Kley HK, Müller WA, et al. Metabolic and hormonal effects of muscular exercise in juvenile type diabetics. *Diabetologia* 13: 355–365, 1977.

17. Bjornstad P, Cree-Green M, Baumgartner A, Maahs DM, Cherney DZ, Pyle L, et al. Renal function is associated with peak exercise capacity in adolescents with type 1 diabetes. *Diabetes Care* 38: 126–131, 2015.

18. Bloch-Damti A, Bashan N. Proposed mechanisms for the induction of insulin resistance by oxidative stress. *Antioxid Redox Signal* 7: 1553–1567, 2005.

19. Boff W, da Silva AM, Farinha JB, Rodrigues-Krause J, Reischak-Oliveira A, Tschiedel B, et al. Superior effects of high-intensity interval vs. moderate-intensity continuous training on endothelial function and cardiorespiratory fitness in patients with type 1 diabetes: a randomized controlled trial. *Front Physiol* 10: 450, 2019.

20. Bogardus C, Thuillez P, Ravussin E, Vasquez B, Narimiga M, Azhar S. Effect of muscle glycogen depletion on in vivo insulin action in man. *J Clin Invest* 72: 1605–1610, 1983.

21. Brazeau A-S, Rabasa-Lhoret R, Strychar I, Mircescu H. Barriers to physical activity among patients with type 1 diabetes. *Diabetes Care* 31: 2108–2109, 2008.

22. Briscoe VJ, Tate DB, Davis SN. Type 1 diabetes: exercise and hypoglycemia. *Appl Physiol Nutr Metab* 32: 576–582, 2007.

23. Brockman NK, Yardley JE. Sex-related differences in fuel utilization and hormonal response to exercise: implications for individuals with type 1 diabetes. *Appl Physiol Nutr Metab* 43: 541–552, 2018.

24. Brod M, Wolden M, Groleau D, Bushnell DM. Understanding the economic, daily functioning, and diabetes management burden of non-severe nocturnal hypoglycemic events in Canada: differences between type 1 and type 2. *J Med Econ* 17: 11–20, 2014.

25. Brownlee M. The pathobiology of diabetic complications: a unifying mechanism. *Diabetes* 54: 1615–1625, 2005.

26. Cabrera SM, Henschel AM, Hessner MJ. Innate inflammation in type 1 diabetes. *Transl Res* 167: 214–227, 2016.

27. Camacho RC, Galassetti P, Davis SN, Wasserman DH. Glucoregulation during and after exercise in health and insulin-dependent diabetes. *Exer Sport Sci Rev* 33: 17–23, 2005.

28. Campbell MD, West DJ, Bain SC, Kingsley MIC, Foley P, Kilduff L, et al. Simulated games activity vs continuous running exercise: a novel comparison of the glycemic and metabolic responses in T1DM patients. *Scand J Med Sci Sports* 25: 216–222, 2015.

29. Campbell PJ, Bolli GB, Cryer PE, Gerich JE. Sequence of events during development of the dawn phenomenon in insulin-dependent diabetes mellitus. *Metab Clin Exp* 34: 1100–1104, 1985.

30. Cartee GD. Mechanisms for greater insulin-stimulated glucose uptake in normal and insulin-resistant skeletal muscle after acute exercise. *Am J Physiol Endocrinol Metab* 309: E949–959, 2015.

31. Chan O, and Sherwin R. Influence of VMH fuel sensing on hypoglycemic responses. *Trends Endocrinol Metab* 24: 616–624, 2013.

32. Chapman NM, Coppieters K, von Herrath M, Tracy S. The microbiology of human hygiene and its impact on type 1 diabetes. *Islets* 4: 253–261, 2012.

33. Charakida M, Masi S, Luscher TF, Kastelein JJ, Deanfield JE. Assessment of atherosclerosis: the role of flow-mediated dilatation. *Eur Heart J* 31: 2854–2861, 2010.

34. Chaturvedi N, Sjoelie AK, Porta M, Aldington SJ, Fuller JH, Songini M, et al. Markers of insulin resistance are strong risk factors for retinopathy incidence in type 1 diabetes. *Diabetes Care* 24: 284–289, 2001.

35. Chetan MR, Charlton MH, Thompson C, Dias RP, Andrews RC, Narendran P. The Type 1 diabetes 'honeymoon' period is five times longer in men who exercise: a case-control study. *Diabetes Med* 2018.

36. Chimen M, Kennedy A, Nirantharakumar K, Pang TT, Andrews R, Narendran P. What are the health benefits of physical activity in type 1 diabetes mellitus? A literature review. *Diabetologia* 55: 542–551, 2012.

37. Codella R, Terruzzi I, Luzi L. Why should people with type 1 diabetes exercise regularly? *Acta Diabetol* 54: 615–630, 2017.

38. Coker RH, Kjaer M. Glucoregulation during exercise: the role of the neuroendocrine system. *Sports Med (Auckland, NZ)* 35: 575–583, 2005.

39. Colberg-Ochs SR. From Froot Loops to fitness: my journey as an educator and person with diabetes. *Diabetes Spectrum* 30: 58–63, 2017.

40. Colberg SR, Sigal RJ, Yardley JE, Riddell MC, Dunstan DW, Dempsey PC, et al. Physical activity/exercise and diabetes: a position statement of the American Diabetes Association. *Diabetes Care* 39: 2065–2079, 2016.

41. Coleman SK, Rebalka IA, D'Souza DM, Hawke TJ. Skeletal muscle as a therapeutic target for delaying type 1 diabetic complications. *World J Diabetes* 6: 1323–1336, 2015.

42. Crowther GJ, Milstein JM, Jubrias SA, Kushmerick MJ, Gronka RK, Conley KE. Altered energetic properties in skeletal muscle of men with well-controlled insulin-dependent (type 1) diabetes. *Am J Physiol Endocrinol Metab* 284: E655–662, 2003.

43. Cryer PE. Hierarchy of physiological responses to hypoglycemia: relevance to clinical hypoglycemia in type I (insulin dependent) diabetes mellitus. *Horm Metab Res* 29: 92–96, 1997.

44. Cryer PE. Hypoglycemia-associated autonomic failure in diabetes. *Handbook of Clinical Neurology* 117: 295–307, 2013.

45. Cryer PE. Mechanisms of hypoglycemia-associated autonomic failure and its component syndromes in diabetes. *Diabetes* 54: 3592–3601, 2005.

46. Cryer PE, Davis SN, Shamoon H. Hypoglycemia in diabetes. *Diabetes Care* 26: 1902–1912, 2003.

47. Dagogo-Jack SE, Craft S, Cryer PE. Hypoglycemia-associated autonomic failure in insulin-dependent diabetes mellitus. Recent antecedent hypoglycemia reduces autonomic responses to, symptoms of, and defense against subsequent hypoglycemia. *J Clin Invest* 91: 819–828, 1993.

48. Davidson MB, Harris MD, Ziel FH, Rosenberg CS. Suppression of sleep-induced growth hormone secretion by anticholinergic agent abolishes dawn phenomenon. *Diabetes* 37: 166–171, 1988.

49. DeRosa MA, Cryer PE. Hypoglycemia and the sympathoadrenal system: neurogenic symptoms are largely the result of sympathetic neural, rather than adrenomedullary, activation. *Am J Physiol Endocrinol Metab* 287: E32–41, 2004.

50. Devendra D, Liu E, Eisenbarth GS. Type 1 diabetes: recent developments. *BMJ* 328: 750–754, 2004.

51. Diaz-Valencia PA, Bougneres P, Valleron AJ. Global epidemiology of type 1 diabetes in young adults and adults: a systematic review. *BMC Public Health* 15: 255, 2015.

52. Donga E, Dekkers OM, Corssmit EPM, Romijn JA. Insulin resistance in patients with type 1 diabetes assessed by glucose clamp studies: systematic review and meta-analysis. *Eur J Endocrinol* 173: 101–109, 2015.

53. Donovan CM, Watts AG. Peripheral and central glucose sensing in hypoglycemic detection. *Physiology (Bethesda, MD)* 29: 314–324, 2014.

54. Dubé MC, Joanisse DR, Prud'homme D, Lemieux S, Bouchard C, Pérusse L, et al. Muscle adiposity and body fat distribution in type 1 and type 2 diabetes: varying relationships according to diabetes type. *Int J Obes* 30: 1721–1728, 2006.

55. Durak EP, Jovanovic-Peterson L, Peterson CM. Randomized crossover study of effect of resistance training on glycemic control, muscular strength, and cholesterol in type I diabetic men. *Diabetes Care* 13: 1039–1043, 1990.

56. Ebeling P, Essén-Gustavsson B, Tuominen JA, Koivisto VA. Intramuscular triglyceride content is increased in IDDM. *Diabetologia* 41: 111–115, 1998.

57. Eckstein ML, Fisher M, Hayes CA, Southerland P, Stettler C, Lagrou PH, et al. Sweet performance: associations of maximum physiological performance and diabetes in a group of world class road cyclists with type 1 diabetes. *American Diabetes Association 79th Scientific Sessions* 2019.

58. Edge JA, Matthews DR, Dunger DB. The dawn phenomenon is related to overnight growth hormone release in adolescent diabetics. *Clin Endocrinol (Oxf)* 33: 729–737, 1990.

59. Ekstrand AV, Groop PH, Grönhagen-Riska C. Insulin resistance precedes microalbuminuria in patients with insulin-dependent diabetes mellitus. *Nephrol Dial Transplant* 13: 3079–3083, 1998.

60. Eshghi SRT, Yardley JE. Morning (fasting) vs. afternoon resistance exercise in individuals with type 1 diabetes: a randomized cross-over study. *J Clin Endocrinol Metab* 2019.

61. Fischer CP. Interleukin-6 in acute exercise and training: what is the biological relevance? *Exerc Immunol Rev* 12: 6–33, 2006.

62. Frid A, Ostman J, Linde B. Hypoglycemia risk during exercise after intramuscular injection of insulin in thigh in IDDM. *Diabetes Care* 13: 473–477, 1990.

63. Fuchsjäger-Mayrl G, Pleiner J, Wiesinger GF, Sieder AE, Quittan M, Nuhr MJ, et al. Exercise training improves vascular endothelial function in patients with type 1 diabetes. *Diabetes Care* 25: 1795–1801, 2002.

64. Gagliardino JJ. Physiological endocrine control of energy homeostasis and postprandial blood glucose levels. *Eur Rev Med Pharmacol Sci* 9: 75–92, 2005.

65. Galassetti P, Mann S, Tate D, Neill RA, Costa F, Wasserman DH, et al. Effects of antecedent prolonged exercise on subsequent counterregulatory responses to hypoglycemia. *Am J Physiol Endocrinol Metab* 280: E908–917, 2001.

66. Galassetti P, Riddell MC. Exercise and type 1 diabetes (T1DM). *Compr Physiol* 3: 1309–1336, 2013.

67. Galassetti P, Tate D, Neill RA, Richardson A, Leu S-Y, Davis SN. Effect of differing antecedent hypoglycemia on counterregulatory responses to exercise in type 1 diabetes. *Am J Physiol Endocrinol Metab* 290: E1109–1117, 2006.

68. Galassetti PR, Iwanaga K, Crisostomo M, Zaldivar FP, Larson J, Pescatello A. Inflammatory cytokine, growth factor and counterregulatory responses to exercise in children with type 1 diabetes and healthy controls. *Pediatr Diabetes* 7: 16–24, 2006.

69. Gastin PB. Energy system interaction and relative contribution during maximal exercise. *Sports Med (Auckland, NZ)* 31: 725–741, 2001.

70. Geelhoed-Duijvestijn PH, Pedersen-Bjergaard U, Weitgasser R, Lahtela J, Jensen MM, Östenson C-G. Effects of patient-reported non-severe hypoglycemia on healthcare resource use, work-time loss, and well-being in insulin-treated patients with diabetes in seven European countries. *J Med Econ* 16: 1453–1461, 2013.

71. Genuth S. Insights from the diabetes control and complications trial/epidemiology of diabetes interventions and complications study on the use of intensive glycemic treatment to reduce the risk of complications of type 1 diabetes. *Endocr Pract* 12(Suppl 1): 34–41, 2006.

72. Giorgino F, Laviola L, Cavallo Perin P, Solnica B, Fuller J, Chaturvedi N. Factors associated with progression to macroalbuminuria in microalbuminuric Type 1 diabetic patients: the EURODIAB Prospective Complications Study. *Diabetologia* 47: 1020–1028, 2004.

73. Goh SY, Cooper ME. Clinical review: The role of advanced glycation end products in progression and complications of diabetes. *J Clin Endocrinol Metab* 93: 1143–1152, 2008.

74. Gomez AM, Gomez C, Aschner P, Veloza A, Munoz O, Rubio C, et al. Effects of performing morning versus afternoon exercise on glycemic control and hypoglycemia frequency in type 1 diabetes patients on sensor-augmented insulin pump therapy. *J Diabetes Sci Technol* 9: 619–624, 2015.

75. Goodpaster BH, He J, Watkins S, Kelley DE. Skeletal muscle lipid content and insulin resistance: evidence for a paradox in endurance-trained athletes. *J Clin Endocrinol Metab* 86: 5755–5761, 2001.

76. Goto K, Higashiyama M, Ishii N, Takamatsu K. Prior endurance exercise attenuates growth hormone response to subsequent resistance exercise. *Eur J Appl Physiol* 94: 333–338, 2005.

77. Gradel AKJ, Porsgaard T, Lykkesfeldt J, Seested T, Gram-Nielsen S, Kristensen NR, et al. Factors affecting the absorption of subcutaneously administered insulin: effect on variability. *J Diabetes Res* 2018:10251021 2018.

78. Graveling AJ, Frier BM. Impaired awareness of hypoglycaemia: a review. *Diabetes Metab* 36(Suppl 3): S64–74, 2010.

79. Gubitosi-Klug RA, Braffett BH, White NH, Sherwin RS, Service FJ, et al, Complications trial/epidemiology of diabetes I, and complications research G. risk of severe hypoglycemia in type 1 diabetes over 30 years of follow-up in the DCCT/EDIC study. *Diabetes Care* 40: 1010–1016, 2017.

80. Guelfi KJ, Jones TW, Fournier PA. The decline in blood glucose levels is less with intermittent high-intensity compared with moderate exercise in individuals with type 1 diabetes. *Diabetes Care* 28: 1289–1294, 2005.

81. Guelfi KJ, Jones TW, Fournier PA. Intermittent high-intensity exercise does not increase the risk of early postexercise hypoglycemia in individuals with type 1 diabetes. *Diabetes Care* 28: 416–418, 2005.

82. Gusso S, Hofman P, Lalande S, Cutfield W, Robinson E, Baldi JC. Impaired stroke volume and aerobic capacity in female adolescents with type 1 and type 2 diabetes mellitus. *Diabetologia* 51: 1317–1320, 2008.

83. Hamann C, Kirschner S, Gunther KP, Hofbauer LC. Bone, sweet bone–osteoporotic fractures in diabetes mellitus. *Nat rev Endocrinol* 8: 297–305, 2012.

84. Hawley JA, Bosch AN, Weltan SM, Dennis SC, Noakes TD. Glucose kinetics during prolonged exercise in euglycaemic and hyperglycaemic subjects. *Pflugers Arch* 426: 378–386, 1994.

85. Hildebrandt P. Subcutaneous absorption of insulin in insulin-dependent diabetic patients. Influence of species, physico-chemical properties of insulin and physiological factors. *Dan Med Bull* 38: 337–346, 1991.

86. Hilsted J. Pathophysiology in diabetic autonomic neuropathy: cardiovascular, hormonal, and metabolic studies. *Diabetes* 31: 730–737, 1982.

87. Hirsch L, Byron K, Gibney M. Intramuscular risk at insulin injection sites–measurement of the distance from skin to muscle and rationale for shorter-length needles for subcutaneous insulin therapy. *Diabetes Technol Ther* 16: 867–873, 2014.

88. Huttunen NP, Käär ML, Knip M, Mustonen A, Puukka R, Akerblom HK. Physical fitness of children and adolescents with insulin-dependent diabetes mellitus. *Ann Clin Res* 16: 1–5, 1984.

89. *IDF Diabetes Atlas* (8th Edition). International Diabetes Federation.

90. International Hypoglycaemia Study G. Glucose concentrations of less than 3.0 mmol/L (54 mg/dL) should be reported in clinical trials: a joint position statement of the American Diabetes Association and the European Association for the Study of Diabetes. *Diabetes Care* 40: 155–157, 2017.

91. Iscoe KE, Campbell JE, Jamnik V, Perkins BA, Riddell MC. Efficacy of continuous real-time blood glucose monitoring during and after prolonged high-intensity cycling exercise: spinning with a continuous glucose monitoring system. *Diabetes Technol Ther* 8: 627–635, 2006.

92. Janghorbani M, Van Dam RM, Willett WC, Hu FB. Systematic review of type 1 and type 2 diabetes mellitus and risk of fracture. *Am J Epidemiol* 166: 495–505, 2007.

93. Jauch-Chara K, Schultes B. Sleep and the response to hypoglycaemia. *Best Pract Res Clin Endocrinol Metab* 24: 801–815, 2010.

94. Jenni S, Oetliker C, Allemann S, Ith M, Tappy L, Wuerth S, et al. Fuel metabolism during exercise in euglycaemia and hyperglycaemia in patients with type 1 diabetes mellitus–a prospective single-blinded randomised crossover trial. *Diabetologia* 51: 1457–1465, 2008.

95. Jimenez CC, Corcoran MH, Crawley JT, Guyton Hornsby W, Peer KS, Philbin RD, et al. National athletic trainers' association position statement: management of the athlete with type 1 diabetes mellitus. *J Athl Train* 42: 536–545, 2007.

96. Kacerovsky M, Brehm A, Chmelik M, Schmid AI, Szendroedi J, Kacerovsky-Bielesz G, et al. Impaired insulin stimulation of muscular ATP production in patients with type 1 diabetes. *J Intern Med* 269: 189–199, 2011.

97. Karvonen M, Tuomilehto J, Libman I, LaPorte R. A review of the recent epidemiological data on the world-wide incidence of type 1 (insulin-dependent) diabetes mellitus. World Health Organization DIAMOND Project Group. *Diabetologia* 36: 883–892, 1993.

98. Kattoor AJ, Pothineni NVK, Palagiri D, Mehta JL. Oxidative stress in atherosclerosis. *Curr Atherosclero Rep* 19: 42, 2017.

99. Kemink SA, Hermus AR, Swinkels LM, Lutterman JA, Smals AG. Osteopenia in insulin-dependent diabetes mellitus; prevalence and aspects of pathophysiology. *J Endocrinol Invest* 23: 295–303, 2000.

100. Kennedy A, Narendran P, Andrews RC, Daley A, Greenfield SM, Group E. Attitudes and barriers to exercise in adults with a recent diagnosis of type 1 diabetes: a qualitative study of participants in the Exercise for Type 1 Diabetes (EXTOD) study. *BMJ Open* 8: e017813, 2018.

101. Kilpatrick ES, Rigby AS, Atkin SL. Insulin resistance, the metabolic syndrome, and complication risk in type 1 diabetes: "double diabetes" in the Diabetes Control and Complications Trial. *Diabetes Care* 30: 707–712, 2007.

102. Komatsu WR, Gabbay MAL, Castro ML, Saraiva GL, Chacra AR, de Barros Neto TL, et al. Aerobic exercise capacity in normal adolescents and those with type 1 diabetes mellitus. *Pediatr Diabetes* 6: 145–149, 2005.

103. Koyama Y, Coker RH, Denny JC, Lacy DB, Jabbour K, Williams PE, et al. Role of carotid bodies in control of the neuroendocrine response to exercise. *Am J Physiol Endocrinol Metab* 281: E742–748, 2001.

104. Krause MP, Riddell MC, Hawke TJ. Effects of type 1 diabetes mellitus on skeletal muscle: clinical observations and physiological mechanisms. *Pediatr Diabetes* 12: 345–364, 2011.

105. Kubiak T, Hermanns N, Schreckling HJ, Kulzer B, Haak T. Assessment of hypoglycaemia awareness using continuous glucose monitoring. *Diabet Med* 21: 487–490, 2004.

106. Laaksonen DE, Atalay M, Niskanen LK, Mustonen J, Sen CK, Lakka TA, et al. Aerobic exercise and the lipid profile in type 1 diabetic men: a randomized controlled trial. *Med Sci Sports Exer* 32: 1541–1548, 2000.

107. Laing SP, Swerdlow AJ, Slater SD, Burden AC, Morris A, Waugh NR, et al. Mortality from heart disease in a cohort of 23,000 patients with insulin-treated diabetes. *Diabetologia* 46: 760–765, 2003.

108. LaPorte RE, Dorman JS, Tajima N, Cruickshanks KJ, Orchard TJ, Cavender DE, et al. Pittsburgh insulin-dependent diabetes mellitus morbidity and mortality study: physical activity and diabetic complications. *Pediatrics* 78: 1027–1033, 1986.

109. LaPorte RE, Tajima N, Akerblom HK, Berlin N, Brosseau J, Christy M, et al. Geographic differences in the risk of insulin-dependent diabetes mellitus: the importance of registries. *Diabetes Care* 8(Suppl 1): 101–107, 1985.

110. Larsen S, Brynjolf I, Birch K, Munck O, Sestoft L. The effect of continuous subcutaneous insulin infusion on cardiac performance during exercise in insulin-dependent diabetics. *Scand J Clin Lab Invest* 44: 683–691, 1984.

111. Lascar N, Kennedy A, Hancock B, Jenkins D, Andrews RC, Greenfield S, et al. Attitudes and barriers to exercise in adults with type 1 diabetes (T1DM) and how best to address them: a qualitative study. *PLOS ONE* 9: e108019, 2014.

112. Leclair E, Liggins RT, Peckett AJ, Teich T, Coy DH, Vranic M, et al. Glucagon responses to exercise-induced hypoglycaemia are improved by somatostatin receptor type 2 antagonism in a rat model of diabetes. *Diabetologia* 59: 1724–1731, 2016.

113. Livingstone R, Boyle JG, Petrie JR. How tightly controlled do fluctuations in blood glucose levels need to be to reduce the risk of developing complications in people with Type 1 diabetes? *Diabet Med* 2019.

114. Lowell BB, Shulman GI. Mitochondrial dysfunction and type 2 diabetes. *Science* 307: 384–387, 2005.

115. Maahs DM, West NA, Lawrence JM, Mayer-Davis EJ. Chapter 1: epidemiology of type 1 diabetes. *Endocrinol Metab Clin North Am* 39: 481–497, 2010.

116. MacLeod KM, Hepburn DA, Frier BM. Frequency and morbidity of severe hypoglycaemia in insulin-treated diabetic patients. *Diabet Med* 10: 238–245, 1993.

117. Magee MF, Bhatt BA. Management of decompensated diabetes. Diabetic ketoacidosis and hyperglycemic hyperosmolar syndrome. *Crit Care Clin* 17: 75–106, 2001.

118. Mäkimattila S, Virkamäki A, Malmström R, Utriainen T, Yki-Jarvinen H. Insulin resistance in type I diabetes mellitus: a major role for reduced glucose extraction. *J Clin Endocrinol Metab* 81: 707–712, 1996.

119. Makura CB, Nirantharakumar K, Girling AJ, Saravanan P, Narendran P. Effects of physical activity on the development and progression of microvascular complications in type 1 diabetes: retrospective analysis of the DCCT study. *BMC Endocr Disord* 13: 37, 2013.

120. Mallad A, Hinshaw L, Schiavon M, Dalla Man C, Dadlani V, Basu R, et al. Exercise effects on postprandial glucose metabolism in type 1 diabetes: a triple-tracer approach. *Am J Physiol Endocrinol Metab* 308: E1106–1115, 2015.

121. Maran A, Pavan P, Bonsembiante B, Brugin E, Ermolao A, Avogaro A, et al. Continuous glucose monitoring reveals delayed nocturnal hypoglycemia after intermittent high-intensity exercise in nontrained patients with type 1 diabetes. *Diabetes Technol Ther* 12: 763–768, 2010.

122. Maser RE, Mitchell BD, Vinik AI, Freeman R. The association between cardiovascular autonomic neuropathy and mortality in individuals with diabetes: a meta-analysis. *Diabetes Care* 26: 1895–1901, 2003.

123. McAuley SA, Horsburgh JC, Ward GM, La Gerche A, Gooley JL, Jenkins AJ, et al. Insulin pump basal adjustment for exercise in type 1 diabetes: a randomised crossover study. *Diabetologia* 59: 1636–1644, 2016.

124. McCarthy MM, Funk M, Grey M. Cardiovascular health in adults with type 1 diabetes. *Prev Med* 91: 138–143, 2016.

125. McGill M, Molyneaux L, Twigg SM, Yue DK. The metabolic syndrome in type 1 diabetes: does it exist and does it matter? *J Diabetes Complicat* 22: 18–23, 2008.

126. Monaco CMF, Hughes MC, Ramos SV, Varah NE, Lamberz C, Rahman FA, et al. Altered mitochondrial bioenergetics and ultrastructure in the skeletal muscle of young adults with type 1 diabetes. *Diabetologia* 61: 1411–1423, 2018.

127. Moser O, Tschakert G, Mueller A, Groeschl W, Pieber TR, Obermayer-Pietsch B, et al. Effects of high-intensity interval exercise versus moderate continuous exercise on glucose homeostasis and hormone response in patients with type 1 diabetes mellitus using novel ultra-long-acting insulin. *PLOS ONE* 10: e0136489, 2015.

128. Mosher PE, Nash MS, Perry AC, LaPerriere AR, Goldberg RB. Aerobic circuit exercise training: effect on adolescents with well-controlled insulin-dependent diabetes mellitus. *Arch Phys Med Rehabil* 79: 652–657, 1998.

129. Moy CS, Songer TJ, LaPorte RE, Dorman JS, Kriska AM, Orchard TJ, et al. Insulin-dependent diabetes mellitus, physical activity, and death. *Am J Epidemiol* 137: 74–81, 1993.

130. Narendran P, Solomon TP, Kennedy A, Chimen M, Andrews RC. The time has come to test the beta cell preserving effects of exercise in patients with new onset type 1 diabetes. *Diabetologia* 58: 10–18, 2015.

131. Nugent AM, Steele IC, al-Modaris F, Vallely S, Moore A, Campbell NP, et al. Exercise responses in patients with IDDM. *Diabetes Care* 20: 1814–1821, 1997.

132. Onkamo P, Vaananen S, Karvonen M, Tuomilehto J. Worldwide increase in incidence of Type I diabetes–the analysis of the data on published incidence trends. *Diabetologia* 42: 1395–1403, 1999.

133. Orchard TJ, Chang Y-F, Ferrell RE, Petro N, Ellis DE. Nephropathy in type 1 diabetes: a manifestation of insulin resistance and multiple genetic susceptibilities? Further evidence from the Pittsburgh Epidemiology of Diabetes Complication Study. *Kidney Int* 62: 963–970, 2002.

134. Orchard TJ, Olson JC, Erbey JR, Williams K, Forrest KYZ, Smithline Kinder L, et al. Insulin resistance-related factors, but not glycemia, predict coronary artery disease in type 1 diabetes: 10-year follow-up data from the Pittsburgh Epidemiology of Diabetes Complications Study. *Diabetes Care* 26: 1374–1379, 2003.

135. Östenson CG, Geelhoed-Duijvestijn P, Lahtela J, Weitgasser R, Markert Jensen M, Pedersen-Bjergaard U. Self-reported non-severe hypoglycaemic events in Europe. *Diabet Med* 31: 92–101, 2014.

136. Patterson CC, Harjutsalo V, Rosenbauer J, Neu A, Cinek O, Skrivarhaug T, et al. Trends and cyclical variation in the incidence of childhood type 1 diabetes in 26 European centres in the 25 year period 1989-2013: a multicentre prospective registration study. *Diabetologia* 62: 408-417, 2019.

137. Perseghin G, Lattuada G, Danna M, Sereni LP, Maffi P, De Cobelli F, et al. Insulin resistance, intramyocellular lipid content, and plasma adiponectin in patients with type 1 diabetes. *Am J Physiol Endocrinol Metab* 285: E1174–1181, 2003.

138. Poortmans JR, Saerens P, Edelman R, Vertongen F, Dorchy H. Influence of the degree of metabolic control on physical fitness in type I diabetic adolescents. *Int J Sports Med* 7: 232–235, 1986.

139. Quirk H, Blake H, Dee B, Glazebrook C. "You can't just jump on a bike and go": a qualitative study exploring parents' perceptions of physical activity in children with type 1 diabetes. *BMC Pediatr* 14: 313, 2014.

140. Ramalho AC, de Lourdes Lima M, Nunes F, Cambuí Z, Barbosa C, Andrade A, et al. The effect of resistance versus aerobic training on metabolic control in patients with type-1 diabetes mellitus. *Diabetes Res Clin Pract* 72: 271–276, 2006.

141. Ratjen I, Weber KS, Roden M, Herrmann ME, Müssig K. Type 1 diabetes mellitus and exercise in competitive athletes. *Exp Clin Endocrinol Diabetes* 123: 419–422, 2015.

142. Robertson RP, Lafferty KJ, Haug CE, Weil R, 3rd. Effect of human fetal pancreas transplantation on secretion of C-peptide and glucose tolerance in type I diabetics. *Transplant Proc* 19: 2354–2356, 1987.

143. Rogers MAM, Kim C, Banerjee T, Lee JM. Fluctuations in the incidence of type 1 diabetes in the United States from 2001 to 2015: a longitudinal study. *BMC Med* 15: 199, 2017.

144. Rogers MAM, Kim C, Banerjee T, Lee JM. Fluctuations in the incidence of type 1 diabetes in the United States from 2001 to 2015: a longitudinal study. *BMC Med* 15: 199, 2017.

145. Ronnemaa T, Koivisto VA. Combined effect of exercise and ambient temperature on insulin absorption and postprandial glycemia in type I patients. *Diabetes Care* 11: 769–773, 1988.

146. Rooijackers HMM, Wiegers EC, Tack CJ, van der Graaf M, de Galan BE. Brain glucose metabolism during hypoglycemia in type 1 diabetes: insights from functional and metabolic neuroimaging studies. *Cell Mol Life Sci* 73: 705–722, 2016.

147. Rosa JS, Flores RL, Oliver SR, Pontello AM, Zaldivar FP, Galassetti PR. Resting and exercise-induced IL-6 levels in children with Type 1 diabetes reflect hyperglycemic profiles during the previous 3 days. *J Appl Physiol* 108: 334–342, 2010.

148. Rosa JS, Oliver SR, Flores RL, Ngo J, Milne GL, Zaldivar FP, et al. Altered inflammatory, oxidative, and metabolic responses to exercise in pediatric obesity and type 1 diabetes. *Pediatr Diabetes* 12: 464–472, 2011.

149. Ruegemer JJ, Squires RW, Marsh HM, Haymond MW, Cryer PE, Rizza RA, et al. Differences between prebreakfast and late afternoon glycemic responses to exercise in IDDM patients. *Diabetes Care* 13: 104–110, 1990.

150. Russell NE, Higgins MF, Amaruso M, Foley M, McAuliffe FM. Troponin T and pro-B-type natriuretic Peptide in fetuses of type 1 diabetic mothers. *Diabetes Care* 32: 2050–2055, 2009.

151. Russell TA. Diabetic nephropathy in patients with type 1 diabetes mellitus. *Nephrol Nurs J* 33: 15–28; quiz 29-30, 2006.

152. Saltiel AR. Insulin signaling in the control of glucose and lipid homeostasis. *Handbook of Experimental Pharmacology* 233: 51–71, 2016.

153. Schmidt MI, Hadji-Georgopoulos A, Rendell M, Margolis S, Kowarski A. The dawn phenomenon, an early morning glucose rise: implications for diabetic intraday blood glucose variation. *Diabetes Care* 4: 579–585, 1981.

154. Scott SN, Cocks M, Andrews RC, Narendran P, Purewal TS, Cuthbertson DJ, et al. Fasted high-intensity interval and moderate-intensity exercise do not lead to detrimental 24-hour blood glucose profiles. *J Clin Endocrinol Metab* 104: 111–117, 2019.

155. Scott SN, Cocks M, Andrews RC, Narendran P, Purewal TS, Cuthbertson DJ, et al. High-intensity interval training improves aerobic capacity without a detrimental decline in blood glucose in people with type 1 diabetes. *J Clin Endocrinol Metab* 104: 604–612, 2019.

156. Seaquist ER, Anderson J, Childs B, Cryer P, Dagogo-Jack S, Fish L, et al. Hypoglycemia and diabetes: a report of a workgroup of the American Diabetes Association and the Endocrine Society. *Diabetes Care* 36: 1384–1395, 2013.

157. Seeger JP, Thijssen DH, Noordam K, Cranen ME, Hopman MT, Nijhuis-van der Sanden MW. Exercise training improves physical fitness and vascular function in children with type 1 diabetes. *Diabetes Obes Metab* 13: 382–384, 2011.

158. Sellmeyer DE, Civitelli R, Hofbauer LC, Khosla S, Lecka-Czernik B, Schwartz AV. Skeletal metabolism, fracture risk, and fracture outcomes in type 1 and type 2 diabetes. *Diabetes* 65: 1757–1766, 2016.

159. Shaw CS, Clark J, Wagenmakers AJM. The effect of exercise and nutrition on intramuscular fat metabolism and insulin sensitivity. *Annu Rev Nutr* 30: 13–34, 2010.

160. Shepherd SO, Cocks M, Meikle PJ, Mellett NA, Ranasinghe AM, Barker TA, et al. Lipid droplet remodelling and reduced muscle ceramides following sprint interval and moderate-intensity continuous exercise training in obese males. *Int J Obes* 41: 1745–1754, 2017.

161. Shulman GI. Ectopic fat in insulin resistance, dyslipidemia, and cardiometabolic disease. *New Engl J Med* 371: 1131–1141, 2014.

162. Sigal RJ, Fisher S, Halter JB, Vranic M, Marliss EB. The roles of catecholamines in glucoregulation in intense exercise as defined by the islet cell clamp technique. *Diabetes* 45: 148–156, 1996.

163. Sigal RJ, Purdon C, Fisher SJ, Halter JB, Vranic M, Marliss EB. Hyperinsulinemia prevents prolonged hyperglycemia after intense exercise in insulin-dependent diabetic subjects. *J Clin Endocrinol Metab* 79: 1049–1057, 1994.

164. Sjoberg KA, Frosig C, Kjobsted R, Sylow L, Kleinert M, Betik AC, et al. Exercise increases human skeletal muscle insulin sensitivity via coordinated increases in microvascular perfusion and molecular signaling. *Diabetes* 66: 1501–1510, 2017.

165. Soedamah-Muthu SS, Fuller JH, Mulnier HE, Raleigh VS, Lawrenson RA, Colhoun HM. High risk of cardiovascular disease in patients with type 1 diabetes in the U.K.: a cohort study using the general practice research database. *Diabetes Care* 29: 798–804, 2006.

166. Sousa GR, Pober D, Galderisi A, Lv H, Yu L, Pereira AC, et al. Glycemic control, cardiac autoimmunity, and long-term risk of cardiovascular disease in type 1 diabetes mellitus: a DCCT/EDIC cohort-based study. *Circulation* 139: 730-743 2019

167. Steffes MW, Sibley S, Jackson M, Thomas W. Beta-cell function and the development of diabetes-related complications in the diabetes control and complications trial. *Diabetes Care* 26: 832–836, 2003.

168. Stettler C, Jenni S, Allemann S, Steiner R, Hoppeler H, Trepp R, et al. Exercise capacity in subjects with type 1 diabetes mellitus in eu- and hyperglycaemia. *Diabetes Metab Res Rev* 22: 300–306, 2006.

169. Tesfaye S, Chaturvedi N, Eaton SEM, Ward JD, Manes C, Ionescu-Tirgoviste C, et al., Group EPCS. Vascular risk factors and diabetic neuropathy. *New Engl J Med* 352: 341–350, 2005.

170. Tielemans SMAJ, Soedamah-Muthu SS, De Neve M, Toeller M, Chaturvedi N, Fuller JH, et al. Association of physical activity with all-cause mortality and incident and prevalent cardiovascular disease among patients with type 1 diabetes: the EURODIAB Prospective Complications Study. *Diabetologia* 56: 82–91, 2013.

171. Trigona B, Aggoun Y, Maggio A, Martin XE, Marchand LM, Beghetti M, et al. Preclinical noninvasive markers of atherosclerosis in children and adolescents with type 1 diabetes are influenced by physical activity. *J Pediatr* 157: 533–539, 2010.

172. Tsalikian E, Mauras N, Beck RW, Tamborlane WV, Janz KF, Chase HP, et al. Impact of exercise on overnight glycemic control in children with type 1 diabetes mellitus. *J Pediatr* 147: 528–534, 2005.

173. Tumova J, Andel M, Trnka J. Excess of free fatty acids as a cause of metabolic dysfunction in skeletal muscle. *Physiol Res* 65: 193–207, 2016.

174. Turner D, Gray BJ, Luzio S, Dunseath G, Bain SC, Hanley S, et al. Similar magnitude of post-exercise hyperglycemia despite manipulating resistance exercise intensity in type 1 diabetes individuals. *Scand J Med Sci Sports* 26: 404–412, 2016.

175. Turner D, Luzio S, Gray BJ, Dunseath G, Rees ED, Kilduff LP, et al. Impact of single and multiple sets of resistance exercise in type 1 diabetes. *Scand J Med Sci Sports* 25: e99–109, 2015.

176. van Herpen NA, Schrauwen-Hinderling VB. Lipid accumulation in non-adipose tissue and lipotoxicity. *Physiol Behav* 94: 231–241, 2008.

177. van Loon LJ. Use of intramuscular triacylglycerol as a substrate source during exercise in humans. *J Appl Physiol (Bethesda, MD: 1985)* 97: 1170–1187, 2004.

178. van Loon LJ, Koopman R, Stegen JH, Wagenmakers AJ, Keizer HA, Saris WH. Intramyocellular lipids form an important substrate source during moderate intensity exercise in endurance-trained males in a fasted state. *J Physiol* 553: 611–625, 2003.

179. Venables MC, Achten J, Jeukendrup AE. Determinants of fat oxidation during exercise in healthy men and women: a cross-sectional study. *J Appl Physiol (Bethesda, MD: 1985)* 98: 160–167, 2005.

180. Veves A, Saouaf R, Donaghue VM, Mullooly CA, Kistler JA, Giurini JM, et al. Aerobic exercise capacity remains normal despite impaired endothelial function in the micro- and macrocirculation of physically active IDDM patients. *Diabetes* 46: 1846–1852, 1997.

181. Vranic M, Kawamori R, Pek S, Kovacevic N, Wrenshall GA. The essentiality of insulin and the role of glucagon in regulating glucose utilization and production during strenuous exercise in dogs. *J Clin Invest* 57: 245–255, 1976.

182. Vranic M, Ross G, Doi K, Lickley L. The role of glucagon-insulin interactions in control of glucose turnover and its significance in diabetes. *Metab* 25: 1375–1380, 1976.

183. Wadén J, Forsblom C, Thorn LM, Saraheimo M, Rosengård-Bärlund M, Heikkilä O, et al., FinnDiane Study G. Physical activity and diabetes complications in patients with type 1 diabetes: the Finnish Diabetic Nephropathy (FinnDiane) Study. *Diabetes Care* 31: 230–232, 2008.

184. Wadén J, Tikkanen HK, Forsblom C, Harjutsalo V, Thorn LM, Saraheimo M, et al, FinnDiane Study G. Leisure-time physical activity and development and progression of diabetic nephropathy in type 1 diabetes: the FinnDiane Study. *Diabetologia* 58: 929–936, 2015.

185. Wagenmakers AJ, Strauss JA, Shepherd SO, Keske MA, Cocks M. Increased muscle blood supply and transendothelial nutrient and insulin transport induced by food intake and exercise: effect of obesity and ageing. *J Physiol* 594: 2207–2222, 2016.

186. Wagenmakers AJ, van Riel NA, Frenneaux MP, Stewart PM. Integration of the metabolic and cardiovascular effects of exercise. *Essays Biochem* 42: 193–210, 2006.

187. Wasserman DH. Four grams of glucose. *Am J Physiol Endocrinol Metab* 296: E11–21, 2009.

188. Wasserman DH, Zinman B. Exercise in individuals with IDDM. *Diabetes Care* 17: 924–937, 1994.

189. Watt MJ, Heigenhauser GJ, LeBlanc PJ, Inglis JG, Spriet LL, Peters SJ. Rapid upregulation of pyruvate dehydrogenase kinase activity in human skeletal muscle during prolonged exercise. *J Appl Physiol (Bethesda, MD: 1985)* 97: 1261–1267, 2004.

190. Weinstock RS, Xing D, Maahs DM, Michels A, Rickels MR, Peters AL, et al., Network TDEC. Severe hypoglycemia and diabetic ketoacidosis in adults with type 1 diabetes: results from the T1D Exchange clinic registry. *J Clin Endocrinol Metab* 98: 3411–3419, 2013.

191. Yardley JE, Iscoe KE, Sigal RJ, Kenny GP, Perkins BA, Riddell MC. Insulin pump therapy is associated with less post-exercise hyperglycemia than multiple daily injections: an observational study of physically active type 1 diabetes patients. *Diabetes Technol Ther* 15: 84–88, 2013.

192. Yardley JE, Kenny GP, Perkins BA, Riddell MC, Balaa N, Malcolm J, et al. Resistance versus aerobic exercise: acute effects on glycemia in type 1 diabetes. *Diabetes Care* 36: 537–542, 2013.

193. Yardley JE, Kenny GP, Perkins BA, Riddell MC, Malcolm J, Boulay P, et al. Effects of performing resistance exercise before versus after aerobic exercise on glycemia in type 1 diabetes. *Diabetes Care* 35: 669–675, 2012.

194. Yardley JE, Sigal RJ, Riddell MC, Perkins BA, Kenny GP. Performing resistance exercise before versus after aerobic exercise influences growth hormone secretion in type 1 diabetes. *Appl Physiol Nutr Metab* 39: 262–265, 2014.

195. Yki-Jarvinen H, DeFronzo RA, Koivisto VA. Normalization of insulin sensitivity in type I diabetic subjects by physical training during insulin pump therapy. *Diabetes Care* 7: 520–527, 1984.

196. Yki-Järvinen H, Koivisto VA. Natural course of insulin resistance in type I diabetes. *New Engl J Med* 315: 224–230, 1986.

197. Zaharieva D, Yavelberg L, Jamnik V, Cinar A, Turksoy K, Riddell MC. The effects of basal insulin suspension at the start of exercise on blood glucose levels during continuous versus circuit-based exercise in individuals with type 1 diabetes on continuous subcutaneous insulin infusion. *Diabetes Technol Ther* 19: 370–378, 2017.

198. Zhong VW, Juhaeri J, Cole SR, Kontopantelis E, Shay CM, Gordon-Larsen P, et al. Incidence and trends in hypoglycemia hospitalization in adults with type 1 and type 2 diabetes in England, 1998-2013: A retrospective cohort study. *Diabetes Care* 40: 1651–1660, 2017.

199. Ziegler D, Zentai CP, Perz S, Rathmann W, Haastert B, Döring A, et al. Prediction of mortality using measures of cardiac autonomic dysfunction in the diabetic and nondiabetic population: the MONICA/KORA Augsburg Cohort Study. *Diabetes Care* 31: 556–561, 2008.

31
BIOCHEMISTRY OF EXERCISE TRAINING: MITIGATION OF CANCERS

Brittany R. Counts, Jessica L. Halle, and James A. Carson

Introduction

The devasting effect of cancer on human health and mortality has been acknowledged for thousands of years (59). Notwithstanding immense breakthroughs in cancer diagnosis and treatment during the modern medical era, it remains the number one or two cause of premature mortality in the industrialized world (31). In the United States 38–42% of men and women are likely to develop a type of cancer during their lifetime (76). Furthermore, the incidence of cancer is rapidly rising worldwide, which is thought to reflect changes in socio-economic development, an increase in the ageing of the population, and the successful treatment of other diseases (13). However, additional changes involving socio-economic status occurring in developing and already developed countries over the past 50 years include increased incidence of obesity and sedentary behaviour, which have the potential to negatively affect the occurrence and treatment of several cancers.

Cancer prevention and treatment are complicated due to disparities between types of cancers. Differences are influenced by distinct genetic and environmental stimuli. Certain cancers are more prevalent in developed countries, while infection-related cancers remain more prominent in low socio-economic areas (13). Based on newly reported cases in 2018, the most prevalent cancer types worldwide were lung, breast, prostate, colon, non-melanoma skin, stomach, and liver (13). The number of reported deaths from cancer worldwide in 2018 closely reflected the reported incidence, with lung cancer by far being the greatest cause of mortality followed by stomach, liver, breast, and colon cancer. Overall, there were 9.6 million deaths attributed to cancer in 2018 (13). While strong relationships for the risk of certain cancer types with either behaviours (i.e., smoking) or environments (i.e., sun exposure) have been established with both epidemiological and basic science evidence, a role for physical activity and exercise behaviours has also been examined. Large epidemiological studies have been able to assess how the incidence and survival of different cancer types are affected by physical activity and exercise (76). Breast and colon cancer risk in the United States was reported to have an inverse relationship with physical activity level over a decade ago (61). As research in this area has continued to increase, more recent analysis has determined that there is strong evidence for physical activity to lower the risk for several additional cancer types, including kidney, endometrium, bladder, and stomach cancer (61). While evidence is rapidly mounting for physical activity and exercise to be associated with the risk for several cancers, further basic research is needed to establish the biological mechanisms responsible for the exercise and physical activity impact on cancer risk.

The heterogeneity that is inherent to different cancer types and humans has contributed to complexities involving the understanding of tumour biology, which has also served as a barrier for the development of successful therapies. Classically, investigating the guiding principles of tumorigenesis has served as the foundation for understating biological mechanisms that drive cell transformation (33). Initially, these traits were termed "Hallmarks of Cancer" and encompassed six cell regulatory processes critically involved in malignant transformation of cells. These processes involved evading apoptosis, sustained angiogenesis, tissue invasion, metastasis, self-sustained growth processes, and limitless replicative potential (33). Furthermore, cell signalling pathways that provided these acquired capabilities in cells are well established. These cellular signalling pathways centred on the regulation of the cell cycle, cell death, DNA damage responses, and associated altered gene expression (33). While these initial observations on a formal process of cellular transformation provided critical insight for understanding tumorigenesis, more recent scientific breakthroughs that have cantered on activating characteristics of cancer cells have provided critical insight into the aetiology of cancer (34). Rather than the prior focus on cancer cells, today there is strong interest in the biology of the entire tumour microenvironment, which involves many cell types. Furthermore, the importance of additional processes involving tumour energy metabolism reprograming, and the evasion of immune destruction have also been acknowledged and widely investigated (34). Defining the critical processes in cellular transformation, the emerging understanding of the tumour microenvironment coupled with tumour metabolic programming, and susceptibility to immune cells has provided additional biological targets for the effect of physical activity and exercise on the prevention, treatment, and recurrence of cancer.

The importance of exercise and physical activity in the prevention of cancer has been widely acknowledged, and exercise prescription for cancer patients and survivors is recommended (61, 75). The scope of this review is to highlight the current understanding of the biological mechanism induced by exercise training that can affect the prevention, treatment, and recurrence of cancer. Furthermore, we provide information on potential next steps, gaps in our current understanding, and potential future research directions for understanding exercise- and physical activity–related biological mechanisms that affect cancer.

Exercise and Cancer Prevention

Tumorigenesis is the process of transforming a normal cell into a malignant cell and has been vigorously studied for decades. While the complexity of this regulation has been well documented (33), instability involving cell growth and survival regulatory genes is an established regulator of the tumorigenesis process. Tumorigenesis can be driven by a variety of endogenous and exogenous stimuli, and the National Cancer Institute defines cancer prevention as an action that lowers the risk of getting cancer. This includes the examination of behaviours, lifestyles, environmental exposure avoidance, and medicines that prevent cancer development. Obesity, diet, alcohol consumption, air pollution, and smoking are well-studied examples of factors that increase the risk of many cancer types (24). Furthermore, advanced age is a critical factor in the development of many cancers and must be factored into the risk associated with other variables (68). Interestingly, ageing is rarely accounted for in pre-clinical cancer prevention studies.

A role for exercise in the prevention of cancer has been widely postulated for decades. There are over 100 identified cancer types, and several types have demonstrated a strong association between decreased risk and increased physical activity at the population level (61, 76). Epidemiological evidence now supports a decreased risk of colon, breast, endometrial, kidney, bladder, oesophageal, and stomach cancers with increasing physical activity level. This list is impactful, as stomach, breast, oesophagus, and colon cancer are also leading causes of cancer deaths worldwide (13). Cancer's continued negative impact on human health has driven the growth of population-level data collection worldwide, and as this forthcoming research on cancer risk becomes available, it is likely that more cancer types will be associated with either exercise level or sedentary behaviour.

Despite the growing association of exercise and physical activity for the risk for some types of cancer, the identification of biological mechanisms involved in the preventive effects of exercise are still being established. The availability and use of appropriate pre-clinical cancer models in controlled exercise studies remain a barrier to our mechanistic understanding of exercise and cancer preventions. A recent comprehensive review of pre-clinical cancer studies investigating the effect of exercise found the published scientific literature in the area to be beset by high heterogeneity related to all aspects of study design and analysis; important recommendations for future rigorous research were warranted (3). There are several underlying complexities related to understanding the mechanistic underpinnings of exercise on cancer prevention. Exercise training can affect cancer risk through changes to the systemic environment and at the cellular level through the prevention of cellular transformation (49). Exercise also has the potential to alter the potency of other identified cancer risk factors, such as obesity. While the majority of pre-clinical studies that examine exercise and cancer focus on tumour growth rather than incidence, we will briefly highlight the direct evidence and current theories for the biological effects of exercise training at the systemic and cellular level that lower cancer risk.

The systemic environment's role in initiating and sustaining tumour growth has been widely acknowledged and researched (52), which also provides a strong premise for exercise training's impact on cancer incidence. Exercise training induces a plethora of health-related systemic changes that have been hypothesized to decrease cancer risk and have recently been reviewed (39, 49). Exercise-induced improvements to the physiological function of the cardiovascular system, glucose homeostasis, lipid metabolism, and immune system can all be connected to plausible reasons for cancer prevention (45). Furthermore, exercise's impact on overall energy balance has been widely implicated in cancer risk (75). Exercise-induced changes in energy balance can encompass more than a reduction in obesity and can be reflected in circulating levels of sex hormones and adipokines (53). Exercise also induces changes in gene expression and signalling pathways in adipose tissue, skeletal muscle, and the liver that positively affect systemic metabolic health (19). Skeletal muscle myokine release that occurs with exercise has also been investigated for the anti-cancer effects of exercise (39). Furthermore, skeletal muscle undergoes metabolic adaptations to exercise that can positively affect systemic metabolism dysfunction associated with cancer risk (3). These exercise adaptations include increased oxidative metabolism, which provides improved metabolic flexibility for the use of lipid and glucose for energy. Improved metabolism in adipocytes has the potential to reduce the production of cytokines such as interleukin-6 (IL-6), which can contribute to chronic inflammation and cancer risk (39). There is a strong premise for systemic exercise adaptations having the capacity to lower cancer risk; however, further mechanistic investigation is warranted to establish which exercise adaptations are critical for suppressing cell transformation of different cancer types and why some cancers have higher sensitivity to certain exercise-induced systemic changes than other types.

Pre-clinical studies examining exercise mechanisms of cancer prevention have been historically limited to the quantification of tumorigenesis in genetic or chemically induced cancer models (64). Therefore, the effect of exercise on tumour growth and metastasis using transplantable tumour models has been more widely investigated (see the next section). Overall, the published literature supports exercise having a suppressive effect on tumour incidence in pre-clinical studies. However, publication bias of positive results should be considered when making this interpretation, as studies with negative findings are more difficult to publish (64). Interestingly, the relatively limited research in this area using genetic cancer models demonstrates the complexity of examining exercise-induced cancer prevention with pre-clinical cancer models. While the majority of pre-clinical studies demonstrate some degree of exercise suppression on tumour incidence, the type of cancer, sex, mode of exercise, and diet all have the capacity to interact with the exercise stimulus. Genetic and chemical pre-clinical breast cancer models employed in exercise studies have generally demonstrated a suppression of tumour incidence; however, an exception was determined with exercise in a female p53-deficient: MMTV-Wnt-1 transgenic model of breast cancer. Interestingly, Colbert et al. (2009) reported in a rigorously designed and carried out study that spontaneous mammary tumorigenesis was increased with treadmill and wheel running exercise (21). Further complexities have been reported, with studies examining the ApcMin mouse, which carries a mutation in the adenomatous polyposis coli gene (*Apc*). The ApcMin mouse is a genetic pre-clinical model that spontaneously develops gastrointestinal tract tumours and has been widely examined for the effects of diet and exercise on tumour incidence (64). Regular treadmill exercise training and ad libitum cage wheel running during the stage of tumorigenesis have been reported to differentially affect tumour incidence in the male ApcMin mouse; treadmill exercise significantly reduced tumour incidence, while ad libitum cage wheel running had no effect (54). Conversely, neither treadmill exercise nor wheel running reduced polyp incidence in the female ApcMin mouse. Diet may also interact with exercise prevention of tumorigenesis. Male ApcMin mice fed a high-fat diet did not reduce tumour incidence with treadmill exercise as did ApcMin mice on a normal chow diet (6). These studies illustrate the complexities of examining mechanisms of cancer prevention in pre-clinical studies that involve the cancer model used, diet, sex, and type of exercise activity. Additional rigorously designed research that examines biologically relevant cancer models and stringently quantifies tumour incidence and a well-conceived exercise stimulus are clearly warranted to establish exercise-induced mechanisms that have the potential to either suppress cell malignant transformation or decrease transformed cell viability.

Exercise and Cancer Treatment

Cancer treatment strives to cure or stop the progression of cancer with a variety of therapeutic approaches (i.e., chemotherapy, radiation, and surgery). The mechanistic understanding of tumour cell growth, physiology, and metabolism has been fundamental in the development of successful treatment strategies for the cancer patient (59). The identification of six hallmarks of tumour cell biology facilitated the initial framework for understanding the complexity of tumour cell biology and growth regulation (33). Processes involving neoplastic cell interaction with the tumour microenvironment have also been widely acknowledged as critical drivers of tumour growth and metastasis (34). In addition to neoplastic cells, the microenvironment includes endothelial, fibroblast, myofibroblast, pericyte, adipocyte, and immune cells that contribute to metabolic, immune, and angiogenic processes vital for sustaining tumour growth (49). Therefore, the tumour microenvironment has become a key focus for understanding the cell interactions that drive tumour growth and provides the basis for additional drivers of tumour growth involving avoidance of immune cell destruction and deregulation of tumour cellular energetics (34).

The systemic environment also has an important role in sustaining tumour growth (52). The tumour can initiate changes to the systemic environment through a variety of tissues and organs, including the spleen, lung, and bone marrow (51). Tumours can mediate these systemic interactions through the release of cytokines, growth factors, and hormones. These factors can manipulate the systemic environment to support tumour growth, including the mobilization of bone marrow cells that can support tumour angiogenesis (52). Systemic changes to hormones, cytokines, and growth factors that are not tumour derived can also provide a stimulus for tumour growth (3). These critical interactions between the tumour and the systemic environment combined with exercise's established capacity to influence the systemic environment provide a strong premise for exercise-induced mechanisms that affect tumour growth. Therefore, further rigorously planned and carried out research is strongly justified to determine if exercise-induced changes to metabolism and immune function through alterations to circulating growth factors, cytokines, and hormones can affect tumour growth. To this end, in vitro studies using conditioned media from exercising humans have demonstrated an ability to decrease the proliferation of several cancer cell lines (39). However, further work is needed to determine the constituents of conditioned media from exercising humans that is sufficient to alter regulation in cancer cells.

The effect of exercise on tumour growth has been widely examined in pre-clinical cancer models (3). The vast majority of pre-clinical studies have studied either breast or colon cancer and used treadmill or wheel running as the exercise stimulus (64). These exercise studies have used genetic, transplantable, and chemical-induced cancer models, and there is tremendous heterogeneity in study design related to the exercise stimulus (3). Exercise treatment heterogeneity in these studies serves to limit strong conclusions on exercise dose involving intensity and duration of the exercise. A consistent tumour growth outcome in these studies is the measurement of tumour volume or size, and despite considerable variability in key study characteristics, most exercise studies have demonstrated an attenuation in tumour growth (64). However, exercise studies do not currently support the elimination of cancer. The attenuation of tumour growth and overall systemic health benefits provide a strong rationale for mechanistic examination of exercise in the overall treatment of the cancer patient. This includes investigating the potential for exercise to minimize chemotherapy treatment side effects and increase chemotherapy efficacy, which could allow for better tolerance of cancer treatments and increased patient survival.

Pre-clinical cancer studies have demonstrated that exercise can regulate tumour intrinsic properties involved in growth and metastasis (39, 49, 73). The mechanistic investigation of tumour growth by exercise has often centred on the regulation of tumour physiology and metabolism (64). Tumour physiology involves mechanisms that sustain tumour growth and dependence on extensive interactions with the microenvironment. Classical tumour physiology needed to sustain growth includes vascularization to supply nutrients and avoidance of immune cell destruction. Both of these properties have been widely hypothesized as mechanisms for exercise attenuation of tumour growth. Other postulated exercise effects that could affect tumour intrinsic properties include increased blood flow, reduced pH, heat production, and sympathetic activation (39, 49). Exercise can increase tumour perfusion and vascularization in several pre-clinical cancer models; decreased tumour hypoxia is associated with a reduction in the aggressiveness of the tumour (11). Exercise also increases the mobilization of natural killer (NK) cells and cytotoxic T cells (64). Well- established exercise-induced immune system changes and increased mobilization involving these cell types have been thought to be a plausible mechanism for exercise effects on tumour growth (39, 49). However, direct evidence for this effect is still needed. A role for exercise regulation through macrophage regulation of the tumour microenvironment involving tumour-promoting (M2) or -suppressing (M1) tumour-associated macrophage phenotypes has been investigated (32). Increased cytotoxicity of tumour-derived macrophages has also been linked to exercise effects on tumour growth (60). Exercise may also affect recruitment of tumour-associated macrophages. Decreased intestinal tumour growth in exercised ApcMIN male mice had fewer macrophages per polyp (5). A critical property of tumours is the ability to evade destruction by infiltrating immune cells, and further work is needed to determine if exercise can alter the susceptibility of tumours to immune cell action. Tumour angiogenesis is also a requirement for growth and requires a variety of cell types, including the mobilization of bone marrow–derived hemopoietic progenitor cells (52). However, the effect of exercise on the tumour's ability to release cytokines, growth factors, and chemokines that could alter vascularization potential has not been established. While the effect of exercise on other cell types within the tumour microenvironment has been recognized (49), further examination of how exercise alters specific cellular interactions in the microenvironment to suppress growth is warranted.

The impact of exercise on established intracellular signalling pathways regulating tumour growth has also been examined (39, 73). The mammalian target of rapamycin (mTOR) and protein kinase B (Akt) signalling networks are key drivers of tumour growth and can be regulated by hormones, growth factors, and the energy status of the cell (73). Furthermore, processes integrated with this network can affect tumour growth through ribosomal biogenesis, protein synthesis, autophagy, ubiquitin proteasome degradation, and apoptosis. Tumours from exercised mice exhibit decreased mTOR signalling, and is hypothesized to be a reduction in circulating growth factors such as IGF-1 that can activate mTOR (73). Intracellular signalling through AMP activated protein kinase (AMPK) has been investigated in tumours. AMPK serves as an energy sensor in cells and can regulate autophagy, protein synthesis, glucose uptake, and oxidative metabolism in cells. Exercise can increase AMPK activity in tumours and implies that exercise can alter tumour metabolism (73). AMPK is also a negative regulator of mTOR and can serve to suppress growth factor and hormone activation of protein synthesis and growth. Despite significant interest in Akt/mTOR and AMPK signalling in tumours, further research is needed to establish if these signalling pathways or the critical processes they regulate are directly involved in the exercise-induced suppression of tumour growth.

Understanding exercise regulation of tumour biology in pre-clinical models has provided important insights on the tumour microenvironment, immune cell function, and systemic environment interactions that regulate growth. However, a more clinically and translatable question is how exercise interacts with cancer treatment (Figure 31.2). Since exercise is not a primary treatment after cancer diagnosis, an important question is determining if exercise can promote cancer patient survival by improving the efficacy and reducing the toxicity of established cancer treatments. While the adverse effects and toxicities of cancer treatment have been well documented (67), exercise during cancer treatment has been found to be safe and contributes to improved patient life quality and decreased fatigue (67). Notwithstanding improvements in cancer patient physical function, exercise has also been investigated for improved cancer treatment efficacy and reduced toxicity. The chemotherapy drug doxorubicin is an anthracycline chemotherapeutic used in the treatment of solid tumours that induces severe side effects related to cardiotoxicity and skeletal muscle myopathy that are related to intracellular reactive oxygen species (ROS) production (69). Pre-clinical studies in non-tumour-bearing mice have demonstrated that exercise training is protective against doxorubicin-induced cardiac toxicity, and improved muscle mitochondria function protects against high ROS levels (47). Several pre-clinical studies have demonstrated that exercise can decrease tumour hypoxia and improve tumour perfusion, which serve to can lessen tumour aggressiveness and improve chemotherapy responsiveness (11, 43, 44). Exercised mice with orthotopically transplanted breast tumours exhibited decreased tumour hypoxia and an increased efficacy of cyclophosphamide treatment (11). There is mounting evidence that justifies rigorously conducted studies that combine relevant pre-clinical cancer models with chemotherapeutic treatments to determine the cellular mechanisms of this multimodal treatment strategy (Figure 31.1).

This knowledge should serve to decrease the overall toxicity of the cancer treatment and possibly improve effectiveness. Either of these outcomes would serve to positively affect the success of many cancer treatments and improve patient survival.

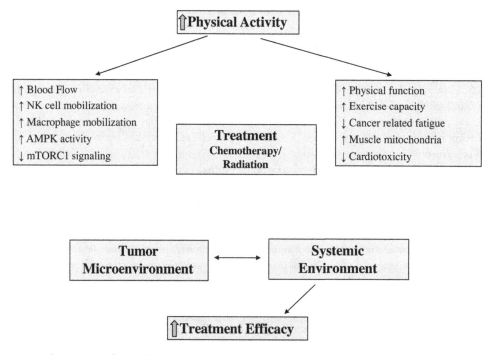

Figure 31.1 Therapeutic efficacy of physical activity during anticancer treatment

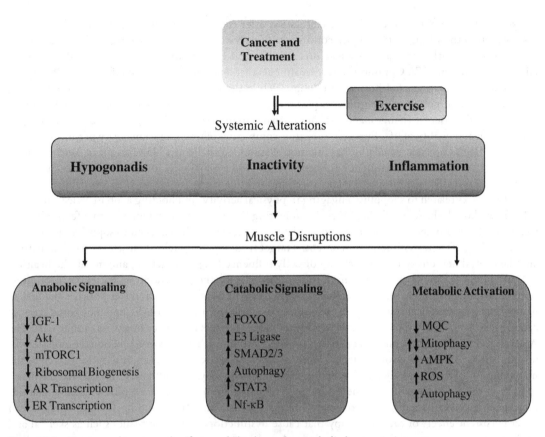

Figure 31.2   Cancer and treatment's effect on skeletal muscle metabolic homeostasis

Exercise and Cancer Survival

Increasing cancer patient survival is an acknowledged objective measure of successful cancer treatment. The percentage of people alive for a defined time period after either diagnosis or the start of treatment for a disease is designated as the survival rate. Improvements in cancer survival rates can reflect advances in both treatment and earlier diagnosis (1). The National Cancer Institute uses a 5-year survival rate after diagnosis as a benchmark for monitoring treatment and early diagnosis success with different cancer types. While the 5-year survival rate for all cancers in the United States has increased over the past 45 years from 49% to 69%, there is considerable variation by individual cancer type. Furthermore, survival outcomes can be affected by other variables such as race (1). The risk for breast, colon, and stomach cancer is associated with physical activity level (61), and have all seen significant improvements in cancer survival in the United States over the past 45 years (1). Beyond associations with cancer incidence rates, the relationship between physical activity level and cancer survival has begun to be investigated. A high level of physical activity post diagnosis has been associated with a reduction in all-cause mortality for breast, colon, and prostate cancer patients (63). Interestingly, prostate cancer risk is not strongly associated with physical activity, which illustrates the differential effects exercise can have for different cancer types for cancer prevention versus survival after cancer diagnosis. In addition to mortality and survival, there is an increased interest in improving the cancer survivor's quality of life. Cancer and its associated treatment can have drastic effects on the ability to maintain physical function, which also serves to increase the risk of developing comorbidities that decrease health and negatively affect cancer survival. This section highlights recent research advances and areas that warrant further investigation to provide a mechanistic understanding of exercise's impact on long-term adverse effects of cancer treatment.

Exercise has the potential to affect rehabilitation after treatment and the prevention of future disease, which both fall under the cancer continuum of survivorship (22). The effects of the cancer and the associated treatments that can affect survivorship and life quality have been termed "persistent effects" of treatment (67). Common cancer treatments that document persistent effects include surgery, chemotherapy, radiation, and hormonal therapy. While the persistent effects vary by treatment type, they include pain, peripheral neuropathy, pulmonary changes, endocrine changes, impaired immune function, cardiovascular changes, and gastrointestinal system dysfunction (67), which can all negatively affect health and quality of life. Furthermore, after completion of treatment a majority of cancer patients still report fatigue and decreased physical function as sustained challenges (25). Fatigue in cancer patients 1 year after completion of treatment has been reported to be a major factor detracting from quality of life (4). Additionally, lingering effects of cancer and treatment are associated with an inability to perform daily tasks related to shopping, engaging in physical activity, and holding a job in cancer survivors (71, 72). Although the scientific literature documenting these persistent and long-term effects of cancer treatment has continued to expand and be validated, further research is needed to supply a mechanistic understanding of these dysfunctions in potential target tissues such as skeletal muscle, heart, vasculature, and the central nervous system, which can directly influence fatigue, function, and metabolic health.

Daily physical activity provides a multitude of benefits for the prevention and attenuated progression of chronic disease (8, 14, 50). Furthermore, exercise in healthy adults induces positive changes to many of the physiological systems (i.e., cardiovascular, immune) that can be disrupted by some types of cancer treatment, which should provide significant health benefits for cancer survivors (Table 31.1). The American Cancer Society endorses exercise for cancer survivors that mirrors the national guidelines for healthy adults: 150 minutes of moderate-intensity exercise weekly. Exercise prescription involves the manipulation of variables related to exercise duration, frequency, and intensity and can have a major impact on the health outcomes achieved by exercise participation. Despite exercise recommendations for cancer survivors, there is an extremely limited mechanistic understanding of how exercise can affect persistent effects of cancer therapy that cause dysfunction in specific tissues such as skeletal and cardiac muscle. At the cellular level exercise-induced improvements in muscle oxidative metabolism could serve as a primary benefit of exercise. Skeletal muscle mitochondrial content, function, and quality control are decreased with cancer cachexia (15, 17). Furthermore, short-term FOLFOX and FOLFIRI chemotherapy administration can suppress muscle mitochondrial biogenesis and content in tumour-free mice (9, 10). Exercise has the potential to mitigate these cancer-induced dysfunctions through improved mitochondrial content, function, and dynamics, which improves the coordination

Table 31.1 Role of physical activity during treatment and survival

Cancer stage	Treatment	Survival	
		Acute effects	*Persistent effects*
Role of physical activity	• Improve chemotherapy efficacy and reduce toxicity	• Improve physical function	• Reduce cardiotoxicity
	• Reduce treatment-associated fatigue	• Decrease the initiation of metabolic disruptions leading to comorbidities	• Reduce cancer-related fatigue
	• Reduce initiation and progression of cachexia	• Improve immune function	• Reduce recurrence
	• Maintain physical function		• Reduce pain
			• Reduce peripheral neuropathy

of mitophagy, mitochondrial fission/fusion, and biogenesis regulation (26, 40, 42). Interestingly, there is an extremely limited understanding of how prior cancer and chemotherapy treatment affects skeletal muscle's cellular response to exercise. Moreover, healthy adult exercise recommendations can be challenging for some cancer survivors. Further research is warranted to determine if lower doses (intensity and duration) of exercise might benefit persistent negative effects of treatment in the cancer survivor.

Future Directions for Cancer Survivors

Cancer cachexia is a debilitating muscle wasting condition that occurs secondary to chronic disease (29). While 50% of all cancer patients will develop cachexia, it attributes to 20–40% of all cancer-related deaths (74). Consequences of cachexia are intolerance to anti-cancer therapy, susceptibility to treatment toxicity, and functional impairments that result in reduced patient life quality (28, 46). The progression of cachexia has been classified as a continuum (pre-cachexia to refractory cachexia), and a worse prognosis resulting in increased energy expenditure, insulin resistance, whole-body catabolism, and hypogonadism occurs with increasing severity (28, 74). Cachectic cancer patients exhibit reduced physical activity, exercise capacity, and muscular strength (35). Pre-clinical models of cancer cachexia also exhibit reduced cage activity, grip strength, and exercise capacity (35). Interestingly, in pre-clinical models of cachexia, voluntary activity declines prior to significant body weight loss, highlighting that decrements in activity might be an early indicator for cachexia's progression (7). Furthermore, physical inactivity that accompanies cachexia progression has been hypothesized to contribute to the condition's progression; therefore, ways to limit physical inactivity are of importance.

Periods of physical inactivity have known consequences on skeletal muscle protein turnover and metabolism (41), which are established drivers of skeletal muscle wasting with cancer cachexia (74) and have been widely investigated in pre-clinical models (2, 17). In skeletal muscle, cancer cachexia disrupts protein turnover regulation through the suppression of protein synthesis and the up-regulation of protein degradation involving the ubiquitin proteasome and lysosomal systems (Figure 31.3). Furthermore, protein synthesis is suppressed in cachectic skeletal muscle through the down-regulation of mTORC1 signalling (77). mTORC1 signalling is affected by the regulation of sex hormones independent of disease and/or cancer status; therefore, it follows that cancer patients that develop cachexia have been strongly associated with hypogonadism (16). Furthermore, reduced circulating testosterone levels have a clear potential to alter inflammation and cancer-induced regulation of the Akt/FOXO/mTORC1 signalling axis (18). Oestrogen can also affect the Akt/FOXO/mTORC1 axis, (56, 70), and female tumour-bearing mice exhibit increased muscle inflammatory signalling when the ovaries are removed (38), which suggests that sex hormones might be protective against the inflammatory environment. Furthermore, muscle mitochondrial dysfunction has been hypothesized to be an important driver of cancer-induced muscle wasting and attributes to the ageing process (2, 17), and sex hormones potentially regulate mitochondria biogenesis and mitophagy through skeletal muscle AMPK activity (70) and mTORC1 signalling (18). Interestingly, increased physical activity has known implications for improving mitochondria function, oxidative metabolism, and protein turnover in skeletal muscle (27). Therefore, increased physical activity has the therapeutic potential to increase skeletal muscle protein synthesis, suppress protein degradation, improve mitochondrial function, and increase circulating sex steroids to aid in maintaining skeletal muscle mass homeostasis.

Over the last decade, maintaining skeletal muscle mass and metabolic homeostasis during cancer's progression has garnered significant scientific interest due to evidence supporting the importance of muscle mass maintenance in late-stage cancer patients (35). For example, late-stage cancer patients with a high muscle mass at diagnosis had a greater survival rate compared to low muscle mass patients, and interestingly those that maintained skeletal muscle mass during anti-cancer treatment had a greater survival rate compared to those that lost muscle mass (20). While the loss of skeletal muscle mass in cachectic cancer patients is complex, the cachectic environment suppresses skeletal muscle protein synthesis, up-regulates protein degradation, impairs oxidative metabolism, and increases production of ROS (37).

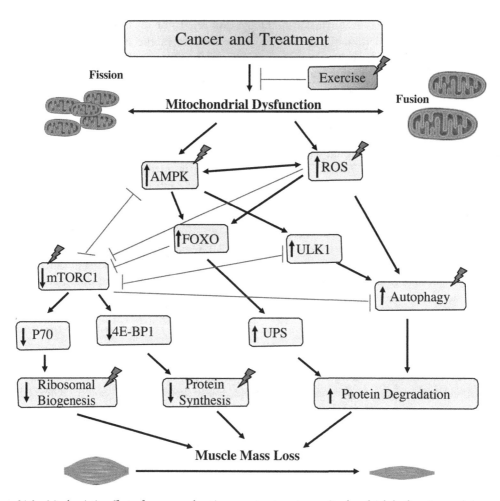

Figure 31.3 Mechanistic effect of cancer and anti-cancer treatment on mitochondrial dysfunction and the control of proteostasis in muscle

In cachectic skeletal muscle, inflammatory signalling induced by cancer can attenuate the magnitude of the muscle protein synthesis induced by stimulated eccentric contractions in tumour-bearing mice (36). Interestingly, contractions were sufficient to overcome the impaired anabolic response to feeding (57), and repeated bouts of eccentric contractions produced a muscle growth response and suppressed AMPK signalling in the presence of the cancer-induced catabolic environment. Therefore, it has been hypothesized that these negative consequences of the systemic environment on skeletal muscle tissue can be reversed or mitigated through increased physical activity. To date, exercise has generally shown beneficial effects in cancer patients; however, clinical trials are currently ongoing to determine the feasibility and efficacy of exercise in late-stage cancer patients. In pre-clinical models, exercise prior to complete tumour development has been sufficient to prevent skeletal muscle mass loss, reduce tumour number, and lower systemic inflammation (54, 65). Future work is needed to determine if exercise during the initiation of cachexia or after significant body weight loss can help mitigate cachexia progression. While additional research is needed to provide the mechanistic basis for exercise prescription in cachectic cancer patients, it would be of interest to hypothesize that exercise interventions can help improve patient physical function, chemotherapy tolerance, and/or chemotherapy potency, leading to a better prognosis and quality of life for the patient.

Cancer-related fatigue (CRF) is defined as a chronic distressing and persistent subjective sense of physical, emotional, and/or cognitive tiredness related to cancer and/or cancer treatment (55). Furthermore, CRF is not the result of fatigue from recent physical activity and was not present prior to cancer diagnosis. Patients commonly report fatigue in the weeks or months following treatment, and it has been reported in one-third of patients for up to 10 years post treatment even if the patient exhibits no signs of disease (58). CRF is diagnosed from self-reports, and severity is categorized by the physician (12). Despite CRF's subjectivity, CRF is the most frequent side effect and complaint of cancer patients before and after anticancer treatment and can often lead to treatment discontinuation (12). Unfortunately, a variety of biological, demographic, medical, psychosocial, and behavioural factors that have been attributed to CRF, which compound the ability to diagnose and treat it. However, dysregulation of the hypothalamic-pituitary-anterior (HPA) pituitary axis, increased systemic inflammation, and muscle metabolism dysregulation are the most common hypothetical mechanisms that contribute to CRF (12). Since persistence of CRF is attributed to reduced patient survival and poor life quality, it is of great interest to reduce fatigue associated with cancer and cancer treatment. Physical activity is routinely discussed as a potential therapeutic option of eliminating or preventing CRF, given that increased physical activity improved life quality and functional outcomes in cancer patients experiencing chronic fatigue (62). Interestingly, cancer patients are often told to reduce their daily physical activity to mitigate CRF symptoms; however, this only seeks to exacerbate their inactivity. There is growing evidence that increased physical activity can improve CRF (23, 30). Aerobic exercise training has demonstrated the greatest reduction in CRF, which is possibly attributed to the longer duration of exercise compared to resistance exercise alone (48). Nonetheless, it is necessary to understand the underlying mechanisms attributed to reduced fatigue, thus providing a non-pharmacological treatment. It has been hypothesized that exercise in cancer patients can reduce chronic systemic inflammation, improve serotonin release thus modifying HPA axis function, and improve muscle metabolism leading to reduced CRF (66). Interestingly, some have suggested that the acute effects of exercise on reduced fatigue are attributed to an improved psychosocial well-being (12), further emphasizing the need to understand the mechanisms behind the relationship between increased physical activity and reduced CRF. Lastly, several studies do not seek to improve CRF, but report fatigue as a secondary outcome; therefore, studies would greatly improve if the cancer patient population in studies targeted fatigued patients.

Summary

The rising incidence of cancer worldwide and the devasting impact on human health and mortality have led to an ever-growing need for successful cancer treatments. In this review, we highlighted the current understanding of the biological mechanisms induced by exercise training that can affect the prevention, treatment, and recurrence of cancer. We also provided information on how exercise can help alleviate the off-target ramifications of cancer by preventing tumour growth, improving drug tolerance, and improving survival. Additional insight is provided for critical areas where future research is clearly needed. Furthermore, research uncovering the mechanistic basis of survivorship issues that negatively affect health after cancer treatment is necessary. We highlight the importance of treating cancer cachexia and CRF. Lastly, we have provided information on potential next steps and highlighted critical gaps in our current understanding of exercise- and physical activity–related biological mechanisms that affect cancer patient survival and health.

References

1. ACS. *Cancer Facts & Figures 2019*. Atlanta, GA: ACS, 2019.
2. Argiles JM, Lopez-Soriano FJ, Busquets S. Muscle wasting in cancer: the role of mitochondria. *Curr Opin Clin Nutr Metab Care* 18: 221–225, 2015.
3. Ashcraft KA, Peace RM, Betof AS, Dewhirst MW, Jones LW. Efficacy and mechanisms of aerobic exercise on cancer initiation, progression, and metastasis: a critical systematic review of in Vivo preclinical data. *Cancer Res* 76: 4032–4050, 2016.

4. Baker F, Denniston M, Smith T, West MM. Adult cancer survivors: how are they faring? *Cancer* 104: 2565–2576, 2005.

5. Baltgalvis KA, Berger FG, Pena MM, Davis JM, Carson JA. Effect of exercise on biological pathways in ApcMin/+ mouse intestinal polyps. *J Appl Physiol (1985)* 104: 1137–1143, 2008.

6. Baltgalvis KA, Berger FG, Pena MM, Davis JM, Carson JA. The interaction of a high-fat diet and regular moderate intensity exercise on intestinal polyp development in Apc Min/+ mice. *Cancer Prev Res (Phila)* 2: 641–649, 2009.

7. Baltgalvis KA, Berger FG, Pena MM, Mark Davis J, White JP, Carson JA. Activity level, apoptosis, and development of cachexia in Apc(Min/+) mice. *J Appl Physiol (1985)* 109: 1155–1161, 2010.

8. Barbaric M, Brooks E, Moore L, Cheifetz O. Effects of physical activity on cancer survival: a systematic review. *Physiother Can* 62: 25–34, 2010.

9. Barreto R, Mandili G, Witzmann FA, Novelli F, Zimmers TA, Bonetto A. Cancer and chemotherapy contribute to muscle loss by activating common signaling pathways. *Front Physiol* 7: 472, 2016.

10. Barreto R, Waning DL, Gao H, Liu Y, Zimmers TA, Bonetto A. Chemotherapy-related cachexia is associated with mitochondrial depletion and the activation of ERK1/2 and p38 MAPKs. *Oncotarget* 7: 43442–43460, 2016.

11. Betof AS, Lascola CD, Weitzel D, Landon C, Scarbrough PM, Devi GR, et al. Modulation of murine breast tumor vascularity, hypoxia and chemotherapeutic response by exercise. *J Natl Cancer Inst* 107: 2015.

12. Bower JE. Cancer-related fatigue–mechanisms, risk factors, and treatments. *Nat Rev Clin Oncol* 11: 597–609, 2014.

13. Bray F, Ferlay J, Soerjomataram I, Siegel RL, Torre LA, Jemal A. Global cancer statistics 2018: GLOBOCAN estimates of incidence and mortality worldwide for 36 cancers in 185 countries. *CA Cancer J Clin* 68: 394–424, 2018.

14. Brown JC, Winters-Stone K, Lee A, Schmitz KH. Cancer, physical activity, and exercise. *Compr Physiol* 2: 2775–2809, 2012.

15. Brown JL, Rosa-Caldwell ME, Lee DE, Blackwell TA, Brown LA, Perry RA, et al. Mitochondrial degeneration precedes the development of muscle atrophy in progression of cancer cachexia in tumour-bearing mice. *J Cachexia Sarcopenia Muscle* 2017.

16. Burney BO, Garcia JM. Hypogonadism in male cancer patients. *J Cachexia Sarcopenia Muscle* 3: 149–155, 2012.

17. Carson JA, Hardee JP, VanderVeen BN. The emerging role of skeletal muscle oxidative metabolism as a biological target and cellular regulator of cancer-induced muscle wasting. *Semin Cell Dev Biol* 54: 53–67, 2016.

18. Carson JA, Manolagas SC. Effects of sex steroids on bones and muscles: similarities, parallels, and putative interactions in health and disease. *Bone* 80: 67–78, 2015.

19. Carson J, Puppa MJ. Biological pathways impacting cancer survival: exercise as a countermeasure for the development and progression of cachexia. In: *Exercise, Energy Balance, and Cancer*, edited by Ulrich CM, Steindorf K, and Berger NA. New York, NY: Springer, 2013, vol. 6, p. 59–82.

20. Cho KM, Park H, Oh DY, Kim TY, Lee KH, Han SW, et al. Skeletal muscle depletion predicts survival of patients with advanced biliary tract cancer undergoing palliative chemotherapy. *Oncotarget* 8: 79441–79452, 2017.

21. Colbert LH, Westerlind KC, Perkins SN, Haines DC, Berrigan D, Donehower LA, et al. Exercise effects on tumorigenesis in a p53-deficient mouse model of breast cancer. *Med Sci Sports Exerc* 41: 1597–1605, 2009.

22. Courneya KS, Friedenreich CM. Physical activity and cancer control. *Semin Oncol Nurs* 23: 242–252, 2007.

23. Cramp F, Byron-Daniel J. Exercise for the management of cancer-related fatigue in adults. *Cochrane Database Syst Rev* 11: CD006145, 2012.

24. Danaei G, Vander Hoorn S, Lopez AD, Murray CJ, Ezzati M. Comparative Risk Assessment Collaborating G. Causes of cancer in the world: comparative risk assessment of nine behavioural and environmental risk factors. *Lancet* 366: 1784–1793, 2005.

25. Denlinger CS, Barsevick AM. The challenges of colorectal cancer survivorship. *J Natl Compr Canc Netw* 7: 883–893; quiz 894, 2009.

26. Ding H, Jiang N, Liu H, Liu X, Liu D, Zhao F, et al. Response of mitochondrial fusion and fission protein gene expression to exercise in rat skeletal muscle. *Biochim Biophys Acta* 1800: 250–256, 2010.

27. Egan B, Zierath JR. Exercise metabolism and the molecular regulation of skeletal muscle adaptation. *Cell Metab* 17: 162–184, 2013.

28. Evans WJ, Morley JE, Argiles J, Bales C, Baracos V, Guttridge D, et al. Cachexia: a new definition. *Clin Nutr* 27: 793–799, 2008.

29. Fearon K, Strasser F, Anker SD, Bosaeus I, Bruera E, Fainsinger RL, et al. Definition and classification of cancer cachexia: an international consensus. *Lancet Oncol* 12: 489–495, 2011.

30. Ferioli M, Zauli G, Martelli AM, Vitale M, McCubrey JA, Ultimo S, et al. Impact of physical exercise in cancer survivors during and after antineoplastic treatments. *Oncotarget* 9: 14005–14034, 2018.

31. Ferlay J, Colombet M, Soerjomataram I, Mathers C, Parkin DM, Pineros M, et al. Estimating the global cancer incidence and mortality in 2018: GLOBOCAN sources and methods. *Int J Cancer* 144: 1941–1953, 2019.

32. Goh J, Kirk EA, Lee SX, Ladiges WC. Exercise, physical activity and breast cancer: the role of tumor-associated macrophages. *Exerc Immunol Rev* 18: 158–176, 2012.

33. Hanahan D, Weinberg RA. The hallmarks of cancer. *Cell* 100: 57–70, 2000.

34. Hanahan D, Weinberg RA. Hallmarks of cancer: the next generation. *Cell* 144: 646–674, 2011.

35. Hardee JP, Counts BR, Carson JA. Understanding the role of exercise in cancer cachexia therapy. *Am J Lifestyle Med* 13: 46–60, 2019.

36. Hardee JP, Counts BR, Gao S, VanderVeen BN, Fix DK, Koh HJ, et al. Inflammatory signalling regulates eccentric contraction-induced protein synthesis in cachectic skeletal muscle. *J Cachexia Sarcopenia Muscle* 9: 369–383, 2018.

37. Hardee JP, Montalvo RN, Carson JA. Linking cancer cachexia-induced anabolic resistance to skeletal muscle oxidative metabolism. *Oxid Med Cell Longev* 2017: 8018197, 2017.

38. Hetzler KL, Hardee JP, LaVoie HA, Murphy EA, Carson JA. Ovarian function's role during cancer cachexia progression in the female mouse. *Am J Physiol Endocrinol Metab* 312: E447–E459, 2017.

39. Hojman P, Gehl J, Christensen JF, Pedersen BK. Molecular mechanisms linking exercise to cancer prevention and treatment. *Cell Metab* 27: 10–21, 2018.

40. Iqbal S, Ostojic O, Singh K, Joseph AM, Hood DA. Expression of mitochondrial fission and fusion regulatory proteins in skeletal muscle during chronic use and disuse. *Muscle Nerve* 48: 963–970, 2013.

41. Jackman RW, Kandarian SC. The molecular basis of skeletal muscle atrophy. *Am J Physiol Cell Physiol* 287: C834–843, 2004.

42. Jheng HF, Tsai PJ, Guo SM, Kuo LH, Chang CS, Su IJ, et al. Mitochondrial fission contributes to mitochondrial dysfunction and insulin resistance in skeletal muscle. *Mol Cell Biol* 32: 309–319, 2012.

43. Jones LW, Antonelli J, Masko EM, Broadwater G, Lascola CD, Fels D, et al. Exercise modulation of the host-tumor interaction in an orthotopic model of murine prostate cancer. *J Appl Physiol (1985)* 113: 263–272, 2012.

44. Jones LW, Viglianti BL, Tashjian JA, Kothadia SM, Keir ST, Freedland SJ, et al. Effect of aerobic exercise on tumor physiology in an animal model of human breast cancer. *J Appl Physiol (1985)* 108: 343–348, 2010.

45. Joyner MJ, Green DJ. Exercise protects the cardiovascular system: effects beyond traditional risk factors. *J Physiol* 587: 5551–5558, 2009.

46. Jung HW, Kim JW, Kim JY, Kim SW, Yang HK, Lee JW, et al. Effect of muscle mass on toxicity and survival in patients with colon cancer undergoing adjuvant chemotherapy. *Support Care Cancer* 23: 687–694, 2015.

47. Kavazis AN, Smuder AJ, Powers SK. Effects of short-term endurance exercise training on acute doxorubicin-induced FoxO transcription in cardiac and skeletal muscle. *J Appl Physiol (1985)* 117: 223–230, 2014.

48. Kessels E, Husson O, van der Feltz-Cornelis CM. The effect of exercise on cancer-related fatigue in cancer survivors: a systematic review and meta-analysis. *Neuropsychiatr Dis Treat* 14: 479–494, 2018.

49. Koelwyn GJ, Quail DF, Zhang X, White RM, Jones LW. Exercise-dependent regulation of the tumour microenvironment. *Nat Rev Cancer* 17: 620–632, 2017.

50. Kushi LH, Doyle C, McCullough M, Rock CL, Demark-Wahnefried W, Bandera EV, et al., American Cancer Society N, Physical Activity Guidelines Advisory C. American Cancer Society guidelines on nutrition and physical activity for cancer prevention: reducing the risk of cancer with healthy food choices and physical activity. *CA Cancer J Clin* 62: 30–67, 2012.

51. McAllister SS, Weinberg RA. Tumor-host interactions: a far-reaching relationship. *J Clin Oncol* 28: 4022–4028, 2010.

52. McAllister SS, Weinberg RA. The tumour-induced systemic environment as a critical regulator of cancer progression and metastasis. *Nat Cell Biol* 16: 717–727, 2014.

53. McTiernan A. Mechanisms linking physical activity with cancer. *Nat Rev Cancer* 8: 205–211, 2008.

54. Mehl KA, Davis JM, Clements JM, Berger FG, Pena MM, Carson JA. Decreased intestinal polyp multiplicity is related to exercise mode and gender in ApcMin/+ mice. *J Appl Physiol (1985)* 98: 2219–2225, 2005.

55. Minton O, Stone P. A systematic review of the scales used for the measurement of cancer- related fatigue (CRF). *Ann Oncol* 20: 17–25, 2009.

56. Montalvo RN, Counts BR, Carson JA. Understanding sex differences in the regulation of cancer-induced muscle wasting. *Curr Opin Support Palliat Care* 12: 394–403, 2018.

57. Montalvo RN, Hardee JP, VanderVeen BN, Carson JA. Resistance exercise's ability to reverse cancer-induced anabolic resistance. *Exerc Sport Sci Rev* 46: 247–253, 2018.

58. Morrow GR, Andrews PL, Hickok JT, Roscoe JA, Matteson S. Fatigue associated with cancer and its treatment. *Support Care Cancer* 10: 389–398, 2002.

59. Mukherjee S. *The Emperor of All Maladies: A Biography of Cancer.* New York, NY: Scribner, 2010, p. xiv.

60. Murphy EA, Davis JM, Brown AS, Carmichael MD, Mayer EP, Ghaffar A. Effects of moderate exercise and oat beta-glucan on lung tumor metastases and macrophage antitumor cytotoxicity. *J Appl Physiol (1985)* 97: 955–959, 2004.

61. PAGAC. *Physical Activity Guidelines Advisory Committee Scientific Report.* Washington, DC: PAGAC, 2018.

62. Patel JG, Bhise AR. Effect of aerobic exercise on cancer-related fatigue. *Indian J Palliat Care* 23: 355–361, 2017.

63. Patel AV, Friedenrichs CM, Hayes SC, Silver JK, Cambell KL, Gerber LH, et al. American College of Sports Medicine Roundtable Report on Physical Activity, Sedentary Behavior, and Cancer Prevention and Control. *Med Sci Sports Exerc* In press: 2019.

64. Pedersen L, Christensen JF, Hojman P. Effects of exercise on tumor physiology and metabolism. *Cancer J* 21: 111–116, 2015.

65. Puppa MJ, White JP, Velazquez KT, Baltgalvis KA, Sato S, Baynes JW, et al. The effect of exercise on IL-6-induced cachexia in the Apc (Min/+) mouse. *J Cachexia Sarcopenia Muscle* 3: 117–137, 2012.

66. Ryan JL, Carroll JK, Ryan EP, Mustian KM, Fiscella K, Morrow GR. Mechanisms of cancer- related fatigue. *Oncologist* 12(Suppl 1): 22–34, 2007.

67. Schmitz KH, Courneya KS, Matthews C, Demark-Wahnefried W, Galvao DA, Pinto BM, et al., American College of Sports M. American College of Sports Medicine roundtable on exercise guidelines for cancer survivors. *Med Sci Sports Exerc* 42: 1409–1426, 2010.

68. Siegel R, Naishadham D, Jemal A. Cancer statistics, 2013. *CA Cancer J Clin* 63: 11–30, 2013.

69. Singal PK, Iliskovic N. Doxorubicin-induced cardiomyopathy. *N Engl J Med* 339: 900–905, 1998.

70. Spangenburg EE, Geiger PC, Leinwand LA, Lowe DA. Regulation of physiological and metabolic function of muscle by female sex steroids. *Med Sci Sports Exerc* 44: 1653–1662, 2012.

71. Stein KD, Syrjala KL, Andrykowski MA. Physical and psychological long-term and late effects of cancer. *Cancer* 112: 2577–2592, 2008.

72. Sweeney C, Schmitz KH, Lazovich D, Virnig BA, Wallace RB, Folsom AR. Functional limitations in elderly female cancer survivors. *J Natl Cancer Inst* 98: 521–529, 2006.

73. Thompson HJ, Jiang W, Zhu Z. Candidate mechanisms accounting for effects of physical activity on breast carcinogenesis. *IUBMB Life* 61: 895–901, 2009.

74. Tisdale MJ. Mechanisms of cancer cachexia. *Physiol Rev* 89: 381–410, 2009.

75. Ulrich CM, Steindorf K, Berger NA. *Exercise, Energy Balance, and Cancer.* New York, NY: Springer, 2013, p. vi.

76. WCRF/AICR. *Diet, Nutrition, Physical Activity and Cancer: A Global Perspective.* WCRF/AICR, 2018.

77. White JP, Baynes JW, Welle SL, Kostek MC, Matesic LE, Sato S, et al. The regulation of skeletal muscle protein turnover during the progression of cancer cachexia in the Apc(Min/+) mouse. *PLOS ONE* 6: e24650, 2011.

32

BIOCHEMISTRY OF EXERCISE TRAINING: EFFECTS ON BONE

Panagiota Klentrou and Rozalia Kouvelioti

Introduction

Osteoporosis is a disease characterized by low bone mass and micro-architectural deterioration of bone tissue leading to enhanced skeletal fragility and increased risk of fracture (26). Osteoporosis is more common among postmenopausal women as a result of hypogonadism (deficiency of reproductive hormones), with one in four women over the age of 50 being diagnosed with this disease. In comparison, only one in eight men suffer from osteoporosis, with 20–30% experiencing osteoporotic-related fractures (114).

Although bone loss is an inevitable part of ageing, the amount of peak bone mass (PBM) attained during growth and the subsequent rate of bone loss determine adult bone mineral status. In fact, achieving a high PBM throughout childhood to late adolescence is considered a critical preventive strategy against developing osteoporosis, whereas low PBM in early adulthood is considered a risk factor for osteoporosis and related fractures later in life (51). Since PBM is established by late adolescence for most sites of the skeleton (99), young adults have the unique opportunity to delay or prevent the onset of osteoporosis; effective preventive measures and positive health practices include sufficient calcium intake and adequate physical activity. Regular exercise in particular has been found to positively correlate with gains in bone mineral density (BMD) among pre-menopausal women. Exercise training has also been shown to have positive effects on bone in post-menopausal women, not only by decreasing the rate of bone loss but also by increasing site-specific (e.g., lumbar spine, femoral neck) BMD (155, 166).

In general, the osteogenic effect of exercise lies in the mechanical loading applied to the bone through the muscle contraction forces. In particular, high-impact activities are most likely to have beneficial effects on bone metabolism and health (73, 105). In high-impact exercise (e.g., running), added loading is also applied from the ground reaction forces, exerting larger mechanical loading on the skeleton compared to low-impact exercise such as swimming and cycling (102). Indeed, numerous studies have reported higher BMD in athletes of high-impact activities (e.g., gymnastics, basketball) compared to athletes of low- or no-impact activities (e.g., swimming, cycling) (73, 105). In addition, low-impact exercise performed at high intensity was recently found as leading to similar bone-related biochemical changes as high-impact exercise in both men and women (76, 77). This chapter will first describe the biochemical characteristics of bone tissue, followed by an examination of the biochemical and metabolic changes that occur in bone as a result of exercise training, which may mitigate the risk of osteoporosis.

Bone Physiology

Two types of bone are found in the body: cortical and trabecular bone. About 75–80% of the makeup of bones consists of compact tissue, while the remaining 20–25% is spongy tissue. Cortical tissue, which surrounds the marrow space of bones, comprises the strongest part of the bone and has supportive and protective properties (21). This type of bone tissue is dense, with well-defined periosteal and endosteal surfaces. The periosteum is the fibrous membrane, which covers the outer surfaces of bones (near the soft tissue), and the endosteum is the membrane that lines the internal cavities of bones (closer to the bone marrow). As a result of the low surface to volume ratio and small surface adjacent to the marrow, there is a low turnover rate in cortical bone (21), despite the cells along the portion of endosteal bone being metabolically active and involved in bone turnover. Cortical bone constantly remodels itself in response to changing mechanical and nonmechanical environmental signals and microdamage. The remodelling process in cortical bone consists of the removal of existing intracortical bone followed by the generation of new osteons (90).

Trabecular, or "spongy," bone is less dense, yet it is considered more metabolically active than compact bone (21). It has a large number of rod- or plate-shaped trabeculae, which form a sponge-like network of small pieces of bone separated by fatty or haematogenous marrow. As a result of the high surface to volume ratio and large surface adjacent to marrow, there is a high turnover rate in trabecular bone (90). Trabecular bone is found in the vertebrae, pelvis, and ends of long bones where more movement occurs, usually referring to the joint cavities.

Bone Cells

Bone is a dynamic tissue, which responds to various signals, including chemical, mechanical, electrical, and magnetic stimuli. Information is transferred across the cell's cytoplasm to the nucleus via binding of a signal ligand to either cell membrane receptors or intracellular receptors (cytoplasmic or nuclear, respectively). There are three types of bone cells: osteoblasts, osteocytes, and osteoclasts. Osteogenic cells are not specialized and derive from mesenchyme embryonic tissue, the tissue from which all connective tissues are formed (69). These cells differentiate into osteoblasts during bone development and repair, in the embryonic stage and in injury, respectively (21). Osteoblasts are the major bone formation cells that initiate calcification, regulate osteoclasts, make the extracellular matrix of bone tissue and produce osteoid, the uncalcified organic matrix of bone. Osteoblasts are approximately 15–30 microns in size and are cuboidal-shaped. They have a large nucleus localized in the bottom half of the cytoplasm, an abundant endoplasmic reticulum, enlarged Golgi apparati, and collagen-containing secretory vesicles. They are responsible for the laying down of new matrix (collagen and hydroxyapatite) on bone surfaces in the process of bone formation and play a critical role in the regulation of bone turnover. They also synthesize and secrete collagen protein to form the osteoid, which then becomes calcified through the depositing of hydroxyapatite by the osteoblasts (90).

Osteoblasts partly originate from the stroma located in the bone marrow adjacent to the endosteum or in the periosteum. Bone is produced as layers (lamellae) of calcified material surrounding blood vessels. Throughout matrix formation, some osteoblasts are left behind and become embedded in the new matrix within cavities called lacunae. These trapped osteoblasts convert into mature bone cells called osteocytes and are nourished by long, slender, cytoplasmic processes that extend from the cells to the blood vessels in canals called canaliculi. These cells can then receive and transmit mechanical signals to other bone cells (neighbouring osteocytes, surface osteoblasts, or lining cells). Osteocytes account for more than 90% of adult bone cells, live the longest (up to 25 years), and as mechanosensitive cells, play an important role in the maintenance of bone mass and structure (28, 127). Both osteoblasts and osteocytes play an active role in mineral homeostasis by helping to release calcium from bone into the blood, which regulates the concentration of calcium in body fluids. The osteocyte lifespan depends on the rate of bone turnover (90).

Osteoclasts, the third major type of bone cells, derive from hemopoietic stem cells and are found in the endosteum. These cells are involved in bone resorption (breakdown of the bone extracellular matrix) by releasing lysosomal enzymes and acids and by doing so breaking down the protein and mineral components of the underlying bone matrix (136). Further, there are multiple functional interconnections of osteocytes, with each other as well as with osteoblasts and osteoclasts and vasculature, allowing the osteocyte network to respond to musculoskeletal-derived mechanical stimuli and thereby affecting bone metabolism (127). The interconnection between osteocytes and bloodstream also allows the exposure of osteocytes to systemic messages from distant tissues. These messages are manifested by extracellular levels of minerals (e.g., inorganic phosphate) and endocrine hormones, mainly oestrogen, parathyroid hormone, and 1,25(OH)2D3 (127).

Bone Growth, Modelling, and Remodelling

Bone growth involves complex processes, which start before birth and continue until bones reach their final size and maturity in early adulthood (34). During childhood, bones grow in width-thickness (appositional growth) and length (interstitial growth) (136). While bones grow, formation exceeds bone resorption; this process ensures bone mass increases in order to reach its peak (82). PBM is an important parameter for skeletal health and relates to the risk of osteoporosis later in life (31, 34). Specifically, the higher the PBM achieved during early adulthood, the lower the risk of osteoporotic fractures later in elderly life. PBM has shown to explain 50% of the variance in BMD in 70-year-old post-menopausal women, while bone loss due to ageing accounts for the other 50%. The increase in bone mass is higher during the first 2 years of life and during puberty, with 25% of the final PBM being achieved over the adolescent growth spurt. PBM is achieved between the twenties and thirties and is higher in males than females (31).

Bone modelling occurs constantly, enabling bones to adapt to changes in (external) biomechanical forces by changing their morphology/shapes (21, 69). Bone remodelling is an ongoing process that takes place during the lifespan to replace old bone tissue and micro-damaged bone (due to normal daily activity) with new tissue (100). Bone remodelling involves the osteoclasts, osteoblasts, and osteocytes within the bone remodelling cavity and consists of cycles of bone resorption and bone formation, namely bone turnover (133). Bone resorption is the first phase in the remodelling cycle, with the osteoclasts synthesizing and releasing proteolytic enzymes. This results in the removal of minerals and collagen fibres from bone and the destruction of bone extracellular matrix osteoclasts. This phase lasts between 2 and 4 weeks in each remodelling cycle, and its duration is regulated by the apoptosis of osteoclasts (100, 133). Bone formation lasts 4 to 6 months with the osteoblasts synthesizing new bone extracellular matrix (133). About 5–10% of total body bone mass is going through this process of remodelling every year with each remodelling cycle lasting between 2 to 8 months (69). About 4% of compact bones and 20% of spongy bones are renewed every year, with different rates of remodelling in different regions of the body. New osteons are produced through this process of remodelling, providing storage of minerals required for various metabolic functions (136).

Bone remodelling sustains the structural integrity and strength of bones and allows the body to respond to external mechanical forces and molecular signals (19). This process controls the mineral density of bones and influences bone strength (21). Normally, there is a balance between bone resorption and bone formation (22, 133). However, when resorption is higher than formation, especially after 50 years of life (69), there is bone mass loss and micro-architectural deterioration. This process of bone remodelling can be assessed by circulating bone turnover (formation and resorption) markers, which will be reviewed later in the chapter.

Bone Turnover and Calcium Homeostasis

In understanding the pathophysiology of osteoporosis, bone turnover is an essential concept because it is this process which governs how bone is replaced, lost, or gained at certain sites and ultimately determines bone's three-dimensional structure (35). Bone turnover is considered a continuous process of constant removal and replacement of volumes of bone tissue, conducted by osteoclasts and osteoblasts, in both cortical and trabecular bone (35). Under normal conditions, the processes of bone formation and resorption are coupled to one another, and the maintenance of skeletal balance is achieved through the action of various hormones and local mediators (140). Osteoclasts burrow into bone, forming cavities where osteoblasts can deposit new bone resulting in the formation of new osteons. This process also results in the liberation of calcium and phosphate into the bloodstream. Bone homeostasis is achieved when the amount of bone resorbed is replaced by a similar amount of newly synthesized bone. A sustained increase in the ratio of osteoclast to osteoblast activity may eventually result in osteoporosis. Therefore, the activity of osteoclasts and osteoblasts is not only important in establishing the calcium and phosphate levels necessary for particular bodily functions but also in maintaining the structural integrity of bone.

Plasma calcium homeostasis is regulated by the activity of three hormones. These hormones include parathyroid hormone (PTH), calcitriol, and calcitonin, which work to regulate the activity of osteoclasts, osteoblasts, and renal/intestinal calcium absorption. PTH, secreted by the parathyroids, and calcitriol, a derivative of vitamin D, both cause an increase in serum calcium concentrations (140). They cause a decrease in osteoblast activity and increases in both osteoclast activity and renal/intestinal calcium absorption. Calcitonin is secreted by the C cells of the thyroid gland and has the opposite effect, in that it results in decreased serum calcium concentrations. Calcitonin increases osteoblast activity and decreases osteoclast activity and renal/intestinal calcium absorption (54).

Activation (conversion of bone surface area from quiescence to an active state) of bone in the adult skeleton can occur approximately every 10 seconds. In bone resorption, osteoclasts travel to sites of activation via circulation and either Volkmann or Haversian canals for intracortical turnover (35). In trabecular turnover, activation occurs at sites exposed to bone marrow. The time of completion of resorption to the initiation of bone formation at a particular site can take approximately 1 to 2 weeks and is known as the reversal phase. Chemotaxis and certain stimulators of proliferation determine whether osteoblasts will appear at the base of the resorption cavity (35). Bone formation, unlike bone resorption, is a two-step process. First, osteoid is synthesized and laid down at specific sites. Following deposition, osteoblasts begin to mineralize the newly formed protein matrix about 5 to 10 days later (35).

Bone Turnover and Oestrogen

Loss of bone mass starts in early adulthood, at approximately 50 years of age, and continues throughout adulthood (23, 33, 94). Bone loss is attributed to the uncoupling of bone resorption and bone formation (23, 33, 60). This decline in bone mass is amplified as women reach menopause (23, 142). Menopause is a natural process that occurs when a woman's menstrual cycle has ceased, leading to a loss of ovarian follicular function (40, 110, 115). Menopause tends to occur around 50 years of age; however, the timing varies among individuals (115). Menopause stems from the reduction or lack of circulating oestrogen (147). Oestrogen plays a crucial role in the development and regulation of the female reproductive system (80, 159). Oestrogen, more specifically oestradiol, is important for bone development and maintenance of BMD throughout various stages in life (80, 81). Oestrogen elicits a protective effect over the development and maintenance of bone through the inhibition of bone resorption (81). Oestrogen deficiency is correlated with longer osteoclast life and shorter osteoblast life (61, 65) Thus, a deficiency in circulating oestrogen in post-menopausal women may cause an increase in bone resorption through the promotion of prolonging osteoclastic activity (65). Oestrogen interacts with and affects multiple mechanisms with respect to bone turnover and development (81). Oestrogen represses osteoclastic cytokine production from immune cells (81, 157), increases osteoblast proliferation (while decreasing osteoblast and osteocyte apoptosis) (75), and induces osteoclast apoptosis (61).

Oestrogen also increases the sensitivity of bone to mechanical loading during the reproductive years, i.e., before menopause, through its influence on osteoblastic cells (39). During menopause, with oestrogen deficiency occurring, women experience an increase in bone resorption; this increase in bone resorption increases bone loss compared to bone replenishment, and therefore, compromises the skeletal structure. In turn, this causes an overall reduction in bone mass and mineralization (39, 66, 115, 147). The compromise to the skeletal system in post-menopausal women causes an increased risk of low BMD and an increased fragility and fracture rate. In short, a decrease in oestrogen lessens bone formation and increases the risk of bone deterioration, which leads to osteoporosis (66, 115). This effect indicates that women have a high risk of developing osteoporosis after menopause (115).

Biochemical Markers of Bone Metabolism

Bone Turnover Markers

Bone turnover markers (BTMs) are biochemical metabolites, including enzymes and non-enzymatic peptides, derived from cellular and non-cellular compartments of bone during the bone remodelling process; BTMs are measured and used in clinical practice. In contrast to other static measures involving imaging techniques such as dual energy x-ray absorptiometry (DXA), BTMs provide dynamic information about the bone status (34). BTMs reflect the metabolic activity of bone during remodelling. as they are quantitative, dynamic indicators of current bone turnover (100).

BTMs can be separated into (1) enzymes or proteins that take part in bone formation and resorption and (2) formation and resorption products (163). Thus, there are different BTMs, which reflect either bone formation or bone resorption (Table 32.1). Bone formation markers show the activity of osteoblasts during different stages of development from the actual formation of bone (collagen and non-collagen bone matrix formation) to the post-osteoid maturation and modification (152). To measure bone resorption, the markers of collagen degradation are most commonly used (152). According to the International Osteoporosis Foundation (IOF), the two bone turnover markers that should be measured in clinical studies in order to assess bone turnover are the amino-terminal propeptide of type I collagen (PINP) and the carboxyl-terminal crosslinking telopeptide of type I collagen (CTX) (152, 163). These markers measure the turnover of type I collagen, with PINP measuring collagen synthesis and CTX measuring collagen breakdown (152).

BTMs can be measured in blood (plasma, serum) and/or urine samples using specific biochemical assays (17, 20, 152). In addition, BTMs can respond to treatment quicker than BMD and thus can be used in shorter clinical trials measuring acute or short-term effects of different interventions, such as diet and exercise (19, 34, 156). The use of BTMs, however, has a few limitations; for example, they cannot be connected to specific skeletal sites (19, 156) and can be affected by a variety of factors such as hormones, nutrition, circadian rhythm, and the sensitivity and specificity of assays (144).

Osteokines and the Signalling Pathways

Osteokines are bone-derived cytokines that are produced by bone cells to regulate the metabolic activity of bone. In particular, osteocytes respond to mechanical loading by producing osteokines, which regulate osteoclast and osteoblast activation/differentiation via specific signalling pathways (165). These osteokines appear to also regulate peripheral tissues (i.e., muscle and adipose) and not just bone (45). The most well-known osteokines measured in humans are sclerostin, osteoprotegerin (OPG), and the receptor activator of nuclear factor kappa B ligand (RANKL).

Sclerostin

In humans, sclerostin is encoded by the *SOST* gene, and before birth, it is expressed in different tissues, e.g., heart and liver (104). Postnatally, the human protein sclerostin is secreted by osteocytes, which as mechanosensitive cells respond to mechanical loading/unloading and produce sclerostin in response to mechanical unloading (119). Studies have shown that sclerostin's expression (mRNA and protein levels)

Table 32.1 Bone turnover markers: Characteristics, role, and function

Bone formation markers*	Characteristics, role, and function
Procollagen I extension peptides: i N-terminal (PINP) ii C-terminal propeptide of type I collagen (PICP)	• Procollagen I extension peptides with either amino terminal (PINP) or carboxyl terminal (PICP) • Generated after proteolytic cleavage of type I collagen secreted from osteoblasts (100) • Reflect bone formation (7)
Bone-specific alkaline phosphatase (BAP)	• An alkaline phosphatase isoform synthesized in osteoblasts (100) • Involved in the mineralization and calcification of newly formed bone
Osteocalcin (OC)	• Produced by osteoblasts (144) and it is the main non-collagen protein found in bone matrix • It shows bone mineralization and bone formation • In some cases, OC may reflect bone resorption, as it is released during bone resorption (59); thus, it can be used as a marker of bone turnover (59)
Crosslinked telopeptides: i C-terminal cross-linking telopeptide of type I collagen (CTX) ii N-terminal cross-linking telopeptide of type I collagen (NTX) Collagen pyridinium crosslinks: i Deoxypyridinoline (Dpd) ii Pyridinoline (Pyr)	• Measure the degradation of collagen products induced by osteoclasts • Breakdown products released with cross-links still attached (carboxyl-terminal collagen cross-linking telopeptide CTX and amino-terminal crosslinking telopeptide NTX) (156) • Collagen crosslinks are small, cyclic amino structures that link collagen molecules via molecular bridges (100) • Dpd found mainly in bone while pyridinoline (Pyr) can also be found in cartilage, vessels, and ligaments • Pyridinium crosslinks are released into the circulatory system and urine during the breakdown of bone matrix and collagen (7, 100)

* (17, 20, 34, 144, 152)

decreases in response to mechanical loading both in vitro, in osteocytes under two-dimensional laminar shear stress for 3 days (141) and in vivo using ulnar loading in mice and rats for 1–2 consecutive days (123). In contrast, sclerostin (mRNA and protein) levels increased in response to mechanical unloading: hindlimb unloading via tail suspension in rodents for 3 consecutive days (123) and in osteocytes being in a simulated microgravity condition for 3 days (141). This osteocyte-specific glycoprotein (127) functions as a bone-specific cytokine (i.e., osteokine) triggering a negative feedback for osteoblast proliferation and function and thus leads to decreased bone formation (25, 104, 143). The main mechanism through which sclerostin exerts its effects is via inhibition of the Wnt canonical signalling pathway in osteocytes and osteoblasts (127). It has also been shown that sclerostin has indirect catabolic effects by promoting osteoclastic bone resorption via the RANK/RANKL pathway (143, 158, 162).

The Canonical Wnt Signalling Pathway

The Wnt signalling pathway is a multifaceted anabolic system that is involved in various organs and tissues, including bone (18, 79). The canonical Wnt signalling pathway is one of two Wnt signalling pathways (the β-catenin–dependent canonical and the independent non-canonical pathways) that play a potential role in bone remodelling/turnover in both physiological and pathological conditions (67, 71, 72). Specifically, Wnt signalling inhibits (-) the differentiation of mesenchymal stem cells (MSCs) into adipocytes and chondrocytes, while it promotes the differentiation of these cells into osteoblasts (67, 82).

Biologically, the canonical Wnt signalling pathway can be defined as a pathway dependent on the stabilization of β-catenin protein (11, 18). Downstream activation of the Wnt pathway begins with the Wnt ligand molecule binding to the low-density lipoprotein-related receptor 5 and low-density lipoprotein-related receptor 6 (LRP5 or LRP6) or a frizzled transmembrane receptor. The binding of the Wnt molecule activates the protein dishevelled (Dsh), triggering downstream phosphorylation of glycogen synthase kinase-3β (GSK-3β), which inhibits GSK-3β from phosphorylating β-catenin (11). The inhibition of GSK-3β facilitates β-catenin to initiate nuclear translocation, which targets gene transcription and leads to bone formation (11, 18). This occurs as β-catenin is building up within the cytoplasm and able to reach its threshold, allowing β-catenin to enter the nucleus of the cell. The Wnt pathway stimulates the process of cell proliferation, renewal of stem cells, stimulation of pre-osteoblast replication, and enhancement of osteoblast activity, increasing the bone mass and functionality of bone cells (11, 79). Thus, the Wnt signalling pathway is a complex anabolic mechanism that is involved in a diverse process to develop bone mass (79). Furthermore, Wnt signalling is an important regulator of the production and secretion of OPG (96), which is secreted by osteoblasts to inhibit the catabolic RANK/RANKL pathway, ultimately reducing osteoclast differentiation, and therefore bone resorption (2, 111).

Wnt signalling can be inhibited by sclerostin, resulting in reduced expression of bone formation genes (67, 82, 103, 121). Briefly, sclerostin binds to LRP 4 (139, 158), LRP 5, and LRP 6, thus preventing the Wnt-LRP 5/6–frizzled interaction. Sclerostin's binding to lipoprotein receptor proteins leads to the release of the GSK3/Axin/APC protein complex into the cytosol, causing the phosphorylation of β-catenin and its degradation by proteasome (67, 82, 103, 121, 143). In contrast, Wnt signalling is active in the absence of sclerostin and other Wnt antagonists. In this case, Wnt glycoproteins bind to frizzled receptors and LRP 5/6 co-receptors to form a complex. This causes recruitment of axin into the intracellular domain of the receptor complex and disruption of the APC–axin–GSK3–catenin complex by Dsh, leading to the accumulation of β-catenin in the cytosol. As explained earlier, β-catenin translocates to the nucleus and in association with the T-cell factor/lymphoid enhancer-binding factor (TCF/LEF), activates the expression of response genes related to bone formation (e.g., OPG) (104, 121).

Sclerostin can also increase the RANKL expression by osteocytes via a RANKL-dependent pathway, leading to increased bone resorption (158). Further, even though sclerostin has been characterized as the strongest antagonist of the Wnt signalling pathway, there are two other antagonist molecules in this pathway: secreted frizzled-related protein (SFRP) and Dickkopf-related protein 1 (DKK1). SFRP binds to LRP 5/6 and Kremen, resulting in the removal of LRP 5/6 from the membrane (104). DKK1 is expressed by both the osteocytes and the osteoblasts, as it regulates the activity of the osteoblastic cells (62, 108). Similarly to sclerostin, DKK1 binds to the LRP-5/6 receptor inhibiting the Wnt molecule from binding (62). However, it is less selective than sclerostin, and its function has been highlighted during bone growth and repair (127). Elevated serum DKK1 concentrations have been observed to enhance osteoclastogenesis, increasing the activity of osteoclastic cells (93). According to a study which examined the mechanical loading effects on Wnt signalling in rodents, sclerostin was mainly reduced after mechanical stimulation in the rodent ulna, while DKK1 showed minimal changes and SFRP expression did not show any changes after the mechanical loading (123). These results indicate that sclerostin responds more to mechanical loading than the other two antagonists of Wnt signalling–related bone formation.

The RANK/RANKL Pathway

The RANKL/RANK pathway is known for its roles in osteoclast maturation, bone modelling, and bone remodelling. Receptor activator of NF-kB (RANK), RANKL, and OPG are the main components of this signalling system. Interestingly, taking part in bone haemostasis is not the only effect of this pathway (13).

RANKL is a homotrimeric protein produced by osteoblasts and other cells, including activated T cells (63, 145, 154). The secreted type of RANKL is a result of proteolytic division or alternative splicing on the membrane form. Matrix metalloproteases (MMP3 or 7) and ADAM (a disintegrin and metalloprotease domain) are responsible for RANKL proteolytic cleavage (55, 95). RANKL, which is secreted by pre-osteoblasts, osteoblasts, osteocytes, and periosteal cells (24, 107, 137), activate RANK that is expressed by osteoclasts and its precursors (58). RANKL has assignments for stimulating pre-osteoclast differentiation (85), adherence osteoclasts to bone tissue and their following activation (85, 88), and maintenance (88).

RANKL is secreted by many tissues, including the osteoclast, and is a marker of bone resorption that is necessary to osteoclast function (60, 74) by promoting differentiation of osteoclast precursors into mature osteocytes (64), as well as through the induction of osteoclast activation (150). When RANKL binds to its associated receptor RANK on osteoclast precursors, it allows osteoclast differentiation and function to be enhanced (2, 111). RANKL stimulates the fusion of osteoclasts to bone and subsequently promotes their activation and survival (74, 111), as well as promoting osteocyte apoptosis (60).

Uninhibited Wnt signalling is an important regulator of the production and secretion of the anabolic OPG (96). OPG prevents osteoclast differentiation and activity and accelerates osteoclast apoptosis by acting as a decoy receptor for RANKL (64, 150). In animal studies, increases in OPG levels have been associated with a decreased osteoclast number, as well as enhanced bone strength and bone density (74). In addition to osteoblasts, there are plenty of cells that could express OPG, such as those in the heart, liver, spleen, and kidney. One study suggested that B cells are in charge of 64% of bone marrow OPG expression (89). OPG belongs to the TNF superfamily, and as such plays an anti-osteoclastogenesis role with binding to RANKL (86). OPG takes part as a decoy receptor for RANKL and inhibits RANKL–RANK binding. In fact, several agents that induce RANKL influence OPG regulation (14, 57). Recent studies have shown increases in plasma OPG levels in post-menopausal women lead to bone mass reinforcement (88).

The ratio of OPG to RANKL is a critical regulator of osteoclast function and bone resorption (2). Although increased levels of RANKL are associated with increased bone resorption, the presence of RANKL alone is insufficient to stimulate resorption independently. In order for bone resorption to be mediated by RANKL, there needs to be an associated decrease in OPG (60), which is secreted by the osteoblasts in order to up-regulate the OPG/RANKL ratio leading to a suppression of osteoclastogenesis (113, 164). Thus, it is suggested that the conclusive determinant of bone turnover is indeed the RANKL/OPG ratio. Most of the time it is both RANKL up-regulation and OPG down-regulation that lead to bone loss (74). In addition, the elimination of RANKL and RANK in animal studies shows a major effect in inhibiting bone mass loss and osteoporosis, while enhancing OPG concentrations in plasma has been shown to lead to increases in BMD in post-menopausal women (138).

Several endogenous factors affect the control of the RANKL to RANK binding, including inflammatory cytokines (TNF- a, IL-1, IL-6, IL-4, IL-11, and IL-17), hormones (vitamin D, oestrogen, glucocorticoids), and mesenchymal transcription factors (57, 106). In addition to the Wnt signalling pathway, OPG is regulated by cytokines, hormones, and growth factors (13, 27, 43, 146).

Exercise and Bone Metabolism

Exercise and Bone Mineral Density

There are various ways to protect the skeleton from disease and resorption, or at least delay the onset of such disorders. For example, physical activity, a healthy diet, and medical intervention can aid in the prevention of age-related bone loss or osteoporosis (126). Several medications, such as bone resorption inhibitors and bone formation stimulators, are indicated in post-menopausal treatment regimens (16). These include bisphosphonates (e.g., alendronate) (10), strontium ranelate, denosumab (a RANKL inhibitor) (50), and PTH (116). A potential limitation for this kind of treatment is the risk of complications such as fever or muscle pain (1, 44). Having a proper regimen that is nutrient-dense is one of the major strategies in saving and augmenting bone mass. Vitamin D, calcium, phosphorus, magnesium, zinc, and copper are some examples of micronutrients that can positively affect bone (87, 128).

Exercise is considered the most influential non-pharmacological method for improving or maintaining bone mass (3, 153). Exercise is both a preventive and a therapeutic strategy to improve BMD and work against the weakening of bone due to natural ageing processes (97). During exercise, the various stresses on the body induce mechanical loading (jumping, running, resistance training etc.), which allows bone to initiate the bone remodelling process. However, not all exercise modalities and intensities are equally efficient in increasing bone mass (41). Furthermore, there are uncertainties with respect to the intensity, duration, and frequency of exercise that elicit an optimal osteogenic exercise response (9). Mechanical strain, as a result of physical activity, causes bone to react and initiate bone remodelling in favour of bone formation. Bone structure and strength must be able to endure the mechanical forces of everyday life to avoid the fracture or deterioration of bone mass (41) and allow bone tissue to experience the higher mechanical forces which increase bone mass during physical activity (48).

It is well established that individuals of all ages and sexes who participate in sports or physical exercise have higher bone mass, bone strength, and a greater osteogenic potential compared to individuals who are not physically active (4, 32, 129). In particular, individuals of all ages and sexes who participate in high-impact dynamic sports which apply various directional impacts have a higher osteogenic response compared to other individuals participating in less impactful exercise (32). For example, plyometric exercise encompasses explosive jumping and mechanical force that can generate force up to seven times an individual's body weight (48). Due to the high mechanical load on bone, which activates bone remodelling, plyometric exercise is considered the most valued modality of exercise for improving bone mass. Previously, one study has shown positive changes in bone mass and reduction in the deterioration of BMD in a population of post-menopausal women as a result of a plyometric exercise intervention (148). However, there are limited data in older populations, including post-menopausal women, on the bone response to acute plyometric exercise protocols.

Exercise and Markers of Bone Turnover

Many observations have been made in terms of acute exercise and its impact on BTMs. These observations have shown that response may vary with respect to type, duration, and intensity of exercise (30, 38, 167). Therefore, the influence that an acute exercise bout has on BTMs is not well understood. Despite variations among studies, some collective conclusions can still be made. The magnitude of stimulation for both osteoclasts and osteoblasts is dependent on mode and intensity, as well as on the duration of exercise, which demonstrates differences in both the immediate and delayed effects of exercise on BTMs (7, 36, 52, 122, 134, 149, 151). Furthermore, sex and age differences are indicated in various studies, showing that exercise does not influence BTMs in the same magnitude amongst different populations. For example, males and females exhibit a different response to an exercise stimulus, while there seems to be an age variation within the same sex in response to the same exercise protocol (30, 38, 48, 76, 77).

In addition, not all exercise protocols and durations elicit the same response even within the same age and sex. Specifically, there is inconsistency regarding the effects of acute resistance exercise, aerobic exercise, and plyometric exercise on BTMs. In response to resistance exercise, there is a general trend for bone formation markers to remain unchanged and bone resorption markers to decrease (6, 124, 160). Endurance running, ranging from 30 minutes to full marathons, typically has been shown to result in increased levels of bone formation and resorption markers (15, 92, 130, 131, 167). Non-weight-bearing exercises, such as cycling, do not have a clear response, with some studies reporting increases in both bone formation and resorption markers and others reporting no changes (49, 118, 125, 155). A few studies examining the effects of a single bout of plyometric exercise on BTMs led to inconsistent results. Lin et al. (91) observed an increase in OC and no change in TRAP, while Rogers et al. (124) observed no change in both BAP and OC and an increase in TRAP and CTX. In addition, a single exercise session consisting of high mechanical loading (144 jumps) in boys and young men reported that although boys demonstrated an increase 24 hours post-exercise, no such increase was observed in men. NTX levels were also higher in boys, with a greater increase over time than in men, suggesting that one session of plyometric exercise stimulated bone turnover in boys, but not in men (68). In general, children demonstrate a clear increase in circulating BTMs in response to high-impact exercise irrespective of sex (30, 68). In contrast, PINP did not change in response to high-intensity interval running or cycling in young adults, although CTX increased following both trials in men, but not in women (76, 77).

In terms of exercise training, results are summarized in Table 32.2. An interesting study by Erickson and Vukovich (36) examined the response of bone markers (BAP and CTX) to two 8-week plyometric training protocols of the same total number of jumps delivered three times per week, but either once a day or twice a day. The results indicated a trend towards the group jumping twice a day to have higher levels of bone formation marker (BAP) suggesting that a recovery period may restore mechanosensitivity and allow for an osteogenic effect (36). However, there was no significant change in the bone resorption marker (CTX) following jumping training. Further, the results are not consistent across studies either in men or women (Table 32.2). For example, Shibata et al. (135) found no changes in osteocalcin (OC) or NTX following 12 months of walking or walking + jumping, but BAP increased in both groups but was much more pronounced in the walking + jumping group (135). Vainionpaa et al. (151) examined the effects of an impact exercise protocol of three times a week over a period of 12 months in middle-aged women and reported no effect on either bone formation or bone resorption markers (151). Likewise, Wieczorek-Baranowska (161) found a decrease in OC after 8 weeks of cycling in postmenopausal women, while Arwadi et al. (5) reported that OC increased after 8 weeks of multimode exercise training in healthy women. Therefore, the bone turnover response to exercise training is highly dependent on the exercise mode, duration, and intensity, as well as on the age and sex of participants.

Exercise and Osteokines

Exercise and Sclerostin

Previous in vivo (animal models) and in vitro studies have shown that mechanical loading results in decreased sclerostin levels, whereas mechanical unloading results in increased levels (123, 141). This decrease in sclerostin after loading is a crucial step to promote osteogenesis. Failure to down-regulate sclerostin after loading impedes the activation of the Wnt pathway and therefore osteoblast activity is not increased (67). In humans, the few studies that have examined the response of sclerostin to exercise-induced mechanical loading provided consistent evidence that sclerostin increases post-exercise (38, 76–78). Specifically, the transient exercise-induced increase in sclerostin was found following both high-impact and low-impact high-intensity exercise in young adults (38, 76–78). In contrast, in spite of having a lower resting concentration, children do not display this post-exercise increase in sclerostin (30, 38, 70); however, children who had excess adiposity have showed a post-exercise increase in sclerostin similar to adults (84). Additionally, it has recently been shown that the acute post-exercise increase in sclerostin appears to be mediated by inflammatory cytokines, and in particular tumour necrosis factor alpha (TNF-α) independent of the impact of exercise (78). Overall, these results highlight the potential role of inflammation on the post-exercise bone homeostasis in humans.

It has also been suggested the post-exercise increase in sclerostin might be related to an acute, transient decrease in the systemic energy availability due to exercise, which would lead to a short-term inhibition of Wnt signalling in bone, as well as in peripheral tissues. Other transient catabolic responses to exercise related to muscle activity, physical stress, and inflammation have also been reported in athletes in relation to sclerostin (46, 83) and in non-athletes in relation to bone formation and resorption markers (101). For example, sclerostin increased consistently and markedly during a 3-week cycling race, suggesting a link between increased muscle activity and increased bone catabolism induced by the physical stress in absence of impact (46). On the other hand, postmenopausal women do not show the

Table 32.2 Studies examining bone turnover markers and osteokine levels in response to exercise training

Reference	Population	Training	Results	Conclusions
(5)	58 healthy women 62 controls	8 weeks of exercise training (including walking, running, cycling etc), 2h/4 d/wk	↓ sclerostin ↑ PINP ↑ BAP ↑ OC ↑ CTX	Exercise training led to a decrease in sclerostin and to increases in bone turnover markers
(8)	48 post-menopausal women 44 controls	1 year of walking 30 min, 3 d/wk +1h aerobic/strength training, 1–2 d/wk	↔ sclerostin ↔ RANKL ↔ CTX ↔ BAP ↑ OPG	Exercise training balanced bone turnover and increased OPG to reduce RANKL signalling
(29)	21 overweight and obese men and women	6 months of aerobic training 4 h/wk	↔ OPG ↔ RANKL ↓ BAP	Exercise training did not lead to changes in OPG or RANKL
(36)	14 young males 7 controls	8 weeks of jumping training (once or twice per day)	↑ BAP ↔ CTX	Exercise training led to an increase in BAP, with greater increase in jumping twice per day, but no changes in CTX
(37)	27 middle aged (40–60 years) males 13 controls	10 weeks of walking training (50 min/day, 5 days/week, high or moderate intensity)	↔ OPG ↓ RANKL	High intensity walking led to significant decrease in RANKL, but no changes in OPG
(98)	47 healthy older men and women (mean age 68.2 years)	32 weeks of resistance exercise training (60 min/day, 3 days/week)	↔ OC ↔ CTX ↔ OPG ↔ RANKL	Exercise training did not lead to changes in OC, CTX, OPG, and RANKL
(97)	47 post-menopausal females 24 controls	8 months of either resistance or aerobic training (60 min/day, 3 days/week)	↔ OPG ↔ RANKL	Exercise training did not lead to changes in OPG and RANKL
(135)	28 healthy pre-menopausal women	12 months of walking or walking and jumping training	↑ BAP ↔ OC ↔ NTX	Exercise training led to an increase in BAP with greater increase in the walking and jogging group, but not changes in OC and NTX
(151)	60 healthy women 60 controls	12 months of high impact exercise (e.g., jumping, running and walking), 1h/3d/wk	↔ PINP ↔ TRACP5b	Exercise training did not lead to changes in PINP, TRACP5b
(161)	27 post-menopausal women	8 weeks on cycle-ergometer 70–80% workload 40 min, 3 d/wk	↔ OPG ↔ CTX ↓ OC	Regular exercise led to a decrease in OC, with no changes in OPG

same post-exercise increase in sclerostin (109), potentially due to ageing-induced changes in the shape and density of the osteocyte lacuna–canalicular network.

Specifically, there is evidence that the osteocyte lacunae become smaller and more spherical and their number density is reduced with ageing. These changes in the morphology and density of the osteocyte lacuna–canalicular network could lead to alterations in the osteocyte mechanosensitivity and response to mechanical loading (53). It is also possible that post-menopausal bones do synthesize sclerostin but have fewer cells or a degraded infrastructure for releasing this sclerostin after exercise. Alternatively, the increase in circulating sclerostin may be related to the recently suggested endocrine role of osteocytes and osteocyte-derived factors in energy and glucose metabolism (112) and in beige adipogenesis (42). In addition, recent findings from our lab show an increase in sclerostin post-exercise in adolescent girls with excess adiposity, while normal-weight girls do not exhibit a sclerostin increase (84). Thus, given the response of sclerostin to increased energy demands at rest and during exhaustive exercise, as well as the increase observed in young girls with excess adiposity, it is also interesting to hypothesize that adiposity may be mediating a potential bone–adipose tissue crosstalk that could be driven by either adiposity, inflammation, or a combination of the two.

Very few exercise training studies have measured sclerostin over time, providing little evidence that sclerostin is affected by various modes of exercise training in men and women (Table 32.2). In fact, the two existing studies reported contradicting results; Arwadi et al. (5) reported that sclerostin increased after 8 weeks of multimode exercise training in healthy women, while Bergström et al. (8) found no changes in sclerostin after 1 year of walking combined with aerobic/strength training in post-menopausal women. One study followed elite female rowers across a training year and showed that when training load (intensity and volume) was highest, serum sclerostin was also highest, and during tapering (low training load), serum sclerostin was the lowest (83). Furthermore, the fluctuation in sclerostin paralleled changes in inflammatory markers, including TNF-α and interleukins 6 and 1β (IL-6, IL-1β). Taken together, this data suggest that in children, the osteogenic response to exercise is mediated by an inhibition of osteoclastogenesis, whereas in adults, intense exercise and periods of intense training can lead to an inhibition of Wnt signalling through the increase in sclerostin, potentially mediated by inflammation.

Exercise, OPG, and RANKL

It has been shown that exercise decreases osteoclastogenesis through changes in the RANK/RANKL pathway (164). For example, treadmill training and vibration stimulation have been shown to result in a decrease in RANKL expression and an increase in OPG expression, leading to an overall reduction in RANKL-induced bone loss in osteoporotic rats (117). However, human studies examining the effects of an acute bout of exercise on OPG and RANKL are limited. Ziegler et al. (167) measured the serum levels of OPG and RANKL following either a 15-km run or a 42-km run, and it was found that OPG increased in those running the longer distance and RANKL decreased in both distances, but to a further extent in the longer distance (167). High-intensity interval cycling has been shown to result in an increase in both OPG and RANKL in young men (101). In addition, while children show an increase in OPG and a decrease in RANKL concentration following acute high-impact exercise, this is not seen in adults (30, 68).

The responsiveness of OPG to exercise training also appears to be exercise mode and sex specific. A study in older adults performing 32 weeks of resistance exercise training 3 days/week found no change in OPG and RANKL (98). Furthermore, Marques et al. (97) also showed that 8 months of either resistance or aerobic training in post-menopausal women resulted in no change in serum levels of OPG or RANKL, albeit BMD increased post-training. In a study that assessed the effect of a walking training programme 50 min/day, 5 days/week for 10 weeks in middle-aged men, no change was found in OPG, but RANKL levels decreased (37). In contrast, a few other studies have shown that OPG does respond to various modes and volumes of exercise training. Bergstrom et al. (8) assessed the effect of moderate training 3 days/week in post-menopausal women and found OPG increased along with BMD at the hip when compared to non-exercising controls. In addition, the increased BMD was only associated with an increase in OPG and was independent of changes in sclerostin or RANKL. In contrast, no change in OPG levels despite positive body composition changes were found following exercise training in obese and overweight patients performing aerobic exercise 4 hours/week for 6 months (29). Also, when post-menopausal women trained on a cycle-ergometer at 70–80% of workload 40 min, 3 days/week for 8 weeks there was no change in OPG levels, although there was a decrease in OC following training (Table 32.2).

Summary and Conclusions

Bone biochemistry involves complex processes, which start before birth and continue until bones reach their final size and maturity in early adulthood. Regular exercise has been associated with higher BMD in men and pre-menopausal women and has been shown to have positive effects on bone in post-menopausal women, mainly by decreasing the rate of bone loss. The osteogenic effect of exercise lies in the mechanical loading applied to the bone through muscle contraction forces. It is well established that individuals of all ages and sexes who participate in sports or physical exercise have higher bone mass, bone strength, and greater osteogenic potential compared to individuals who are not physically active. In addition, high-impact exercise is believed to have augmented beneficial effects on bone metabolism due to the added loading from ground reaction forces, exerting larger mechanical loading on the skeleton compared to low-impact activities. This high mechanical load on bone activates bone remodelling, which can be assessed by measuring the circulating levels of BTMs. However, not all exercise protocols and durations will elicit the same response even within the same age and sex. Specifically, there is inconsistency regarding the effects of acute resistance exercise, aerobic exercise, and plyometric exercise on BTMs, although the general trend is for bone formation markers to remain unchanged and bone resorption markers to decrease, which is why no one particular exercise regimen is recommended above others for the mitigation of osteoporosis. In fact, walking continuous to be the simpler, safest, and more economic exercise recommendation for older adults, while plyometrics should remain part of the exercise recommendations for younger populations. Likewise, exercise training has been shown to decrease osteoclastogenesis through changes in the RANK/RANKL pathway, but the results are age and sex dependent. Other factors, including energy availability, calcium stores, and oestrogen, may influence the bone adaptation to exercise, but more research is needed to shed light on these effects and the cellular mechanisms associated with bone turnover.

References

1. Alami S, Hervouet L, Poiraudeau S, Briot K, Roux C. Barriers to effective postmenopausal osteoporosis treatment: a qualitative study of patients' and practitioners' views. *PLOS ONE* 11(6), 2016.
2. An J, Yang H, Zhang Q, Liu C, Zhao J, Zhang L, et al. Natural products for treatment of osteoporosis: the effects and mechanisms on promoting osteoblast-mediated bone formation. *Life Sciences* 147: 46–58, 2016.
3. Arab Ameri E, Dehkhoda MR, Hemayattalab R. Bone mineral density changes after physical training and calcium intake in students with attention deficit and hyper activity disorders. *Res Dev Disabil* 33(2): 594–599, 2012.
4. Arasheben A, Barzee KA, Morley CP. A meta-analysis of bone mineral density in collegiate female athletes. *JABFM* 24(6): 728–734, 2011.
5. Ardawi MSM, Rouzi AA, Qari MH. Physical activity in relation to serum sclerostin, insulin-like growth factor-1, and bone turnover markers in healthy premenopausal women: a cross-sectional and a longitudinal study. *J Clin Endocrinol Metab* 97(10): 3691–3699, 2012.
6. Ashizawa N, Ouchi G, Fujimura R, Yoshida Y, Tokuyama K, Suzuki M. Effects of a single bout of resistance exercise on calcium and bone metabolism in untrained young males. *Calcif Tissue Int* 62(2): 104–108, 1998.
7. Banfi G, Lombardi G, Colombini A, Lippi G. Bone metabolism markers in sports medicine. *Sports Med* 40(8): 697–714, 2010.
8. Bergström I, Parini P, Gustafsson SA, Andersson G, Brinck J. Physical training increases osteoprotegerin in postmenopausal women. *J Bone Miner Metab* 30(2): 202–207, 2012.
9. Bielemann RM, Martinez-Mesa J, Gigante DP. Physical activity during life course and bone mass: a systematic review of methods and findings from cohort studies with young adults. *BMC Musculoskelet Disord* 14(1): 77, 2013
10. Boivin GY, Chavassieux PM, Santora AC, Yates J, Meunier PJ. Alendronate increases bone strength by increasing the mean degree of mineralization of bone tissue in osteoporotic women. *Bone* 27(5): 687–694, 2000.
11. Bonewald LF, Johnson ML. Osteocytes, mechanosensing and Wnt signaling. *Bone* 42(4): 606–615, 2008.
12. Boyce BF, Xing L. Biology of RANK, RANKL, and osteoprotegerin. *Arthritis Res Ther* 9 (Suppl 1): S1, 2007.

13. Boyce BF, Xing L. Functions of RANKL/RANK/OPG in bone modeling and remodeling. *Arch Biochem Biophys* 473(2): 139–146, 2008.

14. Boyle WJ, Simonet WS, Lacey DL. Osteoclast differentiation and activation. *Nature* 423(6937): 337–342, 2003.

15. Brahm H, Piehl-Aulin K, Ljunghall S. Biochemical markers of bone metabolism during distance running in healthy, regularly exercising men and women. *Scand J Med Sci Sportss* 6(1): 26–30, 2007.

16. Brar KS. Prevalent and emerging therapies for osteoporosis. *Med J Armed Forces India* 66(3): 249–254, 2010.

17. Brown JP, Albert C, Nassar BA, Adachi JD, Cole D, Davison KS, et al. Bone turnover markers in the management of postmenopausal osteoporosis. *Clin Biochem* 42(10–11): 929–942, 2009.

18. Burgers TA, Williams BO. Regulation of Wnt/beta-catenin signaling within and from osteocytes. *Bone* 54(2): 244–249, 2013.

19. Calvo M, Eyre D, Gundberg C. Molecular basis and clinical application of biological markers of bone turnover. *Endocr Rev* 17(4): 333–368, 1996.

20. Civitelli R, Armamento-Villareal R, Napoli N. Bone turnover markers: understanding their value in clinical trials and clinical practice. *Osteoporos Int* 20(6): 843–851, 2009.

21. Clarke, B. Normal bone anatomy and physiology. *Clin J Am Soc Nephrol* 13 Suppl 3: S131–139, 2008.

22. Clowes JA, Riggs BL, Khosla, S. The role of the immune system in the pathophysiology of osteoporosis. *Immuno Rev* 208(1): 207–227, 2005.

23. Cohn SH, Vaswani A, Zanzi I, Ellis KJ. Effect of aging on bone mass in adult women. *Am J Physiol* 230(1): 143–148, 1976.

24. Collin-Osdoby P. Regulation of vascular calcification by osteoclast regulatory factors RANKL and osteoprotegerin. *Circ Res* 95(11): 1046–1057, 2004.

25. Compton JT, Lee FY. A review of osteocyte function and the emerging importance of sclerostin. *J Bone Joint Surg Am* 96(19): 1659–1668, 2014.

26. Consensus development conference: prophylaxis and treatment of osteoporosis. *Osteoporos Int* 1(2): 114–117, 1991.

27. Cundy T, Hegde M, Naot D, Chong B, King A, Wallace R, et al. A mutation in the gene TNFRSF11B encoding osteoprotegerin causes an idiopathic hyperphosphatasia phenotype. *Hum Mol Genet* 11(18): 2119–2127, 2002.

28. Datta HK, Ng WF, Walker JA, Tuck SP, Varanasi SS. The cell biology of bone metabolism. *J Clin Pathol* 61(5): 577–587, 2008.

29. Davenport C, Kenny H, Ashley DT, O'Sullivan EP, Smith D, O'Gorman DJ. The effect of exercise on osteoprotegerin and TNF-related apoptosis-inducing ligand in obese patients. *Eur J Clin Invest* 42(11): 1173–1179, 2012.

30. Dekker J, Nelson K, Kurgan N, Falk B, Josse A, Klentrou P. Wnt signaling-related osteokines and transforming growth factors before and after a single bout of plyometric exercise in child and adolescent females. *Pediatr Exer Sci* 22: 1–29, 2017.

31. Dennison EM, Harvey NC, Cooper C. Programming of osteoporosis and impact on osteoporosis risk. *Clin Obstet Gynecol* 56(3): 549–555, 2013.

32. Dias Quiterio AL, Canero EA, Baptista FM, Sardinha LB. Skeletal mass in adolescent male athletes and nonathletes: Relationships with high-impact sports. *J Strength Cond Res* 25(12): 3439–3447, 2011.

33. Emaus N, Berntsen GKR, Joakimsen RM, Fønnebø V. Longitudinal changes in forearm bone mineral density in women and men aged 25-44 years: The Tromsø study: a population-based study. *Am J Epidemiol* 162(7): 633–43, 2005.

34. Eapen E, Grey V, Don-Wauchope A, Atkinson SA. Bone health in childhood: usefulness of biochemical biomarkers. *EJIFCC* 19(2): 123–136, 2008.

35. Einhorn TA. Bone strength: the bottom line. *Calcif Tissue Int* 51(5): 333–339, 1992.

36. Erickson CR, Vukovich MD. Osteogenic index and changes in bone markers during a jump training program: a pilot study. *Med Sci Sports Exer* 42(8): 1485–1492, 2010.

37. Esen H, Bueyuekyazi G, Ulman C, Taneli F, Ari Z, Goezluekaya F, et al. Do walking programs affect C-reactive protein, osteoprotegerin and soluble receptor activator of nuclear factor-kappaβ ligand? *Turkish K Biochem* 34: 178–186, 2009.

38. Falk B, Haddad F, Klentrou P, Ward W, Kish K, Mezil Y, et al. Differential sclerostin and parathyroid hormone response to exercise in boys and men. *Osteoporos Int* 27(3): 1245–1249, 2016.

39. Fonseca H, Moreira-Gonçalves D, Amado F, Esteves JL, Duarte JA. Skeletal deterioration following ovarian failure: can some features be a direct consequence of estrogen loss while others are more related to physical inactivity? *J Bone Min Metab* 33(6): 605–614, 2014.

40. Freedman MA. Quality of life and menopause: the role of estrogen. *J Womens Health* 11(8): 703–718, 2002.

41. Frost HM. Bone's mechanostat: A 2003 update. *The Anatomical Record Part A: Discoveries in Molecular, Cellular, and Evolutionary Biology* 275(2): 1081–1101, 2003.

42. Fulzele K, Lai F, Dedic C, Saini V, Uda Y, Shi C, et al. Osteocyte-secreted Wnt signaling inhibitor sclerostin contributes to beige adipogenesis in peripheral fat depots. *J Bone Min Resh* 32(2): 373–384, 2017.

43. Glass DA, Bialek P, Ahn JD, Starbuck M, Patel MS, Clevers H, et al. Canonical Wnt signaling in differentiated osteoblasts controls osteoclast differentiation. *Dev Cell* 8(5): 751–764, 2005.

44. Gonzalo-Encabo P, McNeil J, Boyne DJ, Courneya KS, Friedenreich CM. Dose-response effects of exercise on bone mineral density and content in postmenopausal women. *Scand J Med Sci Sports*, 29, 1121–1129, 2019.

45. Gorski JP, Price JL. Bone muscle crosstalk targets muscle regeneration pathway regulated by core circadian transcriptional repressors DEC1 and DEC2. *Bonekey Rep* 5, 27–32, 2016.

46. Grasso D, Corsetti R, Lanteri P, Di Bernardo C, Colombini A, et al. Bone-muscle unit activity, salivary steroid hormones profile, and physical effort over a 3-week stage race. *Scand J Med Sci Sportss* 25(1): 70–80, 2015.

47. Guadalupe-Grau A, Fuentes T, Guerra B, Calbet JA. Exercise and bone mass in adults. *Sport Med* 39(6): 439–468, 2009.

48. Guadalupe-Grau A, Perez-Gomez J, Olmedillas H, Chavarren J, Dorado C, Santana A, et al. Strength training combined with plyometric jumps in adults: sex differences in fat-bone axis adaptations. *J Appl Physiol* 106(4): 1100–1111, 2009.

49. Guillemant J, Accarie C, Peres G, Guillemant S. Acute effects of an oral calcium load on markers of bone metabolism during endurance cycling exercise in male athletes. *Calcif Tissue Int* 74(5): 407–414, 2004.

50. Hanley DA, Adachi JD, Bell A, Brown V. Denosumab: mechanism of action and clinical outcomes. *Int J Clin Pract* 66(12): 1139–1146, 2012.

51. Hansen MA, Overgaard K, Riis BJ, Christiansen C. Potential risk factors for development of postmenopausal osteoporosis — Examined over a 12-year period. *Osteoporos Int* 1: 95–102, 1991.

52. Haryono IR, Tulaar A, Sudoyo H, Purba A, Abdullah M, Jusman SW, et al. Comparison of the effects of walking and bench-step exercise on osteocalcin and ctx-1 in post-menopausal women with osteopenia. *J Musculoskelet Res* 20(2): 1–11, 2017.

53. Hemmatian H, Bakker AD, Klein-Nulend J, van Lenthe GH. Aging, osteocytes, and mechanotransduction. *Curr Osteoporos Rep* 15(5): 401–411, 2017.

54. Henriksen K, Bay-Jensen AC, Christiansen C, Karsdal MA. Oral salmon calcitonin–pharmacology in osteoporosis. *Expert Opin Biol Ther* 10(11): 1617–29, 2010.

55. Hikita A, Yana I, Wakeyama H, Nakamura M, Kadono Y, Oshima Y, et al. Negative regulation of osteoclastogenesis by ectodomain shedding of receptor activator of NF-kappaB ligand. *J Biol Chem* 281(48): 36846–36855, 2006.

56. Hofbauer LC, Heufelder AE. Role of receptor activator of nuclear factor-kappaB ligand and osteoprotegerin in bone cell biology. *J Mol Med* 79(5-6): 243–253, 2001.

57. Hofbauer LC, Schoppet, M. Clinical implications of the osteoprotegerin/RANKL/RANK system for bone and vascular diseases. *JAMA* 292(4): 490–495, 2004.

58. Hsu H, Lacey DL, Dunstan CR, Solovyev I, Colombero A, Timms E, et al. Tumor necrosis factor receptor family member RANK mediates osteoclast differentiation and activation induced by osteoprotegerin ligand. *Proc Natl Acad Sci U S A* 96(7): 3540–3545, 1999.

59. Ivaska KK, Hentunen TA, Vääräniemi J, Ylipahkala H, Pettersson K, Väänänen HK. Release of intact and fragmented osteocalcin molecules from bone matrix during bone resorption in vitro. *J Biol Chem* 279(18): 18361–18369, 2004.

60. Jilka RL, O'Brien CA. The role of osteocytes in age-related bone loss. *Curr Osteoporos Rep* 14(1): 16–25, 2016.

61. Kameda T, Mano H, Yuasa T, Mori Y, Miyazawa K, Shiokawa M, et al. Estrogen inhibits bone resorption by directly inducing apoptosis of the bone-resorbing osteoclasts. *J Exp Med* 186(4): 489–95, 1997.

62. Ke HZ, Richards WG, Li X, Ominsky MS. Sclerostin and dickkopf-1 as therapeutic targets in bone diseases. *Endocr Rev* 33(5): 747–83, 2012.

63. Kearns AE, Khosla S, Kostenuik PJ. Receptor activator of nuclear factor kappaB ligand and osteoprotegerin regulation of bone remodeling in health and disease. *Endocr Rev* 29(2): 155–192, 2008.

64. Khosla S. *Minireview: The OPG/RANKL/RANK System* 142: 5050–5055, 2001.

65. Khosla S. Update on estrogens and the skeleton. *J Clin Endocrinol Metab* 95(8): 3569–3577, 2010.

66. Kim DG, Huja SS, Navalgund A, D'Atri A, Tee B, Reeder S, et al. Effect of estrogen deficiency on regional variation of a viscoelastic tissue property of bone. *J Biomech* 46(1): 110–115, 2013.

67. Kim JH, Liu X, Wang J, Chen X, Zhang, H. Kim, et al. Wnt signaling in bone formation and its therapeutic potential for bone diseases. *Ther Adv Musculoskelet Dis* 5(1): 13–31, 2013.

68. Kish K, Mezil Y, Ward WE, Klentrou P, Falk B. Effects of plyometric exercise session on markers of bone turnover in boys and young men. *Eur J Appl Physiol* 115(10): 2115–2124, 2015.

69. Kini U, Nandeesh BN. Physiology of bone formation, remodeling, and metabolism. In *Radionuclide and Hybrid Bone Imaging*. Berlin: Springer Berlin Heidelberg, 2012, p. 29–57.

70. Klentrou P, Angrish K, Awadia N, Kurgan N, Kouvelioti R, Falk B. Wnt signaling–related osteokines at rest and following plyometric exercise in prepubertal and early pubertal boys and girls. *Pediatr Exer Sci* 30(4): 457–465, 2018.

71. Kobayashi Y, Maeda K, Takahashi N. Roles of Wnt signaling in bone formation and resorption. *Jpn Dent Sci Rev* 44(1): 76–82, 2008.

72. Kobayashi Y, Maeda K, Uehara S, Yamashita T, Takahashi N. Regulatory mechanism of osteoclastogenesis by Wnt signaling. *Inflamm Regen* 31(5): 413–419, 2011.

73. Kohrt WM, Barry DW, Schwartz RS. Muscle forces or gravity: what predominates mechanical loading on bone? *Med Sci Sports Exer* 41(11): 2050–2055, 2009.

74. Kostenuik PJ. Osteoprotegerin and RANKL regulate bone resorption, density, geometry and strength. *Curr Opin Pharmacol* 5: 618–625, 2005.

75. Kousteni S, Chen JR, Bellido T, Han L, Ali AA, O'Brien CA, et al. Reversal of bone loss in mice by nongenotropic signaling of sex steroids. *Science* 298: 843–846, 2002.

76. Kouvelioti R, Kurgan N, Falk B, Ward WE, Josse AR, Klentrou P. Response of sclerostin and bone turnover markers to high intensity interval exercise in young women: does impact matter? *BioMed Res Int* 8: 4864952, 2018.

77. Kouvelioti R, LeBlanc P, Falk B, Ward WE, Josse AR, Klentrou P. Effects of high-intensity interval running versus cycling on sclerostin, and markers of bone turnover and oxidative stress in young men. *Calcif Tissue Int* 104(6): 582–590, 2019.

78. Kouvelioti R, Kurgan N, Falk B, Ward WE, Josse AR, Klentrou P. Cytokine and sclerostin response to high-intensity interval running versus cycling. *Med Sci Sports Exer*, 51: 2458–2464, 2019.

79. Krishnan V, Bryant HU, Macdougald OA. Regulation of bone mass by Wnt signaling. *J Clin Invest* 116(5): 1202–1209, 2006.

80. Krum SA, Miranda-Carboni GA, Hauschka PV, Carroll JS, Lane TF, Freedman LP, et al. Estrogen protects bone by inducing Fas ligand in osteoblasts to regulate osteoclast survival. *EMBO Journal* 27(3): 535–545, 2008.

81. Krum SA. Direct transcriptional targets of sex steroid hormones in bone. *J Cell Biochem* 112(2): 401–408, 2011.

82. Kubota T, Michigami T, Ozono K. Wnt signaling in bone metabolism. *J Bone Miner Metab* 27(3): 265–271, 2009.

83. Kurgan N, Logan-Sprenger H, Falk B, Klentrou P. Bone and inflammatory responses to training in female rowers over an olympic year. *Med Sci Sports Exer* 50(9): 1810–1817, 2018.

84. Kurgan N, McKee K, Calleja M, Josse AR, Klentrou P. Differences in inflammatory cytokines, adipokines and bone markers at rest and in response to plyometric exercise between obese and normal weight adolescent females. *Front Endocrinol* in review, 2020.

85. Lacey DL, Timms E, Tan HL, Kelley MJ, Dunstan CR, Burgess T, et al. Osteoprotegerin ligand is a cytokine that regulates osteoclast differentiation and activation. *Cell* 93(2): 165–176, 1998.

86. Lala R, Matarazzo P, Bertelloni S, Buzi F, Rigon F, de Sanctis C. Pamidronate treatment of bone fibrous dysplasia in nine children with McCune-Albright syndrome. *Acta Paediatr* 89(2): 188–193, 2000.

87. Levis S, Lagari VS. The role of diet in osteoporosis prevention and management. *Curr Osteoporos Rep* 10(4): 296–302, 2012.

88. Li J, Sarosi I, Yan XQ, Morony S, Capparelli C, Tan HL, et al. RANK is the intrinsic hematopoietic cell surface receptor that controls osteoclastogenesis and regulation of bone mass and calcium metabolism. *Proc Natl Acad Sci U S A* 97(4): 1566–1571, 2000.

89. Li Y, Toraldo G, Li A, Yang X, Zhang H, Qian WP, et al. B cells and T cells are critical for the preservation of bone homeostasis and attainment of peak bone mass in vivo. *Blood* 109(9): 3839–3848, 2007.

90. Li XJ, Jee WSS. Integrated bone tissue anatomy and physiology. *Curr Topics Bone Biol* 11–56, 2005.

91. Lin CF, Huang TH, Tu KC, Lin LL, Tu YH, Yang RS. Acute effects of plyometric jumping and intermittent running on serum bone markers in young males. *Eur J Appl Physiol* 112(4): 1475–1484, 2012.

92. Lippi G, Schena F, Montagnana M, Salvagno GL, Banfi G, Guidi GC. Acute variation of osteocalcin and parathyroid hormone in athletes after running a half-marathon. *Clin Chem* 54(6): 1093–1095, 2008.

93. Liu W, Zhang L. Receptor activator of nuclear factor-[kappa] B ligand (RANKL)/RANK/Opsteoprotegerin system in bone and other tissues. *Mol Med Rep* 11(5): 3212–3218, 2015.

94. Lukert BP. Osteoporosis - a review and update. *Arch Phys Med Rehab* 63: 480–487, 1982.

95. Lynch CC, Hikosaka A, Acuff HB, Martin MD, Kawai N, Singh RK, et al. MMP-7 promotes prostate cancer-induced osteolysis via the solubilization of RANKL. *Cancer Cell* 7(5): 485–496, 2005.

96. Manolagas SC. Wnt signaling and osteoporosis. *Maturitas* 78(3): 233–237, 2014.

97. Marques EA, Wanderley F, Machado L, Sousa F, Viana JL, Moreira- Gonçalves D, et al. Effects of resistance and aerobic exercise on physical function, bone mineral density, OPG and RANKL in older women. *Exp Gerontol* 46(7): 524–532, 2011.

98. Marques EA, Mota J, Viana JL, Tuna D, Figueiredo P, Guimarães JT, et al. Response of bone mineral density, inflammatory cytokines, and biochemical bone markers to a 32-week combined loading exercise programme in older men and women. *Arch Gerontol Geriatr* 57(2): 226–33, 2013.

99. Matkovic V, Jelic T, Wardlaw GM, Ilich JZ, Goel PK, Wright JK, et al. Timing of peak bone mass in Caucasian females and its implication for the prevention of osteoporosis. Inference from a cross-sectional model. *J Clin Invest* 93(2): 799–808, 1994.

100. McCullough M, Goss A. Abnormal laboratory results: Bone turnover markers. *Aust Prescr* 35(5): 156–158, 2012.

101. Mezil YA, Allison D, Kish K, Ditor D, Ward WE, Tsiani E, et al. Response of bone turnover markers and cytokines to high-intensity low-impact exercise. *Med Sci Sports Exer* 47(7): 1495–1502, 2015.

102. Milgrom C, Finestone A, Levi Y, Simkin A, Ekenman I, Mendelson S, et al. Do high impact exercises produce higher tibial strains than running? *Br J Sports Med* 34(3):195–199, 2000.

103. Mödder U, Clowes J, Hoey K, Peterson J, McCready L, Oursler M, et al. Regulation of circulating sclerostin levels by sex steroids in women and in men. *J Bone Min Res* 26(1): 27–34, 2011.

104. Moester MJC, Papapoulos SE, Löwik CWGM, van Bezooijen RL. Sclerostin: current knowledge and future perspectives. *Calcif Tissue Int* 87(2), 99–107, 2010.

105. Morseth B, Emaus N, Jørgensen L. Physical activity and bone: The importance of the various mechanical stimuli for bone mineral density. A review. *Norsk Epidemiologi* 20(2)173–178: 2011.

106. Nardone V, D'Asta F, Brandi ML. Pharmacological management of osteogenesis. *Clinics* 69(6): 438–446, 2014.

107. Nakashima T, Hayashi M, Fukunaga T, Kurata K, Oh-Hora M, Feng JQ, et al. Evidence for osteocyte regulation of bone homeostasis through RANKL expression. *Nat Med* 17(10): 1231–1234, 2011.

108. Nayir E. Pathogenesis of bone metastasis. *J Oncol Sci* 1: 9–12, 2016.

109. Nelson K, Kouvelioti R, Theocharidis A, Falk B, Tiidus P, Klentrou P. Effects of plyometric exercise on Wnt signaling-related osteokines and bone turnover markers in pre and postmenopausal women. *Can J Physiol Pharmacol* in review, 2020.

110. Nikpour S, Haghani H. The effect of exercise on quality of life in postmenopausal women referred to the bone densitometry centers of Iran University of Medical Sciences. *J Midlife Health* 5(4):176–179, 2014.

111. Niu T, Rosen CJ. The insulin-like growth factor-I gene and osteoporosis: A critical appraisal. *Gene* 361(1-2): 38–56, 2005.

112. Oldknow KJ, MacRae VE, Farquharson C. Endocrine role of bone: recent and emerging perspectives beyond osteocalcin. *J Endocrinol* 225(1): 1–19, 2015.

113. Ominsky MS, Li X, Asuncion FJ, Barrero M, Warmington KS, Dwyer D, et al. RANKL inhibition with osteoprotegerin increases bone strength by improving cortical and trabecular bone architecture in ovariectomized rats. *J Bone Mineral Res* 23(5): 672–682, 2008.

114. Osteoporosis Canada. http://www.osteoporosis.ca/osteoporosis-and-you/osteoporosis-facts-and-statistics/. 2012.

115. Palacios S, Neyro JL, Fernández de Cabo S, Chaves J, Rejas J. Impact of osteoporosis and bone fracture on health-related quality of life in postmenopausal women. *Climacteric* 17(1): 60–70, 2014.

116. Pazianas, M. Anabolic effects of PTH and the 'anabolic window'. *Trend Endocrinol Metab* 26(3): 111–113, 2015.

117. Pichler K, Loreto C, Leonardi R, Reuber T, Weinberg AM, Musumeci, G. RANKL is downregulated in bone cells by physical activity (treadmill and vibration stimulation training) in rat with glucocorticoid-induced osteoporosis. *Histol Histopathol* 28(9): 1185–1196, 2013.

118. Pomerants T, Tillmann V, Karelson K, Jurimae J, Jurimae, T. Impact of acute exercise on bone turnover and growth hormone/insulin-like growth factor axis in boys. *J Sport Med Phys Fit*48(2): 266–271, 2008.

119. Prideaux M, Findlay DM, Atkins GJ. Osteocytes: The master cells in bone remodelling. *Curr Opin Pharmacol* 28: 24–30, 2016.

120. Purves WK, Orians GH, Heller HC, Sadava, D. *Life: The Science of Biology* (5th Edition). Sunderland, MA and Salt Lake City, UT: Sinauer Associates and W.H. Feeman and Company, 1998.

121. Ralston SH, de Crombrugghe, B. Genetic regulation of bone mass and susceptibility to osteoporosis. *Gene Dev* 20(18): 2492–2506, 2006.

122. Rantalainen T, Heinonen A, Linnamo V, Komi PV, Takala TES, Kainulainen H. Short-term bone biochemical response to a single bout of high-impact exercise. *J Sport Sci Med* 8(4): 553–559, 2009.

123. Robling AG, Niziolek PJ, Baldridge LA, Condon KW, Allen MR, Alam I, et al. Mechanical stimulation of bone *in Vivo* reduces osteocyte expression of sost/sclerostin. *J Biol Chem* 283(9): 5866–5875, 2008.

124. Rogers RS, Dawson AW, Wang Z, Thyfault JP, Hinton PS. Acute response of plasma markers of bone turnover to a single bout of resistance training or plyometrics. *J Appl Physiol* 111(5): 1353–1360, 2011.

125. Rudberg A, Magnusson P, Larsson L, Joborn H. Serum isoforms of bone alkaline phosphatase increase during physical exercise in women. *Calcif Tissue Int* 66(5): 342–347, 2000.

126. Santos L, Elliott-Sale KJ, Sale C. Exercise and bone health across the lifespan. *Biogerontology* 18(6): 931–946, 2017.

127. Sapir-Koren R, Livshits G. Osteocyte control of bone remodeling: is sclerostin a key molecular coordinator of the balanced bone resorption–formation cycles? *Osteoporos Int* 25(12): 2685–2700, 2014.

128. Seem SA, Yuan YV, Tou JC. Chocolate and chocolate constituents influence bone health and osteoporosis risk. *Nutrition* 65: 74–84, 2019.

129. Scott A, Khan KM, Duronio V, Hart DA. Mechanotransduction in human bone. In vitro cellular physiology that underpins bone changes with exercise. *Sport Med* 38(2): 139–160, 2008.

130. Scott JPR, Sale C, Greeves JP, Casey A, Dutton J, Fraser WD. The effect of training status on the metabolic response of bone to an acute bout of exhaustive treadmill running. *J Clin Endocrinol Metab* 95(8): 3918–3925, 2010.

131. Scott JPR, Sale C, Greeves JP, Casey A, Dutton J, Fraser WD. The role of exercise intensity in the bone metabolic response to an acute bout of weight-bearing exercise. *J Appl Physiol* 110(2): 423–432, 2011.

132. Scott JP, Sale C, Greeves JP, Casey A, Dutton J, Fraser WD. Effect of recovery duration between two bouts of running on bone metabolism. *Med Sci Sports Exer* 45(3): 429–438, 2013.

133. Seibel MJ. Biochemical markers of bone turnover: part I: biochemistry and variability. *Clin Biochem Rev* 26(4): 97–122, 2005.

134. Sherk VD, Chrisman C, Smith J, Young KC, Singh H, Bemben MG, et al. Acute bone marker responses to whole-body vibration and resistance exercise in young women. *J Clin Densitom* 16(1):104–109, 2013.

135. Shibata Y, Ohsawa I, Watanabe T, Miura T, Sato Y. Effects of physical training on bone mineral density and bone metabolism. *J Physiol Anthropol Applied Hum Sci* 22(4): 203–208, 2003.

136. Shipman P, Walker A, Bichell D. *Human Skeleton*. Cambridge MA: Harvard University Press, 1984.

137. Silvestrini G, Ballanti P, Patacchioli F, Leopizzi M, Gualtieri N, Monnazzi P, et al. Detection of osteoprotegerin (OPG) and its ligand (RANKL) mRNA and protein in femur and tibia of the rat. *J mol Histol* 36(1-2): 59–67, 2005.

138. Simonet WS, Lacey DL, Dunstan CR, Kelley M, Chang MS, Luthy R, et al. Osteoprotegerin: a novel secreted protein involved in the regulation of bone density. *Cell* 89(2): 309–319, 1997.

139. Sims NA, Chia LY. Regulation of sclerostin expression by paracrine and endocrine factors. *Clin Rev Bone Miner Metab* 10(2), 98–107, 2012.

140. Song L. Calcium and bone metabolism indices. *Adv Clin Chem* 82: 1–46, 2017.

141. Spatz J, Wein M, Gooi J, Qu Y, Garr J, Liu S, et al. The Wnt inhibitor sclerostin is up-regulated by mechanical unloading in osteocytes in vitro. *J Biol Chem* 290(27): 16744–16758, 2015.

142. Stieglitz J, Beheim BA, Trumble BC, Madimenos FC, Kaplan H, Gurven M. Low mineral density of a weight-bearing bone among adult women in a high fertility population. *Am J Phys Anthropol* 156(4): 637–648, 2015.

143. Suen PK, Qin L. Sclerostin, an emerging therapeutic target for treating osteoporosis and osteoporotic fracture: A general review. *J Orthop Translat* 4: 1–13, 2016.

144. Szulc P, Seeman E, Delmas PD. Biochemical measurements of bone turnover in children and adolescents. *Osteoporos Int* 11(4): 281–294, 2000.

145. Takayanagi, H. Osteoimmunology: shared mechanisms and crosstalk between the immune and bone systems. *Nat Rev Immunol* 7(4): 292–304, 2007.

146. Theoleyre S, Wittrant Y, Tat SK, Fortun Y, Redini F, Heymann, D. The molecular triad OPG/RANK/RANKL: involvement in the orchestration of pathophysiological bone remodeling. *Cytokine Growth Factor Rev* 15(6): 457–475, 2004.

147. Todd H, Galea GL, Meakin LB, Delisser PJ, Lanyon LE, Windahl SH, et al. Wnt16 is associated with age-related bone loss and estrogen withdrawal in murine bone. *PLOS ONE* 10(10): 1–17, 2015.

148. Tolomio S, Ermolao A, Travain G, Zaccaria M. Short-term adapted physical activity program improves bone quality in osteopenic/osteoporotic postmenopausal women. *J Phys Act Health* 5(6): 844–853, 2008.

149. Tosun A, Bölükbaşi N, Çingi E, Beyazova M, Ünlü M. Acute effects of a single session of aerobic exercise with or without weight-lifting on bone turnover in healthy young women. *Mod Rheumatol* 16(5): 300–304, 2006.

150. Tyrovola JB, Odont XX. The "mechanostat theory" of frost and the OPG/RANKL/RANK System. *J Cell Biochem* 116(12): 2724–2729, 2015.

151. Vainionpää A, Korpelainen R, Väänänen HK, Haapalahti J, Jämsä T, Leppäluoto J. Effect of impact exercise on bone metabolism. *Osteoporos Int* 20(10): 1725–1733, 2009.

152. Vasikaran S, Eastell R, Bruyère O, Foldes AJ, Garnero P, Griesmacher A. Bone Marker Standards Working Group. Markers of bone turnover for the prediction of fracture risk and monitoring of osteoporosis treatment: a need for international reference standards. *Osteoporos Int* 22(2): 391–420, 2011.

153. Vicente-Rodriguez G. How does exercise affect bone development during growth? *Sport Med* 36(7): 561–569, 2006.

154. Wada T, Nakashima T, Hiroshi N, Penninger JM. RANKL-RANK signaling in osteoclastogenesis and bone disease. *Trend Mol Med* 12(1): 17–25, 2006.

155. Wallace BA, Cumming RG. Systematic review of randomized trials of the effect of exercise on bone mass in pre-and postmenopausal women. *Calcif Tissue Int* 67(1): 10–18, 2000.

156. Watts NB. Clinical utility of biochemical markers of bone remodeling. *Clin Chem* 45(8): 1359–1368, 1999.

157. Weitzmann MN, Pacifici R. Estrogen regulation of immune cell bone interactions. *Ann N Y Acad Sci* 1068(1): 256–274, 2006.

158. Weivoda MM, Oursler MJ. Developments in sclerostin biology: regulation of gene expression, mechanisms of action, and physiological functions. *Curr Osteoporos Rep* 12(1): 107–114, 2014.

159. Wend K, Wend P, Krum SA. Tissue-specific effects of loss of estrogen during menopause and aging. *Front Endocrinol* 3: 19, 2012.

160. Whipple TJ, Le BH, Demers LM, Chinchilli VM, Petit MA, Sharkey N, et al. Acute effects of moderate intensity resistance exercise on bone cell activity. *Int J Sports Med* 25(7): 496–501, 2004.

161. Wieczorek-Baranowska A, Nowak A, Pilaczyńska-Szcześniak L. Osteocalcin and glucose metabolism in postmenopausal women subjected to aerobic training program for 8 weeks. *Metabolism* 61(4): 542–545, 2012.

162. Wijenayaka AR, Kogawa M, Lim HP, Bonewald LF, Findlay DM, Atkins GJ. Sclerostin stimulates osteocyte support of osteoclast activity by a RANKL-dependent pathway. *PLOS ONE* 6(10): e20900, 2011.

163. Yap CY, Aw TC. Bone turnover markers. *Proc Singapore Healthc* 19(3): 273–275, 2010.

164. Yuan Y, Chen X, Zhang L, Wu J, Guo J, Zou D, et al. The roles of exercise in bone remodeling and in prevention and treatment of osteoporosis. *Prog Biophys Mol Biol* 122(2): 122–130, 2016.

165. Zagrodna A, Józków P, Mędraś M, Majda M, Słowińska-Lisowska M. Sclerostin as a novel marker of bone turnover in athletes. *Biol Sport* 33(1): 83–87, 2016.

166. Zehnacker CH, Bemis-Dougherty A. Effect of weighted exercises on bone mineral density in post menopausal women a systematic review. *J Geriatr Phys Ther* 30(2): 79–88, 2007.

167. Ziegler S, Niessner A, Richter B, Wirth S, Billensteiner E, Woloszczuk W, et al. Endurance running acutely raises plasma osteoprotegerin and lowers plasma receptor activator of nuclear factor κ B ligand. *Metabolism* 54(7): 935–8, 2005.

33

METABOLIC EFFECTS OF EXERCISE ON CHILDHOOD OBESITY

Kristi B. Adamo, Taniya S. Nagpal, and Danilo F. DaSilva

Introduction

Childhood Obesity Prevalence

The prevalence of obesity continues to increase and is recognized as a global epidemic (17). Broadly defined, obesity is characterized as excess adiposity and is most commonly classified as having a body mass index (BMI) ≥ 30.0 kg/m^2 (17). More recently, BMI has been criticized as an inappropriate measure of obesity, as it does not accurately measure the percentage of adiposity (82). However, using BMI classification remains the most accessible surrogate measurement of excess adiposity at the population level, and therefore epidemiological studies have relied mostly on the ≥ 30.0 kg/m^2 BMI cut-off to measure and report the global prevalence of obesity for all age groups (4, 50). In addition, for children and adolescents obesity is measured as BMI above the 95th percentile (curves generated from the 1963–1965 and 1966–1970 National Health and Nutrition Surveys) (99).

It has been estimated that over 124 million children and youth (<18 years of age) worldwide have obesity (3). Trends in childhood obesity have been relatively stable since 2000 for high-income English-speaking and Asia-Pacific regions. In Eastern and South Asian regions, the trend seems to have accelerated (3). Globally since 1975, there has been an approximate 5% increase in childhood obesity, and it is predicted that if post-2000 trends continue, by 2022, the prevalence of childhood obesity will surpass statistics of moderate and severe underweight BMI (3). Despite a plateau in trajectory in high-income English-speaking countries, the nationwide prevalence of childhood obesity remains high and is a significant health concern in many regions (5), including Canada, the United States, and the UK (29, 49, 86).

In Canada, approximately one in seven children and youth (age 2–17 years) have obesity (86). In the United States, the prevalence is even higher, with nearly one in five children and youth having obesity (ages 2–19 years) (49). Similarly, in the UK, one in five children has obesity (ages 4–11 years) (29). Across all three high-income countries, the prevalence of childhood obesity over the last decade has stabilized (3). However, the already high and stagnant percentage of affected children is a major health concern and may be indicative of a lack of resources being allocated towards addressing childhood obesity aetiology and implementation of effective prevention and treatment initiatives (51).

Aetiology

Fundamentally, obesity in childhood is the result of positive energy balance (4, 62). It is a widely held belief that reduced physical activity and/or increased sedentary behaviour is implicated in the aetiology of childhood obesity and its associated conditions (20). However, obesity in children (as in adults) is the consequence of an interaction between a myriad of factors that are related to the environment, genetics, and metabolism, as well as lifestyle and eating habits, which can be driven by socio-economic status (62). Therefore the aetiology of childhood obesity can be a combination of modifiable and unmodifiable factors that may contribute to a positive energy balance and reduced effectiveness of prevention and treatment interventions. Examples of modifiable factors include individual lifestyle behaviours (physical inactivity, poor nutrition habits, sedentary behaviour, excessive screen time, lack of sleep), socio-economic status (family income, parents working schedule and lack of availability), and environment (sedentary time in school, neighbourhood outdoor safety, access to unhealthy food options, food marketing, promotion of sedentary behaviours) (51). Non-modifiable factors include genetic predisposition to obesity, genetic syndromes, medications, hormonal disorders, and exposures in the intrauterine (excessive gestational weight gain, gestational diabetes, poor placental function, epigenetics) and early postpartum environment (macrosomia, feeding behaviours) (38, 105).

Children who have an overweight BMI have higher risks for numerous health conditions, and children who have obesity before the age of 6 are likely to have obesity later in childhood and as adults (67). Physical inactivity is also associated with an increased risk of several chronic diseases, including obesity and heart disease (89, 104). Taken together, children with obesity and low activity levels may be at an increased risk for later-life chronic conditions. Physical activity introduced early in the preschool years is associated with improved body composition and decreased risk for cardiovascular consequences (lower total cholesterol, lower resting heart rate, and sub-maximal heart rate during exercise) (85). It is essential to intervene early to prevent and treat childhood obesity, as longitudinal studies have shown that established weight trajectories are difficult to change. Although intervening during childhood is important and necessary, it should be acknowledged that an abundance of evidence also exists suggesting that obesity may be "programmed" in utero.

Developmental Origins of Health and Disease

Epidemiological, animal model, and experimental studies have provided strong evidence implicating pregnancy in downstream child obesity. A healthy intrauterine environment is a vital factor in establishing the best start to life and promoting the long-term health of a child. The late David Barker, whose seminal work guided the Developmental Origins of Health and Disease (DOHaD) concept, advocated that "the womb may be more important than the home" (10) and championed research examining foetal programming and the role of the intrauterine environment on downstream child health. Among the many factors contributing to obesity in children, there are two influential maternal contributors: high maternal BMI and exceeding the Institute of Medicine (IOM) gestational weight gain guidelines (2).

Excess gestational weight gain, independent of maternal BMI, is predictive of high birth weight, and the combination of high BMI and exceeding the gestational weight gain guidelines results in significantly greater odds of having a large-for-gestational-age neonate (35). Sub-group analyses looking at different developmental stages (preschool, children, and adolescents) have shown that high birth weight is associated with increased risk of obesity from preschool to adulthood. Body composition, or the proportion and distribution of fat mass and lean mass, and pattern of weight gain during infancy are also important contributors to obesity risk. It was recently shown that compared to mothers who gained within IOM guidelines, normal-weight mothers with excessive gestational weight gain had infants with 50% higher fat mass (53). Infants who are at the highest end of the distribution for weight or who grow rapidly during infancy are at increased risk of subsequent obesity. The velocity of weight gain, particularly between birth and 6 months of age, is a key determinant of future obesity development (13, 31, 88) (Figure 33.1).

Developmental Programming of Physical Activity

There is also evidence to suggest that early life exposures can alter our tendency to be physically active in later life. Maternal gestational weight gain has also shown to be independently associated with elevated levels of leptin in foetal cord blood (68). Subsequently, leptin has been linked to the

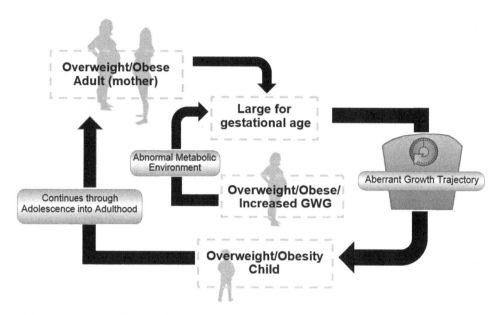

Figure 33.1   Intergenerational cycle of obesity

developmental programming of energy balance regulation (15) and regulation of physical activity (44). A study that evaluated the relationship between maternal gestational weight gain and physical activity behaviours in children found that maternal gestational weight gain was independently associated with preschool-age offspring total physical activity in a sex-dependent manner. Specifically, in boys, greater gestational weight gain was associated with decreased activity levels independent of maternal pre-pregnancy BMI status (35).

The exact mechanisms for sex differences in developmental programming remain to be determined. These differences may be related to differences in placenta function (21). Work by Adamo et al. has demonstrated differential expression of placental nutrient transporters in male offspring of women who are obese vs. lean and those who exceed gestational weight gain guidelines (16). Also, maternal obesity has been linked to the sex-specific methylation of the placenta *LEP* gene, which has also been positively associated with neurobehavioral profiles marked by lethargy, hypotonicity, non-optimal reflexes, and low excitability in males (65). In animal studies, maternal obesity and overfeeding have been directly linked to hypothalamic leptin resistance, reduced leptin signalling, and altered hypothalamic neurodevelopment towards orexigenic pathways (101), each having been associated with regulation of physical activity (44). Collectively, the literature demonstrates that there is considerable sexual dimorphism in the placentas, suggesting that placentas from male and female offspring behave differently, although the exact mechanisms behind the developmental programming of physical activity remain to be determined.

Metabolic and Physiological Impact of Childhood Obesity

Although paediatric obesity is not always associated with physiological changes that may lead to cardiometabolic risk factors (48), there are several metabolic consequences as a result of excessive body weight in children and adolescents, which may be aggravated during adulthood if not treated (58). Insulin resistance is known as a major consequence of paediatric obesity (80) and is strongly associated with other metabolic conditions/diseases, such as type 2 diabetes, polycystic ovarian syndrome, vascular dysfunctions, and cardiovascular diseases (48, 58). Several mechanisms are proposed to explain the link between obesity and insulin resistance. Increased adipose-derived cytokines, impaired glucose transport associated with deficient insulin signalling, and reduced insulin clearance due to increased free fatty acids are the most common explanatory factors (56, 80). Together, these alterations lead to peripheral and hepatic insulin resistance (91), increased ectopic (liver and visceral) fat deposition, intraperitoneal adipose depots, and abdominal subcutaneous fat. These factors may influence the release of inflammatory markers, reduce insulin sensitivity, and cause dyslipidaemia and insulin resistance (91).

Insulin resistance is the trigger for a clustering of physiological alterations referred to as metabolic syndrome. Metabolic syndrome is associated with glucose intolerance, hypertension, hypertriglyceridemia, abdominal obesity, and low high-density lipoprotein cholesterol (HDL-c) levels (1). Although this constellation of factors is more commonly observed in adults, a systematic review revealed that the prevalence of metabolic syndrome is 3.3% in the normal-weight paediatric population and increases to 29.2% in children who have obesity (39).

There is a positive linear relationship between blood pressure and BMI (18), and this is independently associated with cardiovascular disease (58). If high blood pressure is developed during childhood, like obesity, it seems to persist into adulthood (18). Moreover, childhood obesity increases the odds of coronary artery calcification (71) and carotid intimal medial thickness (26). Increased carotid intimal medial thickness is a consequence of increased levels of serum lipids, particularly, low-density lipoprotein cholesterol (LDL-c) (55). Dyslipidaemia—which represents increased levels of LDL-c, triglycerides, and decreased HDL-c—is more frequently observed in children living with obesity and is associated with risk factors for atherosclerosis (1).

Ectopic fat accumulation in both the liver and the visceral region is linked with glucose intolerance and later development of type 2 diabetes (12). Two main pathophysiological aspects commonly featured in the development of type 2 diabetes in children and adolescents are insulin resistance and reduced insulin secretion (18). As β-cell function declines faster in youth who develop type 2 compared to adult-onset (102) diabetes, preventive actions are crucial.

Since the discovery of the endocrine and paracrine functions of adipose tissue, the interest in the association between adiposity and pro- and anti-inflammatory markers has increased. Some of the pro-inflammatory markers known to be derived from the adipocytes are leptin, resistin, visfatin, IL-6, and TNF-α and are known to be associated with insulin resistance (80). Conversely, adiponectin and IL-10 are associated with insulin sensitivity (103).

There is a strong relationship between childhood obesity, markers of oxidative stress, and liver diseases. Both oxidative stress and liver disease are moderated by insulin resistance, higher levels of free fatty acids, and visceral fat accumulation. Changes in free fatty acids can trigger increased reactive oxygen species, and thus generate greater oxidative stress responses (73). The increased oxidative stress can result in hepatocyte damage (93). Additionally, excessive abdominal fat increases the risk for non-alcoholic fatty liver disease (54).

Another physiological system that can be affected by childhood obesity is renal function (23, 69). Children living with obesity presented a lower estimated glomerular filtration rate (eGFR) compared to the non-obese group (23). This level of renal function impairment during childhood may predispose one to the development of kidney disease in later life (45, 69). In addition, other systems whose function may be impaired due to excess body weight include the respiratory (e.g., expiratory flow limitations and lower resting expiratory reserve volume) (46, 76) and reproductive systems (e.g., polycystic ovary syndrome) (80).

Figure 33.2 illustrates (1) organs and systems impaired by childhood obesity (e.g., gastrointestinal, reproductive, respiratory, hepatic, renal, and vascular) and markers associated with this impairment; (2) some common physiological and metabolic responses (e.g., inflammatory and oxidative stress responses), and (3) metabolic parameter alterations due to excess body weight (e.g., hyperlipidaemia and insulin resistance).

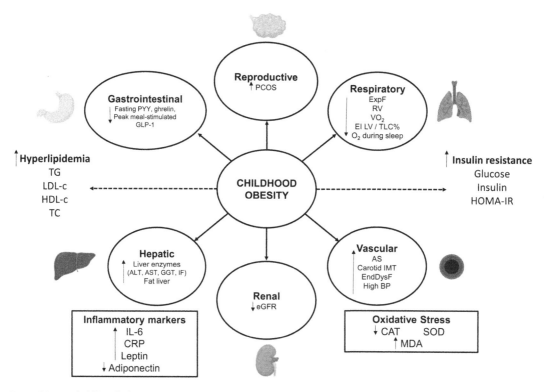

Figure 33.2 Childhood obesity consequences

Exercise as a Mode of Management

Hyperlipidaemia

Exercise interventions in children and adolescents living with obesity can increase energy expenditure (84), and both aerobic and combined (e.g., aerobic + resistance) exercise improves cardiorespiratory fitness (24, 32, 43). Improved performance in a cardiorespiratory fitness test, particularly in the 6-minute walk test, is linked to increased use of fat as an energy substrate in children with obesity (72). The metabolic changes mediated by increased energy expenditure and better substrate utilization are linked to improvements in lipid profile (84).

A recent systematic review of meta-analyses (43) aimed to answer if exercise-based interventions are effective at improving metabolic and physiological parameters, such as lipid profile. One of the meta-analyses included in this review concluded that aerobic exercise improves LDL-c and triglycerides if performed three times per week for 60 minutes at an intensity ≤75% of maximal heart rate (HRmax). If the exercise modality involves combining aerobic and resistance training for ≥60 minutes and >75% HRmax, concomitant improvements in HDL-c may be realized (32). Another systematic review found that compared to aerobic training only, concurrent training enhanced the magnitude of reduction in LDL-c (42). Lipids are considered the main fuel for maintaining a moderate-intensity exercise bout; however, light-intensity exercise is also beneficial for lipid profile changes in the long term, particularly for sedentary obese adolescents (61). The reduction of fat mass in the visceral region appears to be related to the improvement in LDL-c, as it is associated with less free fatty acids and consequently decreased lipoprotein formation (108).

A systematic review reporting on the effects of exercise cessation on the lipid profile of children living with obesity showed that HDL-c and total cholesterol were unaltered 12–48 weeks after completion of the exercise programme; the duration of the exercise programmes was roughly 36–48 weeks (40). Although this review was based on only five studies, the results are encouraging, as some of the benefits from exercise (e.g., sports practice, aerobic and resistance training) are preserved even when the intervention is complete. It is likely that some of the lifestyle changes established during the intervention were maintained by the children, thus supporting the maintenance of the improved lipid profile, although this requires further investigation (40).

Insulin Resistance

Garcia-Hermoso et al. (2019) systematically reviewed other systematic reviews and meta-analyses and found that both aerobic and resistance training is effective in reducing insulin resistance (i.e., HOMA-IR) in children and adolescents with an overweight BMI. When these two different exercise modalities are combined, results are consistent (43). Other indices associated with insulin resistance (e.g., fasting insulin and glucose levels) are also reduced after the same exercise interventions, highlighting exercise as a potential tool to improve insulin resistance in youth living with obesity (43).

Besides insulin sensitivity, insulin secretion has been shown to improve after aerobic exercise training performed for 12 weeks (92). It is worth mentioning that to achieve this benefit, the exercise frequency was five times per week for 40 min/session. Exercising more frequently increases the magnitude of change for insulin resistance–related parameters (43). Exercise benefits also extend to β-cell function, thereby reducing the risk for chronic conditions such as diabetes (63).

Besides exercise frequency, another exercise prescription principle that should be highlighted to achieve improvements in markers of insulin resistance is exercise volume (i.e., frequency per week multiplied by session duration) Overweight or obese children exercising 5 times/week for 40 minutes each session, saw greater improvements in insulin sensitivity, as measured by an oral glucose tolerance test, compared to a group exposed to a lower volume of exercise (5 times/week for only 20 minutes) (25). Intervention programme duration between 4 and 12 weeks is sufficient to promote significant change in markers of insulin resistance, such as insulin sensitivity, and programmes lasting more than 12 weeks did not show additional improvements (43).

The mechanisms associated with improvements in insulin resistance, particularly in the aerobic exercise groups, can be partially explained by increases in lean mass following the training programme. Given the large interindividual variability in these data explained by growth and maturation, these findings should be interpreted with caution (74), knowing that insulin-stimulated glucose disposal improves as body weight, total body fat, and ectopic fat in the liver and muscle are reduced in children and adolescents (64). Consequently, aerobic exercise may be preferable if the intervention goal is to reduce type 2 diabetes risk. The benefits of resistance training were previously attributed to increased muscle contraction that was capable of stimulating the translocation of glucose transporter proteins to the cell membrane (64, 84).

Insulin resistance is associated with polycystic ovarian syndrome (PCOS), and the prevalence of PCOS is higher among girls who have obesity (19). The combination of PCOS and insulin resistance increases the risk of type 2 diabetes. On the other hand, it is known that weight loss, independent of exercise, can decrease the hyperandrogenaemia commonly observed in PCOS (59). As exercise is a useful method to manage weight, including sustaining weight loss, exercise may be an effective prescription for girls who have PCOS (59). Weekly dance classes in overweight girls at risk of PCOS improved waist circumference, triglycerides, and metabolic syndrome severity. Forty per cent of the girls improved free testosterone levels after 6 months of intervention (59). Long-term exercise routines (~5 years) can protect against the occurrence of PCOS in adolescent and adult women, and moderate-intensity physical activity is particularly helpful in avoiding subsequent PCOS (107).

Inflammatory and Oxidative Stress Markers

Both inflammatory and oxidative stress responses are associated with cardiovascular disease risk factors (78). Hyperlipidaemia and insulin resistance frequently develop in response to an increase in the release of inflammatory markers in children (19). Body mass index was positively associated with high-sensitivity C-reactive protein (CRP) (22), which is a sensitive low-grade inflammatory marker. At rest, BMI is inversely associated with antioxidant markers and directly related to pro-oxidant markers (33). The changes in the oxidative stress profile (e.g., increased reactive oxygen and nitrogen species) due to a reduction in antioxidants are linked to low-grade inflammation (36).

With regard to oxidative stress and antioxidant responses to exercise in childhood obesity, the literature is quite scarce. Murphy et al. (2009) found that 12 weeks of aerobic exercise (i.e., Dance Dance Revolution; 5 times/week) did not change asymmetric dimethylarginine (79), an L-arginine analogue shown to inhibit nitric oxide (NO) synthesis and impair endothelial function. Similarly, Tjonna et al. (2009) did not find changes in ox-LDL after 1 year of aerobic interval training (2 times/week; 4 × 4-min intervals at 90–95% HRmax) (98). However, when the exercise approach (30 min fitness + 30 min games and running, 3 times/week for 6 weeks) is combined with a diet intervention (i.e., dietary advice), oxidative stress markers (e.g., ox-LDL, malonaldehyde, and conjugated diene) were reduced in adolescents living with obesity (57). Roberts et al. (2007) found similar results with an even shorter intervention (i.e., 2 weeks duration) combining daily aerobic exercise (2 h to 2 h, 30 min sports and gym) with restrictive food intake and nutritional education. The oxidative markers myeloperoxidase, 8 hydroxy 2′deoxyguanosine, O^{2-}, and H_2O_2 were reduced after the intervention in adolescents with obesity (87). Together, these data suggest that combining exercise with dietary interventions is needed to improve markers of oxidative stress (78). These results are relevant, given that obesity reduces antioxidant capacity, which can increase systemic oxidative stress in children living with obesity (8). The changes in oxidative stress are likely related to growth hormone–dependent mechanisms that can be influenced by excess body weight. Thus adolescence represents a critical intervention target, as puberty can increase oxidative stress markers (78).

As for inflammatory markers, 3 months of moderate-intensity aerobic exercise (3 times/week, 45 minutes/session, brisk walking) combined with behavioural intervention improved CRP in obese adolescents (9). A reduction in CRP seems to be associated with a decrease in body fat and improved vascular function measured by flow-mediated dilation (6, 9, 77).

A systematic review probing the effects of exercise on adipokines in paediatric obesity revealed that adiponectin, a known anti-inflammatory marker, increases after exercise training (43). Leptin, visfatin, and resistin levels seem to be reduced as a chronic result of exercise interventions, but more research is needed regarding the responses of these three markers. The two main factors implicated in the improvement in inflammatory markers are (1) longer duration of the exercise programme and (2) a decrease in body fat. The change in adiponectin levels is physiologically relevant because higher levels of this inflammatory marker can reduce the atherogenic process through changes in macrophages and endothelial function (14).

Mello et al. (2011) found that adolescents with obesity might improve their levels of adiponectin more when aerobic and resistance training is combined (vs. aerobic training only) (28). A systematic review confirmed this finding and advocates for combined aerobic and resistance training to attenuate the inflammatory effects of obesity in the paediatric population (41).

The review of systematic reviews and meta-analyses performed by Garcia-Hermoso et al. (2019) found that adiponectin was higher in the circulation after exercise programmes (43). However, the pooled study analyses did not allow authors to provide a specific exercise dose or type to achieve these benefits, and this is a gap that needs addressing in future studies. Furthermore, the bulk of research focuses on short-term exercise programmes, and therefore further investigation is required to test the effect of more prolonged and sustained exercise interventions. In terms of individual session duration, at least 60 minutes is recommended (43).

Hepatic Function

Non-alcoholic fatty liver disease (NAFLD) is the most common liver disease in children with obesity and is estimated to be present in one out of five Canadian children with overweight or obesity (48). The accumulation of fat in the liver can lead to increased inflammation and a more severe liver disease called non-alcoholic steatohepatitis (NASH). The development of NAFLD starts with excessive accumulation of triglycerides in the liver, followed by hepatic oxidative stress (i.e., high levels of reactive oxygen species [ROS]), lipid peroxidation, and finally hepatocyte damage (96). Although a liver biopsy is the gold standard for diagnosis and grading of NAFLD, biopsies are not routinely performed in children. Less invasive assessments, including blood tests for liver enzymes (alanine aminotransferase [ALT], aspartate aminotransferase [AST], and gamma-glutamyl transferase [GGT]), and abdominal ultrasonography to measure intrahepatic fat, are more common. More costly examinations using proton magnetic resonance or magnetic resonance imaging can also be used.

NAFLD in the paediatric population is a substantial public health concern because of its association with insulin resistance and components of metabolic syndrome, thus elevating the risk of type 2 diabetes and cardiovascular disease. Aerobic training, known to affect blood lipids, glucose, and insulin sensitivity in a positive manner, is suggested to be preventive and effective in the control of NAFLD. Evidence from adults indicates exercise-induced improvements in peripheral insulin resistance reduces the excess delivery of free fatty acids and glucose for free fatty acid synthesis to the liver. In the liver, exercise increases fatty acid oxidation, decreases fatty acid synthesis, and prevents mitochondrial and hepatocellular damage through a reduction of the release of damage-associated molecular patterns (see Figures 33.3 and 33.4).

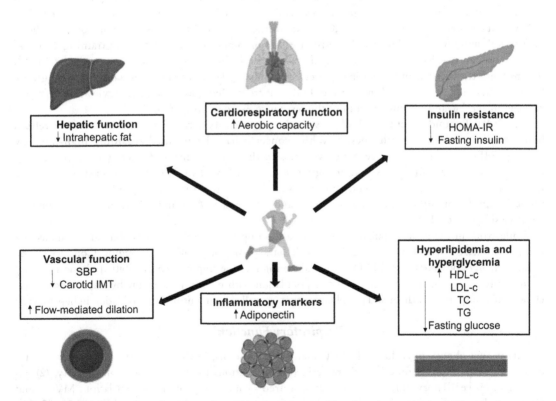

Figure 33.3 Main metabolic/physiological variables that improve after chronic exercise in children and adolescents living with obesity

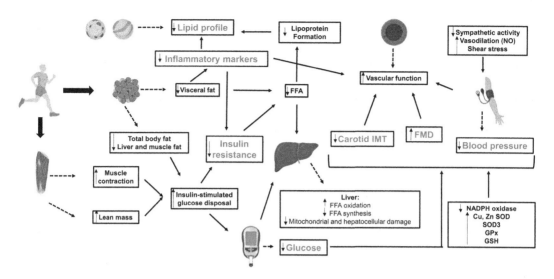

Figure 33.4 Potential mechanisms involved in the metabolic changes promoted by exercise in childhood obesity

Data from a meta-analysis of over 1,200 youth illustrate that exercise is associated with a significant reduction in visceral, subcutaneous, and intrahepatic fat, as well as GGT (47). A second meta-analysis by Medrano and colleagues aiming to determine the effect of type, intensity, volume, and duration of exercise necessary to reduce hepatic fat content and prevalence in NAFLD in children and adolescents concluded that both aerobic and resistance training, at vigorous or moderate-to-vigorous intensities, with a volume ≥60 min/session and a frequency ≥3 sessions/week, reduced hepatic fat content in youth (75).

A recent randomized control trial (RCT) examining outcomes in adolescents with overweight or obesity following 6 months of aerobic, resistance, or combined aerobic + resistance training (3 d/wk, 180 min/wk at 50–65% of peak VO$_2$) found an increase in insulin-stimulated glucose disposal in all groups, with the increase in the aerobic exercise group being larger than the resistance exercise group, but not different from the combined group. Different from Medrano's systematic review, liver fat was reduced in aerobic and combined, but not the resistance exercise group (64).

A 2017 RCT found benefits for both low- and high-intensity aerobic training on NAFLD-related biomarkers in adolescents with obesity. While concerns have been raised regarding high-intensity training (HIT) inducing excessive oxidative stress in those with hepatic damage (70), this study by deLira and colleagues illustrates that engaging in either 12 weeks of isocaloric energy expenditure (350 kcal) of HIT (3 times/wk at ventilatory threshold) or low-intensity training (LIT; 20% below VT) results in significant improvement in lipid profile and a decrease in ALT and AST in adolescents without negative side effects (27).

While work in the adult population examining the impact of aerobic exercise on various molecular pathways linked to NAFLD is ongoing (100), work in the paediatric population is lagging. Collectively, the positive changes observed in NAFLD biomarkers reinforces the importance of habitual physical activity to moderate hepatic damage in the paediatric population with obesity presumably by improving reverse cholesterol transport in the liver and peripheral tissues, as well as augmenting lipid oxidation in hepatocytes.

Respiratory Function

We know that obesity in childhood affects many body systems; in the case of the respiratory system, it can impair pulmonary function; characterized by reductions in (1) lung diffusion capacity, (2) gas exchange, (3) ventilatory muscle endurance (measured by maximal voluntary ventilation; MVV), and (4) airway diameter (as measured by reductions in forced expiratory volume in 1 s [FEV1]) (30, 52, 83). Collectively, these deficiencies result in reduced exercise tolerance.

Available evidence indicates that adolescents with obesity, particularly trunk fat mass, have decreased ventilatory responses compared with their age-matched normal-weight peers, particularly in lung volume and expiratory flow limitation at sub-maximal exercise (76). Furthermore, lung capacities and functional exercise, as measured by the 6-min walk test, are lower in children with obesity compared to non-obese peers (83), and lung function in the paediatric population, measured as the ratio of FEV1 to forced vital capacity (FVC), decreases with increasing BMI (37). This lower FEV1/FVC ratio is driven by a disproportionate increase in FVC vs. FEV1 (60), suggesting that childhood obesity is associated with an imbalance between ventilation and airway flow. Higher cardiorespiratory fitness appears to offer protection and is associated with an improved FEV1/FVC ratio in children with obesity (60).

As such, a 12-week supervised moderate-to-vigorous aerobic exercise training programme, consisting of two 60-min and one 120-min sessions per week was found to decrease exertional dyspnoea and improve inspiratory muscle strength, operating lung volumes, breathing pattern, and cardiorespiratory fitness in adolescents with obesity (76). Likewise, Inselman and colleagues (1993) reported significant improvements in FVC, FEV_1, and MVV following 24 weeks (3 d/wk, ~30 min/d) of continuous tread-mill running at 75–85% maximal HR (52). Given these indices of heightened lung function, one could assert that engaging in regular physical activity has the potential to improve patterns of lung function and attenuate exertional symptoms in children with obesity. It should be noted that there is evidence supporting the role of weight loss in normalizing lung function parameters.

Neural/Gastrointestinal Responses

As previously mentioned, childhood obesity results when energy balance favours intake over expenditure. Food intake is known to be regulated by a network of overlapping homeostatic (metabolic driven) and non-homeostatic (pleasure-driven) mechanisms reinforcing food reward and the motivation to eat (66). While much of our understanding comes from the adult population, there is evidence illustrating an interaction between acute and chronic exercise and the neurocognitive pathways involved in the regulation of food intake in children and adolescents with obesity.

Evidence illustrates that acute exercise (30 min at 70% max capacity) can reduce daily food intake in children with obesity (94). In follow-up work, an acute bout of exercise (45 minutes at 65% of maximal capacity) resulted in a decreased neural response to food cues in adolescents who are obese vs. those who are lean. This distinct response is suggestive of a weight-related effect of exercise on the neural processing of food cues (34). A set of review papers by Thivel et al. summarizes that acute intensive exercise reduces the desire to eat and thus short-term food intake in children with obesity (95). Acute exercise presumably modulates the orexigenic (ghrelin) and anorexigenic signals (GLP-1, PYY, CCK) acting in the arcuate nucleus, thereby transiently affecting energy intake. The impact of chronic physical activity on peripheral and neurocognitive pathways is less clear (90), but any impact would likely be through its effects on body composition.

Renal Function

Limited research has focused on testing the effect of structured exercise interventions or physical activity levels on renal function among children living with obesity. One study, as part of a larger intervention designed to test the effect of soccer compared to traditional activity programmes on body composition, examined the influence of physical activity on renal function among boys (8–12 years of age) who had obesity. Thirty-six boys were divided into one of three groups for a 6-month intervention: soccer, traditional physical activity, and a no-activity control group. The soccer group and the traditional physical activity groups participated in three 60-to 90-minute sessions per week. Changes in renal function were assessed by blood samples collected after an overnight fast at baseline and the end of the 6-month intervention period. To estimate glomerular filtration rate, plasma creatinine and plasma cystatin C levels were evaluated. Overall the results of this study suggested that a 6-month activity programme did not have a significant effect on renal function among boys who have obesity (69).

A recent review paper highlighted the detrimental health effects on renal function as a result of childhood obesity, including an increased risk for later-life kidney disease (23). The authors of this review acknowledged that, to date, a long-term successful physical activity intervention had not been developed and tested to improve renal function markers. However, based on research among youth and adult populations, a healthy lifestyle, including physical activity, should be offered to strengthen and protect renal function in all populations (23).

Vascular Function

The most common vascular outcome measured in paediatric obesity intervention programmes is blood pressure. A systematic review of meta-analyses (43) found that exercise can improve systolic blood pressure (SBP), but the same significant results were not observed for diastolic blood pressure (DBP). Intervention duration between 4 and 12 weeks was enough to promote changes in SBP; paradoxically, interventions longer than 12 weeks showed no effect (43).

Garcia-Hermoso et al. (2016) reviewed the literature and found that high-intensity interval training is more effective than other exercise intensities/modalities (e.g., moderate-intensity continuous and interval training, low-intensity interval training) to improve SBP in youth with overweight and obesity (41). Some physiological mechanisms that could explain these results are (1) the greater decrease in sympathetic nervous system activity, (2) higher vasodilatation mediated by NO, and (3) shear stress promoted by high-intensity exercise that may improve vasodilation. However, these are mostly speculations and deserve further investigation (41, 97).

Supervised exercise seems to be more efficient than non-supervised exercise in increasing flow-mediated dilation (43). This improvement can be achieved with 4–12 weeks of training, frequency >3 times/week, and session duration ≥60 min. Similarly, exercise programmes lasting for 4–12 weeks, with more than 60 min/session and a total exercise time ≥1,500 min may benefit carotid intima-media thickness.

The potential physiological mechanisms contributing to exercise effects on vascular function include (1) the up-regulation of endothelial NO synthase activity that would decrease the expression of nicotinamide adenine dinucleotide phosphate oxidase and stimulate copper/zinc-containing superoxide dismutase, extracellular superoxide dismutase, glutathione peroxidase, and glutathione (7, 43); (2) reduced endothelial dysfunction associated with the increase in adiponectin (i.e., anti-inflammatory marker) and/or decrease in visfatin (81) that would attenuate atherogenic processes via vascular endothelial cells (14, 41); and (3) better blood glucose control resulting in enhanced vascular function (106) (Figure 33.4).

Conclusion

Main Research Limitations and Future Directions

One of the principal research limitations identified in the studies reviewed is the large heterogeneity between exercise programmes (42, 43). Overall there is a lack of consistency in previous research for exercise intensity, duration, and type. Additionally, the literature should be evaluated separately for children (e.g., ages 5–9 years of age) and adolescents (e.g., ages 10–19 years of age), as there would be variation in growth, maturation status, and metabolic and musculoskeletal development (43).

Data related to some metabolic/physiological parameters, such as renal function and oxidative stress, do not allow for more robust conclusions regarding the benefits of exercise. Research in these fields is still limited and should be targeted in future studies.

Summary of the Metabolic Effects of Exercise on Childhood Obesity

Several organs, tissues, and biomarkers are improved with exercise in children and adolescents living with obesity. Figure 33.3 outlines the effects of exercise on the central metabolic/physiological variables in childhood obesity according to the core studies (systematic reviews and meta-analyses) described in this chapter.

Although further research is needed to elucidate the biochemical and physiological pathways through which exercise promotes metabolic change in paediatric obesity, Figure 33.4 summarizes some of the mechanisms currently considered logical.

Evidence-Based Exercise Prescription

Recent systematic reviews with meta-analyses have concluded that an individual exercise prescription that allows children and adolescents living with obesity to achieve the general exercise recommendations (i.e., daily physical activity at moderate-to-vigorous intensity for 60 min, mainly aerobic with some resistance training) as the exercise programme progresses are the most appropriate exercise-based approaches. Following specialized literature in the field of metabolic effects of exercise in childhood obesity (32, 43, 74, 106) and World Health Organization (11) recommendations, we outlined the effects of exercise on the main metabolic/physiological variables in childhood obesity (Figure 33.3). Children and adolescents who have obesity should engage in daily physical activity to realize the metabolic and physiological benefits linked to reduced cardiometabolic risk.

Additionally, Table 33.1 was designed to summarize aspects that should be considered to optimize exercise prescription for youth populations living with obesity, to achieve significant results in the treatment of metabolic outcomes related to excess body weight. We strongly suggest exercise professionals apply the available exercise prescription recommendations to optimize the health of children living with obesity.

Table 33.1 Exercise prescription based on FITT principles to treat known adverse metabolic effects of childhood obesity

Metabolic/physiological marker improved	Frequency	Intensity[b]	Time	Type
TG	>3×/week	Moderate-vigorous	≥1,500 min programme volume[c]	Aerobic
LDL-c	3×/week	Moderate-vigorous	60 min/session	Aerobic
HDL-c	3×/week	Vigorous	≥60 min/session	Aerobic + resistance
Fasting glucose*	3×/week	Moderate-vigorous	60 min/session	Aerobic
Fasting insulin*#	3×/week	Moderate-vigorous	60 min/session	Aerobic
HOMA-IR*	3×/week	Moderate-vigorous	60 min/session	Aerobic
Aerobic capacity	>3×/week	Moderate-vigorous	≥60 min/session	Aerobic
SBP#	3×/week	Moderate-vigorous	60 min/session	Aerobic + resistance[d]
Flow-mediated dilation	>3×/week	Moderate-vigorous	≥60 min/session	Aerobic + resistance[d]
Carotid intima-media thickness	3×/week	Moderate-vigorous	≥60 min/session	Aerobic + resistance[d]
Adiponectin	4–12 weeks programme length[a]	Moderate-vigorous	60 min/session	Aerobic + resistance[d]
Intrahepatic fat	3×/week	Moderate-vigorous	≥60 min/session	Aerobic + resistance[d]

Expert committee recommendation to treat childhood obesity

	Daily	Moderate-vigorous	60 min/session	Aerobic + resistance

* Greater improvements are achieved with greater exercise frequency
\# Greater improvements are achieved with longer exercise duration
a Exercise frequency was not significantly associated with improvements in this outcome, only programme length
b Systematic reviews and meta-analysis did not include specific suggestions. Expert committee recommends moderate-to-vigorous intensity (Barlow; Expert Committee, 2007). High-intensity interval training improves more CRF and SBP compared to other intensities (moderate-intensity interval training, moderate-intensity continuous training, light-intensity interval training) (41)
c Exercise time was not significantly associated with improvements in this outcome, only programme volume
d Type was not pre-defined in the systematic reviews for these specific variables, so we followed the expert committee recommendations (mainly aerobic combined with resistance training)

References

1. (IDF) International Diabetes Foundation. *The IDF Consensus Definition of the Metabolic Syndrome in Children and Adolescents*. Brussels, Belgium: IDF, 2007.
2. (IOM) Institute of Medicine. *Weight Gain During Pregnancy: Reexamining the Guidelines*. Washington, DC: The National Academies Press, 2009.
3. (NCD-RisC) NCD Risk Factor Collaboration. Worldwide trends in body-mass index, underweight, overweight, and obesity from 1975 to 2016: a pooled analysis of 2416 population-based measurement studies in 128.9 million children, adolescents, and adults. *Lancet (London, England)* 390: 2627–2642, 2017.
4. (WHO) World Health Organization. Obesity and overweight https://www.who.int/news-room/factsheets/detail/obesity-and-overweight. [Accessed on October 23 2019].
5. Adamo KB, Ferraro ZM, Brett KE. Can we modify the intrauterine environment to halt the intergenerational cycle of obesity? *Int J Environ Res Public Health*. 9: 1263–1307, 2012.
6. Alberga AS, Frappier A, Sigal RJ, Prud'homme D, Kenny GP. A review of randomized controlled trials of aerobic exercise training on fitness and cardiometabolic risk factors in obese adolescents. *Phys Sportsmed* 41: 44–57, 2013.
7. Ashor AW, Lara J, Siervo M, Celis-Morales C, Mathers JC. Effects of exercise modalities on arterial stiffness and wave reflection: a systematic review and meta-analysis of randomized controlled trials. *PLOS ONE* 9: e110034, 2014.
8. Avloniti A, Chatzinikolaou A, Deli CK, Vlachopoulos D, Gracia-Marco L, Leontsini D, et al. Exercise-induced oxidative stress responses in the pediatric population. *Antioxidants (Basel, Switzerland)* 6: 6–21, 2017.
9. Balagopal P, George D, Patton N, Yarandi H, Roberts WL, Bayne E, et al. Lifestyle-only intervention attenuates the inflammatory state associated with obesity: a randomized controlled study in adolescents. *J Pediatr* 146: 342–348, 2005.
10. Barker DJ. The fetal and infant origins of adult disease. *BMJ (Clinical Res Ed)* 301: 1111, 1990.
11. Barlow SE. Expert committee recommendations regarding the prevention, assessment, and treatment of child and adolescent overweight and obesity: summary report. *Pediatrics* 120(Suppl 4): S164–192, 2007.
12. Bennett CJ, Walker RE, Blumfield ML, Gwini SM, Ma J, Wang F, et al. Interventions designed to reduce excessive gestational weight gain can reduce the incidence of gestational diabetes mellitus: A systematic review and meta-analysis of randomised controlled trials. *Diabetes Clin Pract* 141:69–79, 2018.
13. Botton J, Heude B, Maccario J, Ducimetiere P, Charles MA. Postnatal weight and height growth velocities at different ages between birth and 5 y and body composition in adolescent boys and girls. *Am J Clin Nutr* 87: 1760–1768, 2008.
14. Bouassida A, Chamari K, Zaouali M, Feki Y, Zbidi A, Tabka Z. Review on leptin and adiponectin responses and adaptations to acute and chronic exercise. *Br J Sports Med* 44: 620–630, 2010.
15. Breton C. The hypothalamus-adipose axis is a key target of developmental programming by maternal nutritional manipulation. *J Endocrinol* 216: R19–31, 2013.
16. Brett KE, Ferraro ZM, Holcik M, Adamo KB. Placenta nutrient transport-related gene expression: the impact of maternal obesity and excessive gestational weight gain. *J Matern Fetal Neonatal Med* 29: 1399–1405, 2016.
17. Caballero B. The global epidemic of obesity: an overview. *Epidemiol Rev* 29: 1–5, 2007.
18. Chen X, Wang Y. Tracking of blood pressure from childhood to adulthood: a systematic review and meta-regression analysis. *Circulation* 117: 3171–3180, 2008.
19. Chung ST, Onuzuruike AU, Magge SN. Cardiometabolic risk in obese children. *Ann N Y Acad Sci* 1411: 166–183, 2018.
20. Cliff DP, Okely AD, Morgan PJ, Jones RA, Steele JR. The impact of child and adolescent obesity treatment interventions on physical activity: a systematic review. *Obes Rev* 11: 516–530, 2010.
21. Clifton VL. Review: Sex and the human placenta: mediating differential strategies of fetal growth and survival. *Placenta* 31(Suppl): S33–39, 2010.
22. Cook DG, Mendall MA, Whincup PH, Carey IM, Ballam L, Morris JE, et al. C-reactive protein concentration in children: relationship to adiposity and other cardiovascular risk factors. *Atherosclerosis* 149: 139–150, 2000.
23. Correia-Costa L, Azevedo A, Caldas Afonso A. Childhood obesity and impact on the kidney. *Nephron* 143: 8–11, 2019.
24. da Silva DF, Bianchini JA, Lopera CA, Capelato DA, Hintze LJ, Nardo CC, et al. Impact of readiness to change behavior on the effects of a multidisciplinary intervention in obese Brazilian children and adolescents. *Appetite* 87: 229–235, 2015.
25. Davis CL, Pollock NK, Waller JL, Allison JD, Dennis BA, Bassali R, et al. Exercise dose and diabetes risk in overweight and obese children: a randomized controlled trial. *JAMA* 308: 1103–1112, 2012.

26. Davis PH, Dawson JD, Riley WA, Lauer RM. Carotid intimal-medial thickness is related to cardiovascular risk factors measured from childhood through middle age: the Muscatine Study. *Circulation* 104: 2815–2819, 2001.

27. de Lira CT, Dos Santos MA, Gomes PP, Fidelix YL, Dos Santos AC, Tenorio TR, et al. Aerobic training performed at ventilatory threshold improves liver enzymes and lipid profile related to non-alcoholic fatty liver disease in adolescents with obesity. *Nutr Health* 23: 281–288, 2017.

28. de Mello MT, de Piano A, Carnier J, Sanches P de L, Correa FA, Tock L, et al. Long-term effects of aerobic plus resistance training on the metabolic syndrome and adiponectinemia in obese adolescents. *J Clin Hyperten* 13: 343–350, 2011.

29. Digital NHS. Statistics on obesity, physical activity and diet https://digital.nhs.uk/data-and-information/publications/statistical/statistics-on-obesity-physical-activity-and-diet. [Accessed on October 23 2019.

30. Durbin C, Egan R, Gervasi K, Nadeau N, Neal E, Reich S, et al. The effects of obesity on pulmonary function in children. *JAAPA* 30: 30–33, 2017.

31. Ekelund U, Ong K, Linne Y, Neovius M, Brage S, Dunger DB, et al. Upward weight percentile crossing in infancy and early childhood independently predicts fat mass in young adults: the stockholm weight development study (SWEDES). *Am J Clin Nutr* 83: 324–330, 2006.

32. Escalante Y, Saavedra JM, Garcia-Hermoso A, Dominguez AM. Improvement of the lipid profile with exercise in obese children: a systematic review. *Prev Med* 54: 293–301, 2012.

33. Faienza MF, Francavilla R, Goffredo R, Ventura A, Marzano F, Panzarino G, et al. Oxidative stress in obesity and metabolic syndrome in children and adolescents. *Horm Res Paediatr* 78: 158–164, 2012.

34. Fearnbach SN, Silvert L, Pereira B, Boirie Y, Duclos M, Keller KL, et al. Reduced neural responses to food cues might contribute to the anorexigenic effect of acute exercise observed in obese but not lean adolescents. *Nutr Res* 44: 76–84, 2017.

35. Ferraro ZM, Barrowman N, Prud'homme D, Walker M, Wen SW, Rodger M, et al. Excessive gestational weight gain predicts large for gestational age neonates independent of maternal body mass index. *J Matern Fetal Neonatal Med* 25: 538–542, 2012.

36. Fisher-Wellman K, Bloomer RJ. Acute exercise and oxidative stress: a 30 year history. *Dynamic Med* 8: 1, 2009.

37. Forno E, Han YY, Mullen J, Celedon JC. Overweight, obesity, and lung function in children and adults-a meta-analysis. *J Allergy Clin Immunol Pract* 6: 570–581 e510, 2018.

38. Freemark M. Determinants of risk for childhood obesity. *New Engl J Med* 379: 1371–1372, 2018.

39. Friend A, Craig L, Turner S. The prevalence of metabolic syndrome in children: a systematic review of the literature. *Metab Syndr Relat Disord* 11: 71–80, 2013.

40. Garcia-Hermoso A, Carmona-Lopez MI, Saavedra JM, Escalante Y. Physical exercise, detraining and lipid profile in obese children: a systematic review. *Arch Argent Pediatr* 112: 519–525, 2014.

41. Garcia-Hermoso A, Cerrillo-Urbina AJ, Herrera-Valenzuela T, Cristi-Montero C, Saavedra JM, Martinez-Vizcaino V. Is high-intensity interval training more effective on improving cardiometabolic risk and aerobic capacity than other forms of exercise in overweight and obese youth? A meta-analysis. *Obes Rev* 17: 531–540, 2016.

42. Garcia-Hermoso A, Ramirez-Velez R, Ramirez-Campillo R, Peterson MD, Martinez-Vizcaino V. Concurrent aerobic plus resistance exercise versus aerobic exercise alone to improve health outcomes in paediatric obesity: a systematic review and meta-analysis. *BJSM* 52: 161–166, 2018.

43. Garcia-Hermoso A, Ramirez-Velez R, Saavedra JM. Exercise, health outcomes, and paediatric obesity: a systematic review of meta-analyses. *J Sci Med Sport* 22: 76–84, 2019.

44. Garland T Jr., Schutz H, Chappell MA, Keeney BK, Meek TH, Copes LE, et al. The biological control of voluntary exercise, spontaneous physical activity and daily energy expenditure in relation to obesity: human and rodent perspectives. *J Exp Biol* 214: 206–229, 2011.

45. Garofalo C, Borrelli S, Minutolo R, Chiodini P, De Nicola L, Conte G. A systematic review and meta-analysis suggests obesity predicts onset of chronic kidney disease in the general population. *Kidney Int* 91: 1224–1235, 2017.

46. Gibson N, Johnston K, Bear N, Stick S, Logie K, Hall GL. Expiratory flow limitation and breathing strategies in overweight adolescents during submaximal exercise. *Int J Obes* 38: 22–26, 2014.

47. Gonzalez-Ruiz K, Ramirez-Velez R, Correa-Bautista JE, Peterson MD, Garcia-Hermoso A. The Effects of exercise on abdominal fat and liver enzymes in pediatric obesity: a systematic review and meta-analysis. *Child Obed* 13: 272–282, 2017.

48. Gurnani M, Birken C, Hamilton J. Childhood obesity: causes, consequences, and management. *Pediatr Clin North Am* 62: 821–840, 2015.

49. Hales CM, Fryar CD, Carroll MD, Freedman DS, Ogden CL. Trends in obesity and severe obesity prevalence in US youth and adults by sex and age, 2007-2008 to 2015-2016. *JAMA* 319: 1723–1725, 2018.

50. Hall DM, Cole TJ. What use is the BMI? *Arch Dis Child* 91: 283–286, 2006.
51. Hruby A, Hu FB. The epidemiology of obesity: a big picture. *PharmacoEconomics* 33: 673–689, 2015.
52. Inselma LS, Milanese A, Deurloo A. Effect of obesity on pulmonary function in children. *Pediatr Pulmon* 16: 130–137, 1993.
53. Josefson JL, Hoffmann JA, Metzger BE. Excessive weight gain in women with a normal pre-pregnancy BMI is associated with increased neonatal adiposity. *Pediatr Obes* 8: e33–36, 2013.
54. Jung TW, Yoo HJ, Choi KM. Implication of hepatokines in metabolic disorders and cardiovascular diseases. *BBA Clinical* 5: 108–113, 2016.
55. Juonala M, Viikari JS, Ronnemaa T, Marniemi J, Jula A, Loo BM, et al. Associations of dyslipidemias from childhood to adulthood with carotid intima-media thickness, elasticity, and brachial flow-mediated dilatation in adulthood: the cardiovascular risk in young finns study. *Arterioscler Thromb Vasc Biol* 28: 1012–1017, 2008.
56. Kahn BB, Flier JS. Obesity and insulin resistance. *J Clin Invest* 106: 473–481, 2000.
57. Kelishadi R, Hashemi M, Mohammadifard N, Asgary S, Khavarian N. Association of changes in oxidative and proinflammatory states with changes in vascular function after a lifestyle modification trial among obese children. *Clin Chem* 54: 147–153, 2008.
58. Kelsey MM, Zaepfel A, Bjornstad P, Nadeau KJ. Age-related consequences of childhood obesity. *Gerontology* 60: 222–228, 2014.
59. King AK, McGill-Meeks K, Beller JP, urt Solorzano CM. Go Girls!-Dance-based fitness to increase enjoyment of exercise in girls at risk for PCOS. *Children (Basel, Switzerland)* 6: 99–112, 2019.
60. Kochli S, Endes K, Bartenstein T, Usemann J, Schmidt-Trucksass A, Frey U, et al. Lung function, obesity and physical fitness in young children: The EXAMIN YOUTH study. *Resp Med* 159: 105813, 2019.
61. Kraus WE, Slentz CA. Exercise training, lipid regulation, and insulin action: a tangled web of cause and effect. *Obesity (Silver Spring, MD)* 17(Suppl 3): S21–26, 2009.
62. Kumar S, Kelly AS. Review of childhood obesity: from epidemiology, etiology, and comorbidities to clinical assessment and treatment. *Mayo Clin Proc* 92: 251–265, 2017.
63. Lee S, Bacha F, Hannon T, Kuk JL, Boesch C, Arslanian S. Effects of aerobic versus resistance exercise without caloric restriction on abdominal fat, intrahepatic lipid, and insulin sensitivity in obese adolescent boys: a randomized, controlled trial. *Diabetes* 61: 2787–2795, 2012.
64. Lee S, Libman I, Hughan K, Kuk JL, Jeong JH, Zhang D, et al. Effects of exercise modality on insulin resistance and ectopic fat in adolescents with overweight and obesity: a randomized clinical trial. *J Pediatr* 206: 91–98.e91, 2019.
65. Lesseur C, Armstrong DA, Murphy MA, Appleton AA, Koestler DC, Paquette AG, et al. J. Sex-specific associations between placental leptin promoter DNA methylation and infant neurobehavior. *Psychoneuroendocrinology* 40: 1–9, 2014.
66. Liu CM, Kanoski SE. Homeostatic and non-homeostatic controls of feeding behavior: Distinct vs. common neural systems. *Physiol Behav* 193: 223–231, 2018.
67. Liu W, Li Q, Li H, Li J, Wang HJ, Li B. 20-year trends in prevalence of overweight and obesity among children aged 0-6 in Harbin, China: A multiple cross-sectional study. *PLOS ONE* 13: e0198032, 2018.
68. Logan CA, Bornemann R, Koenig W, Reister F, Walter V, Fantuzzi G, et al. Gestational weight gain and fetal-maternal adiponectin, leptin, and CRP: results of two birth cohorts studies. *Sci Rep* 7: 41847, 2017.
69. Lousa I, Nascimento H, Rocha S, Catarino C, Reis F, Rego C, et al. Influence of the 6-month physical activity programs on renal function in obese boys. *Pediatr Res* 83: 1011–1015, 2018.
70. Mahdiabadi J, Gaeini AA, Kazemi T, Mahdiabadi MA. The effect of aerobic continuous and interval training on left ventricular structure and function in male non-athletes. *Biol Sport* 30: 207–211, 2013.
71. Mahoney LT, Burns TL, Stanford W, Thompson BH, Witt JD, Rost CA, et al. Coronary risk factors measured in childhood and young adult life are associated with coronary artery calcification in young adults: the Muscatine Study. *J Am Coll Cardiol* 27: 277–284, 1996.
72. Makni E, Moalla W, Trabelsi Y, Lac G, Brun JF, Tabka Z, et al. Six-minute walking test predicts maximal fat oxidation in obese children. *Int J Obes* 36: 908–913, 2012.
73. Marseglia L, Manti S, D'Angelo G, Nicotera A, Parisi E, Di Rosa G, et al. Oxidative stress in obesity: a critical component in human diseases. *Int J Mol Sci* 16: 378–400, 2014.
74. Marson EC, Delevatti RS, Prado AK, Netto N, Kruel LF. Effects of aerobic, resistance, and combined exercise training on insulin resistance markers in overweight or obese children and adolescents: A systematic review and meta-analysis. *Prev Med* 93: 211–218, 2016.
75. Medrano M, Cadenas-Sanchez C, Alvarez-Bueno C, Cavero-Redondo I, Ruiz JR, Ortega FB, et al. Evidence-based exercise recommendations to reduce hepatic fat content in youth- a systematic review and meta-analysis. *Prog Cardiovasc Dis* 61: 222–231, 2018.
76. Mendelson M, Michallet AS, Esteve F, Perrin C, Levy P, Wuyam B, et al. Ventilatory responses to exercise training in obese adolescents. *Respir Physiol Neurobiol* 184: 73–79, 2012.

77. Meyer AA, Kundt G, Lenschow U, Schuff-Werner P, Kienast W. Improvement of early vascular changes and cardiovascular risk factors in obese children after a six-month exercise program. *J Am Coll Cardiol* 48: 1865–1870, 2006.

78. Montero D, Walther G, Perez-Martin A, Roche E, Vinet A. Endothelial dysfunction, inflammation, and oxidative stress in obese children and adolescents: markers and effect of lifestyle intervention. *Obes Rev* 13: 441–455, 2012.

79. Murphy EC, Carson L, Neal W, Baylis C, Donley D, Yeater R. Effects of an exercise intervention using Dance Dance Revolution on endothelial function and other risk factors in overweight children. *Int J Pediatr Obes* 4: 205–214, 2009.

80. Nathan BM, Moran A. Metabolic complications of obesity in childhood and adolescence: more than just diabetes. *Curr Opin Endocrinol Diabetes Obes* 15: 21–29, 2008.

81. Northcott JM, Yeganeh A, Taylor CG, Zahradka P, Wigle JT. Adipokines and the cardiovascular system: mechanisms mediating health and disease. *Can J Physiol Pharmacol* 90: 1029–1059, 2012.

82. Ortega FB, Sui X, Lavie CJ, Blair SN. Body mass index, the most widely used but also widely criticized index: would a criterion standard measure of total body fat be a better predictor of cardiovascular disease mortality? *Mayo Clin Proc* 91: 443–455, 2016.

83. Ozgen IT, Cakir E, Torun E, Gules A, Hepokur MN, Cesur Y. Relationship between functional exercise capacity and lung functions in obese chidren. *J Clin Res Pediatr Endocrinol* 7: 217–221, 2015.

84. Paes ST, Marins JC, Andreazzi AE. [Metabolic effects of exercise on childhood obesity: a current view]. *Rev Paul Pediatr* 33: 122–129, 2015.

85. Parizkova J, Mackova E, Mackova J, Skopkova M. Blood lipids as related to food intake, body composition, and cardiorespiratory efficiency in preschool children. *J Pediatr Gastroenterol Nutr* 5: 295–298, 1986.

86. Rao DP, Kropac E, Do MT, Roberts KC, Jayaraman GC. Childhood overweight and obesity trends in Canada. *Health Promot Chronic Dis Prev Can* 36: 194–198, 2016.

87. Roberts CK, Chen AK, Barnard RJ. Effect of a short-term diet and exercise intervention in youth on atherosclerotic risk factors. *Atherosclerosis* 191: 98–106, 2007.

88. Rooney BL, Mathiason MA, Schauberger CW. Predictors of obesity in childhood, adolescence, and adulthood in a birth cohort. *Matern Child Nutr* 15: 1166–1175, 2011.

89. Saakslahti A, Numminen P, Varstala V, Helenius H, Tammi A, Viikari J, et al. Physical activity as a preventive measure for coronary heart disease risk factors in early childhood. *Scand J Med Sci SPorts* 14: 143–149, 2004.

90. Schwartz C, King NA, Perreira B, Blundell JE, Thivel D. A systematic review and meta-analysis of energy and macronutrient intake responses to physical activity interventions in children and adolescents with obesity. *Pediatr Obes* 12: 179–194, 2017.

91. Shah RV, Murthy VL, Abbasi SA, Blankstein R, Kwong RY, Goldfine AB, et al. Visceral adiposity and the risk of metabolic syndrome across body mass index: the MESA Study. *JACC Cardiovasc Imag* 7: 1221–1235, 2014.

92. Shih KC, Kwok CF. Exercise reduces body fat and improves insulin sensitivity and pancreatic beta-cell function in overweight and obese male Taiwanese adolescents. *BMC Pediatr* 18: 80, 2018.

93. Tangvarasittichai S. Oxidative stress, insulin resistance, dyslipidemia and type 2 diabetes mellitus. *World J Diabetes* 6: 456–480, 2015.

94. Thivel D, Isacco L, Rousset S, Boirie Y, Morio B, Duche P. Intensive exercise: a remedy for childhood obesity? *Physiol Behav* 102: 132–136, 2011.

95. Thivel D, Rumbold PL, King NA, Pereira B, Blundell JE, Mathieu ME. Acute post-exercise energy and macronutrient intake in lean and obese youth: a systematic review and meta-analysis. *Int J Obes* 40: 1469–1479, 2016.

96. Tilg H, Moschen AR. Evolution of inflammation in nonalcoholic fatty liver disease: the multiple parallel hits hypothesis. *Hepatology (Baltimore, MD)* 52: 1836–1846, 2010.

97. Tinken TM, Thijssen DH, Hopkins N, Dawson EA, Cable NT, Green DJ. Shear stress mediates endothelial adaptations to exercise training in humans. *Hypertension (Dallas, TX: 1979)* 55: 312–318, 2010.

98. Tjonna AE, Stolen TO, Bye A, Volden M, Slordahl SA, Odegard R, et al. Aerobic interval training reduces cardiovascular risk factors more than a multitreatment approach in overweight adolescents. *Clin Sci (London, England: 1979)* 116: 317–326, 2009.

99. Troiano RP, Flegal KM. Overweight children and adolescents: description, epidemiology, and demographics. *Pediatrics* 101: 497–504, 1998.

100. van der Windt DJ, Sud V, Zhang H, Tsung A, Huang H. The Effects of physical exercise on fatty liver disease. *Gene Expr* 18: 89–101, 2018.

101. Wang H, Ji J, Yu Y, Wei X, Chai S, Liu D, et al. Neonatal overfeeding in female mice predisposes the development of obesity in their male offspring via altered central leptin signalling. *J Neuroendocrinol* 27: 600–608, 2015.

102. Weinstock RS, Drews KL, Caprio S, Leibel NI, McKay SV, Zeitler PS. Metabolic syndrome is common and persistent in youth-onset type 2 diabetes: Results from the TODAY clinical trial. *Obesity (Silver Spring, MD)* 23: 1357–1361, 2015.
103. Weiss R, Taksali SE, Tamborlane WV, Burgert TS, Savoye M, Caprio S. Predictors of changes in glucose tolerance status in obese youth. *Diabetes Care* 28: 902–909, 2005.
104. Wells JC, Ritz P. Physical activity at 9-12 months and fatness at 2 years of age. *Am J Hum Biol* 13: 384–389, 2001.
105. Woo Baidal JA, Morel K, Nichols K, Elbel E, Charles N, Goldsmith J, et al. Sugar-sweetened beverage attitudes and consumption during the first 1000 days of life. *Am J Public Health* 108: 1659–1665, 2018.
106. Zguira MS, Slimani M, Bragazzi NL, Khrouf M, Chaieb F, Saiag B, et al. Effect of an 8-week individualized training program on blood biomarkers, adipokines and endothelial function in obese young adolescents with and without metabolic syndrome. *Int J Environ Res Public Health* 16: 751–762, 2019.
107. Zhang J, Zhou K, Luo L, Liu Y, Liu X, Xu L. Effects of exercise and dietary habits on the occurrence of polycystic ovary syndrome over 5 years of follow-up. *Int J Gynaecol Obstet* 142: 329–337, 2018.
108. Zimmermann R, Lass A, Haemmerle G, Zechner R. Fate of fat: the role of adipose triglyceride lipase in lipolysis. *Biochim Biophys Acta* 1791: 494–500, 2009.

INDEX

Note: Page numbers in *italics* indicate figures and **bold** indicates tables in the text.

acetyl-CoA 6
Achilles tendon pathology 225
acidosis 211, 334
acute exercise: and habitual exercise, relationship between 436–437; skeletal muscle glucose disposal: during 434–436; after 436
Adamo, K. B. 534
adenosine receptor antagonism 369–370
adenosine triphosphate (ATP) 5; breakdown 6; regeneration 6; synthesis 6
β adrenergic signalling 131–132
Aengevaeren, V. L. 466
aerobic energy production, regulation: substrates, mitochondria in 23; TCA cycle 23–24
aerobic exercise 481; energy provision during: fat oxidation, maximal rates of 23; fuel use *22, 23*; fuel utilization 22; oxidative metabolism of CHO and fat 22
aerobic metabolism 7; ATP use, by-products 26
Ahmadi Angali, K. 326
Akerblom, H. K. 489
β-alanine: effects on performance 330; food sources **330**; supplementation 329; effects of 340; exercise performance, effects on 340–341; influence of 340; muscle buffering capacity *339*; side effects 341; strategies 339–340
Albers, P. H. 181
Ali, A. 366
Alizadeh, A. 326
Allsopp, A. J. 326
al-Modaris, F. 489
Alzheimer disease (AD) 401
American Journal of Cardiology 471
amino acids (AAs): oxidation, experimental data 5
AMP-activated protein kinase (AMPK) 146
AMP-dependent protein kinase (AMPK) 73

AMPK signalling 128–129
anaerobic glycolysis 6
Andel, M. 487
Anderson, J. M. 99
Andersson, G. 524
An, P. 222
antecedent hypoglycaemia 482–483
anterior cruciate ligament (ACL) injury 225
Antunes, M. 328
Anwander, H. 340
anxiety 376
apoptosis 400
Aragon, A. A. 327
Ardawi, M. S. M. 522, 524
Areta, J. L. 327
Armstrong, D. D. 94
Armstrong, L. E. 99
Armstrong, R. A. 326
Ashton, K. J. 248
Asp, S. 36
Åstrand, Per-Olof 220
athletes: dietary recommendation: CHO intake 10; dietary fat intake 10; energy intake 9; exercise training load 9; macronutrient intake 9–10; phenylalanine oxidation *11*; protein needs 10; performance, biochemical and metabolic limitations: anaerobic and aerobic respiration, by-products of 209–211; elongated mitochondria *209*; exercise performance 207; future areas of research 213; historical milestones 205–206; intense exercise-induced build-up of ionic by-products *210*; oxygen requirement, ability to 208–209; post-exercise glycogen supercompensation *206*; readily available fuel or metabolites 211–212
Auria Biobank 219
autonomic neuropathy 487

Baba, O. 181
Babcock, L. 197

Babraj, J. 326
Badenhorst, C. 366
Baker, K. M. 339
Baker, S. K. 102
Bamman, M. 253
Barker, D. J. 533
Baumgartner, A. 487
Baylis, C. 538
beetroot: blood flow 328; dietary nitrate, sources of 328; nitric oxide production from *329*
Bellamy, L. M. 250
Bellinger, P. M. 341
Beloni, R. 346
Benatti, F. B. 340, 346
Bergström, I. 524
Bergström, J. 206, 212
Berrigan, D. 501
biguanide drug metformin 441–442; exercise and treatment for T2D, interactions between **442**
Billensteiner E. 524
Billman, G. E. 457
Birk, J. B. 181
Bjornstad, P. 487
Blair, S. N. 286
Blanco, C. E. 195
Blomstrand, E. 94
Blundell, J. E. 286, 541
body mass index (BMI) 4
body weight: energy balance, influence of: dietary intake on 283; exercise training on 282–283
bone formation marker (BAP) 517; characteristics, role, and function **518**
Bonen, A. 253
bones: bone mineral density (BMD) 513; cells: osteoblasts 514; osteoclasts 515; osteocytes 514; growth, modelling, and remodelling 515; metabolism: biochemical markers 517; exercise and 520–522; physiology, types of 514; turnover and calcium homeostasis 515–516
Boobis, L. H. 181, 330, 340
Bouchard, C. 220, 222
Boushel, R. 300
Braber, T. L. 466
Braun, B. 440
breathing process 260
Brehm, A. 488
Brett, K. E. 534
Breuckmann, F. 466
Brinck, J. 524
Broad, E. M. 327
Bröcker-Preuss, M. 466
Brogan, R. J. 222
Brooks, S. 181
Brouwers, B. 253
Buehler, T. 340
Burd, N. A. 102
Burke, L. M. 327
Burkholder, T. J. 94
Busing, F. 286
Byrne, N. M. 285

caffeine: adenosine receptor antagonism 369–370; affinity of 370; and anxiety 376; consumption 363–364; dose, timing, and administration 367–368; exercise performance 366–367; impacts of 369; mechanisms of action 368–369; metabolism and excretion 365, *365*; negative side effects 368; performance, interindividual responses 376–377; pharmacokinetics, absorption 364–365; source of 363
Calabria, E. 89
calcineurin signalling 96
calcitonin 516
calcium signalling 146
calmodulin 96
calmodulin-dependent protein kinase (CaMK) 127
Camera, D. M. 102, 327
Campbell, B. I. 326
Campbell, N. P. 489
Campos, H. O. 329
cAMP-response element-binding protein (CREB) 96
cancer: cancer cachexia 507; cancer-related fatigue (CRF) 509; cellular signalling pathways 500; cellular transformation, processes in 500–501; chemotherapy drug doxorubicin 504; effect of 499; epidemiological studies 499; exercise and physical activity, for prevention: biological mechanisms 500–501; epidemiological evidence 500; factors and risk 500; pre-clinical studies 501; skeletal muscle myokine 501; exercise and survival 505, 507; daily physical activity 506; effects of 506; exercise and treatment 504–505; neoplastic cell interaction 502; physical activity during, therapeutic efficacy *504*; pre-clinical models 502–503; systemic environment 502; tumour microenvironment 502; hallmarks of 500; reported cases 499; survivors, future directions: cachectic skeletal muscle 508; mitochondrial dysfunction control of proteostasis, effect of *508*; oestrogen 507; periods of physical inactivity 507; skeletal muscle metabolic homeostasis, treatment effect on *505*; treatment and survival, role of physical activity **506**
carbohydrate: components of 5; energy 5; exercise fuel source 5; humans, stores in **5**; and lipid storage 295; and nutraceutical compounds 113–314
carbohydrate oxidation, regulation: glucose transport: active form, enzyme to 24; muscle glycogen: liver glucose 24; skeletal muscle glucose, facilitated diffusion 24
carboxyl-terminal crosslinking telopeptide of type I collagen (CTX) 517
cardiovascular autonomic neuropathy 487
cardiovascular disease (CVD): accelerated coronary artery calcification 466; atherosclerotic CAD 468; atrial fibrillation (AF) and exercise 467–468; potential mechanisms and associated sequelae for *468*; cardiac ischemic injury, mechanisms of 459–460; cardiac pre-conditioning 460–462; phenomenology of exercise *463*; study design for ischemic pre-conditioning research *461*; coronary heart disease (CHD) 455; exercise

pre-conditioning: biochemical mechanisms 464–465; cardioprotection, approach 462–463; characteristic aspects 463; clinical verification 465; time course 463; training specifications 463; exercise training volume and cardiovascular health: dose-response association between *468*; high-volume and high-intensity endurance training and potential: adverse cardiovascular maladaptations 465–466; physical activity (PA) 455; regular physical activity, cardioprotective benefits of: antiarrhythmic effects 457; anti-atherosclerotic effects 456; anti-ischemic effects 456–457; antithrombotic effects 457–458; biochemical cardiac pre-conditioning 458; moderate-to-vigorous exercise training, mechanisms *456*; potential underlying mechanisms 456; psychologic effects 458; risk factors, cardiorespiratory fitness and physical activity: comparative benefits 458–459; sedentary death syndrome 455; sudden cardiac death 468–470; United States, risk 469–470; transient cardiac dysfunction and increased myocardial fibrosis 466–467; vigorous and moderate-intensity physical activity, cardioprotective benefits of 458

Carnier, J. 538
carnosine 339
Carr, A. J. 344
Carson, L. 538
Ca²⁺ signalling 124–127
Caudwell, P. 285
Cavalcante, E. F. 328
cell: cellular stress 113; signalling: glycogen in, role of 295–296
cells: division 401
central fatigue 71, 75–77; intracellular processes 76; tetanic contractions 76
Cerrillo-Urbina, A. J. 542
Cheetham, M. E. 181
Chen, C. 322
Cherney, D. Z. 487
childhood obesity: aetiology 532; modifiable and non-modifiable factors 533; physical activity and inactivity 533; developmental origins 533; intergenerational cycle of *534*; metabolic and physiological impact: carotid intimal medial thickness 535; consequences *536*; excess body weight, function impaired due to 535; high blood pressure 535; insulin resistance 534–535; metabolic/physiological variables *539*; metabolic syndrome 535; pathophysiological aspects 535; renal function 535; mode of management, exercise: hepatic function 539–540; hyperlipidaemia 536–537; inflammatory and oxidative stress markers 538; insulin resistance 537; physical activity, developmental programming 533–534; prevalence of: body mass index (BMI) 532; in Canada 532; in UK 532; in United States 532
Chinnaiyan, K. M. 467
Chiu, L. Z. F. 99
Chmelik, M. 488
chronic fatigue syndrome (CFS) 405

chronic obstructive pulmonary disease (COPD) 404
chronic resistance exercise 88–89
Church, D. D. 339
Churchward-Venne, T. A. 102
citric acid cycle 6
Clark, J. 487
Coakley, J. 330
Coffey, V. G. 102
Colbert, L. H. 501
Colley, R. 285
Conlee, R. K. 94
Conway, G. E. 321
Cooper, J. A. 326
Coqueiro, A. Y. 321
Cornnell, H. H. 253
Correa, F. A. 538
creatine phosphate 212
creatine supplementation: bone, effect on 357–359; chemical structure of *354*; mechanisms *357, 358*; muscle energy supply with, enhancement of 353–355; muscle protein: degradation, effect of 356–357; synthesis with, enhancement of 355–356; shuttle system *354*
Cree-Green, M. 487
Cribb, P. J. 326
CRISPR–Cas9 system 227
Cristi-Montero, C. 542
Crohn disease 405
cross-bridge cycling 72
Cross, J. 253
Cryer, P. E. 485
Cuenca, E. 329
Cui, X. 253
cyanide-exposed single soleus fibres 75
cyclooxygenase 2 (COX-2) inhibitors 97
cytokines 97
cytokine signalling 132–133

Damas, F. 251
da Mata Godois, A. 321
Danna, M. 488
da Silva, R. P. 340, 346
Davey, T. 326
Dawson, A. W. 521
De Cobelli, F. 488
Decombaz, J. 340
deJong, A. T. 467
Dela, F. 300
delayed-onset muscle soreness (DOMS) 382
de Mello, M. T. 538
de Oliveira, L. F. 340, 346
de Oliveira, O. M. Jr. 340, 346
de Piano, A. 538
Detroit Free Press Flagstar Marathon 469
De Vito, G. 321
Devlin, B. L. 300
Diabetes Control and Complications Trial (DCCT) 487
diabetic nephropathy 487
dichotomous classification methods 244

dietary recommendations and dietary requirements 9
dihydroethidium (DHE) 54
D'Lugos, A. 197
DNA methylation 233
Doevendans, P. A. 466
Domínguez, R. 329
Donaghue, V. M. 489
Donehower, L. A. 501
Donley, D. 538
Dorchy, H. 489
Douglas, P. S. 466
Dreyer, H. C. 195
Drummond, L. R. 329
Drummond, M. J. 94
Duchenne (DMD) and Becker (BMD) muscular
    dystrophies 404
Dunnett, M. 330
Dwyer, D. B. 344
dystrophin–glycoprotein complex 94–95

eccentric exercise 94
Edelman, R. 489
Egger, A. 340
Ehlers–Danlos syndrome 225
Ekblom, B. 94
electron transport chain (ETC) 143
electron transport system (ETS) 55, 393–394
Elfegoun, T. 94
Eliasson, J. 94
ENCODE project 219
endocrine 98–99
endocrine regulators during exercise: adipose tissue
    (adipokinome) 38–40; liver (hepatokinome) 40–43;
    skeletal muscle (myokinome) 36–38
endothelial nitric oxide synthase (eNOS) 55
energy: intake 277; metabolism: aerobic 73; anaerobic
    72–73; production, pathways 292–293; provision
    during aerobic exercise: aerobic ATP production,
    major substrates 22; fuel use during exercise 22–23;
    fuel utilization 22–23; storage 278; regulation 282;
    see also energy expenditure
energy balance, regulation: energy intake, regulation
    of 280; homeostatic signals 279–280; metabolic
    adaptation 278–279; resting energy expenditure
    280–281
energy expenditure 278, *285*; regulation: exercise
    energy expenditure 281–282; non-exercise activity
    thermogenesis 281; resting energy expenditure 281;
    thermic effect of feeding 281
Epstein, D. 217
Eroshkin, A. M. 253
erythrocytosis 224–225
erythropoietin (EPO) 224; production 262
Escano, M. 197
essential and non-essential amino acids 311
Esser, K. A. 94
Estrem, S. T. 251
exercise: benefits of: epidemiological and experimental
    studies 433; long term and short term, risk 434;
    pre-diabetes 433; exercise-induced autophagy 133;

exercise-induced hepcidin elevation 323; exercise-
    induced PKA regulation 133; fuel selection:
    carbohydrate loading 8–9; factors 7; muscle
    glycogen use and time 8; metabolism 3; *see also*
    acute exercise
exercise training 9; analysing individual, responses
    to: responders and low-responders, classifying
    243; variation influencing, sources of 243; bone
    turnover markers and osteokine levels **523**;
    individual response variability, investigating
    mechanisms of 245; interindividual variability,
    analysing: quantifying interindividual variability
    244; variation influencing, sources of 243–244;
    labelling individuals as non-responders, concerns
    with 244–245
extensor digitorum longus (EDL) 117
extracellular matrix (ECM) 92
extracellular signal–regulated kinase (ERK) 88, 308
Eynon, N. 248

Faigenbaum, A. D. 340
fat: and carbohydrate metabolism, relationship
    between: aerobic ATP contribution 27; ATGL
    and IMTG breakdown 27; FFA transport 27;
    energy store and supply 4; location of 3; obesity,
    and 4; oxidation *4*; oxidation, regulation: AMPK
    phosphorylates 25; mitochondria, FA transport
    25–26; muscle, breakdown of IMTG 25; transport
    proteins 25; percentage 3
fatigue 73; adaptations 79–80; central fatigue 75–77;
    intracellular processes *76*; tetanic contractions *76*;
    peripheral fatigue 77–79; pH: biochemistry of 335–
    336; buffering systems 337–338; intracellular and
    extracellular 338; pKa of ionizable groups of amino
    acids **338**; titration curves *337*; rate of development
    75; recovery 79; repeated tetanic stimulation *74*
Fernandes, R. R. 328
Ferraro, Z. M. 534
Fett, C. A. 321
fibronectin domain–containing protein 5 (FNDC5) 38
focal adhesion kinase (FAK) protein 91
Forsblom, C. 487
Franklin, B. A. 467
free fatty acids (FFAs): mobilized and released 3
Friedman, J. M. 39
Fry, A. C. 99, 102

Gagnon, J. 222
Gallagher, M. J. 467
Galpin, A. J. 99
Galvani, L. 85
García-Fernández, P. 329
Garcia-Hermoso, A. 537, 538, 542
gastrointestinal (GI) dysfunction 405
gene expression, epigenetics and control 232; DNA
    methylation 233; epigenetic mechanisms 234;
    exercise and exercise training, epigenetic responses
    to 234–236; histone modifications and variants
    233–234; unanswered questions 237–238
generalized signalling response 101

gene therapy, clinical trial 227
genetic limitations and athletic performance 217;
    ACTN3 R577X genotype frequencies *224*;
    candidate gene studies 225–226; champion, as
    221; complexity of nature 218–219; complexity
    of nurture 218; complex performance traits 220;
    elite human performance 226–227; endurance
    performance, heritable aspects of 220–221; gene
    doping 227–228; genetic traits, simple and complex
    219–220; importance of genetics *221*; limits of
    performance 228; non-responders to exercise 222;
    physiology within *218*; rare and common genetic
    variants, injury risk 225; rare genetic variants
    224–225; VO$_2$ max 222–224
1000 Genomes Project 219
genome-wide association study (GWAS)
    225–226
Gerrard, D. E. 89
GEUVADIS project 219
Giurini, J. M. 489
glucocorticoid receptor 99
glycogenolysis 5
glycogen, super-compensation 206
glycolysis 5–6
Goldstein, J. A. 467
Goto, K. 323
Graef, J. L. 341
Granados, K. 440
Grant, A. 89
Grant, M. C. 326
Grobbee, D. E. 466
Grubb, A. 250
Gustafsson, S. A. 524

Haapalahti, J. 522
habitual exercise: glucoregulatory benefits of 437–438;
    oxidative metabolic adaptations to 438; *see also* acute
    exercise
Hackney, K. 466
Hagele, F. A. 286
Haines, D. C. 501
Halle, M. 466
Hamilton, M. T. 440
Hand, G. A. 286
Hannon, K. 89
Hansen, C. N. 300
hard-stop pathway 113–114
Harjutsalo, V. 487
Harris, B. D. 340
Harris, R. C. 330, 340, 344
Harris Rosenzweig, P. 324
Hasler, M. 286
Hawley, J. A. 102
Hayashi, N. 323
Haymond, M. W. 485
Heady, J. A. 455
Health, Risk factors, exercise Training
    And Genetics (HERITAGE) Family Study
    220, 222, 226
heat shock factor 1 (HSF1) 113

heat shock proteins (HSP) 112–113; canonical HSP
    functions *113*; cell survival and intracellular
    signalling 113–114; chronic disease and 115;
    exercise, and 115; expression, fibre type specific
    117; HSF1, PGC1α, in coordinating MitoQC
    118; initiation 113; intensity, primary driver of,
    response to exercise 116; involvement in, muscular
    remodelling 116–117; mitochondrial import 115;
    mitochondrial quality control, and 117–118, *119*;
    mitophagy, and 118; oxidative capacity, and 117;
    post-exercise, functions of *116*; protein folding and
    degradation 114; response, dependent on training
    status 116
Heden, T. D. 441
Heffernan, S. M. 321
Heigenhauser, G. J. F. 253
He, K. 322
Helge, J. W. 300
Helvering, L. M. 251
hepatokines 40; angiopoietin-like protein-4
    (ANGPTL4) 42–43; fibroblast growth factor 21
    (FGF21) 41; follistatin (FST) 41–42
heritability 220
Herrera-Valenzuela, T. 542
hexokinase 400
high-intensity interval training (HIIT) protocol 37,
    154, 341, 414, 485
high-intensity, short-term exercise 17; aerobic ATP
    contribution, time 20–21; aerobic pathways 17;
    capacity of energy 17–19; covalent and allosteric
    regulation, combination of 17; direct measurements
    17; important aspect of 21; phosphorylase, activate
    directly 17
high-intensity training (HIT) 439
Hill, C. A. 340
Hiller, W. D. 466
Hills, A. P. 285
Hinton, P. S. 521
Hoffman, J. R. 339, 340
Hoffman, N. J. 300
Holcik, M. 534
Holloszy, J. 232, 292
Holloway, G. P. 253
Hopkins, M. 285
Hornberger, T. A. 94
Horner, K. 321
Huang, T. H. 521
Hultman, E. 206, 212
Human Genome Project (HGP) 219
human lung cancer models 406
Huntington disease (HD) 401
Huttunen, N. P. 489
Hwang, H. 323
hypertrophy 88–89

Iceland deCODE project 219
immune and inflammatory responses
    97
individual patterns of response
    244

individual responses to exercise, genetic influence on: acute changes and training adaptations: chronic skeletal muscle changes 253–254; mechanisms associated 254; multiomic approaches 254–255; pathways 250–251; skeletal muscle mRNA 250–251; skeletal muscle protein synthesis 251–252; animal studies, evidence from 245–246; exercise training responses, quantitative trait loci mapping for 246; inbred strains/lines 245–246; low and high responses to exercise training, selective breeding for 246; biological mechanisms 249–250; current perspectives and future directions 248–249; human studies, evidence from: genetic variants *248*; studies 247; twin and family studies 246–247; molecular basis *249*

inflammatory bowel disease (IBD) 405

inheritance 219–220

injury risk 225–226

insulin-like effect on muscle glucose 5

insulin-like growth factor-1 (IGF-1) 88

interval training 176, *177*, 179; cellular adaptations 179; limitations to studies of 184; fibre type–specific adaptations 186; influence of continuity, on mitochondrial adaptations to 185; novel mechanisms, in mitochondrial biogenesis 186; session *178*; sex-based differences 185; skeletal muscle capillarization 183–184; substrate transport, oxidation, and storage 183

intraindividual variability 244

iron 322–324, 377; food sources **323**; *HFE* genes 378; homeostasis 323; iron-deficiency anaemia 324; *TMPRSS6, TF, and TFR2* genes 378

isolated type 1 fibres 74

Jäger, R. 326

Jahanshahi, A. 326

Jämsä, T. 522

Jannig, P. R. 251

Joanisse, S. 250

Judelson, D. A. 99

Juszczak, D. 324

Käär, M. L. 489

Kacerovsky-Bielesz, G. 488

Kacerovsky, M. 488

Kanaley, J. A. 441

Kang, J. 340

Kasai, N. 323

Keller, C. 37

Kelly, B. M. 222

Kendall, K. L. 341

Kerksick, C.M. 326

Kim, H. J. 330, 340

Kim, P. 330

King, J. C. 325

King, N. A. 285, 541

Kistler, J. A. 489

Knip, M. 489

Köhnke, R. 94

Koh, T. J. 94

Kojima, C. 323

Korpelainen, R. 522

Kortas, J. 324

Kraemer, W. J. 99

Kreis, R. 340

Kristensen, D. E. 181

Krogh, A. 205, 207

lactate: production and transport 379; *SLC16A1* gene 379

lactic acid production 7

Laframboise, M. A. 330

La Gerche, A. 466

Lally, J. 253

La Monica, M. B. 339

Lanham-New, S. A. 326

Lattuada, G. 488

Leckey, J. J. 300

left anterior descending (LAD) 460

Lehmann, N. 466

Leppäluoto, J. 522

Leveritt, M. D. 328

Libardi, C. A. 251

Lilja, M. 222

Li, M. 327

Lin, C. F. 521

Lindhard, J. 205, 207

linker of the nucleoskeleton and cytoskeleton (LINC) complex 86

Lin, L. L. 521

lipid source fuelling aerobic energy metabolism 73

Little, J. P. 248

Liu, F. 327

Liu, W. 322

Lixandrao, M. E. 251

Lockwood, C. M. 341

Lomo, T. 89

long-acting thyroid stimulator (LATS) 91

Lowe, N. M. 325

Lozano-Estevan, M. C. 329

Luden, N. 197

Lundby, C. 222

Lysenko, E. A. 101

Maahs, D. M. 487

Machado, F. S. M. 329

Machado, L. 524

macrovascular complication 486

Madden, R. F. 321

Maffi, P. 488

magnesium 321–322; food sources of **322**

Mäntyranta, E. 224–225

MAPK signalling 129–130

Marley, A. 326

Marques, E. A. 524

Marsh, H. M. 485

Martinez-Vizcaino, V. 542

Mata-Ordonez, F. 329

Maté-Munoz, J. L. 329
Mathieu, M. E. 541
matrix metalloproteinases (MMPs) 94
Mayer, B. 323
Mayer, J. 286
McKay, B. R. 250
McMahon, N. F. 328
McNaughton, L. R. 344, 345
mechanical tension 90
mechanistic target of rapamycin complex 1
    (mTORC1) 86–87
mechanotransduction: biophysical 86; cellular *93*;
    cellular communication 86; evolution of 86; forms
    of 87; nutrition and dietary supplementation
    100–101; physiological systems, integration with:
    endocrine 98–99; immune and inflammatory
    responses 97; metabolism and energy 99–100;
    muscle disruption and damage 97–98; neural 96–97;
    resistance exercise stimulus, type of 102; sex 102;
    training status 100–101; transmembrane proteins 86;
    see also resistance exercise
Medline database 322
metabolic pathways 5–7
Meyer, C. 253
Micielska, K. 324
microvascular dysfunction 486
mild hypoglycaemia 480
Minahan, C. L. 341
Mitchell, C. J. 102, 250
mitochondria: acute molecular responses to exercise
    181–182; adaptations to training and their influence
    on exercise performance 152–153; adaptive response
    of 413; ageing, exercise benefits for: mitochondria,
    impact on 424; muscle, impact on 424; cancer
    406; cardiovascular system 402, 404; chronic
    diseases, abnormalities associated with **403**; content
    413; content in, training-induced changes 153;
    dynamics: fission and fusion 397; mitochondrial
    biogenesis 398; mitochondrial transport 397–398;
    dysfunction *402*, 422; mitochondrial-mediated
    apoptosis 400, 423–424; pathology of 401; potential
    role in ageing and chronic disease 399–400;
    endocrine system 405–406; energy production,
    and 413; gastrointestinal system 405; genetics:
    mitochondrial DNA 396, 423; genome 143–144;
    impact of ageing on muscle and: muscle atrophy
    and dysfunction 420, 422; import and effects
    of exercise: effect of 419–420; mitophagy 419;
    molecular pathways regulating mitophagy 419;
    intensity, acute metabolic responses to exercise
    180–181; intermembrane space 395; interval
    training, induced changes in content 182–183;
    intracellular calcium 417; metabolic homeostasis
    394; mitochondrial biogenesis *180*; exercise-
    mediated *416*; mitochondrial genome in, regulation
    of 414–415; nuclear genome in, regulation of 414;
    p53, regulation of 415; role of exercise 415–417;
    mitochondrial matrix 395–396; musculoskeletal
    system 404–405; neurodegenerative disease

401; optimal exercise prescription 154–155;
    outer mitochondrial membrane (OMM) 395;
    PGC1-α expression, exercise and regulation 418;
    physiology: anatomy of 393; inner mitochondrial
    membrane (IMM) 393–395; quality control
    422–423; mitophagy 398–399; reactive oxygen
    species (ROS) 417–418; remodelling on exercise
    performance, impact of training-induced:
    increased fat utilization 156; increased sensitivity of
    respiratory control 155; reduced glycogen depletion
    155–156; respiratory function in, training-induced
    changes 154; respiratory system 404; structure and
    function within skeletal muscle 143; terminology:
    mitochondrial biogenesis 144; respiratory function
    144
mitochondria-associated membranes (MAMs) 395
mitochondrial biogenesis *180*; exercise-mediated
    416; intracellular signalling pathways involved in:
    AMPK 146; calcium signalling 146; endogenous
    gases 147; p38 MAPK 146–147; SIRT1/GCN5
    147; mitochondrial genome in, regulation of
    414–415; molecular regulation of exercise-induced:
    current dogma 144; molecular events *145*; nuclear
    genome in, regulation of 414; p53, regulation of
    415; role of exercise 415–417; transcription factors
    and co-activators involved in 147–148; emerging
    regulatory proteins 150; NRF-1/2 148; p53 149;
    PGC-1a 148–149; TFAM 148; underexplored
    regulatory events beyond transcription: post-
    transcriptional control of mRNA stability 151;
    protein trafficking and import 152; translational
    control of mitochondrial protein synthesis 151–152;
    see also mitochondria
mitochondrial permeability transition pore (MPTP)
    400
mitochondrial quality control (MitoQC) 117
mitochondrial ROS: during contraction 56–57; in
    oxidative phosphorylation 55
mitochondrial-specific superoxide (MitoSOX) 54
mitogen activated protein kinase (MAPK) pathway 88
mitophagy 118, 419
Miura, T. 522
moderate-intensity continuous training (MICT) 154
modifiable resistance training: contraction mode 164;
    factors and effects on MPS 162–163; mechanistic
    regulation of MPS: amino acid and resistance
    exercise–induced rates of MPS *168*; mTORC1-
    dependent mechanisms 165–167; mTORC1-
    independent mechanisms 167–168; skeletal muscle
    protein synthesis *166*; resistance exercise: load 163;
    volume 163–164; ribosomal biogenesis 168–170
Mohammadshahi, M. 326
Möhlenkamp, S. 466
molecular chaperones *see* heat shock proteins (HSP)
molecular switch 98
Molecular Transducers of Physical Activity
    Consortium (MoTrPAC) 255
Montero, D. 222
Moon, J. R. 341

Moore, A. 489
Moore, C. A. 99
Moreira- Gonçalves, D. 522
Morris, D. 346
Morris, D. L. 222
Morris, J. N. 455
Mosier, E. M. 102
Mosterd, A. 466
mTORC1: activation 307–309; central integration point 307; downstream signaling targets of 309
Muller, M. J. 286
Mullooly, C. A. 489
Murach, K. 197
Murgia, M. 89
Murphy, E. C. 538
muscle protein breakdown (MPB) 162
muscle protein synthesis (MPS) 162; dietary components influencing 310
muscles: contraction 75; damage 382–383; *ACTN3* (rs1815739) gene 382–383; disruption and damage 97–98; fatigue 334; fibre 71–72; fuel selection 7; growth–related genes 94
Mustonen, A. 489
myoblast determination protein 1 (MyoD) 355
myogenic factor 4 and 5 (Myf4 and Myf5) 355–356
myogenic regulatory factors 355
myogenin 355–356
myokines: interleukin-6 (IL-6) 36–37; interleukin-15 (IL-15) 37–38; irisin 38; release during exercise, regulation 134
myopathy 404
myosin heavy chain (MHC) 71; isoform 72, 89; types 72
myostatin: adipokines 38; adiponectin 39–40; leptin 38–39; transforming growth factor $\beta2$ (TGF$\beta2$) 40

Nabuco, H. C. G. 328
Nas, A. 286
Nassenstein, K. 466
National Health Service (NHS) centres 219
Neal, W. 538
Neufer, P. D. 37, 55
Nicholls, D. 55
Nicoll, J. X. 99
Nicoll, J.X. 102
nicotinamide adenine dinucleotide (NADH) 6
Niessner, A. 524
Nilsson, J. 94
Nindl, B. C. 99
nitric oxide (NO) 55
non-exercise activity thermogenesis (NEAT) 278
non-responders 242–243
non-steroidal anti-inflammatory drugs (NSAIDs) 97
Nordic walking training 324
NOX-derived superoxide, contraction and exercise 57–58
nuclear factor of activated T-cells (NFAT) 125
nuclear pore complex (NPC) 92
Nugent, A. M. 489
nutraceutical compounds 113–314

nutrition 305, 375; caffeine, performance, interindividual responses 376–377; dietary factors or biological molecules **383–384**; iron 378; lactate production and transport 379; muscle damage 382–383; sport, genes associated with 376; vitamin A 380–381; vitamin B_{12} 380; vitamin C and collagen 381; vitamin D and bone health 381–382

obesity 4; consequences of 277; prevalence of, among Americans **4**; *see also* childhood obesity; weight loss
Oduoza, U. 326
oestrogen-related receptor (ERR) family 150
Ohsawa, I. 522
oncometabolites 406
Osada, T. 37
osteoblast-induced bone formation 357–358
osteokines 517
osteoporosis 513
osteoprotegerin (OPG) 517
Ostrowski, K. 36
O'Toole, M. L. 466
overweight 4
oxidative capacity 117
oxidative phosphorylation 6; ATP regeneration rate 7
oxidative stress 401, 480

Padilla, J. 440
Painelli, V. S. 340, 346
Pallafacchina, G. 89
Parcell, A. C. 94
Parini, P. 524
Parkinson disease (PD) 401
Parks, J. W. 455
Parnell, J. A. 321
Parr, E. B. 300
Pavey, T.G. 328
peak bone mass (PBM) 513
Pedersen, B. K. 36, 37
Pereira, B. 541
peripheral fatigue 71, 77–79; decreased SR Ca^{2+} release via RyR1 77–78; glycogen depletion 78; impaired action potential propagation 77; impaired myofibrillar function 78–79; reduced SR Ca^{2+} available for release 78
Perkins, S. N. 501
peroxisome proliferator–activated receptor-γ (PPARγ) 38, 150
Perry, C. G. R. 253
Perseghin, G. 488
Pettit-Mee, R. 440
Phillips, B. E. 222
Phillips, S. M. 102, 250, 251
phosphagens 5–6
phosphocreatine (PCr) 5, 354
physical activity energy expenditure (PAEE) 278
physical exercise 401
Pilegaard, H. 37
Pires, W. 329
plasma calcium homeostasis: turnover and oestrogen 516–517

Ponce-González, J. G. 222
Poortmans, J. R. 489
Popov, D. V. 101
post-translation modifications 92
Prakken, N. H. J. 466
Prats, C. 181
pre-sleep protein ingestion 312
primer on redox biology 52; superoxide-producing sites and hydrogen peroxide *53*
Prior, D. L. 466
pro-apoptotic cascade 406
prolonged aerobic exercise: CHO oxidation 28; fuel use *28*;.muscle glycogen and FFA, oxidation of 27; muscle PDH activity 29; plasma free fatty acid (FFA) concentrations *28*; pyruvate dehydrogenase (PDHa) activation *29*
proteins: components of 5; dietary requirements 5; distribution 312–313; energy 5; feeding pattern *312*; individual dose and total protein intake 310–311; source 311–312; synthesis: cellular signalling pathways *309*; molecular mechanisms underpinning 307; turnover: daily protein feeding pattern *306*; skeletal muscle mass regulation 306–307
Prusik, K 324
public health concern 245
pulmonary arterial hypertension (PAH) 404
putative cell signalling cascades activated through exercise *297*
Puukka, R. 489
Pyle, L. 487

Qari, M. H. 522, 524
Qian, H-R. 251
Quesnele, J. J. 330

Rabelo, T. 340, 346
Raffle, P. A. 455
Raizel, R. 321
Ramezani Ahmadi, A. 326
Ramirez-Velez, R. 537, 538
ramped-up training signal 295
ras homologue enriched in brain (Rheb) 91
Ratamess, N. A. 340
Raue, U. 251
reactive oxygen–nitrogen species (RONS) 73
reactive oxygen species (ROS) 51; muscle function during exercise 52; regulation of 53–60; ROS-mediated post-translational modifications during exercise 133; signalling 130–131; and exercise-induced autophagy 133
Ready, S. 440
redox buffering, effects of exercise on: glutathione and thioredoxin *60*; redoxome *61*; regulation 60
redox-sensitive transcription factor Nrf2 150
redox signalling 52; acute and chronic responses, to exercise in muscle 63
Reichek, N. 466
renin–angiotensin system 223

resistance exercise *95*; acute and chronic training variables 87; training–related variables *88*; acute response of SCs and impact *194*; adaptations to: fibre composition 89; hypertrophy 88–89; myonuclei 89–90; ribosome biogenesis 90; biochemical mechanotransduction 90; heterogeneity of response to, responders and non-responders 165; hypertrophic responses to, sex differences in MPS and 164; intensity on mechanotransduction, role of 95–96; mechanotransduction responses to 90; performance variables 87; sarcomeric mechanotransduction 92; satellite cell mechanotransduction 94–95; skeletal muscle force transmission 92, 94
respiratory training device 260–261
responders 242–243
Restaino, R. 440
resting energy expenditure (REE) 278
ribosome-associated co-chaperones (MPP1 and HSPA14) 114
ribosome biogenesis 90, 101
Rice, T. 222
Richter, B. 524
Ricome, A. 89
Rizza, R. A. 485
Roberts, C. G. 455
Rodrigues, Q. T. 329
Rogers, R. S. 521
Rohde, T. 36
Ross, M. L. 327
Ross, R. 340
Rouzi, A. A. 522, 524
Ruegemer, J. J. 485
Rumbold, P. L. 541
Rutherfurd-Markwick, K. 366

Saavedra, J. M. 537, 538, 542
Saerens, P. 489
Sale, C. 340, 344
Saltin, B. 37
Saouaf, R. 489
Saraheimo, M. 487
sarcomere 92
sarcopenia 405
satellite cells 89; activation in response, acute exercise 194–195; acute response, aerobic exercise 197; impact of exercise training, on content 198; training and content 198, **199**, 200; acute response to resistance exercise 195, 197; biology 193; exercise training, acute response 200–201; mechanotransduction 94–95; resistance exercise: acute response to 195, 197; studies examining, impact of *196*; training and content 198
Sato, Y. 522
Sattler, F. R. 195
Saunders, B. 344
Schiaffino, S. 89
Schmid, A. I. 488
Schoenfeld, B. J. 327
Schroeder, E. T. 195

Schumann, U. 323
Schwartz, P. J. 457
secreted frizzled-related protein (SFRP) 519
Serairi Beji, R. 321
Sereni, L. P. 488
Serrano, A. L. 89
severe hypoglycaemia 480
Sharova, A. P. 101
Shaw, C. S. 487
Shearer, J. 321
Shibata, Y. 522
Shi, H. 89
signalling pathways: AMPK signalling 128–129; β adrenergic signalling 131–132; Ca^{2+} signalling 124–127; cytokine signalling 132–133; intracellular signalling events *126*; MAPK signalling 129–130; ROS signalling 130–131
Silva, H. H. 321
Silva, M. G. 321
skeletal muscle: fat energy 4; hypertrophy 310; metabolic pathways *294*
Skeletal Muscle Adaptive Response to Training (SMART) study 255
skeletal muscle during exercise, regulation of ROS generation in: experimental approaches 53–54; NADPH oxidases and mitochondria 54–58; sources and approaches 58–60
skeletal muscle energy: adenosine triphosphate (ATP) 15; muscle cells, characteristic of 15; ATP content and free inorganic phosphate *19*; fat and carbohydrate metabolism, relationship 27; fat oxidation, regulation 25; free adenosine diphosphate (ADP) and adenosine monophosphate (AMP) accumulation *20*; lactate accumulation and phosphocreatine use *18*; metabolism and fuel 15; respiratory and cardiovascular systems 17; skeletal muscle, energy-producing pathways *16*, **16**; phosphocreatine, anaerobic glycolysis, and oxidative phosphorylation *21*; prolonged aerobic exercise 27–29; pyruvate dehydrogenase (PDH) activation *21*
Skinner, J. S. 222
Skovbro, M. 300
Skwiat, T. M. 326
sleep low model 298
slow- and fast-twitch muscle fibres 95–96
Smith, A. E. 341
Smith, R. C. 251
sodium and calcium lactate: exercise performance, effects on 346; side effects 347; supplementation strategies 346
sodium bicarbonate supplementation 341; exercise performance, effects on 343–344; extracellular buffers *342*; side effects 344; strategies 342–343
sodium citrate: exercise performance, effects on 345; supplementation strategies 344–345
sodium-glucose cotransporter-2 inhibitors (SGLT2i) 443
soft tissue injuries 225
Sousa, F. 524
Southward, K. 366

Spiering, B. A. 99
The Sports Gene: Talent, Practice and the Truth about Success 217
Spriet, L. L. 253
sprint interval training (SIT) 154, 439
Squires, R. W. 485
Stec, M. 253
Steele, I. C. 489
Steensberg, A. 37
Steinacker, J. M. 323
Stellingwerff, T. 340
Stephens, B. R. 440
Stephens, N. A. 253
Stepto, N. K. 300
Sterczala, A. J. 99
Stites, A. W. 94
Stone, H. L. 457
Stout, J. R. 340
Study of Underlying Genetic Determinants of Vitamin D and Highly Related Traits (SUNLIGHT) 382
Sugihara, Junior P. 328
Sumi, D. 323
Sunderland, C. 344
systemic hypoxia: aerobic exercise adaptations: acclimation to 264; aerobic adaptations, training under 263–264; aerobic performance benefits of 264–265; negative adaptations, independent of exercise 262–263; positive adaptations, independent of exercise 261–262; anaerobic/resistance exercise adaptations: anaerobic/resistance performance benefits of 266; independent of exercise, negative adaptations to 265; independent of exercise, positive adaptations to 265; positive adaptations to performing 265–266; enhance training adaptations, strategies for 261; hypoxic environment, creating 260–261; local blood flow restriction: with aerobic exercise 269; with anaerobic exercise 270; application of 267; differentiating 267; with high-load resistance exercise 271; impact of applying *268*; with low-load resistance exercise 270–271
Szendroedi, J. 488

Tallon, M. J. 330
t-cell factor/lymphoid enhancer-binding factor (TCF/LEF) 519
ten-eleven translocation (TET) 233
Thalacker-Mercer, A. 253
thermic effect of food (TEF) 278
Thivel, D. 541
Thomason, D. B. 99
Thorn, L. M. 487
three-bout upper-body Wingate test 346
Thyfault, J. P. 521
thyroid hormone 323–324
Tikkanen, H. K. 487
Tirapegui, J. 321
tissue inhibitors of metalloproteinases (TIMPs) 94
Tock, L. 538
Todd, K. 197
Tomeleri, C. M. 328

training adaptation 293, 295; nutritional strategies, glycogen status: fasted training 296, 298; low-carbohydrate, high-fat diets 299–300; periodized carbohydrate availability 298–299; training twice per day 296
training, exercise interaction and 314
transcription factor A mitochondrial (TFAM) 235
translocase of outer membrane (TOM) protein complex 395
translocase receptor TOM70 115
Trappe, T. A. 251
Treff, G. 323
Trewin, A. J. 300
Trivax, J. E. 467
Trnka, J. 487
true response to exercise training (TRUE) 243
tuberous sclerosis complex 2 (TSC2) 91
Tu, K. C. 521
tumorigenesis 500
Tumova, J. 487
Tu, Y. H. 521
type 2 diabetes mellitus (T2DM) 405
type 1 diabetes (T1D): acute complications 479; causes of 479; endocrine responses during exercise 480–482; types of exercises *482*; factors to consider 482–485; blood glucose trends, different types of exercise *482*; glucoregulatory responses to moderate-intensity exercise without T1D *483*; glucoregulatory responses to moderate-intensity exercise with T1D *484*; glucose homeostasis, importance of: hyperglycaemia 480; living with 480, *481*; long-term complications 479; physical performance, and 489–490; regular exercise in people with, importance of 485–489; benefits of regular exercise with T1D *486*; diabetic neuropathies 487; morbidity and mortality study 487; protective mechanisms 487
type 2 diabetes (T2D) and exercise: acute exercise 436–437; American Diabetes Association (ADA), data on 433; clinical considerations: molecular clocks 440–441; pharmacology 441–444; diabetes prevention program (DPP) 437; exercise adaptations, continuum of *434*; exercise, benefits of 433–434; exercise mode/intensity/duration/volume, impact of 439; habitual exercise 437–438; insulin resistance (IR) 434; physical activity and breaking up sedentary behaviour 439; physical activity recommendations 433

ubiquitin conjugating enzyme E2 N (UBE2N) 114
UK Biobank 219
uncoupling protein 1 (UCP1) 38
upper- and lower- body Wingates or YoYo performance 340
Urinary 3-methyl histidine 356
Urwin, C. S. 344

Väänänen, H. K. 522
Vainionpää, A. 522
Vallely, S. 489

Varanoske, A. N. 339
Vechin, F. C. 251
Vepkhvadze, T. F. 101
Vertongen, F. 489
Veves, A. 489
Viana, J. L. 524
Vinogradova, O. L. 101
vitamin A 381; *BCMO1* gene 380
vitamin B$_{12}$: *FUT2* gene 380
vitamin C: and collagen 381; *GSTT1* gene 381
vitamin D: and bone health 381–382; bone metabolism in 325; *GC* and *CYP2R1* genes 381–382; metabolism *326*; supplementation 326
vitamins and ROS 59–60
Volek, J. S. 99
Volpe, S. L. 324, 325
Volta, A. 85
voltage-dependent anion channel (VDAC) proteins 395
Voltarelli, F. A. 321

Wadén, J. 487
Wagenmakers, A. J. M. 487
Walsh, L. 440
Walter, A. A. 341
Wanderley, F. 524
Wang, R. 322, 339
Wang, Z. 521
Wanner, S. P. 329
Warburg effect 406
Watanabe, T. 522
weight loss: diet and exercise interventions on, interactions between 283–284; biochemical and physiological compensatory responses 284–286; potential mechanisms 284
weight maintenance and regain 286–287
Weiss, L. W. 99
Wells, G. D. 330
Wells, S. D. 326
West, D. W. 102, 327
Westerlind, K. C. 501
whey protein 326; amount of 327; consuming, effects of 328; muscle protein synthesis 327; myofibrillar protein synthesis, and *327*; resistance training 328
white adipose tissue (WAT) 38
William, C. R. 471
Williams, C. 181
Williams, C. J. 248
Williams, M. G. 248
Wilmore, J. H. 222
Windham, S. 253
Winkert, K. 323
Winn, N. 440
Wirth, S. 524
Wisløff, U. 248
Wiswell, R. A. 195
within-subject variability (WS) 243
Wofford, H. 346
Wojtaszewski, J. F. P. 181
Woloszczuk, W. 524

Wong, J. J. 330
Woodhouse, L. R. 325
Woolstenhulme, M. T. 94
World Anti-Doping Agency (WADA) 227, 262, 364

xanthine oxidase (XO) 58–59
Xun, P. 322

Yang, R. S. 521
Yeater, R. 538
yes-associated protein (YAP) 91
Yi, F. 253

Zacho, M. 36
Zderic, T. W. 440
Zeng, C. 89
Zhou, T. 322
Ziegler, S. 524
Ziemann, E. 324
Zierath, J. 235
zinc 324; deficiency 325; food sources **324**;
   homeostasis 325; supplementation 325
Zügel, M. 323

Printed in the United States
By Bookmasters